11th EDITION

CLINICAL PROCEDURES

for Medical Assistants

KATHY BONEWIT-WEST, BS, MEd

Professor Emeritus
Medical Assistant Program
Hocking College
Nelsonville, Ohio;
Former Member, Curriculum Review Board of the American Association of Medical Assistants

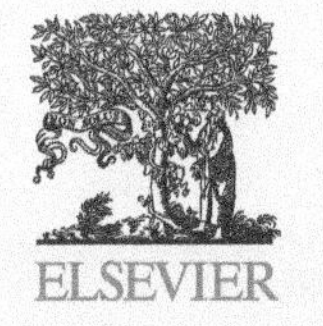

Elsevier
3251 Riverport Lane
St. Louis, Missouri 63043

CLINICAL PROCEDURES FOR MEDICAL ASSISTANTS, ELEVENTH EDITION ISBN: 978-0-323-75858-1

Content Strategist: Laura Klein
Senior Content Development Specialist: Rae Robertson
Publishing Services Manager: Julie Eddy
Senior Project Manager: Rachel E. McMullen
Design Direction: Renee Duenow

Printed in the United States of America

Last digit is the print number: 9 8 7 6 5 4 3 2 1

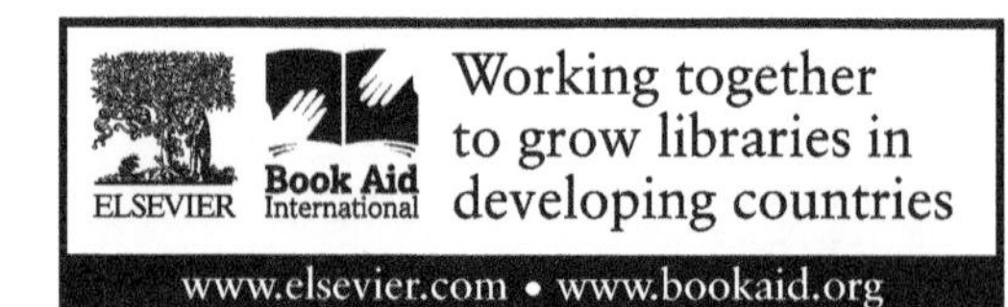

For my daughter Tristen,
You light up my life.

Editorial Consultants and Review Board

Preface

Medical assistants, for many years an integral part of physicians' offices, now fulfill an ever-expanding and varied role in the medical office, both clinically and administratively. With increased responsibilities has come a greater need for professional knowledge and skills. This text has been designed to meet this need.

The underlying principle of the text is to provide a format for the achievement of professional competency in clinical skills performed in the medical office and the understanding of their application to real-life or on-the-job situations. When professional competency is achieved in the classroom, less of a gap should exist between the academic world and the real world, and thus the transition from student to practicing medical assistant is made more easily.

Although I have emphasized the book's usefulness to students in medical assisting programs, the practicing medical assistant will also find this text helpful as a learning and reference source. The organization of the text lends itself well to individualized instruction and convenient reference use.

NEW FEATURES IN THIS EDITION

In this eleventh edition, the text has been expanded to encompass additional theory and clinical procedures. This new material will help students and instructors meet the demand for the increasing number and variety of clinical skills required of the practicing medical assistant by providing the most current and up-to-date procedures performed in the medical office. The reader will find that nearly every chapter incorporates new information to assist in the educational process.

IMPORTANT ADDITIONS INCLUDE THE FOLLOWING

- Over 200 newly updated photographs
- Current information on the OSHA Bloodborne Pathogens Standard
- Information on the types of gloves and glove sizing
- Updated information on the autoclave
- New procedure on the non-contact forehead thermometer
- New procedure on the automated method of measuring blood pressure
- New information on gynecologic infections
- New procedure on a patient-collected vaginal specimen
- Updated pediatric immunization schedule
- Information on topical tissue adhesives
- Comprehensive, updated pharmacology drug table of medications commonly administered and prescribed in the medical office
- Information of the electronic prescribing of medication
- Information on asthma action plans
- Information and procedure on the Cologuard FIT-DNA test
- New information on coagulation tests
- New procedure for performing a CLIA-waived blood glucose test
- Information on a glucose continuous monitoring device
- Information on COVID-19

STANDARD PEDAGOGICAL FEATURES IN THIS EDITION

Other very important features to the eleventh edition are the inclusion of some valuable learning aids:

- The organizational format of this edition facilitates the learning process by providing students and educators with detailed objectives and an in-depth study of the most current and up-to-date clinical procedures performed in the medical office. Presented at the beginning of each chapter are **Learning Outcomes** and **Related Procedures**, a **Chapter Outline**, and **Key Terms.** The learning outcomes address the cognitive knowledge required to perform the procedures. Procedures coincide with the outcomes to delineate the task or skill to be mastered by the student. (In the student *Study Guide*, the procedures are expanded into detailed performance objectives, including outcomes, and conditions and standards of acceptable performance.) The chapter outline provides a quick reference of the cognitive knowledge included in that chapter. The Key Terms list designates the terms that should be mastered for each chapter.

8 The Gynecologic Examination and Prenatal Care

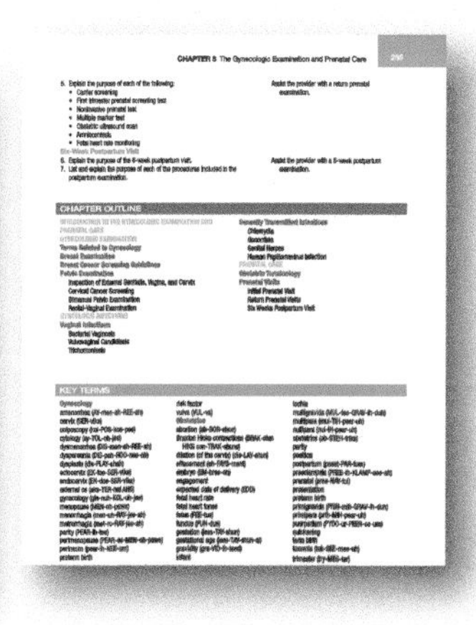

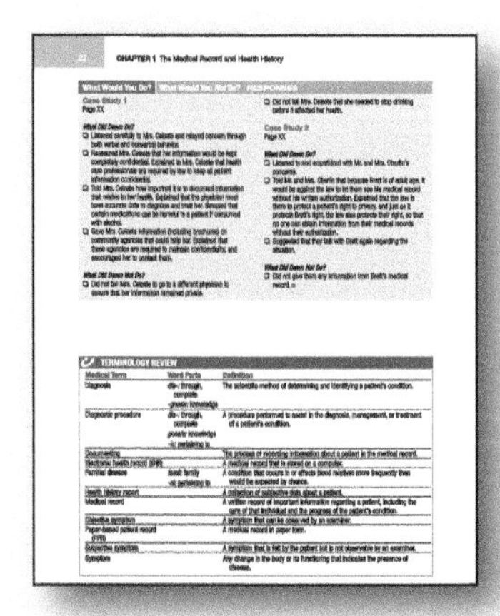

- The **knowledge** or **theory** that the student must acquire to perform each skill is presented in a clear and concise manner. **Numerous illustrations** accompany the theory section to aid the student in acquiring the knowledge relating to each skill.
- **Procedures** for each skill follow the theory section and are designed to help the student perform the skill with the level of competency required on the job. Each procedure is presented in an organized step-by-step format, with underlying principles and illustrations accompanying the techniques. A documentation example follows each procedure to provide the student with a guide for documenting his or her own procedure. Students should find it much easier to acquire competency in documenting with these examples.

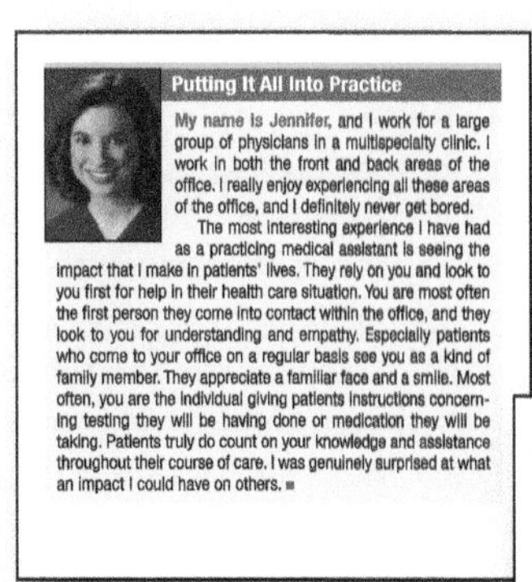

Putting It All Into Practice

My name is Jennifer, and I work for a large group of physicians in a multispecialty clinic. I work in both the front and back areas of the office. I really enjoy experiencing all these areas of the office, and I definitely never get bored.

The most interesting experience I have had as a practicing medical assistant is seeing the impact that I make in patients' lives. They rely on you and look to you first for help in their health care situation. You are most often the first person they come into contact within the office, and they look to you for understanding and empathy. Especially patients who come to your office on a regular basis see you as a kind of family member. They appreciate a familiar face and a smile. Most often, you are the individual giving patients instructions concerning testing they will be having done or medication they will be taking. Patients truly do count on your knowledge and assistance throughout their course of care. I was genuinely surprised at what an impact I could have on others. ■

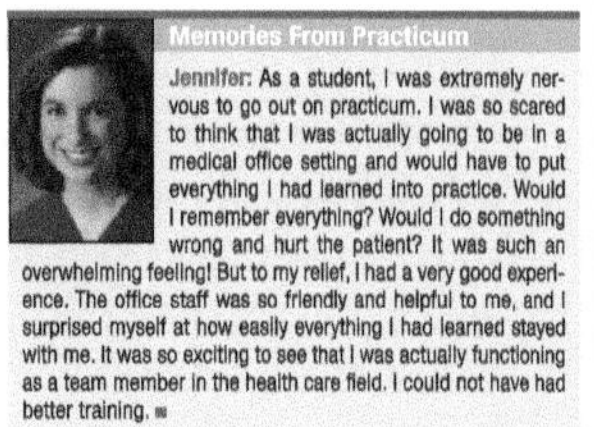

Memories From Practicum

Jennifer: As a student, I was extremely nervous to go out on practicum. I was so scared to think that I was actually going to be in a medical office setting and would have to put everything I had learned into practice. Would I remember everything? Would I do something wrong and hurt the patient? It was such an overwhelming feeling! But to my relief, I had a very good experience. The office staff was so friendly and helpful to me, and I surprised myself at how easily everything I had learned stayed with me. It was so exciting to see that I was actually functioning as a team member in the health care field. I could not have had better training. ■

- The unique and memorable medical assistant biographical profiles (**Memories From Practicum** and **Putting It All Into Practice**) help students "connect" with their future beyond the classroom. The MAs featured are real people sharing their fears, likes, hopes, and aspirations, providing a "real-world" feel to the book and an inspiration for the student.

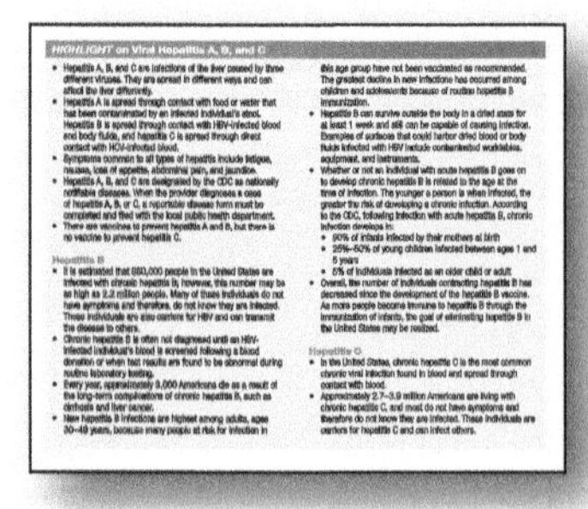

- **Highlight Boxes** feature unique information related to topics included in the textbook. This provides the student with additional and interesting information for a better understanding of each chapter.

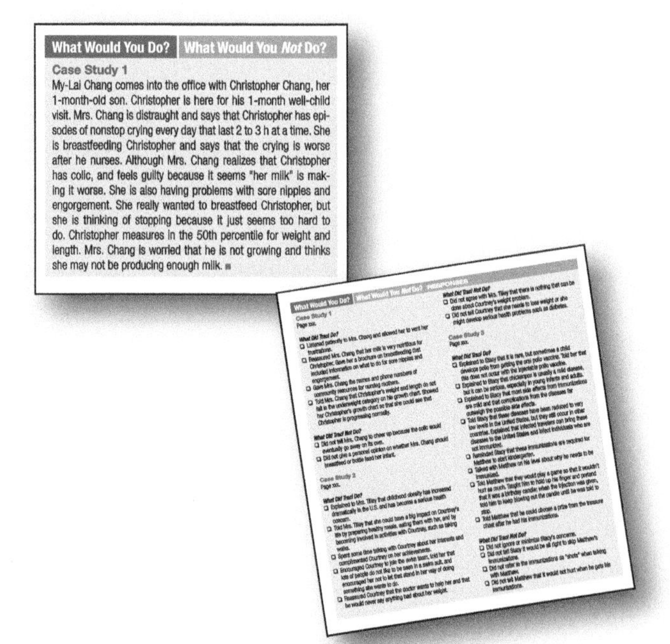

What Would You Do? What Would You *Not* Do?

Case Study 1

My-Lai Chang comes into the office with Christopher Chang, her 1-month-old son. Christopher is here for his 1-month well-child visit. Mrs. Chang is distraught and says that Christopher has episodes of nonstop crying every day that last 2 to 3 h at a time. She is breastfeeding Christopher and says that the crying is worse after he nurses. Although Mrs. Chang realizes that Christopher has colic, and feels guilty because it seems "her milk" is making it worse. She is also having problems with sore nipples and engorgement. She really wanted to breastfeed Christopher, but she is thinking of stopping because it just seems too hard to do. Christopher measures in the 50th percentile for weight and length. Mrs. Chang is worried that he is not growing and thinks she may not be producing enough milk. ■

- **Case Studies** are designed to assist the student in responding to "real-life" situations that occur in the medical office. A practitioner's response is given for each case study, too, as a means of comparison for the student.

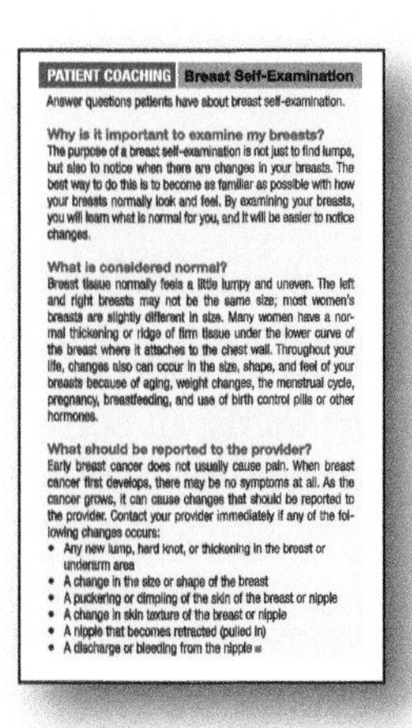

PATIENT COACHING Breast Self-Examination

Answer questions patients have about breast self-examination.

Why is it important to examine my breasts?
The purpose of a breast self-examination is not just to find lumps, but also to notice when there are changes in your breasts. The best way to do this is to become as familiar as possible with how your breasts normally look and feel. By examining your breasts, you will learn what is normal for you, and it will be easier to notice changes.

What is considered normal?
Breast tissue normally feels a little lumpy and uneven. The left and right breasts may not be the same size; most women's breasts are slightly different in size. Many women have a normal thickening or ridge of firm tissue under the lower curve of the breast where it attaches to the chest wall. Throughout your life, changes also can occur in the size, shape, and feel of your breasts because of aging, weight changes, the menstrual cycle, pregnancy, breastfeeding, and use of birth control pills or other hormones.

What should be reported to the provider?
Early breast cancer does not usually cause pain. When breast cancer first develops, there may be no symptoms at all. As the cancer grows, it can cause changes that should be reported to the provider. Contact your provider immediately if any of the following changes occurs:

- Any new lump, hard knot, or thickening in the breast or underarm area
- A change in the size or shape of the breast
- A puckering or dimpling of the skin of the breast or nipple
- A change in skin texture of the breast or nipple
- A nipple that becomes retracted (pulled in)
- A discharge or bleeding from the nipple ■

- **Patient Coaching** boxes emphasize this important aspect of the medical assistant's job and present it in context to make it more relevant, thereby making it more memorable.

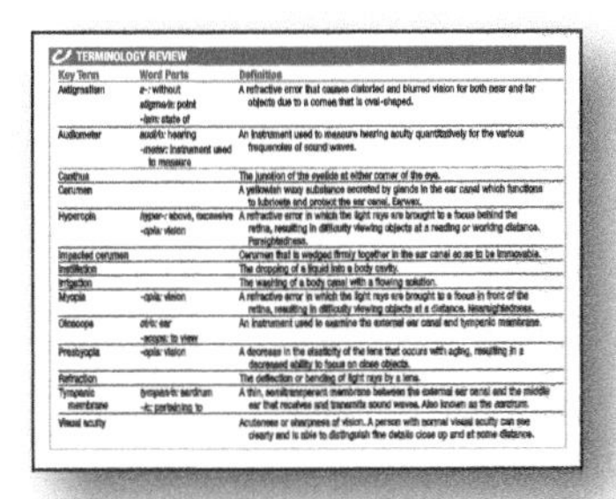

TERMINOLOGY REVIEW

Key Term	Word Parts	Definition
Astigmatism	a-: without stigmat/o: point -ism: state of	A refractive error that causes distorted and blurred vision for both near and far objects due to a cornea that is oval-shaped.
Audiometer	audi/o: hearing -meter: instrument used to measure	An instrument used to measure hearing acuity quantitatively for the various frequencies of sound waves.
Canthus		The junction of the eyelids at either corner of the eye.
Cerumen		A yellowish waxy substance secreted by glands in the ear canal which functions to lubricate and protect the ear canal. Earwax.
Hyperopia	hyper-: above, excessive -opia: vision	A refractive error in which the light rays are brought to a focus behind the retina, resulting in difficulty viewing objects at a reading or working distance. Farsightedness.
Impacted cerumen		Cerumen that is wedged firmly together in the ear canal so as to be immovable.
Instillation		The dropping of a liquid into a body cavity.
Irrigation		The washing of a body canal with a flowing solution.
Myopia	-opia: vision	A refractive error in which the light rays are brought to a focus in front of the retina, resulting in difficulty viewing objects at a distance. Nearsightedness.
Otoscope	ot/o: ear -scope: to view	An instrument used to examine the external ear canal and tympanic membrane.
Presbyopia	-opia: vision	A decrease in the elasticity of the lens that occurs with aging, resulting in a decreased ability to focus on close objects.
Refraction		The deflection or bending of light rays by a lens.
Tympanic membrane	tympan/o: eardrum -ic: pertaining to	A thin, semitransparent membrane between the external ear canal and the middle ear that receives and transmits sound waves. Also known as the eardrum.
Visual acuity		Acuteness or sharpness of vision. A person with normal visual acuity can see clearly and is able to distinguish fine details close up and at some distance.

- **Key Terms** identified at the beginning of the chapter are defined at the end of the chapter in the **Terminology Review**, providing students with a valuable terminology overview for each chapter. Word parts (prefixes, suffixes, and combining forms) for the medical terms are also included in the Terminology Review sections of some chapters to help the student understand the meaning of the medical term through its word parts.

EXTENSIVE SUPPLEMENTAL RESOURCES

PROCEDURAL VIDEOS

The most impressive feature to this book is the inclusion of clinical procedural videos on the Evolve site, which present many of the skills outlined in the textbook. An icon VIDEO is placed within the procedural title bar of the procedures in this text that have accompanying procedural videos. Students will have the invaluable opportunity to watch the procedures at home or at school, using any computer or internet connection. This should greatly enhance the learning of these clinical procedures and provide the medical assistant graduate with competence and confidence in performing clinical procedures in the medical office.

EVOLVE RESOURCES

An Evolve site accompanies the textbook and is designed for students to apply the theory and procedures learned throughout the textbook. Organized by chapter, the site includes **Apply Your Knowledge** questions (multiple-choice questions that give students an opportunity to "apply the knowledge" they learned in that particular chapter). **Procedure Videos, Video Evaluations** (True/False questions that quiz students on their knowledge of the procedures shown in the procedure videos). **Practicum Activities** for your practicum, and various games and interactive activities (i.e., "Quiz Show" and "Road to Recovery") to provide entertainment while learning important concepts related to selected chapters, matching exercises, labeling exercises, identification exercises, and other helpful activities for the student. Lastly, **SimChart for the Medical Office** activities and four **Medical Assisting Credentialing Practice Examinations** (CMA-AAMA, RMA, CMAC, and CCMA) are also offered on the Evolve site. An icon is placed at the beginning of each chapter to prompt students to access the site and see what each chapter has to offer.

STUDY GUIDE

The ***Study Guide*** that accompanies the textbook greatly enhances the learning value of the textbook. Included are extensive exercises for each chapter, practice for competency worksheets, and performance evaluation checklists. Pretests and posttests help better prepare students for chapter tests. Study Guide assignment sheets are incorporated into the study guide for documenting completion of assignments and calculating points earned for each assignment. Laboratory assignment sheets allow the student to keep track of performance of procedures. Included in this edition are video evaluation sheets, which assess the student's knowledge of key points in the clinical skills presented in the procedural videos accompanying the textbook. In addition, its outcome-based approach meets the criteria required for outcome-based program accreditation as stipulated by the Commission on Accreditation of Allied Health Education Programs (CAAHEP) and the Medical Assisting Education Review Board (MAERB) of the American Association of Medical Assistants (AAMA).

CONTINUING EDUCATION

Continuing education is of utmost importance in such a rapidly changing profession. New techniques and developments in the field of medicine have a direct influence on the medical assisting profession. Continuing education helps the medical assistant to maintain and improve existing skills and to learn new skills. The AAMA is a professional organization for medical assistants that is dedicated to continuing education. Information on the AAMA can be obtained by contacting:

American Association of Medical Assistants
20 N. Wacker Dr., No.1575
Chicago, IL 60606–2903
312-899-1500
www.aama-ntl.org

It is the author's hope that individuals who use this approach to medical assisting will view this text not as a stopping place but as a means of opening doors to new paths to be explored in the medical assisting profession.

Kathy Bonewit-West, BS, MEd

Acknowledgments

The completion of the eleventh edition of this text permits the opportunity to relay appreciation to the medical assisting educators who so eagerly and enthusiastically use and enjoy this text. To them I am also indebted for their helpful assistance and suggestions for the eleventh edition.

The following professionals served as invaluable consultants and reviewers and deserve special recognition and appreciation:

Sharlene K. Aasen, CMA (AAMA), Globe College, Oakdale, Minnesota.

Diana Bennett, RN, BSN, MAT, Indiana Vocational Technical College, Indianapolis, Indiana.

Julie A. Benson, AS, RMA, RPhbt, EKG, Medical Program Director, Platt College, Tulsa, Oklahoma.

Lisa Breitbard, AA, LVN, Maric College of Medical Careers, San Diego, California.

Carol S. Champagne, RMA, CMA (AAMA), ICEA, CCE, Clearwater Family Practice Clinic, Clearwater, Kansas; Chairperson, RMA, Continuing Education Committee; Certified Childbirth Education, Private Practice.

Gary A. Clarke, PhD, Assistant Professor of Biology, Roanoke College, Salem, Virginia.

Beverly G. Dugas, TN, Douglas College, New Westminster, British Columbia, Canada.

Julie D. Franklin, MT (ASCP), MHE, Former Program Director, Medical Office Assisting, Chattanooga State Technical Community College, Chattanooga, Tennessee.

Cathy Goodwin, CMA (AAMA), Medical Assistant, San Diego, California.

Jeanne Howard, CMA (AAMA), AAS, Medical Assisting Technology, El Paso Community College, El Paso, Texas.

Gail I. Jones, MS, MT (ASCP), Dettman-Connell School of Medical Technology, Fort Worth, Texas.

Richard W. Kocon, PhD, Laboratory Director, Damon Medical Laboratory, Inc., Needham Heights, Massachusetts.

Louis Komarmy, MD, Clinical Pathologist, Children's Hospital, San Francisco, California.

Albert B. Lowenfels, MD, Associate Director of Surgery, Westchester County Medical Center, Valhalla, New York.

Susan J. Matthews, RN, BSN, MEd, Watterson College, Louisville, Kentucky.

Sharon McCaughrin, CMA (AAMA), Corporate Director of Education, Ross Medical Education Centers, Warren, Michigan.

Deborah Montone, BS, RN, RMA, LLS-P, RCS, Dean of Academics, Hohokus School of Medical Sciences, Ramsey, New Jersey.

Sally A. Murdock, BSN, MS, RN, California Public Health Nursing Certification, Medical Assisting, San Diego Mesa College, San Diego, California.

Kathryn L. Murphy, RN, CMA (AAMA), Medical Program Director, Department Chair, and Instructor, Springfield College, Springfield, Missouri.

Donna F. Otis, LPN, Medical Instructor, MAA Program, Metro Business College, Rolla, Missouri.

Raymond E. Phillips, MD, FACP, Senior Attending Physician, Phelps Memorial Hospital, North Tarrytown, New York.

Vicki Prater, CMA (AAMA), Concorde Career Institute, San Bernardino, California.

Linda Reed, Indiana Vocational Technical College, Indianapolis, Indiana.

Marjorie J. Reif, PA-C, CMA (AAMA), Rochester Community College, Rochester, Minnesota.

Alan M. Rosich, Instructor of Radiologic Technology, Lorain County Community College, Elvira, Ohio.

Kimberly Rubesne, MA, Median School of Allied Health Careers, Pittsburgh, Pennsylvania.

Lynn G. Slack, CMA (AAMA), ICM School of Business and Medical Careers, Pittsburgh, Pennsylvania.

Robin Snider-Flohr, MBA, RN, CMA (AAMA), Jefferson Community College, Steubenville, Ohio.

Edward R. Stapleton, EMT-P, Assistant Clinical Professor and Director of Prehospital Care and Education, Department of Emergency Medicine, School of Medicine, University Hospital and Medical Center, State University of New York, Stony Brook, New York.

Sandra E. Sterling, MT (ASCP), Boulder Valley Vocational-Technical School, Boulder, Colorado.

Marie Thomas, CLT (NCA), Berdan Institute, Totowa, New Jersey.

Joan K. Werner, PT, PhD, Director, Physical Therapy Program, University of Wisconsin, Madison, Wisconsin.

The photographs in the textbook were taken by Brian Blauser and Jack Foley, professional photographers. I am indebted to them for their careful precision and patience in taking and editing the photographs, thus greatly enhancing the learning value of this text.

A very special thanks to Marlene Donovan, Dawn Shingler, Lori Jarvis Cline, and Janice Smith for their dedication and hard work, not only on this edition but for also in the field of medical assisting education as a whole. They have contributed immensely to the recognition of medical assisting students and practitioners as valued members of the health care community.

I would like to gratefully acknowledge the following practicing medical assistants for contributing many hours to be photographed for demonstration of the clinical procedures in the text: Dawn Shingler, Megan Baer, Danielle Brown, Theresa Cline, Marlyne Cooper, Dori Glover,

Jennifer Hawk, Kevin Hickey, Cammie Lindner, Judy Markins, Korey McGrew, Natalie Morehead, Amber Nelson, Traci Powell, Emma Schmeltzer, Latisha Sharpe, Michelle Shockey, Michelle Villers, Huang Ying, Linda O'Nail, Heidi Hopstetter, Anitra Martin, Alexandra Schostek, Abby Erdy, and David Hopkins.

I would also like to acknowledge the following individuals who portrayed patients in the photographs in the text: Brian Adevc, David Arnold, Connie Arthur, Jessica Bennett, Kim Bingham, Pamela Bitting, Adrian Bolin, Caitlin Brennan, Hollie Bonewit-Cron, LeAnn Brown, Phillip Carr, Chloe Cline, Angie Coffin, Dawn Decaminada, Bonnie Dennis, Aja Fox, Jennifer Gardner, Markly Georges, Connie Hazlett, Gary Hazlett, Kyra Horn, Isabella Ipacs, Joey Ipacs, Susan Ipacs, Braylin Kemp, Charles Larimer, Pam Larimer, Christopher Mace, Mickey Midkiff, Deborah Murray, Delaney Murray, Michael Nkrumah, Heather Pike, Dawn Shingler, Jan Six, Megan Skidmore, Colton Smith, Sydney Smith, Clinton Swart, Melanie Walker, Tristen West, Lynn Witkowski, Toni Cooper, Maxden Cooper, Jade Model, Kimberly Ephlin, Sam Coppoletti, Kayla Smith, Lauren Tacosik, Taylor Cossin, Martha Cooper, Doris Wilderman, Dianne Ridenour, Molly Stephens, Haylee Golden, Madison Camp, and Bill Finnearty.

I would like to extend my appreciation to the authors, publishers, and equipment companies who have granted me permission to use their illustrations.

The publication of the eleventh edition was accomplished through the capable guidance of many talented individuals at Elsevier. Many thanks to Rachel McMullen, Senior Project Manager, for her outstanding production work. This edition could not have attained this level of excellence without the exceptional capabilities of Rae Robertson, Senior Content Development Specialist. I also want to relay a very special thank you to Kristin Wilhelm, Executive Content Strategist, for her dedication to quality medical assisting education and her encouragement in helping me achieve my very best in this edition.

With warm regard, I would like to recognize those very important individuals—the medical assisting students, graduates, and practicing medical assistants—who continually strive for excellence in meeting the demands and ever-increasing requirements of such a challenging profession. A quote by an unknown author really says it better: "Celebrate your talents, for they are what make you unique."

Kathy Bonewit-West, BS, MEd

Contents

Clinical Procedure Icons

The OSHA Bloodborne Pathogens Standard must be followed when performing many of the clinical procedures presented in this text. To assist the student in following the OSHA Standard, icons have been incorporated into the procedures. An illustration of each icon, along with its description, is outlined below.

HAND HYGIENE is an important medical aseptic practice and is crucial in preventing the transmission of pathogens in the medical office. The medical assistant should sanitize the hands frequently, using proper techniques. When performing clinical procedures, the hands should always be sanitized before and after patient contact, before applying gloves and after removing gloves, and after contact with blood or other potentially infectious materials.

CLEAN DISPOSABLE GLOVES should be worn when it is reasonably anticipated that the medical assistant will have hand contact with the following: blood and other potentially infectious materials, mucous membranes, nonintact skin, and contaminated articles or surfaces.

BIOHAZARD CONTAINERS are closable, leakproof, and suitably constructed to contain the contents during handling, storage, transport, or shipping. The containers must be labeled or color coded and closed before removal to prevent the contents from spilling.

APPROPRIATE PROTECTIVE CLOTHING such as gowns, aprons, and laboratory coats should be worn when gross contamination can reasonably be anticipated during performance of a task or procedure.

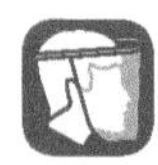

FACE SHIELDS OR MASKS IN COMBINATION WITH EYE-PROTECTION DEVICES must be worn whenever splashes, spray, spatter, or droplets of blood or other potentially infectious materials may be generated, posing a hazard through contact with the medical assistant's eyes, nose, or mouth.

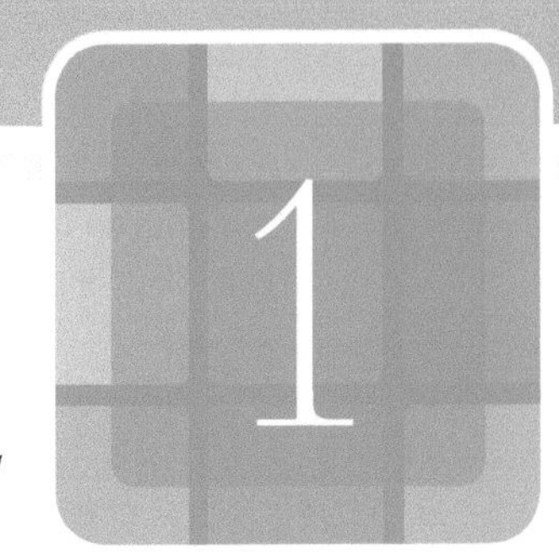

The Medical Record and Health History

Check out the Evolve site at http://evolve.elsevier.com/Bonewit to access additional interactive activities and exercises to help you study and prepare for success.

LEARNING OUTCOMES

Components of the Medical Record

1. List and describe functions served by the medical record.
2. Describe the following categories of documents or reports included in the medical record: administrative documents, clinical documents, laboratory reports, diagnostic procedure reports, therapeutic service reports, hospital documents, and consent documents.

Types of Medical Records

3. Explain the difference between a paper-based patient record (PPR) and an electronic health record (EHR).
4. List the general functions of EHR software.
5. Explain the advantages of EHRs.

Health History

6. List and describe the seven sections of the health history.
7. List the guidelines that should be followed in documenting the chief complaint.

Documentation in the Medical Record

8. List and describe the guidelines to follow to ensure accurate and concise documentation.
9. List and describe the types of progress notes that are documented by the medical assistant.
10. Explain the difference between a subjective and objective symptom, and list examples of each.
11. List and describe common symptoms.

PROCEDURES

Assist a patient in completing a health history form.

Document the following in a paper-based medical record:

- Procedures
- Administration of medication
- Specimen collection
- Laboratory tests
- Progress notes
- Instructions given to the patient
- Obtain and document patient symptoms.

CHAPTER OUTLINE

Procedures
Administration of Medication
Specimen Collection
Diagnostic Procedures and Laboratory Tests
Results of Laboratory Tests
Patient Instructions

KEY TERMS

diagnosis (dye-ag-NOE-sis)
diagnostic procedure
documenting
electronic health record (EHR)
familial (fah-MIL-yul) disease
health history report
medical record
objective symptom
paper-based patient record (PPR)
subjective symptom
symptom (SIMP-tum)

Introduction to the Medical Record

Medical records are a crucial part of a medical practice. A **medical record** is a written record of the important information regarding a patient, including the care of that individual and the progress of his or her condition.

The patient's medical record serves many important functions. The provider uses the information in the medical record as a basis for decisions regarding the patient's care and treatment. The medical record documents the results of treatment and the patient's progress. The medical record provides an efficient and effective method by which information can be communicated to authorized personnel in the medical office.

The medical record also serves as a legal document. The law requires that a record be maintained to document the care and treatment being received by a patient. If something goes wrong, good documentation works to protect the provider and the medical staff legally. Incomplete records could be used as evidence in court to show that a patient did not receive the quality of care that meets generally accepted standards.

The medical assistant must always keep in mind that the information contained in a patient's medical record is strictly confidential and must not be read by or discussed with anyone except the provider or medical staff involved with the care of the patient (see the box Highlight on the HIPAA Privacy Rule).

COMPONENTS OF THE MEDICAL RECORD

A medical record consists of numerous documents. Each document in the medical record has a specific function or purpose. Medical record documents can be classified into categories. Each of these categories is listed and described as follows along with the specific documents or reports included in each.

MEDICAL OFFICE ADMINISTRATIVE DOCUMENTS

Administrative documents contain information necessary for the efficient (record-keeping) management of the medical office and include the following:

- Patient registration record
- Notice of Privacy Practices (NPP) acknowledgment form
- Correspondence

MEDICAL OFFICE CLINICAL DOCUMENTS

Medical office clinical documents include a variety of records and reports that assist the provider in the care and treatment of the patient and include the following:

- Health history report
- Physical examination report
- Progress notes
- Medication record
- Consultation report
- Home health care report

LABORATORY REPORTS

A laboratory report is a report of the analysis or examination of body specimens. Its purpose is to relay the results of laboratory tests to the provider to assist in diagnosing and treating disease. Laboratory reports include the following:

- Hematology report
- Clinical chemistry report
- Immunology report
- Urinalysis report
- Microbiology report
- Parasitology report
- Cytology report
- Histology report

DIAGNOSTIC PROCEDURE REPORTS

A **diagnostic procedure** is a type of procedure performed to assist in the diagnosis, management, or treatment of a patient's condition. Diagnostic procedure reports consist of a narrative description and interpretation of a diagnostic procedure and include the following:

- Electrocardiogram report
- Holter monitor report
- Colonoscopy report
- Spirometry report
- Radiology report
- Diagnostic imaging report

THERAPEUTIC SERVICE REPORTS

Therapeutic service reports document the assessments and treatments designed to restore a patient's ability to function and include the following:

- Physical therapy report
- Occupational therapy report
- Speech therapy report

HOSPITAL DOCUMENTS

Hospital documents assist the patient's provider in reviewing the patient's hospital visit and in providing follow-up care. Hospital documents are prepared by the provider responsible for the care of a patient while at the hospital and include the following:

- History and physical report
- Operative report
- Discharge summary report
- Pathology report
- Emergency department report

CONSENT DOCUMENTS

Consent forms are legal documents required to perform certain procedures or to release information contained in the patient's medical record and include the following:

- Consent to treatment form
- Release of medical information form

HIGHLIGHT on the HIPAA Privacy Rule

What is the HIPAA Privacy Rule?

The acronym HIPAA stands for the Health Insurance Portability and Accountability Act. HIPAA is a federal law consisting of several components, one of which contains provisions to protect a patient's privacy, known as the HIPAA Privacy Rule.

The HIPAA Privacy Rule went into effect on April 14, 2003. The primary purpose of this rule is to provide patients with better control over the use and disclosure of their health information. All health care providers, health plans, and health care clearinghouses (e.g., billing services) that use, store, maintain, or transmit health information must comply with this rule.

What is included in the HIPAA Privacy Rule?

The HIPAA Privacy Rule is outlined here as it relates to the medical office:

1. The medical office must develop a written document known as a Notice of Privacy Practices (NPP). The NPP must explain to patients how their protected health information (PHI) will be used and protected by the medical office. PHI includes health information in any form (written, electronic, or oral) that contains patient-identifiable information (e.g., name, social security number, telephone number). The medical office must make a reasonable effort to provide an NPP to each patient and to obtain a signed acknowledgment from the patient that he or she has received an NPP.
2. A patient's written consent is not required for the use or disclosure of PHI for the following:
   - Medical treatment: *Examples:*
     (1) Patient referral to a specialist
     (2) Emergency care provided at a hospital
     (3) Tests on a patient performed by the laboratory
   - Payment: *Examples:*
     (1) Determination of eligibility for insurance benefits
     (2) Review of services provided for medical necessity
     (3) Utilization review activities
   - Health care operations: *Examples:*
     (1) Quality assessment activities
     (2) Contacting patients with information about care or treatment
     (3) Employee review activities
     (4) Training of health care students
   - Legally mandated reports. *Examples:*
     (1) Reports of child or elder abuse
     (2) Reportable diseases
     (3) Reports of injuries that may be a result of a crime
3. Patients have the right to access their medical records and to request changes to the records if they believe them to be inaccurate.
4. To prevent unnecessary or inappropriate access to PHI, the medical office must make an effort to limit the use of, disclosure of, and requests for PHI to the minimum necessary to accomplish the intended purpose (e.g., a request from an insurance company for procedures performed on a patient). However, this requirement does not apply to the use of PHI for the routine practice of medicine within the medical office.
5. Patients have a right to request an accounting of the transfer of their information for purposes other than treatment, payment, or health care operations.
6. Business associates to whom the medical office may disclose PHI must respect the HIPAA Privacy Rule. The medical office must execute a written agreement with each business associate to handle PHI in accordance with HIPAA. Business associates may include the following organizations and firms:

continued

HIGHLIGHT on the HIPAA Privacy Rule—cont'd

- Medical laboratories
- Transcription services
- Law firms
- Accounting firms
- Software and hardware consultants
- Billing services

7. The medical office must implement for all employees a basic training program on privacy and security of PHI.
8. The medical office is required to put in place appropriate administrative, physical, and technical security safeguards to protect the privacy of PHI from accidental use or disclosure or violation of the above-listed requirements.
9. The medical office is required to notify affected individuals following a breach of unsecured PHI.

What if a medical office does not comply with the HIPAA Privacy Rule?

There are severe penalties if a medical office fails to comply with the HIPAA Privacy Rule, which can include civil and criminal penalties.

Where can more information on the HIPAA Privacy Rule be found?

The following website contains current information on HIPAA: www.hhs.gov/hipaa

What Would You Do? What Would You *Not* Do?

Case Study 1

Moira Celeste, an account executive for a large insurance company, comes to the office complaining of insomnia and depression. Three months ago, her husband of 27 years left, and now they are legally separated. Since then, Moira has had a lot of trouble sleeping at night. She also feels lethargic during the day and has not been eating much. Moira says that she has been having some problems with alcohol. She wants to know of any community agencies that could help her with her problem but that would be sure to keep the information confidential. She has a very responsible job with her firm and does not want anyone to know about her alcohol problem. She also does not want any information about her problem put in her medical record, and she especially does not want the physician to know about it because he is friends with many of her colleagues at work. ■

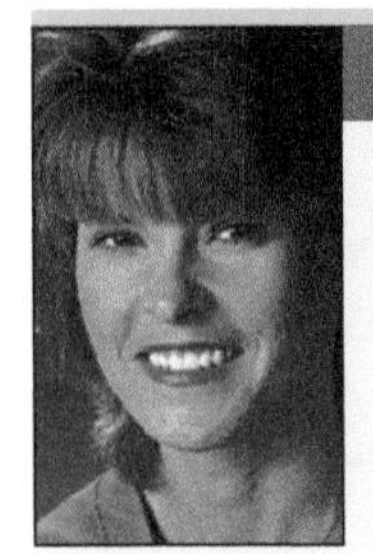

Putting It All into Practice

My Name is Dawn, and I work for an orthopedic surgeon. I work in both the clinical and the administrative areas of the office. In the administrative area, I work as a supervisor in billing and collections.

Working in billing and collections is very challenging and sometimes stressful. It can even be embarrassing. We are a new practice, and when we opened, there was no collection system. When it came time to review our accounts, we realized that, like every other business, we needed a collection system. We immediately jumped in and took charge.

The primary physician at our office is from New York, and we were unfamiliar with his family members. One day he walked into our office with a very puzzled look. I asked him what was wrong. He replied, "You guys are doing a great job with our collection rate. I asked you to be stern, but thoughtful, when sending out patient collection letters, but did you have to send one to my mother-in-law?!" Needless to say, we fixed the error immediately. This incident prompted us to restructure our collection system, and we added a comment screen to our computer system on all of our patients' accounts. Going into a medical office that already has a system in place may be easier, but you can learn a lot more by setting up an office system yourself.

Types of Medical Records

There are two types of medical records; these include the paper-based patient record (PPR) and the electronic health record (EHR), which are described in more detail as follows.

PAPER-BASED PATIENT RECORD

Medical offices may rely on the use of paper medical records, known as **paper-based patient records (PPRs).** Although most of the medical record is paper based, some patient data are maintained on the computer; these include patient registration information and patient charges and payments. Many of the documents included in a PPR consist of preprinted forms that contain specific information documented by the patient, the medical assistant, or the provider. Examples of these forms include the patient registration form, health history form, and the medication record form.

ELECTRONIC HEALTH RECORD

The **electronic health record (EHR)** is a computerized record of the important health information regarding a patient, including the care of that individual and the progress of the patient's condition. As technology has advanced, most offices have converted, either partially or fully, to an EHR for

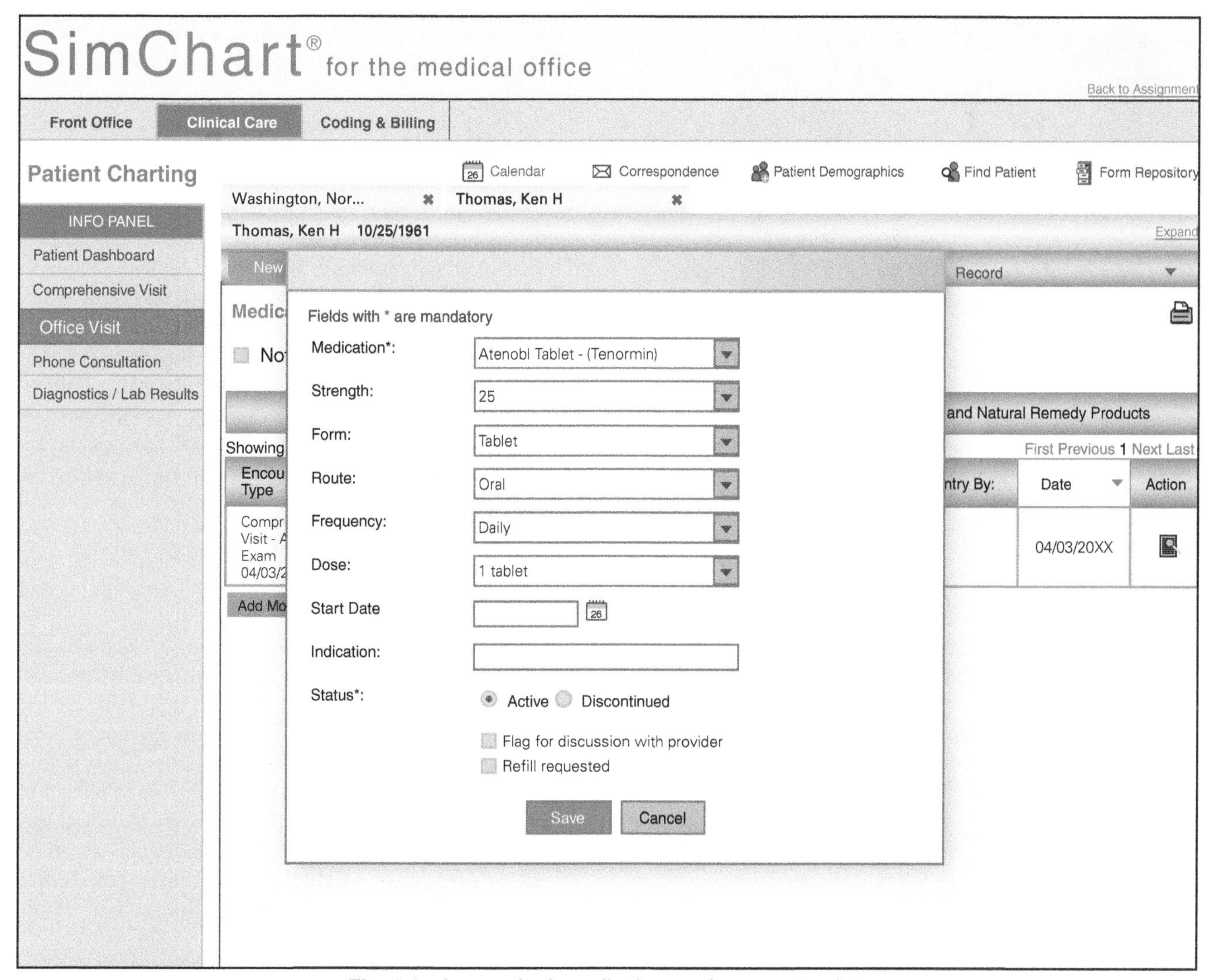

Fig. 1.1 An example of a medication record computer template.

maintaining patient health information. With an EHR, the entire record is stored in a database on the computer, including the health history report and physical examination report, medication record, progress notes, laboratory and diagnostic reports, hospital reports, and consent documents.

EHR software programs allow for the creation, storage, organization, editing, and retrieval of medical records on a computer. The EHR program also incorporates practice management software for scheduling, billing, and filing insurance claims. This allows the EHR to include more information than a paper-based medical record.

Many of the documents in an EHR consist of forms (known as *templates*) that are displayed on the computer screen and are filled out in much the same way as a paper form. Each computer template includes spaces (known as *fields*) in which information is entered by health care personnel. Fig. 1.1 illustrates an example of a medication record computer template with fields for entering information relative to a patient's medication.

ADVANTAGES OF THE ELECTRONIC HEALTH RECORD

The incorporation of an EHR in the medical office leads to better-quality patient care through improved communication, faster access to data, and clearer and better documentation. These advantages are accomplished as described in the following section.

Speed and Productivity

One of the principal advantages of an EHR is that the computer can retrieve requested documents from a patient's record very quickly (Fig. 1.2). Documents received from outside facilities, such as laboratory reports, can be stored very quickly in the EHR. EHRs do not need to be filed, as with a paper-based record. This saves considerable time and frees up the office space required to store paper records. Paper costs are also reduced, and time is saved in not having to look for lost records.

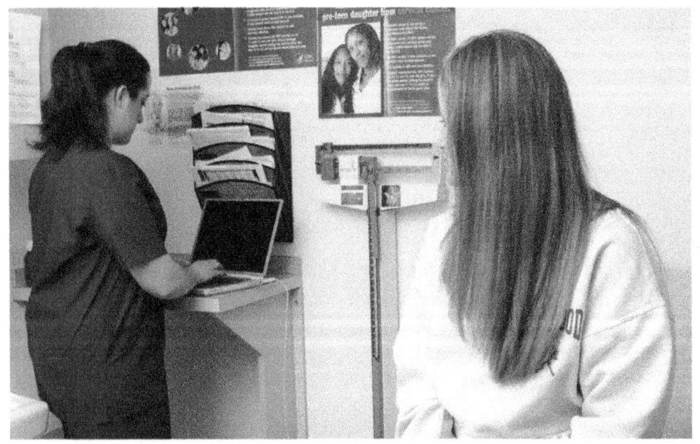

Fig. 1.2 An electronic health record allows for the rapid storage and retrieval of data in the patient's record.

Efficiency

EHR software programs facilitate the entry of data into the patient's medical record. To assist in entering data, EHR programs use point and click technology, such as radio buttons, drop-down menus, and free text entry. (Note: *Radio buttons* consist of a series of on-screen buttons that allow only one selection to be made from a list of options.) EHR programs also have the capability to print certain documents for the patient following a medical office visit such as a patient health visit summary and customized patient education instructions. One of the principal advantages of an EHR is the ability to generate prescriptions, as described in detail in Chapter 11.

Provider Accessibility

The EHR provides immediate access to the patient's medical record by the provider and health care personnel to review patient information such as current medications, allergies, immunizations, and laboratory and diagnostic test results. A patient's EHR can be accessed from any EHR-accessible device with an internet connection such as a computer, tablet, or smartphone. The provider also has ready access to a patient's EHR from a remote location such as a hospital, an extended care facility, and the provider's home.

Patient Accessibility

A growing number of medical offices allow patients to access their health information through a patient portal. A *patient portal* is a secure online website that provides patients with 24-hour access to their personal health information through an internet connection. Using a secure username and password, patients can view and print health information such a summary of a medical office visit, educational materials, current medications, immunizations, allergies, and laboratory and diagnostic test results. A patient portal often allows the patient to interact with the medical office to perform the following tasks: request prescription refills, schedule nonurgent appointments, check benefits and coverage, make payments, complete forms, update contact information, and communicate with medical office personnel through e-mail. A patient portal allows the patient to become more involved with their health care and facilitates the workflow of the medical office.

Health History Report

The **health history report** is a collection of subjective data about the patient. Most of this information is obtained by having the patient complete a preprinted form that is then reviewed for completeness by the medical assistant. Some of the information included in the health history is obtained by the provider or medical assistant by interviewing the patient. A quiet, comfortable room that allows for privacy encourages the patient to communicate honestly and openly. Showing genuine interest in and concern for the patient reduces apprehension and facilitates the collection of data.

A thorough history is taken for each new patient, and subsequent office visits provide information regarding changes in the patient's illness or treatment. Along with the physical examination and laboratory and diagnostic tests, the health history is used for the following reasons: to determine the patient's general state of health, to arrive at a diagnosis and to prescribe treatment, and to document any change in a patient's illness after treatment has been instituted. The term **diagnosis** refers to the scientific method of determining and identifying a patient's condition.

In an office with an EHR, the patient may complete a health history paper-and-pencil form, and the medical assistant then enters these data and/or scans the health history form into the patient's medical record. An alternative is for the medical assistant to enter the information directly into the computer while asking the patient questions related to his or her health status. Although not yet in widespread use, computer-guided questionnaires are available for a patient to complete the health history at a *kiosk* in the medical office or online through a secure medical office website. If the

Memories *from* Practicum

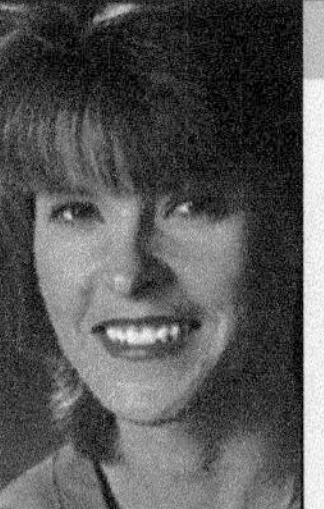

Dawn: During my practicum as a medical assisting student, I was placed in a family practice clinic. I was very nervous my first day, wondering how in the world I would be able to remember everything I had learned in school. My first patients were an elderly couple. The wife was there for some test results for cancer. I looked at the results, and they were positive. After the physician relayed the results, the husband broke down. He had just lost his granddaughter to a heart attack and his son-in-law to a stroke. You could tell that he just could not bear losing his wife too.

One week later, the elderly man's wife was placed in a nursing home. He came into our office for an appointment. As I was working him up, he was telling me stories about himself and his wife when they were first married. He looked so sad. I sat with him for a few minutes after completing his work-up and gave his stories my full attention. As I was leaving the room, a smile came across his face, and he thanked me for listening to him. I realized that working in a physician's office is more than just knowing what I learned in school. Compassion and showing patients you really do care about them are just as important. I felt good about myself that day. ■

patient completes this questionnaire at the medical office, a quiet and private area for the patient to complete it must be provided, and the medical assistant must be available to answer questions.

What Would You Do? What Would You *Not* Do?

Case Study 2

Brett Oberlin is 21 years old and lives at home. He commutes to a local college and is a junior majoring in art education. His mother and father have come to the medical office and ask to see his medical record. The physician is attending a medical conference and will not return for another 4 days. Mr. and Mrs. Oberlin found some medications in Brett's room and looked them up on the Internet. They found out that they are used to treat human immunodeficiency virus (HIV) infection. Brett would not talk to them about the medications and told them he is an adult and it is none of their business. Mr. and Mrs. Oberlin are very concerned about Brett. They also are worried about other members of the family being exposed to HIV. They say that because they are supporting him, they should be allowed to see his record. ■

COMPONENTS OF THE HEALTH HISTORY

The health history is taken before the physical examination is performed, allowing the provider the opportunity to compare findings. The health history consists of seven parts or sections.

IDENTIFICATION DATA

The identification data section is included at the beginning of the health history form to obtain basic demographic data on the patient (Fig. 1.3A). The patient is usually responsible for completing the identification data section.

CHIEF COMPLAINT

The chief complaint (CC) identifies the patient's reason for seeking care (i.e., the symptom that is causing the patient the most trouble). The CC is used as a foundation for the more detailed information obtained for the present illness (PI) and review of systems (ROS) sections of the health history. The medical assistant is usually responsible for obtaining the CC from the patient and documenting it in the patient's medical record. This information may be documented on a preprinted, lined form (see Fig. 1.3F) or entered directly into an EHR (refer to Procedure 1.1). Certain guidelines must be followed in obtaining and documenting the CC, as follows:

- An open-ended question should be used to elicit the CC from the patient: What seems to be the problem? How can we help you today? What can we do for you today?
- The CC should be limited to one or two symptoms and should refer to a specific, rather than vague, symptom.
- The CC should be documented concisely and briefly, using the patient's own words as much as possible.
- The duration of the symptom (onset) should be included in the CC.
- The medical assistant should avoid using names of diseases or diagnostic terms to document the CC.

Documenting Chief Complaints

Following are correct and incorrect examples of documenting CCs.

Correct Examples

- Burning during urination that has lasted for 2 days.
- Pain in the shoulder that started 2 weeks ago.
- Shortness of breath for the past month.

Incorrect Examples

- Has not felt well for the past 2 weeks. (This statement refers to a vague, rather than a specific, complaint.)
- Ear pain and fever. (The duration of the symptoms is not listed.)
- Pain upon urination indicative of a urinary tract infection. (Names of diseases should not be used to document the CC; the duration of the symptom is not listed.)

PRESENT ILLNESS

The PI is an expansion of the CC and includes a full description of the patient's current illness from the time of its onset. The medical assistant is often responsible for completing this section of the health history, which is documented on the same form as the CC (see Fig. 1.3F) or entered directly into the EHR. To complete this section of the health history, the medical assistant asks the patient questions to obtain a detailed description of the symptom causing the greatest problem. A general guide for obtaining further information on symptoms is presented in Procedure 1.1, and a more thorough study for analyzing a symptom is included in Chapter 1 of the *Study Guide for Students.*

PAST HISTORY

The past medical history is a review of the patient's past medical status (see Fig. 1.3B). Obtaining information on past medical care assists the provider in providing optimal care for the current problem. Most medical offices ask the patient to complete this section of the health history through a checklist type of form. The medical assistant should assist the patient with this section as necessary by offering to answer any questions regarding the information required. The past history includes the following areas:

- Major illnesses
- Childhood diseases
- Unusual infections
- Accidents and injuries

PATIENT HEALTH HISTORY

A

IDENTIFICATION DATA Please print the following information.

Today's date ____

Name ____ ___ Male ___ Female

Address ____ ___ Married ___ Separated ___ Divorced ___ Widowed ___ Single

____ Date of Birth ____

Telephone ____ ____

Home number Work number

B

PAST HISTORY

Have you ever had the following: (Circle "no" or "yes", leave blank if uncertain)

Measles ____ no yes	Heart Disease ____ no yes	Diabetes ____ no yes	Hemorrhoids ____ no yes
Mumps ____ no yes	Arthritis ____ no yes	Cancer ____ no yes	Asthma ____ no yes
Chickenpox ____ no yes	Sexually Transmitted Disease ____ no yes	Polio ____ no yes	Allergies ____ no yes
Whooping Cough ____ no yes	Anemia ____ no yes	Glaucoma ____ no yes	Eczema ____ no yes
Scarlet Fever ____ no yes	Bladder Infections ____ no yes	Hernia ____ no yes	AIDS or HIV+ ____ no yes
Diphtheria ____ no yes	Epilepsy ____ no yes	Blood or Plasma Transfusions ____ no yes	Infectious Mono ____ no yes
Pneumonia ____ no yes	Migraine Headaches ____ no yes	Back Trouble ____ no yes	Bronchitis ____ no yes
Rheumatic Fever ____ no yes	Tuberculosis ____ no yes	High Blood Pressure ____ no yes	Mitral Valve Prolapse no yes
Stroke ____ no yes	Ulcer ____ no yes	Thyroid Disease ____ no yes	Any other disease ____ no yes Please list: ____
Hepatitis ____ no yes	Kidney Disease ____ no yes	Bleeding Tendency ____ no yes	____

MAJOR HOSPITALIZATIONS: If you have ever been hospitalized for any major medical illness or operation, write in your most recent hospitalizations below.

Hospitalizations	Year	Operation or illness	Name of hospital	City and state
1st Hospitalization				
2nd Hospitalization				
3rd Hospitalization				
4th Hospitalization				

TESTS AND IMMUNIZATIONS: Mark an X next to those that you have had.

Tests:

- ☐ TB Test
- ☐ Rectal/Hemoccult
- ☐ Sigmoidoscopy
- ☐ Colonoscopy
- ☐ Electrocardiogram
- ☐ Chest x-ray
- ☐ Mammogram
- ☐ Pap Test

Immunizations:

- ☐ Influenza
- ☐ Hepatitis B
- ☐ Tetanus
- ☐ MMR
- ☐ Polio

CURRENT MEDICATIONS: List the following that you are currently taking: Prescription medications, over-the-counter (OTC) medications, vitamin supplements, and herbal supplements. ☐ None

Medication	Frequency

ALLERGIES: List all allergies (foods, drugs, environment). ☐ None

____

____

____

____

ACCIDENTS/ INJURIES: Describe all serious accidents, severe injuries, head injury, or fractures. Include the date each occurred. ☐ None

Accident/Injury:	Date:

Fig. 1.3 Health history form.

C

FAMILY HISTORY

For each member of your family, follow the purple or blue line across the page and check boxes for:
1. His or her present state of health
2. Any illnesses he or she has had

	Good Health	Poor Health	Deceased	If deceased, write in age and cause of death.	Allergies or Asthma	Diabetes	Heart Disease	Stroke	Cancer	High Blood Pressure	Glaucoma	Arthritis	Ulcer	Kidney Disease	Mental Health Problems	Alcohol/Drug Abuse	Obesity	High Cholesterol	Thyroid Disease
Father:																			
Mother:																			
Brothers/Sisters:																			

D

SOCIAL HISTORY

EDUCATION ______ High school ______ College ______ Postgraduate

Occupation ______ Years ______

Previous occupations ______ Years ______

______ Years ______

Have you ever been exposed to any of the following in your environment?

☐ Excess dust (coal, lime, rock) ☐ Cleaning fluids/solvents ☐ Radiation ☐ Other toxic materials
☐ Sand ☐ Hair spray ☐ Insecticides
☐ Chemicals ☐ Smoke or auto exhaust fumes ☐ Paints

Please answer the following questions by placing an X in the box in front of the word Yes or No, except where you are asked for specific information. This information is obviously highly confidential and will be released to other health care professionals or insurance carriers ONLY with your consent.

DIET:
- Do you eat a good breakfast? ☐ Yes ☐ No
- Do you snack between meals (soft drinks, chips, candy bars)? ☐ Yes ☐ No
- Do you eat fresh fruits and vegetables each day? ☐ Yes ☐ No
- Do you eat whole grain breads and cereals? ☐ Yes ☐ No
- Is your diet high in fat content? ☐ Yes ☐ No
- Is your diet high in cholesterol content? ☐ Yes ☐ No
- Is your diet high in salt content? ☐ Yes ☐ No
- Are you allergic to any foods? ☐ Yes ☐ No
- How many glasses of water do you drink each day? ______
- How would you describe your overall eating habits? ☐ Excellent ☐ Good ☐ Fair ☐ Poor

PERSONAL HISTORY:
- Do you find it hard to make decisions? ☐ Yes ☐ No
- Do you find it hard to concentrate or remember? ☐ Yes ☐ No
- Do you feel depressed? ☐ Yes ☐ No
- Do you have difficulty relaxing? ☐ Yes ☐ No
- Do you have a tendency to worry a lot? ☐ Yes ☐ No
- Have you gained or lost much weight recently? ☐ Yes ☐ No
- Do you lose your temper often? ☐ Yes ☐ No
- Are you disturbed by any work or family problems? ☐ Yes ☐ No
- Are you having sexual difficulties? ☐ Yes ☐ No
- Have you ever considered committing suicide? ☐ Yes ☐ No
- Have you ever desired or sought psychiatric help? ☐ Yes ☐ No

EXERCISE:
- Do you exercise on a regular basis? ☐ Yes ☐ No
- Does your job require strenuous, sustained physical work? ☐ Yes ☐ No

SLEEP PATTERNS:
- Do you seem to feel exhausted or fatigued most of the time? ☐ Yes ☐ No
- Do you have difficulty either falling asleep or staying asleep? ☐ Yes ☐ No

USE OF TOBACCO/ALCOHOL/CAFFEINE/DRUGS: Amt:
- How much do you smoke per day? ☐ Cigarettes __ ☐ Cigars/pipes __ ☐ Don't smoke
- Do you take two or more alcoholic drinks per day? ☐ Yes ☐ No
- Do you drink six or more cups of coffee or tea per day? ☐ Yes ☐ No
- Are you a regular user of sleeping pills, marijuana, tranquilizers, pain killers, etc? ☐ Yes ☐ No
- Have you ever used heroin, cocaine, LSD, PCP, etc? ☐ Yes ☐ No

List any country outside the USA you have visited in the past six months. ______

When did you have your last physical examination? ______

Fig. 1.3, cont'd

Patient's Name________________________________

E

REVIEW OF SYSTEMS

HEAD AND NECK
____ Frequent headaches
____ Neck pain
____ Neck lumps or swelling

EYES
____ Wears glasses
____ Blurry vision
____ Eyesight worsening
____ Sees double
____ Sees halo
____ Eye pain or itching
____ Watery eyes
____ Eye trouble

EARS
____ Hearing difficulties
____ Earaches
____ Running ears
____ Buzzing in ears
____ Motion sickness

MOUTH
____ Dental problems
____ Swelling on gums or jaws
____ Sore tongue
____ Taste changes

NOSE AND THROAT
____ Congested nose
____ Running nose
____ Sneezing spells
____ Head colds
____ Nosebleeds
____ Sore throat
____ Enlarged tonsils
____ Hoarse voice

RESPIRATORY
____ Wheezes or gasps
____ Coughing spells
____ Coughs up phlegm
____ Coughed up blood
____ Chest colds
____ Excessive sweating, night sweats

CARDIOVASCULAR
____ High blood pressure
____ Racing heart
____ Chest pains
____ Dizzy spells
____ Shortness of breath
____ Shortness of breath at night
____ More pillows to breathe
____ Swollen feet or ankles
____ Leg cramps
____ Heart murmur

DIGESTIVE
____ Heartburn
____ Bloated stomach
____ Belching
____ Stomach pains
____ Nausea
____ Vomited blood
____ Difficulty swallowing
____ Constipation
____ Loose bowels
____ Black stools
____ Grey stools
____ Pain in rectum
____ Rectal bleeding

URINARY
____ Night frequency
____ Day frequency
____ Wets pants or bed
____ Burning on urination
____ Brown, black, or bloody urine
____ Difficulty starting urine
____ Urgency

MALE GENITAL
____ Weak urine stream
____ Prostate trouble
____ Burning or discharge
____ Lumps on testicles
____ Painful testicles

FEMALE GENITAL
__/__/__ Last menstrual period
__/__/__ Last Pap test
____ Postmenopausal or hysterectomy
____ Noticed vaginal bleeding
____ Abnormal LMP
____ Heavy bleeding during periods
____ Bleeding between periods
____ Bleeding after intercourse
____ Recent vaginal itching/discharge
____ No monthly breast exam
____ Lump or pain in breasts
____ Complications with birth control

OBSTETRIC HISTORY
____ Gravida
____ Para
____ Preterm
____ Miscarriages
____ Stillbirths
____ Has had an abortion

MUSCULOSKELETAL
____ Aching muscles
____ Swollen joints
____ Back or shoulder pains
____ Painful feet
____ Disability

SKIN
____ Skin problems
____ Itching or burning skin
____ Bleeds easily
____ Bruises easily

NEUROLOGICAL
____ Faintness
____ Numbness
____ Convulsions
____ Change in handwriting
____ Trembles

F

PROGRESS NOTES

Date	

Fig. 1.3, cont'd

- Hospitalizations and operations
- Previous medical tests
- Immunizations
- Allergies
- Current medications

FAMILY HISTORY

The family history is a review of the health status of the patient's blood relatives (see Fig. 1.3C). This section of the health history focuses on diseases that tend to be familial. A **familial disease** is a condition that occurs in or affects blood relatives more frequently than would be expected by chance. Examples of familial diseases include hypertension, heart disease, allergies, and diabetes mellitus. The patient usually completes this section of the health history and is asked to provide the following information about each blood relative:

- State of health
- Presence of any significant disease
- If deceased, cause of death

SOCIAL HISTORY

The social history section of the health history includes information on the patient's lifestyle, such as health habits and living environment (see Fig. 1.3D). The social history is important because the patient's lifestyle may have an impact on his or her condition and may influence the course of treatment chosen by the provider. The social history also provides the provider with information regarding the effect that the illness may have on the patient's daily living pattern. If it is necessary for the individual to make a major lifestyle adjustment (e.g., stop smoking, reduce working hours), the provider may recommend support services to assist in this transition. This section of the history is usually completed by the patient and includes the following areas:

- Education
- Occupation (past and present)
- Living environment
- Diet
- Personal history
- Exercise

Yan, Tai I 04/07/1956 Expand

New Patient Visit 04/05/2014 ▼ Add New | Record ▼

General	○ Yes	● No	HEENT	○ Yes	● No	HEEN T/2	○ Yes	● No
Fever	○	●	HA	○	●	Blurred Vision	●	○
Chills	○	●	Vision Changes	○	●	Ringing	○	●
Sweats	○	●	Dizziness	●	○	Deafness	○	●
Fatigue	○	●	Ear Ache	○	●	Vertigo	○	●
Weight Gain	○	●	Sore Throat	○	●	Epistaxis	○	●
Weight Loss	○	●	Discharge	○	●	Hoarse	○	●
Cardiac	**○ Yes**	**● No**	**Resp**	**○ Yes**	**● No**	**GI**	**○ Yes**	**● No**
Chest Pain	○	●	Cough	○	●	Constipation	○	●
Palpitations	○	●	Congestion	○	●	Dysphagia	○	●
DOE	○	●	Expectoration	○	●	N/V	○	●
Edema	○	●	Wheezing	○	●	Abdominal Pain	○	●
PND	○	●	SOB	○	●	Heart Burn	○	●
Diaphoresis	○	●	Hemoptysis	○	●	Diarrhea	○	●
GU	**○ Yes**	**● No**	**MS**	**○ Yes**	**● No**	**Hem/Skin**	**○ Yes**	**● No**
Dysuria	○	●	Myalgia	○	●	Anemia	○	●
Incontinence	○	●	Back Pain	○	●	Adenopathy	○	●
Frequency	○	●	Radiation	○	●	Rashes	○	●
Nocturia	○	●	Joint Pain	○	●	Leg Ulcer	○	●
Sexual Dysfunction	○	●	Joint Swelling	○	●	Bruising	○	●
Irregular Menses	○	●	Injury	○	●	Itching	○	●

Fig. 1.4 Review of systems computer template.

REVIEW OF SYSTEMS

A ROS is a systematic review of each body system to detect any symptoms that have not yet been revealed. The importance of the ROS is that it assists in identifying symptoms that might otherwise remain undetected. The provider usually completes the ROS by asking a series of detailed and direct questions related to each body system; the results of this section of the health history assist the provider in a preliminary assessment of the type and extent of physical examination required. Fig. 1.3E shows an example of an ROS paper-based form, and Fig. 1.4 illustrates an example of an ROS computer template.

Documentation in the Medical Record

Documenting is the process of recording information about a patient in the medical record and is performed by medical office personnel who are directly involved with the health care of the patient. The medical record is considered a legal document; the information must be documented as completely and accurately as possible. Developing good documenting skills requires a thorough knowledge of documentation guidelines combined with much repeated practice. To provide guidance in attaining this important skill, general guidelines for documentation are presented in this section for both the PPR and EHR, followed by guidelines specific only to the PPR. With an EHR, the medical assistant enters information into a computer using radio buttons, drop-down menus, and free text entry.

The medical assistant should always take the time to document properly in the patient's medical record. Good documentation helps to coordinate efforts in the medical office and leads to high-quality health care.

GENERAL GUIDELINES FOR DOCUMENTATION

To ensure accurate and concise documentation, specific guidelines must be followed. These are listed and described as follows:

1. *Check the name and date of birth on the medical record before making an entry, to ensure you have the correct record.* If the medical assistant documents in the wrong patient's record by mistake, information such as a procedure that was performed on a patient may be excluded from the correct patient's record. From a legal standpoint, a procedure not documented was not performed.
2. *Document information accurately, using clear and concise phrases.*
   - The medical assistant should be brief but thorough and should avoid vagueness and duplication of information.
   - It is not necessary to include the patient's name in the entry because the entire medical record centers on one patient; it is assumed the information refers to that patient.
   - Each phrase should begin with a capital letter and end with a period.
   - Standard abbreviations, medical terms, and symbols can be used to help save time and space. It is *crucial* that the medical assistant first check the office policy to determine the abbreviations, medical terms, and symbols that are used in that office. Using commonly accepted terminology avoids confusing others who read the record. A list of abbreviations and symbols commonly used in medical offices is presented in Table 1.1.
3. *Spell correctly.* Correct spelling is essential for accuracy in documentation. If you are in doubt about the spelling of a word, consult a dictionary.
4. *Document immediately after performing a procedure.* When a procedure has been performed, it should be documented without delay. If a time lapse occurs between performing the procedure and documenting it, the medical assistant may not remember certain aspects of the procedure, such as the results of the treatment or the patient's reaction. It is important to note that procedures should never be documented in advance.
5. *Never document for someone else.* The individual performing the procedure should be the one to document it.

DOCUMENTING IN THE PAPER-BASED PATIENT RECORD

Additional guidelines for documenting in the PPR are listed and described as follows:

1. *Use black ink to make entries in the patient's record.* Black ink must be used to provide a permanent record. In addition, entries made in black ink are easier to reproduce when a record must be duplicated for insurance company purposes and patient referral.
2. *Write in legible handwriting.* For the medical record to be meaningful to others, the medical assistant must document information legibly. If the medical assistant's cursive script is not legible, the information should be printed.
3. *Begin each new entry on a separate line, and do not leave blank space.* Each new entry should begin on a separate line and be dated with the month, day, year, and time (either AM/PM or military time). If part of the line is not needed, draw a single line through unneeded space so that nothing can be added at a later date.
4. *Each entry should be signed by the person making it.* The signature should include the medical assistant's first initial, full last name, and title (e.g., D. Bennett, CMA [AAMA]). The following title abbreviations are often used for medical assistants:

   CMA (AAMA): certified medical assistant (American Association of Medical Assistants)

Table 1.1 Abbreviations and Symbols Commonly Used in the Medical Office[a]

Abbreviations Used to Document Symptoms and Procedures	
āā	of each
Ab	abortion
abs	absent
ac	before meals
ad lib	as desired
admin	administer
AM or a.m.	before noon
amt	amount
AP	apical pulse
approx	approximately
appt	appointment
ASA	acetylsalicylic acid (aspirin)
ASAP	as soon as possible
BA	backache
b/c	because
BC	birth control
Bid	twice a day
BM	bowel movement
BP	blood pressure
BPM	beats per minute
BS	blood sugar
BSE	breast self-examination
$\overline{C}$	with
caps	capsules
Cath	catheter, catheterize
CC	chief complaint
chemo	chemotherapy
CMA (AAMA)	certified medical assistant (American Association of Medical Assistants)
c/o	complains of
CS	cesarean section
Cx	cervix
D	day
/d	per day
d/c	discontinue
disch	discharge
DNKA	did not keep appointment
DOB	date of birth
DRE	digital rectal examination
DSD	dry, sterile dressing
DTaP	diphtheria and tetanus toxoids and acellular pertussis vaccine
DVA	distance visual acuity
ED	emergency department
EDD	expected date of delivery
Fe	iron
F/U	follow-up
Fx	fracture
GYN	gynecology
h or hr	hour
H/A	headache
HBP	high blood pressure
HC	head circumference
Hep B	hepatitis B vaccine
H_2O	water
HR	heart rate
HRT	hormone replacement therapy
Ht	height
ID	intradermal
IM	intramuscular
IPV	inactivated polio vaccine
IV	intravenous
Lab	laboratory
Lac	laceration
Lat	lateral
LB	lower back
LBP	lower back pain
LMP	last menstrual period
med, meds	medication, medications
min	minute
MMR	measles, mumps, and rubella
mod	moderate
N/A	not applicable
NB	newborn
N/C	no complaints
neg	negative
NICU	newborn intensive care unit
NKA	no known allergies
NKDA	no known drug allergies
NS	normal saline
N&V	nausea and vomiting
NVA	near visual acuity
OB	obstetrics
occ	occasionally
oint	ointment
OR	operating room
OT	occupational therapy
OTC	over-the-counter (nonprescription medication)
OV	office visit
P	pulse
Pap	Pap test
path	pathology
pc	after meals
peds	pediatrics
PEN	penicillin
per	by or through
pharm	pharmacy
PM or p.m.	afternoon
PMS	premenstrual syndrome

Continued

Table 1.1 Abbreviations and Symbols Commonly Used in the Medical Office[a]—cont'd

po or PO	by mouth
pos	positive
postop	postoperative (after surgery)
preop	preoperative (before surgery)
prep	preparation
prn	as needed
PT	physical therapy, prothrombin time
Pt or pt	patient
Qh	every hour
q(2,3,4)h	every (2,3,4) hours
Qid	4 times a day
QNS	quantity not sufficient
QS	quantity sufficient
quad	quadriplegic
R	respiration
Reg	regular
rehab	rehabilitation
RMA	registered medical assistant
Rx	prescription
$\bar{s}$	without
subcut	subcutaneous
S/E	side effects
Sl	slight
SOB	shortness of breath
Sol	solution
spec	specimen
STAT	immediately
surg	surgery
T	temperature
tab, tabs	tablet, tablets
temp	temperature
Tid	3 times a day
TLC	total lung capacity, tender loving care
TPR	temperature, pulse, and respiration
Tr	trace
TSE	testicular self-examination
Vit	vitamin
VO	verbal order
VS	vital signs
Wk	week
WNL	within normal limits
WO	written order
w/o	without
Wt	weight

Abbreviations Used to Document Body Parts and Locations

abd	abdomen
EENT	eye, ear, nose, and throat
GI	gastrointestinal
GU	genitourinary
Ⓛ or lt	left
ⓁⒶ	left arm
ⓁⓁ	left leg
LLQ	lower left quadrant
LRQ	lower right quadrant
LUQ	left upper quadrant
Ⓡ or rt	right
ⓇⒶ	right arm
ⓇⓁ	right leg
RLQ	right lower quadrant
RUQ	right upper quadrant

Abbreviations Used to Document Measurement

C	Celsius
cm	centimeter
dL	deciliter
F	Fahrenheit
g	gram
kg	kilogram
l	liter
Lb	pound
M	meter
mcg	microgram
mg	milligram
mL	milliliter
mm	millimeter
Oz	ounce
Pt	pint
Qt	quart
T	tablespoon
tsp	teaspoon

Miscellaneous Abbreviations

Patient Examination

Dx	diagnosis
H/O	history of
H&P	history and physical
Hx	history
PE or Px	physical examination
Sx	symptoms
Tx	treatment

Conditions

BPH	benign prostatic hyperplasia
CA	cancer
CAD	coronary artery disease
CHF	congestive heart failure
COPD	chronic obstructive pulmonary disease
CRC	colorectal cancer
CVA	cerebrovascular accident

Table 1.1 Abbreviations and Symbols Commonly Used in the Medical Office[a]—cont'd

DM	diabetes mellitus
DVT	deep vein thrombosis
Fe def	iron deficiency
GC	gonorrhea
GDM	gestational diabetes mellitus
HTN	hypertension
IBS	irritable bowel syndrome
MI	myocardial infarction
MS	multiple sclerosis
OA	osteoarthritis
OM	otitis media
PID	pelvic inflammatory disease
RA	rheumatoid arthritis
RF	rheumatic fever
STD (STI)	sexually transmitted disease (sexually transmitted infection)
TB	tuberculosis
URI	upper respiratory infection
UTI	urinary tract infection

Diagnostic Procedures

CT, CAT	computed axial tomography
CXR	chest x-ray
ECG	electrocardiogram
Echo	echocardiogram
EEG	electroencephalogram
FOBT	fecal occult blood test
IVP	intravenous pyelogram
LP	lumbar puncture
MRI	magnetic resonance imaging
NST	nonstress test
PET	positron emission tomography
PFT	pulmonary function test
TRUS	transrectal ultrasound
US	ultrasound

Laboratory Tests

ABG	arterial blood gas
BG	blood glucose
Bx	biopsy
CBC	complete blood count
C&S	culture and sensitivity
diff	differential
ESR	erythrocyte sedimentation rate
FBG	fasting blood glucose
FBS	fasting blood sugar
GCT	glucose challenge test
GTT	glucose tolerance test
Hct	hematocrit
Hgb	hemoglobin
OGTT	oral glucose tolerance test
PPBS	postprandial blood sugar
PSA	prostate-specific antigen
PT, PT/INR	prothrombin time
RBC	red blood cell
RBS	random blood sugar
SG	specific gravity
trig	triglycerides
UA	urinalysis
WBC	white blood cell

Symbols

Ø	none, no
✓	check
↑	increase
↓	decrease
♀	female
♂	male
°	degree
×	times
$\overline{p}$	after
#	number
1°	primary
2°	secondary
Ⓡ	rectal temperature
Ⓐ	axillary temperature
″	inches
′	feet

[a]This table follows The Joint Commission (TJC)'s list of "Do Not Use" abbreviations and symbols. TJC's requirements do not currently apply to preprogrammed health information technology systems such as electronic health records.

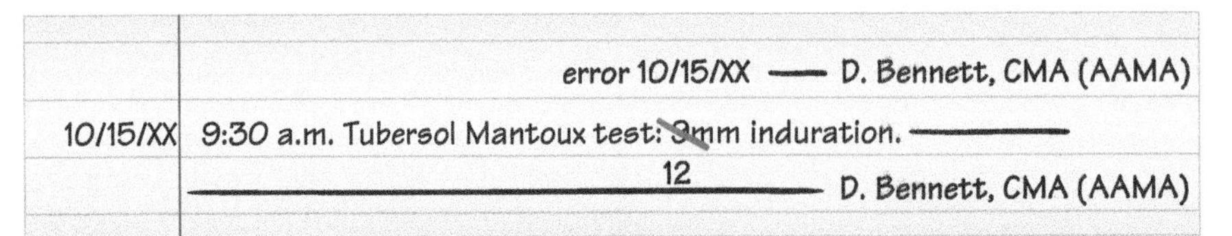

Fig. 1.5 Proper method for correcting an error in a patient's medical record.

RMA: registered medical assistant
MA: medical assistant
SMA: student medical assistant

5. *Never erase or obliterate an entry.* If a documenting error is made, the medical assistant must never erase or obliterate it. Should the provider or medical staff be involved in litigation, erased or obliterated entries tend to reduce credibility. If incorrect information is documented, the medical assistant should draw a single line through the incorrect information, permitting it to remain legible. The word *error* is then written above the incorrect data, including the date and the medical assistant's first initial, last name, and credentials. Some medical offices may request that the reason for the change also be documented. The correct information is then inserted next to the error (Fig. 1.5).

DOCUMENTING PROGRESS NOTES

After completion of the initial health history, a system is needed to update the medical record with new information each time the patient visits the medical office. Most offices use progress notes to fulfill this function. Progress notes document the patient's health status and the care and treatment being received by the patient in chronologic order. Progress notes provide effective communication among medical office personnel and serve as a legal document.

The medical assistant is frequently responsible for documenting progress notes in the medical record. In the PPR, they are usually documented on special preprinted lined sheets known as *progress note sheets*. These sheets have a column for the date and time and a column for documenting information (see Fig. 1.3F). In the EHR, progress notes are documented by the medical assistant on a *progress notes template* screen. Types of progress notes that are often documented by the medical assistant are presented next, along with an example of each.

DOCUMENTING PATIENT SYMPTOMS

The medical assistant takes patient symptoms during office visits and telephone conversations. Information conveyed during a telephone conversation helps the medical assistant determine whether the patient needs to be seen and the immediacy of the situation.

A **symptom** is any change in the body or its functioning that indicates the presence of disease. Symptoms can be classified as subjective or objective. A **subjective symptom** is one that is felt by the patient and cannot be observed by another person. Pain, pruritus, vertigo, and nausea are examples of subjective symptoms. An **objective symptom** is one that can be observed by another person and by the patient. Rash, coughing, and cyanosis are objective symptoms. The medical assistant should have a thorough knowledge of common symptoms and should be able to recognize them. Table 1.2 lists and describes common symptoms.

Taking patient symptoms during an office visit consists of the following:

1. Obtaining a CC
2. Obtaining additional information about the CC

If the patient complains of pain in the abdomen that has lasted for 2 days (CC), additional information is needed to describe the pain, including its type, specific location, onset, intensity, precipitating factors, and duration. The procedure for taking patient symptoms during an office visit is outlined in Procedure 1.1. Additional skills and practice on taking patient symptoms are included in Chapter 1 of the *Study Guide*.

OTHER ACTIVITIES THAT NEED TO BE DOCUMENTED

PROCEDURES

The medical assistant frequently documents procedures performed on the patient, including vital signs, weight and height, visual acuity, and ear irrigations. Procedures should be documented immediately after they are performed; from a legal standpoint, a procedure that is not documented was not performed. In general, the following information should be included: the date and time, the type of procedure, the outcome, and the patient reaction (Fig. 1.6).

The specific information to be documented is included with each procedure presented in this textbook.

ADMINISTRATION OF MEDICATION

Documenting medications and immunizations administered to the patient is an important responsibility in the medical office. The documentation should include the date and time, the name of the medication, the lot number (if required), the dosage given, the route of administration, the injection site used (for parenteral medication), and any significant observations or patient reactions (Fig. 1.7).

Table 1.2 Common Symptoms

Symptom	Definition
Integumentary System	
Diaphoresis	Excessive perspiration.
Flushing	A red appearance to the skin, which generally affects the face and neck. A flushed appearance is commonly present with a fever.
Jaundice	A yellow appearance to the skin, first evident in the whites of the eyes.
Rash	An eruption on the skin.
Circulatory System	
Bradycardia	An abnormally slow pulse rate.
Dehydration	A decrease in the amount of water in the body. The patient has a flushed appearance, dry skin, and decreased output of urine.
Edema	The retention of fluid in the tissues, resulting in swelling. Skin over the area is tight. Edema is most easily observed in the extremities.
Tachycardia	An abnormally fast pulse rate.
Gastrointestinal System	
Anorexia	A loss of appetite and a lack of interest in food.
Constipation	A condition in which the stool becomes hard and dry, resulting in difficult passage from the rectum. The consistency of the stool, rather than the frequency of defecation, is used as a guide in determining the presence of constipation. (Frequency of bowel movements varies with the individual; some people have a bowel movement only every 2–3 days but are not constipated.) Other symptoms of constipation include headache, nausea, and general malaise.
Diarrhea	The passage of an increased number of loose, watery stools. The fecal material moves rapidly through the intestinal tract, resulting in decreased absorption by the body of water, electrolytes, and nutrients. Other symptoms usually associated with diarrhea are intestinal cramping and general weakness.
Flatulence	The presence of excessive gas in the stomach or intestines.
Nausea and vomiting	Nausea is a sensation of discomfort in the stomach with a feeling that vomiting may occur. Vomiting is the ejection of the stomach contents through the mouth, also known as ***emesis.*** The ejected content is known as ***vomitus.***
Respiratory System	
Cough	An involuntary and forceful exhalation of air followed by a deep inhalation. A cough may be productive (meaning a discharge is produced) or nonproductive (no discharge is present).
Cyanosis	A bluish discoloration of the skin due to lack of oxygen.
Dyspnea	Labored or difficult breathing.
Epistaxis	Hemorrhaging from the nose (nosebleed).
Nervous System	
Chills	A feeling of coldness accompanied by shivering. Chills are generally present with a fever.
Convulsions	Involuntary contractions of the muscles.
Fever or pyrexia	A body temperature that is higher than normal.
Headache	A feeling of pain or aching in the head. It is a common symptom that accompanies many illnesses. Tension, fatigue, and eyestrain can result in a headache.
Malaise	A vague sense of body discomfort, weakness, and fatigue, often marking the onset of a disease and continuing through the course of the illness.
Pain	Irritation of pain receptors, resulting in a feeling of distress or suffering. Pain is an important indication that a part of the body is not working properly.
Pruritus	Severe itching.
Vertigo	A feeling of dizziness or light-headedness.

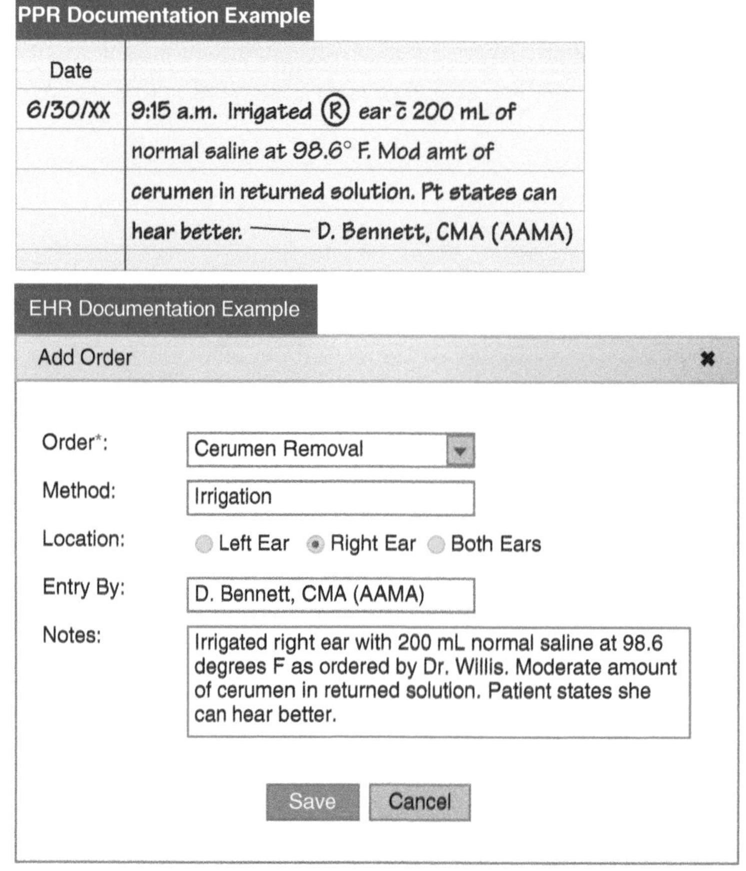

Fig. 1.6 Proper method for documenting a procedure in the medical record.

SPECIMEN COLLECTION

Each time a specimen is collected from a patient, the medical assistant should document the date and time of the collection, the type of specimen, and the area of the body from which the specimen was obtained. If the specimen is to be sent to an outside laboratory for testing, this information also should be documented, including the tests requested, the date the specimen was sent, and where it was sent (Fig. 1.8). In this way, the provider would know that the specimen was collected and sent to the laboratory when test results are not back yet.

DIAGNOSTIC PROCEDURES AND LABORATORY TESTS

Diagnostic procedures and laboratory tests ordered for a patient should always be documented in the medical record. If the patient does not undergo the test, documented proof exists that the test was ordered. Documenting diagnostic procedures and laboratory tests ordered by the provider protects the provider legally and refreshes the provider's memory of the procedures and tests being run on the patient when results are not yet back from the testing facility. Information to include in the entry consists of the date and time, the type of procedure or test ordered, the scheduling date, and where it is being performed (Fig. 1.9).

RESULTS OF LABORATORY TESTS

With a PPR, it is not necessary to document results from laboratory reports returned from outside laboratories because the report itself is filed in the patient's record. In case of a STAT request or critical findings, the test results may be telephoned to the medical office, requiring the medical assistant to document the results on a report form. Careful documentation is essential to avoid errors, which could affect the patient's diagnosis. Results of laboratory tests performed by the medical assistant in the office should be documented in the medical record and must include the date and time, name of the test, and test results (Fig. 1.10).

Many medical offices communicate with outside laboratories electronically using a computer system that interfaces with the computer system in the outside laboratory. Once the patient's tests have been completed, the laboratory test results are sent electronically to the medical office. After the provider reviews the laboratory report and places his or her electronic signature on the report, the report is electronically filed in the patient's EHR. If an office using an EHR is not networked through computers with an outside laboratory, the laboratory reports received by the office must be scanned into the computer and electronically filed in the patient's EHR.

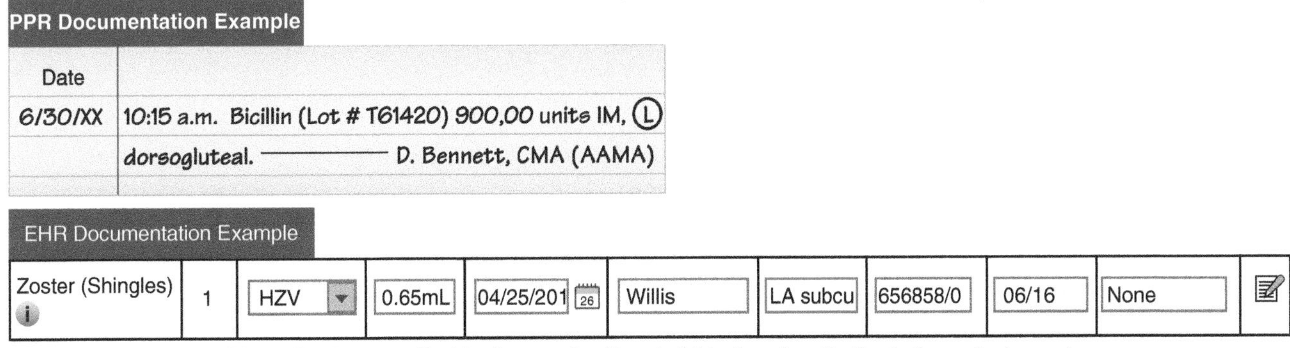

PPR Documentation Example

Date	
6/30/XX	10:15 a.m. Bicillin (Lot # T61420) 900,00 units IM, Ⓛ
	dorsogluteal. ——— D. Bennett, CMA (AAMA)

EHR Documentation Example

Zoster (Shingles)	1	HZV	0.65mL	04/25/201	Willis	LA subcu	656858/0	06/16	None	

Fig. 1.7 Proper method for documenting the administration of medication in the medical record.

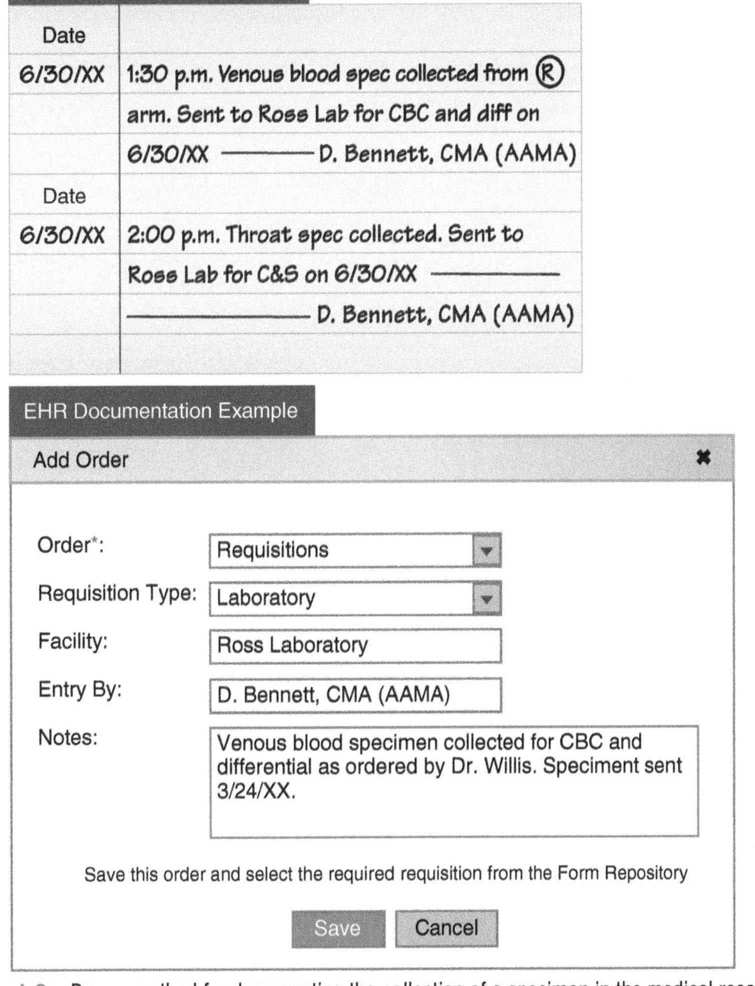

PPR Documentation Example

Date	
6/30/XX	1:30 p.m. Venous blood spec collected from Ⓡ
	arm. Sent to Ross Lab for CBC and diff on
	6/30/XX ——— D. Bennett, CMA (AAMA)
Date	
6/30/XX	2:00 p.m. Throat spec collected. Sent to
	Ross Lab for C&S on 6/30/XX ———
	——— D. Bennett, CMA (AAMA)

EHR Documentation Example

Add Order

Order*: Requisitions

Requisition Type: Laboratory

Facility: Ross Laboratory

Entry By: D. Bennett, CMA (AAMA)

Notes: Venous blood specimen collected for CBC and differential as ordered by Dr. Willis. Speciment sent 3/24/XX.

Save this order and select the required requisition from the Form Repository

Save Cancel

Fig. 1.8 Proper method for documenting the collection of a specimen in the medical record.

PATIENT INSTRUCTIONS

It often is necessary to relay instructions to a patient regarding medical care (e.g., wound care, cast care, care of sutures). The medical assistant should document this information, taking care to include the date and time and the type of instructions relayed to the patient. Many medical offices have printed instruction sheets that are given to the patient. The patient is asked to sign a form, which is filed or scanned into the patient's record, indicating that he or she has read and understands the instructions (Fig. 1.11). The form also should be signed by the medical assistant, who functions as a signature witness. This protects the provider legally in the event that the patient fails to follow the instructions and causes further harm or damage to a body part.

Other areas that the medical assistant is responsible for documenting in the medical record include missed or canceled appointments, telephone calls from patients (Fig. 1.12), medication refills, and changes in medication or dosage by the provider.

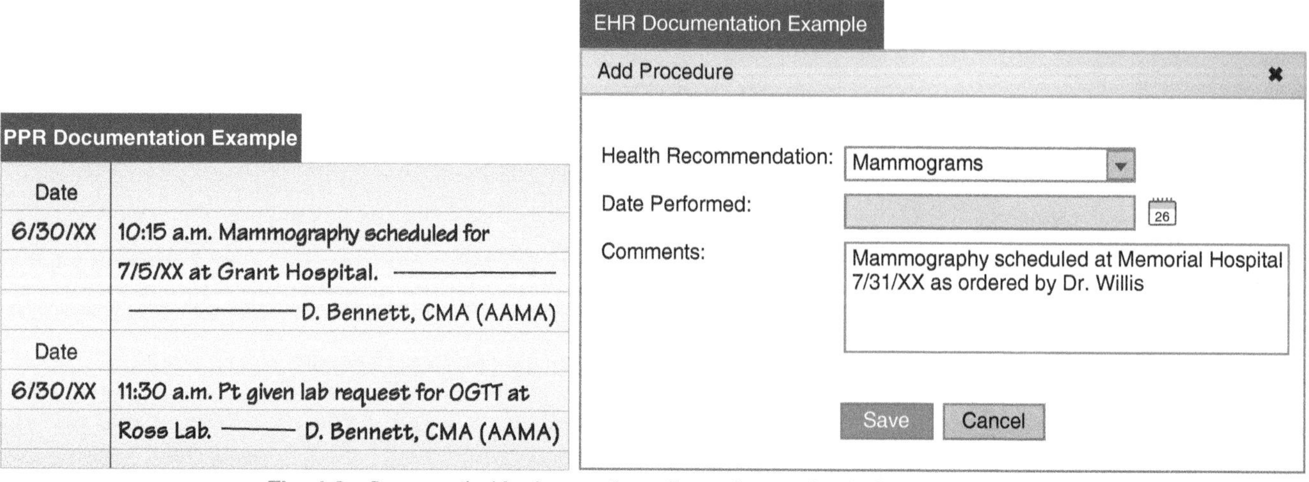
PPR Documentation Example

Date	
6/30/XX	10:15 a.m. Mammography scheduled for
	7/5/XX at Grant Hospital. ————
	———— D. Bennett, CMA (AAMA)
Date	
6/30/XX	11:30 a.m. Pt given lab request for OGTT at
	Ross Lab. ——— D. Bennett, CMA (AAMA)

EHR Documentation Example

Add Procedure

Health Recommendation: Mammograms

Date Performed:

Comments: Mammography scheduled at Memorial Hospital 7/31/XX as ordered by Dr. Willis

Save Cancel

Fig. 1.9 Proper method for documenting a diagnostic procedure in the medical record.

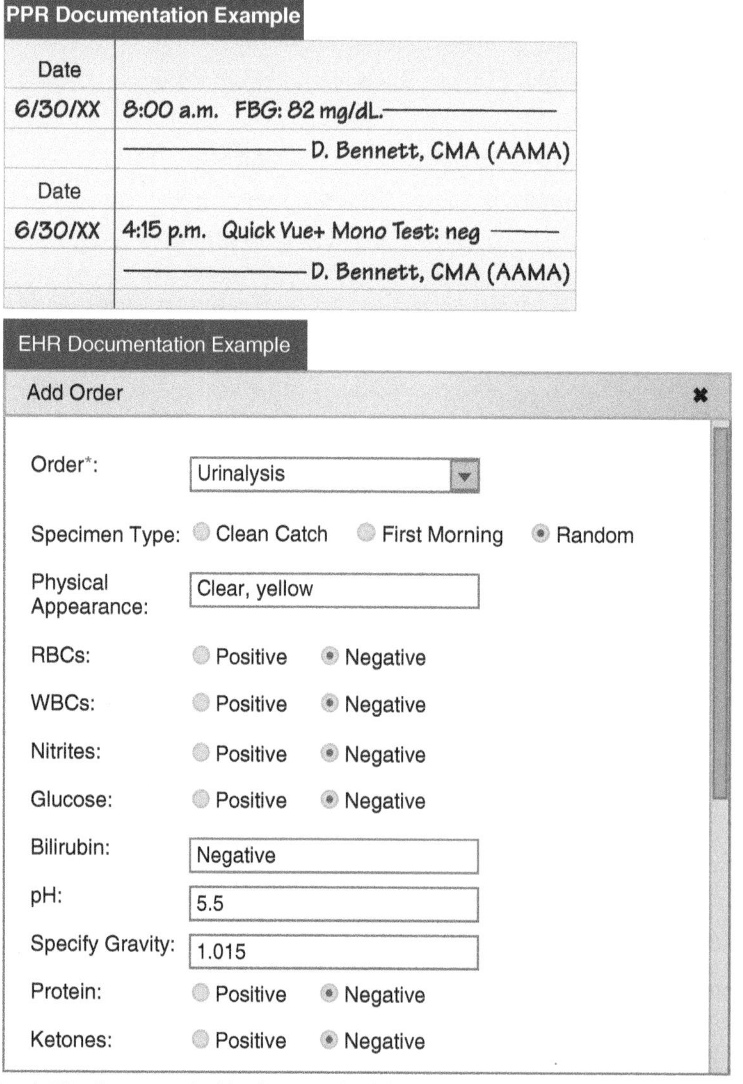
PPR Documentation Example

Date	
6/30/XX	8:00 a.m. FBG: 82 mg/dL.————
	———— D. Bennett, CMA (AAMA)
Date	
6/30/XX	4:15 p.m. Quick Vue+ Mono Test: neg ———
	———— D. Bennett, CMA (AAMA)

EHR Documentation Example

Add Order

Order*: Urinalysis

Specimen Type: Clean Catch / First Morning / Random (selected)

Physical Appearance: Clear, yellow

RBCs: Positive / Negative (selected)

WBCs: Positive / Negative (selected)

Nitrites: Positive / Negative (selected)

Glucose: Positive / Negative (selected)

Bilirubin: Negative

pH: 5.5

Specify Gravity: 1.015

Protein: Positive / Negative (selected)

Ketones: Positive / Negative (selected)

Fig. 1.10 Proper method for documenting laboratory test results in the medical record.

PATIENT INSTRUCTIONS FOR WOUND CARE

Name of patient: ______________________________

Follow the instructions indicated below for care of your wound:

1. Use ice bag and elevate to reduce swelling and pain. Elevate higher than your heart.
2. You may take aspirin/Tylenol for pain.
3. Keep the dressing clean and dry.
4. Replace the dressing within __________ days.
5. Discard the dressing within __________ days.
6. Cleanse the wound daily as instructed.
7. Stitches should be removed in __________ days.
8. Despite the greatest of care, any wound can become infected. If your wound becomes red or swollen, shows pus or red streaks, or feels more sore instead of less sore, contact the physician **immediately.**

I have received and understand the above instructions:

Patient (or representative): ______________________________

Relationship to patient: ______________________________

Witness: ______________________________ Time and date: ______________

Fig. 1.11 Instruction sheet for patients.

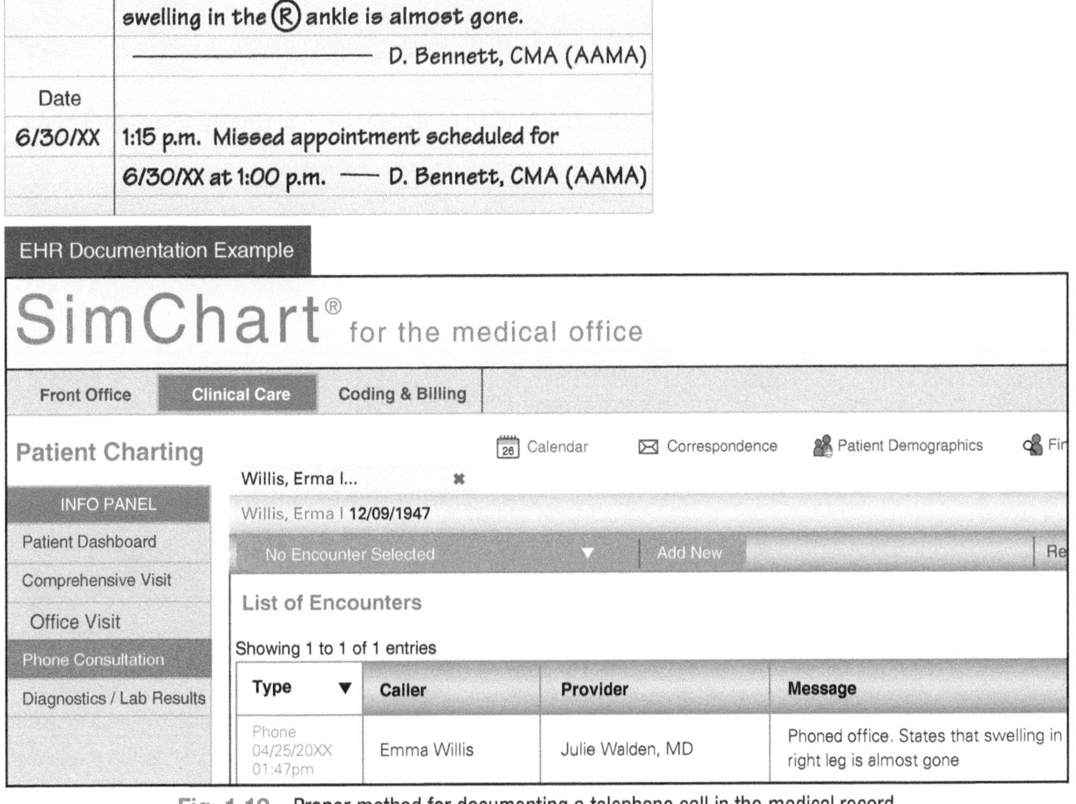

PPR Documentation Example

Date	
6/30/XX	11:15 a.m. Phoned office. States that
	swelling in the Ⓡ ankle is almost gone.
	———————— D. Bennett, CMA (AAMA)
Date	
6/30/XX	1:15 p.m. Missed appointment scheduled for
	6/30/XX at 1:00 p.m. —— D. Bennett, CMA (AAMA)

Fig. 1.12 Proper method for documenting a telephone call in the medical record.

What Would You Do? What Would You *Not* Do? RESPONSES

Case Study 1
Page 4

What Did Dawn Do?

- ❑ Listened carefully to Mrs. Celeste and relayed concern through both verbal and nonverbal behavior.
- ❑ Reassured Mrs. Celeste that her information would be kept completely confidential. Explained to Mrs. Celeste that health care professionals are required by law to keep all patient information confidential.
- ❑ Told Mrs. Celeste how important it is to document information that relates to her health. Explained that the physician must have accurate data to diagnose and treat her. Stressed that certain medications can be harmful to a patient if consumed with alcohol.
- ❑ Gave Mrs. Celeste information (including brochures) on community agencies that could help her. Explained that these agencies are required to maintain confidentiality, and encouraged her to contact them.

What Did Dawn Not Do?

- ❑ Did not tell Mrs. Celeste to go to a different physician to ensure that her information remained private.
- ❑ Did not tell Mrs. Celeste that she needed to stop drinking before it affected her health.

Case Study 2
Page 7

What Did Dawn Do?

- ❑ Listened to and empathized with Mr. and Mrs. Oberlin's concerns.
- ❑ Told Mr. and Mrs. Oberlin that because Brett is of adult age, it would be against the law to let them see his medical record without his written authorization. Explained that the law is there to protect a patient's right to privacy, and just as it protects Brett's right, the law also protects their right, so that no one can obtain information from their medical records without their authorization.
- ❑ Suggested that they talk with Brett again regarding the situation.

What Did Dawn Not Do?

- ❑ Did not give them any information from Brett's medical record. ■

TERMINOLOGY REVIEW

Medical Term	Word Parts	Definition
Diagnosis	*dia-:* through, complete *-gnosis:* knowledge	The scientific method of determining and identifying a patient's condition.
Diagnostic procedure	*dia-:* through, complete *gnos/o:* knowledge *-ic:* pertaining to	A procedure performed to assist in the diagnosis, management, or treatment of a patient's condition.
Documenting		The process of recording information about a patient in the medical record.
Electronic health record (EHR)		A medical record that is stored on a computer.
Familial disease	*famil:* family *-al:* pertaining to	A condition that occurs in or affects blood relatives more frequently than would be expected by chance.
Health history report		A collection of subjective data about a patient.
Medical record		A written record of important information regarding a patient, including the care of that individual and the progress of the patient's condition.
Objective symptom		A symptom that can be observed by an examiner.
Paper-based patient record (PPR)		A medical record in paper form.
Subjective symptom		A symptom that is felt by the patient but is not observable by an examiner.
Symptom		Any change in the body or its functioning that indicates the presence of disease.

PROCEDURE 1.1 Obtaining and Documenting Patient Symptoms

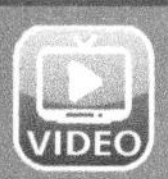

Outcome Obtain and document patient symptoms.

Equipment/Supplies

- Medical record of the patient to be interviewed
- Pen with black ink

1. **Procedural Step.** Assemble the equipment. Ensure that you have the correct patient's record in the form of either a paper-based record or an electronic record. If using a paper record, make sure you have a pen with black ink for documenting patient symptoms.
   Principle. Black ink must be used in a paper-based patient record (PPR) to provide a permanent record.
2. **Procedural Step.** Go to the waiting room and ask the patient to come back.
3. **Procedural Step.** Escort the patient to a quiet, comfortable room, such as an examination room, that allows for privacy.
   Principle. Patient symptoms should be taken in a room that encourages communication and maintains patient privacy.
4. **Procedural Step.** In a calm and friendly manner, greet the patient and introduce yourself. Identify the patient by his or her full name and date of birth.
   Principle. A warm introduction sets a positive tone for the remainder of the interview.
5. **Procedural Step.** Ask the patient to be seated. You should seat yourself so that you face the patient at a distance of 3 to 4 feet.
   Principle. This type of seating arrangement facilitates open communication and respects the patient's personal boundaries.
6. **Procedural Step.** Use good communication skills to interact with the patient. These include the following:
   a. Use the patient's name of choice.
   b. Show genuine interest and concern for the patient.
   c. Maintain appropriate eye contact.
   d. Use terminology the patient can understand.
   e. Listen carefully and attentively to the patient.
   f. Pay attention to the patient's nonverbal messages.
   g. Avoid judgmental comments.
   h. Avoid rushing the patient.
   i. Use reflection, restatement, and clarification techniques as needed.
7. **Procedural Step.** Locate the progress note sheet in the PPR or the chief complaint template screen in the electronic health record (EHR). If using a PPR, document the date and time and the abbreviation for chief complaint (CC).
8. **Procedural Step.** Use an open-ended question to elicit the chief complaint, such as "What seems to be the problem?"
   Principle. An open-ended question allows the patient to verbalize freely.
9. **Procedural Step.** Document the chief complaint.
   a. ***PPR:*** Document the chief complaint following the documentation guidelines outlined on pages 12 to 16. In addition, these guidelines should be followed:
      1. Limit the chief complaint to one or two symptoms, and refer to a specific rather than a vague symptom.
      2. Document the chief complaint concisely and briefly, using the patient's own words as much as possible.
      3. Include the duration of the symptom (onset) in the chief complaint.
      4. Avoid using names of diseases or diagnostic terms to document the chief complaint.
   b. ***EHR:*** Document the chief complaint by completing each field of the chief complaint template using radio buttons, drop-down menus and free text entry.
10. **Procedural Step.** Obtain additional information regarding the chief complaint.
   a. ***PPR:*** Obtain additional information using *what, when, and where* questions, which are outlined as follows. Following proper documentation guidelines, document this information after the chief complaint in the PPR.

What Questions

- What exactly have you been experiencing?
- Does the symptom occur suddenly or gradually?
- Does anything make it worse?

Where Question

- Where is the symptom located?

When Questions

- When did the symptom first occur?
- How long does it last?
- Does anything cause it to occur?

   b. ***EHR:*** Complete the following fields on the progress notes template: location, quality, severity, duration, timing, context, modifying factors, and associated signs and symptoms.

Continued

PROCEDURE 1.1 Obtaining and Documenting Patient Symptoms—cont'd

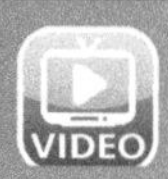

Principle. Obtaining additional information provides a complete description of the CC.

11. **Procedural Step.** Thank the patient, and proceed to the next step in the patient work-up. (This usually includes measuring vital signs and height and weight, and preparing the patient as needed for the physical examination [see Chapters 4 and 5].)
12. **Procedural Step.** Inform the patient approximately how long he or she will need to wait for the provider.
13. **Procedural Step.** If using a PPR, place the patient's medical record where it can be reviewed by the provider (as designated by the medical office policy).
    Principle. The provider will want to review the patient's record before examining the patient.

PPR Documentation Example

Date	
6/30/XX	3:15 p.m. CC: Intense pain in the Ⓛ ear for the
	past 2 days. Pt states pain is sharp and
	continuous. Pt noted sl yellow discharge
	from Ⓛ ear. Fever of 101° F began last night
	about 9 p.m. Took Tylenol 2 tabs at 8 a.m.
	——————— D. Bennett, CMA (AAMA)

EHR Documentation Example

Chief Complaint *: Dizziness when standing up X 2 weeks

History of Present Illness

Location:	Generalized	Timing:	"It happens when I stand up"
Quality:	"I feel dizzy and weak"	Context:	"If I have been sitting or lying down"
Severity:	Moderate dizziness for a few seconds	Modifying Factors:	"It is worse if I stand up fast"
Duration:	2 weeks	Associated Signs and Symptoms:	None

PROCEDURE 1.1

Medical Asepsis and the OSHA Standard

Check out the Evolve site at http://evolve.elsevier.com/Bonewit/today/ to access additional interactive activities and exercises to help you study and prepare for success.

LEARNING OUTCOMES / PROCEDURES

Microorganisms and Medical Asepsis

1. Define microorganism and give examples of types of microorganisms.
2. Explain the difference between a nonpathogen and a pathogen.
3. Define medical asepsis.
4. List the six basic requirements for growth and multiplication of microorganisms.
5. Outline the infection process cycle, including the following:
   - Give examples of the means of entry of microorganisms into the body.
   - Give examples of the means of transmission of microorganisms from one person to another.
   - Give examples of the means of exit of microorganisms from the body.
6. List and explain the protective mechanisms the body uses to prevent the entrance of microorganisms.
7. Explain the difference between resident flora and transient flora.
8. State when each of the following is performed: handwashing, antiseptic handwashing, and use of an alcohol-based hand sanitizer.
9. Explain the difference between surgical gloves and exam gloves and when each should be worn.
10. State the advantages and disadvantages of the following types of gloves: latex, nitrile, and vinyl.
11. Explain why it is important to wear the correct size gloves.
12. Identify medical aseptic practices that should be followed in the medical office.

Procedures:
- Handwashing.
- Application of an alcohol-based hand sanitizer.
- Determination of glove size.
- Application and removal of disposable exam gloves.

OSHA Bloodborne Pathogens Standard

13. Explain the purpose of the Occupational Safety and Health Administration (OSHA).
14. List and describe the elements that must be included in the OSHA exposure control plan.
15. Explain the purpose of the following OSHA requirements: labeling requirements and sharps injury log.
16. List the steps that must be performed following an exposure incident.
17. Define and provide examples of each of the following: engineering controls, work practice controls, personal protective equipment, and housekeeping procedures.
18. Identify the guidelines for use of personal protective equipment.

Procedures:
- Adhere to the OSHA Bloodborne Pathogens Standard.

Regulated Medical Waste

19. List examples of medical waste and explain how to discard each type of waste.
20. Explain how to handle and dispose of regulated medical waste.

Procedures:
- Prepare regulated waste for pickup by an infectious waste service.

Bloodborne Diseases

21. Explain the differences between acute and chronic hepatitis B and C.
22. List the means of transmission for hepatitis B and C.
23. Describe the treatment for hepatitis B and C.
24. State the recommendations for hepatitis B vaccination.
25. Describe postexposure prophylaxis for hepatitis B.
26. Explain what occurs when HIV gains entrance into the body.
27. List the means of transmission for HIV.
28. List and describe the three types of HIV tests.
29. Describe the treatment for HIV-infected individuals.

CHAPTER OUTLINE

KEY TERMS

acute infection
aerobe (AIR-obe)
anaerobe (AN-er-obe)
antiseptic
chronic infection
cilia (SIL-ee-ah)
hand hygiene
infection
medical asepsis
microorganism (MYE-kroe-OR-gan-iz-um)
nonintact (NON-in-takt) skin
nonpathogen (non-PATH-oh-jen)
opportunistic (OP-pore-tune-IS-tik) infection
optimum (OP-tuh-mum) growth temperature
parenteral (pare-EN-ter-al)
pathogen (PATH-oh-jen)
postexposure prophylaxis (proe-fil-ACKS-is)
regulated medical waste
resident flora (FLOE-ruh)
transient (TRAN-zee-ent) flora

INTRODUCTION TO MEDICAL ASEPSIS AND THE OSHA STANDARD

Medical asepsis and infection control are crucial in preventing the spread of disease. The medical assistant should always practice good medical aseptic techniques to provide a safe and healthy environment in the medical office. The Occupational Safety and Health Administration (OSHA) Bloodborne Pathogens Standard is important for infection control. The federal government requires this standard to reduce the exposure of health care employees to infectious diseases. This chapter presents a thorough discussion of medical asepsis, infection control, the OSHA Bloodborne Pathogens Standard, and the bloodborne diseases that are the biggest threats to the medical assistant.

MICROORGANISMS AND MEDICAL ASEPSIS

Microorganisms are tiny living plants or animals that cannot be seen with the naked eye, but instead must be viewed with a microscope. Common types of microorganisms include bacteria, viruses, protozoa, fungi, and animal parasites. Most microorganisms are harmless and do not cause disease. They are termed **nonpathogens**. Other microorganisms, known as **pathogens**, are harmful to the body and can cause disease.

In the medical office, practices must be employed to inhibit the growth and hinder the transmission of pathogenic microorganisms to prevent the spread of infection. These practices are known as *medical asepsis*. **Medical asepsis** means that an object or area is clean and free from disease-producing microorganisms. Nonpathogens would still be present on a clean or medically aseptic object or surface, but all the pathogens would have been eliminated.

GROWTH REQUIREMENTS FOR MICROORGANISMS

For microorganisms to survive, certain growth requirements must be present in the environment, as follows:

1. *Proper nutrition.* Microorganisms that use inorganic or nonliving substances as sources of food are known as *autotrophs.* Microorganisms that use organic or living substances for food are known as *heterotrophs.*
2. *Oxygen.* Most microorganisms need oxygen to grow and multiply and are termed **aerobes**. Other microorganisms, known as **anaerobes**, grow best in the absence of oxygen.

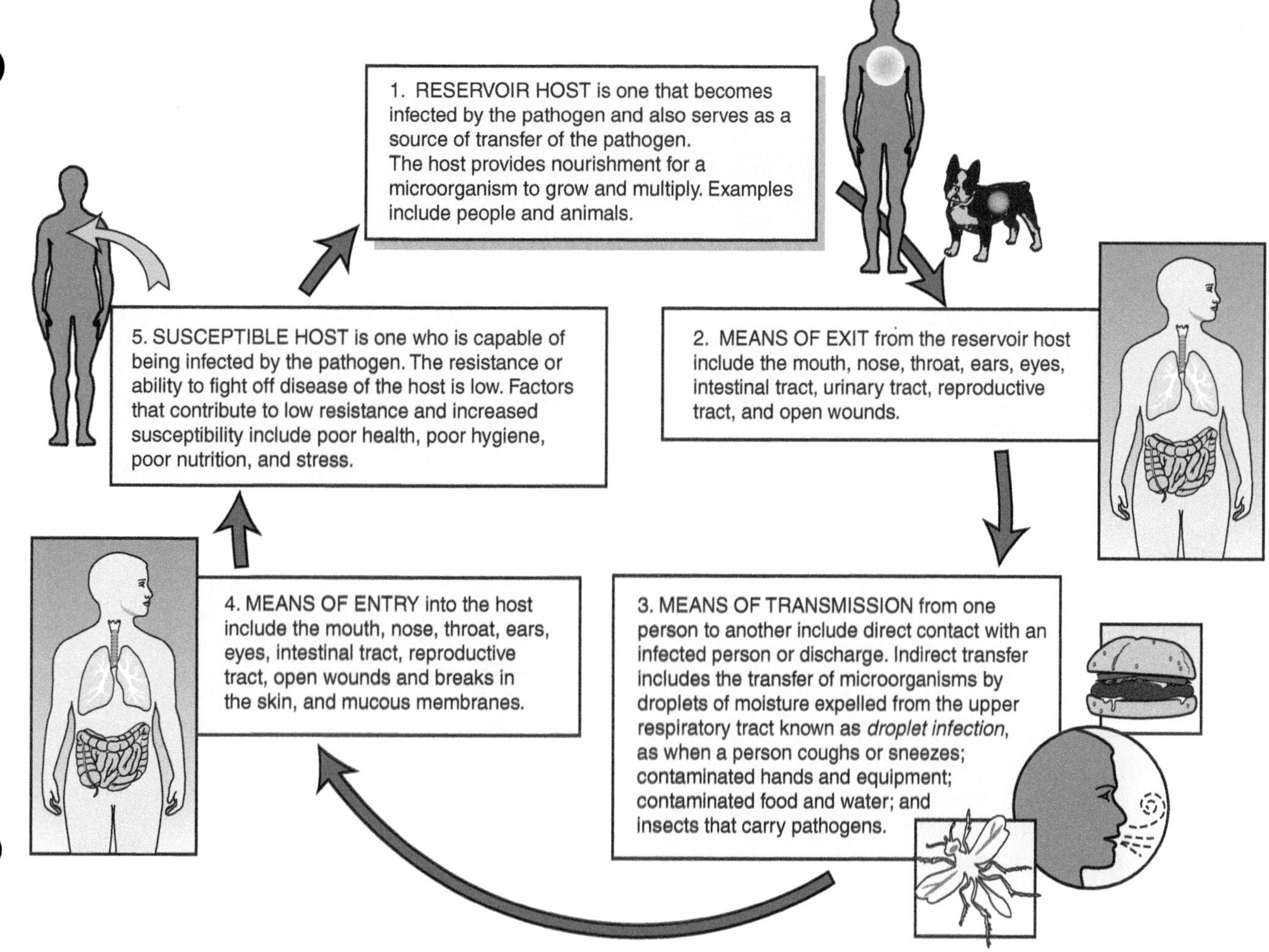

Fig. 2.1 The infection process cycle.

3. *Temperature.* Each microorganism has a temperature at which it grows best, known as the **optimum growth temperature**. Most microorganisms grow best at 98.6°F (37°C), the human body temperature.
4. *Darkness.* Microorganisms grow best in darkness.
5. *Moisture.* Microorganisms need moisture for cell metabolism and to carry away wastes.
6. *pH.* The pH is the degree to which a solution is acidic or basic. Most microorganisms prefer a neutral pH. If the environment of the microorganisms becomes too acidic or too basic, they die.

If growth requirements are taken away from the environment of pathogenic microorganisms, they are unable to survive. Eliminating these conditions is one way to reduce the growth and transmission of pathogens in the medical office.

INFECTION PROCESS CYCLE

Infection is the condition in which the body, or part of it, is invaded by a pathogen. For a pathogen to survive and produce disease, a continuous cycle must be followed; this is known as the *infection process cycle* (Fig. 2.1). If the cycle is broken at any point, the pathogen dies. The medical assistant has a responsibility to help break this cycle in the medical office by practicing good techniques of medical asepsis. These techniques are discussed in the next section.

PROTECTIVE MECHANISMS OF THE BODY

The body has protective mechanisms to help prevent the entrance of pathogens. These mechanisms help to break the infection process cycle and include the following:

1. The skin is the body's most important defense mechanism; it serves as a protective barrier against the entrance of pathogens.
2. The mucous membranes of the body, which line the nose and throat and respiratory, gastrointestinal, and genital tracts, help protect the body from invasion by pathogens.
3. Mucus and **cilia** in the nose and respiratory tract fight off pathogens. Mucus traps pathogens that enter the body, and the hairlike cilia constantly beat toward the outside to remove them from the body.
4. Coughing and sneezing help force pathogens from the body.

BOX 2.1 CDC Guidelines for Hand Hygiene in Health Care Settings

Wash Hands With Soap and Water
- When the hands are visibly soiled
- After caring for a person with known or suspected infectious diarrhea
- After known or suspected exposure to spores (e.g., *Bacillus anthracis, Clostridium difficile* outbreaks)
- Before eating
- After using the restroom

Apply an Alcohol-Based Hand Sanitizer (or Wash Hands)
- Immediately before touching a patient
- Before performing an aseptic task or handling invasive medical devices
- Before moving from work on a soiled body site to a clean body site on the same patient
- After touching a patient or the patient's immediate environment
- After contact with blood, body fluids, or contaminated surfaces if the hands are not visibly soiled
- Immediately after glove removal

5. Lysozyme is an enzyme present in tears, saliva, and sweat that destroys bacteria that attempt to enter the body.
6. Urine and vaginal secretions are acidic. Pathogens cannot grow in an acidic environment.
7. The stomach secretes hydrochloric acid, which helps in the process of digestion. This acidic environment discourages the growth of pathogens that enter the stomach.

MEDICAL ASEPSIS IN THE MEDICAL OFFICE

There are many important medical aseptic practices employed in the medical office to prevent the spread of infection. The most important of these practices are hand hygiene and the use of medical gloves discussed in this section.

Hand Hygiene

Hand hygiene refers to the process of cleansing or sanitizing the hands. Hand hygiene is considered the most important medical aseptic practices in the medical office for preventing the spread of infection. Specific techniques for sanitizing the hands in the medical office include the following:
- Handwashing with plain soap and water
- Handwashing with an antimicrobial soap and water
- Applying an alcohol-based hand sanitizer

The Centers for Disease Control and Prevention (CDC) has established recommendations for hand hygiene in health care settings. The purpose of these guidelines is to promote improved hand hygiene practices and to reduce transmission of pathogenic microorganisms to patients and employees in health care settings. The CDC guidelines for hand hygiene as they apply to the medical office are outlined in Box 2.1.

Resident and Transient Flora

Microorganisms residing on the hands can be classified into the following categories: resident flora and transient flora. **Resident flora** (also known as *normal flora*) normally resides and grows in the epidermis and deeper layers of the skin known as the *dermis*. Resident flora is usually harmless and nonpathogenic. Because resident flora is attached to the deeper skin layers, it is difficult to remove from the skin.

Transient flora lives and grows on the superficial skin layers, or epidermis. It is picked up on the hands during daily activities. In the medical office, this may include contact with an infected patient, contaminated equipment, or contaminated surfaces. Transient flora is often pathogenic, but because it is attached loosely to the skin, it can be removed easily from the hands with proper hand hygiene techniques.

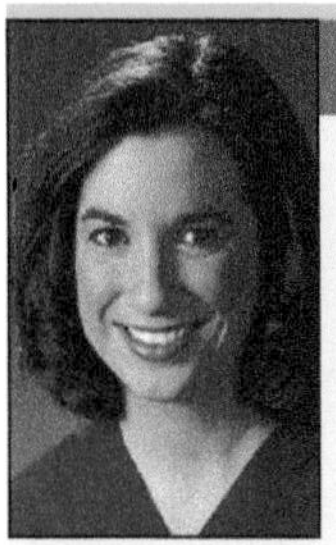

Putting It All Into Practice

My name is Jennifer, and I work for a large group of physicians in a multispecialty clinic. I work in both the front and back areas of the office. I really enjoy experiencing all these areas of the office, and I definitely never get bored.

The most interesting experience I have had as a practicing medical assistant is seeing the impact that I make in patients' lives. They rely on you and look to you first for help in their health care situation. You are most often the first person they come into contact within the office, and they look to you for understanding and empathy. Especially patients who come to your office on a regular basis see you as a kind of family member. They appreciate a familiar face and a smile. Most often, you are the individual giving patients instructions concerning testing they will be having done or medication they will be taking. Patients truly do count on your knowledge and assistance throughout their course of care. I was genuinely surprised at what an impact I could have on others. ■

Hand Hygiene Techniques

Hand hygiene techniques are essential in preventing the spread of disease in the medical office. It is important to follow the hand hygiene procedures exactly to ensure the removal of dirt and transient flora from the hands.

Handwashing

Handwashing refers to washing the hands with plain soap and water. Plain soap contains agents that help break down and emulsify dirt and oil present on the skin. Soap sanitizes the hands through the physical removal of dirt and transient flora. It is important to use adequate friction during handwashing to ensure the removal of all transient flora. The CDC recommends that the hands be rubbed together vigorously for at least 20 seconds, making sure to cover all surfaces and to focus on the fingertips and fingernails. Procedure 2.1 outlines the handwashing procedure.

The CDC hand hygiene guidelines recommend that handwashing be performed when the hands are visibly soiled

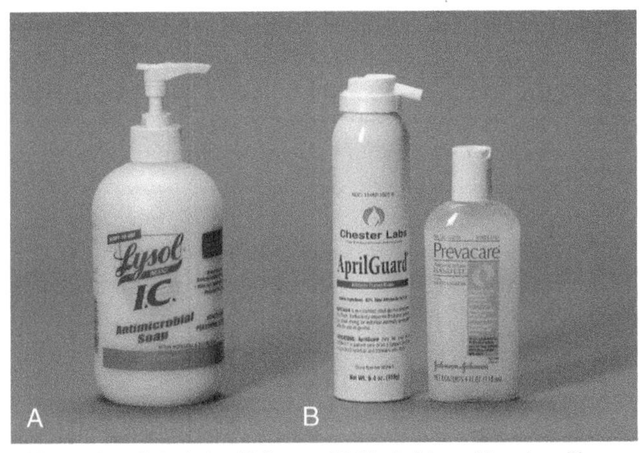

Fig. 2.2 (A) Antimicrobial soap. (B) Alcohol-based hand sanitizers.

with dirt or body fluids, before eating, and after using the restroom (see Box 2.1). If the hands are not visibly soiled, the CDC recommends that an alcohol-based hand sanitizer, rather than handwashing, be used to sanitize the hands. This is because repeated handwashing tends to dry out the hands, leading to irritation, chapping, and dermatitis.

Antiseptic Handwashing

Washing the hands with an antimicrobial soap is termed *antiseptic handwashing.* Antimicrobial soaps contain an **antiseptic**, which is an agent that functions to kill or inhibit the growth of microorganisms (Fig. 2.2A). Antiseptic handwashing sanitizes the hands through the mechanical scrubbing action and through the action of the antiseptic. Proper handwashing with an antimicrobial soap removes all soil and transient flora from the hands. Most antimicrobial soaps also deposit an antibacterial film on the skin that discourages bacterial growth. The medical assistant should perform antiseptic handwashing before performing a sterile procedure or assisting with minor office surgery. Examples of antiseptics contained in antimicrobial soaps include chlorhexidine, chloroxylenol, hexachlorophene, iodine, quaternary ammonium compounds, and triclosan.

Alcohol-Based Hand Sanitizers

CDC guidelines recommend the use of an alcohol-based hand sanitizer (ABHS) for cleansing the hands when they are not visibly soiled (see Box 2.1). ABHSs, also known as *alcohol-based hand rubs,* consist of 60% to 95% alcohol (ethanol, isopropanol, or n-propanol) and come in the forms of gels, foams, and sprays (see Fig. 2.2B). Studies have shown that ABHSs are more effective than traditional soap and water handwashing in removing transient flora and reducing bacterial counts on the hands. The advantages that ABHSs offer over traditional handwashing are as follows:

- ABHSs are usually more accessible than sinks.
- ABHSs do not require rinsing and hand drying with a towel.
- Less time is required to perform hand hygiene. It takes approximately 30 seconds to sanitize the hands with an ABHS compared with 1 to 2 minutes to perform proper handwashing.
- ABHSs are less damaging to the skin, resulting in less dryness and irritation. Most ABHSs contain emollients, which help prevent the skin of the hands from over drying. As the alcohol dries in the ABHS, protective fats and oils remain on the hands.

ABHSs have several disadvantages. They are more expensive than plain soap. They also cause a brief stinging sensation if they are applied to broken skin, such as a cut or abrasion on the hand. Procedure 2.2 describes the proper steps for sanitizing the hands with an ABHS.

Medical Gloves

Medical gloves are essential in protecting health care workers and patients from infectious diseases. Gloves provide a physical barrier to protect against infection; this is known as barrier protection. The CDC recommends that medical gloves be worn when the health care worker is likely to come in contact with blood and other potentially infectious materials (OPIM); mucous membranes or nonintact skin; when performing vascular access procedures; and when handling or touching contaminated surfaces or items.

Medical gloves consist of durable layer of material that forms a physical barrier between the health care worker's hands and the patient and/or contaminants. The glove material must be flexible, free from holes, breaches, and cracks, and strong enough to prevent breakage during normal use.

Medical gloves used to be available in both powdered and nonpowdered forms. Powdered gloves reduce friction between the hands and gloves, making it easier to put on and take off the gloves. However, the use of powder on gloves was found to result in significant risks to health care workers and patients. These risks include severe airway inflammation, respiratory allergic reactions, wound inflammation, and postoperative complications. Because of this, the Food and Drug Administration banned powdered gloves in January 2017.

Glove Categories

There are two categories of gloves used in the medical office, which include surgical gloves and exam gloves. The type of glove used depends on the procedure being performed. In general, surgical gloves are used for sterile procedures while exam gloves are used for aseptic procedures.

Surgical Gloves

Surgical gloves are disposable and sterile, meaning they are free of all microorganisms. They are designed to fit each hand separately and are manufactured to a higher standard than exam gloves to offer superior comfort, fit, strength, and flexibility. The medical assistant uses surgical gloves to perform sterile procedures (e.g., sterile dressing change) and to assist the provider during minor office surgery. They help prevent the patient from developing an infection following a sterile procedure and reduce the risk of exposure of the medical assistant to blood and body fluids. Surgical gloves are discussed in more detail in Chapter 10.

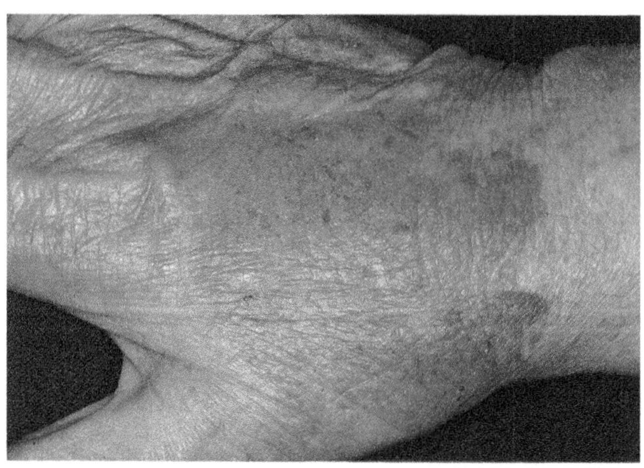

Fig. 2.3 Latex glove allergy. (From Goodman CC: *Pathology: implications for the physical therapist*, ed 3, St Louis: Saunders; 2010.)

Exam Gloves

Exam gloves are disposable, nonsterile, and ambidextrous, meaning the same design is used for both hands. They are used to protect against infection when performing certain procedures such as administering an injection, performing a venipuncture, or performing a urinalysis. Exam gloves are also worn to protect the medical assistant from pathogens when handling or touching contaminated surfaces or items such as cleaning up a blood spill or sanitizing contaminated instruments. Procedure 2.3 presents the proper method for applying and removing disposable exam gloves.

Types of Exam Gloves

There are three types of exam gloves commonly used in the medical office. They are categorized by their material and include latex, nitrile, and vinyl.

Latex Gloves: Latex gloves are made from natural rubber latex (NRL), which is a milky liquid that is extracted from rubber trees. Latex gloves offer many advantages. They are highly durable and flexible, provide a high level of touch sensitivity, offer good barrier protection and are cost-effective. Latex gloves fit like a second skin, which makes them comfortable to wear for an extended period.

The primary disadvantage of latex gloves is that they can cause an allergic reaction in individuals with a hypersensitivity to latex. A mild allergic reaction to latex causes the following symptoms: redness of the skin, urticaria (hives), and itching (Fig. 2.3). A more severe allergic reaction causes sneezing, itchy red eyes, runny nose, and asthma symptoms (shortness of breath, coughing, and wheezing). Symptoms typically begin within minutes after contact with the latex.

Anyone with frequent exposure to latex, such as health care workers, is at a greater risk for developing a hypersensitivity to latex. The incidence of latex allergy in the general population tends to be low (1% to 6%); however, the risk for health care workers developing a hypersensitivity to latex ranges from 8% to 12%. Because of this, most medical offices now use latex-free gloves. This protects both health care workers and patients with a hypersensitivity to latex.

Nitrile Gloves: Nitrile gloves are made from a synthetic rubber that does not contain latex. They are highly durable, have a comfortable fit, are puncture resistant, provide good barrier protection, and have a long shelf life. Based on these qualities, nitrile gloves are an ideal alternative when latex allergies are of a concern. The primary disadvantage of nitrile gloves is that they are more expensive than either latex or vinyl gloves.

Vinyl Gloves: Vinyl gloves are made of polyvinyl chloride and were the first latex-free alternative to become available for health care workers with a latex allergy. They are easy to put on and take off and are low in cost. However, vinyl gloves have some disadvantages. They are not as elastic and flexible as latex and nitrile gloves. This causes them to fit loosely, resulting in less comfort and dexterity when performing procedures. Vinyl gloves are also not as durable as other types of gloves, making them susceptible to tearing and puncturing when put under stress. Because of this, the barrier protection of vinyl gloves is not as reliable as latex and nitrile gloves. Based on these disadvantages, it is recommended that vinyl gloves be used for short-term procedures in which the medical assistant is not likely to come into contact with blood, or OPIM.

Glove Sizing

Gloves are required for many procedures performed in the medical office. To ensure adequate barrier protection when wearing gloves, it is essential that the medical assistant determine his or her correct glove size. Gloves that fit correctly feel comfortable and allow the medical assistant to perform a procedure in the same way the procedure could be performed with bare hands. Gloves that are too small may rip as they are applied or may become uncomfortable to wear. Gloves that are too large may make it difficult to perform procedures because the excess material will get in the way.

Surgical gloves are sized more precisely than exam gloves because they are usually worn for a longer period to perform procedures requiring exceptional dexterity. Surgical gloves come in numerical sizes that range from 5.5 to 9.0. Exam gloves come in the following lettered sizes: XS, S, M, L, XL.

Glove size is determined through a two-part process. The circumference of the widest part of the dominant hand is first measured to obtain an individual's approximate glove size. Next, the fit of the gloves in the approximate size is assessed to determine the exact glove size for that individual. The correct glove size may end up being a size larger or smaller than the approximate size obtained through the hand measurement. This is because glove size can vary based on other factors, such as the shape of the hand, shape and length of the fingers, material making up the glove, and the brand of the glove. The procedure for determining glove size is presented in Box 2.2.

Glove Guidelines

The medical assistant should adhere to the following glove guidelines to ensure proper barrier protection:

BOX 2.2 Determination of Glove Size

1. Extend the dominant hand and lay it on a flat surface with the fingers together and the hand relaxed. The dominant hand is preferred because the muscles in this hand are more developed, resulting in a larger measurement than the nondominant hand.
2. Measure the circumference in inches of the widest part of the palm of your hand by placing a cloth tape measure around the hand just below your knuckles. The circumference of the hand shown below is 8 inches. A cloth tape measure should be used because it will not stretch during the measurement. (*Note:* It may be easier to ask another individual to perform this step of the procedure.)

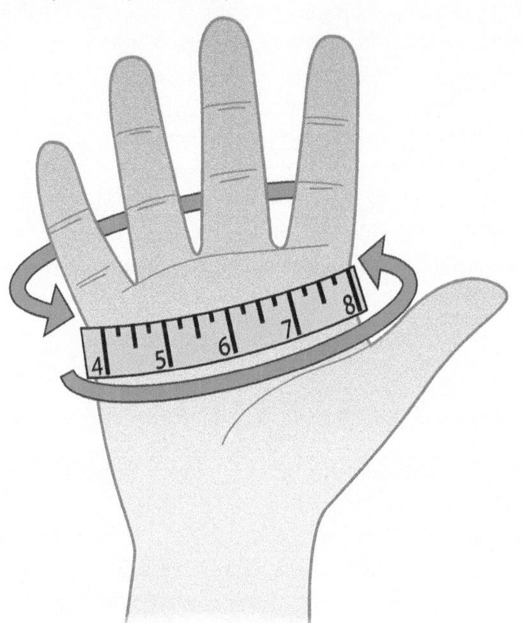

3. Determine your approximate glove size as follows:
   A. **Surgical gloves:** Round the hand measurement to the nearest whole or half-inch and convert it to a decimal number. *(For example, 7¼ inches is rounded to 7½ inches and converted to 7.5; therefore, 7.5 is the approximate glove size.)*
   B. **Exam gloves:** Round the number to the nearest whole inch. Translate this number to the appropriate letter size using the General Exam Glove Sizing Chart provided here. *(For example, 7 ½ inches is rounded to 8 inches which translates to an M glove size.)*

   (*Note:* If the manufacturer includes a brand-specific sizing chart on their glove box or on their website, it should be used instead of the General Chart.)
4. Don a pair of gloves in the approximate size determined through the hand measurement.
5. Perform the following assessment to determine your correct glove size:
   A. Correctly Fitted Gloves:
   If the fit of your gloves meets these criteria, this is your correct glove size:
   - The gloves are snug on your hand without restricting movements.
   - The gloves are comfortable and fits like a second skin.
   - You can move your fingers normally without stretching the gloves too much as you move and flex your fingers.

   B. Gloves are Too Large:
   If your gloves are too large, one or more of the criteria listed below will be evident. Obtain the next size smaller and repeat the assessment. If necessary, repeat this step until you have determined your correct glove size.
   - When applying the gloves, they do not have to stretch very much to fit your hands.
   - Wrinkles are observed around your palms and the rest of the glove bunches up around your wrists.
   - Your fingertips do not reach the end of the gloves, leaving material dangling at the end of each finger.

   C. Gloves are Too Small:
   If your gloves are too small, one or more of the criteria listed below will be evident. Obtain the next size larger and repeat the assessment. If necessary, repeat this step until you have determined your correct glove size.
   - When applying the gloves, they must stretch significantly for your hands to fit inside.
   - The fingertips of the gloves press against your fingers and may even puncture through the gloves.
   - The gloves are uncomfortable, and movements are stifled by the glove.

General Exam Glove Sizing Chart

Hand Measurement (In Inches)	Exam Glove Size
6	XS
7	S
8	M
9	L
10	XL

1. Wear the correct size glove to ensure a snug and comfortable fit and to avoid hand fatigue.
2. Wear gloves if contact with blood or OPIM, mucous membranes, and nonintact skin could occur.
3. Keep fingernails trimmed short (less than 1/4-inch long) to reduce the risk of tearing the gloves during application and use.
4. If gloves become contaminated, torn, or punctured, they must be replaced as soon as practical.
5. Remove gloves after caring for a patient. Do not wear the same pair of gloves for the care of more than one patient.
6. Sanitize the hands after removing gloves regardless of whether or not the gloves are visibly contaminated. Pathogens may gain access to the medical assistant's hands

through small defects in the gloves or by contamination of the hands during glove removal.
7. Do not store gloves in areas where there are extremes in temperatures (e.g., near a heater or an air conditioner). These conditions can cause deterioration of the gloves resulting in glove defects which, in turn, may not provide adequate barrier protection.

Infection Control

In addition to hand hygiene and glove protection, other good aseptic practices to control infection in the medical office include the following:

1. Follow the OSHA Bloodborne Pathogens Standard (presented in this chapter).
2. Keep the medical office free from dirt and dust, which can collect and carry microorganisms.
3. Ensure that the reception area and examining rooms are well ventilated. Stuffy rooms encourage microorganisms to settle on objects.
4. Keep the reception area and examining rooms bright and airy. Light discourages the growth of microorganisms.
5. Eliminate insects. Insects are a means of transmission of pathogens.
6. Carefully dispose of wastes, such as urine, feces, and respiratory secretions; all wastes should be handled as though they contain pathogens.
7. Do not let soiled items touch clothing.
8. Avoid coughs and sneezes of patients. Moisture droplets expelled from the lungs with coughing and sneezing may contain pathogens.
9. Use discretion in the amount of jewelry worn; wear minimal jewelry or no jewelry at all. Microorganisms can become lodged in the grooves and crevices of jewelry and serve as a means of transmission of pathogens.
10. Teach patients aseptic practices to control the spread of infection at home.

OSHA BLOODBORNE PATHOGENS STANDARD

PURPOSE OF THE STANDARD

The federal government established OSHA to assist employers in providing a safe and healthy working environment for their employees. To provide a safe working environment for health care workers, OSHA developed a comprehensive set of regulations known as the *OSHA Occupational Exposure to Bloodborne Pathogens Standard.* These regulations went into effect in 1992 and are designed to reduce the risk to employees of exposure to infectious diseases.

The OSHA Bloodborne Pathogens Standard must be followed by any employee with occupational exposure to pathogens, regardless of the place of employment. In addition to medical assistants, employees with occupational exposure include providers, nurses, dentists, dental hygienists, medical laboratory personnel, and emergency medical technicians. Employees who may have less obvious occupational exposure are correctional and law enforcement officers, firefighters, hospital laundry workers, morticians, and custodians.

Failure by employers to comply with the OSHA standard could result in a citation carrying a maximum penalty of $7000 for each violation and a maximum penalty of $70,000 for repeat violations.

What Would You Do? What Would You *Not* Do?

Case Study 1

Petra Meyer has come in for her annual gynecologic examination. Because Petra has been feeling tired and run-down, the provider orders blood to be drawn for a complete blood count (CBC) and a comprehensive blood chemistry profile. Petra indicates that she wears rubber latex gloves when housecleaning to protect her hands from the chemicals in her cleaning solution. Petra says that the last two times she cleaned her house, she experienced redness and itching of her hands along with a runny nose and red itchy eyes. She wants to know if this might be caused by breathing in the cleaning solution or getting some of it on her hands after taking off her gloves. Petra says she also experienced redness and itching of her feet the last time she wore her rubber flip-flops. ■

OSHA TERMINOLOGY

The following definitions help clarify terms related to the OSHA Bloodborne Pathogens Standard.

Occupational exposure: Occupational exposure is reasonably anticipated skin, eye, mucous membrane, or parenteral contact with blood or OPIM that may result from the performance of an employee's duties.

Sharps: Sharps are objects that can penetrate the skin, including (but not limited to) needles, lancets, scalpels, broken glass, and glass capillary tubes.

Parenteral: **Parenteral** refers to the piercing of the skin barrier or mucous membranes, such as through needlesticks, human bites, cuts, and abrasions.

Blood: Blood means human blood, human blood components, and products made from blood. Blood components include plasma, serum, platelets, and serosanguineous fluid (e.g., exudates from wounds). An example of a blood product is a medication derived from blood, such as immune globulins.

Bloodborne pathogens: Bloodborne pathogens are pathogenic microorganisms in human blood that can cause disease in humans. Bloodborne pathogens include, but are not limited to, hepatitis B virus (HBV), hepatitis C virus (HCV), and human immunodeficiency virus (HIV).

Other potentially infectious materials: OPIM include the following:

- Semen and vaginal secretions
- Cerebrospinal, synovial, pleural, pericardial, peritoneal, and amniotic fluids

- Any body fluid that is visibly contaminated with blood
- Any body fluid that has not been identified
- Saliva in dental procedures
- Any unfixed human tissue
- Any tissue culture, cells, or fluid known to be HIV infected

Contaminated: Contaminated is defined as the presence or reasonably anticipated presence of blood or OPIM on an item or surface.

Decontamination: Decontamination is the use of physical or chemical means to remove, inactivate, or destroy pathogens on a surface or item to the point where they are no longer capable of transmitting infectious particles, and the surface or item is rendered safe for handling, use, or disposal.

Nonintact skin: **Nonintact skin** is skin that has a break in the surface. It includes, but is not limited to, skin with dermatitis, abrasions, cuts, burns, hangnails, chapping, and acne.

Exposure incident: An *exposure incident* is defined as a specific eye, nose, mouth, or other mucous membrane, nonintact skin, or parenteral contact with blood or OPIM that results from an employee's duties.

COMPONENTS OF THE OSHA STANDARD

The OSHA Bloodborne Pathogens Standard is presented on the following pages as it pertains to the medical office and includes the following categories:

- Exposure control plan
- Labeling requirements
- Communication of hazards to employees
- Record keeping

Exposure Control Plan

The OSHA standard requires that the medical office develop an exposure control plan (ECP) (Fig. 2.4). The ECP is a written document stipulating the protective measures that must be followed in that medical office to eliminate or minimize employee exposure to bloodborne pathogens and OPIM. The ECP must be made available for review by all medical office staff. The ECP must include the following elements:

1. *An exposure determination.* The purpose of this section of the ECP is to identify employees who must receive training, protective equipment, hepatitis vaccination, and other protections required by the OSHA Bloodborne Pathogens Standard. The exposure determination must include (1) a list of all job classifications in which *all* employees are likely to have occupational exposure, such as providers, medical assistants, and laboratory technicians, and (2) a list of job classifications in which only *some* employees have occupational exposure, such as custodians. For the second classification of jobs, the determination must include a list of tasks in which occupational exposure may occur, such as emptying the trash.

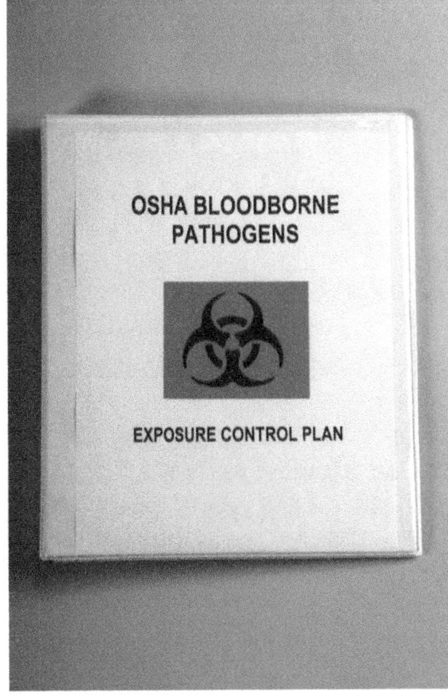

Fig. 2.4 Example of an exposure control plan.

2. *The method of compliance.* The method of compliance section of the ECP must document the specific health and safety control measures that are taken in the medical office to eliminate or minimize the risk of occupational exposure. These measures are extremely important in reducing the risk of infectious disease for the medical assistant and are discussed in greater detail later in this section (see the section Control Measures).
3. *Postexposure evaluation and follow-up procedures.* Postexposure evaluation and follow-up must specify the procedures to follow in the event of an exposure incident in the medical office, including the method of documenting and investigating an exposure incident and the postexposure evaluation, medical treatment, and follow-up that would be made available to the employee (Box 2.3).

OSHA requires employers to review and update their ECP at least annually to ensure that the plan remains current with the latest information on eliminating or reducing exposure to bloodborne pathogens. The ECP also must be updated whenever necessary to reflect new or modified tasks and procedures performed in the medical office that affect occupational exposure.

Labeling Requirements

The OSHA Bloodborne Pathogens Standard requires that containers and appliances containing biohazardous materials be labeled with a *biohazard warning label.* The biohazard warning label must be fluorescent orange or orange-red and must contain the biohazard symbol and the word *BIOHAZARD* in a contrasting color (Fig. 2.5A).

A warning label must be attached to the following: (1) containers of regulated waste; (2) refrigerators and freezers

BOX 2.3 OSHA Postexposure Evaluation and Follow-Up Procedures

An exposure incident is a specific eye, nose, mouth, or other mucous membrane, nonintact skin, or parenteral contact with blood or other potentially infectious materials that results from an employee's duties. In case of exposure involving bloodborne pathogens or other potentially infectious materials (OPIM), OSHA requires the following steps to be performed:

1. Perform initial first aid measures immediately (e.g., wash a needlestick injury thoroughly with soap and water).
2. Document the route of exposure and the conditions and circumstances of the exposure incident. This includes such information as the engineering controls, the work practice controls, and personal protective equipment being used at the time of the incident.
3. Identify and document the source individual (unless the employer can establish that identification is not feasible or is prohibited by state or local law). A *source individual* is any person, living or dead, whose blood or OPIM may be a source of occupational exposure to the health care worker.
4. Obtain consent to test the source individual's blood. Test it as soon as possible to determine hepatitis B virus (HBV), hepatitis C virus (HCV), and human immunodeficiency virus (HIV) infectivity. The following guidelines apply to this requirement:
   - If consent is not obtained, the employer must document that legally required consent cannot be obtained.
   - If the source individual's consent is not required by law, the source individual's blood (if available) must be tested and the results documented.
   - If the source individual is already known to be infected with HBV, HCV, or HIV, testing does not need to be repeated.
5. Provide the exposed employee with the source individual's test results. Inform the employee of applicable laws and regulations concerning disclosure of the identity and infectious status of the source individual.
6. Obtain consent to test the employee's blood. Collect and test the blood of the employee as soon as possible for HBV, HCV, and HIV.
7. When medically indicated, provide the employee with appropriate postexposure prophylaxis, as recommended by the U.S. Public Health Service.

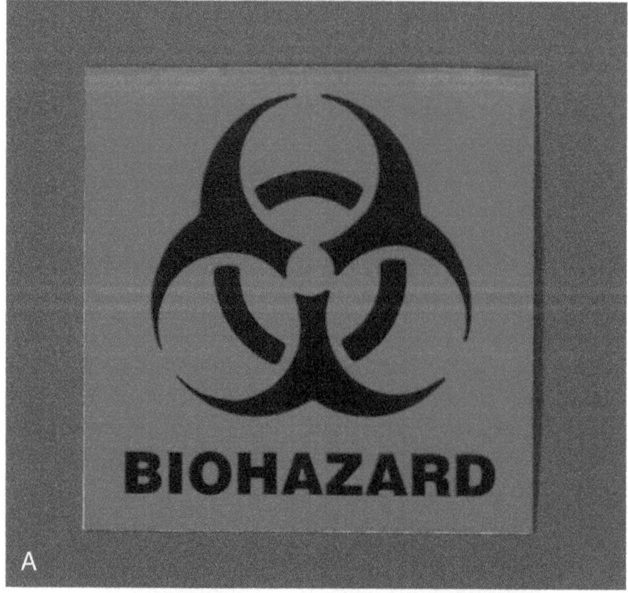

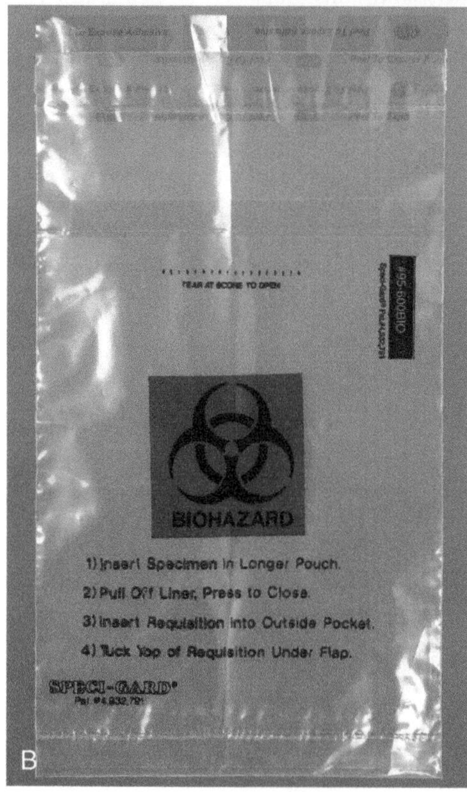

Fig. 2.5 (A) Biohazard warning label. (B) Biohazard bag used to hold and transport blood or other potentially infectious materials.

used to store blood and OPIM; and (3) containers and bags used to store, transport, or ship blood or OPIM (see Fig. 2.5B). Red bags or red containers may be substituted for biohazard warning labels. The labeling requirement is designed to alert employees to possible exposure, particularly in situations in which the nature of the material or contents is not readily identifiable as blood or OPIM.

Communicating Hazards to Employees

According to the OSHA standard, employers must ensure that all medical office employees with risk of occupational exposure participate in a training program. This program must present the ECP for the medical office while focusing on the measures that employees must take for their safety. Training must be provided at the time an employee is initially assigned to tasks in which occupational exposure may occur and at least annually thereafter.

The employer must maintain records of the training sessions, which must include presentation dates, session content, names and qualifications of the trainers, and names and job titles of employees who attended. These records must be maintained for 3 years from the date of the training session.

Record Keeping

The OSHA Bloodborne Pathogens Standard requires that the following records be maintained:

1. *OSHA medical record.* The OSHA standard requires that the employer maintain an accurate OSHA record of every medical office employee at risk for occupational exposure. These records must be kept confidential except for review by OSHA officials and as required by law. The record must include the following: employee's name; Social Security number; hepatitis B vaccination status, including dates of vaccination; results of any postexposure examinations, medical testing, and follow-up procedures; and a written evaluation of any exposure incident along with a copy of the exposure incident report.
2. *Sharps injury log.* Employers with more than 10 employees at risk for occupational exposure are required to maintain a log of injuries from contaminated sharps. The log must be maintained in a way that protects the confidentiality of injured employees (e.g., removal of personal identification). The purpose of the log is to help employers and employees keep track of all needlestick injuries. This tracking helps in identifying problem areas that need attention and ineffective devices that need to be replaced. The sharps injury log must contain the following information:
   - Type and brand of device involved in the injury
   - Location of the incident (i.e., work area)
   - Explanation of how the incident occurred

CONTROL MEASURES

OSHA requires specific health and safety control measures to eliminate or minimize the risk of occupational exposure in the medical office. These measures are divided into five categories: engineering controls, work practice controls, personal protective equipment, housekeeping, and hepatitis B vaccination.

Engineering Controls

The medical office must use engineering controls to eliminate or minimize the risk of occupational exposure. *Engineering controls* include all measures and devices that isolate or remove the bloodborne pathogens hazard from the workplace. Engineering controls must be examined and maintained or replaced as required to ensure their effectiveness. Examples of engineering controls include the following:

- Readily accessible handwashing facilities
- Safer medical devices
- Biohazard sharps containers and biohazard bags
- Autoclaves

Safer Medical Devices

Safer medical devices are an example of an engineering control. A *safer medical device* is a device that, based on reasonable judgment, would make an exposure incident involving a contaminated sharp less likely. *Reasonable judgment* refers to the judgment of the health care worker who would be using the device.

Safer medical devices include sharps with engineered sharps injury protection and needleless systems. A *sharp with engineered sharps injury protection (SESIP)* is a non-needle sharp or a needle device with a built-in safety feature used for procedures that involve the risk of sharps injury. Examples of SESIPs include safety-engineered syringes and phlebotomy devices (Fig. 2.6).

A *needleless system* is a device that does not use a needle for (1) the administration of medication or other fluids, (2) the collection or withdrawal of body fluids after initial access to a vein or artery has been established, or (3) any other procedure involving the potential for occupational exposure to bloodborne pathogens because of percutaneous injuries from contaminated sharps. An example of a needleless system is a jet injection syringe, which uses compressed air rather than a needle to administer an injection.

Work Practice Controls

Work practice controls reduce the likelihood of exposure by altering the way the technique is performed. It is important that the medical assistant consistently adhere to these safety rules, which include the following:

1. Perform all procedures involving blood or OPIM in a manner that minimizes splashing, spraying, spattering, and generation of droplets of these substances.
2. Observe warning labels on biohazard containers and appliances. Bags or containers that bear a biohazard warning label or are color-coded red indicate that they hold blood or OPIM. Refrigerators, freezers, and other appliances that contain hazardous materials also must bear a biohazard warning label.
3. Bandage cuts and other lesions on the hands before gloving.
4. Sanitize the hands after removing gloves, regardless of whether or not the gloves are visibly contaminated.
5. If your hands or other skin surfaces come in contact with blood or OPIM, thoroughly wash the area as soon as possible with soap and water.
6. If your mucous membranes (e.g., eyes, mouth, nose) come in contact with blood or OPIM, flush them with water as soon as possible.
7. Do not break or shear contaminated needles.
8. Do not remove, recap, or bend a contaminated needle. (*Note:* Sterile needles may be recapped, such as after the withdrawal of medication from a vial or ampule.)
9. Immediately after use, place contaminated sharps in a puncture-resistant, leakproof container that is appropriately labeled or color-coded. *Contaminated sharps* are contaminated objects that can penetrate the skin, including (but not limited to) needles, lancets, scalpels, broken glass, and capillary tubes.

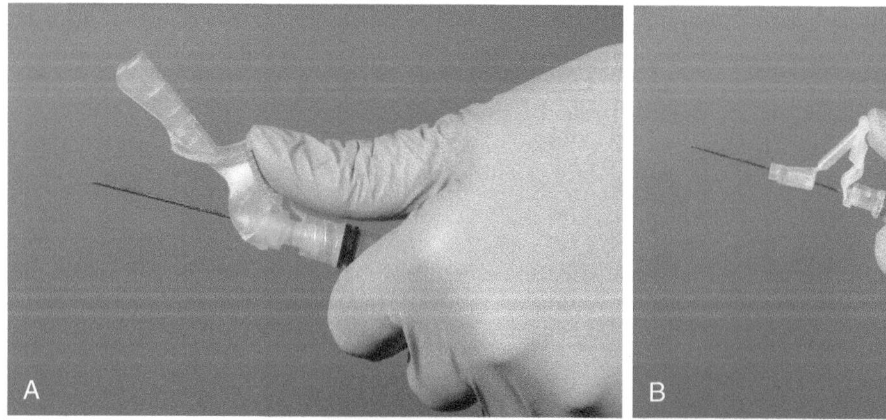

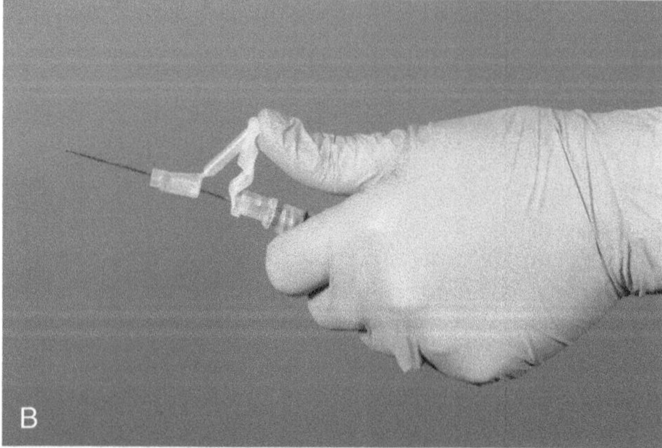

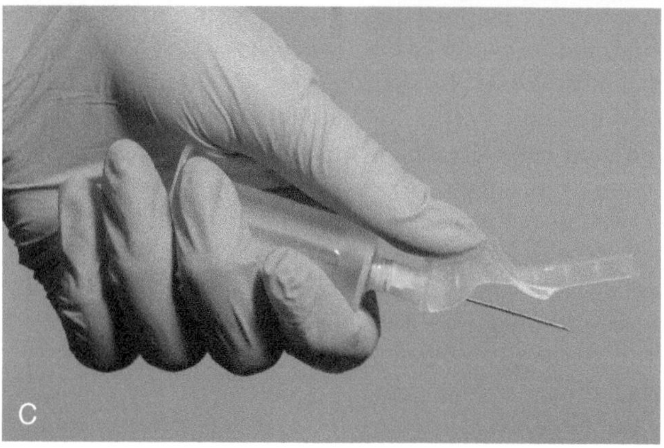

Fig. 2.6 Safer medical devices. (A and B) Safety-engineered syringes. (C) Safety-engineered phlebotomy device.

10. Do not eat, drink, smoke, apply cosmetics or lip balm, or handle contact lenses in areas where you may be exposed to blood or OPIM.
11. Do not store food or drinks in refrigerators, freezers, or cabinets or on shelves or countertops where blood or OPIM are present.
12. Place blood specimens or OPIM in containers that prevent leakage during collection, handling, processing, storage, transport, or shipping. Ensure that the containers are closed before they are stored, transported, or shipped, and are labeled or color-coded for easy identification.
13. Before any equipment that might be contaminated is serviced or shipped for repair or cleaning, such as a centrifuge, it must be inspected for blood or OPIM. If such material is present, the equipment must be decontaminated. If it cannot be decontaminated, it must be appropriately labeled to clearly indicate the contamination site, to enable those coming into contact with the equipment to take appropriate precautions.
14. If you are exposed to blood or OPIM, perform first aid measures immediately (e.g., wash a needlestick injury thoroughly with soap and water). After taking these measures, report the incident to your provider-employer as soon as possible so that postexposure procedures can be instituted (see Box 2.3). The most obvious exposure incident is a needlestick, but any eye, mouth, or other mucous membrane, nonintact skin, or parenteral contact with blood or OPIM constitutes an exposure incident and should be reported.

Personal Protective Equipment

The OSHA standard specifies that personal protective equipment must be used in the medical office whenever occupational exposure remains after engineering and work practice controls have been instituted. *Personal protective equipment* is clothing or equipment that protects an individual from contact with blood or OPIM; examples include gloves, chin-length face shields, masks, protective eyewear, laboratory coats, and gowns. The type of protective equipment appropriate for a given task depends on the degree of exposure that is anticipated, as outlined here:

1. Wear gloves when it is reasonably anticipated that your hands will have contact with blood and OPIM, mucous membranes, or nonintact skin; when performing vascular access procedures; and when handling or touching contaminated surfaces or items. Gloves cannot prevent a needlestick or other sharps injury, but they can prevent a pathogen from entering the body through a break in the skin, such as a cut, abrasion, burn, or rash.
2. Wear chin-length face shields or masks in combination with eye-protection devices whenever splashes, spray, spatter, or droplets of blood or OPIM may be generated, posing a hazard through contact with the eyes, nose, or mouth (e.g., removing a stopper from a tube of blood, transferring serum from whole blood) (Fig. 2.7).

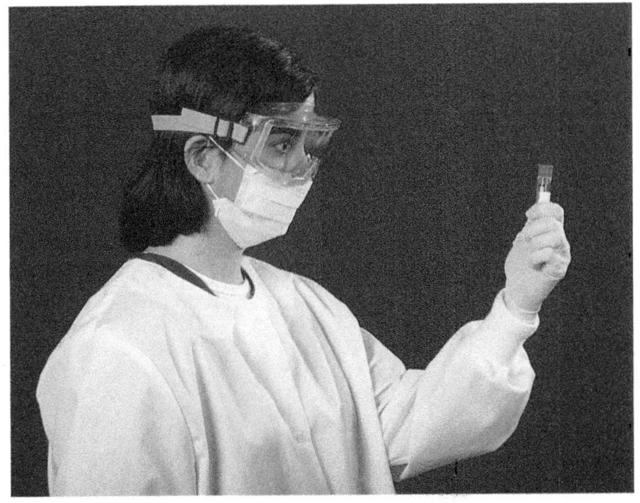

Fig. 2.7 Jennifer wears a combination mask and eye protection device and a laboratory coat to protect against splashes, spray, spatter, and droplets of blood.

3. Wear appropriate protective clothing, such as gowns, aprons, and laboratory coats, when gross contamination can reasonably be anticipated during performance of a task or procedure (e.g., laboratory testing procedure). The type of protective clothing needed depends on the task and degree of exposure anticipated.

Personal Protective Equipment Guidelines

Certain guidelines must be followed when using protective equipment:

1. Protective equipment must not allow blood or OPIM to pass through or reach the skin, underlying garments (e.g., scrubs, street clothes, undergarments), eyes, mouth, or other mucous membranes under normal conditions of use and for the time the protective equipment is used.
2. The employer must provide appropriate personal protective equipment at no cost to the health care worker. The employer is responsible for ensuring that the equipment is available in appropriate sizes, is readily accessible, and is used correctly. In addition, the employer must ensure that the equipment is cleaned, laundered, repaired, replaced, or disposed of as necessary to ensure its effectiveness.
3. If the medical office uses latex gloves, latex-free alternatives must be provided for employees who are allergic to latex gloves. Examples of alternatives include nitrile and vinyl gloves.
4. If gloves become contaminated, torn, or punctured, replace them as soon as practical.
5. All eye protection devices must have solid side shields; chin-length face shields, goggles, and glasses with solid side shields are acceptable (Fig. 2.8); standard prescription eyeglasses are unacceptable as eye protection.
6. If a garment is penetrated by blood or OPIM, it must be removed as soon as possible and placed in an appropriately designated container for washing.

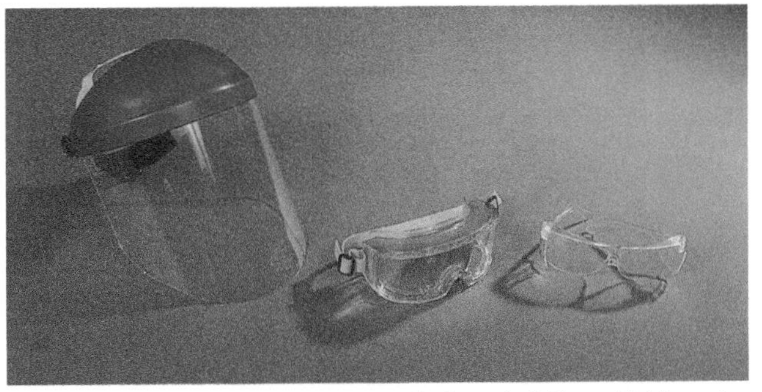

Fig. 2.8 Examples of eye protection devices. *Left,* Face shield; *center,* goggles; *right,* glasses with solid side shields.

7. All personal protective equipment must be removed before you leave the medical office.
8. When protective equipment is removed, it must be placed in an appropriately designated area or container for storage, washing, decontamination, or disposal.
9. Utility gloves may be decontaminated and reused unless they are cracked, peeling, torn, or punctured or no longer provide barrier protection.
10. If you believe that using protective equipment would prevent proper delivery of health care or would pose an increased hazard to your safety or that of a coworker, in extenuating circumstances you may temporarily and briefly decline its use. After such an incident, the circumstances must be investigated to determine whether the situation could be prevented in the future.

Housekeeping

The OSHA standard requires that specific housekeeping procedures be followed to ensure that the work site is maintained in a clean and sanitary condition. The medical office must develop and implement a written schedule for cleaning and decontaminating each area where exposure occurs. The cleaning and decontamination method must be specified for each task and should be based on the type of surface to be cleaned, the type of soil present, and the tasks or procedures being performed in that area. Housekeeping procedures include the following:

1. Clean and decontaminate equipment and work surfaces after completing procedures that involve blood or OPIM. Cleaning is accomplished using plain soap, and decontamination is performed using an appropriate disinfectant (Fig. 2.9).
2. Clean and decontaminate all equipment and work surfaces as soon as possible after exposure to blood or OPIM. For decontamination of blood spills, OSHA recommends the use of a 10% solution of sodium hypochlorite (household bleach) in water (1 part bleach to 9 parts water).
3. Inspect and decontaminate all reusable receptacles, such as bins, pails, and cans, on a regular basis. If contamination is visible, the item must be cleaned and decontaminated as soon as possible.
4. Do not pick up broken, contaminated glassware with the hands, even if gloves are worn. Use mechanical means,

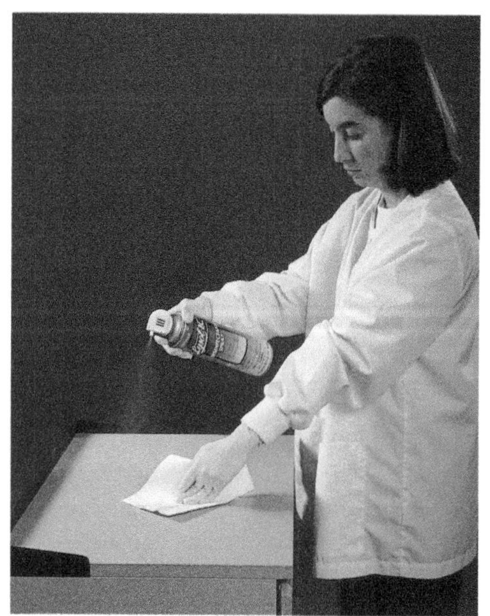

Fig. 2.9 Clean and decontaminate work surfaces with an appropriate disinfectant after completing procedures involving blood and other potentially infectious materials.

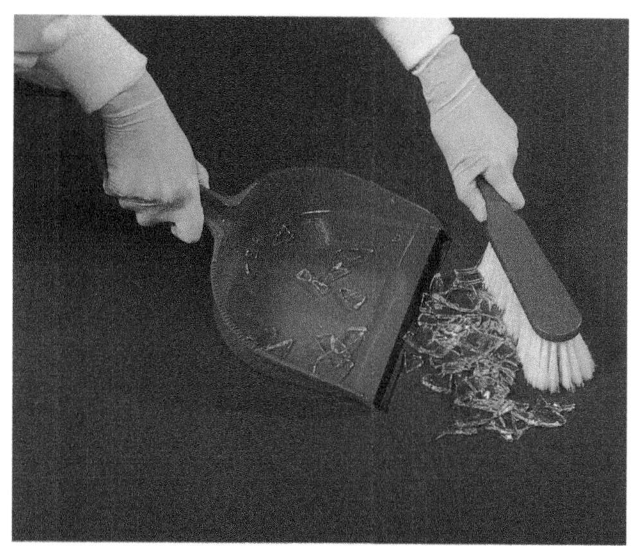

Fig. 2.10 Use mechanical means to pick up broken contaminated glass.

such as a brush and dustpan, tongs, and forceps (Fig. 2.10).

5. Protective coverings, such as plastic wrap and aluminum foil, may be used to cover work surfaces or equipment, but they must be removed or replaced if contamination occurs.
6. Handle contaminated laundry as little as possible and with appropriate personal protective equipment. Place all contaminated laundry in leakproof bags that are properly labeled or color-coded. Contaminated laundry must not be sorted or rinsed at the medical office.
7. If the outside of a biohazard container becomes contaminated, it must be placed in a second suitable container.
8. Biohazard sharps containers (Fig. 2.11) must be closable, puncture resistant, and leakproof. They must bear a biohazard warning label and must be color-coded red

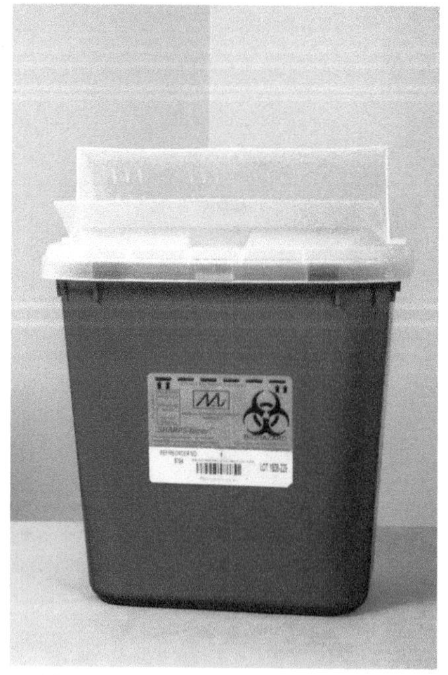

Fig. 2.11 Biohazard sharps container.

to ensure identification of the contents as hazardous. To ensure effectiveness, the following guidelines must be observed:

- Locate the sharps container as close as possible to the area of use to avoid the hazard of transporting a contaminated needle through the workplace.
- Maintain sharps containers in an upright position to keep liquid and sharps inside.
- Do not reach into the sharps container with your hand.
- Replace sharps containers on a regular basis, and do not allow them to overfill. (It is recommended that sharps containers be replaced when they are three-quarters full.)

What Would You Do? What Would You *Not* Do?

Case Study 2

Tracy Smith is pregnant and is at the medical office to have her blood drawn for a prenatal profile. Tracy says she has been reading information about the hepatitis B vaccine because she knows her baby will be given this vaccine soon after birth. She wants to know why it is recommended that an infant be immunized for hepatitis B. Tracy says that infants are not at risk for contracting hepatitis B because the way it is transmitted is mostly through sexual contact and illegal drug use. ■

Hepatitis B Vaccination

The OSHA standard requires employers to offer the hepatitis B vaccination series free of charge to all medical office personnel who have occupational exposure. The vaccination must be offered within 10 working days of initial assignment to a position with occupational exposure, unless the

HEPATITIS B DECLINATION FORM

I understand that due to my occupational exposure to blood or other potentially infectious materials, I may be at risk of acquiring hepatitis B virus (HBV) infection. I have been given the opportunity to be vaccinated with hepatitis B vaccine at no charge to myself. However, I decline hepatitis B vaccination at this time. I understand that by declining this vaccine I continue to be at risk of acquiring hepatitis B, a serious disease. If in the future I continue to have occupational exposure to blood or to other potentially infectious materials and I want to be vaccinated with hepatitis B vaccine, I can receive the vaccination series at no charge to me.

____
Employee Name (printed)

______________________________ ____________
Employee Signature Date

______________________________ ____________
Witness Signature Date

Fig. 2.12 Hepatitis B declination form. This form must be signed by an employee with occupational exposure who declines hepatitis B vaccination.

following factors exist: (1) the individual has previously received the hepatitis B vaccination series, (2) antibody testing has revealed that the individual is immune to hepatitis B, or (3) the vaccine is contraindicated for medical reasons.

Medical office personnel who decline vaccination must sign a hepatitis B waiver form documenting refusal. This form must be filed in the employee's OSHA record (Fig. 2.12). Employees who decline vaccination may request the vaccination later; the employer must then provide it, according to the aforementioned criteria.

Approximately 5% of the population does not form antibodies to the hepatitis B vaccine. Because of this, the CDC recommends that an antibody titer test be performed on all health care workers between 1 and 2 months after the last dose of the hepatitis B vaccine. The titer test is performed to determine if the health care worker has developed protective antibodies against HBV and is immune to infection. Health care workers who do not respond to the primary vaccination series, as indicated by a negative titer test, must be revaccinated with a second three-dose vaccination series and then undergo a repeat titer test. If the titer test is still negative, this means that the health care worker probably lacks immunity to HBV infection.

HANDLING REGULATED MEDICAL WASTE

Regulated medical waste (RMW) is medical waste that may contain infectious materials posing a threat to health and safety. Regulated medical waste (RMW) must be handled carefully to prevent an exposure incident. The OSHA Bloodborne Pathogens Standard outlines specific actions to take when handling RMW, as follows:

1. Separate regulated waste from the general refuse at its point of origin. Disposable items containing RMW should be placed directly into biohazard containers and should not be mixed with the regular trash (Box 2.4).
2. Ensure that biohazard containers are closable, leakproof, and suitably constructed to contain the contents during handling, storage, and transport. These containers include biohazard bags and sharps containers.
3. To prevent spillage or protrusion of the contents, close the lid of a sharps container before removing it from an examining room. Never open, empty, or clean a contaminated sharps container. If there is a chance of leakage from the sharps container, the medical assistant should place it in a second container that is closable, leakproof, and appropriately labeled or color-coded.
4. Securely close biohazard bags before removing them from an examining room. To provide additional protection, some medical offices double-bag by placing the primary bag inside a second biohazard bag.
5. Transport full biohazard containers to a secured area away from the general public, using personal protective equipment (e.g., gloves).

DISPOSAL OF REGULATED MEDICAL WASTE

Each state is responsible for developing policies for disposal of RMW. To avoid noncompliance, it is important for the medical office to keep current with the specific regulated waste policies and guidelines set forth in their state.

Most medical offices use a commercial medical waste service to dispose of RMW. This service is responsible for picking up and transporting the medical waste to a treatment facility for incineration (or other means) to destroy pathogens and render them harmless. The waste can then be safely disposed of in a sanitary landfill. Regulated waste

BOX 2.4 Guidelines for Discarding Medical Waste in the Medical Office

Regular Waste Container

The following items that have been used for health care *are not* considered regulated medical waste and can be discarded in a covered waste container lined with a regular trash bag.

- Disposable drapes
- Disposable patient gowns
- Examining table paper
- Disposable clean or sterile gloves
- Gauze tinged with blood or other body fluids
- Disposable probe covers for thermometers
- Tongue depressors
- Tissues with respiratory secretions
- Disposable ear speculums
- Empty urine containers
- Urine testing strips
- Disposable diapers
- Feminine hygiene products

Biohazard Sharps Container

The following items are sharps. They *are* considered regulated medical waste and must be discarded in a biohazard sharps container.

- Hypodermic syringes and needles
- Venipuncture needles
- Lancets
- Razor blades
- Scalpel blades
- Suture needles
- Blood tubes
- Capillary pipets
- Microscope slides and coverslips
- Broken glassware

Biohazard Bag Waste Container

The following items *are* considered regulated medical waste. They are not sharps and can be discarded in a covered waste container lined with a biohazard bag.

- Any item saturated or dripping with blood or other potentially infectious materials (OPIM) (e.g., dressings, gauze, cotton balls, paper towels, tissues that are saturated or dripping with blood)
- Any item caked with dried blood or OPIM, such as dressings and sutures
- Disposable clean or sterile gloves contaminated with blood or OPIM
- Disposable vaginal speculums and collection devices (e.g., swabs, spatulas, brushes)
- Tissue or fluid removed during minor office surgery
- Microbiologic waste, such as specimen cultures and collection devices
- Discarded live and attenuated vaccines

Sanitary Sewer

Disposal of small quantities of blood and other body fluids to the sanitary sewer is considered a safe method of disposing of these waste materials. The following fluids can be carefully poured down a utility sink, drain, or toilet. (*Note:* State regulations may dictate the maximum volume allowable for discharge of blood or body fluids into the sanitary sewer.)

- Blood
- Body excretions such as urine
- Body secretions such as sputum

treatment facilities must be licensed and hold permits issued by the Environmental Protection Agency (EPA), allowing them to dispose of RMW.

A series of steps must be followed for preparing and storing RMW for pickup by the service. Although these steps may vary slightly from state to state, general measures required by most states include the following:

1. Place biohazard bags and sharps containers into a receptacle provided by the medical waste service. The receptacle is usually a cardboard box (Fig. 2.13). The box should be securely sealed with packing tape, and a biohazard warning label must appear on two opposite sides of the box.
2. Store the biohazard boxes in a locked room inside the facility or in a locked collection container outside for pickup by the medical waste service. This step is aimed at preventing unauthorized access to items such as needles and syringes. The regulated waste storage area should be labeled with one of the following:
   - "Authorized Personnel Only" sign
   - International biohazard symbol
3. Many states require that a tracking record be completed when the waste is picked up by the medical waste service. This form includes such information as the type and quantity of waste (weighed in pounds) and where it is being sent. The form must be signed by a representative of the medical waste service and the medical office. After the waste has been destroyed at the regulated waste treatment facility, a record documenting its disposal is transmitted to the medical office.

What Would You Do? What Would You *Not* Do?

Case Study 3

Giles Lee is at the medical office. In 1988, he was in a serious car accident and had to have a blood transfusion. Giles says that he donated blood for the first time 2 months ago. Last week, he received a letter saying that the blood he donated tested positive for hepatitis C and that he should see his provider. Giles says that he must have gotten hepatitis C from the blood transfusion he received many years ago. He does not understand how that could have happened because he thought the blood supply was tested for hepatitis C. Giles wants to know why he has not had any symptoms of hepatitis C and wants to know if he can give hepatitis C to his wife. ■

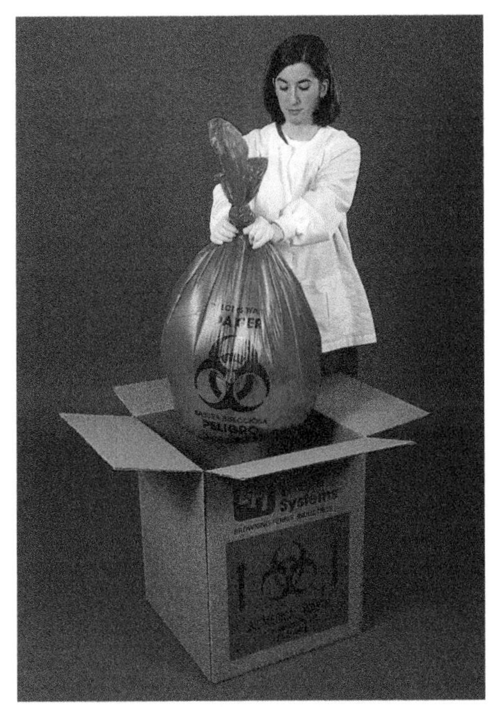

Fig. 2.13 Jennifer places a biohazard bag inside a cardboard box in preparation for pickup by the medical waste service.

BLOODBORNE DISEASES

A **bloodborne disease** is any disease caused by a pathogen spread through direct contact with blood or other body fluids. The most common route of transmission of bloodborne pathogens to a health care worker is through accidental needlesticks and other sharps-related injuries. There are more than 20 bloodborne pathogens that can infect a health care worker. The bloodborne pathogens that are the biggest threats to health care workers include the hepatitis B virus (HBV), hepatitis C virus (HCV), and human immunodeficiency virus (HIV), which is discussed in greater detail in this section.

Hepatitis B is much easier to transmit than HIV. After a needlestick exposure to HBV-infected blood, health care workers not immune to hepatitis B have a 6% to 30% chance of developing it. The risk of a hepatitis C infection following a needlestick exposure to HCV-infected blood is approximately 2%. After a needlestick exposure to HIV-infected blood, a health care worker has a 0.3% chance of being infected with HIV and a 0.1% chance of being infected after a mucous membrane exposure of the eyes, nose, or mouth. Studies show that most exposures of health care workers to HBV, HBC, and HIV do not result in infection.

HEPATITIS B

Hepatitis B is an infection of the liver caused by the hepatitis B virus that can result in serious liver damage. The virus is found in the blood and in certain body fluids (e.g., semen and vaginal secretions) of HBV-infected individuals. The hepatitis B virus can cause both acute and chronic infections. A newly acquired infection is known as an acute infection. An **acute infection** is an infection that develops suddenly and lasts for a short period of time. A **chronic infection** is an infection that develops slowly and may worsen over an extended period of time. Some acute infections (which include both hepatitis B and C) can persist in the body and then develop into chronic infections.

ACUTE HEPATITIS B

Hepatitis B is classified as acute if the infection lasts for 6 months or less. Many individuals do not experience any symptoms with acute hepatitis B. Individuals who develop symptoms usually experience them for several weeks, but in some cases, they may continue for as long as 6 months. On an average, these symptoms appear 3 months after exposure but can appear any time between 2 and 5 months following exposure. Symptoms of acute HBV hepatitis B are often mild and flu-like and may be mistaken for another condition, such as influenza. These symptoms usually include a mild fever, fatigue, loss of appetite, abdominal pain, and muscle and joint pain. Because of a lack of symptoms or only mild symptoms, many people with acute hepatitis B do not know they are infected. Some HBV-infected individuals may experience more severe symptoms such as nausea, vomiting, dark urine, dark clay-colored bowel movements, and jaundice, often prompting them to seek medical care. Many people (especially adults) can clear the virus from their system and recover completely. These people become immune to hepatitis B and cannot get infected again.

CHRONIC HEPATITIS B

Patients who are unable to fight off acute hepatitis B remain infected and may go on to develop chronic hepatitis B. Infants and young children are more likely to develop a chronic infection, while most adults (95%) are able to fight off the virus and do not develop chronic hepatitis B.

Many individuals with chronic hepatitis B are not aware of being infected. This is because chronic hepatitis B does not typically exhibit any symptoms until it causes serious HBV-related health problems. During the asymptomatic period, which may last for decades or more, the virus may be slowly damaging the liver; in addition, the individual is a carrier for hepatitis B during this time and can infect others. Chronic hepatitis B can eventually lead to serious liver disease, which includes cirrhosis, liver cancer, and liver failure.

Transmission

HBV is found in the blood and body fluids of infected individuals and is mostly transmitted through unprotected sexual contact, sharing needles, syringes, or drug preparation equipment, and perinatally from an infected mother to her infant during birth. Other modes of transmission include direct contact with blood or open sores of an infected

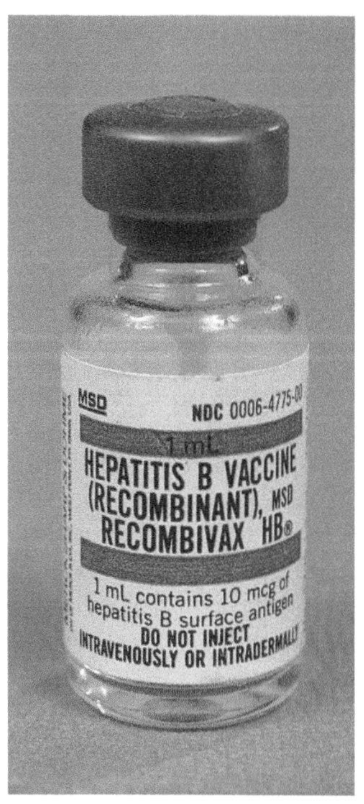

Fig. 2.14 Hepatitis B vaccine.

individual, getting a tattoo or body piercing with contaminated instruments, and the sharing of items such as razors or toothbrushes with an infected individual. Hepatitis B is not spread by food, water, breastfeeding, sneezing, coughing, hugging, kissing, or sharing eating utensils or drinking glasses.

The most common means of transmitting hepatitis B to a health care worker is through blood and blood components (e.g., plasma and serum) transferred through accidental needlesticks and other sharps-related injuries. The virus is also spread to health care workers, but less effectively, through blood splashes to the eyes, mouth, and nonintact skin. Fortunately, the number of health care workers who contract hepatitis B in the workplace has declined dramatically since the development of the OSHA standard and the hepatitis B vaccine.

Hepatitis B Vaccine

The best means of preventing hepatitis B is by administering the hepatitis B vaccine, which is produced from genetically altered yeast cells. The hepatitis B vaccine (Fig. 2.14) is an active immunizing agent, meaning the body is actively stimulated to produce antibodies against HBV. The vaccine is administered intramuscularly in a series of three doses; brand names are *Recombivax HB* and *Engerix-B*. After the first dose is administered, the second dose is given 1 month after the first dose, and the third dose is administered 6 months after the first dose (i.e., 0, 1 month, and 6 months). There is a new hepatitis B vaccine available for adults that consist of a series of two doses administered intramuscularly 1 month apart. The brand name of this vaccine is *Heplisav-B*. The hepatitis B vaccine is well tolerated by most patients. The most common side effect is soreness at the injection site, including induration, erythema, and swelling. Occasionally, a low-grade fever, headache, and dizziness occur.

As previously discussed, the OSHA standard recommends that all health care workers receive the hepatitis B vaccine as a preventive measure against hepatitis B. Following an exposure incident, a health care worker who has previously been vaccinated probably would not require further treatment.

Recommendations for Vaccination

The CDC has developed recommendations for hepatitis B vaccination, which include the following: all infants within 24 hours of birth and all children and adolescents 18 years old or younger who have not been previously vaccinated. The vaccine is further recommended for adults older than 18 years who are at an increased risk for developing hepatitis B; examples include the following:

- Employees with occupational exposure (e.g., health care workers, public safety personnel)
- People who live with someone who has HBV
- Anyone with a sexually transmitted infection (including HIV)
- Sexual partners of someone with HBV
- Individuals with multiple sex partners
- Men who have sex with men
- Injection drug users
- Individuals with chronic liver disease
- Residents and staff in institutions for the developmentally disabled
- People who travel to countries where hepatitis B is common

Treatment

There is no specific treatment for patients diagnosed with acute hepatitis B. In most cases, care is focused on measures to help the body fight off the infection, which include a healthy diet, drinking plenty of fluids, and rest. The provider usually orders regular HBV testing to determine if the virus is still in the patient's body.

A chronic hepatitis B infection can be treated with antiviral medications. These medications slow the replication of the virus and can prevent or delay liver disease; however, they rarely completely rid the body of the virus. Once a patient begins antiviral medication therapy, he or she must continue it for life. If liver disease develops, treatments are available based upon the type and severity of the liver disease.

Postexposure Prophylaxis

Postexposure prophylaxis (PEP) refers to treatment administered to an individual after exposure to an infectious disease, to reduce the risk of developing that disease. PEP may be employed in situations that result in exposure to HBV-infected blood or body fluids such as occupational exposure, unprotected sex, sexual assault, and sharing needles, syringes, and drug preparation equipment. Infants exposed prenatally to HBV during birth require PEP, which is 85% to 95% effective in preventing an HBV infection in the infant.

The PEP for unvaccinated or incompletely vaccinated individuals exposed to HBV is the administration of the first dose of the hepatitis B vaccine series, an active immunizing agent. In addition, a passive immunizing agent is administered known as *hepatitis B immune globulin (HBIG). HBIG* is prepared from the plasma of healthy individuals with high levels of hepatitis B antibodies. HBIG provides temporary immunity to hepatitis B for 3 to 6 months, giving the active immunizing agent a chance to take effect. It is important to administer both agents as soon as possible after an exposure incident—preferably within 24 hours, but no later than 7 days. The remaining dose(s) of the hepatitis vaccine series should then be administered following the appropriate vaccine schedule.

If an exposed individual has been vaccinated for hepatitis B, a blood test will be performed to determine the level of HBV antibodies present in his or her blood. An individual exposed to HBV with adequate antibody protection does not require PEP.

HEPATITIS C

Hepatitis C is an infection of the liver caused by the hepatitis C virus that can result in serious liver damage. The virus is found in the blood of an individual infected with hepatitis C. The hepatitis C virus can cause both acute and chronic infections. Most individuals with acute hepatitis C have no symptoms; if symptoms do occur, they typically last 2 weeks to 3 months. The symptoms are usually mild and flulike and similar to those of acute hepatitis B.

Approximately 15% to 25% of individuals with acute hepatitis C can clear the virus from their system within 6 months after infection and recover completely. The remaining 75% to 85% of individuals remain infected and go on to develop chronic hepatitis C. Approximately 20 to 30 years following infection, 10% to 20% of individuals with chronic hepatitis C develop serious liver disease, such as cirrhosis or liver cancer. Ultimately, 1% to 5% of individuals with chronic hepatitis C die from liver failure.

For reasons not yet completely understood, individuals born between 1945 and 1965 (often referred to as "baby boomers") are five times more likely to have chronic hepatitis C compared with adults born in other years. These HCV-infected baby boomers account for about 75% of all cases of chronic hepatitis C in the United States.

Transmission

An HCV infection can be transmitted when blood from an infected individual enters the bloodstream of someone who is not infected. The most common route of transmission is by sharing needles, syringes, or drug preparation equipment with an HCV-infected individual. Less commonly, HCV can be transmitted by getting a tattoo or body piercing with HCV-contaminated instruments and from an HCV-infected mother to her infant during birth. Unlike hepatitis B, hepatitis C is rarely transmitted through sexual contact with an HCV-infected individual. Hepatitis C is not spread by food, water, breastfeeding, sneezing, coughing, hugging, kissing, or sharing eating utensils or drinking glasses.

A test to determine the presence of hepatitis C in donor blood did not exist until 1992. Up until this time, a significant number of people contracted the disease from HCV-infected blood transfusions and organ transplants and are now living with chronic hepatitis C. Routine HCV testing of the US blood supply since 1992 now makes it rare for someone to contract hepatitis C in this way.

The most common means of transmitting hepatitis C to a health care worker is through HCV-infected blood or blood components transferred through accidental needlesticks and other sharps-related injuries. The chance of contracting hepatitis C by a health care worker is much lower than that of contracting hepatitis B.

Treatment

There is no specific treatment for an individual diagnosed with acute hepatitis C. In most cases, care is focused on measures to help the body fight off the infection, which include a healthy diet, drinking plenty of fluids, and rest. The provider usually orders regular HCV testing to determine if the virus is still in the body.

The treatment for chronic hepatitis C has evolved substantially since the development of highly effective antiviral medications. Treatment usually involves the daily administration of antiviral medications for a period of 12 weeks. These medications attack the virus and cure the disease in more than 95% of infected individuals, thereby preventing serious liver damage and possible death. Unfortunately, most people with chronic hepatitis C do not know they are infected and therefore, do not receive the needed antiviral medication therapy.

PEP for hepatitis C with immune globulin is not effective in reducing the risk of a hepatitis C infection and therefore is not currently recommended. At present, there is no vaccine available to prevent hepatitis C; however, research in this area is ongoing. HCV reinfection can occur in individuals who have been infected with HCV and cleared the virus from their body and in individuals who have been cured with antiviral medications. The best way to prevent reinfection is by avoiding high-risk situations and behaviors that can spread the disease, such as injection drug use with contaminated needles and syringes.

HCV Testing Recommendations

Chronic hepatitis C is known as a "silent disease." This is because more than 50% of infected individuals have no symptoms and do not know they are infected. These individuals are also carriers for HCV and can infect others. Individuals with chronic hepatitis C can be infected for years or even decades before symptoms first begin to appear. During this time, the virus may be slowly attacking the liver, eventually resulting in serious liver damage and possible death. To identify individuals with chronic hepatitis C, the CDC recommends a screening test for individuals with a greater risk of being infected with HCV, which include:

- Any individual born between 1945 and 1965
- Current or former injection drug users (including those who injected only once many years ago)
- Recipients of blood transfusions or organ transplants prior to July 1992
- Individuals with hemophilia who received clotting factor concentrates made before 1987, when less advanced methods for manufacturing those products were used
- Individuals who received a tattoo or body piercing with unsterile equipment
- Individuals who have undergone long-term hemodialysis treatments
- Health care workers exposed to HCV-infected blood through accidental needlesticks or other sharps injuries or mucous membrane exposure
- People with HIV infection
- Infants born to HCV-infected mothers

Memories From Practicum

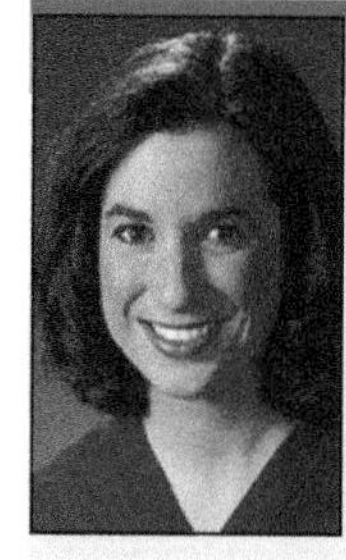

Jennifer: As a student, I was extremely nervous to go out on practicum. I was so scared to think that I was actually going to be in a medical office setting and would have to put everything I had learned into practice. Would I remember everything? Would I do something wrong and hurt the patient? It was such an overwhelming feeling! But to my relief, I had a very good experience. The office staff was so friendly and helpful to me, and I surprised myself at how easily everything I had learned stayed with me. It was so exciting to see that I was actually functioning as a team member in the health care field. I could not have had better training. ■

HIGHLIGHT on Viral Hepatitis A, B, and C

- Hepatitis A, B, and C are infections of the liver caused by three different viruses. They are spread in different ways and can affect the liver differently.
- Hepatitis A is spread through contact with food or water that has been contaminated by an infected individual's stool. Hepatitis B is spread through contact with HBV-infected blood and body fluids, and hepatitis C is spread through direct contact with HCV-infected blood.
- Symptoms common to all types of hepatitis include fatigue, nausea, loss of appetite, abdominal pain, and jaundice.
- Hepatitis A, B, and C are designated by the CDC as nationally notifiable diseases. When the provider diagnoses a case of hepatitis A, B, or C, a reportable disease form must be completed and filed with the local public health department.
- There are vaccines to prevent hepatitis A and B, but there is no vaccine to prevent hepatitis C.

Hepatitis B

- It is estimated that 850,000 people in the United States are infected with chronic hepatitis B; however, this number may be as high as 2.2 million people. Many of these individuals do not have symptoms and therefore, do not know they are infected. These individuals are also carriers for HBV and can transmit the disease to others.
- Chronic hepatitis B is often not diagnosed until an HBV-infected individual's blood is screened following a blood donation or when test results are found to be abnormal during routine laboratory testing.
- Every year, approximately 3,000 Americans die as a result of the long-term complications of chronic hepatitis B, such as cirrhosis and liver cancer.
- New hepatitis B infections are highest among adults, ages 30–49 years, because many people at risk for infection in this age group have not been vaccinated as recommended. The greatest decline in new infections has occurred among children and adolescents because of routine hepatitis B immunization.
- Hepatitis B can survive outside the body in a dried state for at least 1 week and still can be capable of causing infection. Examples of surfaces that could harbor dried blood or body fluids infected with HBV include contaminated worktables, equipment, and instruments.
- Whether or not an individual with acute hepatitis B goes on to develop chronic hepatitis B is related to the age at the time of infection. The younger a person is when infected, the greater the risk of developing a chronic infection. According to the CDC, following infection with acute hepatitis B, chronic infection develops in:
  - 90% of infants infected by their mothers at birth
  - 25%–50% of young children infected between ages 1 and 5 years
  - 5% of individuals infected as an older child or adult
- Overall, the number of individuals contracting hepatitis B has decreased since the development of the hepatitis B vaccine. As more people become immune to hepatitis B through the immunization of infants, the goal of eliminating hepatitis B in the United States may be realized.

Hepatitis C

- In the United States, chronic hepatitis C is the most common chronic viral infection found in blood and spread through contact with blood.

HIGHLIGHT on Viral Hepatitis A, B, and C—cont'd

- Approximately 2.7–3.9 million Americans are living with chronic hepatitis C, and most do not have symptoms and therefore do not know they are infected. These individuals are carriers for hepatitis C and can infect others.
- Sharing contaminated needles, syringes for injection drug use is known to play a major role in HCV transmission. According to the CDC, there has been a dramatic increase in new cases of hepatitis C among young adults between the ages of 18 and 39 years who inject heroin and prescription opioids.
- Chronic hepatitis C is a leading cause of liver cirrhosis and liver transplantation in the United States.
- New screening efforts and more effective treatments for hepatitis C are helping providers identify and cure more people with the disease. As a result, hepatitis C may become less common in the future. Researchers estimate that hepatitis C could be a rare disease in the United States by 2036.

ACQUIRED IMMUNODEFICIENCY SYNDROME

Acquired immunodeficiency syndrome (AIDS) is a chronic disorder of the immune system that eventually destroys the body's ability to fight off infection. AIDS is caused by a retrovirus known as *human immunodeficiency virus (HIV)*. The following description helps to clarify the difference between these terms. The viral infection of the body with HIV is known as *HIV infection,* whereas the term *AIDS* is used to refer to the last stage of HIV infection. Simply put, the terms *HIV infection* and *AIDS* refer to different stages of the same disease.

AIDS was first reported in the United States in 1981, but most likely it existed here and in other parts of the world for many years before that. More than 1.1 million individuals have HIV in the United States, and approximately 14% of these individuals do not know that they are infected.

When HIV gains entrance into the body, it begins to attack and destroy certain white blood cells known as *CD4⁺ T cells,* which are involved in protecting the body against viral, bacterial, fungal, and protozoal infections. Without treatment, more and more CD4⁺ T cells are destroyed, and the immune system is gradually weakened. After a period of time, which typically lasts about 10 years, the body's immune system becomes so weakened by the attack that it is unable to fight off the diseases and infections associated with AIDS. Once an individual reaches the AIDS stage of the infection, life expectancy is about 3 years.

AIDS is characterized by the presence of severe and life-threatening opportunistic infections and unusual cancers that occur due to advanced HIV infection and are known as *AIDS-defining conditions.* An **opportunistic infection** takes advantage of an opportunity not normally available, such as the weakened immune system of an HIV-infected individual. Opportunistic infections occur more often and are more severe with a weakened immune system than with a healthy immune system. The CDC has developed a list of AIDS-defining conditions; some examples of these include pneumonia, tuberculosis, herpes simplex 1 virus, candidiasis (thrush), salmonella infection, cryptococcal meningitis, toxoplasmosis, cytomegalovirus, anal cancer, and Kaposi's sarcoma, which is characterized by slightly elevated pink, brown, or reddish purple blotches or bumps anywhere on the skin (Fig. 2.15).

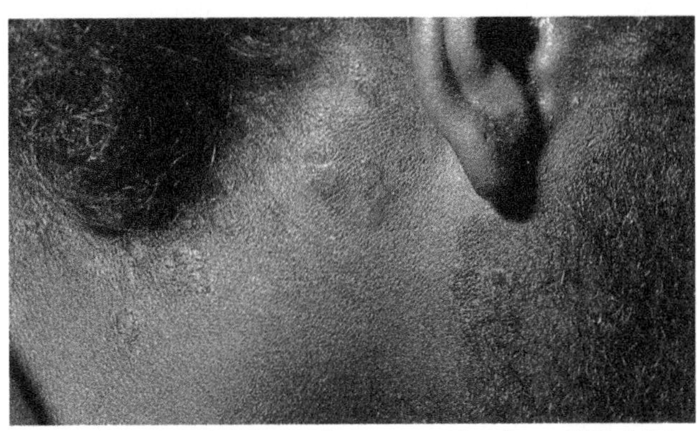

Fig. 2.15 Kaposi sarcoma is an example of an AIDS-defining condition. (From Forbes CD: *Color atlas and text of clinical medicine,* ed 3, St Louis: Mosby; 2003.)

According to the CDC definition, a patient has AIDS if they have a positive HIV test result and have one or more of the following:

- $CD4^+$ T-cell count below 200 cells/mm^3 (normal $CD4^+$ T-cell count for a healthy individual ranges from 500 to 1500 cells/mm^3
- CD4+ T-cell percentage of total lymphocytes of less than 14%
- Presence of an AIDS-defining condition

TRANSMISSION

In the general population, HIV is spread primarily through sexual contact with an infected person and by sharing drug injection needles with someone who is infected. An untreated HIV-infected mother can transmit the virus to her baby during pregnancy or birth. HIV also can be spread to infants through the breast milk of infected mothers. Because of this, the CDC recommends that HIV testing be included in the routine panel of prenatal screening tests for all pregnant women at the first visit. Treatment of the mother early in the pregnancy can almost completely eliminate transmission of HIV to the fetus.

Scientific evidence shows that HIV is not spread through casual, everyday contact. There is no evidence that HIV is spread by sharing facilities or equipment, such as telephones, computers, food utensils, bedding, doorknobs, and bathrooms.

Because HIV is not passed through the air, it is not spread through coughing and sneezing. HIV also is not spread through saliva, tears and sweat, or by shaking hands and hugging, or by mosquitoes, ticks, and other blood-sucking insects.

Because HIV is not easily transmitted, the risk to health care workers is quite low. Since reporting began in 1985, the CDC has received reports of 58 documented cases of HIV infection from occupational exposure to health care workers. Despite the low risk of infection, the serious nature of HIV infection warrants the use of the OSHA Bloodborne Pathogens Standard by all health care workers. Precautions minimizing the risk of exposure to blood and body fluids also are recommended as a means of protection against other bloodborne pathogens, such as hepatitis B, hepatitis C, and syphilis.

HIV TESTING

The only way to know for sure if an individual is infected with HIV is to be tested. The CDC recommends HIV testing for all patients between the ages of 13 and 64 at least once as part of routine health care. Patients should be notified that HIV testing will be performed; however, patients have the option of declining the testing (known as *opt-out testing*). The CDC further recommends that individuals at high risk for HIV infection undergo HIV testing at least annually. Examples of high-risk behaviors include having sex with an HIV-infected individual and the sharing needles and syringes with an infected person. If the HIV test result is positive, a follow-up test that is more specific is always performed to confirm the test results.

A negative HIV test is not always conclusive for the absence of HIV infection. Once an individual has been infected with HIV, it takes time for the HIV antigens and antibodies to be produced and reach a level that can be detected by HIV tests. The time between HIV infection and when an HIV test can provide an accurate test result is known as the *window period*, which varies from person to person and the type of test being used. If an individual has recently been infected with HIV, the test may yield a false-negative result, and the individual should be retested after the window period for that test has been reached.

Types of Tests

Several different types of tests can be used to screen for the presence of HIV. Most tests require a blood specimen obtained through a venipuncture or finger puncture, although some screening tests can be performed on oral fluid. The types of tests used to screen for HIV include the following:

1. ***Antibody/Antigen Tests:*** Antibody/antigen tests are the most commonly used HIV screening tests ordered by a provider in a medical office setting. The window period needed to provide an accurate test result is between 2 and 6 weeks following exposure. Antigen/antibody tests check for the presence of both HIV antibodies and antigens and are usually performed at an outside medical laboratory with the results being sent to the provider.
2. ***Antibody tests:*** Antibody tests check the blood only for the presence of HIV antibodies and, because of this, are less sensitive than other types of screening tests. The window period for antibody tests is between 3 and 12 weeks after exposure. The ELISA (enzyme-linked immunosorbent assay) test is usually the first test ordered by the provider to screen for the presence of HIV. Alternatively, rapid CLIA-waived HIV antibody testing kits are now available that can be performed by the medical assistant in the medical office. The results from a rapid test can be obtained in 30 minutes or less. Brand names of rapid antibody tests include *Uni-Gold Recombigen HIV*, *Clearview HIV*, and *OraQuick Advance*. Several rapid antibody tests are now available in drugstores or online and can be performed by an individual at home.
3. ***NAT:*** The nucleic acid test (NAT) is the most sensitive test and can detect HIV sooner than other types of tests. It uses DNA technology to detect the presence of HIV. The window period for the NAT is 1 to 4 weeks after exposure. This test is expensive and therefore not routinely used for screening individuals for HIV unless they have recently had a high-risk exposure or a possible exposure and have early symptoms of HIV.

TREATMENT

There is no known cure for AIDS and there is no vaccine to prevent HIV infection; however, it can be controlled with proper medical care. Powerful antiretroviral medications have been developed that prevent the reproduction of the virus, thereby reducing the viral load and increasing the CD4+ T-cell count. Viral load refers to the amount of HIV present in the blood of an infected individual. The daily administration of a combination of these medications is known as *antiretroviral therapy* or *ART*.

If ART is followed as prescribed, HIV patients can get and keep a viral load so low that the virus cannot be detected in their blood, known as an *undetectable viral load*. An undetectable viral load dramatically delays HIV from progressing to full-blown AIDS, thereby allowing patients to live longer and healthier lives. In fact, patients who receive early effective ART following an HIV diagnosis can expect to live a near normal lifespan. An undetectable viral load also makes it virtually impossible to transmit the virus to others. Unfortunately, even with effective medication therapy, HIV cannot be completely eliminated from the body. Once infected, an individual is infected for life; therefore it is very important that an HIV-infected individual carefully follow his or her prescribed ART regimen to prevent HIV from reproducing and destroying $CD4^+$ T-cells.

Numerous treatments are also available to treat the opportunistic infections and cancers that occur with AIDS. Medications used to treat opportunistic infections include antivirals, antibiotics and antifungal medications. The type of medication used depends on which opportunistic infection has been contracted by the patient.

What Would You Do? What Would You *Not* Do? RESPONSES

Case Study 1
Page 32

What Did Jennifer Do?
- ❑ Told Petra that the physician would need to determine what is causing her symptoms.
- ❑ Documented Petra's symptoms in her medical record. Made sure to document that Petra's symptoms occur after she has contact with rubber latex gloves and rubber flip-flops.
- ❑ Used latex-free gloves and tourniquet when drawing Petra's blood.
- ❑ If Petra is diagnosed with a latex allergy, documented this information in her medical record.
- ❑ If instructed to do so by the physician, provided Petra with latex allergy education and guidelines.

What Did Jennifer Not Do?
- ❑ Did not tell Petra that she has a latex allergy, because only the physician is qualified to make a diagnosis.

Case Study 2
Page 38

What Did Jennifer Do?
- ❑ Told Tracy that having her infant immunized for hepatitis B is an investment in her child's future. Explained that her child could be exposed to the virus anytime in his or her life. Stressed that if a young child becomes infected with hepatitis B, the child has a higher risk of developing chronic hepatitis, which can cause liver problems later in life.
- ❑ Gave Tracy a brochure on hepatitis B to take home.

What Did Jennifer Not Do?
- ❑ Did not needlessly alarm Tracy regarding the complications of hepatitis B.

Case Study 3
Page 40

What Did Jennifer Do?
- ❑ Explained to Giles that the blood supply was not tested for hepatitis C until 1992 because a test to detect the presence of hepatitis C in the blood supply was not developed until then.
- ❑ Told Giles that it is possible for someone to have hepatitis C and not exhibit any symptoms.
- ❑ Told Giles that he should ask the physician his question about giving hepatitis C to others.

What Did Jennifer Not Do?
- ❑ Did not automatically assume that Giles had hepatitis C, because he had not yet been seen by the physician. It would be up to the physician to make a diagnosis of hepatitis C.
- ❑ Did not tell Giles about the serious complications of hepatitis C. If Giles is diagnosed with hepatitis C, it would be the physician's responsibility to relay this information.

TERMINOLOGY REVIEW

Key Term	Word Parts	Definition
Acute infection		An infection that develops suddenly and lasts for a short period of time.
Aerobe	*aer/o:* air	A microorganism that needs oxygen to live and grow.
Anaerobe	*an-:* without *aer/o:* air	A microorganism that grows best in the absence of oxygen.
Antiseptic	*anti-:* against *-septic:* infection	An agent that inhibits the growth of or kills microorganisms.
Chronic infection		An infection that develops slowly and may worsen over an extended period of time.
Cilia		Slender, hairlike projections that constantly beat toward the outside to remove microorganisms from the body.
Hand hygiene		The process of cleansing or sanitizing the hands.
Infection		The condition in which the body, or part of it, is invaded by a pathogen.
Medical asepsis	*a-:* without *sepsis:* infection	Practices that are employed to inhibit the growth and hinder the transmission of pathogenic microorganisms to prevent the spread of infection.
Microorganism	*micro-:* small *organism:* organism	A microscopic plant or animal.
Nonintact skin	*non-:* not	Skin that has a break in the surface. It includes, but is not limited to, abrasions, cuts, hangnails, paper cuts, and burns.
Nonpathogen	*non-:* not *path/o:* disease *-gen:* producing	A microorganism that does not normally produce disease.

Continued

TERMINOLOGY REVIEW—cont'd

Key Term	Word Parts	Definition
Opportunistic infection		An infection that takes advantage of an opportunity not normally available such as the weakened immune system of an HIV-infected individual.
Optimum growth temperature		The temperature at which an organism grows best.
Parenteral	*para-:* apart from *enter/o:* intestine *-al:* pertaining to	Piercing of the skin barrier or mucous membranes, such as through needlesticks, human bites, cuts, and abrasions.
Pathogen	*path/o:* disease *-gen:* producing	A disease-producing microorganism.
Postexposure prophylaxis	*post-:* after *pro-:* before *phylaxis:* prevention of disease	Treatment administered to an individual after exposure to an infectious disease to prevent the disease.
Regulated medical waste		Medical waste that may contain infectious materials posing a threat to health and safety.
Resident flora		Harmless, nonpathogenic microorganisms that normally reside on the skin and usually do not cause disease. Also known as *normal flora.*
Transient flora		Microorganisms that reside on the superficial skin layers and are picked up during daily activities. They are often pathogenic but can be removed easily from the skin by sanitizing the hands.

PROCEDURE 2.1 Handwashing

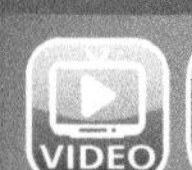

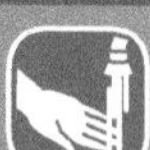

Outcome Perform handwashing.

Equipment/Supplies

- Liquid soap
- Paper towels
- Waste container

1. **Procedural Step.** Remove your watch or push it up on the forearm so that the wrist is clear. Avoid wearing rings. If you wear rings, remove all except a plain wedding band and put them in a safe place.
   Principle. Microorganisms can lodge in the crevices and grooves of rings.
2. **Procedural Step.** Stand at the sink, making sure clothing does not touch the sink.
   Principle. The sink is considered contaminated, and if the uniform touches the sink, it may pick up microorganisms and transfer them.
3. **Procedural Step.** Turn on the faucets, using a paper towel.
   Principle. The faucets are considered contaminated because they harbor microorganisms.

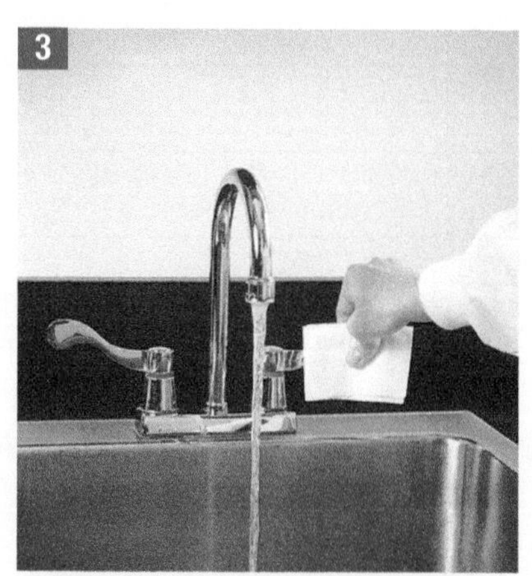

Turn on the faucet using a paper towel.

PROCEDURE 2.1 Handwashing—cont'd

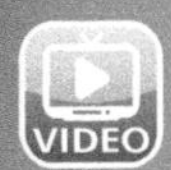

4. **Procedural Step.** Adjust the water temperature. The water should be warm to make the best suds.
   Principle. Water that is too hot or too cold tends to dry the skin, causing chapping and cracking and making it easy for pathogens to enter the body or be transferred to patients.
5. **Procedural Step.** Discard the paper towel in the waste container.
   Principle. The paper towel is considered contaminated after touching the faucets.
6. **Procedural Step.** Wet the hands and forearms thoroughly with water. The hands should be always held lower than the elbows. Do not touch the inside of the sink because it is also contaminated.
   Principle. When you hold the hands lower than the elbows, bacteria and debris are carried away from the arms and body and into the sink.
7. **Procedural Step.** Apply soap to the hands. Apply 1 teaspoon of liquid soap (approximately the size of a nickel) to the palm of one hand.

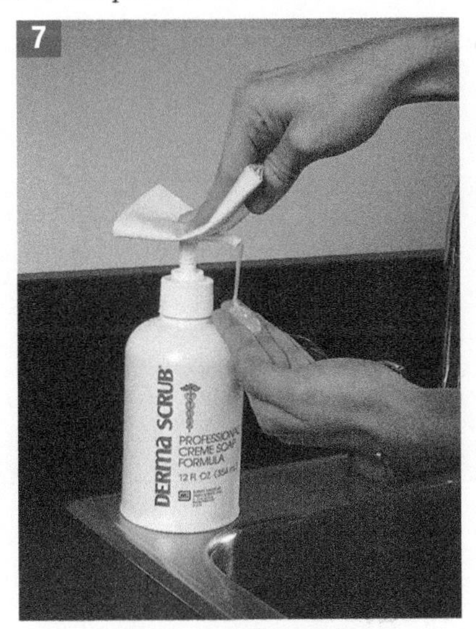

Apply soap to the hands.

8. **Procedural Step.** Wash the palms and backs of the hands with 10 circular motions. The CDC recommends that the hands be rubbed together vigorously for at least 20 s, making sure to cover all surfaces. Use friction along with the circular motions to wash the palm and back of each hand.
   Principle. Friction helps to dislodge and remove microorganisms from the hands.

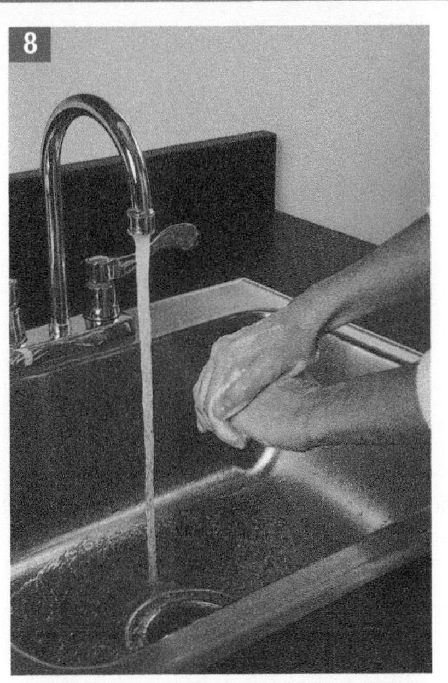

Wash the palms and backs of the hands.

9. **Procedural Step.** Wash the fingers with 10 circular motions while focusing on the fingertips and fingernails. Interlace the fingers and thumbs and use friction and circular motions while rubbing the fingers back and forth.
   Principle. This kind of movement helps remove microorganisms and debris that have accumulated between the fingers.

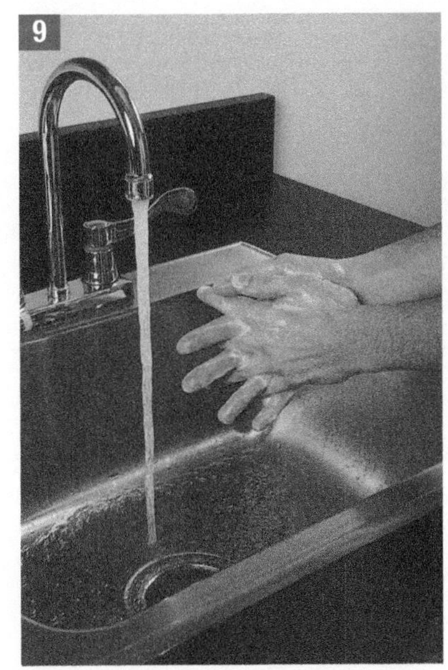

Interlace the fingers and thumbs and use friction.

10. **Procedural Step.** Rinse well, making sure to hold the hands lower than the elbows.
    Principle. Running water helps to rinse away dirt and microorganisms.

Continued

PROCEDURE 2.1 Handwashing—cont'd

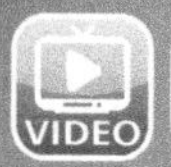

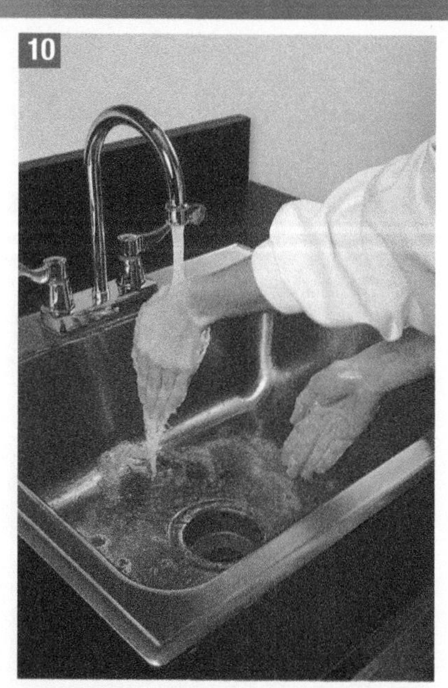

Rinse well, holding the hands lower than the elbows.

11. **Procedural Step.** Wash the wrists and forearms, using friction along with circular motions.
    (*Note:* The hands are washed first because they are the most contaminated; microorganisms and dirt are washed away and do not spread to the wrists and forearms.)

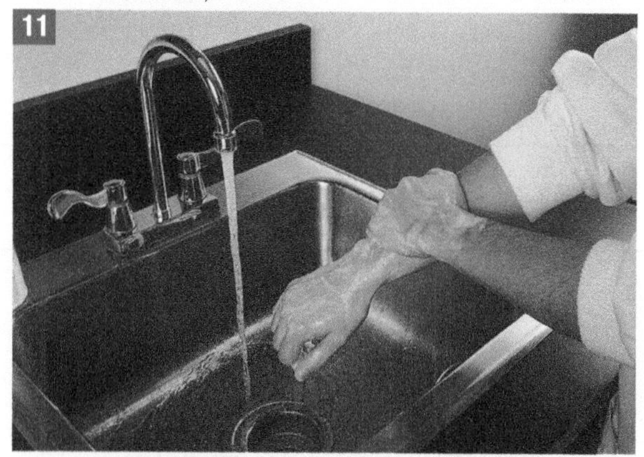

Wash wrists and forearms using friction.

12. **Procedural Step.** Clean the fingernails with a manicure stick. The fingernails should be cleaned at least once daily, preferably during initial handwashing (i.e., handwashing performed just after arriving at the medical office to begin your day).
    Principle. The area under the fingernails is likely to harbor large amounts of microorganisms.
13. **Procedural Step.** Rinse the arms and hands.
    Principle. The running water rinses away the dirt and microorganisms.
14. **Procedural Step.** Repeat the handwashing procedure. For initial handwashing or when the hands come into contact with blood or other potentially infectious materials, the handwashing procedure should be repeated to ensure removal of all pathogens.
15. **Procedural Step.** Dry the hands gently and thoroughly and discard the paper towel.
    Principle. Gently drying the hands prevents them from becoming chapped. Microorganisms can lodge in the crevices of chapped hands. Ensure that the hands are completely dried, because wet skin also may cause chapping.

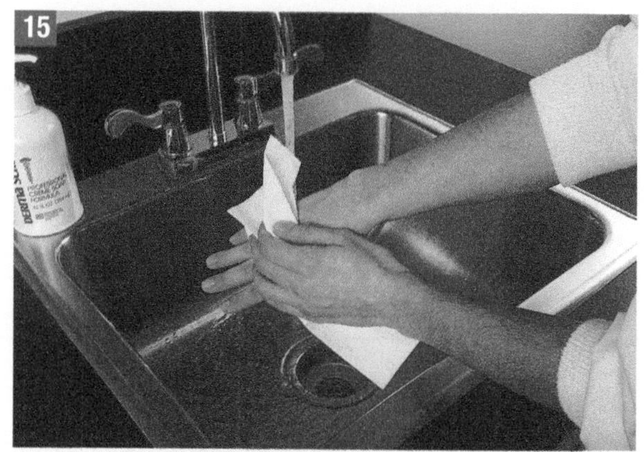

Dry the hands gently and thoroughly.

16. **Procedural Step.** Turn off the water, using a paper towel, and discard the paper towel in a waste container.
    Principle. The faucet is considered contaminated, whereas the hands are medically aseptic or clean.
17. **Procedural Step.** Do not touch the sink with the bare hands.
    Principle. The hands are now medically aseptic, and the sink is considered contaminated.

PROCEDURE 2.2 Applying an Alcohol-Based Hand Sanitizer

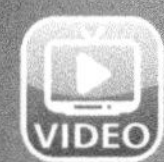

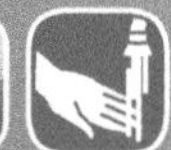

Outcome Apply an alcohol-based hand sanitizer.

Equipment/Supplies

- Alcohol-based hand sanitizer

1. **Procedural Step.** Inspect the hands to ensure that they are not visibly soiled. Hands that are visibly soiled must be washed with soap and water.
   Principle. Alcohol-based hand sanitizers are not intended for the removal of visible soil.
2. **Procedural Step.** Remove your watch or push it up on the forearm. Avoid wearing rings. If you wear rings, remove all except a plain wedding band and put them in a safe place.
   Principle. Microorganisms can lodge in the crevices and grooves of rings.
3. **Procedural Step.** Apply the alcohol-based hand sanitizer to the palm of one hand as follows:
   a. *Gel:* Apply approximately 1 mL of the gel to the palm of one hand; this amount is approximately equal to the size of a dime.

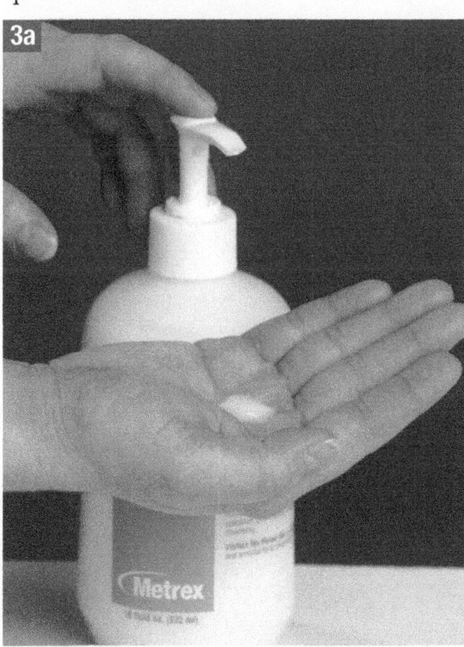

Apply gel equal to the size of a dime.

   b. *Foam.* Apply 3 grams of foam to the palm of one hand; this amount is approximately equal to the size of a walnut.
   Principle. The proper amount of hand sanitizer must be applied to ensure coverage of all surfaces of both hands. Using more than the recommended amount results in a prolonged (and unnecessary) period of time for your hands to dry.

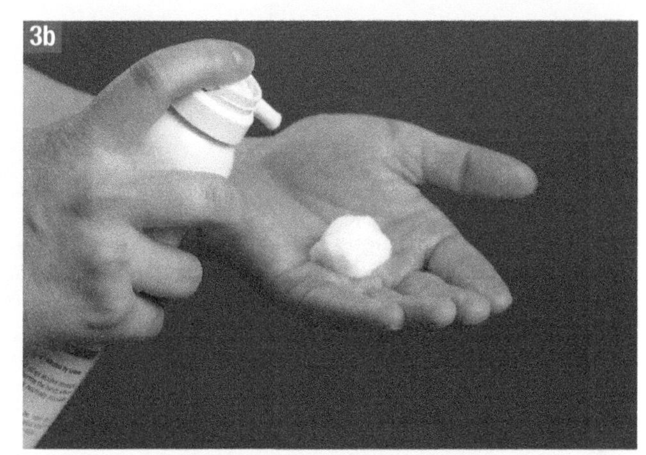

Apply foam equal to the size of a walnut.

4. **Procedural Step.** Thoroughly spread the hand sanitizer over all surfaces of both hands (and fingers) up to 1/2 inch above the wrist. Spread the hand sanitizer around the fingertips and around and under your fingernails.
   Principle. Failure to cover all surfaces can leave areas of the hands contaminated. Microorganisms tend to collect around and underneath the fingernails.
5. **Procedural Step.** Rub the hands together until they are dry; this usually takes up to 30 s. Allow your hands to dry completely before touching anything. The hands are now medically aseptic.
   Note: After cleaning your hands 5–10 times with a hand sanitizer, a buildup of emollients may occur on your hands. The emollients can be easily removed by washing your hands with soap and water.
   Principle. If you have applied a sufficient amount of hand sanitizer, it should take up to 30 s for your hands to feel dry. Your hands will still feel a little wet at first. Let them dry completely before touching anything.

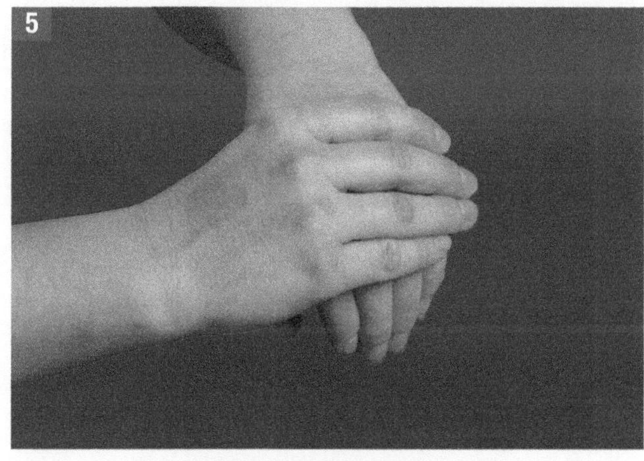

Rub the hands together until they are dry.

PROCEDURE 2.3 Application and Removal of Disposable Exam Gloves

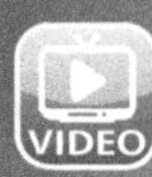

Outcome Apply and remove disposable exam gloves.

Equipment/Supplies

- Disposable exam gloves

Applying Disposable Exam Gloves

No special technique is required when disposable exam gloves are applied. This is because both the hands and the gloves are clean; the medical assistant can touch any part of the gloves during application without contaminating them.

1. **Procedural Step.** Remove all rings and sanitize your hands. Handwashing should be performed if the hands are visibly soiled. If this is not the case, use an alcohol-based hand sanitizer to sanitize the hands. Ensure that your hands are completely dry.
   Principle. Rings may cause the gloves to tear. The warm, moist environment inside gloves provides ideal growing conditions for the multiplication of transient microorganisms present on the hands. Sanitizing the hands removes these microorganisms and prevents the transmission of pathogens. Moisture encourages the growth of microorganisms.
2. **Procedural Step.** Choose the appropriate size of gloves; they should not be too small or too large. The gloves should fit snugly but not be too tight. Apply the gloves and adjust them so they fit comfortably.
   Principle. If your gloves are too small, they may rip as you are applying them or may become uncomfortable to wear. If they are too large, you may find it difficult to perform your tasks.

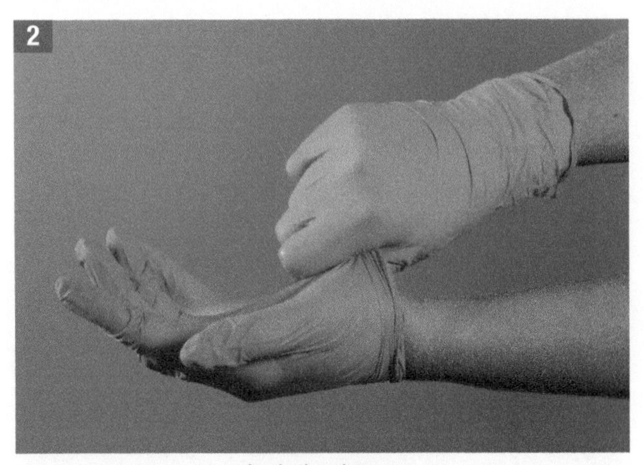

Apply the gloves.

3. **Procedural Step.** Inspect the gloves for tears. If a tear is present, remove the torn glove and apply a new one.

Removing Disposable Exam Gloves

Gloves must be removed in a manner that protects the medical assistant from contaminating his or her clean hands with pathogens that may be present on the outsides of the gloves. This is accomplished by not allowing the bare hands to come in contact with the outsides of the gloves.

1. **Procedural Step.** Grasp the outside of the left glove 1–2 inches from the top with your gloved right hand.
   (*Note:* It does not matter which glove is removed first. You may start with the right glove if you prefer.)

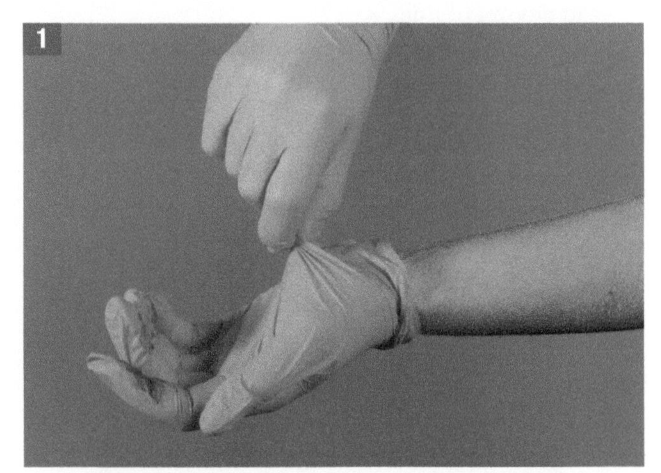

Grasp the glove 1 to 2 inches from the top of the glove.

2. **Procedural Step.** Slowly pull the left glove off the hand. It will turn inside out as it is removed from your hand.
3. **Procedural Step.** Pull the left glove free and scrunch it into a ball with your gloved right hand.

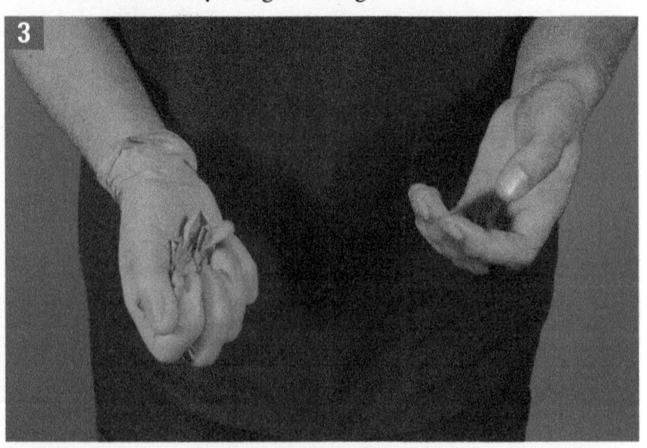

Scrunch the glove into a ball.

4. **Procedural Step.** Place the index and middle fingers of the left hand on the inside of the right glove. Do not allow your clean hand to touch the outside of the glove.

PROCEDURE 2.3 Application and Removal of Disposable Exam Gloves—cont'd

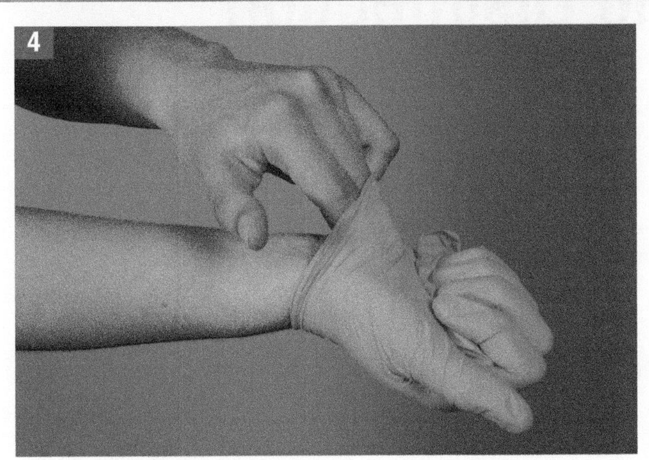

Place the index and middle fingers inside the glove.

5. Procedural Step. Pull the glove off the right hand. It will turn inside out as it is removed from your hand, enclosing the balled-up left glove. Discard both gloves in an appropriate container. If your gloves are visibly contaminated with blood or other potentially infectious materials, discard them in a biohazard waste container. Otherwise, they can be discarded in a regular waste container.

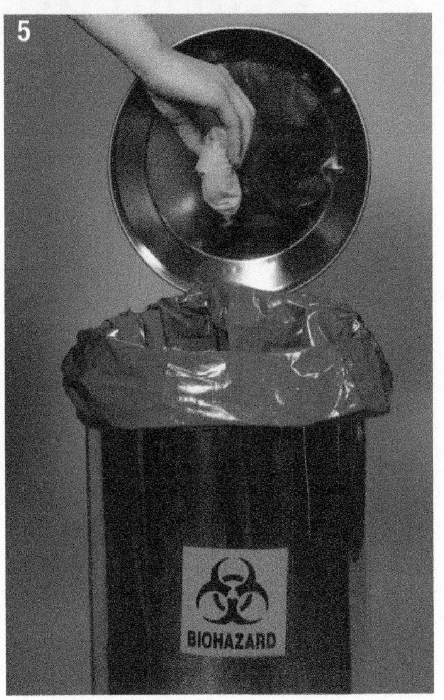

Discard both gloves in an appropriate container.

6. Procedural Step. Sanitize your hands to remove any microorganisms or other contaminants that may have come in contact with your hands during glove removal.

3 Sterilization and Disinfection

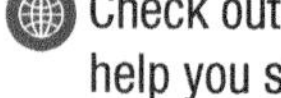

Check out the Evolve site at http://evolve.elsevier.com/Bonewit/today/ to access additional interactive activities and exercises to help you study and prepare for success.

LEARNING OUTCOMES	PROCEDURES
Hazard Communication Standard	
1. Explain the purpose of the Hazard Communication Standard.	Read and interpret an SDS.
2. List and describe the information that must be included on the label of a hazardous chemical.	
3. List and describe the information that must be included in a safety data sheet (SDS).	
Sanitization	
4. State the purpose of sanitization.	Sanitize instruments.
5. State the advantages of using an ultrasonic cleaner.	
6. List and describe the guidelines for sanitizing instruments.	
Disinfection	
7. Describe the three levels of disinfection: high, intermediate, and low.	
8. Describe the following: critical item, semicritical item, and noncritical item.	
9. List and describe the guidelines for disinfecting items.	
10. List and describe use of disinfectants commonly employed in the medical office.	
Sterilization	
11. Explain how the autoclave functions to sterilize items.	
12. List the components of a sterilization monitoring program.	
13. List and describe the various types of sterilization indicators.	
14. Identify the advantages of sterilization paper and sterilization pouches.	Wrap an item with sterilization paper. Wrap an item with a sterilization pouch.
15. List and describe the guidelines for loading the autoclave.	
16. Identify the steps in the autoclave cycle.	Sterilize items in an autoclave.
17. Explain the importance of drying the sterilized load.	
18. Explain how to handle and store sterilized packs.	
19. Identify the daily, weekly, and monthly autoclave maintenance.	Maintain the autoclave.
Other Sterilization Methods	
20. State the primary use of the following sterilization methods: dry heat, ethylene oxide gas, chemicals, and radiation.	

CHAPTER OUTLINE

INTRODUCTION TO STERILIZATION AND DISINFECTION
DEFINITION OF TERMS
HAZARD COMMUNICATION STANDARD
Hazard Communication Program
Inventory of Hazardous Chemicals
Labeling of Hazardous Chemicals
  Container Label Requirements
Safety Data Sheets
  Safety Data Sheet Requirements
Employee Information and Training
SANITIZATION
Sanitizing Instruments
  Cleaning Instruments
Guidelines for Sanitizing Instruments
DISINFECTION
Levels of Disinfection
  High-Level Disinfection
  Intermediate-Level Disinfection
  Low-Level Disinfection
Types of Disinfectants
  Glutaraldehyde
  Alcohol

KEY TERMS

autoclave (AU-toe-klave)
critical item
decontamination
detergent
disinfectant (dis-in-FEK-tant)
hazardous chemical
health hazard
incubate (IN-kyoo-bate)
load
noncritical item
physical hazard
Safety Data Sheet (SDS)
sanitization (san-ih-tih-ZAY-shun)
semicritical item
spore
sterilization (stare-ill-ih-ZAY-shun)

Introduction to Sterilization and Disinfection

The air and all objects around us contain microorganisms. The medical assistant is responsible for helping to reduce and eliminate microorganisms to prevent the spread of disease. This can be accomplished by practicing good techniques of medical and surgical asepsis.

Physical and chemical methods are used to destroy microorganisms in the medical office. The method selected depends on the intended use of the item. Items that penetrate sterile tissue or the vascular system, such as surgical instruments, must be sterilized, typically with the use of an autoclave (physical method). Items that come in contact with the skin, such as stethoscopes, blood pressure cuffs, and percussion hammers, should be disinfected (chemical method).

Sanitization, disinfection, and autoclave maintenance involve the use of hazardous chemicals. It is essential for the medical assistant to know the precautions that are required when working with hazardous chemicals.

Definitions of Terms

Terms that aid in understanding this chapter are listed and defined here.

Sanitization Sanitization is a series of steps designed to remove debris from an item and reduce the number of microorganisms to a safe level. Sanitization removes all organic and inorganic debris from an item, such as blood, body fluids, tissue, and soil. For items that are used in examinations, treatments, and office surgery to be properly sterilized or disinfected, they must first be sanitized.

Decontamination Decontamination refers to the use of physical or chemical means to remove pathogens on an item so that it is no longer capable of transmitting disease; this makes the item safe to handle.

Detergent A detergent is an agent that cleanses by emulsifying dirt and oil.

Disinfectant A disinfectant is an agent used to destroy pathogenic microorganisms; however, it does not kill the resistant spores. The most common disinfectants used in the medical office consist of chemical agents. Chemical disinfectants are used on inanimate objects and surfaces in contrast to antiseptics, which are used on living tissue.

Spore A spore is a hard, thick-walled capsule that some bacteria form by losing moisture and condensing their contents to contain only the essential parts of the protoplasm of the bacterial cell. Spores represent a resting and protective stage of bacteria and are more resistant to drying, sunlight, heat, and disinfectants than vegetative bacteria. Spores cannot reproduce, whereas vegetative bacteria are alive and can reproduce. Favorable conditions cause spores to germinate into vegetative bacteria again, capable of reproducing. Two examples of species of bacteria that form spores are *Clostridium botulinum,* which causes botulism, and *Clostridium tetani,* which causes tetanus.

Sterilization Sterilization is the process of destroying all forms of microbial life, including spores. An item that is *sterile* is free of all living microorganisms and spores. There can be no relative degrees of sterility—An item is either sterile or not sterile. The method most commonly used to sterilize items in the medical office is steam under pressure using an autoclave.

Hazard Communication Standard

The Hazard Communication Standard (HCS) is a requirement of the Occupational Safety and Health Administration (OSHA). The purpose of the HCS is to ensure that employees are informed of the hazards associated with chemicals in their workplace and the precautions to take to protect themselves when working with hazardous chemicals. A **hazardous chemical** is any chemical that is a health or a physical hazard. A **health hazard** is defined as the potential of the chemical to cause acute toxicity, skin corrosion or irritation, serious eye damage or irritation, respiratory or skin sensitization, germ cell mutagenicity, cancer, or reproductive toxicity or to be an aspiration hazard. A **physical hazard** is defined as the potential of the chemical to catch fire, explode, or react with other chemicals or materials.

The HCS uses the Globally Harmonized System of Classification and Labeling of Chemicals (GHS) set forth by the United Nations. The GHS is an international standard that provides consistency in the classification and labeling of chemicals. The GHS classifies chemicals according to their health and physical hazards. The GHS also requires the use of a standardized format for labeling containers and for the development of safety data sheets (SDSs).

The GHS enable employees to quickly obtain and more easily understand information regarding the safe handling, use, and disposal of hazardous chemicals. This assists in preventing injury and illness associated with exposure to hazardous chemicals.

In the medical office, sanitization, disinfection, and autoclave maintenance require the use of hazardous chemicals; the medical assistant must have a thorough knowledge of the HCS. The HCS consists of the following components:

- Development of a hazard communication program
- Inventory of hazardous chemicals
- Labeling requirements
- SDS requirements
- Employee information and training

HAZARD COMMUNICATION PROGRAM

As part of the HCS, employers are required to develop a hazard communication program. The hazard communication program consists of a written plan that describes what the facility is doing to meet the requirements of the HCS. The information in the plan must be made available and communicated to all employees who work with hazardous chemicals.

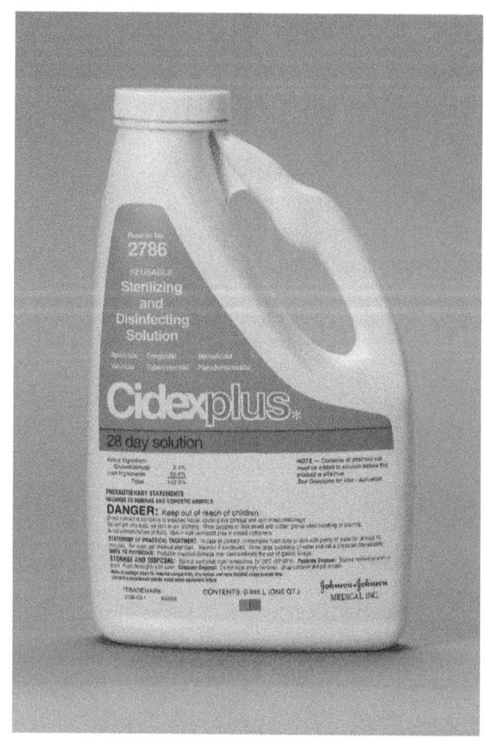

Fig. 3.1 Hazardous chemical used as a disinfectant in the medical office.

INVENTORY OF HAZARDOUS CHEMICALS

The employer must develop and maintain a list of hazardous chemicals that are used and stored in the workplace. The list must be updated as new chemicals are introduced into the workplace. In the medical office, hazardous chemicals typically include the following:

- Products for sanitization, disinfection, and autoclave maintenance (e.g., chemical disinfectants, instrument cleaners, autoclave cleaners) (Fig. 3.1)
- Chemicals for laboratory testing (e.g., testing reagents, developing solutions, controls)
- Pharmaceutical products such as local anesthetics (e.g., lidocaine [Xylocaine])
- Front office supplies (e.g., copier and printer toners)
- Cleaning products (e.g., drain cleaner, household bleach)

LABELING OF HAZARDOUS CHEMICALS

The HCS requires that a hazardous chemical container be labeled by the manufacturer with a warning to alert the user that the chemical is dangerous. This label must include the

PRODUCT IDENTIFIER
Code: 7489
Product Name: Glutaraldehyde Solution

SUPPLIER IDENTIFICATION
Poston Corporation
2010 East Main Street
Camden, New Jersey 08106

PRECAUTIONARY STATEMENTS
Do not breathe dust/fumes/gas/mist/vapors/spray
Avoid release to the environment
Wear protective gloves/ eye protection/ face protection
IF ON SKIN: Wash with plenty of soap and water
IF ON EYES: Rinse cautiously with water for several minutes. Remove contact lenses, if present and easy to do. Continue rinsing
IF SWALLOWED: Immediately call a POISON CENTER or doctor/physician

HAZARD PICTOGRAMS

SIGNAL WORD
DANGER

HAZARD STATEMENTS
Toxic if swallowed
May be harmful in contact with skin
Causes skin irritation
Causes serious eye damage
May cause allergy or asthma symptoms or breathing difficulties
May cause respiratory irritation
Very toxic to aquatic life

SUPPLEMENTAL INFORMATION
Storage: Store at room temperature
Disposal: Discard residual solution in drain. Flush thoroughly with water

Expiration Date: 10/15/xx

Fig. 3.2 Hazardous chemical container label following the Globally Harmonized System of Classification and Labeling of Chemicals.

possible hazards of the chemical and the steps that can be taken to protect against those risks and must not be removed or defaced. If a label falls off a product or is damaged or obscured, a replacement label must be applied. If a chemical is transferred to a new container, a label with the required information must be attached to the new container.

CONTAINER LABEL REQUIREMENTS

The HCS requires that manufacturers label the containers of hazardous chemicals they produce according to GHS guidelines. The information on the container label allows the user of the chemical to tell at a glance the hazards of using the chemical and how to prevent or lessen exposure to the chemical (Fig. 3.2). Information required on the label of a hazardous chemical container includes the following:

- *Product Identifier:* The product identifier specifies how the chemical is identified. This can be (but is not limited to) the chemical name and the code number or batch number.
- *Supplier Identification:* Supplier information includes the name, address, and telephone number of the chemical manufacturer.
- *Precautionary Statement(s):* A precautionary statement is a phrase that describes recommended measures to be taken to minimize or prevent adverse effects resulting from exposure to the chemical or improper storage or handling (e.g., if on skin, wash with plenty of soap and water, do not eat, drink, or smoke while using this produce; keep container tightly closed).
- *Hazard Pictograms:* Hazard pictograms consist of standardized graphic symbols allowing users to quickly identify the types of hazards associated with the chemical. There are eight different pictograms representing the health and physical hazards covered in the GHS (Fig. 3.3).
- *Signal Word:* A signal word indicates the relative degree of severity of the chemical. There are two signal words under GHS:
  Danger: Denotes a more severe hazard possible
  Warning: Denotes a less serious hazard possible but potentially harmful
- *Hazard Statement(s):* A hazard statement is a phrase that describes the nature and (when appropriate) the degree of hazard associated with the chemical (e.g., toxic if swallowed; causes severe skin burns and eye damage).
- *Supplementary Information:* The manufacturer may provide additional information such as directions for use and the expiration date of the chemical.

SAFETY DATA SHEETS

A **safety data sheet (SDS)** is a document that provides more detailed information than the container label regarding the chemical, its hazards, and measures to take to prevent injury and illness when handling the chemical (Fig. 3.4). Manufacturers of hazardous chemicals are required to develop and make available an SDS for each hazardous chemical they produce according to GHS guidelines.

The HCS requires that a current SDS be kept on file for each hazardous chemical used or stored in the workplace. In the event of an accidental exposure, information on the SDS must be readily available as a reference for emergency treatment. It is important that the medical assistant thoroughly review the SDS of a hazardous chemical before using it.

PICTOGRAM	MEANING OF PICTOGRAM	TYPE OF HAZARD(S) (Associated with this pictogram)
Health Hazard 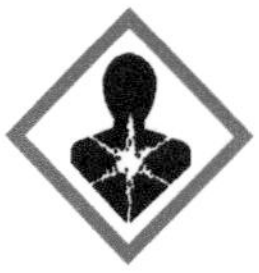	The chemical is a risk to health if used improperly	• Carcinogen • Mutagenicity • Reproductive Toxicity • Respiratory Sensitizer • Target Organ Toxicity • Aspiration Toxicity
Severe Toxic 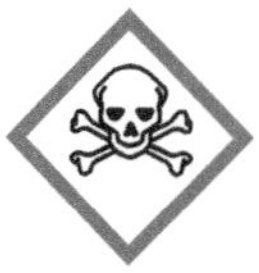	The chemical is a serious health or physical hazard or poison. It will produce adverse effects following a single dose. This pictogram is usually used in combination with the Health Hazard Pictogram.	• Acute Toxicity (fatal or toxic) if inhaled or swallowed, or if it comes in contact with the skin.
Acute Toxic 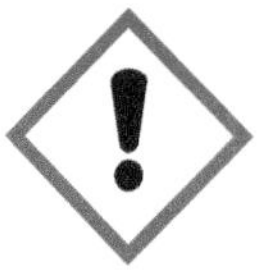	The chemical may cause immediate, serious health effects but it is less severe than the Severe Toxic pictogram (skull and crossbones). This pictogram is usually used in combination with the Health Hazard Pictogram.	• Irritant (skin and eye) • Skin Sensitizer • Acute Toxicity • Narcotic Effects • Respiratory Tract Irritant
Flammable 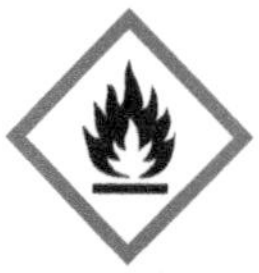	The chemical may burst into flame. Be careful to keep away from ignition sources and combustible materials.	• Flammables • Pyrophorics • Self-Heating • Emits Flammable Gas • Self-Reactive • Organic Peroxides
Corrosive 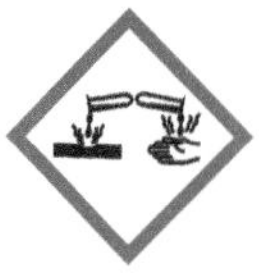	The chemical is a physical or health hazard that can easily damage skin or eyes. Be aware of PPE and storage requirements.	• Skin Corrosion/Burns • Eye Damage • Corrosive to Metals
Oxidizer 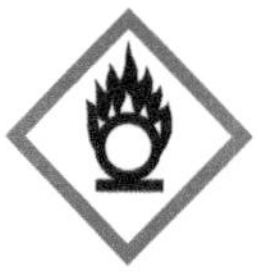	The chemical may cause other materials to ignite or burn faster. It can create an increased fire risk in work or storage environment.	• Oxidizers
Gas Under Pressure 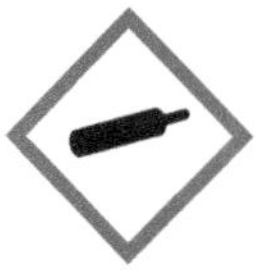	This chemical consists of pressurized gas that would explode, rocket, or damage health if heated, ruptured or leaking.	• Gases Under Pressure
Explosive 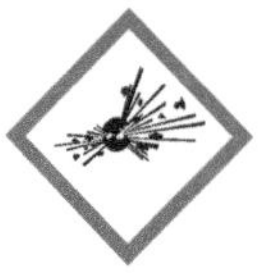	This material can blow up or otherwise create an uncontrolled reaction. Should be treated with extreme caution.	• Explosives • Self-Reactives • Organic Peroxides

Fig. 3.3 Globally Harmonized System of Classification and Labeling of Chemicals Hazard Pictograms. (Pictograms from the US Department of Labor, Occupational Safety and Health Administration.)

SAFETY DATA SHEET
(SDS)

SECTION 1: IDENTIFICATION

Product name: Glutaraldehyde Solution	**Telephone:** 1 (800) 331-0766
Brand: Aldecyde	**Emergency phone number:** 1 (800) 773-8690
Manufacturer: Poston Corporation, 2010 East Main Street, Camden, New Jersey 08106	**Recommended Use:** High Level Disinfectant
	Restrictions on Use: Not recommended for drug, food, or household use.

SECTION 2: HAZARDS IDENTIFICATION

Hazard Classification

Acute toxicity, oral:	GHS Category 3	Respiratory sensitization:	GHS Category 1
Skin irritation:	GHS Category 2	Skin sensitization:	GHS Category 1
Serious eye damage:	GHS Category 1	Acute aquatic toxicity:	GHS Category 1

Signal Word

Danger

Hazard Statements

H301	Toxic if swallowed
H313	May be harmful in contact with skin
H315	Causes skin irritation
H318	Causes serious eye damage
H334	May cause allergy or asthma symptoms or breathing difficulties if inhaled
H335	May cause respiratory irritation
H400	Very toxic to aquatic life

Hazard Pictograms

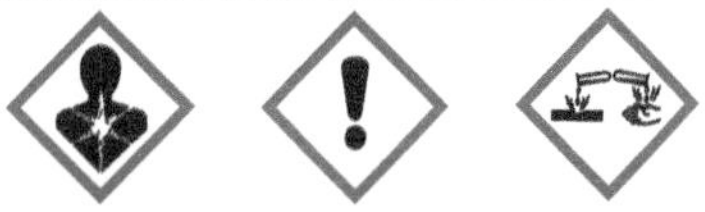

	Precautionary Statements
P260	Do not breathe dust/fumes/gas/mist/vapors/spray
P273	Avoid release to the environment
P280	Wear protective gloves/eye protection/face protection
P302 + P352	IF ON SKIN: Wash with plenty of soap and water
P305 + P351 + P338	IF ON EYES: Rinse cautiously with water for several minutes. Remove contact lenses, if present and easy to do. Continue rinsing.
P310	IF SWALLOWED: Immediately call a POISON CENTER or doctor/physician

SECTION 3: COMPOSITION/INFORMATION ON INGREDIENTS

CAS NUMBER	CHEMICAL NAME OF INGREDIENTS	PERCENT
111-30-8	Glutaraldehyde	2.5
7732-18-5	Water	97.4
7632-00-0	Sodium Nitrite	<1

SECTION 4: FIRST AID MEASURES

Skin Contact: Rinse with water. Remove contaminated clothing and wash before reuse. Consult a physician if skin redness or irritation persist.

Eye Contact: Immediately flush with water for 15 minutes. Seek medical attention.

Inhalation: Remove to fresh air immediately. If experiencing difficulty breathing, seek medical attention.

Ingestion: Call a physician or Poison Control Center immediately. Do not ingest emetic.

SECTION 5: FIRE FIGHTING MEASURES

Suitable Extinguishing Media: Use extinguishing agent which is suitable for the surrounding fire.

Hazardous Combustion Products: Carbon monoxide and carbon dioxide.

Special Protective Equipment for Firefighters: Wear self-contained breathing apparatus for fire fighting if necessary.

Fig. 3.4 Safety data sheet (SDS).

(Continued)

SAFETY DATA SHEET
(SDS)

SECTION 6: ACCIDENTAL RELEASE MEASURES

Personal Precautions: Ventilate area. Avoid breathing vapors or mist. Wear eye and skin protection while handling material for cleanup.

Cleanup Procedures: Contain spill by placing suitable absorbent material around the edges of the spill and work inward. Carefully scoop up into waste container for disposal. Dispose of in accordance with applicable Federal, State and Local regulations.

SECTION 7: HANDLING AND STORAGE

Precautions for Safe Handling: Use in a well-ventilated area. Avoid breathing vapors or mist. Avoid contact with skin, eyes, and clothing. Remove contaminated clothing and launder before use.

Conditions for Safe Storage: Store in a cool, dry area (59-86º F) away from direct sunlight or sources of intense heat. Keep container tightly closed when not in use.

SECTION 8: EXPOSURE CONTROLS/PERSONAL PROTECTION

Exposure Control Limits

PEL: 0.2 ppm
TLV: 0.2 ppm

Engineering Controls and Personal Protective Equipment

Ventilation: Ensure adequate ventilation.

Respiratory Protection: None normally required for routine use.

Skin Protection: Wear protective chemical-resistant gloves. Wear suitable protective clothing.
Eye Protection: Eye protection required.

SECTION 9: PHYSICAL AND CHEMICAL PROPERTIES

APPEARANCE: Bluish-green liquid	BOILING POINT: 212º F
PHYSICAL STATE: Liquid	EVAPORATION RATE: 0.98
ODOR: Sharp odor	VAPOR PRESSURE (mm Hg): 0.20 at 20º C
ODOR THRESHOLD: 0.04 ppm	VAPOR DENSITY (AIR = 1): 1.1
pH: 7.5-8.5	SPECIFIC GRAVITY: 1.004
FREEZING POINT: 32º F	SOLUBILITY IN WATER: Complete (100%)

SECTION 10: STABILITY AND REACTIVITY

STABILITY: Stable under recommended storage conditions.

CONDITIONS TO AVOID: Avoid temperatures above 200º F

INCOMPATIBILITY (MATERIAL TO AVOID): Strong acids, bases, and oxidizing agents.

HAZARDOUS DECOMPOSITION BYPRODUCTS: None

HAZARDOUS POLYMERIZATION: Will not occur

SECTION 11: TOXICOLOGICAL INFORMATION

Acute Health Hazards

Inhalation: Inhalation of mist or vapors may be severely irritating to the nose, throat, and lungs.

Skin Contact: May cause skin irritation. May aggravate pre-existing dermatitis.

Eye Contact: Severe irritant and corrosive to the eyes.

Ingestion: Ingestion of this material may cause oral thrush, nausea, vomiting, epigastric distress, diarrhea, headache, fatigue, dizziness, insomnia, mental confusion, and impairment.

Chronic Health Hazards

No adverse effects expected based on the available data.

Medical Conditions Aggravated By Exposure

Inhalation of vapor may cause asthma-like symptoms (chest discomfort and tightness, difficulty with breathing) as well as aggravate pre-existing asthma and inflammatory or fibrotic pulmonary disease.

Carcinogen

None of the components is listed as a carcinogen or potential carcinogen by NTP, IARC, or OSHA.

SECTION 12: ECOLOGICAL INFORMATION

This product is classified as toxic to the aquatic environment.

Fig. 3.4, **cont'd**

SAFETY DATA SHEET (SDS)	
SECTION 13: DISPOSAL CONSIDERATIONS	
Container must be triple rinsed and disposed of in accordance with Federal, State, and/or Local regulations. Used solution should be flushed thoroughly with water into sewage disposal in accordance with Federal, State, and/or Local regulations.	
SECTION 14: TRANSPORT INFORMATION	
Restrictions:	None. Not regulated.
UN Number:	None
UN Proper Shipping Name:	N/A
Transport Hazard Class:	N/A
Packing Group Number:	N/A
SECTION 15: REGULATORY INFORMATION	
EPA SARA 311/312 Hazard Classification:	Acute Health, Chronic Health
SECTION 16: OTHER INFORMATION	
Issue Date:	4/28/02
Revision Date:	10/10/2022

Fig. 3.4, **cont'd**

If an SDS is missing, it must be replaced. This is accomplished by contacting the manufacturer of the chemical for a replacement or by going to the manufacturer's website; most manufacturers post their SDSs on their websites for easy access.

What Would You Do? What Would You *Not* Do?

Case Study 1

Elba Cordera has brought her daughter Maria in for a well-baby visit. Maria is 9 months old and is just starting to crawl. Mrs. Cordera is taking precautions to baby-proof her house to protect Maria from accidents. Mrs. Cordera wants to know how to tell whether a cleaning product is poisonous. She also wants to know what she should do if Maria gets into a cleaning product and spills it on herself or swallows it. ■

SAFETY DATA SHEET REQUIREMENTS

The GHS guidelines require that the information on an SDS of a hazardous chemical (see Fig. 3.4) be presented using a standardized 16-section format that follows a specified sequence as outlined:

1. *Identification:* This section provides information used to identify the chemical and must include the product name and brand name and the name, address, phone number, and emergency phone number of the manufacturer. This section must also include the recommended use of the chemical and any restrictions on use.
2. *Hazards Identification:* This section includes the hazards of the chemical and the appropriate warning information associated with those hazards and includes the following:
   - Hazard classification of the chemical
   - Signal word
   - Hazard statement(s)
   - Hazard pictograms
   - Precautionary statement(s)
3. *Composition/Information on Ingredients:* This section provides a list of the ingredients in the chemical.
4. *First-Aid Measures:* This section describes the initial care that an untrained responder can provide to an individual who has been exposed to the chemical. It is subdivided according to the different routes of exposure (e.g., skin contact, inhalation).
5. *Fire-Fighting Measures:* Some hazardous chemicals may cause a fire if used improperly. This section provides recommendations for fighting a fire caused by the chemical, including suitable extinguishing agents.
6. *Accidental Release Measures:* This section provides recommendations on the appropriate response to spills, leaks, or releases, including containment and cleanup practices to prevent or minimize exposure to people, properties, or the environment. It also identifies the personal precautions that should be taken during the cleanup such as wearing skin and eye protection.
7. *Handling and Storage:* This section identifies precautions for the safe handling of the chemical and conditions for the safe storage of the chemical.
8. *Exposure Controls/Personal Protection:* This section indicates the exposure control limits, engineering controls, and personal protective measures that should be used to protect oneself from the chemical.
9. *Physical and Chemical Properties:* This section lists the physical and chemical properties associated with the chemical such as appearance, physical state, odor, pH, and boiling point.

10. *Stability and Reactivity:* Some chemicals react when combined with other chemicals or materials. This section lists the substances and conditions that the chemical should be kept away from to prevent a dangerous reaction.
11. *Toxicologic Information:* This section identifies the toxicologic effects that can result from overexposure to the chemical and includes the following:
    - Route of entry, which indicates how the chemical can enter the body, including inhalation, skin contact, eye contact, and ingestion
    - Signs and symptoms of overexposure (e.g., skin irritation, eye damage, lung damage) categorized according to acute and chronic health hazards
    - Medical conditions that are aggravated by exposure to the chemical (e.g., asthma, dermatitis)
    - Indication of whether the chemical has been identified as a potential carcinogen
12. *Ecologic Information:* This section provides information to help determine the environmental impact of the chemical if it were released into the environment.
13. *Disposal Considerations:* This section provides guidance on proper disposal of the chemical.
14. *Transport Information:* This section provides guidance to suppliers for shipping and transporting the chemical.
15. *Regulatory Information:* This section identifies the safety, health, and environmental regulations specific for the chemical that is not indicated anywhere else on the SDS.
16. *Other Information:* This section includes other important information related to the chemical such as when the SDS was prepared or when the last known revision was made.

Putting It All into Practice

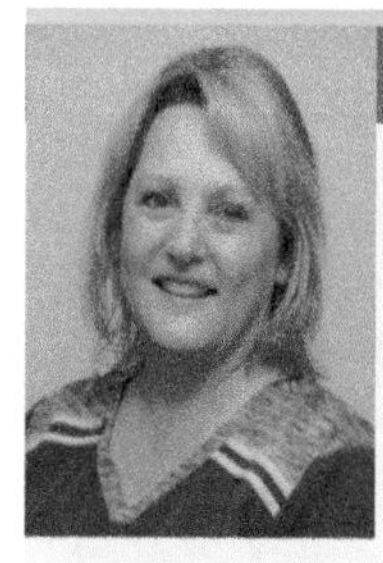

My name is Linda, and I work for two physicians in a family practice medical office. As a medical assistant, one of the situations you deal with on an almost-daily basis is drug representatives who come to the office to promote their products. Their job is anything but easy. The waiting and the frequent rejections would make most people think twice before applying for the job.

One winter day, I am sure I made one drug representative really think twice about his career choice. As the representative stopped at our office, he, being a polite young man, let a patient wearing wet, snow-covered boots enter the building first. Trying to make a good impression with a new suit and dress shoes, he soon found himself doing a "Spanish fandango" while trying to maintain his balance and eventually crashed to the floor.

I thought I would help by mopping up the snow-tracked floor. What I did not know was the mop had wax on it. Needless to say, when he returned with the requested drug samples, we were not able to keep him from falling a second time! ■

EMPLOYEE INFORMATION AND TRAINING

The HCS requires that employees be provided with information and training regarding hazardous chemicals in the workplace. The training session must be offered at the time of an employee's initial assignment to a work area where hazardous chemicals are present and whenever a new chemical hazard is introduced into the work area. The training program must be an ongoing activity, and each training session must be documented.

Sanitization

Sanitization consists of a series of steps that removes debris from an item and reduces the number of microorganisms to a safe level (Procedure 3.1). Debris may consist of organic or inorganic material such as blood, body fluids, body tissue, and soil. Debris on the surface of an item can result in incomplete sterilization or disinfection. This is because the debris acts as a physical barrier preventing the physical or chemical agent from reaching the surface of the item to kill microorganisms.

SANITIZING INSTRUMENTS

The items most frequently sanitized in the medical office are medical and surgical instruments. The general steps in the sanitization procedure of instruments are as follows:

1. *Rinse* the instruments immediately after use to prevent debris from drying on the instruments, making it harder to remove later.
2. *Decontaminate* the instruments with a chemical disinfectant to remove pathogenic microorganisms, making the instrument safe to handle.
3. *Clean* the instruments with an instrument cleaner to remove all organic and inorganic debris. An instrument cleaner contains a detergent and may also be combined with an enzymatic cleaner which can break down organic matter such as blood and tissue.
4. *Thoroughly rinse* the instruments to remove all loosened debris and cleaning solution residue.
5. *Dry* the instruments to prevent stains on the instruments.
6. *Inspect each instrument* for defects and working condition.
7. *Lubricate* hinged instruments to make the instruments function well and last longer.

CLEANING INSTRUMENTS

Two methods can be used to clean instruments: the manual method and the ultrasound method.

Manual Method

The manual method involves the cleaning of instruments manually with an instrument cleaner and a brush. Manual

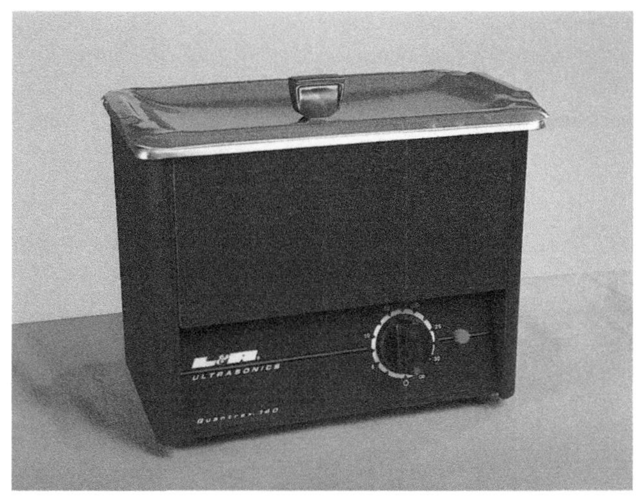

Fig. 3.5 Ultrasonic cleaner.

cleaning is recommended for delicate instruments because vibrations that occur with the ultrasound method may damage these instruments.

Ultrasound Method

The ultrasound method involves the use of an *ultrasonic cleaner* (Fig. 3.5) and an instrument cleaner. The ultrasound method offers a safety advantage in that instruments do not have to be handled during the cleaning process. This decreases the incidence of an accidental puncture or cut from a sharp instrument. An ultrasonic cleaner works by converting sound waves into mechanical energy, which creates small bubbles all over the instruments. When the bubbles burst, vibrations occur that loosen and remove debris from the instruments. Ultrasonic cleaners are especially good at removing debris from hard-to-reach areas, such as box locks of hemostats and screw locks of scissors.

Before the instruments are placed in the ultrasonic cleaner, they should be separated according to the type of metal (e.g., stainless steel, aluminum, brass). Instruments made of dissimilar metals should not be cleaned together in the ultrasonic cleaner. When different metals are in close contact, the ions from one metal can flow to another. This may result in a permanent blue-black stain on an instrument, which can be removed only by having the instrument refinished.

GUIDELINES FOR SANITIZING INSTRUMENTS

The following guidelines should be followed when sanitizing surgical instruments:

1. *Wear gloves during the sanitization process.* The medical assistant should wear disposable gloves during the entire sanitization procedure. This protects the medical assistant from bloodborne pathogens and other potentially infectious materials. The medical assistant should be especially careful when working with hazardous chemicals and when handling sharp instruments. Heavy-duty utility gloves should be worn over the disposable gloves to provide protection from the irritating effects of chemical agents and accidental punctures or cuts from sharp instruments.
2. *Handle instruments carefully.* Instruments are expensive and delicate, yet durable and can last for many years if handled and maintained properly. Dropping an instrument on the floor or throwing an instrument into a basin may damage it. Instruments should never be piled in a heap because they may become entangled and may be damaged when separated. Keep sharp instruments separate from other instruments to prevent damaging or dulling the cutting edge. In addition, keep delicate instruments separate to protect them from damage.
3. *Follow instructions on labels of chemical agents.* Before using a chemical agent (e.g., chemical disinfectant, instrument cleaner), check the expiration date on the container label. Chemicals have a tendency to lose potency over time and should not be used past their expiration date. Thoroughly review the SDS of the chemical agent and carefully read the label on the container to determine the use, mixing, and storage of the chemical agent. Follow the precautions listed on the label regarding personal safety, such as the use of gloves and eye protection.
4. *Use a proper cleaning agent.* A low-sudsing instrument cleaner with a neutral pH should be used to clean the instruments. Commercially available instrument cleaners meet these criteria (Fig. 3.6). Instrument cleaners often come in a concentrated form and must be diluted with water before use. Never substitute any other type of cleaner, such as dishwasher detergent or laundry detergent; these detergents may not be low-sudsing or may not have the proper pH for sanitizing instruments. If an instrument cleaner with an alkaline pH is used and is not completely rinsed off, it could leave a residue on the instrument. This could result in an orange-brown stain on the instrument that resembles rust. Using an acid instrument cleaner also can cause staining and permanent corrosion.
5. *Use proper cleaning devices.* Proper cleaning devices should be used for the manual cleaning of surgical instruments. A stiff nylon brush should be used to clean the surface of the instrument. A stainless-steel wire brush can be used to clean grooves, crevices, or serrations. A stain on an instrument often can be removed by using a commercial instrument stain remover (see Fig. 3.6). Never use steel wool or other abrasives to remove stains because damage to the instrument could occur.
6. *Carefully inspect each instrument for defects and proper working condition.* After cleaning, rinsing, and drying the instrument, it is important to check it for defects and proper working condition as follows:
   - The blades of an instrument should be straight and not bent.
   - The tips of an instrument should approximate tightly and evenly when the instrument is closed.

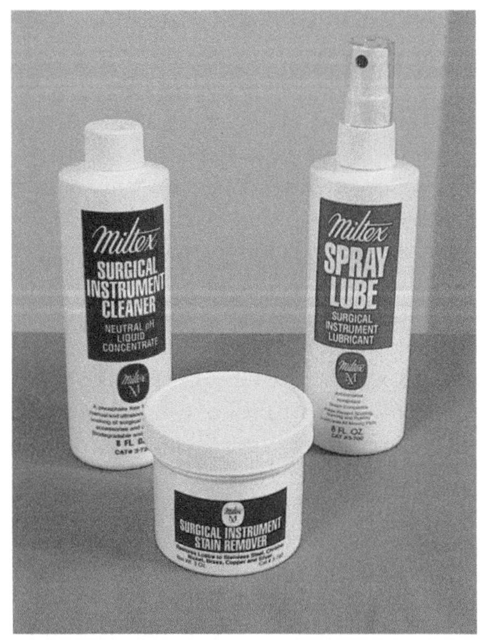

Fig. 3.6 Commercially available instrument cleaners. *Left,* Instrument cleaner; *center,* stain remover; *right,* spray lubricant.

- An instrument with a box lock (e.g., hemostatic forceps, needle holders) should move freely but must not be too loose. The pin that holds the box lock together should be flush against the instrument.
- An instrument with a spring handle (e.g., thumb and tissue forceps) should have sufficient tension to grasp objects tightly.
- The cutting edge of a sharp instrument should be smooth and devoid of nicks.
- Scissors should cut cleanly and smoothly. To test for this, the medical assistant should cut into a thin piece of gauze. The scissors are in proper working condition if they cut all the way to the end of the blade without catching on the gauze.

7. *Lubricate hinged instruments.* Lubricate box locks, screw locks, scissor blades, and any other moving part of each instrument. The lubricant makes the instrument function better and last longer. Use a lubricant that can be penetrated by steam, such as a commercial spray lubricant or a lubricant bath (see Fig. 3.6). Lubricate after performing the final rinse (and drying of the instrument); otherwise, the lubricant would be rinsed off the instrument. Never use industrial oils or silicon sprays. These substances are not steam penetrable and can build up on the instrument, affecting its working condition.

Disinfection

Disinfection is the process of destroying pathogenic microorganisms, but it does not kill spores. Disinfection is accomplished in the medical office through the use of liquid chemical agents. Chemical disinfection has been discussed with respect to its role in the sanitization process to decontaminate instruments and make them safe to handle. This section discusses the use of chemical disinfection to disinfect semicritical and noncritical items so they can be used for patient care.

LEVELS OF DISINFECTION

Based on killing action, disinfection can be classified according to three levels.

HIGH-LEVEL DISINFECTION

High-level disinfection is a process that destroys all microorganisms with the exception of spores. High-level disinfection is used to disinfect semicritical items. A **semicritical item** is an item that comes in contact with nonintact skin or intact mucous membranes, such as a flexible fiberoptic sigmoidoscope. Examples of high-level disinfectants include 2% glutaraldehyde (e.g., Cidex, MetriCide) and ortho-phthalaldehyde (e.g., Cidex OPA and MetriCide OPA).

INTERMEDIATE-LEVEL DISINFECTION

Intermediate-level disinfection is a process that inactivates tubercle bacilli (the causative agents of tuberculosis), all vegetative bacteria, most viruses, and most fungi, but it does not kill spores. Intermediate-level disinfection is used to disinfect noncritical items. **Noncritical items** are items that come in contact with intact skin but not with mucous membranes, including stethoscopes, blood pressure cuffs, tuning forks, percussion hammers, and crutches. A common intermediate-level disinfectant is isopropyl alcohol, which is frequently used in the form of alcohol wipes.

LOW-LEVEL DISINFECTION

Low-level disinfection is a process that kills most bacteria, some viruses, and some fungi, but it cannot be relied on to kill resistant microorganisms, such as tubercle bacilli, and it cannot kill spores. Low-level disinfectants typically are used to disinfect surfaces such as examining tables, laboratory countertops, walls, furniture, and floors. Low-level disinfectants used in the medical office include sodium hypochlorite (household bleach), phenolics, and quaternary ammonium compounds.

TYPES OF DISINFECTANTS

The disinfectants used most frequently in the medical office are described next. Table 3.1 lists these disinfectants, along with the level of disinfection, common names, and uses for each.

Table 3.1 Disinfectants Used in the Medical Office

Disinfectant	Level of Disinfection	Common Names	Use in the Medical Office
Glutaraldehyde	High-level disinfection	Cidex MetriCide ProCide Omnicide Wavicide	Disinfection of flexible fiberoptic sigmoidoscopes. Decontamination of surgical instruments during the sanitization procedure.
Alcohol	Intermediate- to low-level disinfection	Isopropyl alcohol	Disinfection of stethoscopes, blood pressure cuffs, tuning forks, and percussion hammers; isopropyl alcohol wipes are used to disinfect rubber stoppers of multiple-dose medication vials.
Chlorine and chlorine compounds	Intermediate-level disinfection	Sodium hypochlorite (household bleach)	Recommended by OSHA for decontamination of blood spills.
Phenolics	Low-level disinfection	Carbolic acid Hydroxybenzene Phenic acid Phenyl hydroxide Phenylic acid	Disinfection of walls, furniture, floors, and laboratory work surfaces.
Quaternary ammonium compounds	Low-level disinfection	Benzalkonium chloride	Disinfection of walls, furniture, floors, and laboratory work surfaces.

OSHA, Occupational Safety and Health Administration.

GLUTARALDEHYDE

Glutaraldehyde is a high-level disinfectant that has a rapid killing action and is not inactivated by the presence of organic material. Because it does not corrode lenses, metal, or rubber, it is often used for semicritical items that cannot be exposed to heat, such as flexible fiberoptic sigmoidoscopes. It is also used to decontaminate surgical instruments during the sanitization procedure to make them safe to handle. Brand names for glutaraldehyde include Cidex and MetriCide.

Glutaraldehyde is highly toxic and can cause harm to the body if not handled properly. When working with glutaraldehyde, the medical assistant must work in an area that is well ventilated. Utility gloves and safety goggles must be worn to protect oneself from the irritating effects of this chemical (Fig. 3.7). If the hands or any other part of the body come in contact with glutaraldehyde, the area should be rinsed thoroughly under running water.

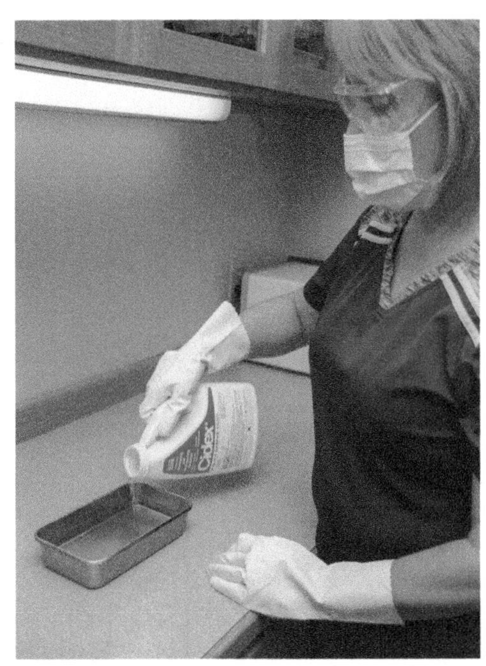

Fig. 3.7 Linda wears utility gloves and safety goggles to protect her from the irritating effects of glutaraldehyde. (From Isihara J: *Tests for color blindness*, Tokyo: Kanehara; 1920.)

ALCOHOL

Alcohol is frequently used as a disinfectant in the medical office. The two most common types are *ethyl alcohol* and *isopropyl alcohol.* The disinfecting action of alcohol is increased by the presence of water; a 70% solution of alcohol is recommended. Stronger concentrations (95% to 100%) are not as effective. A disadvantage of alcohol is that it tends to dissolve the cement from around the lenses of instruments.

Ethyl alcohol and isopropyl alcohol provide intermediate- to low-level disinfection and can be used to disinfect stethoscopes, blood pressure cuffs, and percussion hammers. Isopropyl alcohol wipes are used to disinfect small surfaces such as the diaphragm of a stethoscope and rubber stoppers on multiple-dose medication vials.

CHLORINE AND CHLORINE COMPOUNDS

Chlorine and chlorine compounds are some of the oldest and most used disinfectants. Their most important use is in the chlorination of water. In the medical office, chlorine is used in the form of liquid sodium hypochlorite (household bleach), which is an intermediate level disinfectant. A 10% solution of household bleach in water (i.e., 1 part bleach to 9 parts water) inactivates tuberculosis bacteria, hepatitis B and C viruses, human immunodeficiency virus, and many bacteria in 10 minutes at room temperature. Because of this, household bleach is recommended by OSHA for the decontamination of blood spills. A disadvantage of this disinfectant is that it can irritate skin and mucous membranes and is highly corrosive to metal.

PHENOLICS

Phenolics are primarily used to disinfect walls, furniture, floors, laboratory work surfaces, and examining tables. This disinfectant is a corrosive poison and tends to be irritating to the eyes and skin. For this reason, eye and skin protective devices should be worn when working with phenolics in the pure form. Many derivatives of phenolics are commonly used and are usually nonirritating, including Lysol and hexachlorophene.

QUATERNARY AMMONIUM COMPOUNDS

The quaternary ammonium compounds (often referred to as *quats*) are used in the medical office for the disinfection of noncritical surfaces, such as floors, furniture, and walls in the waiting room and examining rooms.

GUIDELINES FOR DISINFECTION

Certain guidelines should be followed when disinfecting items with a chemical agent.

SANITIZE SEMICRITICAL ITEMS BEFORE DISINFECTING THEM

Before disinfecting a semicritical item, it must first be thoroughly sanitized and checked for proper working order. It is important to remove all organic and inorganic debris from the item before it is disinfected. If debris is still present on the item after it is sanitized, the chemical disinfectant will be unable to reach all surfaces of the item to kill microorganisms. In addition, with some disinfectants, organic matter can absorb the chemical disinfectant and inactivate it. The item should be thoroughly rinsed after cleaning because detergent residue may interfere with the disinfecting process. The item must be completely dry before placing it in the disinfectant, because water dilutes the chemical and decreases its effectiveness.

OBSERVE SAFETY PRECAUTIONS

The medical assistant should carefully read the SDS and the container label before using a chemical disinfectant. All safety precautions should be followed when using the chemical to protect against illness or injury from a hazardous chemical.

PROPERLY PREPARE AND USE THE DISINFECTANT

It is important that the manufacturer's directions on preparation, dilution, and use of the chemical disinfectant be followed carefully. The disinfectant should be prepared exactly as indicated on the container label. Some disinfectants are used at their full strength, whereas others require dilution. Some disinfectants (e.g., glutaraldehyde) require the addition of an activator before they can be used. Properly preparing the disinfectant ensures the destruction of microorganisms. A disinfectant must be applied for a certain length of time to kill microorganisms. The medical assistant must be sure to disinfect for the length of time indicated on the container label.

PROPERLY STORE THE DISINFECTANT

Chemical disinfectants should be closed tightly and stored properly under the storage conditions recommended by the manufacturer. Because chemical disinfectants lose their potency over time, the medical assistant should strictly adhere to the manufacturer's recommendations for the shelf life, use life, and reuse life. Each of these terms is defined next as it relates to chemical disinfectants.

Shelf life Shelf life is the length of time a chemical disinfectant may be stored before use and still retain its effectiveness. The shelf life is indicated by an expiration date on the container. The expiration date should always be checked before using the chemical. Outdated disinfectants should not be used.

Use life Some disinfectants must be combined with another chemical to be activated before they are used. Use life is the period of time a disinfecting solution is effective after it has been activated. Cidex Plus (Johnson & Johnson, New Brunswick, NJ) is effective for 28 days after activation. At the end of this time, any chemical remaining in the container must be discarded. When a chemical

Memories *from* Practicum

Linda: During my practicum experience, I was placed in a pediatrician's office. I wanted to go to a pediatric site because I love being around children. One day I was in the examining room with my patient, a 4-year-old boy who was there with his mother. It was standard procedure at this office to take every patient's temperature. I started getting out our electronic thermometer to take his temperature when I noticed he looked a little frightened. He was looking at the thermometer funny, and he said, "Can you do it in my ear?" I said I was sorry but we didn't have that kind of thermometer. I told him I could do it under his arm or under his tongue. His mom looked at him, and he said, "But I want it in my ear." He finally agreed to let me do it under his arm. When I was finished taking his temperature, he smiled and said, "You are so nice!"■

disinfectant is activated, the date on which it will expire should be written on the label of the container.

Reuse life Reuse life is the maximum number of days a reusable chemical disinfectant is effective. For example, Cidex Plus can be reused for 28 days to disinfect items. At the end of this time, the disinfectant must be discarded. The name of the disinfectant and the date when the disinfectant must be discarded should be written on an adhesive label and affixed to the container into which the disinfectant will be poured.

Sterilization

Sterilization is the process of destroying all forms of microbial life, including spores. An item that is sterile is free of all living microorganisms and spores. Sterilization must be used to process all critical items. A **critical item** is an item that comes in contact with sterile tissue or the vascular system such as surgical instruments.

As previously described, a semicritical item (one that comes in contact with nonintact skin or with intact mucous membranes) can be chemically disinfected with a high-level disinfectant. Most offices prefer instead to sterilize semicritical items (e.g., vaginal specula, nasal specula) in the autoclave. The autoclave provides a convenient, efficient, safe, and inexpensive method for destroying microorganisms. Chemical disinfectants not only are more expensive to use but also are more hazardous and create problems regarding their proper disposal. The exception is a semicritical item that is heat sensitive. Flexible fiberoptic sigmoidoscopes would be damaged by the heat of an autoclave and must be chemically disinfected.

STERILIZATION METHODS

Sterilization can be accomplished using physical and chemical methods. The method used to achieve sterility depends primarily on the nature of the item to be sterilized. The most common physical and chemical sterilization methods include the following:

Physical Methods
Autoclave (steam under pressure)
Dry heat oven (hot air)
Radiation

Chemical Methods
Ethylene oxide gas
Cold sterilization (chemical agents)

The most common method for sterilizing items in the medical office is steam under pressure using an autoclave. The autoclave is discussed in detail in this chapter; the other methods of sterilization are briefly described.

AUTOCLAVE

The **autoclave** is dependable, efficient, and economical and is used to sterilize items that are not harmed by moisture or high temperature, such as surgical and medical instruments. An autoclave consists of an outer jacket surrounding an inner sterilizing chamber. Under pressure, water is converted into steam, which fills the inner sterilizing chamber. The pressure plays no direct part in killing microorganisms; rather, it functions to attain a higher temperature than could be reached by the steam from boiling water (212°F [100°C]). As the steam enters the chamber, the cooler, drier air present in the chamber is forced out through a valve.

During an autoclave cycle, steam penetrates the articles placed in the chamber. The articles are cooler, causing the steam to condense into moisture and transfer its heat to each article, killing all microorganisms and spores present on the article.

The autoclave must be operated at a pressure of at least 15 pounds of pressure per square inch (psi) and a temperature of at least 250°F (121°C). Vegetative forms of most microorganisms are killed in a few minutes at temperatures ranging from 130°F to 150°F (54°C to 65°C), but certain spores can withstand a temperature of 240°F (115°C) for longer than 3 hours. However, no organism can survive direct exposure to saturated steam at 250°F (121°C) for 15 minutes or longer.

The sterilization process using an autoclave is discussed in this section (with the exception of sanitizing items, which was already presented). The sterilization process consists of the following components:

- Monitoring program
- Sanitizing items
- Wrapping items
- Loading the autoclave
- Operating the autoclave (autoclave cycle)
- Handling and storing packs
- Maintaining the autoclave

MONITORING PROGRAM

The Centers for Disease Control and Prevention (CDC) recommends that medical offices establish and maintain a monitoring program to ensure that autoclaved items are sterile. The monitoring program consists of quality control measures that include the following:

1. Written policies and procedures for each step of the sterilization process
2. Sterilization indicators to ensure that minimum sterilizing conditions have been achieved (described in more detail in this section).
3. Records for each autoclave cycle, maintained in an autoclave log (see Fig. 3.8). Some autoclaves have recorders that automatically print out most of this information at the end of the cycle (Fig. 3.9). The information that

AUTOCLAVE LOG						
Date/Time	Description of the Load	Cycle Time (min)	Temperature (° F)	Indicator* (+/–)	Initials	Comments
7/25/XX 4:00 PM	Surgical instruments	20	250	–	KV	
7/26/XX 3:00 PM	MOS tray setups	30	250	–	KV	
*Indicator Interpretation: Positive (+): Spores not killed, indicating sterilization conditions have not been met. Negative (–): Spores killed, indicating sterilization conditions have been met.						
MAINTENANCE: (Indicate date, vendor name, service, etc.)						

Fig. 3.8 Example of an autoclave log.

should be documented for each autoclave cycle includes the following:

- Date and time of the cycle
- Description of the load
- Exposure time
- Exposure temperature and pressure
- Results of the sterilization indicator
- Initials of the operator

Sterilization Indicators

Articles processed in an autoclave must be exposed to steam at a time, temperature, and pressure that will result in sterilization. Sterilization indicators are available to determine the effectiveness of each autoclave cycle and to check against improper wrapping of items, improper loading of the autoclave, and faulty operation of the autoclave.

An item in a wrapped pack is not considered sterile unless the steam has penetrated to the center of the pack; therefore a sterilization indicator should be placed in the center of each pack. The medical assistant should carefully read the instructions that come with the sterilization indicators. The most reliable indicators check for the attainment of the proper temperature and indicate the duration of the temperature.

If an indicator does not change properly, a problem may be present in the sterilization technique or in the working condition of the autoclave. The manufacturer's guidelines for proper sterilization techniques should be reviewed and the items should be resterilized, following these guidelines. If the indicator still does not change properly, the autoclave is in need of repair and should not be used until it has been serviced.

Sterilization indicators should be stored in a cool, dry area. Excessive heat or moisture can damage the indicator. The most common sterilization indicators are chemical indicators and biologic indicators, which are described next.

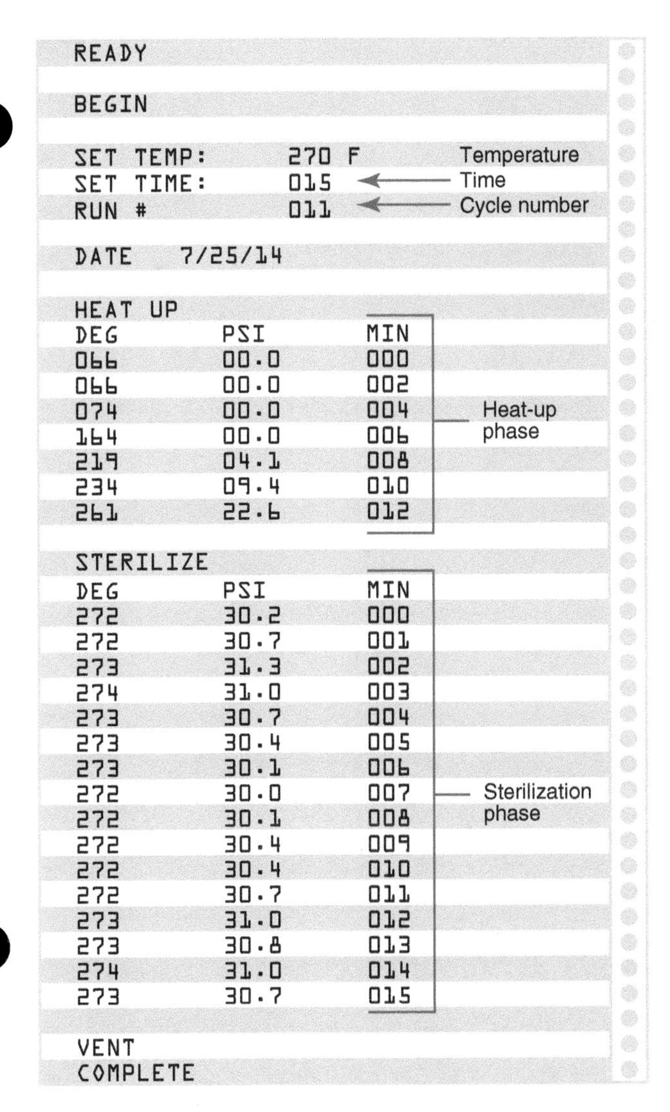
READY

BEGIN

SET TEMP:	270 F	
SET TIME:	015	
RUN #	011	

DATE 7/25/14

HEAT UP

DEG	PSI	MIN
066	00.0	000
066	00.0	002
074	00.0	004
164	00.0	006
219	04.1	008
234	09.4	010
261	22.6	012

STERILIZE

DEG	PSI	MIN
272	30.2	000
272	30.7	001
273	31.3	002
274	31.0	003
273	30.7	004
273	30.4	005
273	30.1	006
272	30.0	007
272	30.1	008
272	30.4	009
272	30.4	010
272	30.7	011
273	31.0	012
273	30.8	013
274	31.0	014
273	30.7	015

VENT
COMPLETE

Fig. 3.9 Example of a printout of an autoclave cycle. (Courtesy GSI [Grayson-Stadler], Milford, NH.)

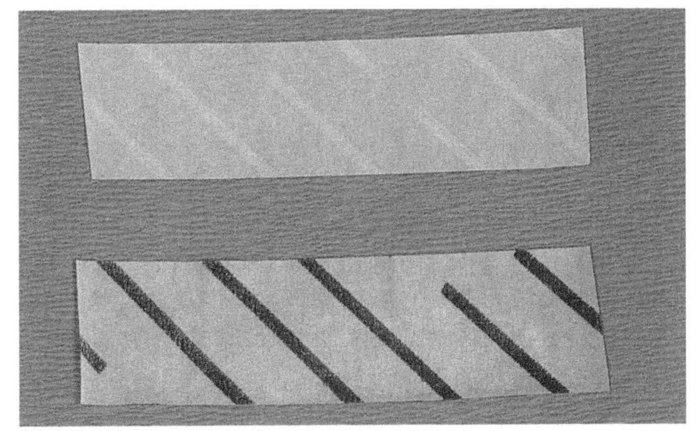

Fig. 3.10 Autoclave tape. *Top,* Autoclave tape as it appears before the sterilization process. *Bottom,* Black diagonal lines appear on the tape indicating the wrapped item has been in the autoclave and subjected to a high temperature. (Courtesy GSI [Grayson-Stadler], Milford, NH.)

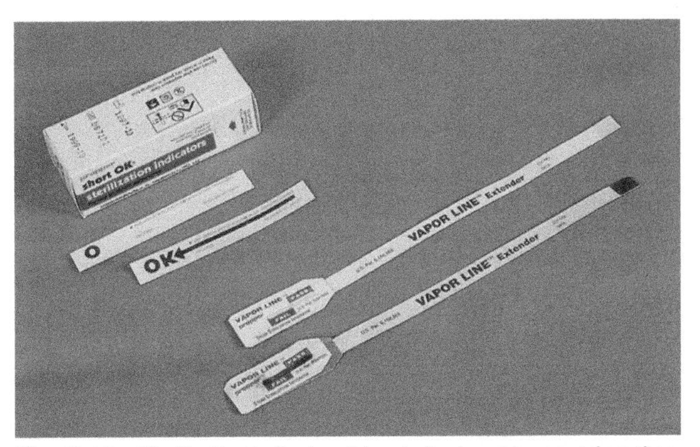

Fig. 3.11 Sterilization indicator strips. Indicator strips contain a thermolabile dye that change color when exposed to steam under pressure for a certain length of time.

Chemical Indicators

Chemical indicators are impregnated with a thermolabile dye that changes color when exposed to the sterilization process. If the chemical reaction of the indicator does not show the expected results, the item may not be sterile and must be resterilized. Chemical indicators include autoclave tape and sterilization indicator strips.

Autoclave Tape

Autoclave tape has diagonal lines containing a chemical which changes color (usually from beige to black) if it has been exposed to steam. Autoclave tape is similar to masking tape; however, it is slightly more adhesive, which allows it to adhere to a hot, moist pack during the autoclave cycle. The tape is available in a variety of colors, can be written on, and is useful for closing and identifying a wrapped item (Fig. 3.10). Autoclave tape has some limitations as an indicator. Because it is placed on the outside of the pack, it cannot ensure that steam has penetrated to the center of the pack. It also does not ensure that the item has been sterilized; it merely indicates that an item has been in the autoclave and that a high temperature has been attained. This helps to differentiate between processed and unprocessed loads.

Sterilization Indicator Strips

Sterilization indicator strips are commercially prepared strips made of paper or plastic that contain a thermolabile dye and that change color when exposed to steam under pressure for a certain length of time (Fig. 3.11). Most indicator strips are designed to change color after being exposed to a temperature of 250°F (121°C) for 15 minutes. The indicator strip should be placed in the center of the wrapped pack, with the end containing the dye placed in an area of the pack considered to be the hardest for steam to penetrate.

Biologic Indicators

Biologic indicators are the best means available for determining the effectiveness of the sterilization procedure. The CDC recommends that medical office personnel use a biologic indicator to monitor all autoclaves at least once a week.

A biologic indicator is a preparation of living bacterial spores. Biologic indicators are commercially available in the

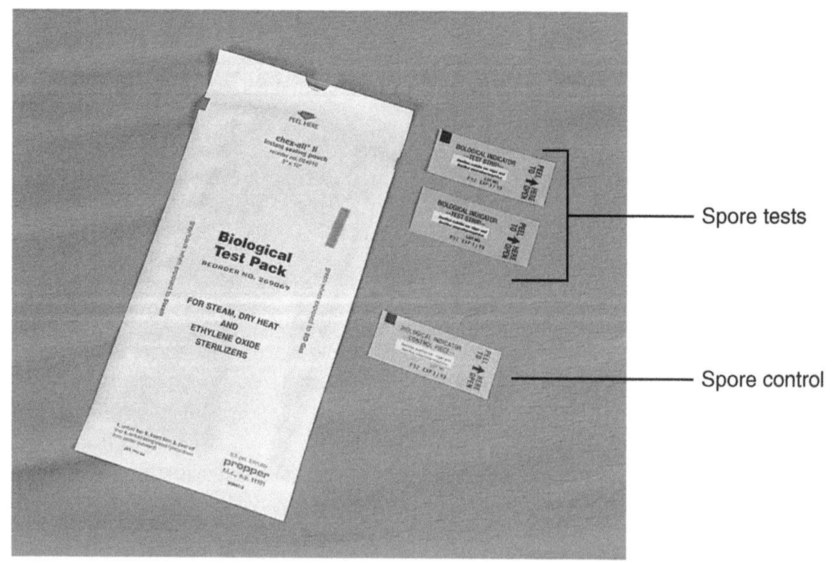

Fig. 3.12 Biologic indicator. A biologic indicator includes two spore tests that are sterilized *(top right)* and one spore control that is not sterilized *(bottom right)*.

form of dry spore strips in small glassine envelopes. Biologic monitoring of an autoclave requires the use of a preparation of spores of *Geobacillus stearothermophilus,* which is a microorganism whose spores are particularly resistant to moist heat and are not harmful to humans.

Each biologic testing unit includes two spore tests that are sterilized and one spore control that is not sterilized (Fig. 3.12). The biologic indicator is placed in the center of two wrapped items. The items are placed in areas of the autoclave that are the least accessible to steam penetration, such as on the bottom tray of the autoclave, near the front of the autoclave, and in the back of the autoclave.

After the indicators have been exposed to sterilization conditions, they must be processed before the results can be obtained. The two methods for processing results are the *in-house method* and the *mail-in method.*

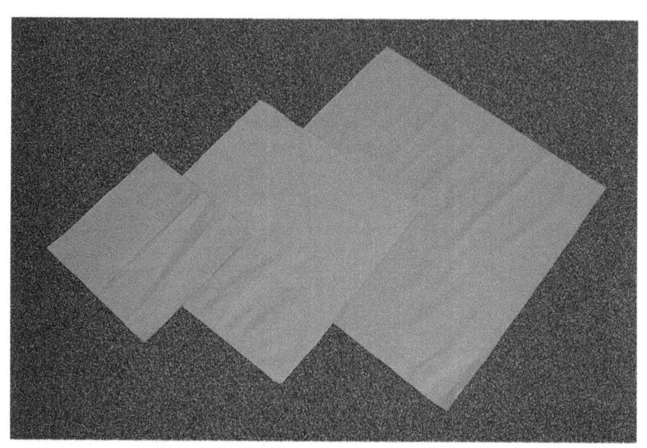

Fig. 3.13 Sterilization wrapping paper. Sterilization wrapping paper consists of square sheets of paper that are available in different sizes.

In-House Method

The in-house method involves processing and interpreting the results at the medical office. After sterilization, the processed spores are **incubated** for 24 to 48 hours. If sterilization conditions have been met, the color or condition of the processed spores is different from those of the control, and the spore test result is interpreted as negative. If sterilization conditions have not been met, the processed spores and the unprocessed control display the same color or condition, and the spore test result is interpreted as positive.

Mail-in Method

With this method, the processed spores and the (unprocessed) control are mailed to a processing laboratory. The test is performed by the laboratory, and the results are returned to the medical office.

If spores are not killed in routine spore tests, the autoclave should be checked immediately for proper use and function, and the spore test should be repeated. If the spore test result remains positive, the autoclave should not be used until it is serviced.

WRAPPING ITEMS

Items to be sterilized in the autoclave must first be thoroughly sanitized (see Procedure 3.1). Next, the items are prepared for autoclaving by wrapping them. The purpose of wrapping items is to protect them from recontamination during handling and storage. Items that are wrapped and handled correctly remain sterile after autoclaving until the package seal is broken.

The wrapping material must be made of a substance that is not affected by the sterilization process and must allow steam to penetrate while preventing contaminants (e.g., dust, insects, microorganisms) from entering during handling and storage. The wrapping material should not tear or puncture easily and should allow the sterilized pack to be opened without contaminating the contents. A wrapper

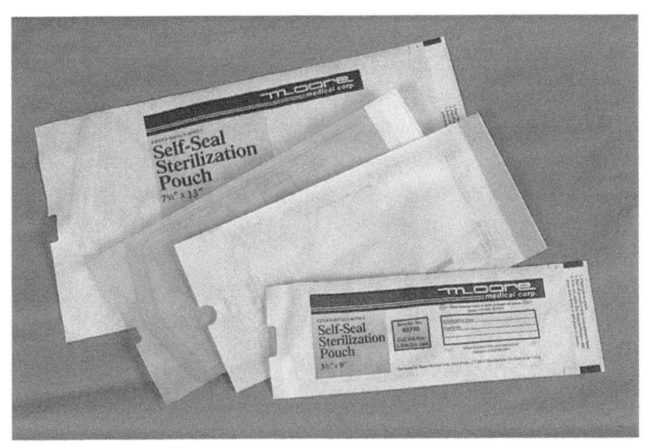

Fig. 3.14 Sterilization pouches. Sterilization pouches consist of a combination of paper and plastic and are available in different sizes.

should not be used if it is torn or has a hole. Examples of good wrapping materials for the autoclave include sterilization paper and pouches described as follows.

Sterilization Paper

Sterilization paper is a disposable and inexpensive wrapping material. It consists of square sheets of paper available in different sizes (Fig. 3.13). The most common sizes (in inches) are 12 × 12, 15 × 15, 18 × 18, 24 × 24, 30 × 30, and 36 × 36. An item must be wrapped in such a way that it does not become contaminated when the pack is opened.

Autoclave tape is used to seal and label the contents of the pack. After removing a wrapped pack from the autoclave, the medical assistant should check the autoclave tape for the proper color change. If the tape does not change to the appropriate color, the pack must be rewrapped and resterilized.

The proper method for wrapping an instrument using sterilization paper is outlined in Procedure 3.2.

The disadvantage of sterilization paper is that it is difficult to spread open for removal of the contents. It has a "memory" and tends to flip back easily, so it may not open flat to provide a sterile field. (*Memory* is the ability of a material to retain a specific shape or configuration.) Because sterilization paper is opaque, it is not possible to view the contents of the pack before opening it.

Sterilization Pouches

Sterilization pouches consist of a combination of paper and plastic; paper makes up one side of the pouch, and a plastic film makes up the other side (Fig. 3.14). Pouches are available in different sizes; the most common sizes (in inches) are 3 × 9, 5 × 10, and 7 × 12.

Pouches have a peel-apart seal on one end used to open the pouch for removal of the sterile item inside. The other end of the pouch is open and is used to insert the item into the pouch during the wrapping procedure. Once the item has been inserted, this end is sealed with an adhesive strip or a heat-sealing device. The proper method for wrapping an instrument using a pouch is outlined in Procedure 3.3.

Pouches provide good visibility of the contents on the plastic side. Most manufacturers include a sterilization indicator on the outside of the pouch. After removing a pouch from the autoclave, the medical assistant should check the indicator for the proper color change. If the indicator does not change to the appropriate color (as specified by the manufacturer), the contents of the pouch must be rewrapped and resterilized.

Loading the Autoclave

Before loading the autoclave, the medical assistant should check the level of water in the water reservoir. Distilled water must be used to fill the water reservoir to the proper level. Normal tap water contains minerals which have a corrosive effect on the stainless-steel chamber of the autoclave. Tap water can also cause mineral deposits that prevent valves from opening or closing properly.

For an item to attain sterility, steam must reach all surfaces of an item at a specified time, temperature, and pressure. To accomplish this, packs must be positioned in the autoclave in such a manner that allows for the free circulation of steam. Proper positioning also facilitates the drying process. The following guidelines should be followed when loading the autoclave:

1. Small packs are best because steam penetrates them more easily; it takes longer for steam to reach the center of a large pack to ensure sterilization. A pack should be no larger than 12 × 12 × 20 inches.
2. To allow for proper steam circulation, packs should be positioned as loosely as possible inside the autoclave, with approximately 1 to 3 inches between small packs and 2 to 4 inches between large packs. Packs should not be allowed to touch surrounding walls, and at least 1 inch should separate the autoclave trays. Placing the packs too close together interferes with the free circulation of steam within the chamber (Fig. 3.15).
3. Pouches should be positioned vertically on their sides in an autoclave rack to maximize steam circulation and to facilitate the drying process. Pouches can also be placed flat on an autoclave tray with the paper side up and the plastic side down. This allows moisture to escape through the paper side during the drying process.

OPERATING THE AUTOCLAVE

The autoclave must be operated according to the manufacturer's instructions. The medical assistant should read the operating manual carefully before operating the autoclave for the first time. Thereafter the manual should be kept in an accessible location so that it is available if needed as a reference. The steps involved in achieving sterilization are known as the *autoclave cycle* and include the following:

1. Water is converted to steam and fills the autoclave chamber.
2. The desired temperature and pressure are reached.
3. The load is sterilized at the proper time, temperature, and pressure.
4. Steam is vented from the chamber.
5. The load is dried.

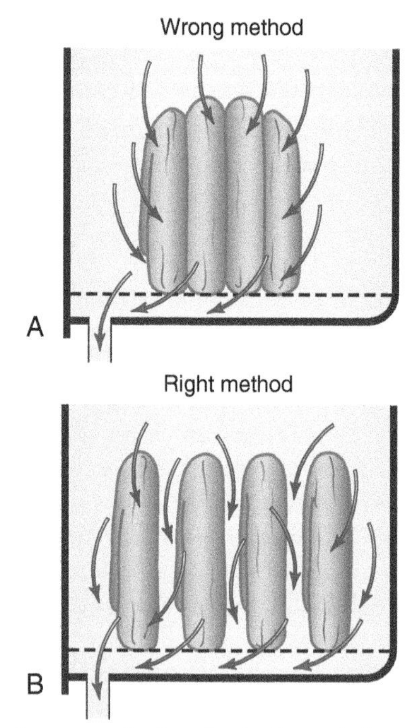

Fig. 3.15 Arrangement of packs in the autoclave. (A) Improper arrangement of packs in the autoclave. This arrangement prevents adequate steam penetration and interferes with proper sterilization. (B) Proper arrangement of packs in the autoclave. The packs are separated from each other, and steam can now penetrate each pack. (Courtesy of and modified from AMSCO/American Sterilizer Company, Erie, PA.)

The proper temperature and pressure must occur during an autoclave cycle to ensure sterilization of the load. A **load** refers to the items being sterilized during an autoclave cycle. The most common sterilization temperature/pressure combinations include 250°F (121°C) at 15 psi and 270°F (132°C) at 27 psi. The sterilizing time is based on the type of load being sterilized. Steam can easily reach the surfaces of hard, nonporous items such as unwrapped instruments (e.g., vaginal specula) to kill microorganisms; these items require a shorter sterilization time. A large minor office surgery pack requires a longer sterilization time because more time is needed for the steam to penetrate to the center of the pack. Sterilizing times typically range from 3 to 30 minutes.

Based on the type of load being sterilized, the medical assistant must select the proper autoclave cycle (Fig. 3.16) which includes one of the following:

- Unwrapped items
- Pouches
- Wrapped items

Once the autoclave cycle is selected, the autoclave automatically begins processing the load. Water is converted into steam under pressure and enters the autoclave chamber. After the desired temperature and pressure are attained, the autoclave begins the time countdown. At the end of the countdown, sterilization is achieved. The steam is then automatically vented from the chamber, causing the pressure to decrease to zero and the chamber to cool.

The sterilized packs are moist and must be allowed to dry before they are removed from the autoclave. This is because microorganisms can move quickly through the moisture on a wet wrap, contaminating the sterile item inside. After the steam is completely vented from the autoclave, the door automatically cracks open approximately (½) inch. This allows moisture on the wet packs to change from a liquid to a vapor and escape through the crack, thus drying the load. The residual heat in the inner chamber also helps dry the load. The load is allowed to dry for 15 to 60 minutes, depending on the type of load. Loads that contain large packs require a longer drying time than loads with smaller packs.

What Would You Do? What Would You *Not* Do?

Case Study 2

Cassie Augusta is in the examining room and is being prepared for the removal of a sebaceous cyst. Cassie is concerned about the instruments that the physician will be using to perform the procedure. She wants to know if they are "safe." Cassie says that her friend Mackenzie got a tattoo several years ago and developed hepatitis C 3 weeks later. Mackenzi thinks she got hepatitis C from the instruments that were used for her tattoo procedure. Cassie wants to know if it is possible for surgical instruments to give someone hepatitis C. She says she heard that hepatitis can cause liver cancer and wants to know if this is true. Cassie also wants to know if there is a vaccine to prevent hepatitis C. ■

HANDLING AND STORING PACKS

Sterilized wrapped items should be handled carefully and as little as possible. If a wrapped item is crushed, compressed, or dropped, the sterility of the contents cannot be assumed, and the pack must be rewrapped and resterilized. This is known as *event-related sterility,* meaning that a sterile pack is considered sterile indefinitely unless an event occurs that interferes with the sterility of the item.

Sterilized packs should be stored in a clean, dry area that is free from dust, insects, and other sources of contamination. Wrapped items should be stored with the most recently sterilized items placed in the back. The medical assistant should inspect each sterilized pack at least twice: before storing it and before using it. If the pack is torn or opened or if it is wet, it is no longer sterile and must be rewrapped and resterilized. Procedure 3.4 outlines a general procedure for sterilizing items in the autoclave.

MAINTAINING THE AUTOCLAVE

To ensure proper operation and maximum lifespan of the autoclave, it must be maintained properly. The manufacturer's operating manual provides specific information on the care and maintenance of the autoclave.

Safety precautions must be followed when performing maintenance procedures. Before proceeding with maintenance, the autoclave must be cool, the pressure gauge at zero, and the power cord disconnected from the wall socket.

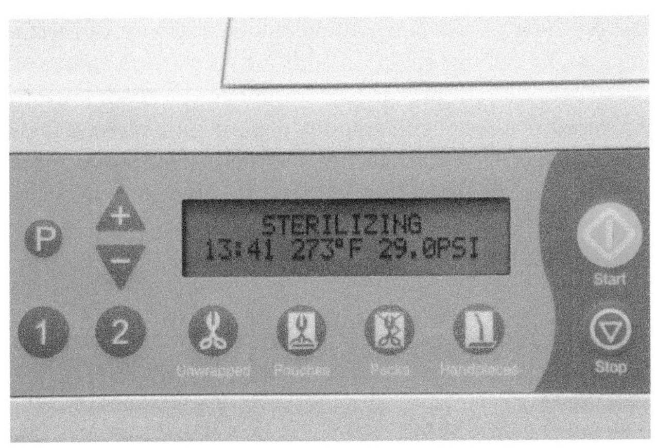

Fig. 3.16 Autoclave cycles used in the medical office: Unwrapped (items), pouches, and packs.

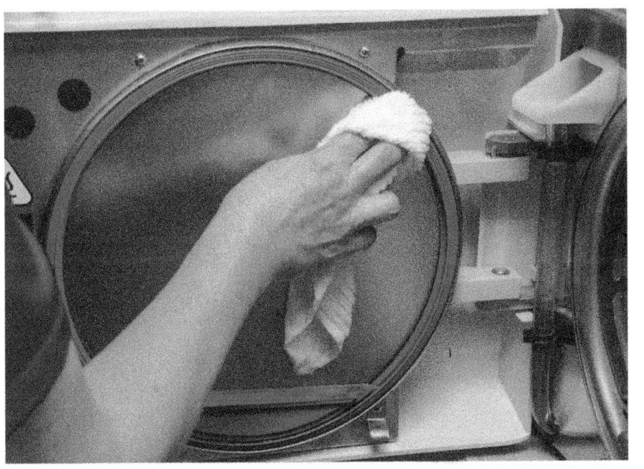

Fig. 3.17 The door gaskets are cleaned with a damp cloth during autoclave maintenance.

Autoclave maintenance should be performed on a daily, weekly, and monthly basis as follows.

Daily Maintenance

1. Wipe the outside of the autoclave with a damp cloth and a mild detergent.
2. Inspect the door gaskets for damage that could prevent a good seal.
3. Clean the rubber gaskets on the inside of the door of the autoclave with a damp cloth (Fig. 3.17).

Weekly Maintenance

1. Drain the water in the reservoir into a container and dispose of it.
2. Clean the inside of the chamber according to the manufacturer's instructions. This usually involves the following steps:
   - Remove the trays, and clean the chamber with a soft cloth or a soft brush and an autoclave cleaner. Do not use steel wool, a steel brush, or other abrasive agents because they can damage the chamber.
   - Rinse the chamber thoroughly with distilled water.
   - Thoroughly dry the chamber.
3. Wash the trays with an autoclave cleaner, and rinse them thoroughly with distilled water.
4. Refill the water reservoir with distilled water, and leave the door open overnight.

Monthly Maintenance

1. Flush the system with an autoclave cleaner to remove any buildup of residue, which could cause corrosion of the chamber lines. Carefully follow the manufacturer's operating manual to perform this procedure.
2. Wash the autoclave chamber and trays with an autoclave cleaner.
3. Remove and clean door gaskets with an autoclave cleaner and a soft brush.
4. Remove and clean filters with an autoclave cleaner and a stiff bristled brush, and rinse with distilled water. The filters prevent debris from causing valve failure.
5. Check the pressure relief valve to make sure it is functioning properly. The purpose of the pressure relief valve is to release excessive steam pressure during the autoclave cycle.

OTHER STERILIZATION METHODS

In addition to the autoclave, other methods can be used to sterilize items. These methods are not typically used in the medical office and are discussed only briefly in this chapter.

DRY HEAT OVEN

Dry heat ovens are used to sterilize items that cannot be penetrated by steam or may be damaged by it. Dry heat is less corrosive than moist heat for instruments with sharp edges; it does not dull their sharp edges. Moist heat sterilization tends to erode the ground-glass surfaces of reusable syringes, whereas dry heat does not.

Dry heat ovens operate similarly to ordinary cooking ovens. A longer exposure period is needed with dry heat because microorganisms and spores are more resistant to dry heat than to moist heat and because dry heat penetrates more slowly and unevenly than moist heat. The most commonly used temperature for dry heat sterilization is 320°F (160°C) for 2 hours or 340°F (170°C) for 1 hour. The recommended wrapping material for dry heat sterilization is aluminum foil because it is a good conductor of heat, and it protects against recontamination during handling and storage. Dry heat sterilization indicators are available to determine the effectiveness of the sterilization process.

ETHYLENE OXIDE GAS STERILIZATION

Ethylene oxide is a colorless gas that is toxic and flammable. It is used to sterilize heat-sensitive items that cannot be sterilized in an autoclave. After items are sterilized with this gas, they must be aerated to remove the toxic residue of the ethylene oxide.

Ethylene oxide sterilization is a more complex and expensive process than steam sterilization. It frequently is used in the medical manufacturing industry for processing prepackaged, disposable items, such as syringes, sutures, catheters, and surgical packs.

COLD STERILIZATION

Cold sterilization involves the use of a chemical agent for an extended length of time. Only chemicals that are designated *sterilants* by the Environmental Protection Agency (EPA) can be used for sterilizing items. If a chemical agent holds this status, the word *sterilant* is printed on the front of the container.

The item to be sterilized must be completely submerged in the sterilant for a long period (6 to 24 hours depending on the type of sterilant). Prolonged immersion of instruments can damage them. In addition, each time an instrument is added to the sterilant container, the clock must be restarted for the entire amount of time. For these reasons and because this method involves the use of a hazardous chemical, cold sterilization should be used only when an autoclave, gas, or a dry heat oven is not indicated or is unavailable.

RADIATION

Radiation uses high-energy ionizing radiation to sterilize items. Medical manufacturers use radiation to sterilize prepackaged surgical equipment and instruments that cannot be sterilized by heat or chemicals.

What Would You Do? What Would You *Not* Do? RESPONSES

Case Study 1

Page 61

What Did Linda Do?

- ❑ Complimented Mrs. Cordera for her concern and efforts to baby-proof her home.
- ❑ Gave Mrs. Cordera a patient information brochure on baby-proofing the home.
- ❑ Told Mrs. Cordera that she should assume that all cleaning products are poisonous. Showed Mrs. Corder a chemical disinfectant container label and pointed out the information on the label that tells what to do in case of an accidental poisoning.
- ❑ Gave the Poison Help Line number (1-800-222-1222) to Mrs. Cordera and told her that is the fastest way to determine what to do in case of accidental poisoning. Told her to keep this number by her phone.

What Did Linda Not Do?

- ❑ Did not take Mrs. Cordera's question lightly.

Case Study 2

Page 72

What Did Linda Do?

- ❑ Told Cassie that her concern was valid.
- ❑ Told Cassie that hepatitis C can be transmitted through contaminated instruments.
- ❑ Reassured Cassie that surgical instruments used in the medical office are properly sterilized in the autoclave and include the use of sterilization indicators to ensure all germs have been killed.
- ❑ Gave Cassie a patient information sheet on hepatitis C. Told her that individuals with chronic hepatitis C can develop liver cancer and that the best way to avoid hepatitis C is through preventative measures and behaviors.
- ❑ Told Cassie that a vaccine is not yet available to prevent hepatitis C; however, there are antiviral medications available to treat hepatitis C that are 95% effective.

What Did Linda Not Do?

- ❑ Did not minimize Cassie's concern about contaminated instruments.
- ❑ Did not overly alarm Cassie about the consequences of chronic hepatitis C.

Terminology Review

Term	Definition
Autoclave	An apparatus for the sterilization of materials, using steam under pressure.
Critical item	An item that comes in contact with sterile tissue or the vascular system.
Decontamination	The use of physical or chemical means to remove pathogens from an item so that it is no longer capable of transmitting disease.
Detergent	An agent that cleanses by emulsifying dirt and oil.
Disinfectant	An agent used to destroy pathogenic microorganisms but not their spores. Disinfectants are usually applied to inanimate objects and surfaces.
Hazardous chemical	Any chemical that is a health or a physical hazard.
Health hazard	The potential of a chemical to cause acute toxicity, skin corrosion or irritation, serious eye damage or irritation, respiratory or skin sensitization, germ cell mutagenicity, cancer or reproductive toxicity, or is an aspiration hazard.
Incubate	To provide proper conditions for growth and development.
Load	The items that are being sterilized.
Noncritical item	An item that comes into contact with intact skin but not with mucous membranes.
Physical hazard	The potential of a chemical to catch fire, explode, or react with other chemicals.
Safety data sheet	A document that provides detailed information on a chemical, its hazards, and measures to take to prevent injury and illness when handling the chemical.
Sanitization	A series of steps designed to removes debris from an item and reduce the number of microorganisms to a safe level.
Semicritical item	An item that comes into contact with nonintact skin or intact mucous membranes.
Spore	A hard, thick-walled capsule formed by some bacteria that contains only the essential parts of the protoplasm of the bacterial cell.
Sterilization	The process of destroying all forms of microbial life, including spores.

PROCEDURE 3.1 Sanitization of Instruments

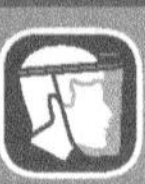

Outcome Sanitize instruments

Equipment/Supplies
- Sink
- Disposable gloves
- Heavy-duty utility gloves
- Contaminated instruments
- High-level disinfectant and safety data sheet (SDS)
- Disinfectant container
- Instrument cleaner and SDS
- Basin
- Stiff nylon brush
- Stainless-steel wire brush
- Paper towels
- Cloth towel
- Instrument lubricant

1. **Procedural Step.** Review the SDS for the hazardous chemicals you will be using in the sanitization process.
   Principle. An SDS provides information regarding a chemical agent, its hazards, and measures to take to prevent injury and illness when handling a chemical agent.
2. **Procedural Step.** Apply disposable gloves. Transport the contaminated instruments to the cleaning area as soon as possible after use. The instruments should be carried in a covered basin from the examining room to the cleaning area.
   Principle. Disposable gloves act as a barrier to protect the medical assistant from infectious materials. Transporting contaminated instruments in a covered basin promotes infection control.
3. **Procedural Step.** Apply heavy-duty utility gloves over the disposable gloves.
   Principle. Utility gloves help protect the hands from the irritating effects of chemical solutions.
4. **Procedural Step.** Separate sharp instruments and delicate instruments from other instruments.
   Principle. Separating sharp instruments from others prevents damage to or dulling of the cutting edge of these instruments. Delicate instruments should be separated to protect them from damage.
5. **Procedural Step.** Immediately rinse the instruments thoroughly under warm, not hot, running water (approximately 110°F [44°C]) to remove debris, such as blood, body fluids, and tissue.
   Principle. Rinsing the instruments as soon as possible prevents debris from drying on the instruments, making it difficult to remove later. Hot water may cause coagulation of organic material, making it more difficult to remove.

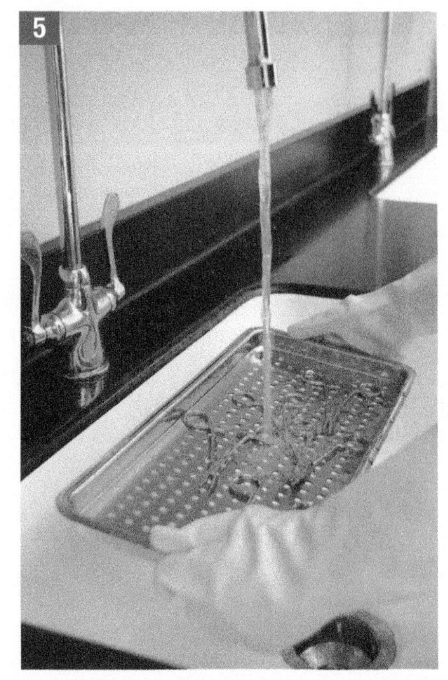

Rinse instruments under warm water to remove debris.

6. **Procedural Step.** Decontaminate the instruments with a high-level chemical disinfectant as follows:
   a. Select the proper chemical disinfectant (e.g., glutaraldehyde), and review the SDS for the disinfectant.
   b. Check the expiration date on the container label.
   c. Review and observe all precautionary statements listed on the label of the disinfectant (e.g., wear protective gloves and eye protection).
   d. Read the manufacturer's instructions for the proper activation, dilution, and use of the disinfectant.
   e. Label the container that will hold the disinfectant with the name of the disinfectant and the date when the disinfectant is no longer effective and must be discarded (reuse life).
   f. Pour the chemical into the disinfectant container, and immerse the items into the disinfectant. Ensure the items are completely submerged in the disinfectant.
   g. Cover the container, and disinfect the items for 10 minutes.

   Principle. Decontamination removes pathogenic microorganisms from the instruments, making them safe to handle. A disinfectant past its expiration date loses its

PROCEDURE 3.1 Sanitization of Instruments—cont'd

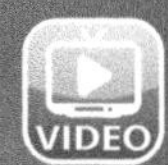

potency and should not be used. The container must be kept covered to prevent the escape of toxic fumes and to prevent evaporation of the disinfectant, which could change its potency.

7. Procedural Step. Clean the instruments. The instruments can be cleaned using the manual method or the ultrasound method as follows.

Manual Method for Cleaning Instruments

a. Obtain the instrument cleaner, and check its expiration date.
b. Review and observe all personal safety precautions listed on the label of the instrument cleaner.
c. Prepare the instrument cleaning solution following the manufacturer's directions for proper mixing and use.
d. Remove the items from the disinfectant, and place them in the basin containing the instrument cleaner.
e. Use a stiff nylon brush to clean the surface of each instrument. Scrub all parts of the instrument thoroughly. Brush delicate instruments carefully to prevent damaging them.

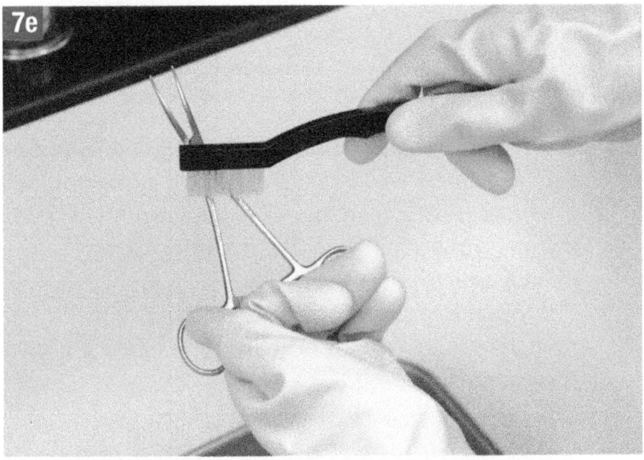

Clean the surface of the instrument with a stiff nylon brush.

f. Use a stainless-steel wire brush to clean grooves, crevices, or serrations where debris such as blood and tissue may collect.

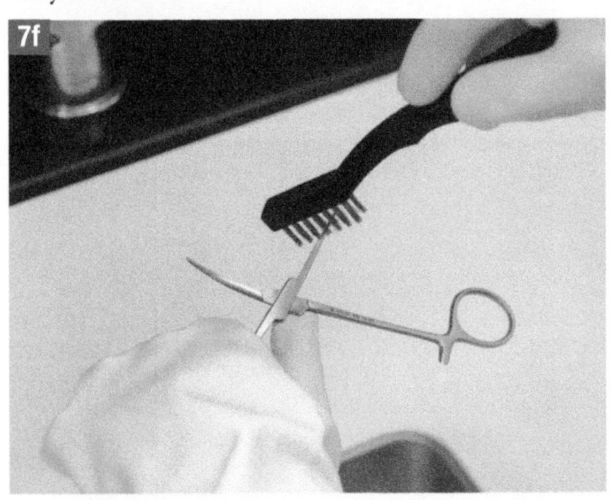

Clean gloves, crevices, or serrations with a wire brush.

g. If there is a stain on the instrument, attempt to remove it with an instrument stain remover.
h. Scrub each instrument until it is visibly clean and free from debris and stains.

Principle. An instrument cleaner past its expiration date loses its potency and should not be used. Taking appropriate precautions with cleaning agents prevents harm to the medical assistant. All debris must be removed from the instruments to ensure proper sterilization.

Ultrasound Method for Cleaning Instruments

a. Using the ultrasonic instrument cleaner recommended by the manufacturer, check the expiration date and prepare the cleaning solution in the ultrasonic cleaner. Observe all personal safety precautions listed on the label.
b. Remove the items from the disinfectant, and separate instruments made of dissimilar metals, such as stainless steel, aluminum, and bronze.
c. Place the instruments in the ultrasonic cleaner with hinged instruments in an open position.
d. Ensure that sharp instruments do not touch other instruments.
e. Ensure that all instruments are fully submerged in the cleaning solution.

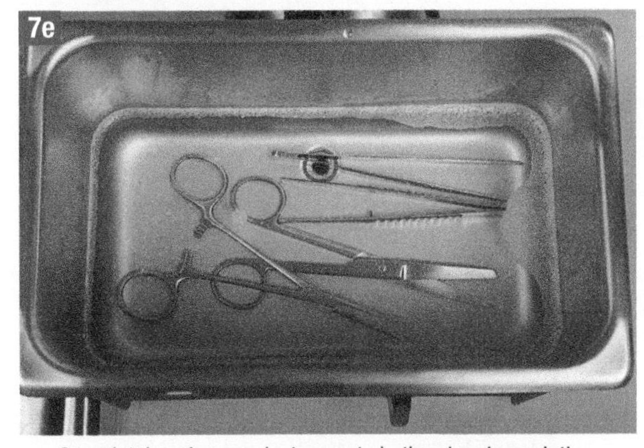

Completely submerge instruments in the cleaning solution.

f. Place the lid on the ultrasonic cleaner.

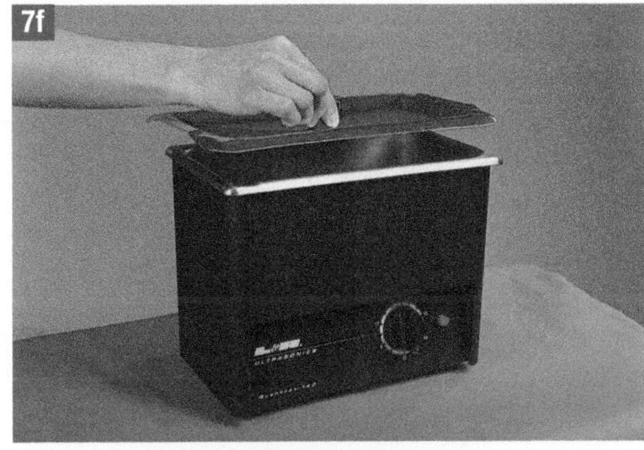

Place the lid on the ultrasonic cleaner.

Continued

PROCEDURE 3.1 Sanitization of Instruments—cont'd

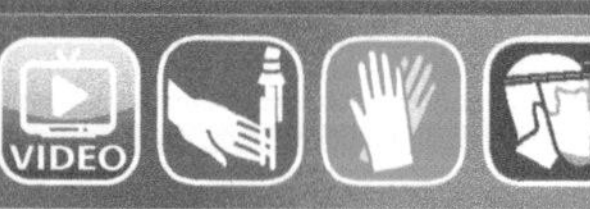

g. Turn on the ultrasonic cleaner, and clean the instruments for the length of time recommended by the manufacturer.
h. After completion of the cleaning cycle, remove the instruments from the machine.

Principle. Taking appropriate precautions with chemical agents prevents harm to the medical assistant from hazardous chemicals. Mixing dissimilar metals together could result in permanent stains on the instruments. Instruments must be completely submerged with hinged instruments in an open position so the solution can reach all parts of the instrument.

8. Procedural Step. Rinse each instrument thoroughly with warm, not hot, water (110°F [44°C]) for at least 20 to 30 seconds to remove all traces of the detergent. Open and close hinged instruments while rinsing to ensure the solution is completely rinsed out of every part of the instrument.

Principle. Detergent residue left on the instrument could cause stains, which could build up and interfere with proper functioning of the instrument. Using warm water helps to remove the cleaning solution and facilitates the drying process.

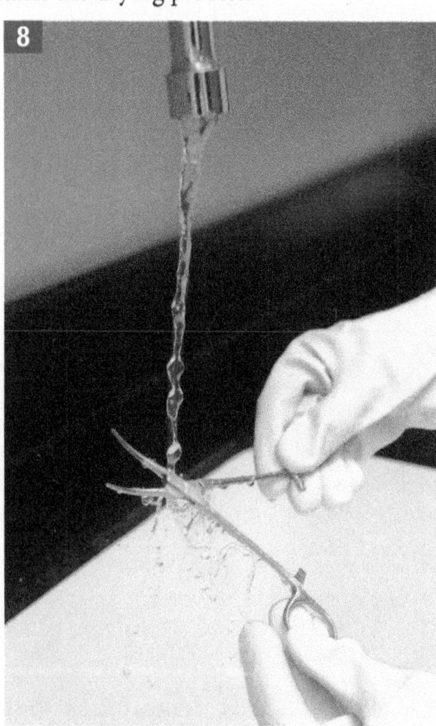

Rinse thoroughly with warm water.

9. Procedural Step. Dry each instrument with a paper towel, and place the instrument on a cloth towel for additional air drying.

Principle. If the instrument is not completely dry, stains may occur on the instrument.

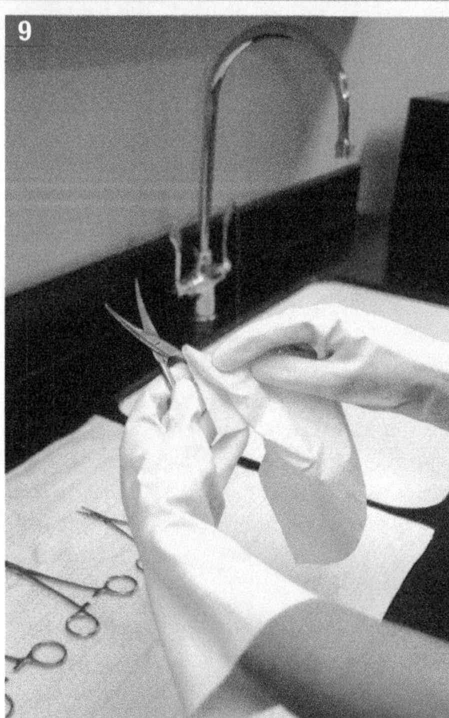

Dry the instrument with a paper towel.

10. Procedural Step. Inspect each instrument for defects and proper working condition. Scissors should cut all the way to the end of a thin piece of gauze without catching. If defects are noted or the instrument is not working properly, it must be discarded or sent to the manufacturer for repair.

Principle. Instruments that have defects or are not in proper working condition are not safe to use during a medical or surgical procedure.

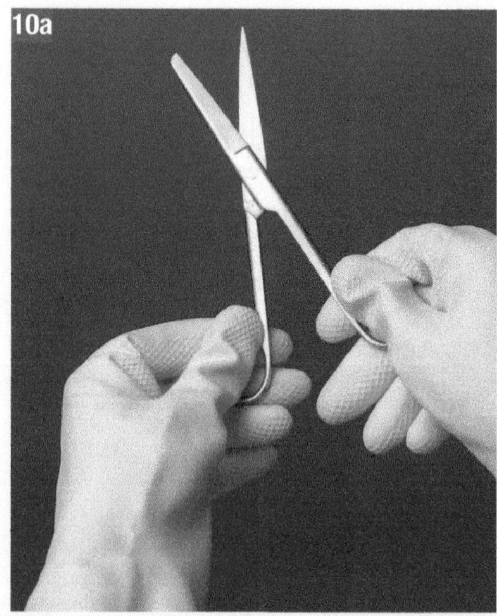

Inspect the instrument for defects and proper working order.

PROCEDURE 3.1 Sanitization of Instruments—cont'd

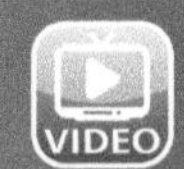
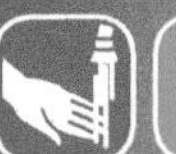

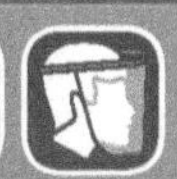

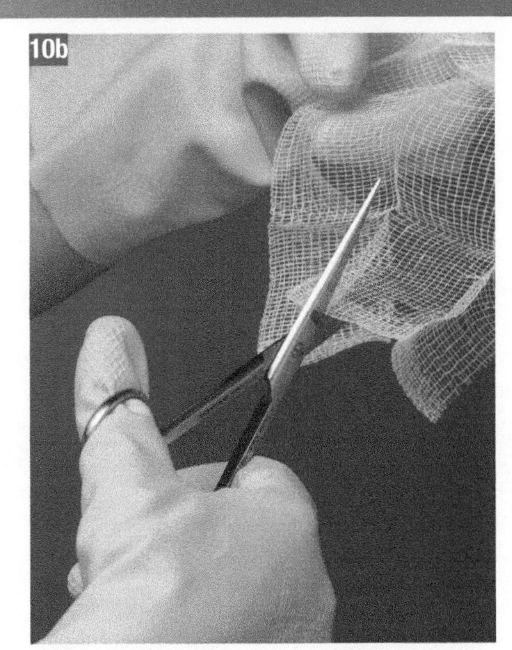

Scissors should cut through gauze without catching.

11. Procedural Step. Lubricate hinged instruments using a steam-penetrable lubricant as follows:

a. Apply the lubricant to a hinged instrument in its open position.

b. Open and close the instrument after applying the lubricant so it reaches all parts of the hinged area.

c. Place the instrument back on the towel, and allow it to drain. Rinsing or wiping is unnecessary.

Principle. Lubricating an instrument makes it function better and last longer.

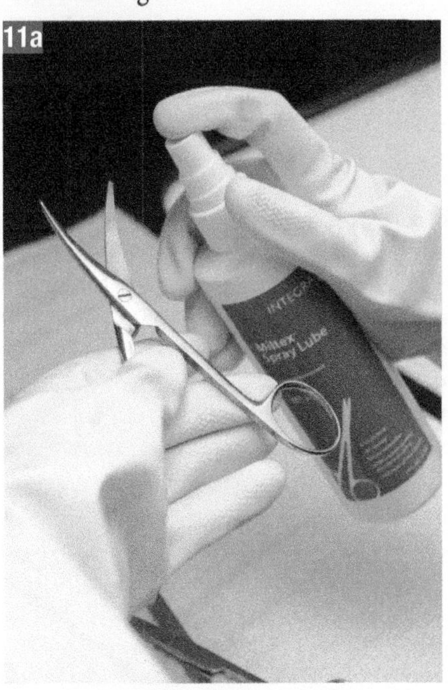

Lubricate hinged instruments.

12. Procedural Step. Dispose of the cleaning solution according to the manufacturer's instructions. Remove both sets of gloves, and sanitize your hands.

13. Procedural Step. Wrap the instruments and sterilize them in the autoclave.

PROCEDURE 3.2 Wrapping an Instrument Using Sterilization Paper

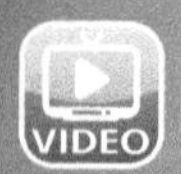

Outcome Wrap an instrument using sterilization paper

Equipment/Supplies
- Sanitized instrument
- Appropriate-sized sterilization wrapping paper
- Sterilization indicator strip
- Autoclave tape
- Permanent marker

1. **Procedural Step.** Sanitize your hands.
2. **Procedural Step.** Assemble the equipment. Select the appropriate-sized wrapping paper for the instrument being wrapped. Check the expiration date on the box of sterilization indicators. If the indicator strips are outdated, do not use them.
   Principle. Instruments are wrapped so they are protected from recontamination following sterilization. Outdated indicator strips may not provide accurate test results.
3. **Procedural Step.** Place the wrapping paper on a clean, flat surface. Turn the wrap in a diagonal position to your body so that it resembles a diamond shape.

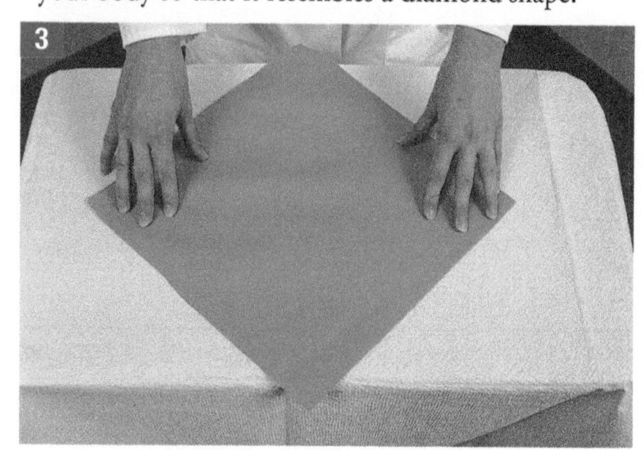

Turn the wrapping paper in a diagonal position.

4. **Procedural Step.** Place the instrument in the center of the wrapping paper with the longest part of the instrument pointing toward the two side corners. If the instrument has a movable joint, place it on the wrap in a slightly open position. If necessary, a gauze square can be used to hold the instrument in an open position.
   Principle. Instruments with movable joints must be in an open position to allow steam to reach all parts of the instrument. If the instrument is in a closed position, heat exposure could cause the instrument to crack at its weakest part, such as the lock area.
5. **Procedural Step.** Place an indicator strip in the center of the wrap next to the instrument.
   Principle. Indicator strips assess the effectiveness of the sterilization process.

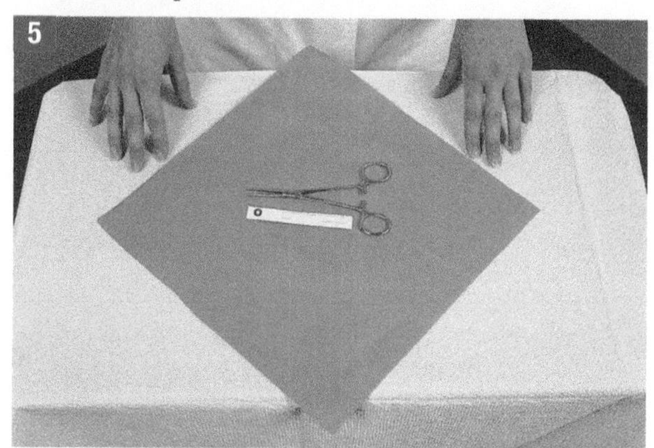

Place an indicator strip in the center of the wrap next to the instrument.

6. **Procedural Step.** Fold the wrapping paper up from the bottom, and double-back a small corner, creating a flap. This flap will later be used to open the sterile pack without contaminating the instrument.

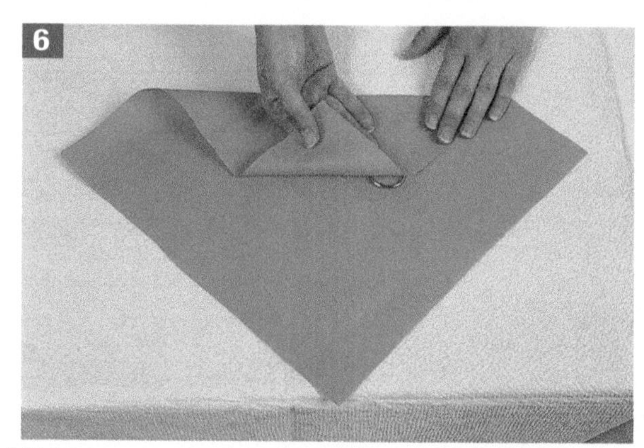

Fold the wrapping paper up from the bottom, and double-back a small corner.

PROCEDURE 3.2 Wrapping an Instrument Using Sterilization Paper—cont'd

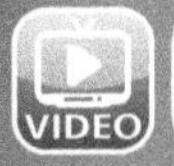

7. **Procedural Step.** Fold over one edge of the wrapping paper, and double-back the corner.
8. **Procedural Step.** Fold over the other edge of the wrapping paper, and double-back the corner.

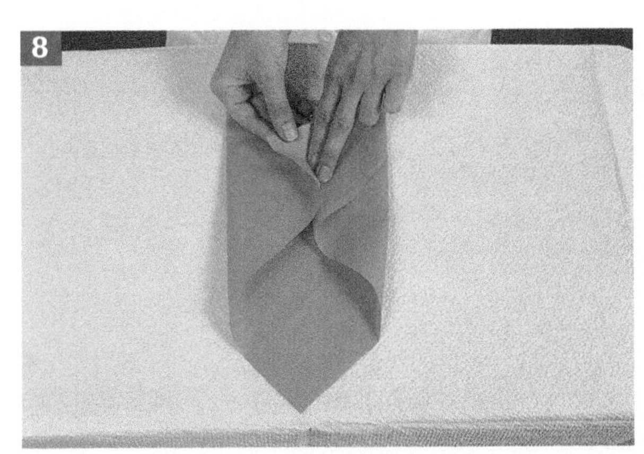

Fold over the other edge of the wrapping paper, and double-back the corner.

9. **Procedural Step.** Fold the wrapping paper up from the bottom, pull the top flap down, and secure it with autoclave tape. Ensure that the pack is firm enough for handling but loose enough to permit proper circulation of steam.
   Principle. An instrument must be wrapped properly to permit full penetration of steam and to prevent contaminating it when the pack is opened. Using autoclave tape indicates that the pack has been through the autoclave cycle and prevents mix-ups with packs that have not been processed.

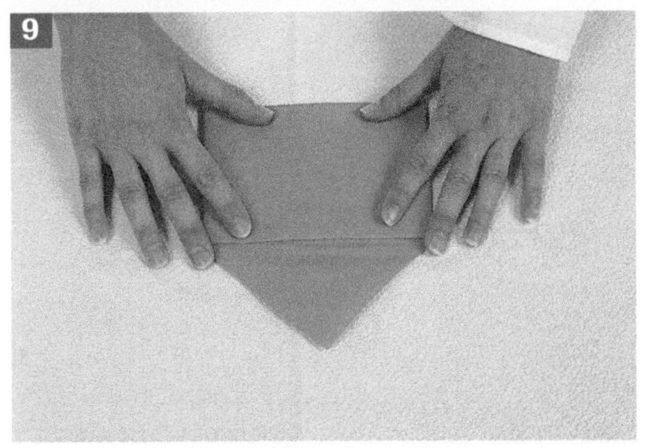

Fold the wrapping paper up from the bottom.

10. **Procedural Step.** Label the pack according to its contents. Mark the pack with the date of sterilization and your initials.
    Principle. Dating the pack helps in ensuring that the most recently sterilized packs are stored behind previously sterilized packs.

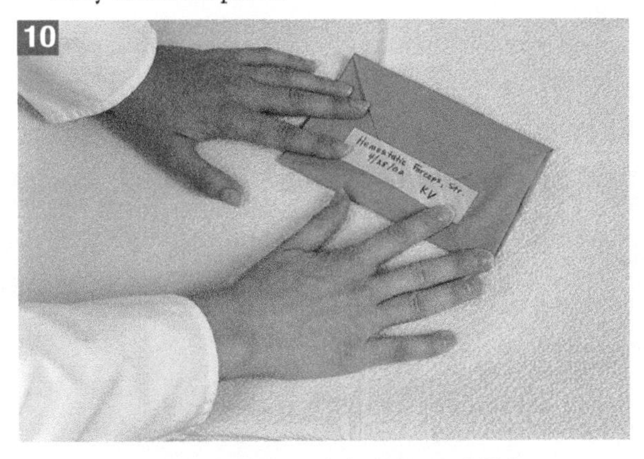

Label and date the pack. Include your initials.

PROCEDURE 3.3 Wrap an Instrument Using a Pouch

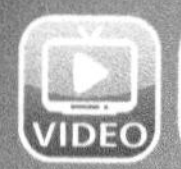

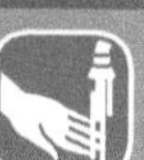

Outcome Wrap an instrument using a pouch

Equipment/Supplies

- Sanitized instrument
- Appropriate-sized sterilization pouch
- Permanent marker

1. **Procedural Step.** Sanitize your hands.
2. **Procedural Step.** Assemble the equipment. Select the appropriate-sized sterilization pouch for the instrument being wrapped. For hinged instruments, use a pouch wide enough so the instrument can be placed in a slightly open position inside the pouch.
   Principle. Instruments are wrapped so they are protected from recontamination following sterilization.
3. **Procedural Step.** Place the pouch on a clean, flat surface.
4. **Procedural Step.** Label the pack according to its contents. Mark the pouch with the date of sterilization and your initials.
   Principle. Dating the pouch helps in ensuring that the most recently sterilized pouches are stored behind previously sterilized pouches.

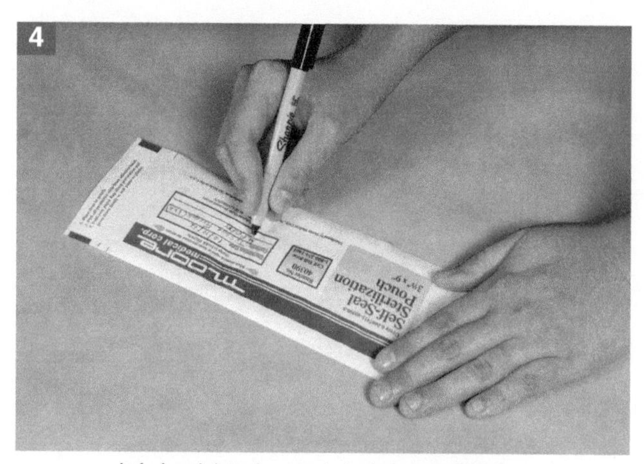

Label and date the pouch. Include your initials.

5. **Procedural Step.** Insert the instrument to be sterilized into the unsealed, open end of the pouch. If the instrument has a movable joint, place it in the pouch in a slightly open position.

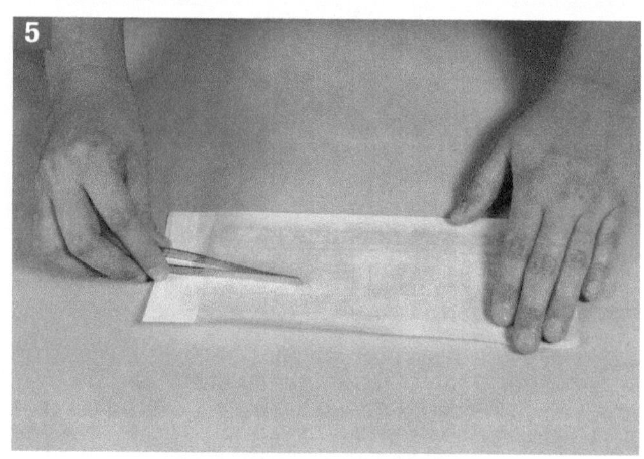

Insert the instrument into the pouch.

6. **Procedural Step.** Seal the open end of the pouch as follows:
   Adhesive Closure. Peel off the paper strip located above the perforated line to expose the adhesive. Fold along the perforated line and press firmly to seal the paper to the plastic. Ensure that the seal is secure by running your fingers back and forth on both sides of the pouch over the entire sealing area.
   Heat Closure. Seal the pouch using a heat-sealing device.

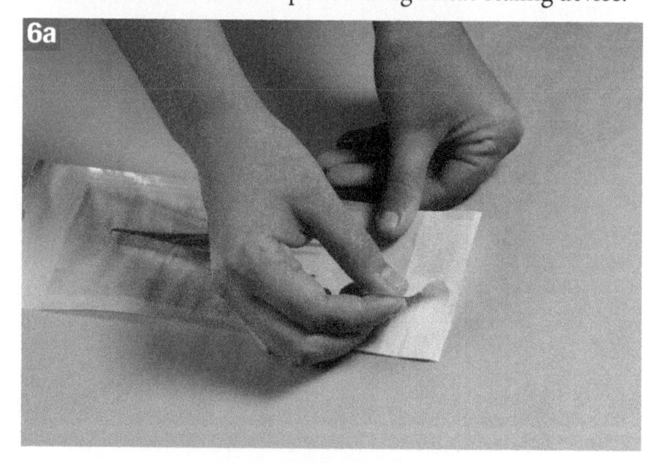

Peel off the paper strip.

PROCEDURE 3.3 Wrap an Instrument Using a Pouch—cont'd

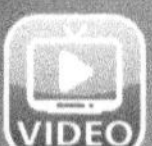

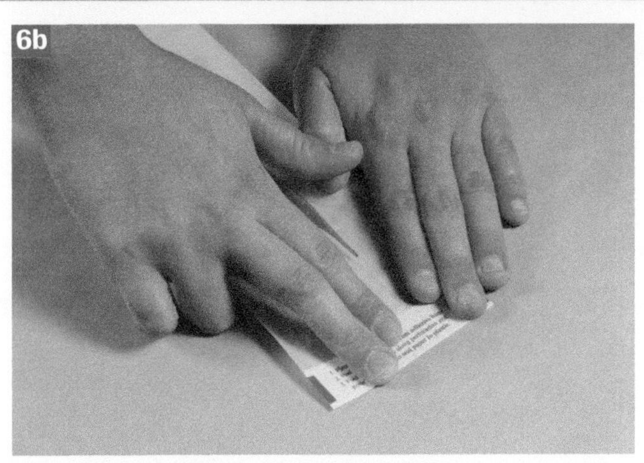

6b

Press firmly to seal the pouch.

7. **Procedural Step.** Sterilize the pouch in the autoclave.

PROCEDURE 3.4 Sterilizing Items in an Autoclave

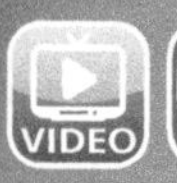

Outcome Sterilize a load in an autoclave

Equipment/Supplies

- Autoclave and operating manual
- Distilled water
- Wrapped items
- Heat-resistant gloves

1. **Procedural Step.** Assemble the equipment.
2. **Procedural Step.** Check the level of water in the water reservoir and add distilled water, if needed.
   Principle. Distilled water is used to prevent corrosion of the stainless-steel chamber of the autoclave.

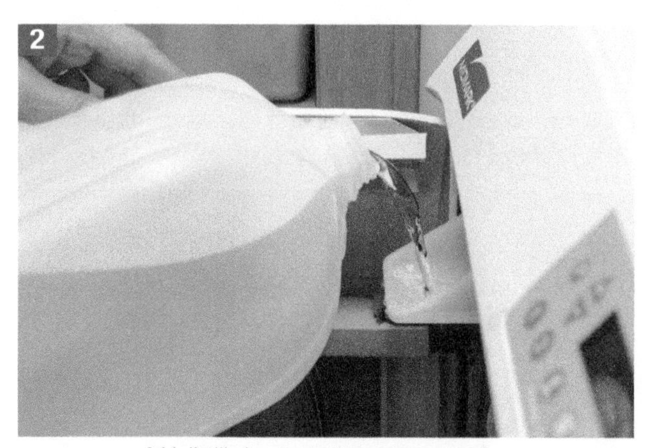
Add distilled water to the water reservoir.

3. **Procedural Step.** Properly load the autoclave following these guidelines:
   a. Place small packs 1–3 inches apart and large packs 2–4 inches apart.
   b. Place pouches vertically on their sides in a metal rack to maximize steam circulation and facilitate drying. As an alternative, pouches can be placed flat on a tray with the paper side up and the plastic side down to allow moisture to escape through the paper side during the drying process.
   c. Do not allow the packs to touch the chamber walls.
   d. Ensure that at least 1 inch separates the autoclave trays.
   Principle. The autoclave must be loaded properly to ensure proper steam circulation and to facilitate the drying process.

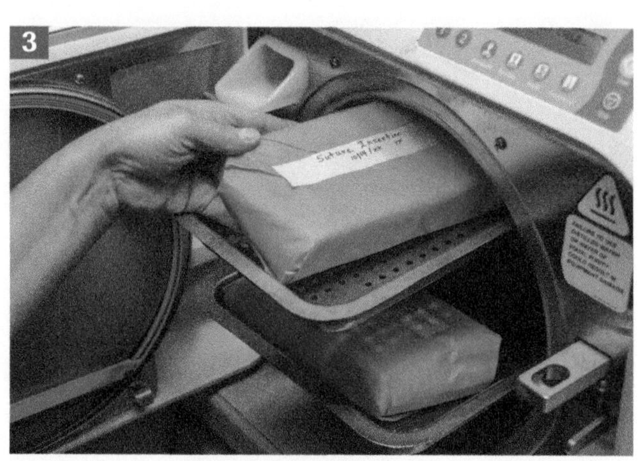
Properly load the autoclave.

4. **Procedural Step.** Operate the autoclave according to the procedure described in the operating manual. A general procedure for autoclave operation is outlined as follows.
   a. Close and latch the door of the autoclave.
   b. Determine the autoclave cycle according to what is being sterilized as follows:
      - Unwrapped items
      - Pouches
      - Wrapped items
   c. Select the desired autoclave cycle by pressing the appropriate button on the autoclave.
   d. Press the start button. A message on the display screen (or indicator light) identifies each stage of the autoclave cycle to tell you what is happening in the autoclave as follows:
      - ***Filling:*** The chamber is filling with water
      - ***Heating:*** The temperature and pressure are increasing until the desired parameters are reached
      - ***Sterilizing:*** The load is being sterilized at the proper time, temperature, and pressure
      - ***Venting:*** Steam is venting from the chamber
      - ***Drying:*** The door cracks and the load is drying
      - ***Ready:*** The autoclave cycle is complete, and the sterilized load can be removed from the autoclave

PROCEDURE 3.4 Sterilizing Items in an Autoclave—cont'd

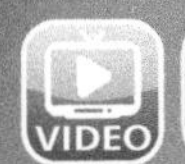

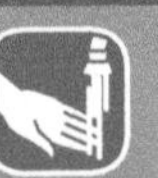

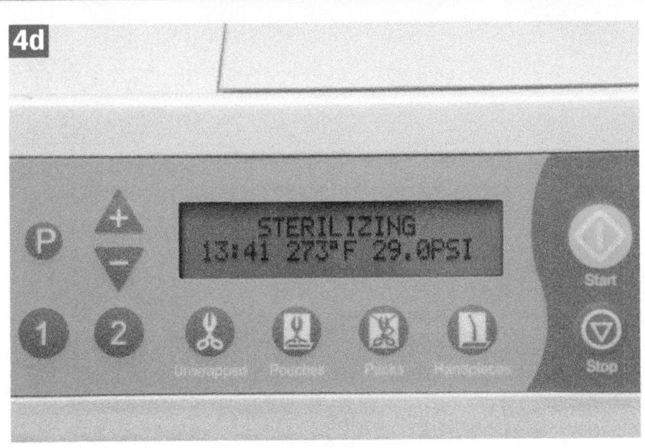

Sterilizing stage.

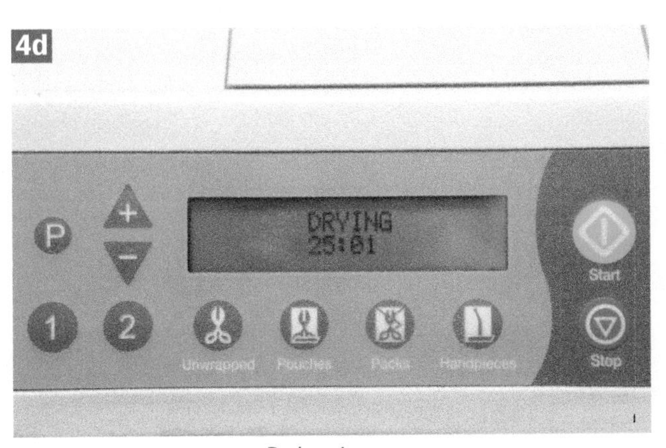

Drying stage.

5. Procedural Step. Turn off the autoclave. Wearing heat-resistant gloves, remove the load from the autoclave. Do not touch the inner chamber of the autoclave with your bare hands.

Principle. Heat-resistant gloves protect the medical assistant's hands when the warm packs from the autoclave are being removed. The chamber of the autoclave is hot and could burn bare skin.

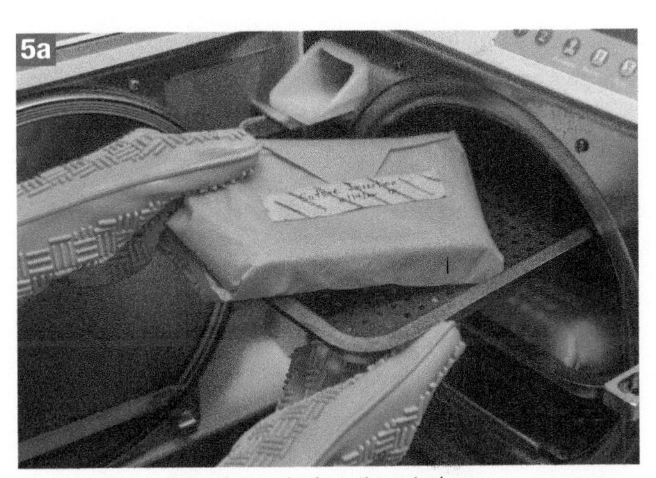

Removing packs from the autoclave.

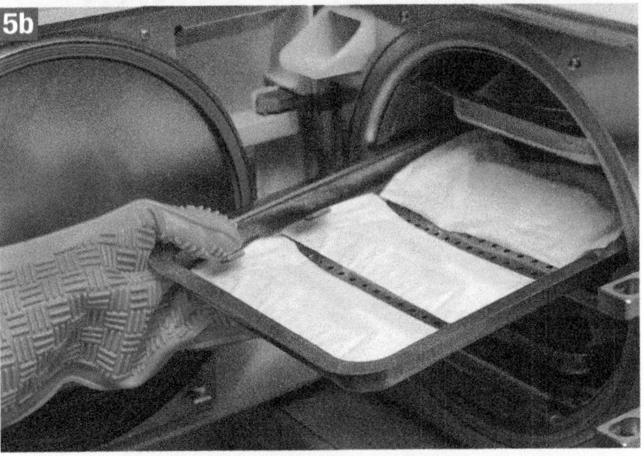

Removing pouches from the autoclave.

6. Procedural Step. Inspect the packs as you take them out of the autoclave. If a pack shows any damage, such as holes or tears, the pack should be rewrapped and resterilized.

7. Procedural Step. Check the autoclave tape on the outside of each pack to ensure the proper response has occurred.

Principle. Autoclave tape indicates only that the item has been through the autoclave cycle; it does not ensure that sterilization has taken place. Sterilization is confirmed when the pack is opened for use and the sterilization indicator strip in the center of the pack is checked for its proper response.

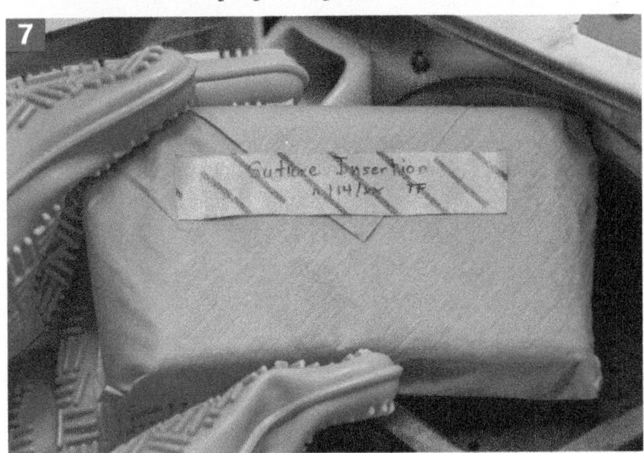

Check the autoclave tape on the outside of the pack.

8. Procedural Step. Document monitoring information in the autoclave log. Include the date and time of the cycle, a description of the load, and the exposure time and temperature. If a biologic indicator has been included in the load, process it according to the medical office policy, and document results on the autoclave log.

9. Procedural Step. Store the packs in a clean, dustproof area with the most recently sterilized packs placed behind previously sterilized packs.

10. Procedural Step. Maintain appropriate daily care of the autoclave, following the manufacturer's recommendations.

4 Vital Signs

 Check out the Evolve site at http://evolve.elsevier.com/Bonewit/today/ to access additional interactive activities and exercises to help you study and prepare for success.

LEARNING OUTCOMES	PROCEDURES
Temperature	
1. Define a vital sign. 2. Explain the reasons for taking vital signs. 3. Explain how body temperature is maintained. 4. List examples of how heat is produced in the body. 5. List examples of how heat is lost from the body. 6. State the normal body temperature range and the average body temperature. 7. List and explain factors that can cause variation in the body temperature. 8. List and describe the three stages of a fever. 9. List the sites for taking body temperature, and explain why these sites are used.	Measure oral body temperature. Measure axillary body temperature. Measure rectal body temperature. Measure aural body temperature. Measure temporal artery body temperature.
Pulse	
10. Explain the mechanism of pulse. 11. List and explain the factors that affect the pulse rate. 12. Identify a specific use for each of the eight pulse sites. 13. State the normal range of pulse rate for each age group. 14. Explain the difference between pulse rhythm and pulse volume.	Measure radial pulse. Measure apical pulse.
Respiration	
15. Explain the purpose of respiration. 16. State what occurs during inhalation and exhalation. 17. State the normal respiratory rate for each age group. 18. List and explain the factors that affect the respiratory rate. 19. Explain the difference between rhythm and depth of respiration. 20. Describe the character of each of the following abnormal breath sounds: crackles, rhonchi, wheezes, and pleural friction rub.	Measure respiration.
Pulse Oximetry	
21. Explain the purpose of pulse oximetry. 22. State the normal oxygen saturation level of a healthy individual. 23. Explain how pulse oximetry results are interpreted. 24. List and describe the functions of the controls, indicators and displays on a pulse oximeter. 25. List and describe factors that may interfere with an accurate pulse oximetry reading.	Perform pulse oximetry.
Blood Pressure	
26. Define blood pressure. 27. Identify the blood pressure categories for an adult. 28. List and describe factors that can temporarily affect the blood pressure. 29. List and describe the risk factors that increase the risk of developing primary hypertension. 30. List and describe the categories of hypotension. 31. Identify and describe the different parts of a stethoscope and a sphygmomanometer. 32. Describe the methods for determining proper cuff size. 33. Describe the five phases of the Korotkoff sounds. 34. State the advantages and disadvantages of an automatic blood pressure monitor. 35. Explain how to prevent errors in blood pressure measurement.	Measure blood pressure. Determine systolic pressure by palpation.

CHAPTER OUTLINE

KEY TERMS

adventitious (ad-ven-TISH-us) sounds
afebrile (uh-FEB-ril)
alveoli (al-VEE-oh-lie)
antecubital (AN-tih-CYOO-bi-tul) space
antipyretic (AN-tih-pye-REH-tik)
aorta (ay-OR-tuh)
apnea (AP-nee-uh)
axilla (aks-ILL-uh)
blood pressure
bounding pulse
bradycardia (BRAY-dee-CAR-dee-uh)
bradypnea (BRAY-dip-NEE-uh)
Celsius (SELL-see-us) scale
conduction (kon-DUK-shun)
convection (kon-VEK-shun)
crisis
cross-contamination
cyanosis (sye-an-OH-sus)
diastole (dye-AS-toh-lee)
diastolic (DYE-uh-STOL-ik) pressure
dyspnea (DISP-nee-uh)
dysrhythmia (dis-RITH-mee-uh)
eupnea (YOOP-nee-uh)
exhalation (EKS-hal-AY-shun)
Fahrenheit (FAIR-en-hite) scale
febrile (FEH-bril)
fever
frenulum linguae (FREN-yoo-lum LIN-gway)
hyperpnea (HYE-perp-NEE-uh)
hyperpyrexia (HYE-per-pye-REK-see-uh)
hypertension (HYE-per-TEN-shun)
hyperventilation (HYE-per-ven-til-AY-shun)
hypopnea (hye-POP-nee-uh)
hypotension (HYE-poe-TEN-shun)
hypothermia (HYE-poe-THER-mee-uh)
hypoxemia (hye-pok-SEE-mee-uh)
hypoxia (hye-POKS-ee-uh)
inhalation (IN-hal-AY-shun)
intercostal (IN-ter-KOS-tul)
Korotkoff (kuh-ROT-kof) sounds
malaise (mal-AYZE)
manometer (man-OM-uh-ter)
orthopnea (orth-OP-nee-uh)
pulse deficit
pulse oximeter
pulse oximetry
pulse pressure
pulse rhythm
pulse volume
radiation (RAY-dee-AY-shun)
Sao_2
sphygmomanometer (SFIG-moe-man-OM-uh-ter)
SpO_2
stethoscope (STETH-uh-skope)
systole (SIS-toh-lee)
systolic (sis-TOL-ik) pressure
tachycardia (TAK-ih-KAR-dee-uh)
tachypnea (TAK-ip-NEE-uh)
thready pulse

Introduction to Vital Signs

Vital signs are objective guideposts that provide data to determine a person's state of health. Vital signs include temperature, pulse, and respiration (collectively called *TPR*), and blood pressure. Another indicator of a patient's health status is pulse oximetry. Some providers order this measurement routinely for all patients, while other providers only order it when the patient complains of respiratory problems (e.g., shortness of breath).

The normal ranges of the vital signs are finely adjusted, and any deviation from normal may indicate disease. During the course of an illness, variations in the vital signs may occur. The medical assistant should be alert to any significant changes and report them to the provider because they indicate a change in the patient's condition. When patients visit the medical office, vital signs are routinely checked to establish each patient's usual state of health and to establish baseline measurements against which future measurements can be compared. The medical assistant should have a thorough knowledge of the vital signs and should attain proficiency in taking them to ensure accurate measurements.

General guidelines that the medical assistant should follow when measuring the vital signs are as follows:

1. Be familiar with the normal ranges for all vital signs. Keep in mind that normal ranges vary based on the different age groups (infant, child, adult, elder).
2. Make sure that all equipment for measuring vital signs is in proper working condition to ensure accurate findings.
3. Eliminate or minimize factors that affect the vital signs, such as physical exercise, food and beverage consumption, tobacco use, and emotional states.

Temperature

REGULATION OF BODY TEMPERATURE

Body temperature is maintained within a fairly constant range by the hypothalamus, which is located in the brain. The hypothalamus functions as the body's thermostat. It normally allows the body temperature to vary by only about 1° to 2° Fahrenheit (F) throughout the day.

Body temperature is maintained through a balance of the heat produced in the body and the heat lost from the body (Fig. 4.1). A constant temperature range must be maintained for the body to function properly. When minor changes in the temperature of the body occur, the hypothalamus senses this and makes adjustments as necessary to ensure that the body temperature stays within a normal and safe range. If an individual is playing tennis on a hot day, the body's heat-cooling mechanism is activated to remove excess heat from the body through perspiration.

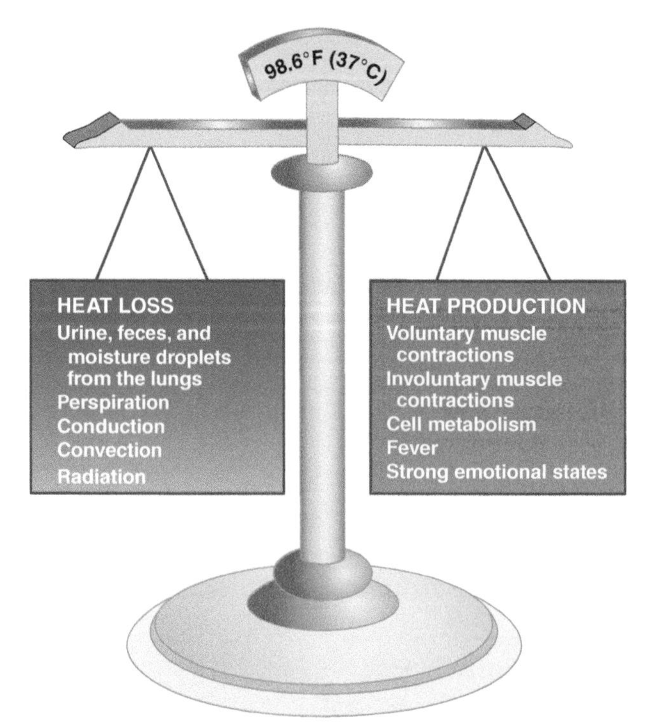

Fig. 4.1 Body temperature represents a balance between the heat produced in the body and the heat lost from the body.

HEAT PRODUCTION

Most of the heat produced in the body is through voluntary and involuntary muscle contractions. Voluntary muscle contractions involve the muscles over which a person has control, for example, the moving of legs or arms. Involuntary muscle contractions involve the muscles over which a person has no control; examples are physiologic processes such as digestion, the beating of the heart, and shivering.

Body heat also is produced by cell metabolism. Heat is produced when nutrients are broken down in the cells. Fever and strong emotional states also can increase heat production in the body.

HEAT LOSS

Heat is lost from the body through the urine, feces, and in water vapor during exhalation. Perspiration also contributes to heat loss. Perspiration is the excretion of moisture through the pores of the skin. When the moisture evaporates, heat is released and the body is cooled.

Radiation, conduction, and convection all cause loss of heat from the body. **Radiation** is the transfer of heat in the form of waves; body heat is continually radiating into cooler surroundings. **Conduction** is the transfer of heat from one object to another by direct contact; heat can be transferred by conduction from the body to a cooler object it touches. **Convection** is the transfer of heat through air currents; cool

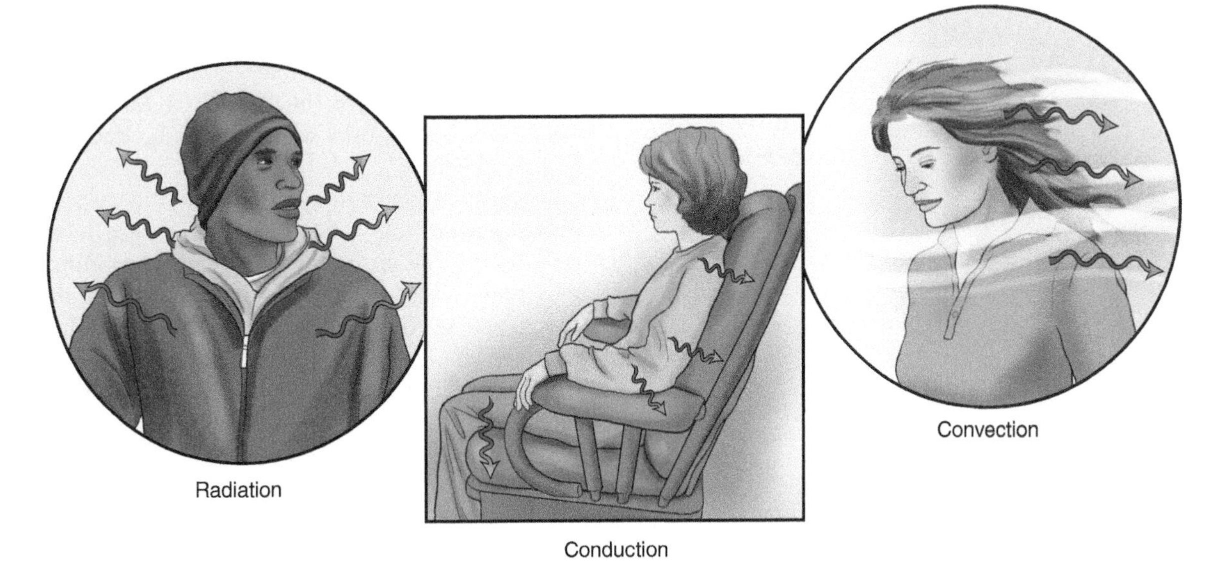

Fig. 4.2 Heat loss from the body. With **radiation,** the body gives off heat in the form of waves to the cooler outside air. With **conduction,** the chair becomes warm as heat is transferred from the individual to the chair. With **convection,** air currents move heat away from the body.

air currents can cause the body to lose heat. These processes are illustrated in Fig. 4.2.

BODY TEMPERATURE RANGE

The purposes of measuring body temperature are to establish the patient's baseline temperature and to monitor an abnormally high or low body temperature. The normal body temperature range is 97°F to 99°F (36.1°C to 37.2°C), with the average temperature being 98.6°F (37°C). Body temperature is usually documented using the Fahrenheit system of measurement. Table 4.1 lists comparable **Fahrenheit** and **Celsius** temperatures and explains how to convert temperatures from one scale to the other.

ALTERATIONS IN BODY TEMPERATURE

A body temperature greater than 100.4°F (38°C) indicates a **fever**, or *pyrexia*. When an individual has a fever, the heat the body is producing is greater than the heat the body is losing. A fever can be caused by many medical conditions ranging from non-serious to life-threatening. A body temperature measurement between 99°F (37.2°C) and 100.4°F (38°C) is known as a *low-grade fever*. A temperature reading greater than 106°F (41.1°C) is known as **hyperpyrexia**. Hyperpyrexia is a serious condition, and a temperature greater than 108 °F (42.2°C) is generally fatal.

A body temperature less than 97°F (36.1°C) is classified as **hypothermia**. This means that the heat the body is losing is greater than the heat it is producing. A person usually cannot survive with a temperature below 70°F (21°C). Terms used to describe alterations in body temperature are illustrated in Fig. 4.3.

Table 4.1 Equivalent Fahrenheit and Celsius Temperatures

Fahrenheit	Celsius
93.2	34
95	35
96.8	36
97.7	36.5
98.6	37
99.5	37.5
100.4	38
101.3	38.5
102.2	39
104	40
105.8	41
107.6	42
109.4	43
111.2	44

Temperature Conversion

1. *Celsius to Fahrenheit:* To convert Celsius to Fahrenheit, multiply by 9/5 and add 32:°F = (°C × 9/5) + 32
2. *Fahrenheit to Celsius:* To convert Fahrenheit to Celsius, subtract 32 and multiply by 5/9:°C = (°F − 32) × 5/9

VARIATIONS IN BODY TEMPERATURE

During the day-to-day activities of an individual, normal body temperature may fluctuate. The body temperature rarely stays the same throughout the course of a day. The medical assistant should take the following points into consideration when evaluating a patient's temperature.

1. *Age.* Infants and young children normally have a higher body temperature than adults because their

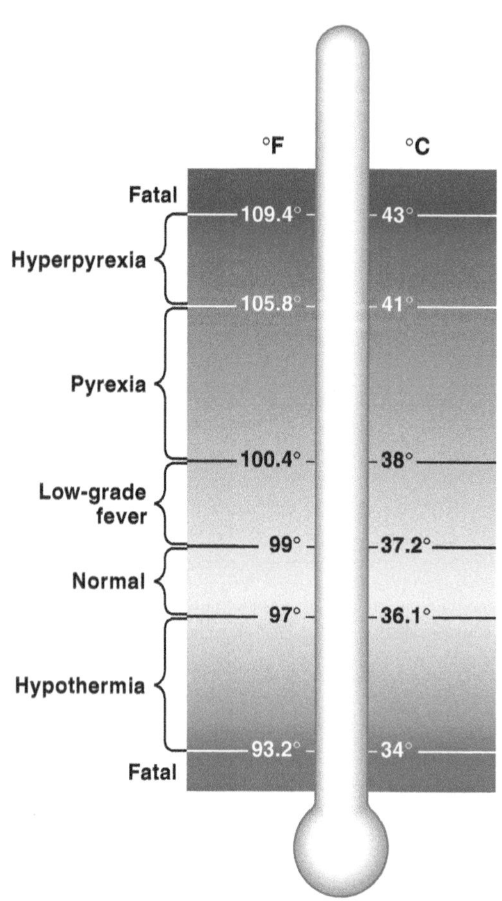

Fig. 4.3 Terms that describe alterations in body temperature (adult oral temperature).

thermoregulatory system is not yet fully established. Elderly individuals usually have a lower body temperature owing to factors such as loss of subcutaneous fat, lack of exercise, and loss of thermoregulatory control.

2. *Diurnal variations.* During sleep, body metabolism slows down, as do muscle contractions. The body's temperature is lowest in the morning before metabolism and muscle contractions begin increasing.
3. *Emotional states.* Strong emotions such as extreme anger and crying can increase the body temperature. This is important to consider when working with young children, who frequently cry during examination procedures or when they are ill.
4. *Environment.* Cold weather tends to decrease the body temperature, whereas hot weather increases it.
5. *Exercise.* Vigorous physical exercise causes an increase in voluntary muscle contractions, which elevates the body temperature.
6. *Patient's normal body temperature.* Some patients normally run a low or high temperature. The medical assistant should review the patient's temperature recordings before taking the patient's temperature.
7. *Pregnancy.* Cell metabolism increases during pregnancy, and this elevates body temperature.

FEVER

Fever, or pyrexia, denotes that a patient's temperature has increased to higher than 100.4°F (38°C). An individual who has a fever is said to be **febrile**; one who does not have a fever is **afebrile.**

Fever is a common symptom of illness, particularly inflammation and infection. When there is an infection in the body, the invading pathogen functions as a *pyrogen,* which is any substance that produces fever. Pyrogens reset the hypothalamus, causing the body temperature to increase to above normal. Fever is not an illness itself, but rather a sign that the body may have an infection. Most fevers are self-limited, that is, the body temperature returns to normal after the disease process is complete.

Stages of a Fever

A fever can be divided into the following three stages:

1. The *onset* is when the temperature first begins to increase. This increase may be slow or sudden, the patient often experiences coldness and chills, and the pulse and respiratory rate increase.
2. During the *course of a fever,* the temperature rises and falls in one of the following three fever patterns: continuous, intermittent, or remittent. Fever patterns are described and illustrated in Table 4.2. During this stage the patient has an increased pulse and respiratory rate and feels warm to the touch. The patient also may experience one or more of the following: flushed appearance, increased thirst, loss of appetite, headache, and malaise. **Malaise** refers to a vague sense of body discomfort, weakness, and fatigue.
3. During the *subsiding stage,* the temperature returns to normal. It can return to normal gradually or suddenly (known as a **crisis**). As the body temperature is returning to normal, the patient usually perspires and may become dehydrated.

ASSESSMENT OF BODY TEMPERATURE

ASSESSMENT SITES

There are five sites for measuring body temperature: mouth, axilla, rectum, ear, and forehead. The locations in which temperatures are taken should have an abundant blood supply so that the temperature of the entire body is obtained, not the temperature of only a part of the body. In addition, the site must be as closed as possible to prevent air currents from interfering with the temperature reading. The site chosen for measuring a patient's temperature depends on the patient's age, condition, and state of consciousness; the type of thermometer available; and the medical office policy.

Table 4.2 Fever Patterns

Pattern	Description	Illustration
Continuous fever	Body temperature fluctuates minimally but always remains elevated. *Occurs with:* Scarlet fever; Pneumococcal pneumonia	98.6°F (37°C)
Intermittent fever	Body temperature alternately rises and falls and at times returns to normal or becomes subnormal. Occurs with: Bacterial infections; Viral infections	98.6°F (37°C)
Remittent fever	Wide range of temperature fluctuations occur, all of which are above normal. Occurs with: Influenza; Pneumonia; Endocarditis	98.6°F (37°C)

HIGHLIGHT on Fever

Although most fevers indicate an infection is present, not all do. Noninfectious causes of fever include heatstroke, drug hypersensitivity, neoplasms, and central nervous system damage.

A fever usually is not harmful if the temperature remains below 102°F (38.9°C). Research suggests that fever may serve as a defense mechanism to destroy pathogens that are unable to survive above the normal body temperature range.

The level of the fever is not related to the seriousness of the infection. A patient with a temperature of 104°F (40°C) may not be any sicker than a patient with a temperature of 102°F (38.9°C).

In children, fever often is one of the first signs of illness and has a tendency to become highly elevated. In contrast, in elderly patients, fever may be elevated to only 1°F–2°F above normal, even with a severe infection.

During a fever, the body's basal metabolism increases by 7% for each degree of temperature elevation. Heart and respiratory rates also increase to meet this metabolic demand.

Chills during a fever result when the hypothalamus has been reset at a higher temperature. In an attempt to reach this temperature, involuntary muscle contractions (chills) occur, which produce heat, causing the temperature of the body to increase. After the higher temperature has been reached, the chills subside, and the individual then feels warm.

Increased perspiration during a fever occurs when the hypothalamus has been reset at a lower temperature, for example, after an individual takes an **antipyretic** medication (drug that reduces fever) or after the cause of the fever has been removed. To cool the body and reach this lower temperature, the body perspires, often profusely; profuse perspiration is known as *diaphoresis.*

Putting It All Into Practice

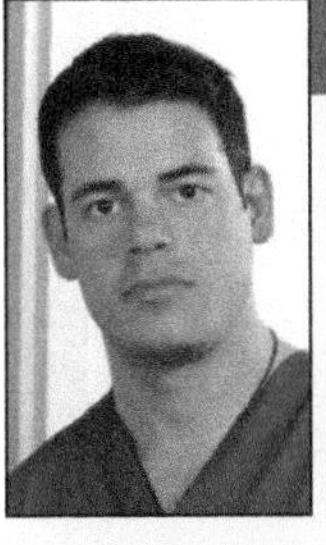

My name is Sergio, and I am a Registered Medical Assistant. I work in a large clinic that is associated with a medical school. At present, I work in the family medicine department, but I also have worked in dermatology and internal medicine. Family medicine is the area I enjoy most because of the wide variety of tasks that are performed. There is rarely a dull moment.

I focus primarily on clinical medical assisting. Taking vital signs is a big part of my job responsibilities. It is routine at my clinic to measure the height, weight, TPR, blood pressure, and pulse oximetry of every patient seen at the clinic, no matter what the reason for his or her visit. I assist the provider with various procedures, examinations, and minor office surgery, and I administer injections, run electrocardiograms, and perform various laboratory tests.

Taking vital signs and length and weight on small children can be very challenging at times. Some children start to cry as soon as they are put on the scale. I try to calm the child as much as possible, and for good behavior, I give a lot of praise. Stickers also are a great reward for cooperative behavior. Usually when small children learn that they can trust you, they are not as frightened by the experience. It is rewarding when a child learns not to be afraid of being evaluated for routine vital signs. ■

Oral Temperature

The oral method is a convenient and one of the most common means for measuring body temperature. When the medical assistant documents a temperature, the provider assumes it has been taken through the oral route unless otherwise noted. There is a rich blood supply under the tongue in the area on either side of the **frenulum linguae**, which is the midline fold that connects the undersurface of the tongue with the floor of the mouth. The thermometer should be placed in this area to obtain the most accurate reading. The patient must keep the mouth closed during the procedure to provide a closed space for the thermometer.

Axillary Temperature

Axillary temperature is recommended as a site for measuring temperature in toddlers and preschoolers. The **axilla** is the space below the shoulder or armpit. The axillary site also should be used for mouth-breathing patients and for patients with oral inflammation or who have had oral surgery.

The temperature obtained through the axillary method measures approximately 1°F lower than the same person's temperature taken through the oral route. The medical assistant should indicate in the patient's medical record that the temperature was taken through the axillary route.

Rectal Temperature

The rectal temperature provides an extremely accurate measurement of body temperature because few factors can alter the results. The rectum is highly vascular and, of the five sites, provides the most closed cavity. The temperature obtained by the rectal route measures approximately 1°F higher than the same person's temperature taken by the oral route. The medical assistant should indicate in the patient's medical record if the temperature has been taken rectally.

In general, the rectal method is used for infants and young children, unconscious patients, and mouth-breathing patients and when greater accuracy in body temperature is desired. The rectal site should not be used with newborns because of the danger of rectal trauma.

Aural Temperature

The aural (ear) site is used with the tympanic membrane thermometer. The ear provides a closed cavity that is easily accessible. Tympanic membrane thermometers provide instantaneous results, are easy to use, and are comfortable for the patient. They make it easier to measure the temperature of children between the ages of 6 months and 6 years, uncooperative patients, and patients who are unable to have their temperatures taken orally. The aural site should not be used for children under 6 months of age because their ear canals are too narrow for proper positioning of the thermometer. The aural temperature reading measures approximately 0.5° F to 1° F (0.3° C to 0.6° C) higher than oral body temperature.

Forehead Temperature

The temporal artery is a major artery of the head that runs laterally across the forehead and down the side of the neck. In the area of the forehead, the temporal artery is located approximately 2 mm below the surface of the skin. Because the temporal artery is located so close to the skin surface and is easily accessible, the forehead provides an ideal site for obtaining a body temperature measurement. In addition, the temporal artery has a constant steady flow of blood, which assists in providing an accurate measurement of the patient's body temperature.

The forehead site can be used to measure body temperature in individuals of all ages (newborns, infants, children, adults, elderly). The results compare in accuracy with other methods used to measure body temperature. The temporal artery temperature reading measures approximately 0.5° F to 1° F (0.3° C to 0.6° C) lower than oral body temperature.

TYPES OF THERMOMETERS

The three types of thermometers most commonly used in the medical office for measuring body temperature are electronic thermometers, tympanic membrane thermometers, and temporal artery thermometers which are described in more detail as follows.

Electronic Thermometer

An electronic thermometer can be used in the medical office to measure body temperature. Electronic thermometers are portable and measure oral, axillary, and rectal temperatures ranging from 84°F to 108°F (28.9°C to 42.2°C).

An electronic thermometer measures body temperature in a brief time—between 4 and 20 seconds depending on the brand of thermometer used. The temperature results are digitally displayed on a liquid crystal diode (LCD) screen. An electronic thermometer consists of interchangeable oral and rectal probes attached to a battery-operated portable unit (Fig. 4.4). The probes are color-coded for ease in identifying them. The oral probe is color-coded with blue on its collar and is used to take oral and axillary temperatures; the rectal probe is color-coded with red on its collar and is used to take rectal temperatures only.

A disposable plastic cover is placed over the probe to prevent the transmission of microorganisms among patients. Depending on the method of taking the temperature, the probe may be inserted into the mouth, axilla, or rectum and is left in place until an audible tone is emitted from the thermometer. When the tone sounds, the patient's temperature in degrees Fahrenheit (or Celsius) is displayed on the screen. The medical assistant ejects the plastic probe cover into a regular waste container.

The casing, probes, and attached cords of the electronic thermometer should be periodically cleaned with a soft cloth slightly dampened with a solution of warm water and a disinfectant cleaner.

Procedures 4.1, 4.2, and 4.3 outline the methods for measuring oral, axillary, and rectal temperatures using an electronic thermometer.

Tympanic Membrane Thermometer

The tympanic membrane thermometer is used at the aural site. The tympanic membrane thermometer functions by detecting thermal energy that is naturally radiated from the body. As with the rest of the body, the tympanic membrane gives off heat waves known as *infrared waves.* The sensor lens

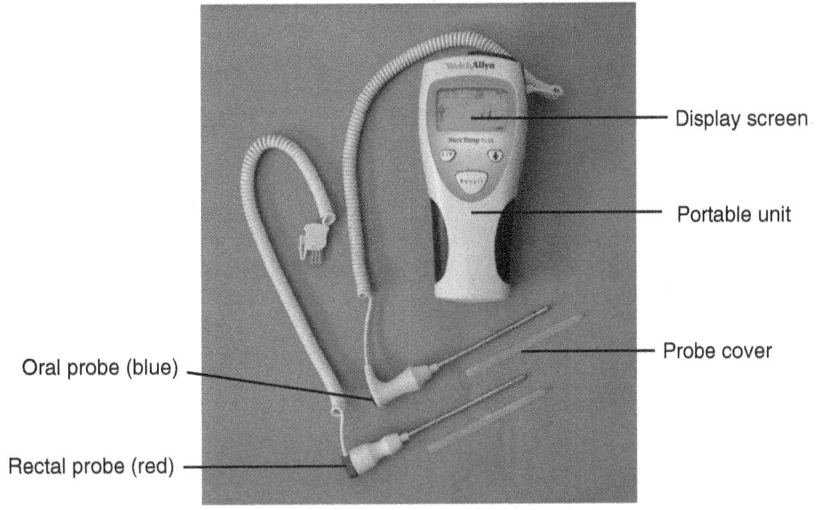

Fig. 4.4 Electronic thermometer.

of a tympanic thermometer functions like a camera by taking a "picture" of these infrared waves, which are considered a documented indicator of body temperature (Fig. 4.5). The thermometer calculates the body temperature from the thermal energy generated by the waves and displays the result on the screen of the thermometer.

The tympanic membrane thermometer is battery operated and consists of a small handheld device with a probe containing a sensor lens (Fig. 4.6). To operate the thermometer, the probe is covered with a disposable soft plastic cover and is placed in the outer third of the external ear canal. An activation button is depressed momentarily, and the results are displayed in 1 to 2 seconds on a digital screen. The probe cover is ejected into a regular waste container. Additional guidelines for using a tympanic membrane thermometer are presented in Box 4.1. The procedure for taking aural body temperature using a tympanic membrane thermometer is presented in Procedure 4.4.

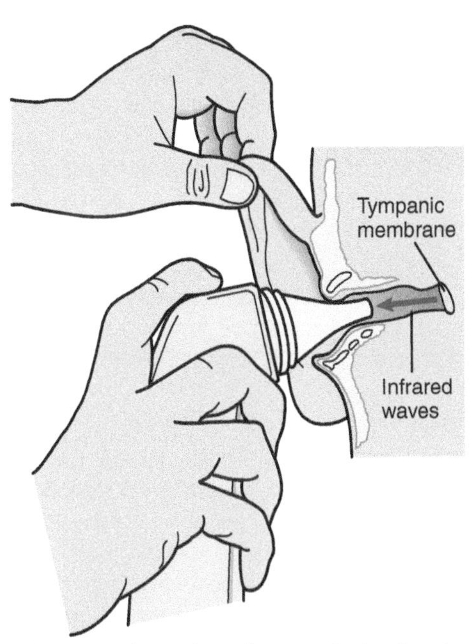

Fig. 4.5 The tympanic membrane thermometer functions by detecting thermal energy that is naturally radiated from the tympanic membrane.

Temporal Artery Thermometer

Use of a temporal artery thermometer is the newest method for assessing body temperature. The temporal artery thermometer is battery operated and consists of a small handheld device with a probe containing a sensor lens.

A temporal artery thermometer works in a similar manner to a tympanic membrane thermometer. The temporal artery gives off infrared waves and the sensor lens captures these thermal waves and calculates the body temperature and displays it on the screen of the thermometer. There are two types of temporal thermometers which include a *contact temporal artery thermometer* (Fig. 4.7A) and a *non-contact temporal artery thermometer* (see Fig. 4.7B). As their names imply, the contact thermometer comes in contact with the patient's skin and the non-contact thermometer does not. A non-contact thermometer poses the lowest risk of cross-contamination among the various types of thermometers. **Cross-contamination** is the process by which microorganisms are unintentionally transferred from one person, object, or place to another which may result in the spread of disease. Guidelines for temporal artery temperature measurement are presented in Box 4.2. The procedure for measuring body temperature with a contact and non-contact temporal artery thermometer is presented in Procedure 4.5.

Earlobe Temperature Measurement

Sweating of the forehead can cause an inaccurate temporal artery temperature reading. This is because perspiration causes the skin of the forehead to cool, resulting in a falsely low temperature reading. Sweating of the forehead occurs when a patient's fever breaks. It also occurs when a patient's

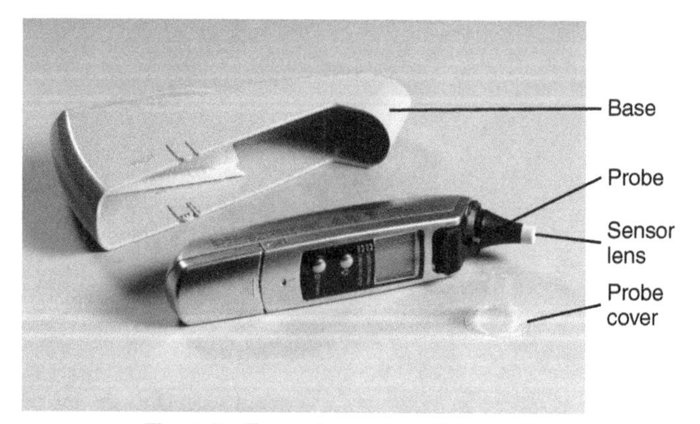

Fig. 4.6 Tympanic membrane thermometer.

BOX 4.1 Guidelines for Using a Tympanic Membrane Thermometer

The following guidelines help ensure accurate aural temperature measurement with a tympanic membrane thermometer.

1. **Determine whether a tympanic thermometer can be used to measure the patient's temperature.** Due to the size of their ear canal, a tympanic thermometer is not recommended for infants under 6 months of age. The tympanic thermometer should not be used on a patient with inflammation of the external ear canal (e.g., otitis externa) or when the ear contains a discharge such as blood or pus. The presence of otitis media and tympanostomy tubes does not significantly affect the temperature reading; a normal amount of cerumen also has no effect. An excessive buildup of cerumen that occludes the ear canal can result in a falsely low temperature reading.
2. **Determine whether external factors are present that may influence the temperature reading.** If any of these factors are present, remove the individual from the situation and wait 20 min before taking the temperature. External factors are present in an individual who has been lying on one ear or the other, who has had the ears covered (e.g., hat, earmuffs), who has been exposed to very hot or very cold temperatures, or who has been recently swimming or bathing. If an individual wears hearing aids, remove the hearing device from one ear and wait 20 min before taking the temperature in that ear.
3. **Select the temperature measurement system desired.** The temperature of a tympanic membrane thermometer can be displayed in degrees Fahrenheit or degrees Celsius. Follow the manufacturer's instructions to change from one measurement to the other.
4. **Place the probe properly in the patient's ear.** The most important factor in obtaining an accurate temperature is proper placement of the probe in the patient's ear, which is outlined as follows:
   - **Straighten the ear canal.** The ear canal has an S shape that obstructs the view of the tympanic membrane. To obtain an accurate temperature measurement, the ear canal must be straightened before inserting the probe. This allows the probe sensor to obtain a clear picture of the tympanic membrane. In adults and children older than 3 years of age, the canal is straightened by gently pulling the ear auricle upward and backward. In children younger than 3 years of age, the canal is straightened by pulling the ear pinna downward and backward.
   - **Seal the opening of the ear.** The probe must be inserted tightly enough to seal the opening of the ear without causing the patient discomfort. If the probe does not seal the ear canal, cooler external air can cause the thermometer to register a lower temperature.
   - **Correctly position the probe.** Position the tip of the probe toward the opposite temple (approximately midway between the opposite ear and the eyebrow). This allows the sensor to obtain the best possible picture of the tympanic membrane. If the tip is positioned incorrectly, it may be aimed at the ear canal, which results in a falsely low reading.
5. **Verify the accuracy of the temperature reading, if needed.** If you need to take the patient's temperature again, you can use the other ear. There are slight but insignificant differences between temperature readings in the right ear and those in the left ear. Before using the same ear, however, you must wait 2 min to allow the aural temperature to stabilize.
6. **Check the probe lens before taking the temperature.** The end of the probe is covered with a lens that is transparent to heat waves. To ensure an accurate temperature measurement, it is extremely important to keep this lens clean, dry, and intact. To protect the lens, always store the thermometer in its storage base when transporting or storing the thermometer. Before taking a temperature, always check to ensure that the lens is shiny and clear. Fingerprints, cerumen, and dust reduce the transparency of the lens, resulting in falsely low temperature readings. If the lens is dirty, it must be cleaned before taking the patient's temperature. If the lens is damaged, the thermometer cannot be used and must be repaired or replaced.
7. **Respond appropriately to digital messages.** A message to alert the user is displayed in the digital screen under the following circumstances:
   - An attempt is made to take a temperature without changing the cover after the last temperature.
   - An attempt is made to take a temperature with no probe cover in place.

Continued

BOX 4.1 Guidelines for Using a Tympanic Membrane Thermometer—cont'd

- The ambient (surrounding) temperature is not within the operating range for the thermometer (50°F [10°C] to 104°F [40°C]).
- The battery is low.
- The thermometer is in need of repair.

8. Care for the tympanic thermometer properly.
   - **Probe lens.** Dust and other minute particles of environmental debris can build up on the probe lens during normal use. The lens should be cleaned as a part of routine maintenance or when it becomes dirty. If the thermometer is placed in the ear without a probe cover, immediately remove the probe and clean the lens. To clean the lens, gently wipe its surface with an antiseptic wipe and allow it to dry. After cleaning, allow at least 5 min before taking a temperature.
   - **Thermometer casing.** Clean the casing of the thermometer periodically by wiping it dry with a soft cloth slightly moistened with alcohol. Never submerge the thermometer in water or a cleaning solution. Do not use an abrasive cleaner on the casing, as this could damage the casing.
9. **Store the thermometer properly.** The thermometer must be stored in its storage base to protect the lens from damage and dirt. Store the thermometer in a clean, dry area within a temperature range of 50°F (10°C) to 104°F (40°C). Keep the thermometer away from temperature extremes, which could damage the thermometer.

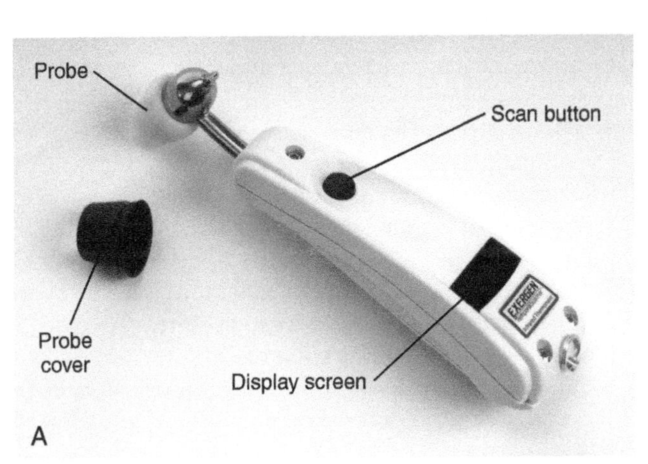

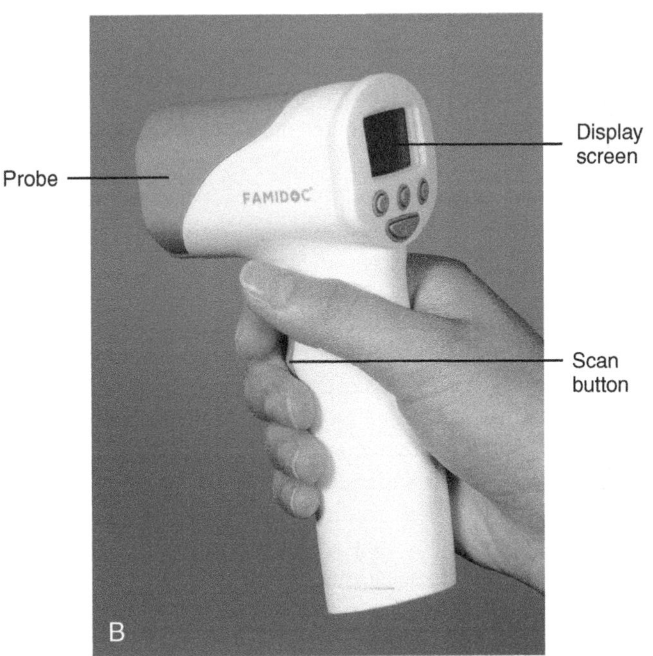

Fig. 4.7 Temporal artery thermometers. (A) Contact thermometer. (B) Noncontact thermometer.

skin is clammy; in this instance, forehead sweating may be present but not readily visible. To avoid this problem, the temperature of the neck area located just behind the earlobe is also measured when taking temperature with a contact temporal artery thermometer.

The area behind the earlobe is less affected by sweating than the forehead. During sweating, the blood vessels behind the earlobe dilate, resulting in a constant, steady flow of blood, which provides an accurate measurement of body temperature. After scanning the forehead with a contact thermometer, the medical assistant should place the probe of the thermometer in the soft depression of the neck just below the mastoid process of the ear. If the patient's forehead has cooled from sweating, the temperature of the neck area behind the earlobe automatically registers as the peak temperature, thereby overriding the forehead temperature. It is important to note that the area behind the earlobe does not normally provide an accurate body temperature measurement and supersedes the forehead measurement only when the patient is in a diaphoretic state.

Manufacturers of non-contact temporal artery thermometers do not recommend the use of the earlobe site when measuring a patient's temperature; if sweating of the forehead is present, it should be removed by wiping the forehead with a soft cloth before taking the patient's temperature.

BOX 4.2 Temporal Artery Thermometer Guidelines

1. The operating environmental temperature for a temporal artery thermometer is 60°F–104°F (15.5°C–40°C).
2. Do not take temperature over scar tissue, open sores, or abrasions.
3. Ensure that the forehead is exposed to the environment. Anything covering the area to be measured (e.g., hair, hat, wig, bandages) traps body heat, resulting in a falsely high reading.
4. Clean the forehead if sweat is present. Sweat on the forehead can result in a falsely low temperature reading.
5. Ensure that the sensor lens is clean and intact. Fingerprints, cerumen, and dust reduce the transparency of the lens, resulting in falsely low temperature readings. If the sensor lens is damaged, the thermometer cannot be used and must be repaired or replaced.

Care and Maintenance

The temporal artery thermometer should be stored in a clean, dry area. The thermometer must be protected from extremes in temperature, direct sunlight, and dust. The casing of the thermometer should be cleaned periodically with a soft cloth moistened with a solution of warm water and a disinfectant cleaner; never splash water on or immerse the unit in water because this could damage the internal components of the thermometer.

To obtain an accurate measurement, the sensor lens must be clean and shiny. Dust and other minute particles of environmental debris can build up on the sensor lens during normal use, preventing the sensor lens from getting an accurate "view" of the heat emitted by the temporal artery and resulting in a falsely low reading. The sensor lens should be cleaned if it becomes dirty and also as a part of routine maintenance. The lens is cleaned by gently wiping its surface with an antiseptic wipe or a cotton-tipped swab moistened with alcohol and allowing it to dry.

Pulse

MECHANISM OF THE PULSE

When the left ventricle of the heart contracts, blood is forced from the heart into the **aorta**, which is the major trunk of the arterial system of the body. The aorta is already filled with blood and must expand to accept the blood being pushed out of the left ventricle. This creates a pulsating wave that travels from the aorta through the walls of the arterial system. This wave, known as the *pulse*, can be felt as a light tap by an examiner. The pulse rate is measured by counting the number of taps, or beats, per minute. The heart rate can be determined by taking the pulse rate.

Table 4.3 Pulse Rates of Various Age Groups

Age Group	Pulse Range (beats/min)	Average Pulse (beats/min)
Infant (birth to 1 year)	120–160	140
Toddler (1– 3 years)	90–140	115
Preschool child (3– 6 years)	80–110	95
School-age child (6– 12 years)	75–105	90
Adolescent (12– 18 years)	60–100	80
Adult (after 18th year)	60–100	80
Adult (after 60th year)	67–80	74
Well-trained athletes	40–60	50

FACTORS AFFECTING PULSE RATE

Pulse rate can vary depending on many factors. The medical assistant should take each of the following into consideration when measuring pulse:

1. *Age.* The pulse varies inversely with age. As age increases, the pulse rate gradually decreases. Table 4.3 lists the pulse rates of various age groups.
2. *Gender.* Women tend to have a slightly faster pulse rate than men.
3. *Physical activity.* Physical activity, such as jogging and swimming, increases the pulse rate temporarily.
4. *Emotional states.* Strong emotional states, such as anxiety, fear, excitement, and anger, temporarily increase the pulse rate.
5. *Metabolism.* Increased body metabolism, such as occurs during pregnancy, increases the pulse rate.
6. *Fever.* Fever increases the pulse rate.
7. *Medications.* Medications may alter the pulse rate. For example, digitalis decreases the pulse rate, and epinephrine increases it.

What Would You Do? What Would You *Not* Do?

Case Study 1

Marcela Mason comes in with Olivia, her 5-year-old daughter. Olivia has had a fever and sore throat for the past 2 days. Sergio takes Olivia's temperature in her left ear with a tympanic membrane thermometer, and it measures 103.3°F. Mrs. Mason says that she has an ear thermometer at home, but when she took Olivia's temperature with it, the readings were always below 97°F. She knew that could not be right because Olivia felt so warm. Mrs. Mason prefers to use her ear thermometer to take Olivia's temperature, but she thinks that it might be broken because of the low readings. ■

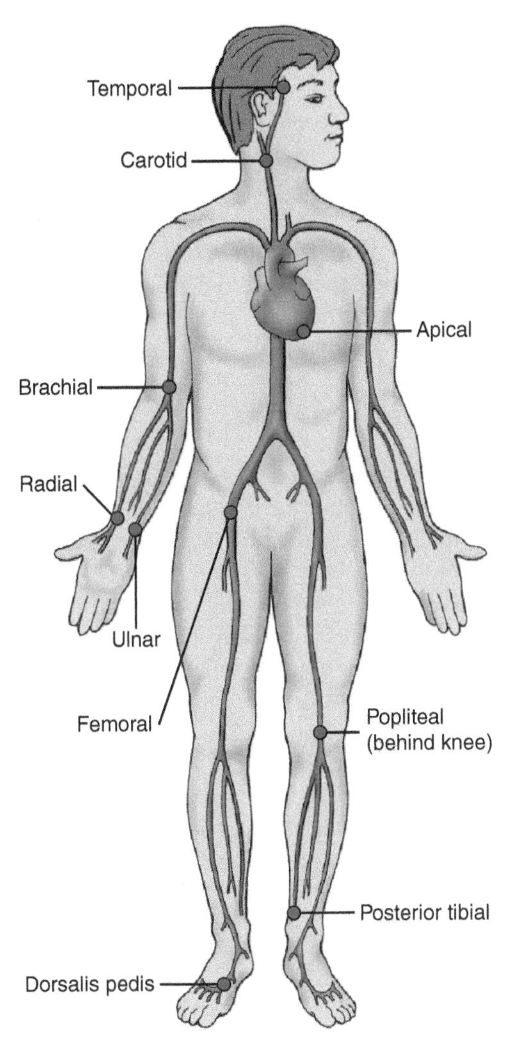

Fig. 4.8 Pulse sites.

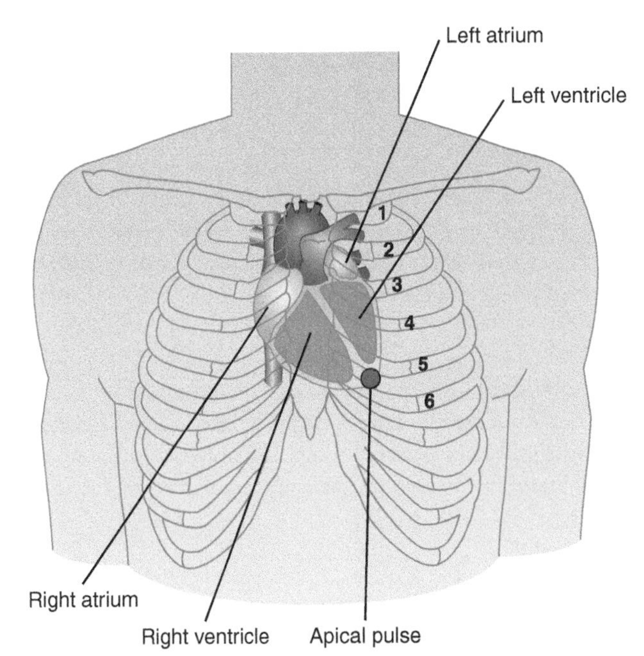

Fig. 4.9 The apical pulse is found over the apex of the heart, which is located in the fifth intercostal space at the junction of the left midclavicular line.

PULSE SITES

The pulse is felt most strongly when a superficial artery is held against a firm tissue, such as bone. The locations of sites used for measuring the pulse are shown in Fig. 4.8 and are described next.

Radial

The most common site for measuring the pulse is the radial artery, which is located in a groove on the inner aspect of the wrist just below the thumb. The radial pulse is easily accessible and can be measured with no discomfort to the patient. This site is also used by individuals at home monitoring their own heart rates, such as athletes, patients taking heart medication, and individuals starting an exercise program. The procedure for measuring radial pulse is outlined in Procedure 4.6.

Apical

The apical pulse has a stronger beat and is easier to measure than the other pulse sites. If the medical assistant is having difficulty feeling the radial pulse, or if the radial pulse is irregular or abnormally slow or rapid, the apical pulse should be taken (Procedure 4.7). This pulse site is often used to measure pulse in infants and in children up to 3 years old because the other sites are difficult to palpate accurately in these age groups. The apical pulse is measured using a stethoscope. The chest piece of the stethoscope is placed lightly over the apex of the heart, which is located in the fifth **intercostal** (between the ribs) space at the junction of the left midclavicular line (Fig. 4.9). A *lub-dup* sound is heard through the stethoscope. The *lub* sound occurs when the cuspid valves of the heart valves of the heart close and the *dup* sound occurs when the semilunar valves of the heart close. Each *lub-dup* is counted as one heartbeat.

Brachial

The brachial pulse is in the **antecubital space**, which is the space located at the front of the elbow. This site is used to take blood pressure, to measure pulse in infants during cardiac arrest, and to assess the status of the circulation to the lower arm.

Ulnar

The ulnar pulse is located on the ulnar (little finger) side of the wrist. It is used to assess the status of circulation to the hand.

Temporal

The temporal pulse is located in front of the ear and just above eye level. This site is used to measure pulse when the radial pulse is inaccessible. It is also an easy access site to assess pulse in children.

Carotid

The carotid pulse is located on the anterior side of the neck, slightly to one side of the midline, and is the best site to find a pulse quickly. This site is used to measure pulse in children and adults during cardiac arrest. The carotid site also is commonly used by individuals to monitor pulse during exercise.

Femoral

The femoral pulse is in the middle of the groin. This site is used to measure pulse in infants and children and in adults during cardiac arrest and to assess the status of circulation to the lower leg.

Popliteal

The popliteal pulse is at the back of the knee and is detected most easily when the knee is slightly flexed. This site is used to measure blood pressure when the brachial pulse is inaccessible and to assess the status of circulation to the lower leg.

Posterior Tibial

The posterior tibial pulse is located on the inner aspect of the ankle just posterior to the ankle bone. This site is used to assess the status of circulation to the foot.

Dorsalis Pedis

The dorsalis pedis pulse is located on the upper surface of the foot, between the first and second metatarsal bones. This site is used to assess the status of circulation to the foot.

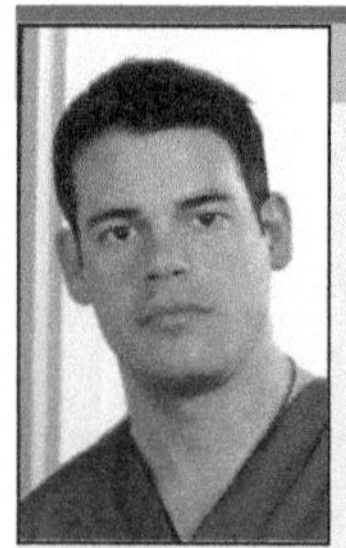

Memories *from* Practicum

Sergio: One experience that really stands out in my memory occurred during my practicum at a family practice medical office. I needed to take the blood pressure of a small 6-year-old boy. After I put the cuff on his arm, his eyes started filling up with tears. I stopped, removed the cuff, and asked him if something was wrong. He said he was afraid that when I started squeezing that thing around his arm, his hand would fall off. I sat down next to him, spent some time talking with him, and reassured him that his hand would be perfectly fine and would not fall off. I put the cuff on my arm and pumped it up to show him that he would be safe. He then agreed to let me take his blood pressure. After I took his blood pressure, he wiggled his hand, gave me a big smile, and said that it didn't hurt at all. That situation made me realize that children may have a lot of fears about what might happen to them at the medical office. Since that experience, I always take the time to explain procedures to children before I perform them. ■

ASSESSMENT OF PULSE

The purpose of measuring pulse is to establish the patient's baseline pulse rate and to assess the pulse rate after special procedures, medications, or disease processes that affect heart functioning. Pulse is measured using palpation at all of the pulse sites except the apical site.

Pulse is palpated by applying moderate pressure with the sensitive pads located on the tips of the three middle fingers. The pulse should not be taken with the thumb because the thumb has a pulse of its own. This could result in measurement of the medical assistant's pulse rather than the patient's pulse. Excessive pressure should not be applied when measuring pulse because this could obliterate, or close off, the pulse. It may not be possible to detect the pulse if too little pressure is applied, however. An accurate assessment of pulse includes determinations of the pulse rate, the pulse rhythm, and the pulse volume.

PULSE RATE

The pulse rate is the number of heart pulsations or heartbeats that occur in 1 minute; therefore pulse rate is measured in beats per minute. Normal pulse rates vary widely in the various age groups, as shown in Table 4.3. For a healthy adult, the normal resting pulse rate ranges from 60 to 100 beats/min, with the average falling between 70 and 80 beats/min.

An abnormally fast heart rate of more than 100 beats/min is known as **tachycardia**. Tachycardia may indicate disease states such as hemorrhaging or heart disease. Tachycardia usually occurs when an individual is involved in vigorous physical exercise or is experiencing strong emotional states.

Bradycardia is an abnormally slow heart rate—less than 60 beats/min. A pulse rate of less than 60 beats/min may occur normally during sleep. Trained athletes often have low pulse rates. If a patient exhibits tachycardia or bradycardia during radial pulse measurement, the apical pulse should also be measured.

PULSE RHYTHM AND VOLUME

In addition to measuring the pulse rate, the medical assistant should determine the rhythm and volume of the pulse. The **pulse rhythm** denotes the time interval between heartbeats; a normal rhythm has the same time interval between beats and is described as regular. Any irregularity in the heart's rhythm is known as a **dysrhythmia** (also termed *arrhythmia*) and is characterized by unequal or irregular intervals between the heartbeats. If a dysrhythmia is present, the provider may order one or more of the following: an apical-radial pulse, an electrocardiogram, or Holter monitoring.

An *apical-radial pulse* is measured to determine whether a pulse deficit is present. Taking an apical-radial pulse involves measuring the apical pulse at the same time as the radial pulse for a duration of 1 full minute. A **pulse deficit** exists when the radial pulse rate is less than the apical pulse rate. If one medical assistant measures an apical pulse rate of 88 beats/min while another medical assistant simultaneously measures a radial pulse rate of 76 beats/min, this results in a pulse deficit of 12 beats. A pulse deficit means that not all of the heartbeats are reaching the peripheral arteries. A pulse deficit is caused by an inefficient contraction of the heart that is not strong enough to transmit a pulse wave to the peripheral pulse site. A pulse deficit frequently occurs with atrial fibrillation, which is a type of dysrhythmia.

The **pulse volume** refers to the strength of the heartbeat. The amount of blood pumped into the aorta by each contraction of the left ventricle should remain constant, making the pulse feel strong and full. If the blood volume decreases, the pulse feels weak and may be difficult to detect. This type of pulse is usually accompanied by a fast heart rate and is described as a **thready pulse**. An increase in the blood volume results in a pulse that feels extremely strong and full, known as a **bounding pulse**.

PATIENT COACHING Aerobic Exercise

Answer questions patients have about aerobic exercise.

What is aerobic exercise?

Aerobic exercise is any type of cardiovascular conditioning. Aerobic means "with oxygen." During aerobic exercise, muscles must work harder which increases the demand for oxygen. This causes the breathing and heart rate to increase to supply the body with enough oxygen. Over time, aerobic exercise strengthens the heart muscle making the heart a more efficient pump resulting in a slower resting heart rate. Aerobic exercise is accomplished through steady, nonstop activity, such as walking, jogging, cycling, or swimming. Each workout should include warm-up and cool-down periods of 5–10 min. This is needed to prevent muscle or joint injuries.

What are the benefits of an aerobic exercise program?

The benefits of an aerobic exercise program include a lower risk of heart disease and stroke, lowering of the blood pressure, reduction of stress, increased energy, reduction of body fat, better sleep, better bone health, and fewer symptoms of depression and anxiety.

How often should aerobic exercise be performed?

The American Heart Association (AHA) recommends that healthy adults get at least 150 minutes per week of *moderate-intensity* aerobic activity or 75 minutes per week of *vigorous intensity* aerobic activity (or a combination of both), preferably spread out through the week. Exercise intensity refers to how hard the body is working during physical activity. Your health and fitness goals, as well as your current level of fitness, will determine your ideal exercise intensity.

How is exercise intensity measured subjectively?

A subjective measurement of exercise intensity is based on how you feel during the exercise.

- **Moderate-intensity aerobic exercise.** When you are engaged in moderate-intensity exercise, your heart beats faster and your breathing is heavier, and you can carry on a conversation but you can't sing. You also develop a light sweat and feel some strain on your muscles. Examples of moderate-intensity exercise include walking at a brisk pace, riding a bike on flat ground, pushing a lawnmower, playing a game of volleyball or badminton, and performing continuous gardening chores (such as weeding and mulching).
- **Vigorous intensity aerobic exercise.** Vigorous intensity exercise is conducted at a higher intensity level and feels more taxing. During vigorous exercise your heart beats much faster, your breathing is deep and rapid and you can't say more than a few words without pausing for breath. Examples of vigorous intensity exercise include running/jogging, racquetball or tennis, swimming laps, biking up a hill, and basketball.

How is exercise intensity measured objectively?

Your target heart rate (THR) range offers a more objective way to measure exercise intensity. Your THR range is a safe and effective exercise range that indicates you are exercising at the right level for your age and for what you are trying to accomplish with exercise (e.g., weight loss, improve fitness, train for a competition). Exercising at a level below your THR range does little to promote fitness; exercising at a level above your THR may not be safe. THR range can be determined using a THR online calculator or through the following formulas:

1. **Moderate-intensity aerobic exercise.** Your THR range during moderate-intensity exercise should be 50%–70% of your maximum heart rate (MHR) which is calculated as follows.
   a. Subtract your age from 220 to determine your MHR, which is the upper limit of what your body can handle during exercise for your age. The MHR of a 40-year-old person is calculated as follows:
      220 − 40 years old = **180** (MHR)
   b. Determine the lower end of your THR range by multiplying your MHR by 0.5. For our example:
      180 × 0.50 = **90** (low end of THR)
   c. Determine the upper end of your THR range by multiplying your MHR by 0.7. For our example:
      180 × 0.70 = **126** (upper end of THR)

   The THR range for moderate-intensity exercise for a 40-year-old individual is a heart rate that falls between 90 and 126 beats/min during physical activity.
2. **Vigorous-intensity aerobic exercise.** Your THR range during vigorous-intensity exercise should be 70%–85% of your MHR which is calculated as follows:
   a. Determine the lower end of your THR range by multiplying your MHR by 0.7. For our example:
      180 × 0.70 = **126** (low end of THR)
   b. Determine the upper end of your THR range by multiplying your MHR by 0.85. For our example:
      180 × 0.85 = **153** (upper end of THR)

   The THR range for vigorous-intensity exercise for a 40-year-old individual is a heart rate that falls between 126 and 153 beats/min during physical activity.

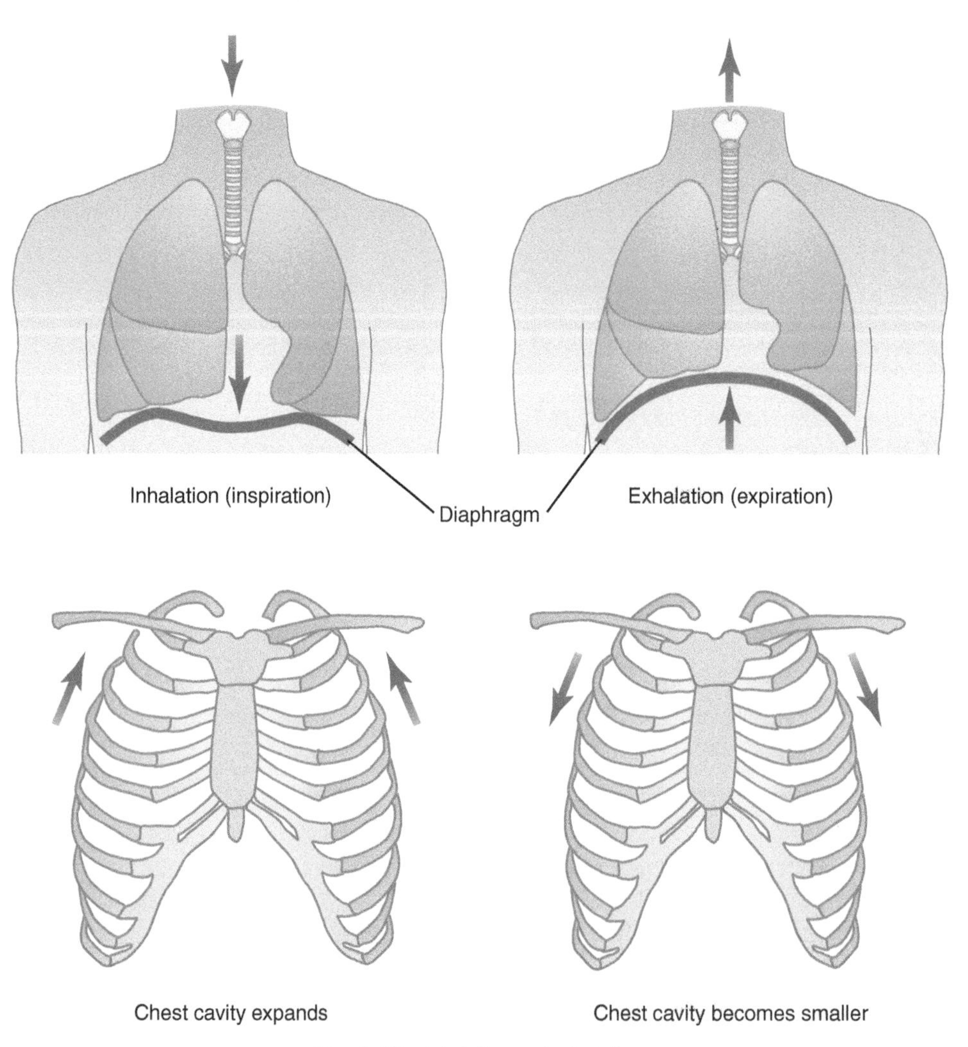

Fig. 4.10 Inhalation and exhalation.

Respiration

MECHANISM OF RESPIRATION

The purpose of respiration is to provide for the exchange of oxygen and carbon dioxide between the atmosphere and the blood. Oxygen is taken into the body to be used for vital body processes, and carbon dioxide is given off as a waste product.

Each respiration is divided into two phases: **inhalation** and **exhalation** (Fig. 4.10). During inhalation, or inspiration, the diaphragm descends and the lungs expand, causing air containing oxygen to move from the atmosphere into the lungs. Exhalation, or expiration, involves the removal of carbon dioxide from the body. The diaphragm ascends, and the lungs return to their original state so that air containing carbon dioxide is expelled. One complete respiration is composed of one inhalation and one exhalation.

Respiration can be classified as *external* or *internal.* External respiration involves the exchange of oxygen and carbon dioxide between the **alveoli** and the blood. **Alveoli** are thin-walled air sacs in the lungs located at the end of the bronchioles (Fig. 4.11). The blood, located in small capillaries, comes in contact with the alveoli, picks up oxygen, and carries it to the cells of the body. At this point, the oxygen is given off to the cells, and carbon dioxide is picked up by the blood to be transported as a waste product to the lungs. The exchange of oxygen and carbon dioxide between the body cells and the blood is known as *internal respiration.*

CONTROL OF RESPIRATION

The medulla oblongata, located in the brain, is the control center for involuntary respiration. A buildup of carbon dioxide in the blood sends a message to the medulla, which triggers respiration to occur automatically.

To a certain extent, respiration is also under voluntary control. An individual can control respiration during activities such as singing, laughing, talking, eating, and crying. Voluntary respiration is ultimately under the control of the medulla oblongata. The breath can be held for only a certain length of time, after which carbon dioxide begins to build up in the body, resulting in a stimulus to the medulla that causes respiration to occur involuntarily. Small children may voluntarily hold their breath during a temper tantrum.

A parent who does not understand the principles of respiration may be concerned that the child might stop breathing. The medical assistant should be able to explain that involuntary respiration would eventually occur and the child would resume breathing.

What Would You Do? What Would You *Not* Do?

Case Study 2

Alex Jacoby is 18 years old and a senior in high school. He comes to the office complaining of severe pain in his left shoulder. His vital signs are as follows: temperature 98.5°F, pulse 48 beats/min, respirations 12 breaths/min, and blood pressure 108/68 mm Hg. Alex is an outstanding competitive swimmer and is currently ranked first in the state in the 100-yard butterfly. Alex has an important swim meet coming up and must do well so that he can get a college athletic scholarship. He says he thinks he can take 2 s off his best time at this meet and he doesn't want anything to interfere with that. Alex wants the physician to do whatever he can to make his shoulder better and thinks that a steroid injection and pain pills might be the answer. Alex also wants to know why his pulse rate is so slow. ■

ASSESSMENT OF RESPIRATION

Because an individual can control his or her respiration, the medical assistant should measure respirations without the patient's knowledge. Patients may change their respiratory rate unintentionally if they are aware that they are being measured. An ideal time to measure respiration is after the pulse is taken. Procedure 4.6 outlines the procedures for taking pulse and respiration in one continuous procedure.

RESPIRATORY RATE

The respiratory rate of a normal healthy adult ranges from 12 to 20 respirations per minute. With most adults, there is a ratio of one respiration for every four pulse beats. If the respiratory rate is 18, the pulse rate would be approximately 72 beats/min. An abnormal increase in the respiratory rate of more than 20 respirations per minute is referred to as **tachypnea.** An abnormal decrease in the respiratory rate of less than 12 respirations per minute is known as **bradypnea.** When measuring the respiratory rate, the medical assistant should take into consideration the following factors:

1. *Age.* As age increases, the respiratory rate decreases. The respiratory rate of a child would be expected to be faster than that of an adult. Table 4.4 provides a chart of the respiratory rates for various age groups.
2. *Physical activity.* Physical activity increases the respiratory rate temporarily.
3. *Emotional states.* Strong emotional states temporarily increase the respiratory rate.
4. *Fever.* A patient with a fever has an increased respiratory rate. One way that heat is lost from the body is through the lungs; a fever causes an increased respiratory rate as the body tries to rid itself of excess heat.
5. *Medications.* Certain medications increase the respiratory rate, and others decrease it. If the medical assistant is unsure of what effect a particular drug may have on the respiratory rate, he or she should consult a drug reference, such as the *Prescribers' Digital Reference* (PDR).

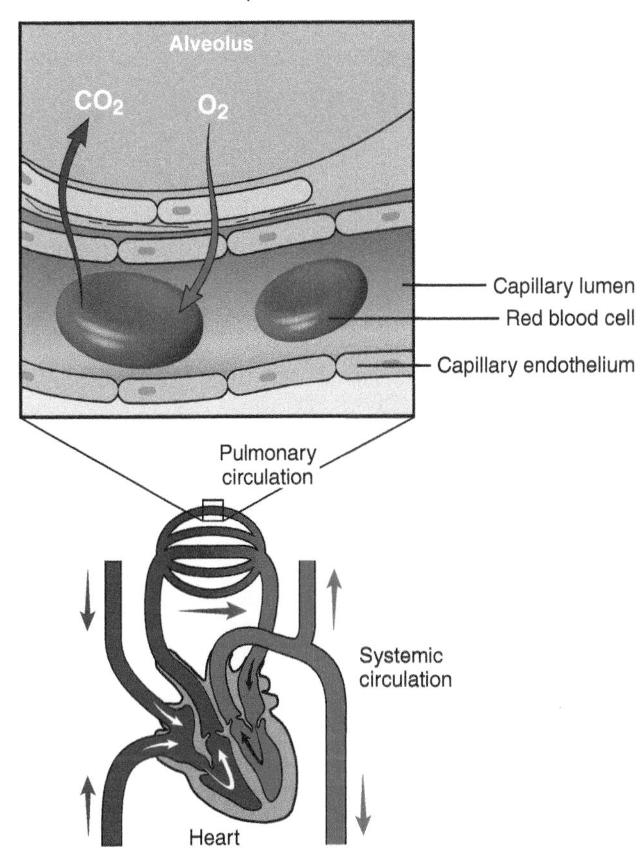

Fig. 4.11 Exchange of oxygen and carbon dioxide between the alveoli of the lungs and the blood.

Table 4.4 Respiratory Rates of Various Age Groups

	Average Respiratory Range, Breaths per Minute	Respiratory Average, Breaths per Minute
Infant (birth to 1 year)	30–60	35
Toddler (1–3 years)	24–40	30
Preschool child (3–6 years)	22–34	25
School-age child (6–12 years)	18–30	22
Adolescent (12–18 years)	12–16	16
Adult (after 18 years)	12–20	16

RHYTHM AND DEPTH OF RESPIRATION

The *rhythm* and *depth* should be noted when measuring respiration. Normally the rhythm should be even and regular, and

PATIENT COACHING **Chronic Obstructive Pulmonary Disease**

Answer questions that patients have about chronic obstructive pulmonary disease (COPD).

What is COPD?

COPD is a chronic airway obstruction that results from emphysema or chronic bronchitis or a combination of these conditions. COPD is a chronic, debilitating, irreversible, and sometimes fatal disease.

How many people have COPD?

More than 16 million Americans have been diagnosed with COPD; however, it is estimated that millions more have the disease but remain undiagnosed. COPD is the third leading cause of death in the United States behind heart disease and cancer. Although COPD is much more common in men than in women, the greatest increase in death rates is occurring in women.

What causes COPD?

Cigarette smoking over a period of many years is the leading cause of COPD. Other causes include air pollution and occupational exposure to irritating inhalants, such as noxious dusts, fumes, and vapors.

What types of tests might the provider order?

Respiratory tests to diagnose COPD include various types of pulmonary function tests. Examples of pulmonary function tests are spirometry, lung volumes, diffusion capacity, arterial blood gas studies, and cardiopulmonary exercise tests.

What treatment might the provider prescribe?

Treatment is focused on improving breathing difficulties and may include bronchodilator drug therapy, breathing exercises, and oxygen therapy.

1. Encourage patients with COPD to comply with the therapy prescribed by the provider.
2. Provide the patient with information about smoking, emphysema, and chronic bronchitis. Educational materials are available from the American Lung Association, the American Heart Association, and the American Cancer Society. ■

the pauses between inhalation and exhalation should be equal. The depth of respiration indicates the amount of air that is inhaled or exhaled during the process of breathing. Respiratory depth is typically described as normal, deep, or shallow and is determined by observing the amount of movement of the chest. For normal respirations, the depth of each respiration in a resting state is approximately the same. Deep respirations are those in which a large volume of air is inhaled and exhaled, whereas shallow respirations involve the exchange of a small volume of air. Normal respiration is referred to as **eupnea**. The rate is approximately 12 to 20 breaths/min, the rhythm is even and regular, and the depth is normal.

Hyperpnea is an abnormal increase in the rate and depth of respirations. A patient with hyperpnea exhibits a very deep, rapid, and labored respiration. Hyperpnea occurs normally with exercise and abnormally with pain and fever. It also can occur with any condition in which the supply of oxygen is inadequate, such as heart disease and lung disease.

Hyperventilation is an abnormally fast and deep type of breathing that is usually associated with acute anxiety conditions, such as panic attacks. An individual who is hyperventilating is "overbreathing," which usually causes dizziness and weakness.

Hypopnea is a condition in which a patient's respirations exhibit an abnormal decrease in rate and depth. The depth is approximately half that of normal respiration. Hypopnea often occurs in individuals with sleep disorders.

COLOR OF THE PATIENT

The patient's color should be observed while the respiration is being measured. A reduction in the oxygen supply to the tissues results in a condition known as **cyanosis**, which causes a bluish discoloration of the skin and mucous membranes. Cyanosis is first observed in the nail beds and lips because in these areas the blood vessels lie close to the surface of the skin. Cyanosis typically occurs in patients with advanced emphysema and in patients during cardiac arrest.

Apnea is a temporary absence of respirations. Some individuals experience apnea during sleep; this condition is known as *sleep apnea.* Apnea can be a serious condition if the individual's breathing ceases for more than 4 to 6 minutes because brain damage or death could occur.

RESPIRATORY ABNORMALITIES

A patient who is having difficulty breathing or shortness of breath has a condition known as **dyspnea.** Dyspnea may occur normally during vigorous physical exertion and abnormally in patients with asthma and emphysema. A patient with dyspnea may find it easier to breathe while in a sitting or standing position. This state is called **orthopnea** and occurs with disorders of the heart and lungs, such as asthma, emphysema, pneumonia, and congestive heart failure.

BREATH SOUNDS

Breath sounds are caused by air moving through the respiratory tract. Normal breath sounds are quiet and barely audible. Abnormal breath sounds are referred to as **adventitious sounds** and typically signify the presence of a respiratory disorder. The causes and characteristics of abnormal breath sounds are presented in Table 4.5.

Table 4.5 Abnormal Breath Sounds

Type	Cause	Character
Crackles[a] (rales)	Air moving through airways that contain fluid	Dry or wet intermittent sounds that vary in pitch (this sound can be duplicated by rubbing hair together next to ear)
Rhonchi*	Thick secretions, tumors, or spasms that partially obstruct air flow through large upper airways	Deep, low-pitched, rumbling sound more audible during expiration
Wheezes	Severely narrowed airways caused by partial obstruction in smaller bronchi and bronchioles; common symptom of asthma	Continuous, high-pitched, whistling musical sounds heard during inspiration and expiration
Pleural friction rub[a]	Inflamed pleurae rubbing together	High, grating sound similar to rubbing leather pieces together, heard on inspiration and expiration

[a]Audible only through a stethoscope.

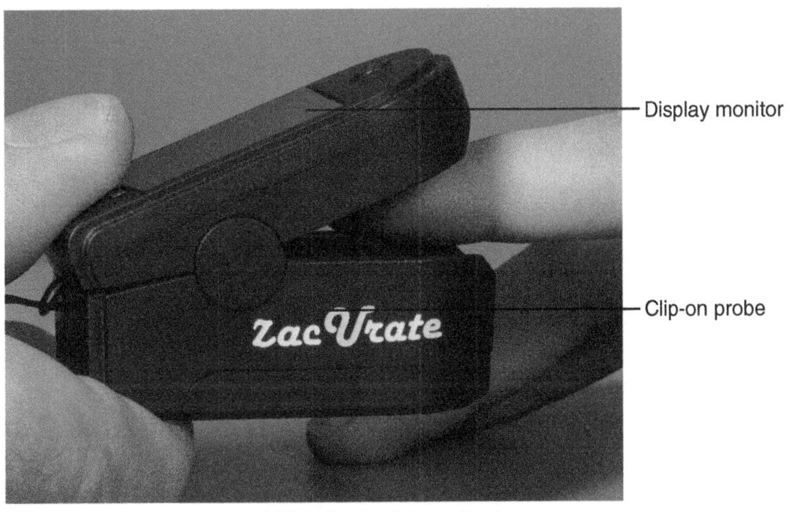

Fig. 4.12 Pulse oximeter.

Pulse Oximetry

Pulse oximetry is a painless and noninvasive procedure used to measure the oxygen saturation of hemoglobin in arterial blood. Hemoglobin is a complex compound found in red blood cells that functions in transporting oxygen in the body. Pulse oximetry provides information on a patient's cardiorespiratory status—in particular, the amount of oxygen being delivered to the tissues of the body. The procedure for performing pulse oximetry is presented in Procedure 4.8.

A **pulse oximeter** is a device used to measure and display the oxygen saturation of the blood. It is a computerized portable device that consists of a display monitor and a two-sided, clip-on probe (Fig. 4.12). A pulse oximeter also measures the patient's pulse rate in beats per minute. Pulse oximeters can be obtained by individuals over the counter or through a provider's prescription for use at home. The measurement of the oxygen saturation of blood by patients at home has increased substantially as a result of the COVID-19 pandemic.

ASSESSMENT OF OXYGEN SATURATION

The clip-on probe of the pulse oximeter must be attached to a peripheral pulsating capillary bed, such as the tip of a finger. One side of the probe contains a *light-emitting diode (LED)* that transmits infrared light and red light through the capillary bed in the patient's finger to a light detector located on the other side of the probe, known as a *light sensor* (Fig. 4.13).

Hemoglobin that is bright red in color has a high oxygen content *(oxygen rich)* and absorbs more of the infrared light emitted by the LED. Hemoglobin that is dark red in color is low in oxygen *(oxygen poor)* and absorbs more of the red light. The computer of the oximeter compares and calculates the light transmitted from the oxygen-rich hemoglobin and the oxygen-poor hemoglobin and from this ratio is able to determine the oxygen saturation of the patient's hemoglobin. This measurement is converted to a percentage and is displayed as a digital readout on the screen of the monitor. Because the pulse oximeter measures the oxygen saturation of peripheral capillaries, the abbreviation **SpO_2** *(saturation of peripheral oxygen)* is used to document the reading.

A more complete but invasive measurement of oxygen saturation is arterial blood gas analysis, which requires drawing a blood specimen from an artery. The abbreviation for this type of arterial oxygen saturation measurement is **SaO_2** *(saturation of arterial oxygen)*.

INTERPRETATION OF RESULTS

The pulse oximetry reading represents the percentage of hemoglobin that is saturated (filled) with oxygen. Each molecule of hemoglobin can carry four oxygen molecules.

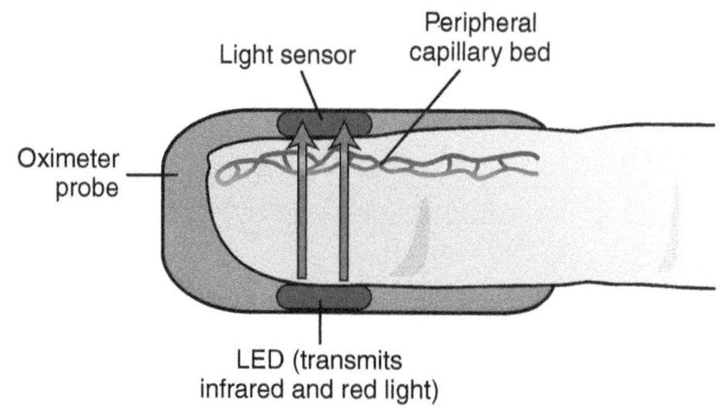

Fig. 4.13 The probe of the pulse oximeter is attached to a peripheral capillary bed in the fingertip. The LED transmits light through the capillary bed to a light sensor located on the other side of the probe to measure the oxygen saturation of hemoglobin.

If 100 molecules of hemoglobin were fully saturated with oxygen, they would be carrying 400 molecules of oxygen, and the oxygen saturation reading would be 100%. If these same 100 molecules of hemoglobin were carrying only 360 molecules of oxygen, however, the oxygen saturation reading would be 90%. The more hemoglobin that is saturated with oxygen, the higher the oxygen saturation of the blood.

The oxygen saturation level of most healthy individuals is 95% to 99%. Because the air we breathe is only 21% saturated with oxygen, it is unusual for an individual's hemoglobin to be fully or 100% saturated with oxygen. Patients on supplemental oxygen sometimes have a reading of 100%, however.

An oxygen saturation level of less than 95% typically results in an inadequate amount of oxygen reaching the tissues of the body, although patients with chronic pulmonary disease are sometimes able to tolerate lower saturation levels. Respiratory failure, resulting in tissue damage, usually occurs when the oxygen saturation decreases to a level between 85% and 90%. Cyanosis typically appears when an individual's oxygen saturation reaches a level of 75%, and an oxygen saturation of less than 70% is life-threatening.

A decrease in the oxygen saturation of the blood (less than 95%) is known as **hypoxemia**. Hypoxemia can lead to a more serious condition known as hypoxia. **Hypoxia** is defined as a reduction in the oxygen supply to the tissues of the body, and if not treated it can lead to tissue damage and death. The first symptoms of hypoxia include headache, mental confusion, nausea, dizziness, shortness of breath, tachycardia, and cyanosis. The tissues most sensitive to hypoxia are the brain, heart, pulmonary vessels, and liver.

PURPOSE OF PULSE OXIMETRY

In the medical office, pulse oximetry is performed on patients complaining of respiratory problems (e.g., dyspnea). A decreased pulse oximetry reading (along with clinical signs and symptoms and further testing) assists in the proper diagnosis and treatment of a patient's condition, which may include drug therapy and oxygen therapy.

Conditions that can cause a decreased SpO_2 value (hypoxemia) include the following:

- Acute pulmonary disease (e.g., pneumonia)
- Chronic pulmonary disease (e.g., emphysema, asthma, bronchitis)
- Cardiac problems (e.g., congestive heart failure, coronary artery disease)

In addition to assisting in the diagnosis of a patient's condition, pulse oximetry is used to assess the following:

- Effectiveness of oxygen therapy
- Patient's tolerance to activity
- Effectiveness of treatment (e.g., bronchodilators)
- Patient's tolerance to analgesia and sedation

In the medical office, pulse oximetry is most often used as a "spot-check" measurement—in other words, as a single measurement of oxygen saturation. Occasionally, pulse oximetry may be used in the medical office for the short-term *continuous monitoring* of a patient experiencing an asthmatic attack or to monitor a patient during minor office surgery.

COMPONENTS OF THE PULSE OXIMETER

Most medical offices use a handheld pulse oximeter, which is portable, lightweight, and battery operated. This is in contrast to a stand-alone oximeter, which is more apt to be used in a hospital setting for the continuous bedside monitoring of a patient's oxygen saturation level and pulse rate. The two main parts of the pulse oximeter—the monitor and the probe—are described in detail next.

Monitor

The monitor of the pulse oximeter contains controls, indicators, and displays (Fig. 4.14). These may vary slightly depending on the brand of oximeter. Those that are found on most handheld pulse oximeters include the following:

1. *Power-on control.* Turns the oximeter on.
2. *SpO_2% display.* A digital display of the patient's oxygen saturation expressed as a percent. This number is updated with every few pulse beats.
3. *Pulse rate display.* This display indicates the patient's pulse rate in beats per minute. This number is updated with each pulse beat.
4. *Pulse strength bar-graph indicator.* This indicator provides a visual display of the patient's pulse strength at the probe placement site. The pulse strength indicator consists of a segmented display of bars. The pulse strength indicator "sweeps" with each pulse beat, and the stronger the pulse, the more segments that light up on the bar graph.
5. *Battery icon display.* The battery icon is used to warn that the battery is getting low. When the battery icon flickers continuously on the LED screen, the battery is low and needs to be replaced.
6. *Power-on self-test.* When the pulse oximeter is turned on, it will take about 4 to 6 seconds before displaying the results. It automatically performs a power-on self-test

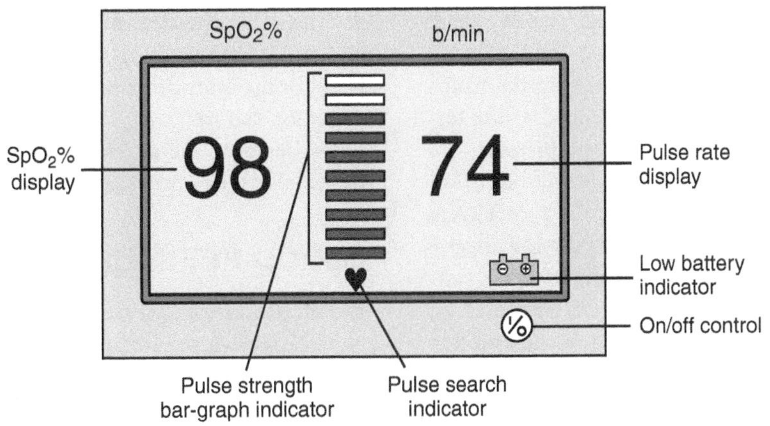

Fig. 4.14 Pulse oximeter monitor: controls, indicators, and displays.

(POST), which takes a few seconds. During the POST, the oximeter checks its internal systems to ensure they are functioning properly. When the POST is completed, the oximeter begins searching for a pulse. It takes several seconds for the oximeter to locate a pulse and to calculate and display the SpO_2 reading. If the oximeter is unable to detect a pulse, or if the pulse is too weak to provide the data needed to calculate oxygen saturation, the oximeter is unable to make a measurement. In this case, the pulse oximeter fails to display the blood oxygen saturation level and/or the pulse rate. If this occurs, the medical assistant should reposition the probe or move the probe to another finger and perform the procedure again.

Clip-on Probe

The clip-on probe must be attached to the patient at a peripheral site that is highly vascular and where the skin is thin. The most common site to apply the probe is the tip of a finger; any finger except for the little finger can be used. Many manufacturers of pulse oximeters recommend the thumb as an application site. Other acceptable probe application sites include the big toe and the earlobe.

FACTORS AFFECTING PULSE OXIMETRY

Although pulse oximetry is an easy procedure to perform, the medical assistant must be aware of certain factors that may interfere with an accurate reading. These factors are listed, along with guidelines for correcting or preventing them.

1. *Incorrect positioning of the probe.* As previously discussed, the oximeter probe consists of two parts: an LED and a light sensor. Because light is transmitted from the LED through the tissues to the light sensor, it is important that LED and light sensor be aligned directly opposite each other during the measurement. In most cases, this automatically occurs when the clip-on probe is applied to the patient's finger. Proper alignment of the probe may be impossible, however, with patients who have very small fingers (e.g., a thin individual and a child) because the probe cannot detect enough blood to make a measurement. To obtain an accurate reading, the probe must be moved to another site, such as the big toe or earlobe.
2. *Fingernail polish or artificial nails.* A dark, opaque coating on the fingernail may result in a falsely low reading. This is because the coating interferes with proper light transmission through the finger. The darker the coating, the more likely that the SpO_2 reading will be affected. Blue, black, and green fingernail polishes tend to cause the most problems. If the patient is wearing dark fingernail polish, it should be removed with acetone or fingernail polish remover. If the patient has long fingernails or artificial fingernails, another site should be used to take the measurement, such as the big toe or earlobe. These situations may obstruct the light sensor and prevent an accurate measurement. Oil, dirt, and grime on the fingertip can also interfere with proper light transmission. If the patient's fingertip is dirty, cleanse the site with soap and water and allow it to dry. Areas with bruises, burns, stains, broken skin, or tattoos should be avoided as a probe placement site. Darkly pigmented skin and jaundice do not usually affect the ability of the oximeter to obtain an accurate reading.
3. *Low pulse bar strength.* The pulse strength bar graph indicator can be used to determine the reliability of a reading. If the height of the pulse bar graph is less than 30%, this indicates signal inadequacy and the displayed SpO_2 and pulse rate readings are potentially incorrect. In this case, the probe should be repositioned on the patient's finger making sure the tip of the finger touches the end of the probe stop and that the LED light and the light sensor are aligned directly opposite to each other.
4. *Poor peripheral blood flow.* A pulse oximeter works best when there is a strong pulse in the finger to which the probe is applied. Poor peripheral blood flow may cause the pulse to be so weak that the oximeter cannot obtain a reading. Conditions resulting in poor blood flow include peripheral vascular disease, vasoconstrictor medications, severe hypotension, and hypothermia. In addition, patients with cold fingers (but who are not hypothermic) may have enough constriction of the peripheral capillaries

that it interferes with obtaining a reading. To solve these problems, the medical assistant should ask the patient to warm his or her hands and fingers by rubbing the hands together. The probe should never be attached to the finger of an arm to which an automatic blood pressure cuff is applied because blood flow to the finger will be cut off when the cuff inflates, resulting in loss of the pulse signal.

5. *Ambient (surrounding) light.* Ambient light shining directly on the probe, such as bright fluorescent light, direct sunlight, or an overhead examination light, may result in an inaccurate reading. This is because some of the ambient light may be picked up by the light sensor and alter the reading. This problem can be corrected by one of the following: turning off the light, moving the patient's hand away from the light source, or covering the probe with an opaque material such as a washcloth.
6. *Finger movement.* Finger movement during the measurement is a common cause of an inaccurate reading. Motion affects the ability of the light to travel from the LED to the light sensor and prevents the probe from picking up the pulse signal. To avoid this problem, it is important that the medical assistant instruct the patient to keep his or her finger stationary during the procedure. Occasionally, movement of the fingers cannot be eliminated, such as when the patient has tremors of the hands. In these instances, the oxygen saturation level should be measured at a site that is less affected by motion, such as the big toe or the earlobe.

CARE AND MAINTENANCE

The pulse oximeter should be cleaned periodically using a cloth slightly dampened with a solution of warm water and a disinfectant cleaner. The medical assistant should make sure that the cloth is not too wet to prevent the solution from running into the oximeter, which could damage the internal components.

The inside of the probe also should be disinfected before and after each patient measurement by wiping it thoroughly with an antiseptic wipe and allowing it to dry. The probe should never be soaked or immersed in a liquid solution because this would damage it. The probe is heat sensitive and cannot be autoclaved. The pulse oximeter should be stored at room temperature in a dry environment.

Blood Pressure

MECHANISM OF BLOOD PRESSURE

Blood pressure is the pressure or force exerted by the circulating blood on the walls of the arteries. Contraction and relaxation of the heart result in two different pressures—systolic pressure and diastolic pressure. Each time the ventricles contract, blood is pushed out of the heart and into the aorta and pulmonary trunk, exerting pressure on the walls of the arteries. This phase in the cardiac cycle is known as **systole**, and it represents the highest point of blood pressure in the body, or the **systolic pressure**. The phase of the cardiac cycle in which the heart relaxes between contractions is referred to as **diastole**. The **diastolic pressure** (documented during diastole) is lower because the heart is relaxed.

BLOOD PRESSURE MEASUREMENT

Blood pressure is measured with a **sphygmomanometer** which is a device that measures the pressure of blood within an artery. There are two types of sphygmomanometers which include the *aneroid* sphygmomanometer and the *digital* sphygmomanometer (more commonly known as an *automatic blood pressure monitor*).

A blood pressure reading consists of two numbers. The top number is the systolic pressure, and the bottom number is the diastolic pressure. The standard unit for measuring blood pressure is millimeters of mercury (mm Hg). A blood pressure reading of 110/70 mm Hg means that there was enough force to raise a column of mercury 110 mm during systole and 70 mm during diastole. These two numbers identify whether a blood pressure reading is healthy or unhealthy. According to the AHA normal healthy blood pressure for an adult is a reading less than 120/80 mm Hg.

Blood pressure should be taken during every office visit to compare a patient's readings over time. This is a good preventive measure in guarding against problems that may occur as a result of high blood pressure. A single blood pressure reading taken on one occasion does not characterize an individual's blood pressure accurately. An average of two or more blood pressure readings taken on two or more separate office visits is recommended to minimize errors and provide a more accurate measurement.

BLOOD PRESSURE CATEGORIES

In 2017, the ACC (American College of Cardiology) and the AHA issued new guidelines for the interpretation of blood pressure in adults. The new guidelines are outlined in Table 4.6 and are described below.

Normal: A blood pressure reading of less than 120/ 80 mm Hg is classified as normal.

Elevated: A systolic reading between 120 and 129 mm Hg *and* a diastolic reading less than 80 mm Hg is classified as elevated. An *elevated* reading means that an individual has an increased risk of developing high blood pressure. Without lifestyle modifications, an individual with a consistently elevated reading is likely to develop high blood pressure.

High blood pressure: The 2017 ACC/AHA guidelines lowered the threshold for the diagnosis of high blood pressure. This is because scientific studies showed that the risk of some complications of high blood pressure begin to develop at a blood pressure reading lower than previously thought. A systolic reading of 130 mm Hg or higher *or* a diastolic reading of 80 mm Hg or higher

Table 4.6 Categories of Blood Pressure in Adults[a]

Blood Pressure Category[b]	Systolic Blood Pressure (mm Hg)		Diastolic Blood Pressure (mm Hg)
Normal	Less than 120	*and*	Less than 80
Elevated	120–129	*and*	Less than 80
Hypertension:			
Hypertension Stage 1	130–139	*or*	80–89
Hypertension Stage 2	140 or higher	*or*	90 or higher

[a]Individuals with a systolic BP and a diastolic BP in two different categories should be designated to the higher BP category.

[b]Based on an average of two or more readings taken on two or more separate occasions.

Reprinted with permission *Hypertension* 2018;71:e13-e115. © 2018 American Heart Association, Inc.

is classified as high blood pressure or *hypertension.* The previous guidelines set the threshold for the diagnosis of high blood pressure at a systolic reading of 140 mm Hg or higher *or* a diastolic reading of 90 mm Hg or higher. The goal of the new guidelines is to allow for intervention of complications caused by high blood pressure (e.g., cardiovascular disease) much earlier than before.

FACTORS TEMPORARILY AFFECTING BLOOD PRESSURE

Blood pressure does not remain at a constant level. A number of factors may temporarily affect blood pressure throughout the course of a day. If possible, the medical assistant should make an attempt to reduce or eliminate these factors if present. This helps to ensure an accurate blood pressure reading.

1. *Diurnal variations.* Fluctuations in an individual's blood pressure are normal during the course of a day. Blood pressure is normally lower at night as a result of decreased metabolism and physical activity during sleep. The blood pressure begins to rise several hours before waking. As metabolism and activity increase during the day, the blood pressure continues to rise, usually peaking in the middle of the afternoon. In the later afternoon and evening, the blood pressure begins dropping again. Patients who are self-monitoring their blood pressure at home should measure their blood pressure at the same time of day.
2. *Emotional states.* Strong emotional states, such as anger, fear, and excitement, increase the blood pressure. If the medical assistant observes such a reaction, an attempt should be made to calm the patient before taking his or her blood pressure.
3. *Physical exercise.* Physical activity temporarily increases the blood pressure. To ensure an accurate reading, a patient who has been involved in physical activity should be given an opportunity to rest for 20 to 30 minutes before blood pressure is measured.
4. *Body position.* The blood pressure of a patient who is in a lying or standing position is usually different from that measured when the patient is sitting. For example, the diastolic pressure of an individual in a sitting position is higher than his or her diastolic pressure in a lying position. A notation should be made in the patient's medical record if the reading was obtained in any position other than sitting, by using the following abbreviations: *L* (lying) and *St* (standing).
5. *Full bladder.* A full bladder can increase the blood pressure as much as 10 to 15 mm Hg. To ensure an accurate reading, a patient should be asked to void before blood pressure is measured.
6. *Tobacco use.* Tobacco products (cigarettes, cigars, smokeless tobacco) contain nicotine which temporarily increases the blood pressure. To ensure an accurate reading, patients should not use tobacco products for 30 minutes before having their blood pressure measured.
7. *Medications.* Certain medications may increase or decrease the blood pressure. For example, OTC cold medications that contain decongestants (e.g., phenylephrine, pseudoephedrine) may cause a temporary increase in the blood pressure. Because of this, it is important to document all prescription and over-the-counter medications patients are taking in their medical records.
8. *Alcohol and caffeine consumption.* Alcohol and caffeine consumption can cause a temporary increase in the blood pressure. A patient should not consume these substances for at least 30 minutes before having blood pressure measured.
9. *Other factors.* Other factors that may temporarily increase the blood pressure include pain and a recent meal.

PULSE PRESSURE

The difference between the systolic pressure and the diastolic pressure is known as the **pulse pressure**. It is determined by subtracting the smaller number from the larger. If the blood pressure is 110/70 mm Hg, the pulse pressure would be 40 mm Hg. A pulse pressure between 30 and 50 mm Hg is considered to be within normal range.

HYPERTENSION

High blood pressure or **hypertension** means the force of the circulating blood against the walls of the blood vessels is consistently above normal. Hypertension is the most common cause of cardiovascular disease-related deaths among Americans. It is estimated that 78 million adult Americans (one in three adults) have high blood pressure but only about half of these (53%) have their high blood pressure under control. The incidence of hypertension in the United

States has increased dramatically as a result of an aging population and an increased incidence of obesity.

If hypertension is not brought under control, over time it can cause severe damage to the blood vessels of vital organs, such as the heart, brain, kidneys, and eyes. This damage increases the risk of a heart attack or heart failure, stroke, aneurysm, kidney damage, and damaged vision. Early detection and treatment of high blood pressure can prevent these complications. High blood pressure is often discovered during a routine medical examination or (less commonly) when an individual experiences one of the complications of hypertension caused by damage to a vital organ.

HYPERTENSION CATEGORIES

The 2017 ACC/AHA guidelines categorize hypertension into the following stages:

1. ***Hypertension Stage 1:*** Hypertension stage 1 is defined as a sustained systolic reading between 130 and 139 mm Hg, *or* a sustained diastolic reading between 80 and 89 mm Hg. At this stage, the provider is likely to prescribe lifestyle modifications and may consider adding blood pressure medication if the patient currently has or is at increased risk for cardiovascular disease.
2. ***Hypertension Stage 2:*** Hypertension stage 2 is defined as a sustained systolic reading of 140 mm Hg or higher, *or* a sustained diastolic reading of 90 mm Hg or higher. At this stage, the provider is likely to prescribe a combination of blood pressure medications and lifestyle modifications.

SYMPTOMS

Hypertension is known as a "silent killer" because there are typically few or no warning signs or symptoms until the sustained increase in the blood pressure has caused significant damage to vital organs resulting in serious complications. Without regular blood pressure measurements, an individual with hypertension may go undiagnosed for many years. Symptoms that may indicate the presence of the serious complications of hypertension include one or more of the following: headaches, dizziness, flushed face, fatigue, epistaxis (nosebleed), excessive perspiration, heart palpitations, chest pain, vision problems, shortness of breath, frequent urination, and leg claudication (cramping in the legs with walking).

PRIMARY HYPERTENSION

In 90% to 95% of cases, the precise cause of hypertension is unknown. This type of hypertension is known as *primary or essential hypertension.* Without treatment, primary hypertension usually worsens over time. Certain factors increase the risk of developing primary hypertension; these are listed and described below.

Uncontrollable Risk Factors

- *Heredity.* A family history of high blood pressure increases an individual's risk of developing high blood pressure.
- *Ethnicity.* In the United States, African-Americans tend to develop hypertension more often than individuals of any other racial background.
- *Age.* Blood pressure normally increases as an individual grows older. For example, a 6-year-old child may have a blood pressure reading of 104/ 68 mm Hg, whereas a young, healthy adult may have a blood pressure reading of 118/ 78 mm Hg, and it would not be unusual for a 60-year-old man to have a reading of 134/ 84 mm Hg. As an individual gets older, there is a loss of elasticity in the walls of the blood vessels, causing this increase in pressure to occur.
- *Gender.* Men are more likely to develop high blood pressure than women until the age of 45 years. Starting at age 65, women usually have a higher blood pressure than men of the same age. (From ages 45 to 65, the risk is equal for both men and women).

Controllable Risk Factors

- *Obesity.* Obesity is one of the biggest risk factors for hypertension, especially in younger people. This is because an increased body mass requires more blood to supply the tissues with oxygen and nutrients. This increased volume of blood circulating through the blood vessels results in an increase in the blood pressure.
- *Sodium intake.* Sodium, found in salt and many processed foods, canned foods, and snack foods, does not cause high blood pressure; however, it can aggravate high blood pressure. As sodium increases in the body, the blood vessels retain more water to try to balance the sodium concentration. This increases the blood volume which causes an increase in the blood pressure. Most Americans consume more sodium than they need. The current AHA recommendation is to consume no more than 2300 mg of sodium per day (equivalent to 1 teaspoon of salt) while an ideal limit is no more than 1500 mg of sodium per day (equivalent to 2/3 teaspoon of salt).
- *Lack of physical exercise.* Physical activity is important for a healthy heart and circulatory system. A sedentary lifestyle increases the chance of developing high blood pressure.
- *Chronic stress.* Research indicates that individuals under continuous stress tend to develop more heart and circulatory problems than people not under stress which can result in an increase in the blood pressure.
- *Tobacco use:* Over time, tobacco use may damage the walls of blood vessels which can result in an increase in the blood pressure.
- *Alcohol consumption.* Heavy and regular alcohol consumption can increase blood pressure.

Treatment

Primary hypertension cannot be cured, but treatments are available to bring it under control. These include lifestyle modifications, such as weight reduction; a healthy diet such as the DASH diet (refer to Chapter 25: Nutrition), lowering sodium (salt) intake and increasing potassium intake;

regular physical exercise; cessation of tobacco use; limitation or elimination of alcohol consumption; and stress management. If lifestyle modifications alone are not enough, medications are available for reducing blood pressure, allowing the patient to lead a normal, healthy, active life. Treatment for essential hypertension is usually life-long. If the patient discontinues lifestyle modifications or stops taking medication, the blood pressure will increase again.

SECONDARY HYPERTENSION

While 90% to 95% of individuals with hypertension have primary hypertension, the remaining 5% to 10% of individuals have *secondary hypertension.* This means that the hypertension is secondary to another medical condition and has a known cause.

Conditions that can result in secondary hypertension include chronic kidney disease, adrenal and thyroid disorders, narrowing of the aorta, steroid therapy, oral contraceptives, diabetes, obstructive sleep apnea, and preeclampsia associated with pregnancy. Once the underlying medical condition is treated, the secondary hypertension usually decreases or even returns to normal.

HYPOTENSION

Hypotension or low blood pressure means the pressure of the circulating blood against the walls of the blood vessels is below normal. Hypotension is defined as a blood pressure reading of less than 90/ 60 mm Hg. Hypotension can be temporary or chronic. Chronic hypotension in healthy individuals without any symptoms usually requires no treatment.

Hypotension may occur as a result of a medical condition, especially when the blood pressure drops suddenly or is accompanied by signs and symptoms such as dizziness or lightheadedness, fainting, blurred vision, nausea, fatigue, and lack of concentration. Medical conditions that cause hypotension include pregnancy, dehydration, heart conditions, endocrine disorders, moderate or severe blood loss, anaphylactic shock, and a severe infection of the bloodstream (septicemia).

Categories of Hypotension

Hypotension is divided into the following categories based upon when the blood pressure drops.

1. ***Orthostatic hypotension:*** Orthostatic hypotension (or postural hypotension) is a drop in blood pressure caused by a sudden change in body position. It occurs most often when an individual is sitting or lying down and then suddenly stands up. After standing up, the patient may experience dizziness and lightheadedness which is often referred to as "seeing stars." Orthostatic hypotension occurs more often in older adults, especially those on antihypertensive medication and/or diuretics. Orthostatic hypotension can be prevented by using slow and gradual movements when standing up.
2. ***Postprandial hypotension:*** Postprandial hypotension is a sudden drop in blood pressure that occurs after eating. Older adults, especially those with Parkinson disease, are more likely to develop this type of hypotension.
3. ***Neurally mediated hypotension***: Neurally mediated hypotension may occur after an individual has been standing or exercising for a long period of time causing dizziness or nausea. It is more commonly seen in children and young adults. Emotionally upsetting or scary events can also cause this type of hypotension.
4. ***Severe hypotension:*** Severe hypotension can occur with shock and is the most extreme form of hypotension. Shock is caused by the failure of the cardiovascular system to deliver enough blood to the body's vital organs to function properly. Shock causes the blood pressure to drop to a dangerously low level and can be life-threatening if not treated promptly. The organs most affected are the heart, brain, and lungs, which can be irreparably damaged in 4 to 6 minutes. The general signs and symptoms of severe shock are weakness, restlessness, anxiety, disorientation, pallor, cold and clammy skin, rapid breathing, and rapid pulse. If not treated, these symptoms can progress rapidly to a significant drop in the blood pressure, cyanosis, loss of consciousness, and death.

What Would You Do? What Would You *Not* Do?

Case Study 3

Tyrone Jackson, 45 years old, is at the medical office to have his blood pressure checked. Six months ago, Tyrone started taking a diuretic and an antihypertensive drug prescribed by the physician to reduce his blood pressure. The last documentation in his medical record indicates that Tyrone's blood pressure decreased from 168/112 mm Hg to 118/78 mm Hg; however, his blood pressure at this visit is 138/98 mm Hg. Tyrone says that he has not been very good at following the lifestyle modifications and medication plan prescribed by the physician. He says it is hard to remember to take his blood pressure pills every day. He says that he felt just fine before being put on blood pressure pills, but when he started taking them, he felt awful. He had to urinate more often; when he got up fast, he felt dizzy; and he also has some problems with headaches. Tyrone says that he decided to cut back on his medication to see if these problems got better, and sure enough, they went away altogether. ■

BLOOD PRESSURE MEASUREMENT: MANUAL METHOD

The manual method requires the medical assistant to perform the steps in the blood pressure procedure manually or by hand; this includes inflation and deflation of the cuff of the sphygmomanometer and determining the blood pressure measurement by listening to the sounds produced by the brachial artery (Korotkoff sounds). The equipment

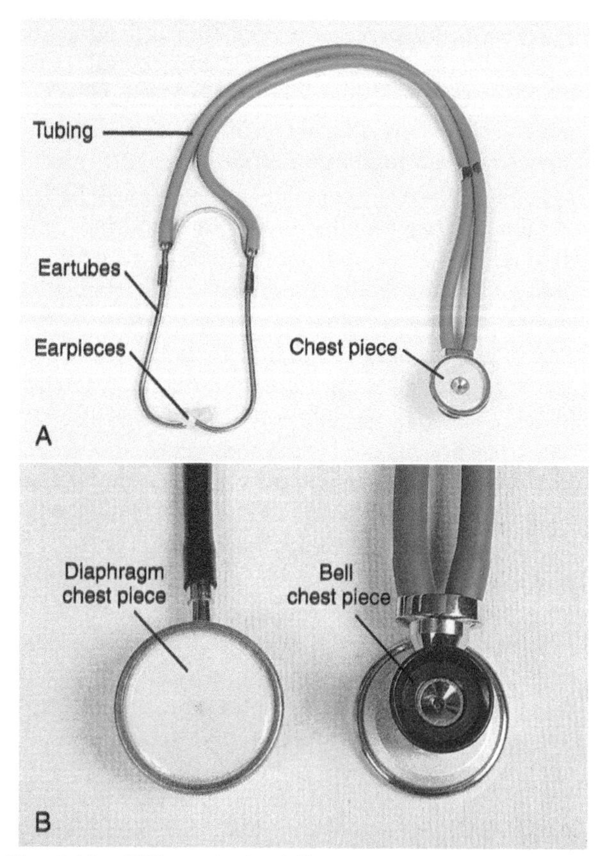

Fig. 4.15 (A) The parts of a stethoscope. (B) Types of chest pieces.

needed to measure blood pressure using the manual method includes a stethoscope and an aneroid sphygmomanometer.

STETHOSCOPE

A **stethoscope** is a medical device that amplifies sounds produced by the body and allows a user to hear them. The stethoscope was first introduced in the 1800s by a French physician named René Laennec. This early stethoscope consisted of a simple wooden tube with a bell-shaped opening at one end.

The most common type of stethoscope used in the medical office is the acoustic stethoscope which consists of the following parts: earpieces, ear tubes, tubing, and a chest piece (Fig. 4.15A). The *earpieces* are made of a soft flexible material to provide a comfortable fit. They should fit snugly in the ear canal to provide for effective auscultation and to keep out unwanted sounds. The *ear tubes* consist of metal tubes that connect the earpieces to the tubing. The ear tubes are angled in a way that allows the earpieces to be directed slightly forward. This allows the earpieces to follow the direction of the ear canal to provide for maximum sound quality. The *tubing* connects the ear tubes to the chest piece. The purpose of the *tubing* is to transfer sounds from the chest piece and relay them to the earpieces. The usual length of the tubing on a stethoscope is 12 to 16 inches (30 to 40 cm). This length provides convenience and ease when placing the chest piece over the brachial artery during blood pressure measurement.

Chest Piece

There are two types of chest pieces: a *diaphragm,* which is a large, flat disc and a *bell,* which has a bowl-shaped appearance and is surrounded by a rubber ring (see Fig. 4.15B). Most health care workers prefer a two-sided chest piece with a diaphragm on one side and a bell on the other side. When using a two-sided chest piece, the medical assistant must ensure that the desired side is rotated into its proper position before use. Failure to do so will prevent the medical assistant from hearing sounds through the earpieces.

The diaphragm chest piece is more useful for hearing medium to high-pitched sounds, such as lung and bowel sounds, whereas the bell chest piece is more useful for hearing low-pitched sounds, such as those produced by the heart and vascular system. Studies have shown that the diaphragm and bell provide similar results when measuring blood pressure and therefore, either one can be used for the reliable measurement of blood pressure. Because the diaphragm is easier to hold firmly in place on the patient's arm and covers a larger area, most health care workers use the diaphragm for measuring blood pressure. However, if the medical assistant is having difficulty hearing sounds from the diaphragm when measuring blood pressure, he or she should switch to the bell.

Care and Maintenance

Stethoscopes must be cared for properly to ensure proper functioning and to prevent the transmission of pathogens in the medical office. The earpieces should be removed and cleaned regularly with a cotton-tipped applicator moistened with alcohol to remove cerumen. The chest piece should be cleaned with an antiseptic wipe to remove dirt, dust, lint, and oils. The tubing should be cleaned with a paper towel using an antimicrobial soap and water. Alcohol should not be used to clean the tubing because it can dry out the tubing and cause it to crack over time.

ANEROID SPHYGMOMANOMETER

A sphygmomanometer is a device that measures the pressure of blood within an artery. An aneroid sphygmomanometer consists of a **manometer** (for registering pressure), an inner inflatable bladder surrounded by a covering known as the *cuff,* and a pressure bulb with a control valve to inflate and deflate the inner bladder (Fig. 4.16). The manometer consists of a gauge with a round scale which is calibrated in millimeters with a needle that points to the calibrations (Fig. 4.17). To ensure an accurate reading, the needle must be positioned initially at zero. At least once a year an aneroid sphygmomanometer should be recalibrated to ensure its accuracy.

Aneroid sphygmomanometers are available in three different designs:

- Portable aneroid sphygmomanometer (see Fig. 4.16)
- Wall-mounted aneroid sphygmomanometer (Fig. 4.18A)
- Mobile floor-stand aneroid sphygmomanometer (see Fig. 4.18B)

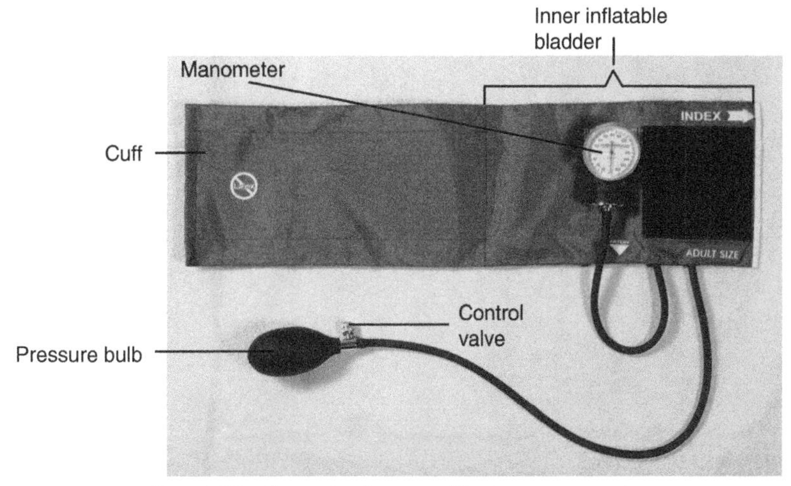

Fig. 4.16 The parts of an aneroid sphygmomanometer.

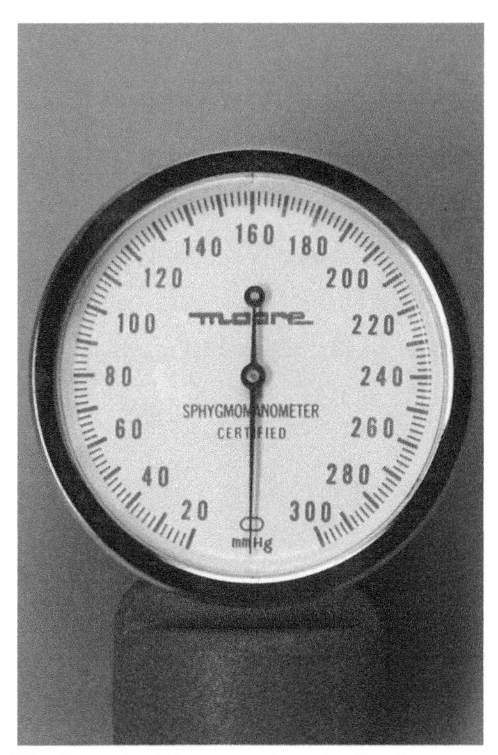

Fig. 4.17 The scale of the gauge of an aneroid sphygmomanometer.

Cuff Sizes

Blood pressure cuffs for adults come in a variety of sizes which include *small adult, adult, large adult,* and *adult thigh* (Fig. 4.19). The adult cuff is typically used for the average-sized adult arm while a small adult cuff is used for adults with thin arms. The thigh cuff is used for taking blood pressure from the thigh or for adults with large arms.

It is essential that the correct cuff size be used to measure blood pressure. If the cuff is too small, the reading may be falsely high, as it would be, for example, when an adult cuff is used on a patient with a large arm. If the cuff is too large, the reading may be falsely low, as it would be when an adult cuff is used on a patient with a thin arm. Prevention of errors is of upmost importance when measuring blood pressure (Box 4.3). Not using the correct cuff size is the most common error made in blood pressure measurement.

In obese patients with an arm circumference greater than 52 cm (20 inches), it may not be possible to fit even an adult thigh cuff around the patient's arm. In this situation the AHA states that the patient's blood pressure can be measured using the forearm and radial artery; however, the AHA further states that this method may result in a falsely high systolic reading. When this method is used, an appropriate-sized cuff should be positioned midway between the elbow and the wrist, with the center of the bladder positioned over the radial pulse. The medical assistant should then place the chest piece of the stethoscope over the radial pulse and should measure the patient's blood pressure using the same technique presented in Procedure 4.9.

Determination of Correct Cuff Size

There are several ways to determine the correct cuff size of a patient to ensure an accurate blood pressure measurement.

1. **Assessment of Bladder Length and Width:** For accurate blood pressure measurement, the cuff size should have an inner bladder length that encircles at least 80% (but not more than 100%) of the arm circumference and a bladder width that is at least 40% of the arm circumference (Fig. 4.20).
2. **Determination of Upper Mid-Arm Circumference:** The correct cuff size can be determined based on the circumference of the upper mid-arm which is located midway between the shoulder and elbow. The circumference of the upper mid-arm should be measured with a flexible centimeter tape measure wrapped evenly around the arm (Fig. 4.21). The measurement is then compared to a table

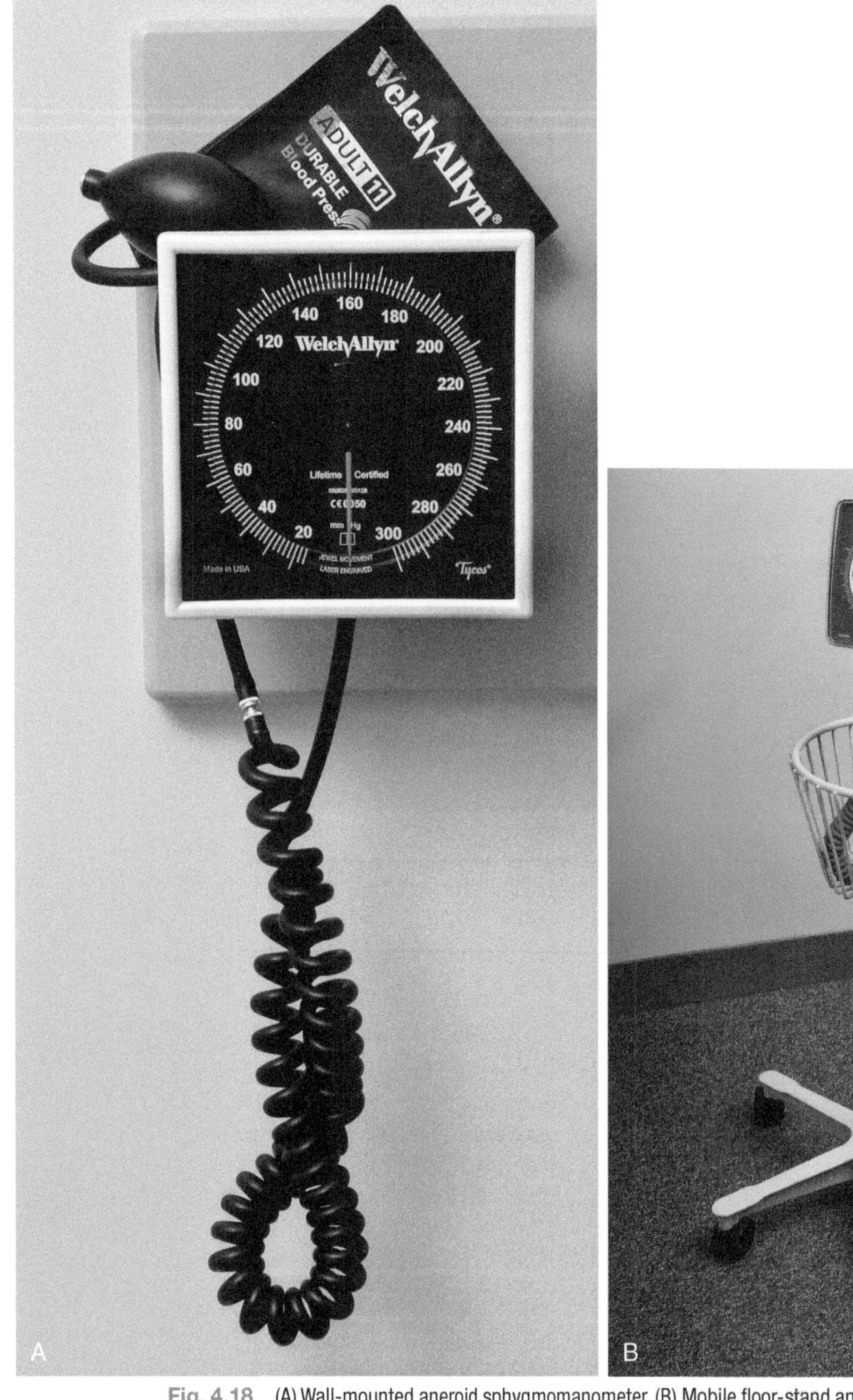

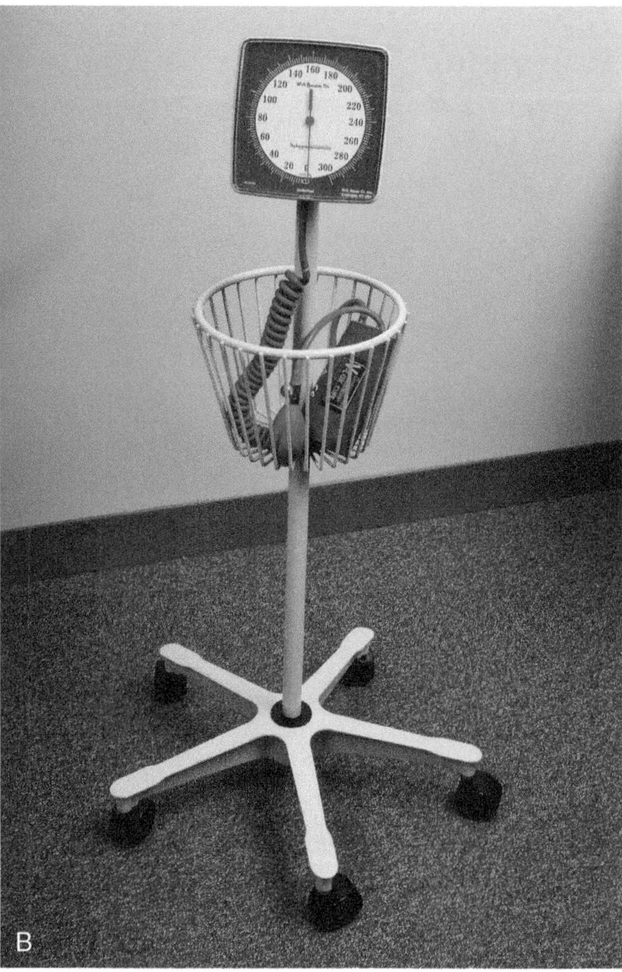

Fig. 4.18 (A) Wall-mounted aneroid sphygmomanometer. (B) Mobile floor-stand aneroid sphygmomanometer. (A, Courtesy Holzer Health Systems, Athens, OH.)

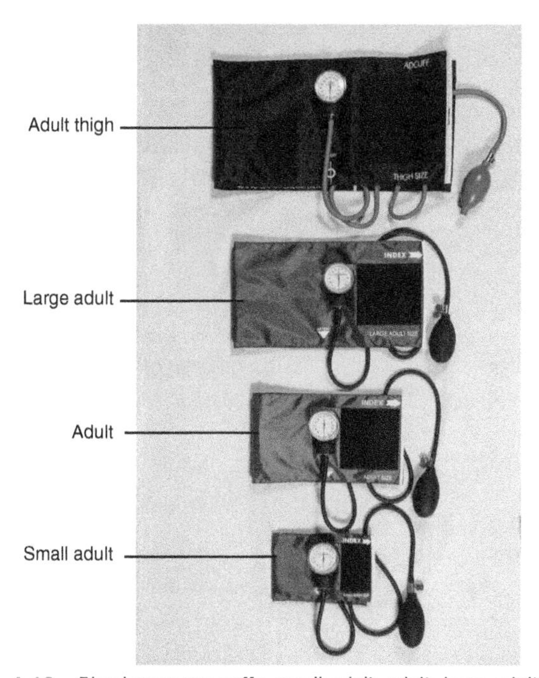

Fig. 4.19 Blood pressure cuffs: small adult, adult, large adult, and thigh.

outlining the cuff sizes and the mid-arm circumference range of each (Table 4.7).

3. **Assessment of Range and Index Lines:** Most blood pressure cuffs are marked with two *range lines* (Fig. 4.22A) and an *index line* located at the end of the cuff. When the correct-sized cuff is applied to the patient's arm, the *index line* should fall between the two range lines (see Fig. 4.22, B). If the index line does not fall within the range lines, the cuff is not a correct fit for that patient and a larger or a smaller cuff must be used.

KOROTKOFF SOUNDS

Korotkoff sounds are used to determine systolic and diastolic blood pressure readings. When the bladder of the cuff is inflated, the brachial artery is compressed so that no audible sounds are heard through the stethoscope. As the cuff is deflated, the sounds become audible until the blood flows freely, at which point the sounds can no longer be heard (Table 4.8). The first clear tapping sound represents the systolic pressure and the point at which the sounds disappear

BOX 4.3 Prevention of Errors in Blood Pressure Measurement

The following guidelines should be followed to prevent errors in blood pressure measurement:

1. *Instruct the patient* not to consume caffeine or alcohol, use tobacco, or exercise for 30 min before blood pressure measurement to prevent a falsely high blood pressure reading.
2. *The patient should be comfortably seated* in a quiet room for at least 5 min before blood pressure is taken. Patient anxiety and apprehension caused by being in a medical office setting can temporarily increase the blood pressure reading by as much as 30 mm Hg. This is known as the "white coat effect," which refers to the white lab coat worn by the provider.
3. *Position the patient properly.* The patient should be seated in a chair with back support with the legs uncrossed (at the knees) and both feet flat on the floor. If the back is not supported (such as when a patient is seated on an examining table), the diastolic reading can be increased by as much as 6 mm Hg. Crossing the legs at the knees can increase the systolic reading by 2– 8 mm Hg. The arm should be positioned at heart level and well supported on a flat surface with the palm facing upward. If the arm is above heart level, the blood pressure reading may be falsely low. If the arm is not supported or is placed below heart level, the blood pressure reading may be falsely high.
4. *Never take blood pressure over clothing.* Taking blood pressure over clothing could result in an inaccurate reading. The patient's sleeve should be rolled up approximately 5 inches above the elbow so that the cuff can be applied to bare skin. If the sleeve is too tight after being rolled up, the arm should be removed from the sleeve. A tight sleeve creates a tourniquet-like effect which causes partial compression of the brachial artery, resulting in a falsely low reading.
5. *Always use the correct cuff size.* Incorrect cuff size is the most common cause of an inaccurate blood pressure measurement. If the cuff is too small, it may come loose as the cuff is inflated, or the reading may be falsely high. If the cuff is too large, the reading may be falsely low.
6. [a]*Correctly position the cuff.* The center of the inner bladder should be positioned directly above the brachial pulse site with the lower edge of the cuff approximately 1–2 inches (2.5–5 cm) above the bend in the elbow. Most cuffs are labeled with arrows indicating the center of the bladder for the right and left arms. Centering the inner bladder above the pulse site allows for complete compression of the brachial artery. The cuff should be placed high enough above the bend in the elbow to prevent the diaphragm of the stethoscope from touching it; otherwise, extraneous sounds may be picked up which could interfere with an accurate measurement.
7. *Wrap the cuff snugly around the patient's arm.* The cuff should be snug but not too tight. To assess the appropriate tightness of the cuff, one finger should slip easily under the cuff.
8. [a]*Position the earpieces so that the sounds can be heard clearly.* The earpieces of the stethoscope should be positioned in the ears with the earpieces directed slightly forward. This allows the earpieces to follow the direction of the ear canal, which facilitates hearing.

Continued

BOX 4.3 Prevention of Errors in Blood Pressure Measurement—cont'd

9. [a]*Position the chest piece properly.* The chest piece should be placed firmly, but gently, over the brachial pulse site to assist in transmission of clear and audible sounds. The chest piece should not be allowed to touch the cuff, to prevent extraneous sounds from being picked up, which could interfere with an accurate measurement.
10. [a]*Rapidly inflate the cuff.* The cuff should be rapidly inflated to a level that is approximately 30 mm Hg above the previously measured or palpated systolic pressure. Overinflation of the cuff is uncomfortable for the patient and could result in a falsely high blood pressure reading.
11. [a]*Release the pressure at a moderate steady rate.* The pressure in the cuff should be released at a rate of 2–3 mm Hg per second to ensure an accurate blood pressure measurement. Releasing the pressure too slowly is uncomfortable for the patient and could cause a falsely high diastolic reading. Releasing the pressure too quickly could cause a falsely low systolic reading.
12. *Wait before taking blood pressure again.* The medical assistant should wait 1–2 min before taking blood pressure again in the same arm to allow the blood flow in the brachial artery to return to normal to ensure an accurate reading.
13. *Measure and document the blood pressure in both arms during the initial blood pressure assessment of a new patient.* There may normally be a small difference in blood pressure between the two arms. During return visits, the blood pressure should be measured in the arm with the higher initial reading.

[a]Applies only to the manual method of measuring blood pressure. (The absence of this footnote applies to both the manual and automatic methods of measuring blood pressure).

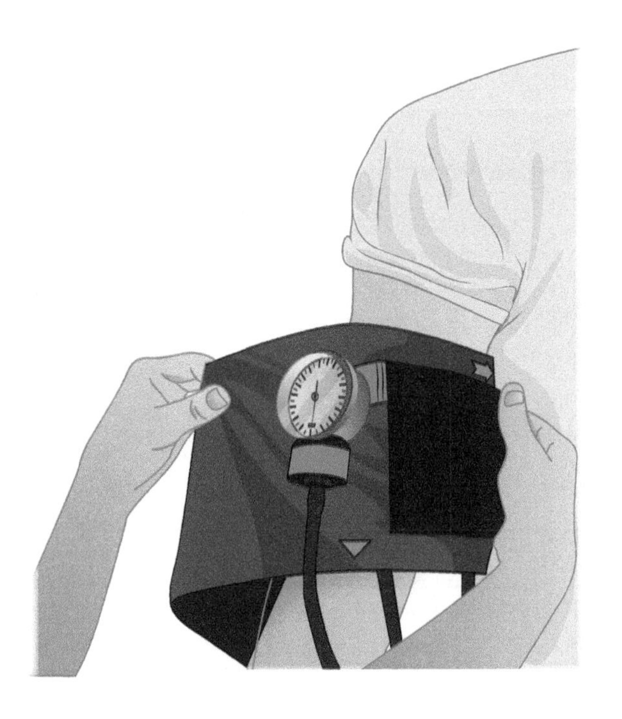

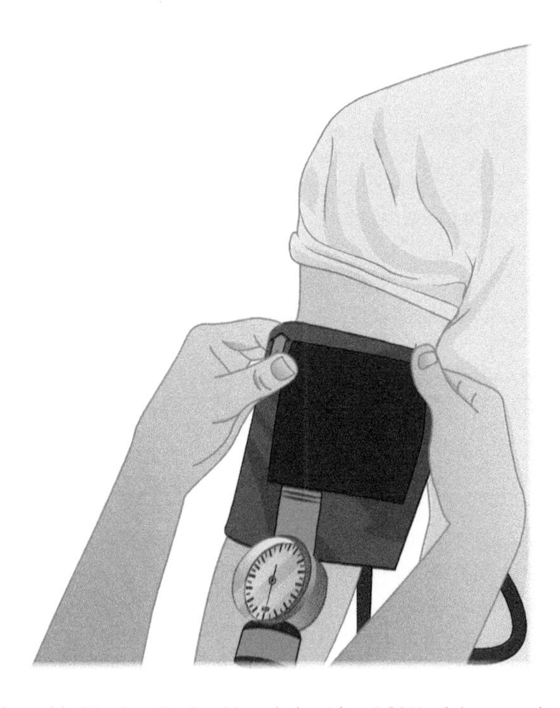

Fig. 4.20 Determination of cuff size using bladder length and width. (A) The inner bladder length should encircle at least 80% of the arm circumference. (B)The bladder width should be at least 40% of the arm circumference.

represents the diastolic pressure. The medical assistant should practice listening to these sounds and should be able to identify the various Korotkoff phases.

Procedure 4.9 outlines the procedure for taking blood pressure using an aneroid sphygmomanometer. Procedure 4.10 outlines the procedure for determining systolic pressure by palpation.

BLOOD PRESSURE MEASUREMENT: AUTOMATIC METHOD

Automatic blood pressure monitors are increasingly being used in medical offices to measure blood pressure. The steps in the procedure are performed automatically by the

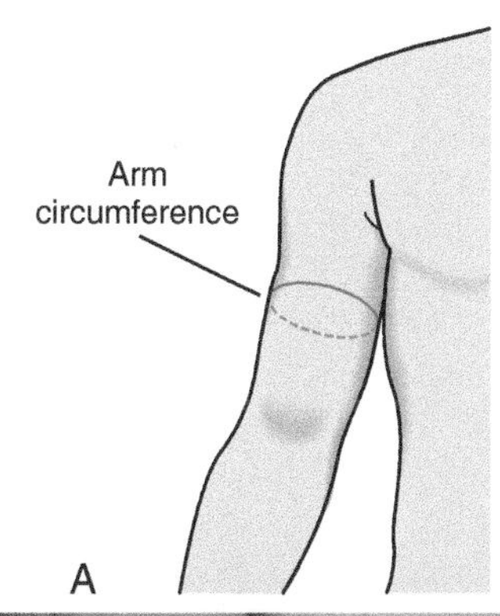

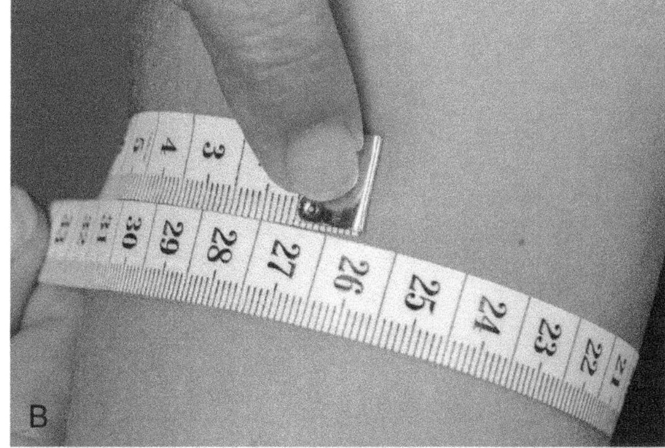

Fig. 4.21 Determination of cuff size using upper mid-arm circumference. (A) Upper mid-arm circumference is located midway between the shoulder and elbow. (B) Upper mid-arm circumference is measured with a centimeter tape measure. The mid-arm circumference of this patient is 25.5 cm, which means a small adult BP cuff is required.

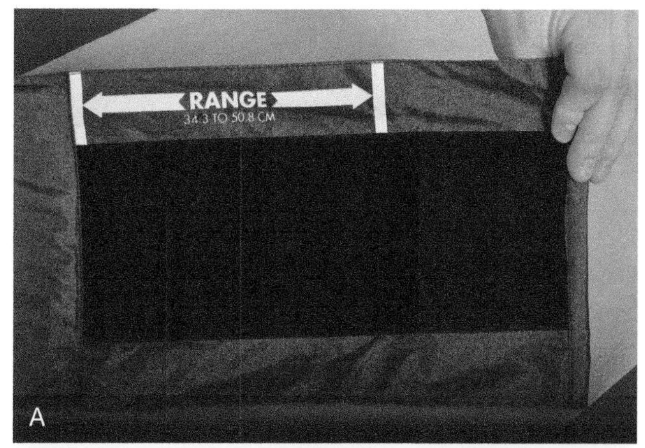

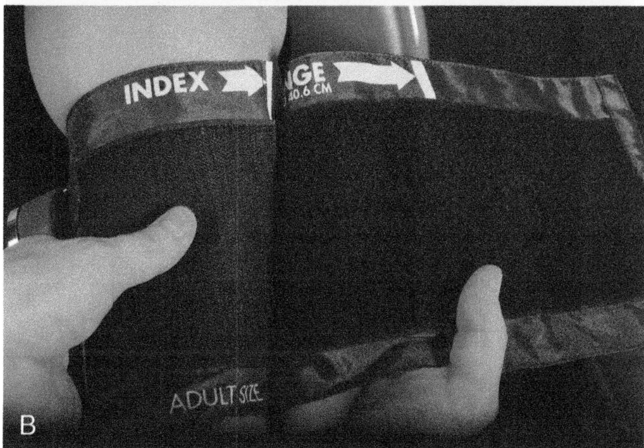

Fig. 4.22 Determination of cuff size using the range and index lines. (A) Range lines on a blood pressure cuff. (B) The index line falls within the range lines, indicating this is the proper-sized cuff for this patient.

Table 4.7 Recommended Cuff Size for Adults

Upper Mid-Arm CircumferenceRange (cm)	Cuff Size
22–26 cm	Small adult
27–34 cm	Adult
35–44 cm	Large adult
45–52 cm	Adult thigh

monitor (Procedure 4.11). The equipment for measuring blood pressure using the automatic method includes an automatic blood pressure monitor (also known as a digital sphygmomanometer). Automatic monitors are especially popular for the home monitoring of blood pressure.

Automatic monitors use an electronic pressure sensor to measure oscillations from the wall of the brachial artery as the cuff gradually deflates. An oscillation is a back-and-forth movement that occurs in the brachial artery as the pulse wave travels through it. The point of maximum oscillation corresponds to the mean arterial pressure, which is an overall index of an individual's blood pressure. A computer in the monitor then uses this information to calculate the systolic blood pressure and the diastolic blood pressure. Results are then displayed digitally on an LED screen. The automatic blood pressure procedure takes approximately 30 seconds to complete from start to finish.

Automatic blood pressure monitors are available in the following designs:

- Portable automatic monitor (Fig. 4.23A)
- Mobile floor-stand automatic monitor (see Fig. 4.23B)

The medical assistant should closely follow the manufacturer's instructions for the particular brand and model of automatic monitor used; these instructions are outlined in the user manual that accompanies the monitor. Many of the guidelines for the accurate measurement of blood pressure using the automatic method are the same as those for the manual measurement of blood pressure (see Box 4.3). The automatic monitor should be calibrated periodically according to the manufacturer's recommendations. Automatic monitors offer certain advantages and disadvantages, described as follows.

Table 4.8 Korotkoff Sounds

Phase	Description	Illustration
	Inflation of cuff compresses and closes off brachial artery so that no blood flows through the artery.	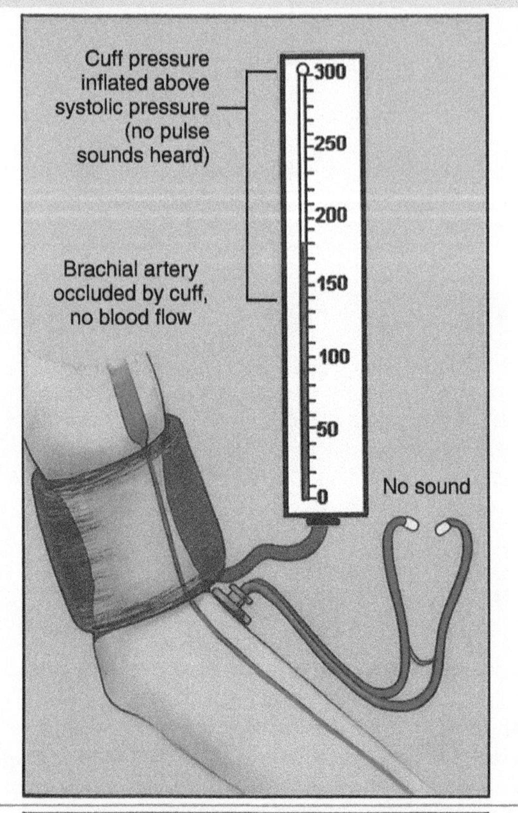
Phase I	First faint but clear tapping sound is heard, and it gradually increases in intensity. First tapping sound is the systolic pressure.	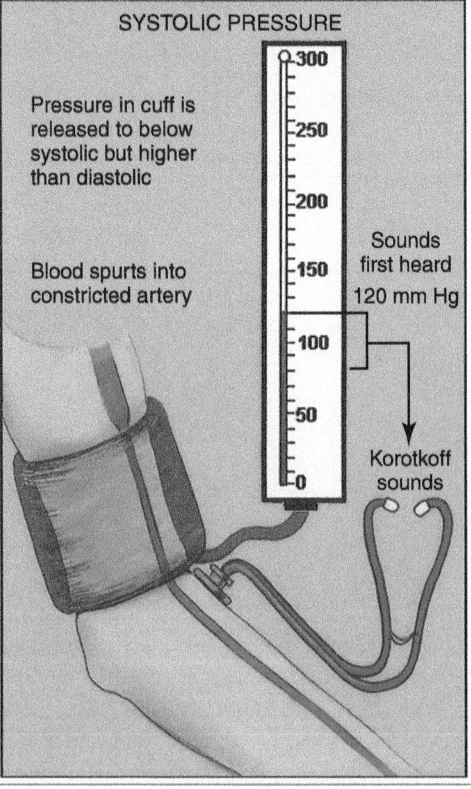

Table 4.8 Korotkoff Sounds—cont'd

Phase	Description	Illustration
Phase II	As cuff continues to deflate, sounds have murmuring or swishing quality.	
Phase III	With further deflation, sounds become crisper and increase in intensity.	
Phase IV	Sounds become muffled and have soft, blowing quality.	
Phase V	Sounds disappear. This is documented as the diastolic pressure.	

ADVANTAGES

1. The cuff does not have to be manually inflated and deflated because this function is performed automatically by the monitor.
2. A stethoscope and user listening skills are not required to obtain the reading because the electronic pressure sensor in the automatic monitor measures oscillations from the wall of the brachial artery to obtain the reading.
3. Automatic monitors are less susceptible to external environmental noise than are manual monitors.
4. The blood pressure measurement is easy to read because the systolic and diastolic readings are shown on a digital display screen.
5. Most automatic monitors allow multiple readings to be taken during the measurement procedure. The monitor automatically calculates averages of these values and displays them on the screen.
6. Automatic monitors measure the pulse rate, which is displayed on the screen along with the blood pressure measurement.
7. Most automatic monitors come equipped with an internal memory for storing multiple blood pressure measurements.

DISADVANTAGES

1. There are certain conditions that may result in an inaccurate reading with an automatic blood pressure monitor. These include preeclampsia, dysrhythmias (such as atrial fibrillation), arteriosclerosis, and a very weak pulse. If any of these conditions are present, an alternative method of blood pressure measurement should be used.
2. Because the monitor relies on brachial artery oscillations to obtain a reading, stiff arteries (especially in older patients) can interfere with obtaining an accurate reading.
3. Automatic monitors designed for use in a medical office setting are more expensive than manual monitors.

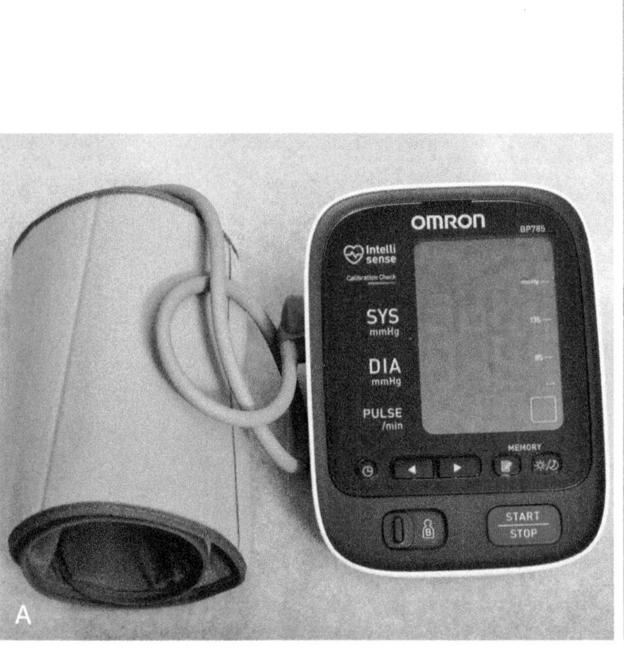

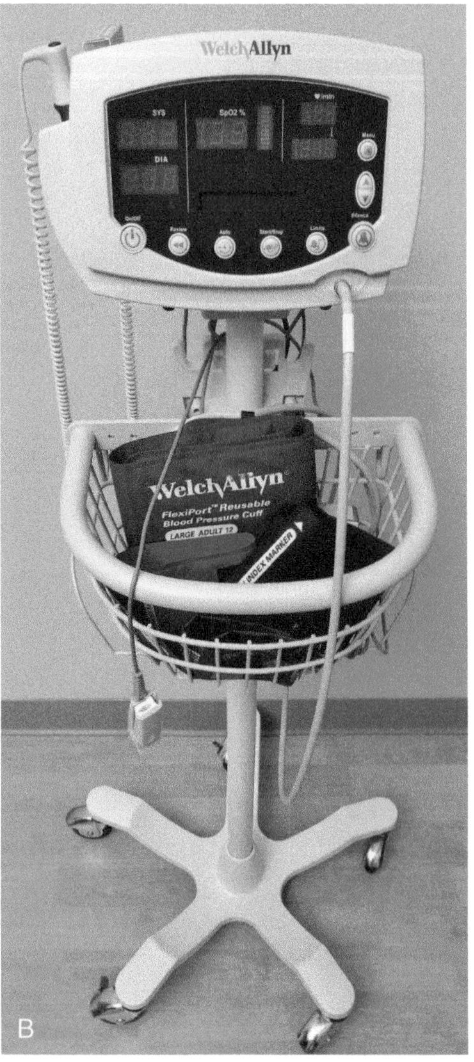

Fig. 4.23 Automatic blood pressure monitors. (A) Portable automatic monitor. (B) Mobile floor-stand automatic monitor (also includes an electronic thermometer and pulse oximeter). (B, Courtesy Holzer Health Systems, Athens, OH.)

What Would You Do? What Would You *Not* Do? RESPONSES

Case Study 1

Page 96

What Did Sergio Do?

- ❑ Told Mrs. Mason that sometimes ear thermometers can be a little tricky to use.
- ❑ Showed Mrs. Mason how to use the ear thermometer and let her practice by taking Olivia's temperature.
- ❑ Explained how to care for and maintain the ear thermometer to prevent inaccurate readings.

What Did Sergio Not Do?

- ❑ Did not ask Mrs. Mason if she had read the directions that came with her ear thermometer.
- ❑ Did not ask Mrs. Mason why she waited so long to bring Olivia to the office.

Case Study 2

Page 101

What Did Sergio Do?

- ❑ Recognized and congratulated Alex on his swimming achievements.
- ❑ Told Alex that it is normal for his pulse to be that slow because of his athletic training and it shows that he is in good shape.
- ❑ Assured Alex that the physician will do everything he can to help Alex.
- ❑ Stressed to Alex how important it is to follow the physician's advice so that his shoulder heals as soon as possible.

What Did Sergio Not Do?

- ❑ Did not comment on Alex's request for a steroid injection or pain pills. Made sure to document the information so that the physician could handle the situation.

What Would You Do? What Would You *Not* Do? RESPONSES—Cont'd

❑ Did not criticize Alex for putting a swim meet before his health.

Case Study 3
Page 109

What Did Sergio Do?

❑ Empathized with Tyrone about having to remember to take his medication. Suggested that he get a daily pill container to help him remember.

❑ Stressed to Tyrone the importance of following his lifestyle modifications and taking his blood pressure medication. Explained to him that high blood pressure is a "silent disease." He may feel fine, but damage to his body organs can still be taking place if he does not follow his treatment plan.

❑ Gave Tyrone a brochure about high blood pressure and went over the long-term effects of hypertension and lifestyle modifications that could help lower blood pressure.

❑ Encouraged Tyrone to call the office when he experiences side effects from medications because the physician may be able to do something to help.

What Did Sergio Not Do?

❑ Did not minimize the importance of following his treatment plan.

TERMINOLOGY REVIEW

Key Term	Word Parts	Definition
Adventitious sounds		Abnormal breath sounds.
Afebrile	*a-:* without	Without fever; the body temperature is normal.
Alveoli	*alveol/o:* air sac	Thin-walled air sacs of the lungs in which the exchange of oxygen and carbon dioxide takes place.
Antecubital space	*ante-:* before cubitum: elbow	The space located at the front of the elbow.
Antipyretic	*anti-:* against *pyr/o:* fever *-ic:* pertaining to	An agent that reduces fever.
Aorta		The major trunk of the arterial system of the body. The aorta arises from the upper surface of the left ventricle.
Apnea	*a-:* without or absence of *-pnea:* breathing	The temporary cessation of breathing.
Axilla		The area under the shoulder or armpit.
Blood pressure		The pressure or force exerted by the circulating blood on the walls of the arteries.
Bounding pulse		A pulse with an increased volume that feels very strong and full.
Bradycardia	brady-: slow cardi/o: heart *-ia:* condition of diseased or abnormal state	An abnormally slow heart rate (less than 60 beats/min).
Bradypnea	brady-: slow *-pnea:* breathing	An abnormal decrease in the respiratory rate of less than 10 respirations per minute.
Celsius scale		A temperature scale in which the freezing point of water is 0° and the boiling point of water is 100°; also called the *centigrade scale.*
Conduction		The transfer of energy, such as heat, from one object to another by direct contact.
Convection		The transfer of energy, such as heat, through air currents.
Crisis		A sudden falling of an elevated body temperature to normal.
Cross-contamination		The process by which microorganisms are unintentionally transferred from one person, object, or place to another.

Continued

TERMINOLOGY REVIEW—cont'd

Key Term	Word Parts	Definition
Cyanosis	cyan/o: blue *-osis:* abnormal condition	A bluish discoloration of the skin and mucous membranes.
Diastole		The phase in the cardiac cycle in which the heart relaxes between contractions.
Diastolic pressure		The point of lesser pressure on the arterial wall, which is recorded during diastole.
Dyspnea	*dys-:* difficult, painful, abnormal *-pnea:* breathing	Shortness of breath or difficulty in breathing.
Dysrhythmia	*dys-:* difficult, painful, abnormal rhythm: rhythm *-ia:* condition of diseased or abnormal state	An irregular rhythm; also termed *arrhythmia.*
Eupnea	*eu-:* normal, good *-pnea:* breathing	Normal respiration. The rate is 16–20 respirations per minute, the rhythm is even and regular, and the depth is normal.
Exhalation	*-ex:* outside, outward	The act of breathing out.
Fahrenheit scale		A temperature scale in which the freezing point of water is 32° and the boiling point of water is 212°.
Febrile		Pertaining to fever.
Fever		A body temperature that is above normal; synonym for *pyrexia.*
Frenulum linguae		The midline fold that connects the undersurface of the tongue with the floor of the mouth.
Hyperpnea	*hyper-:* above, excessive *-pnea:* breathing	An abnormal increase in the rate and depth of respirations.
Hyperpyrexia	*hyper-:* above, excessive *pyr/o:* fever *-ia:* condition of diseased or abnormal state	An extremely high fever.
Hypertension	*hyper-:* above, excessive *-tension:* pressure	The force of the circulating blood against the walls of the blood vessels is consistently above normal.
Hyperventilation	*hyper-:* above, excessive	An abnormally fast and deep type of breathing, usually associated with acute anxiety conditions.
Hypopnea	*hypo-:* below, deficient *-pnea:* breathing	An abnormal decrease in the rate and depth of respirations.
Hypotension	*hypo-:* below, deficient *tension:* pressure	The pressure of the circulating blood against the walls of the blood vessels is below normal.
Hypothermia	*hypo-:* below, deficient therm/o: heat *-ia:* condition of diseased or abnormal state	A body temperature that is below normal.
Hypoxemia	*hypo-:* below, deficient *ox/i:* oxygen *-emia:* blood condition	A decrease in the oxygen saturation of the blood. Hypoxemia may lead to hypoxia.

TERMINOLOGY REVIEW—cont'd

Key Term	Word Parts	Definition
Hypoxia	*hypo-:* below, deficient *ox/i:* oxygen *-ia:* condition of diseased or abnormal state	A reduction in the oxygen supply to the tissues of the body.
Inhalation	*in-:* in, into	The act of breathing in.
Intercostal	*inter-:* between cost/o: rib *-al:* pertaining to	Between the ribs.
Korotkoff sounds		Sounds heard during the measurement of blood pressure that are used to determine the systolic and diastolic blood pressure readings.
Malaise	-mal: bad	A vague sense of body discomfort, weakness, and fatigue that often marks the onset of a disease and continues through the course of the illness.
Manometer	*-meter:* instrument used to measure	An instrument for measuring pressure.
Orthopnea	*orth/o:* straight *-pnea:* breathing	The condition in which breathing is easier when an individual is in a sitting or standing position.
Pulse oximeter	*ox/i:* oxygen *-meter:* instrument used to measure	A device used to measure the oxygen saturation of arterial blood.
Pulse oximetry	*ox/i:* oxygen *-metry:* measurement	The use of a pulse oximeter to measure the oxygen saturation of arterial blood.
Pulse pressure		The difference between the systolic and diastolic pressures.
Pulse rhythm		The time interval between heartbeats.
Pulse volume		The strength of the heartbeat.
Radiation		The transfer of energy, such as heat, in the form of waves.
SaO_2 (saturation of arterial oxygen)		Abbreviation for the percentage of hemoglobin that is saturated with oxygen in arterial blood.
Sphygmomanometer	sphygm/o: pulse *-meter:* instrument used to measure	A device that measures the pressure of blood within an artery.
SpO_2 (saturation of peripheral oxygen)		Abbreviation for the percentage of hemoglobin that is saturated with oxygen in arterial blood as measured by a pulse oximeter.
Stethoscope	*steth/o:* chest *-scope:* to view, to examine	An instrument used for amplifying and hearing sounds produced by the body.
Systole		The phase in the cardiac cycle in which the ventricles contract, sending blood out of the heart and into the aorta and pulmonary trunk.
Systolic pressure		The point of maximum pressure on the arterial walls, which is recorded during systole.
Tachycardia	*tachy-:* fast, rapid cardi/o: heart *-ia:* condition of diseased or abnormal state	An abnormally fast heart rate (more than 100 beats/min).
Tachypnea	tachy-: fast *-pnea:* breathing	An abnormal increase in the respiratory rate of more than 20 respirations per minute.
Thready pulse		A pulse with a decreased volume that feels weak and thin.

PROCEDURE 4.1 Measuring Oral Body Temperature—Electronic Thermometer

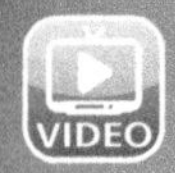

Outcome Measure oral body temperature.

Equipment/Supplies

- Electronic thermometer
- Oral probe (blue collar)
- Plastic probe cover
- Waste container

1. **Procedural Step.** Sanitize your hands and assemble the equipment.
2. **Procedural Step.** Remove the thermometer unit from its storage base, and attach the oral (blue collar) probe to it. This is accomplished by inserting the latching plug (at the end of the coiled cord of the oral probe) to the plug receptacle on the thermometer unit until it clicks into place. Insert the probe into the face of the thermometer.
   Principle. The oral probe is color-coded with a blue collar for ease in identifying it.

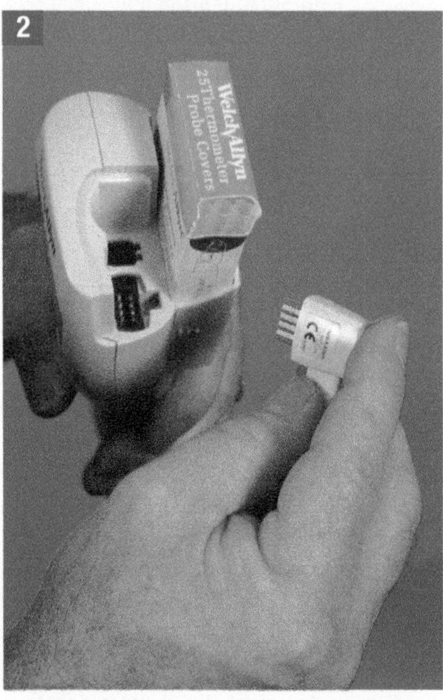

Attach the oral probe to the thermometer.

3. **Procedural Step.** Greet the patient and introduce yourself. Identify the patient and explain the procedure. If the patient has recently ingested hot or cold food or beverages or has been smoking, you must wait 15–30 min before taking the temperature.
   Principle. Ingestion of hot or cold food or beverages and smoking change the temperature of the mouth, which could result in an inaccurate reading.
4. **Procedural Step.** Grasp the probe by the collar, and remove it from the face of the thermometer. Slide the probe into a disposable plastic probe cover until it locks into place.
   Principle. Removing the probe from the thermometer automatically turns on the thermometer. The probe cover prevents the transfer of microorganisms from one patient to another.

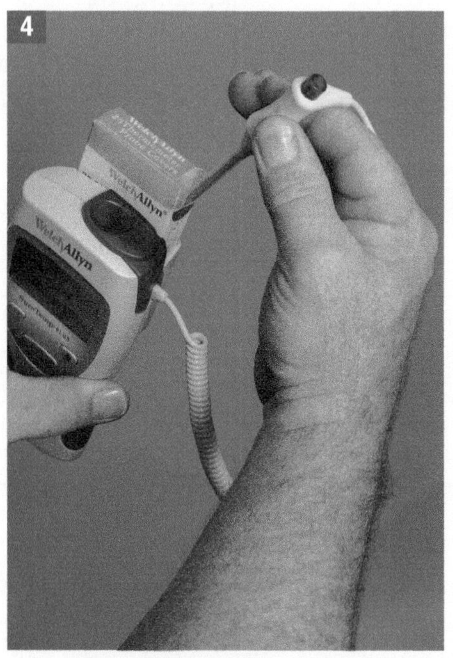

Slide the probe into a probe cover.

5. **Procedural Step.** Take the patient's temperature by inserting the probe under the patient's tongue in the pocket located on either side of the frenulum linguae. Instruct the patient to keep the mouth closed.
   Principle. There is a good blood supply in the tissue under the tongue. The mouth must be kept closed to prevent cooler air from entering and affecting the temperature reading.

PROCEDURE 4.1 Measuring Oral Body Temperature—Electronic Thermometer—cont'd

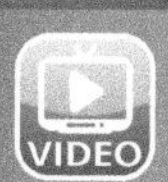

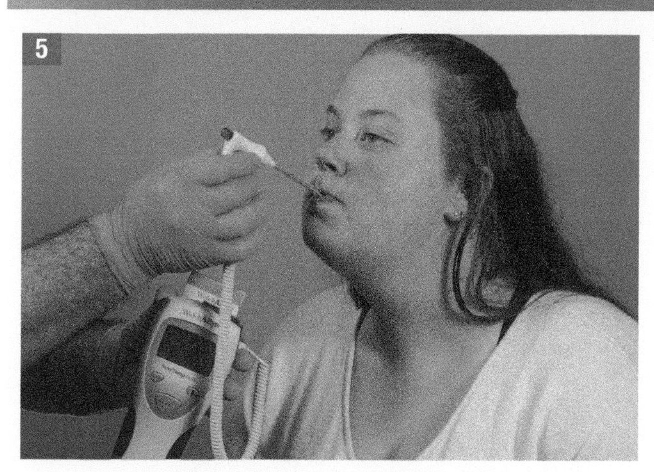

Insert the probe under the patient's tongue.

6. Procedural Step. Hold the probe in place until you hear the tone. At that time, the patient's temperature appears as a digital display on the screen. Make a mental note of the temperature reading. (The temperature indicated on this thermometer is 98.5°F [36.9°C].)

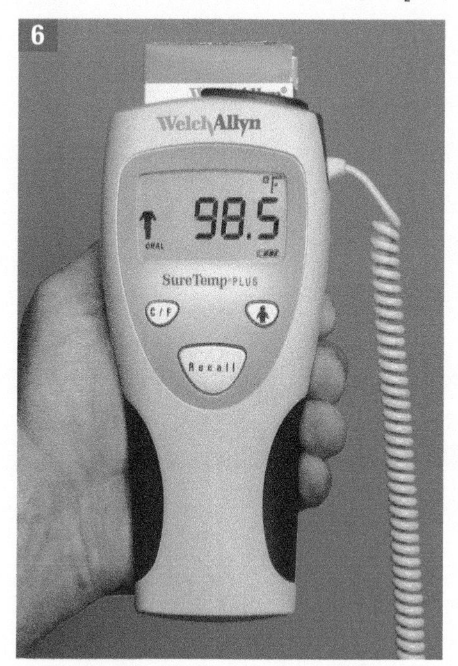

The temperature appears as a digital display on the screen.

7. Procedural Step. Remove the probe from the patient's mouth. Discard the probe cover by firmly pressing the ejection button while holding the probe over a regular waste container. Do not allow your fingers to come in contact with the probe cover.

Principle. The probe cover should not be touched, to prevent the transfer of microorganisms from the patient to the medical assistant. Saliva is not considered regulated medical waste; the probe can be discarded in a regular waste container.

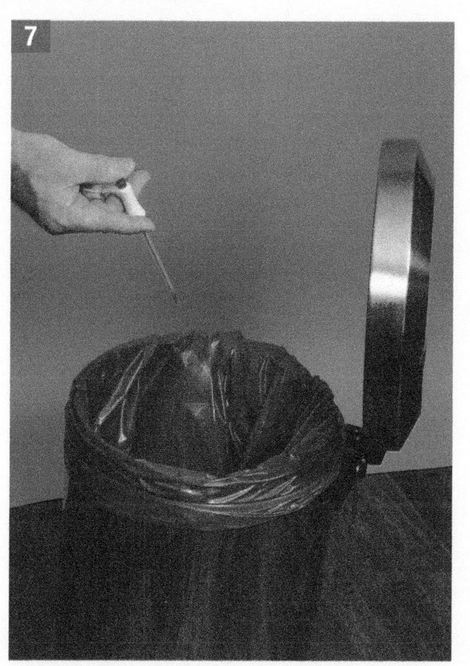

Discard the probe cover by pressing the ejection button.

8. Procedural Step. Return the probe to its stored position in the thermometer unit. Return the thermometer unit to its storage base.

Principle. Returning the probe to the unit automatically turns off and resets the thermometer.

9. Procedural Step. Sanitize your hands.

10. Procedural Step. Document the results in the patient's medical record.

a. *Electronic health record:* In SimChart for the Medical Office, document the temperature reading and site using textboxes, drop-down menus, and/or radio buttons. The temperature can be documented in either Fahrenheit or Celsius, and the software will convert the temperature so that both are displayed (refer to the SimChart® example).

b. *Paper-based patient record:* Document the date, the time, and the temperature reading.

Principle. Patient data must be documented properly to aid the provider in the diagnosis and to provide future reference.

Continued

PROCEDURE 4.1 Measuring Oral Body Temperature—Electronic Thermometer—cont'd

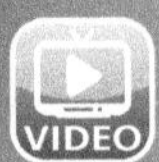

Add Vital Signs

Temperature

Fahrenheit: 98.5

Celsius: 36.9

Site: -Select-
-Select-
Forehead
Oral
Rectal
Tympanic

Pulse

Pulse:

Site: -Select-

Respiration

Respiration:

Blood Pressure

Systolic: Site: -Select-

Diastolic: Mode: -Select-

Position: -Select-

Oxygenation

Saturation%: Site: -Select-

Oxygen Delivery: ○ Room Air

PPR Documentation Example

Date	
10/15/XX	2:15 p.m. T: 98.5° F.—S. Martinez, RMA

PROCEDURE 4.2 Measuring Axillary Body Temperature—Electronic Thermometer

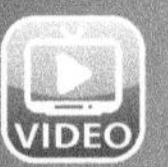

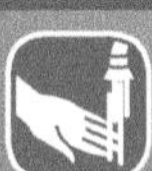

Outcome Measure axillary body temperature. *Note:* Many of the principles for taking a temperature already have been stated and are not included in this procedure.

Equipment/Supplies

- Electronic thermometer
- Oral probe (blue collar)
- Plastic probe cover
- Waste container

1. **Procedural Step.** Sanitize your hands, and assemble the equipment.
2. **Procedural Step.** Remove the thermometer unit from its storage base, and attach the oral (blue collar) probe to it. This is accomplished by inserting the latching plug (on the end of the coiled cord of the oral probe) to the plug receptacle on the thermometer unit until it locks into place. Insert the probe into the face of the thermometer.
3. **Procedural Step.** Greet the patient and introduce yourself. Identify the patient and explain the procedure.
4. **Procedural Step.** Remove clothing from the patient's shoulder and arm. Ensure that the axilla is dry. If it is wet, pat it dry with a paper towel or a gauze pad. ***Principle.*** Clothing removal provides optimal exposure of the axilla for proper placement of the thermometer. Rubbing the axilla causes an increase in the

PROCEDURE 4.2 Measuring Axillary Body Temperature—Electronic Thermometer—cont'd

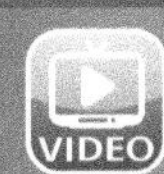

temperature in that area owing to friction, resulting in an inaccurate temperature reading.

5. **Procedural Step.** Grasp the probe by the collar, and remove it from the face of the thermometer. Slide the probe into a disposable probe cover until it locks into place.
6. **Procedural Step.** Take the patient's temperature by placing the probe in the center of the patient's axilla. Instruct the patient to hold the arm close to the body. Hold the arm in place for small children and other patients who cannot maintain the position themselves.
Principle. Interference from outside air currents is reduced when the arm is held in the proper position.

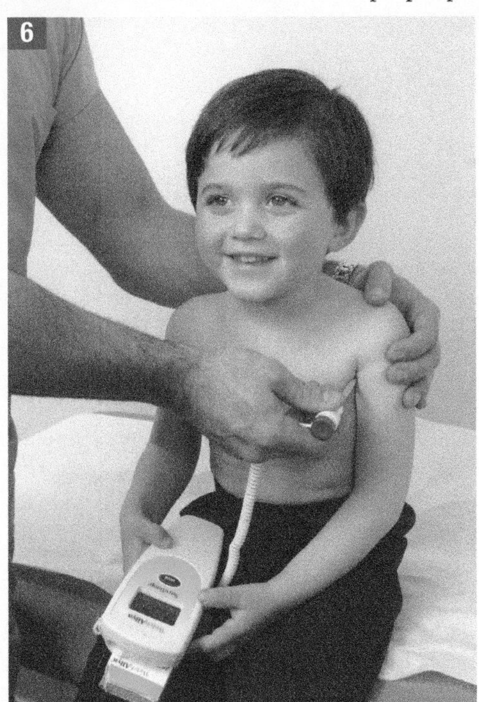

Place the probe in the center of the patient's axilla.

7. **Procedural Step.** Hold the probe in place until you hear the tone. At that time, the patient's temperature appears as a digital display on the screen. Make a mental note of the temperature reading.
8. **Procedural Step.** Remove the probe from the patient's axilla. Discard the probe cover by firmly pressing the ejection button while holding the probe over a regular waste container. Do not allow your fingers to come in contact with the probe cover.
9. **Procedural Step.** Return the probe to its stored position in the thermometer unit. Return the thermometer unit to its storage base.

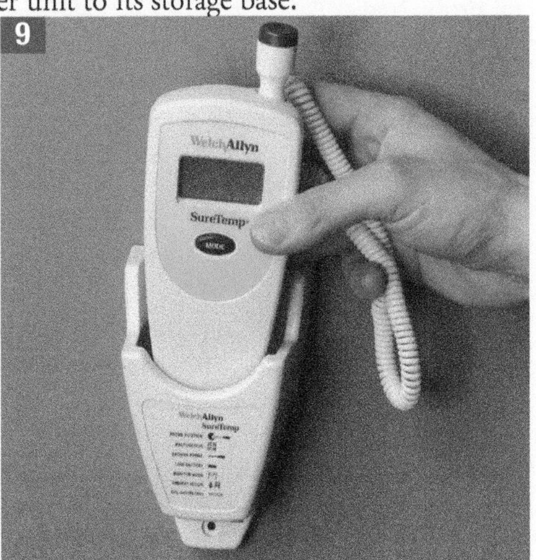

Return the thermometer to its base.

10. **Procedural Step.** Sanitize your hands.
11. **Procedural Step.** Document the results in the patient's medical record.
    a. *Electronic health record:* In SimChart for the Medical Office, document the temperature reading and site using textboxes, drop-down menus, and/or radio buttons. The temperature can be documented in either Fahrenheit or Celsius and the software will convert the temperature so that both are displayed.
    b. *Paper-based patient record:* Document the date, the time, and the axillary temperature reading. The symbol Ⓐ must be documented next to the temperature reading to tell the provider that an axillary reading was taken.

PPR Documentation Example

Date	
10/15/XX	9:30 a.m. T: 97.4° F Ⓐ –S. Martinez, RMA

Procedure 4.2

PROCEDURE 4.3 Measuring Rectal Body Temperature—Electronic Thermometer

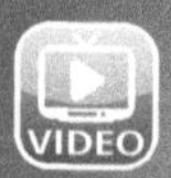

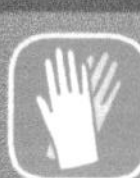

Outcome Measure rectal body temperature.

Equipment/Supplies

- Electronic thermometer
- Rectal probe (red collar)
- Plastic probe cover
- Lubricant
- Disposable gloves
- Tissues
- Waste container

1. **Procedural Step.** Sanitize your hands, and assemble the equipment.
2. **Procedural Step.** Remove the thermometer unit from its storage base. Attach the rectal (red collar) probe to it. This is accomplished by inserting the latching plug (on the end of the coiled cord of the rectal probe) to the plug receptacle on the thermometer unit. Insert the probe into the face of the thermometer.
   Principle. The rectal probe is color-coded with a red collar for ease in identifying it.
3. **Procedural Step.** Greet the patient and introduce yourself. Identify the patient and explain the procedure. If the patient is a child or an adult, provide him or her with a patient gown. Instruct the patient to remove enough clothing to provide access to the anal area and to put on the gown with the opening in the back. If the patient is an infant, ask the parent to remove the infant's diaper.
   Principle. It is important to explain what you will be doing, because body temperature may be higher in a fearful or apprehensive patient. The patient gown provides the patient with modesty and comfort.
4. **Procedural Step.** Apply gloves. Position the patient. *Adults and children:* Position the patient in the modified left lateral recumbent position, and drape the patient to expose only the anal area. *Infants:* Position the infant on his or her abdomen.
   Principle. Gloves protect the medical assistant from microorganisms in the anal area and feces. Correct positioning allows clear viewing of the anal opening and provides for proper insertion of the thermometer. Draping reduces patient embarrassment and provides warmth.
5. **Procedural Step.** Grasp the probe by the collar, and remove it from the face of the thermometer. Slide the probe into a disposable plastic probe cover until it locks into place. Apply a lubricant to the tip of the probe cover up to a level of 1 inch.
   Principle. A lubricated thermometer can be inserted more easily and does not irritate the delicate rectal mucosa.

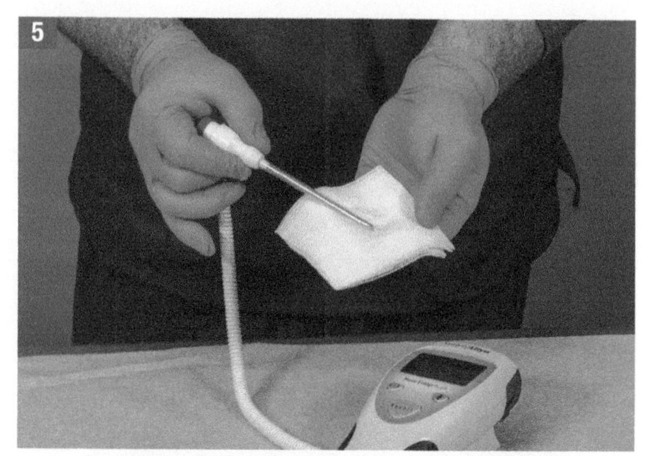

5 Apply a lubricant to the tip of the probe cover.

6. **Procedural Step.** Instruct the patient to lie still. Separate the buttocks to expose the anal opening, and gently insert the thermometer probe approximately 1 inch into the rectum of an adult, 5/8 inch in children, and 1/2 inch in infants. Do not force insertion of the probe. Hold the probe in place until the temperature registers.
   Principle. The probe must be inserted correctly to prevent injury to the tissue of the anal opening. The probe should be held in place to prevent damage to the rectal mucosa.

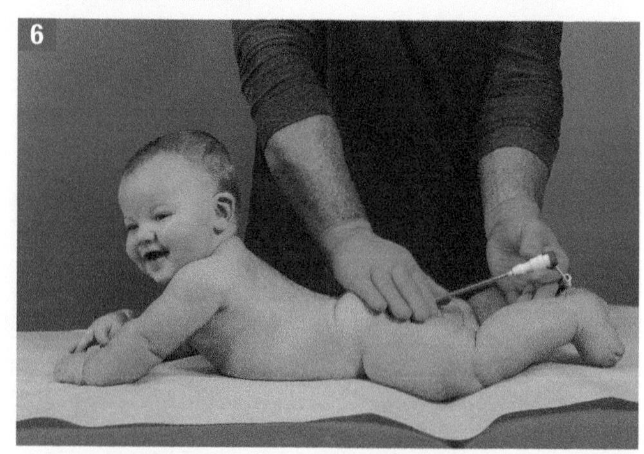

6 Gently insert the probe into the rectum.

PROCEDURE 4.3 Measuring Rectal Body Temperature—Electronic Thermometer—cont'd

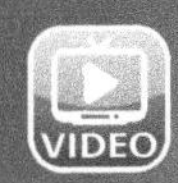

7. **Procedural Step.** Hold the probe in place until you hear the tone. At that time, the patient's temperature appears as a digital display on the screen. Make a mental note of the temperature reading.
8. **Procedural Step.** Gently remove the probe from the rectum in the same direction as it was inserted. Avoid touching the probe cover. Discard the probe cover by firmly pressing the ejection button while holding the probe over a regular waste container. Return the probe to its stored position in the thermometer unit. Return the thermometer unit to its storage base.
   Principle. Fecal material is not considered regulated medical waste; the probe can be discarded in a regular waste container.
9. **Procedural Step.** Wipe the patient's anal area with tissues to remove excess lubricant. Dispose of the tissues in a regular waste container.
   Principle. Wiping the anal area makes the patient more comfortable.
10. **Procedural Step.** Remove gloves, and sanitize your hands.
11. **Procedural Step.** Document the results in the patient's medical record.
    a. *Electronic health record:* In SimChart for the Medical Office, document the temperature reading and site using textboxes, drop-down menus, and/or radio buttons. The temperature can be documented in either Fahrenheit or Celsius and the software will convert the temperature so that both are displayed.
    b. *Paper-based patient record:* Document the date, the time, and the rectal temperature reading. The symbol (R) must be documented next to the temperature reading to tell the provider that a rectal reading was taken.

PPR Documentation Example

Date	
10/15/xx	3:00 p.m. T: 99.8° F, (R) ————
	———— S. Martinez, RMA

PROCEDURE 4.4 Measuring Aural Body Temperature

Outcome Measure aural body temperature.

Equipment/Supplies

- Tympanic membrane thermometer
- Probe cover
- Waste container

1. **Procedural Step.** Sanitize your hands, and assemble the equipment.
   Principle. Your hands should be clean and free from contamination.
2. **Procedural Step.** Greet the patient and introduce yourself. Identify the patient and explain the procedure.
   Principle. It is important to explain what you will be doing, because body temperature may be higher in a fearful or apprehensive patient.
3. **Procedural Step.** Remove the thermometer from its storage base. Ensure that the sensor lens is clean and intact. If the lens is dirty, gently wipe it with an antiseptic wipe or cotton swab moistened with alcohol and allow it to dry. After cleaning, allow at least 5 min before taking the temperature. If the lens is damaged, the thermometer cannot be used and must be repaired or replaced.
   Principle. A dirty sensor lens reduces the transparency of the lens and may result in a falsely low temperature reading.
4. **Procedural Step.** Attach a cover on the probe by pressing the probe tip straight down into the cover box. You will be able to see and feel the cover snap securely into place on the probe. This procedure automatically turns on the thermometer.

Continued

PROCEDURE 4.4 Measuring Aural Body Temperature—cont'd

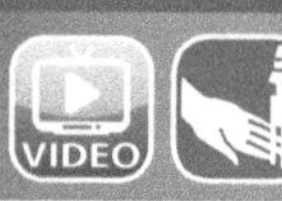

Principle. The probe cover protects the sensor lens and provides infection control. The cover must be seated securely on the probe to activate the thermometer.

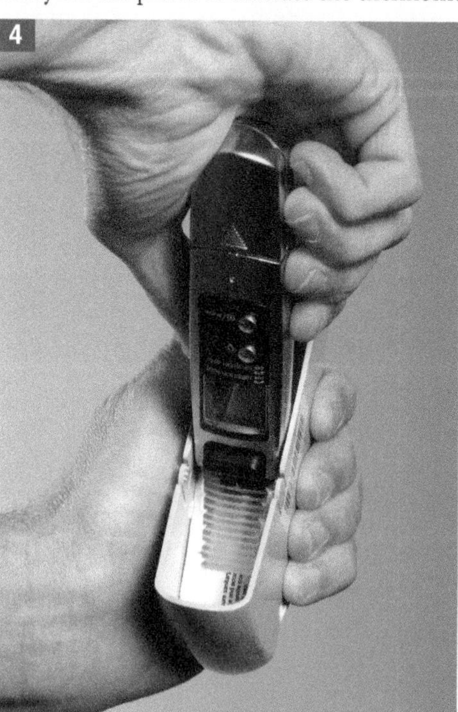

Place a cover on the probe.

5. **Procedural Step.** Pull the probe straight up from the cover box. Look at the digital display to see if the thermometer is ready to use. The °F (or °C) icon flashes when the thermometer is ready to use.

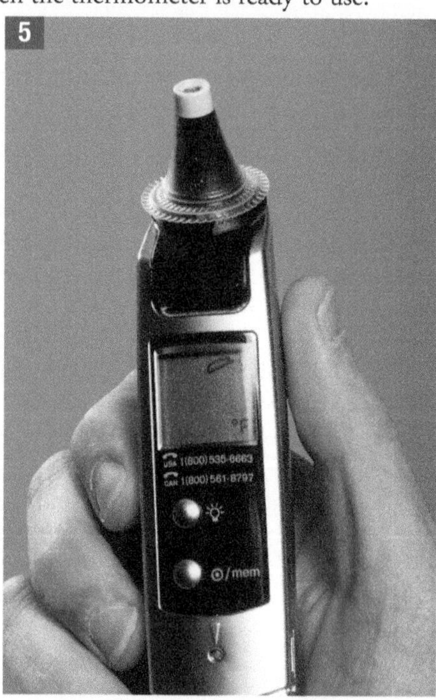

Look to see if the thermometer is ready for use.

6. **Procedural Step.** Hold the thermometer in your dominant hand. If you are right-handed, you should take the temperature in the patient's right ear. If you are left-handed, take the temperature in the patient's left ear.

   Principle. Taking the temperature with the dominant hand assists in the proper placement of the probe in the patient's ear.

7. **Procedural Step.** Straighten the patient's external ear canal with your nondominant hand, as follows:

   Adults and children older than 3 years: Gently pull the ear auricle upward and backward.

   Children younger than 3 years: Gently pull the ear pinna downward and backward.

   Principle. Straightening the ear canal allows the probe sensor to obtain a clear picture of the tympanic membrane, resulting in an accurate temperature measurement.

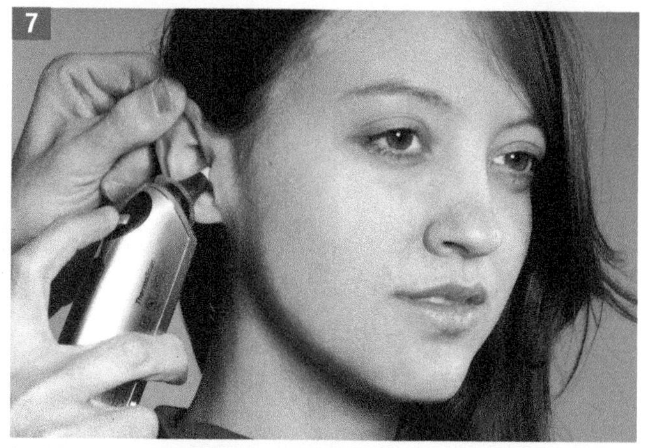

Straighten the canal of adults and children older than 3 years by pulling the ear auricle upward and backward.

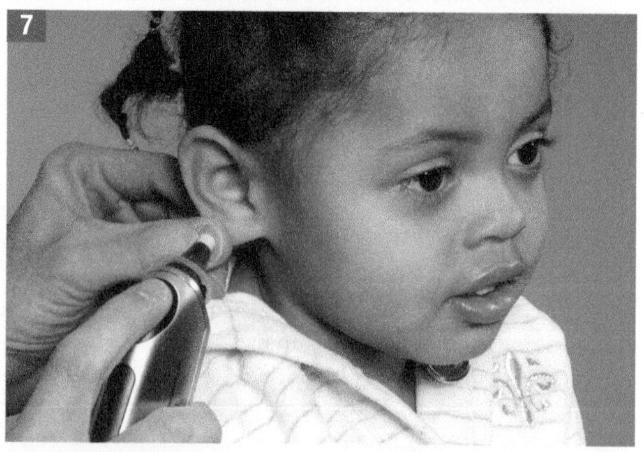

Straighten the canal of children younger than 3 years by pulling the ear auricle downward and backward.

8. **Procedural Step.** Insert the probe into the patient's ear canal tightly enough to seal the opening, but without

PROCEDURE 4.4 Measuring Aural Body Temperature—cont'd

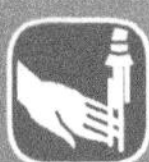

causing patient discomfort. Point the tip of the probe toward the opposite temple (approximately midway between the opposite ear and eyebrow).

Principle. Sealing the ear canal prevents cooler external air from entering the ear, which could result in a falsely low reading. Correct positioning of the probe optimizes the view of the tympanic membrane by the sensor lens, leading to an accurate temperature reading.

9. **Procedural Step.** Ask the patient to remain still. Hold the thermometer steady, and depress the activation button. Depending on the brand of the thermometer, perform one of the following:
   a. Hold the button down for 1 full second and then release it, or
   b. Hold down the button down until an audible tone is heard.

   Principle. The thermometer cannot take a temperature unless the activation button is depressed for 1 full second. When the button is depressed, the sensor lens scans the thermal energy radiated by the tympanic membrane.

10. **Procedural Step.** Remove the thermometer from the ear canal. Turn the digital display of the thermometer toward you, and read the temperature. Make a mental note of the temperature reading. If the temperature seems to be too low, repeat the procedure to ensure that you have used the proper technique. The temperature indicated on this thermometer is 99.8°F (37.7°C). The temperature remains on the display screen for 30–60 s or until another cover is inserted on the probe (whichever occurs first).

    Principle. Improper technique can result in a falsely low temperature reading.

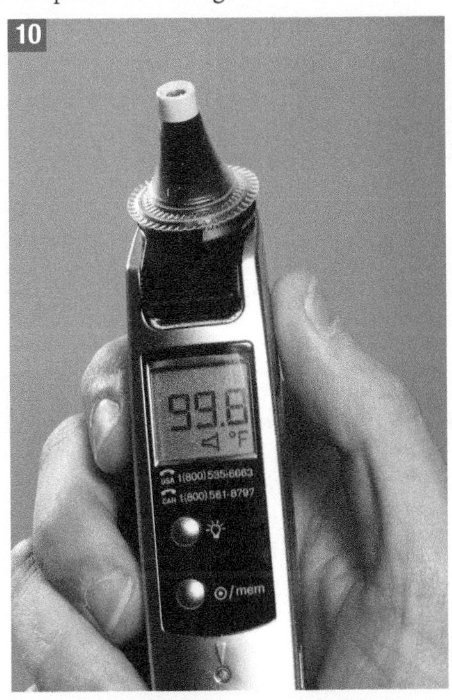

Read the temperature on the digital display.

11. **Procedural Step.** Dispose of the probe cover by ejecting it into a regular waste container. Wipe the sensor lens with an antiseptic.

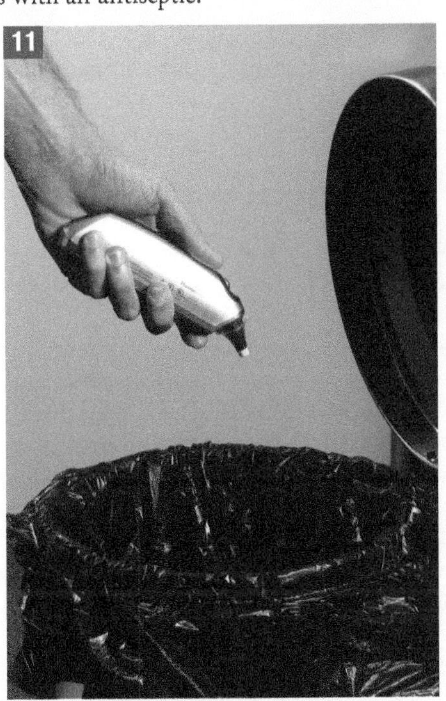

Dispose of the probe cover.

12. **Procedural Step.** Replace the thermometer in its storage base.

    Principle. The thermometer should be stored in its base to protect the sensor lens from damage and dirt.

13. **Procedural Step.** Sanitize your hands.
14. **Procedural Step.** Document the results in the patient's medical record.
    a. *Electronic health record:* In SimChart for the Medical Office, document the temperature reading and site using textboxes, drop-down menus, and/or radio buttons. The temperature can be documented in either Fahrenheit or Celsius and the software will convert the temperature so that both are displayed.
    b. *Paper-based patient record:* Document the date, the time, the aural temperature reading, and which ear was used to take the temperature. Indicating which ear was used alerts the provider that the temperature was taken through the aural route.

PPR Documentation Example

Date	
10/15/XX	3:00 p.m. T: 99.8° F, Ⓡ ear ————
	———— S. Martinez, RMA

Continued

PROCEDURE 4.5 Measuring Temporal Artery Body Temperature

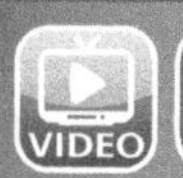

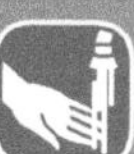

Outcome Measure temporal artery body temperature.

Equipment/Supplies

- Contact temporal artery thermometer and probe cover
- Noncontact temporal artery thermometer
- Antiseptic wipe or cotton swab moistened with alcohol
- Waste container

1. **Procedural Step.** Sanitize your hands, and assemble the equipment.
2. **Procedural Step.** Greet the patient and introduce yourself. Identify the patient and explain the procedure.
3. **Procedural Step.** Examine the sensor lens of the thermometer to ensure that the lens is clean and intact, making sure not to touch it with your fingers. If the sensor lens is dirty, clean it with an antiseptic wipe or a cotton swab moistened with alcohol and allow it to dry. If the lens is damaged, the thermometer cannot be used and must be repaired or replaced.
   Principle. A dirty sensor lens reduces the transparency of the lens and may result in a falsely low temperature reading.
4. **Procedural Step.** Place a disposable cover over the probe. If the thermometer does not use disposable covers, clean the sensor lens with an antiseptic wipe or a cotton swab moistened with alcohol, and allow it to dry *(Note: This cleansing step does not need to be performed if it was previously performed in Step 3).*
   Principle. Applying a probe cover or cleaning the probe with an antiseptic prevents cross-contamination.
   Contact temporal artery thermometer measurement:

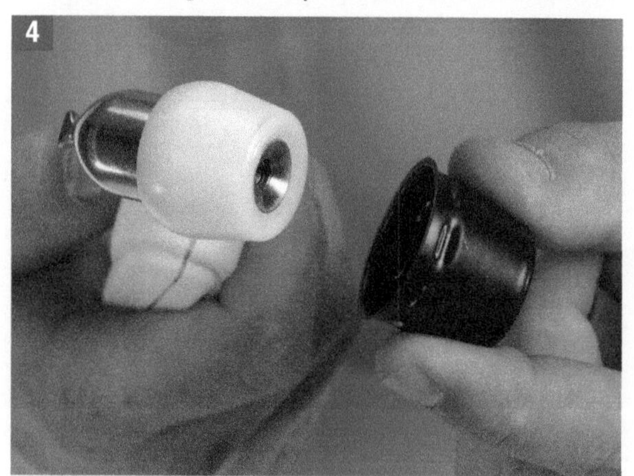

Place a disposable probe cover on the thermometer.

5. **Procedural Step.** Select an appropriate site; the right or left side of the forehead can be used. The site selected should be fully exposed to the environment.
   Principle. The temporal artery is located in the center of the forehead, approximately 2 mm below the surface of the skin.
6. **Procedural Step.** Prepare the patient by brushing away any hair that is covering the side of the forehead to be scanned and the area behind the earlobe on the same side.
   Principle. Hair covering the area to be measured traps body heat, resulting in a falsely high temperature reading.
7. **Procedural Step.** Hold the thermometer in your dominant hand with your thumb on the scan button.
8. **Procedural Step.** Gently position the probe of the thermometer on the center of the patient's forehead, midway between the eyebrow and the hairline.

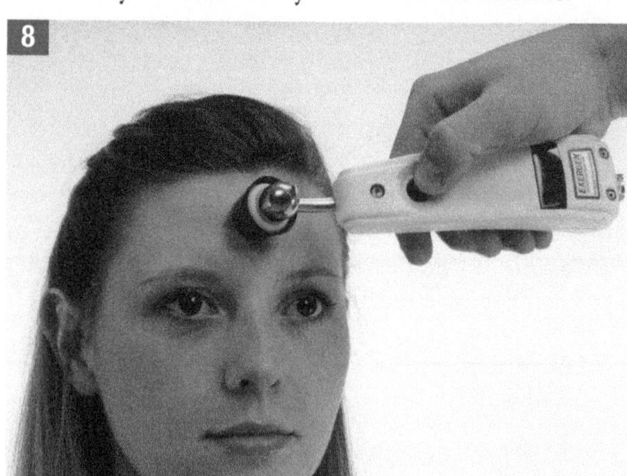

Position the probe on the center of the patient's forehead.

9. **Procedural Step.** Depress the scan button, and keep it depressed for the entire measurement.
   Principle. Not keeping the scan button depressed can result in a falsely low temperature reading.
10. **Procedural Step.** Slowly and gently slide the probe straight across the forehead, midway between the eyebrow and the upper hairline. Continue until the hairline is reached. Keep the scan button depressed and the probe flush (flat) against the forehead. During this time, a beeping sound occurs and a red light blinks to indicate that a measurement is taking place. Rapid beeping and blinking indicate a rise to a higher temperature. Slow beeping indicates that

PROCEDURE 4.5 Measuring Temporal Artery Body Temperature—cont'd

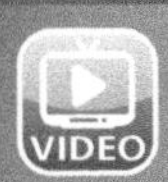

the thermometer is still scanning but is not finding a higher temperature.

Principle. The thermometer continually scans for the peak temperature as long as the scan button is depressed. The probe must be held flat against the forehead to ensure accurate scanning of the temporal artery.

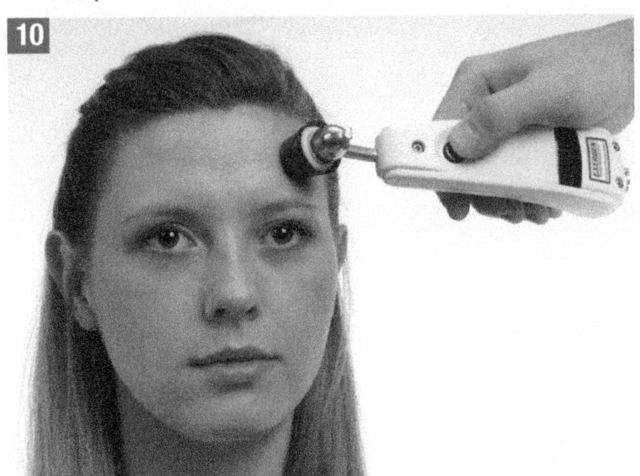

Slowly slide the probe straight across the patient's forehead.

11. Procedural Step. Keeping the button depressed, lift the probe from the forehead, and gently place the probe behind the earlobe in the soft depression of the neck just below the mastoid process. Hold the probe in place for 1–2 s.

Principle. Taking the patient's temperature behind the earlobe prevents an error in temperature measurement in the event that the patient's forehead is sweating.

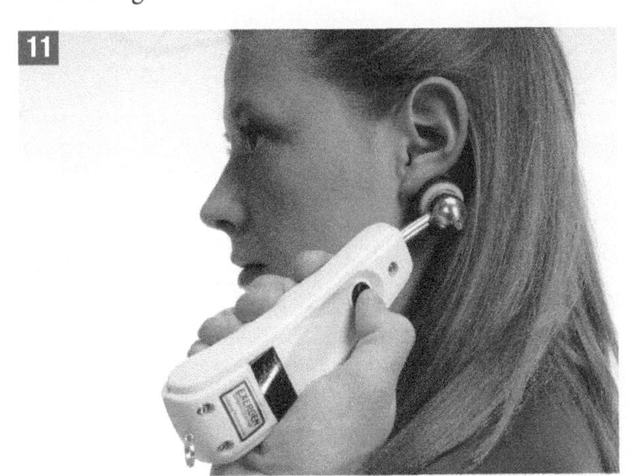

Place the probe behind the earlobe.

12. Procedural Step. Release the scan button, and read the temperature on the display screen. Make a mental note of the temperature reading. (The temperature indicated on this thermometer is 99.1°F [37.3°C].) The reading remains on the display for approximately 15–30 s after the scan button is released. The thermometer shuts off automatically after 30 s. If the patient's temperature needs to be taken again, wait 60 s or use the opposite side of the forehead.

Principle. Taking a measurement cools the skin, and taking another measurement too soon may result in an inaccurate reading.

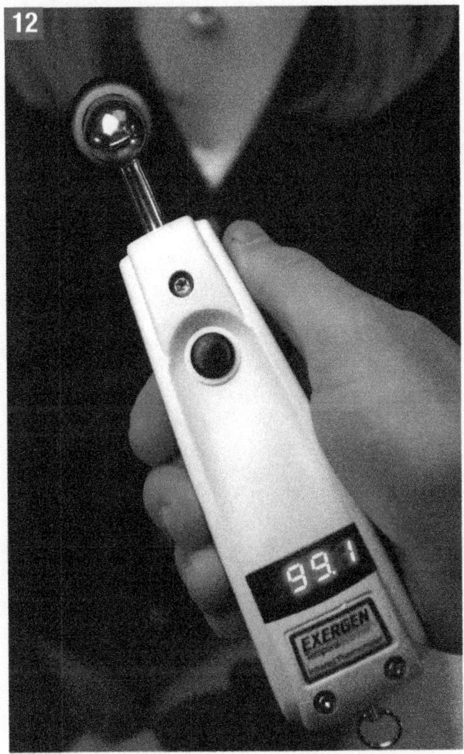

Read the temperature on the display screen.

13. Procedural Step. Dispose of the probe cover by pushing it off the probe with your thumb and ejecting it into a regular waste container. Wipe the sensor lens with an antiseptic wipe.

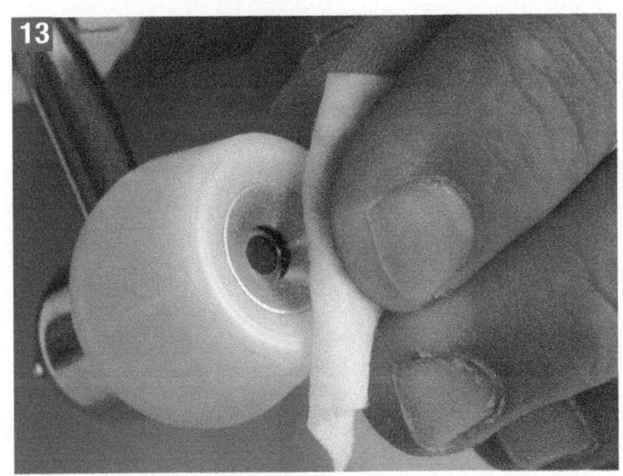

Wipe the probe with an antiseptic wipe.

Continued

PROCEDURE 4.5 Measuring Temporal Artery Body Temperature—cont'd

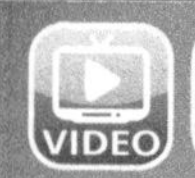

Noncontact temporal artery thermometer measurement

14. **Procedural Step.** Prepare the patient by brushing away any hair covering the forehead. If sweat is present on the patient's forehead, remove it by wiping the forehead with a soft cloth.
    Principle. Sweating of the forehead may result in a falsely low temperature reading.
15. **Procedural Step.** Hold the thermometer in your dominant hand and position the probe of the thermometer 2 inches (5 cm) away from the center of the patient's forehead (between the eyebrows).
    Principle. If the thermometer is positioned more than 2 inches away from the forehead, a falsely low temperature reading may occur.

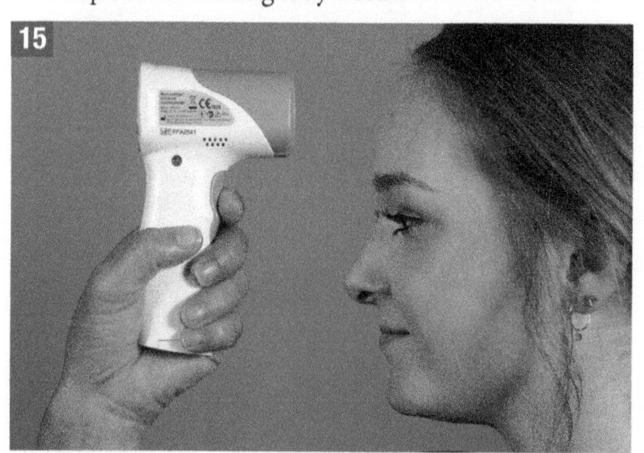

Position the probe of the thermometer.

16. **Procedural Step.** Holding the thermometer steady, press the scan button until an audible tone is heard. Release the scan button, and read the temperature on the display screen. Make a mental note of the temperature reading. (The temperature indicated on this thermometer is 98.1° F [36.7° C].) The reading remains on the display for approximately 15–30 s after the scan button is released. The thermometer shuts off automatically after 30 s. If the patient's temperature needs to be taken again, wait 60 s.
    Principle. When the scan button is depressed, the sensor lens scans the thermal energy radiated by the temporal artery. Moving the thermometer during the measurement may result in an inaccurate measurement.

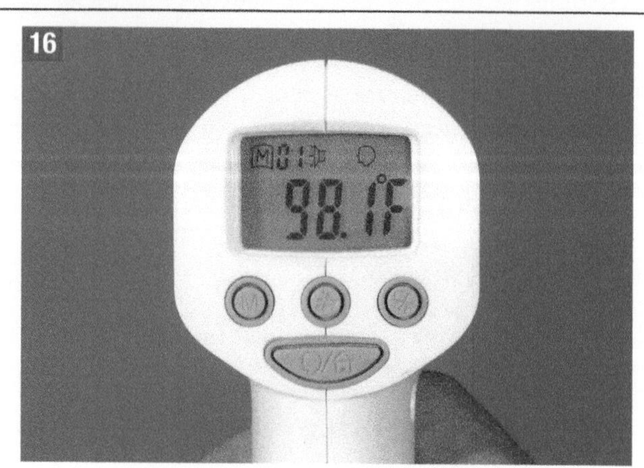

Read the temperature on the display screen.

17. **Procedural Step.** Wipe the sensor lens with a cotton swab moistened with alcohol.

    Complete both procedures as follows:
18. **Procedural Step.** Sanitize your hands.
19. **Procedural Step.** Document the results in the patient's medical record.
    a. *Electronic health record:* In SimChart for the Medical Office, document the temperature reading and site using textboxes, drop-down menus, and/or radio buttons. The temperature can be documented in either Fahrenheit or Celsius and the software will convert the temperature so that both are displayed.
    b. *Paper-based patient record:* Document the date, the time, and the temperature reading. The symbol Ⓣⓐ must be documented next to the temperature reading to tell the provider that a temporal artery reading was taken.
20. **Procedural Step.** Store the thermometer in a clean, dry area.

PPR Documentation Example

Date	
10/15/XX	9:15 a.m. T: 98.1° F (TA) ————
	———————— S. Martinez, RMA

PROCEDURE 4.6 Measuring Pulse and Respiration

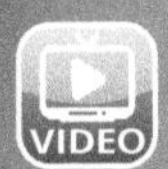

Outcome Measure pulse and respiration.

Equipment/Supplies

- Watch with a second hand

1. **Procedural Step.** Sanitize your hands. Greet the patient and introduce yourself. Identify the patient and explain the procedure. Observe the patient for any signs that might affect the pulse or respiratory rate.
   Principle. Pulse rate can vary according to the factors listed on page 96.
2. **Procedural Step.** Have the patient sit down. Position the patient's arm in a comfortable position. The forearm should be slightly flexed to relax the muscles and tendons over the pulse site.
   Principle. Relaxed muscles and tendons over the pulse site make it easier to palpate the pulse.
3. **Procedural Step.** Place your three middle fingertips over the radial pulse site. Never use your thumb to take a pulse. The radial pulse is located in a groove on the inner aspect of the wrist just below the thumb.
   Principle. The thumb has a pulse of its own; using the thumb results in measurement of the medical assistant's pulse and not the patient's pulse.

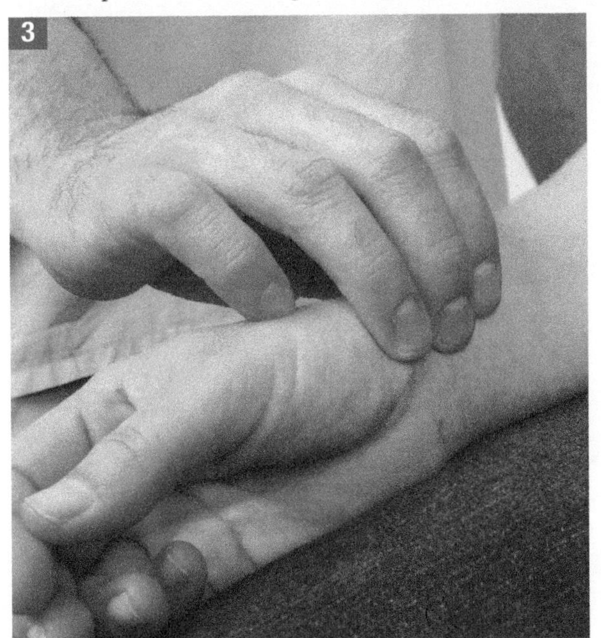

Place the three middle fingers over the radial pulse site.

4. **Procedural Step.** Apply moderate, gentle pressure directly over the site until you feel the pulse. If you cannot feel the pulse, this may be caused by:
   a. Incorrect location of the radial pulse: Move your fingers to a slightly different location in the groove of the wrist until you feel the pulse.
   b. Applying too much pressure or not enough pressure: Vary the depth of your hold until you can feel the pulse.
   Principle. A normal pulse can be felt with moderate pressure. The pulse cannot be felt if not enough pressure is applied, whereas too much pressure applied to the radial artery closes it off, and no pulse is felt.
5. **Procedural Step.** Count the pulse for 30 s and make a mental note of this number. Note the rhythm and volume of the pulse. If abnormalities are present in the rhythm or volume, count the pulse for 1 full minute.
   Principle. A longer time ensures an accurate assessment of abnormalities.

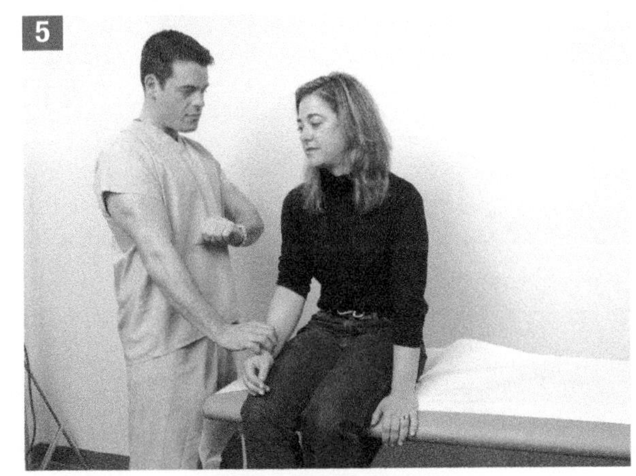

Count the pulse for 30 seconds.

6. **Procedural Step.** After taking the pulse, continue to hold three fingers on the patient's wrist with the same amount of pressure, and measure the respirations. This helps to ensure that the patient is unaware that respirations are being monitored.
   Principle. If the patient is aware that respiration is being measured, the breathing may change.

Procedure 4.6

Continued

PROCEDURE 4.6 Measuring Pulse and Respiration—cont'd

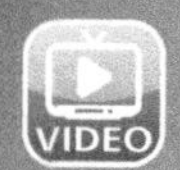
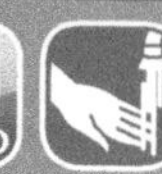

6

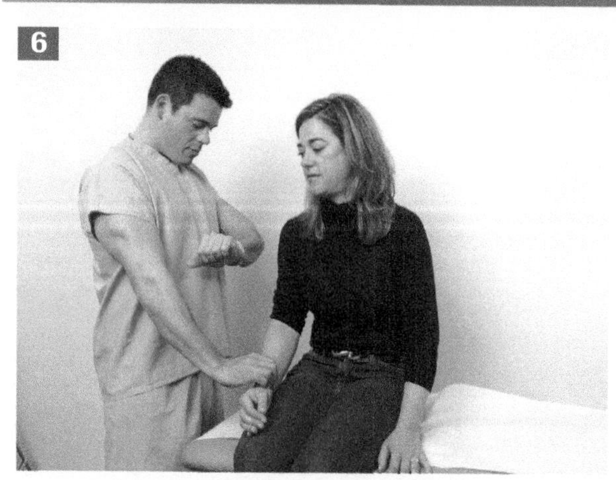

Count the number of respirations for 30 seconds.

7. **Procedural Step.** Observe the rise and fall of the patient's chest as the patient inhales and exhales.
   Principle. One complete respiration includes one inhalation and one exhalation.
8. **Procedural Step.** Count the number of respirations for 30 s and make a mental note of this number; note the rhythm and depth of the respirations. Also observe the patient's color. If abnormalities are present in rhythm or depth, count the respiratory rate for 1 full minute.
9. **Procedural Step.** Sanitize your hands.
10. **Procedural Step.** Document the results in the patient's medical record. If you counted the pulse and respirations for 30 s, multiply each of the numbers counted by 2. This will give you the pulse rate and respiratory rate for 1 full minute.
    a. *Electronic health record:* In SimChart for the Medical Office, document the pulse rate, rhythm, volume, and site for taking the pulse; and the respiratory rate, rhythm, and depth using textboxes, dropdown menus, and/or radio buttons.
    b. *Paper-based patient record:* Document the date; the time; the pulse rate, rhythm, and volume; and the respiratory rate, rhythm, and depth.

PPR Documentation Example

Date	
10/15/XX	2:30 p.m. P: 74. Reg and strong. R: 18.
	Even and reg.————S. Martinez, RMA

Procedure 4.7

PROCEDURE 4.7 Measuring Apical Pulse

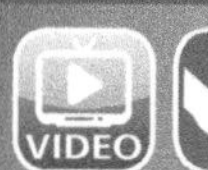
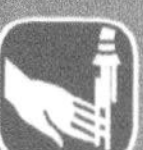

Outcome Measure apical pulse.

Equipment/Supplies

- Watch with a second hand
- Stethoscope
- Antiseptic wipe

1. **Procedural Step.** Sanitize your hands. Greet the patient and introduce yourself. Identify the patient and explain the procedure. Observe the patient for any signs that might increase or decrease the pulse rate.
2. **Procedural Step.** Assemble the equipment. If the stethoscope's chest piece consists of a diaphragm and a bell, rotate the chest piece to the bell position. Clean the earpieces and chest piece of the stethoscope with an antiseptic wipe.
   Principle. The bell position allows better auscultation of heart sounds. Cleaning the earpieces helps prevent the transmission of microorganisms.
3. **Procedural Step.** Ask the patient to unbutton or remove his or her shirt. Have the patient sit or lie down (supine).
   Principle. A sitting or supine position allows access to the apex of the heart.
4. **Procedural Step.** Warm the chest piece of the stethoscope with your hands. Insert the earpieces of the stethoscope into your ears, with the earpieces directed slightly forward, and place the chest piece over the apex of the patient's heart. The apex of the heart is located in the fifth intercostal space at the junction of the left midclavicular line.
   Principle. Warming the chest piece reduces the discomfort of having a cold object placed on the chest. In addition, a cold chest piece could startle the patient, resulting in an increase in pulse rate. The earpieces should be directed forward to follow the direction of the ear canal, which facilitates hearing.

PROCEDURE 4.7 Measuring Apical Pulse—cont'd

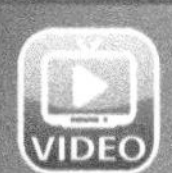

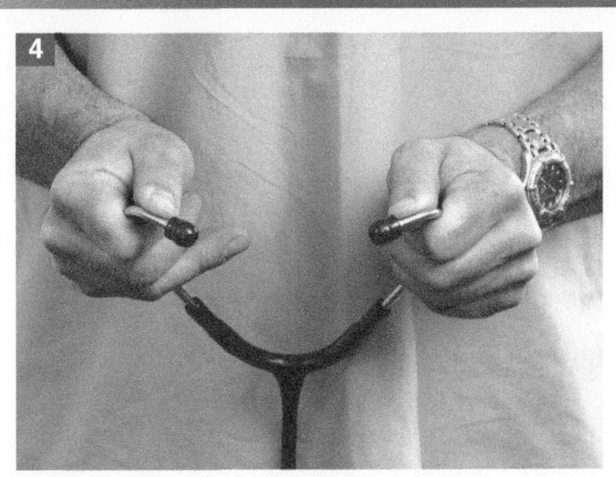

Insert the earpieces into your ears with the earpieces directed slightly forward.

5. **Procedural Step.** Listen for the heartbeat, and count the number of beats for 30 s (and multiply by 2) if the rhythm and volume are normal or if the apical pulse of an infant or child is being taken. If abnormalities are present in the rhythm or volume, count the pulse for 1 full minute. You will hear a *lub-dup* sound through the stethoscope. This sound is the closing of the valves of the heart. Each *lub-dup* is counted as one beat.

5

Count the number of beats for 30 seconds, and multiply by 2.

6. **Procedural Step.** Sanitize your hands.
7. **Procedural Step.** Document the results in the patient's medical record.
   a. *Electronic health record:* In SimChart for the Medical Office, document the rate, rhythm, and volume and the site for taking the pulse using textboxes, drop-down menus, and/or radio buttons.
   b. *Paper-based patient record:* Document the date, the time, and the apical pulse rate, rhythm, and volume.
8. **Procedural Step.** Clean the earpieces and the chest piece of the stethoscope with an antiseptic wipe.

PPR Documentation Example

Date	
10/15/XX	10:15 a.m. AP: 68. Reg and strong. ______
	______ S. Martinez, RMA

PROCEDURE 4.8 Performing Pulse Oximetry

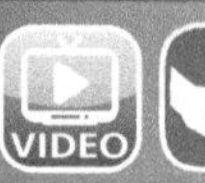

Outcome Perform pulse oximetry.

Equipment/Supplies

- Handheld pulse oximeter
- Antiseptic wipe

1. **Procedural Step.** Sanitize your hands.
2. **Procedural Step.** Assemble the equipment. Handle the pulse oximeter carefully, and perform the following:
   a. Carefully inspect the probe to ensure it opens and closes smoothly. Inspect the probe windows (LED and light sensor) to ensure they are clean and free of lint.
   b. Disinfect the probe windows and surrounding platforms with an antiseptic wipe, and allow them to dry.

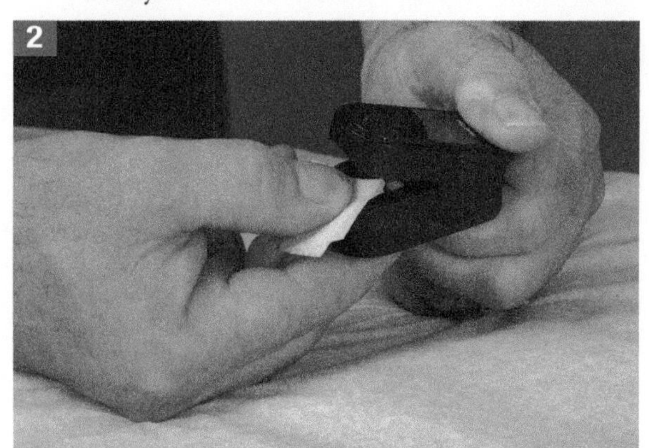

Disinfect the probe with an antiseptic wipe.

   Principle. Misuse or improper handling of the pulse oximeter could damage it. Dirt or lint on the probe windows could interfere with proper light transmission, leading to an inaccurate reading. Cross-contamination between patients is prevented by disinfecting the probe.
3. **Procedural Step.** Greet the patient and introduce yourself. Identify the patient and explain the procedure. Explain to the patient that the clip-on probe does not hurt and feels similar to a clothespin attached to the finger.
4. **Procedural Step.** Seat the patient comfortably in a chair with the lower arm firmly supported just below heart level and the palm facing down.
   Principle. Supporting the lower arm helps prevent patient movement during the procedure. Placing the lower arm just below heart level helps to ensure an accurate reading.
5. **Procedural Step.** Select an appropriate finger to apply the probe. Use the tip of the patient's index, middle, ring finger, or thumb. If the patient's fingers are small and the probe cannot seem to be aligned properly, use the big toe or earlobe to take the measurement. If the patient exhibits tremors of the hands, use the earlobe to obtain the reading.
   Principle. The probe must be applied to a peripheral site with thin skin that is highly vascular. Small fingers may not allow for proper positioning of the probe on the finger.
6. **Procedural Step.** Observe the patient's fingernail. If the patient is wearing dark fingernail polish, ask him or her to remove it with acetone or nail polish remover. If the patient has long nails or is wearing artificial nails, choose another probe site, such as the big toe or earlobe.
   Principle. An opaque coating on the fingernail may interfere with proper light transmission through the finger, leading to an inaccurate reading. Long nails or artificial nails may obstruct the light sensor and prevent an accurate measurement.
7. **Procedural Step.** Check to ensure that the patient's fingertip is clean. If it is dirty, cleanse the site with soap and water, and allow it to dry. Ensure that the patient's finger is not cold. If it is cold, ask the patient to rub his or her hands together.
   Principle. Oils, dirt, or grime on the finger can interfere with proper light transmission through the finger, leading to an inaccurate reading. Sometimes patients with cold fingers may have enough constriction of the capillaries that it interferes with obtaining a reading.
8. **Procedural Step.** Ensure that ambient light does not interfere with the measurement. Position the probe securely on the fingertip as follows:
   a. Ensure that the probe window is fully covered by placing the finger over the LED window, with the fleshy tip of the finger covering the window. The tip of the finger should touch the end of the probe stop.

PROCEDURE 4.8 Performing Pulse Oximetry—cont'd

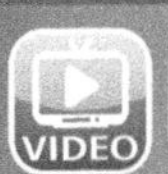

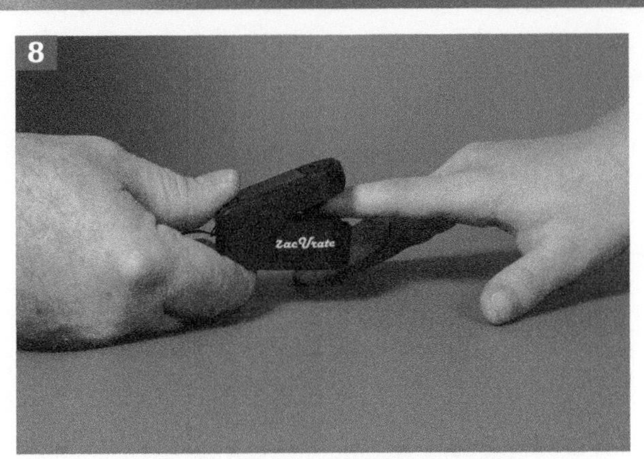

Position the probe securely on the fingertip.

b. Ensure that the LED and the light sensor are aligned opposite to each other.

Principle. Ambient light can be picked up by the probe and alter the reading. Proper alignment of the LED and light sensor is necessary for an accurate reading.

9. **Procedural Step.** Instruct the patient to keep his or her finger stationary and to breathe normally. Turn on the oximeter by pressing the power-on control. Wait while the oximeter goes through its power-on self-test (POST).

Principle. Finger movement may lead to an inaccurate reading. The monitor automatically conducts a POST to ensure that it is functioning properly.

10. **Procedural Step.** Allow several seconds for the pulse oximeter to detect the pulse and calculate the oxygen saturation of the blood. Ensure that the pulse strength indicator fluctuates with each pulsation and that the pulse signal is strong. If the oximeter is unable to locate a pulse, reposition the probe on the patient's finger or move the probe to another finger, and perform the procedure again.

Principle. The reading takes 4–6 s to display. The pulse strength indicator provides a quick assessment of pulse quality. If the oximeter is unable to locate a pulse, it will be unable to obtain a reading.

11. **Procedural Step.** Leave the probe in place until the oximeter displays a reading. Read the oxygen saturation value and pulse rate, and make a mental note of these readings. On this pulse oximeter, the oxygen saturation reading is 97% and the pulse rate is 88. If the SpO_2 reading is less than 95%, reposition the probe on the finger or move the probe to a different finger, and perform the procedure again.

Principle. A low SpO_2 reading may be caused by improper positioning of the probe on the finger.

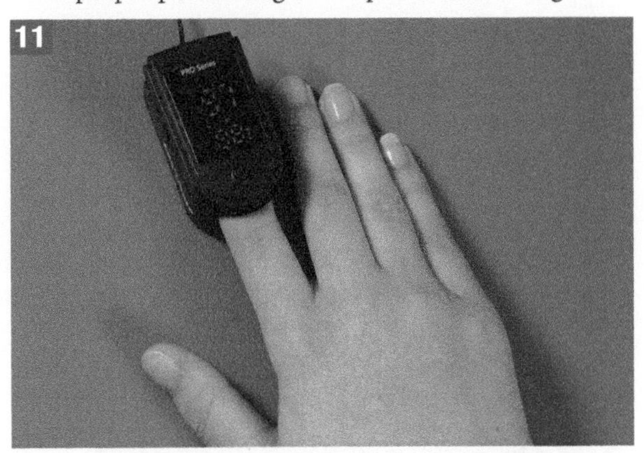

Read the oxygen saturation value and pulse rate.

12. **Procedural Step.** Remove the probe from the patient's finger. The pulse oximeter will automatically shut down after the finger is removed from the probe.
13. **Procedural Step.** Sanitize your hands.
14. **Procedural Step.** Document the results in the patient's medical record.

   a. *Electronic health record:* In SimChart for the Medical Office, enter the SpO_2 reading and the pulse rate using textboxes, drop-down menus, and/or radio buttons.

   b. *Paper-based patient record:* Document the date, the time, the SpO_2 reading, and the pulse rate.
15. **Procedural Step.** Disinfect the probe with an antiseptic wipe. Properly store the monitor in a clean, dry area.

PPR Documentation Example

Date	
10/15/XX	2:30 p.m. SpO_2: 97%. P: 88. ———
	——— S. Martinez, RMA

Procedure 4.8

PROCEDURE 4.9 Measuring Blood Pressure: Manual Method

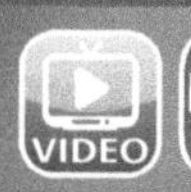
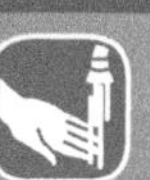

Outcome Measure blood pressure using the manual method.

Equipment/Supplies

- Stethoscope
- Portable aneroid sphygmomanometer
- Antiseptic wipe

1. **Procedural Step.** Sanitize your hands, and assemble the equipment. If the chest piece consists of a diaphragm and a bell, rotate it to the diaphragm position. Clean the earpieces and diaphragm of the stethoscope with the antiseptic wipe.
Principle. The diaphragm must be rotated to the proper position for sound to be heard through the earpieces.

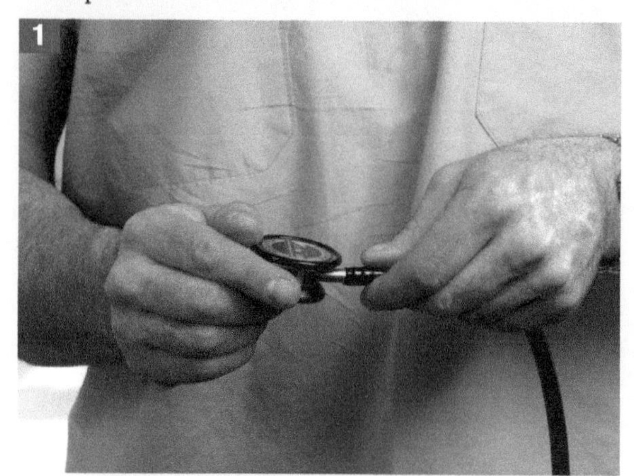

Rotate the chest piece to the diaphragm position.

2. **Procedural Step.** Greet the patient and introduce yourself. Identify the patient and explain the procedure. Ask the patient to empty the bladder. Observe and question the patient for factors that might influence the blood pressure reading (e.g., emotional states, physical activity). If it is not possible to reduce or eliminate these factors, document them in the patient's medical record. Determine how high to pump the cuff by checking the patient's medical record for the previously measured systolic reading, or determine the patient's systolic pressure by palpation (see Procedure 4.10).
Principle. A full bladder can increase the blood pressure reading. An inaccurate reading may occur if factors are present that could influence the reading.
3. **Procedural Step.** Instruct the patient to sit quietly in a comfortable position with the legs uncrossed at the knees and the feet flat on the floor. The patient should be allowed to relax in a sitting position for at least 5 min before the blood pressure measurement.
Principle. Patient anxiety can cause a significant increase in blood pressure.
4. **Procedural Step.** Roll up the patient's sleeve approximately 5 inches above the elbow so that the cuff can be applied to bare skin. If the sleeve does not roll up or is too tight after being rolled up, remove the arm from the sleeve. The arm should be positioned at heart level and well supported on a flat surface, with the palm facing upward.
Principle. Clothing can result in an inaccurate blood pressure reading. A tight sleeve causes partial compression of the brachial artery, resulting in an inaccurate reading. Placing the arm above heart level may cause the reading to be falsely low. Not supporting the arm or placing it below heart level and crossing the legs at the knees may cause the reading to be falsely high.
5. **Procedural Step.** Determine the patient's correct cuff size. Make sure the cuff is completely deflated so that there is no residual air in the bladder of the cuff.
Principle. The correct-sized cuff must be used to ensure an accurate measurement. If the cuff is too small, it may come loose as the cuff is inflated, or the reading may be falsely high. If the cuff is too large, the reading may be falsely low.
6. **Procedural Step.** Making sure the arm is well-extended, locate the brachial pulse with the index and middle fingertips. The brachial pulse is located near the center of the antecubital space but slightly toward the little finger–side of the arm. Center the inner bladder above the brachial pulse site with the lower edge of the cuff approximately 1–2 inches (2.5–5 cm) above the bend in the elbow. Most cuffs are labeled with arrows indicating the center of the bladder for the right and left arms.
Principle. A well extended arm allows easier palpation of the brachial pulse. Centering the inner bladder above the pulse site allows complete compression of the brachial artery. The cuff should be placed high enough above the bend in the elbow to prevent the diaphragm of the stethoscope from touching it;

PROCEDURE 4.9 Measuring Blood Pressure: Manual Method—cont'd

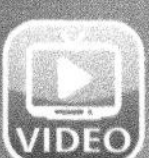

otherwise, extraneous sounds may be picked up which could interfere with an accurate measurement.

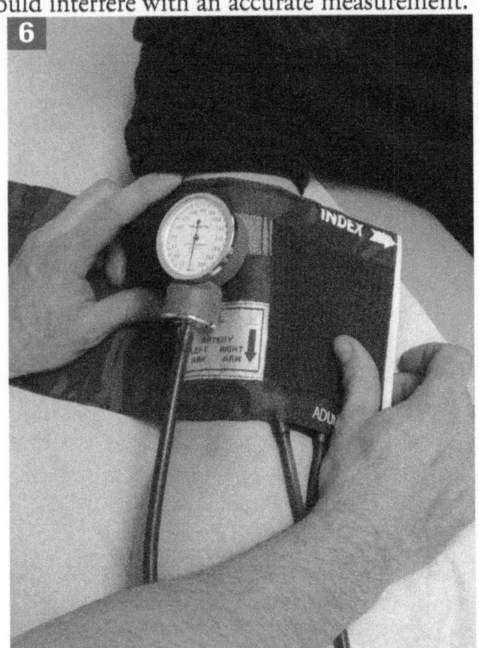

Center the inner bladder above the brachial pulse site.

7. **Procedural Step.** Wrap the cuff smoothly and snugly around the patient's arm, and secure the end of it. The cuff should be snug but not too tight. To assess the appropriate tightness of the cuff, one finger should slip easily under the cuff. Position the manometer for direct viewing and at a distance of no more than 3 feet.

   Principle. Applying the cuff properly facilitates the application of equal pressure over the brachial artery. The medical assistant may have trouble seeing the scale on the manometer if it is placed more than 3 feet away.

8. **Procedural Step.** Instruct the patient to relax as much as possible and not to talk or move during the procedure. Place the earpieces of the stethoscope in your ears, with the earpieces directed slightly forward. During the blood pressure measurement, the tubing of the stethoscope should hang freely and should not be permitted to rub against any object.

   Principle. Patient talking or movement can result in a falsely high reading. The earpieces should be directed forward, permitting them to follow the direction of the ear canal, which facilitates hearing. If the stethoscope tubing rubs against an object, extraneous sounds may be picked up which could interfere with an accurate measurement.

9. **Procedural Step.** Locate the brachial pulse again, and place the diaphragm of the stethoscope over the brachial pulse site. The diaphragm should be positioned to make a tight seal against the patient's skin. Do not allow the diaphragm to touch the cuff.

   Principle. Proper positioning of the diaphragm and good contact of the diaphragm with the skin help transmit clear and audible Korotkoff sounds through the earpieces of the stethoscope to ensure an accurate measurement.

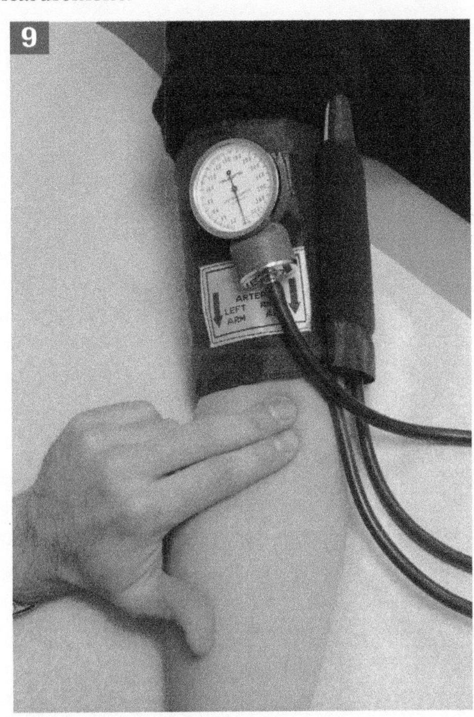

Locate the brachial pulse again before placing the diaphragm over the site.

10. **Procedural Step.** Close the control valve on the bulb by turning the thumbscrew clockwise (to the right) with the thumb and forefinger of your dominant hand until it feels tight but can still be loosened when you need to deflate the cuff. Pump air into the cuff as rapidly as possible to approximately 30 mm Hg above the previously measured or palpated systolic pressure. Do not overinflate the cuff.

    Principle. Inflation of the cuff compresses and closes off the brachial artery so that no blood flows through the artery. Over inflation of the cuff is uncomfortable for the patient and may result in a falsely high blood pressure reading.

Continued

PROCEDURE 4.9 Measuring Blood Pressure: Manual Method—cont'd

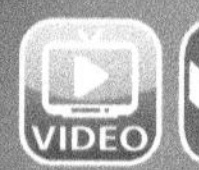

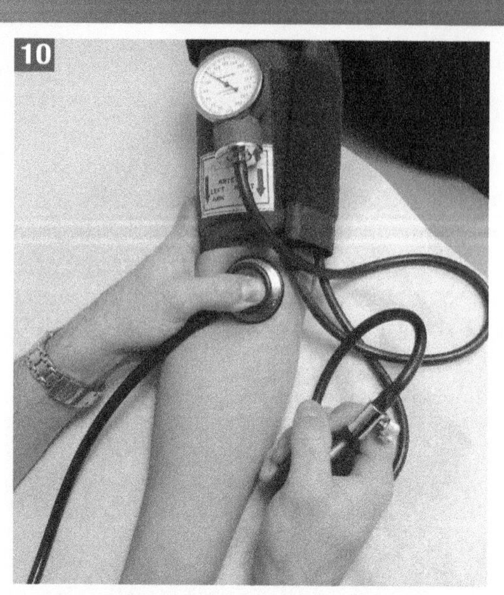

Pump air into the cuff as rapidly as possible.

11. **Procedural Step.** Release the pressure at a moderately steady rate of 2– 3 mm Hg/sec by slowly turning the thumbscrew counterclockwise (to the left) with the thumb and forefinger. This opens the control valve and allows the air in the cuff to escape slowly. Listen for the first clear tapping sound (phase I of the Korotkoff sounds). This represents the systolic pressure. Note this point on the scale of the gauge.
Principle. Releasing the pressure too slowly is uncomfortable for the patient and could cause a falsely high diastolic reading. Releasing the pressure too quickly could cause a falsely low systolic reading and a falsely high diastolic reading.

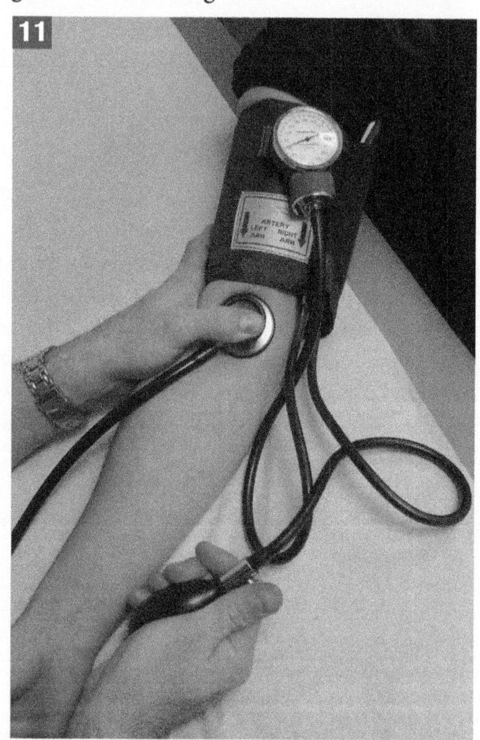

Release the pressure at a moderately steady rate.

12. **Procedural Step.** Continue to deflate the cuff while listening to the Korotkoff sounds. Listen for the onset of the muffled sound that occurs during phase IV. Continue to deflate the cuff, and note the point on the scale of the gauge at which the sound ceases (phase V). This represents the diastolic pressure. Continue to steadily deflate the cuff for another 10 mm Hg to ensure that there are no more sounds. Quickly and completely deflate the cuff to zero.
13. **Procedural Step.** If you are taking two or more blood pressure readings or if you could not obtain an accurate blood pressure reading, wait 1–2 min before taking another measurement from the same arm.
Principle. Waiting 1–2 min allows the blood flow in the brachial artery to return to normal.
14. **Procedural Step.** Remove the earpieces of the stethoscope from your ears, and carefully remove the cuff from the patient's arm.
15. **Procedural Step.** Sanitize your hands.
16. **Procedural Step.** Calculate an average of the readings if two or more blood pressure readings were taken. Document the results in the patient's medical record.
    a. *Electronic health record:* In SimChart for the Medical Office, enter the blood pressure reading, which arm was used, and what position the patient was in when the blood pressure was taken using textboxes, drop-down menus, and/or radio buttons.
    b. *Paper-based patient record:* Document the date, the time, and the blood pressure reading. Make a notation in the patient's medical record if the lying or standing position was used to take blood pressure. Abbreviations that can be used are *L* (lying) and *St* (standing).
17. **Procedural Step.** Clean the earpieces and the chest piece of the stethoscope with an antiseptic wipe, and replace the equipment properly.

PPR Documentation Example

Date	
10/20/XX	2:30 p.m. BP: 106/74 _S. Martinez, RMA

PROCEDURE 4.10 Determining Systolic Pressure by Palpation

Outcome Determine systolic pressure by palpation.

Equipment/Supplies

- Sphygmomanometer

1. **Procedural Step.** Sanitize your hands, and assemble the equipment.
2. **Procedural Step.** Locate the brachial pulse with the fingertips. Place the cuff on the patient's arm so that the inner bladder is centered over the brachial pulse site.
3. **Procedural Step.** Wrap the cuff smoothly and snugly around the patient's arm, and secure the end of it.
4. **Procedural Step.** Position the manometer for direct viewing and at a distance of no more than 3 feet.
5. **Procedural Step.** Locate the radial pulse with your fingertips.
6. **Procedural Step.** Close the valve on the bulb, and pump air into the cuff until the pulsation ceases.
7. **Procedural Step.** Release the valve at a moderate rate of 2– 3 mm Hg per heartbeat while palpating the artery with your fingertips.
8. **Procedural Step.** Document the point at which the pulsation reappears as the palpated systolic pressure.
9. **Procedural Step.** Deflate the cuff completely and wait 15–30 s before taking the patient's blood pressure.

PROCEDURE 4.11 Measuring Blood Pressure: Automatic Method

Outcome Measure blood pressure using the automatic method.

Equipment/Supplies

- Automatic blood pressure monitor

1. **Procedural Step.** Sanitize your hands, and assemble the equipment. Connect the air tube to the monitor by plugging the air plug into the air jack on the monitor.
2. **Procedural Step.** Greet the patient and introduce yourself. Identify the patient and explain the procedure. Ask the patient to empty the bladder. Observe and question the patient for factors that might influence the blood pressure reading (e.g., emotional states, physical activity). If it is not possible to reduce or eliminate these factors, document them in the patient's medical record.
3. **Procedural Step.** Instruct the patient sit quietly in a comfortable position with the legs uncrossed at the knees and the feet flat on the floor. The patient should be allowed to relax in a sitting position for at least 5 min before the blood pressure measurement.
4. **Procedural Step.** Using the left arm, roll up the patient's sleeve approximately 5 inches above the elbow so that the cuff can be applied to bare skin. If the sleeve does not roll up or is too tight after being rolled up, remove the arm from the sleeve. The arm should be positioned at heart level and well supported on a flat surface, with the palm facing upward.
5. **Procedural Step.** Determine the correct cuff size.
6. **Procedural Step.** Making sure the arm is well-extended, locate the brachial pulse with the index and middle fingertips. The brachial pulse is located near the center of the antecubital space but slightly toward the little finger–side of the arm. Position the lower edge of the cuff approximately 1 inch (2.5 cm) above the bend in the elbow with the artery position indicator (consisting of a stripe or an arrow) placed above the brachial pulse site.

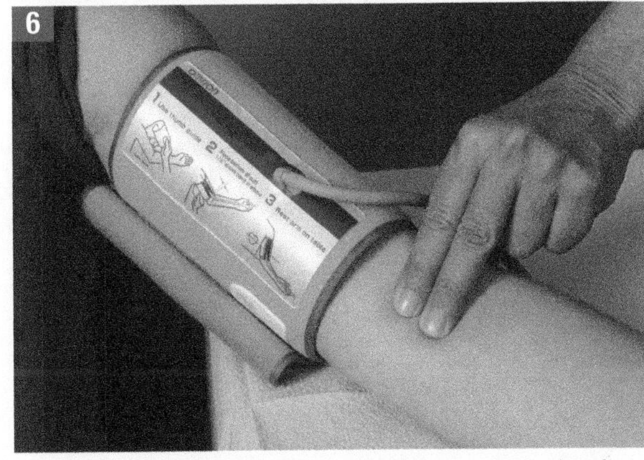

Place the artery position indicator above the brachial pulse site.

Continued

PROCEDURE 4.11 Measuring Blood Pressure: Automatic Method—cont'd

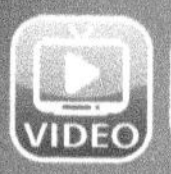

7. Procedural Step. Wrap the cuff smoothly and snugly around the patient's arm, and secure the end of it. The cuff should be snug but not too tight. To assess the appropriate tightness of the cuff, one finger should slip easily under the cuff. Position the digital display screen for direct viewing and at a distance of no more than 3 feet.

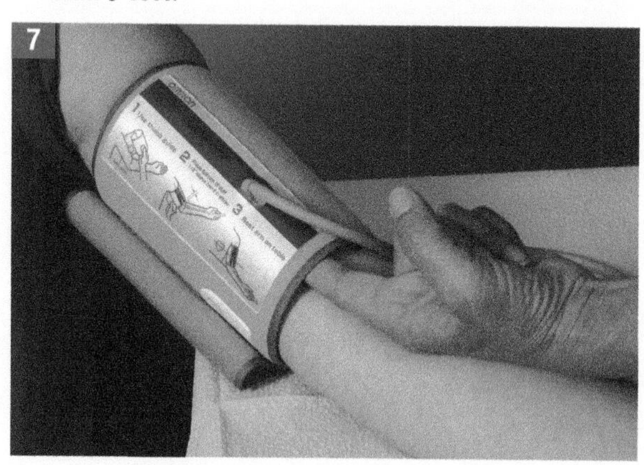

One finger should slip easily under the cuff.

8. Procedural Step. Instruct the patient to relax as much as possible and not to talk or move during the procedure. Make sure the patient's arm does not rest on the air tube.

Principle. Talking or moving can result in an error message on the display screen indicating the monitor was unable to obtain a reading. The patient's arm resting on the air tube restricts the flow of air to the cuff.

9. Procedural Step. Press the START/STOP button. All symbols temporarily appear on the display screen followed by the automatic inflation of the cuff. The monitor determines how much the cuff should be inflated to reach a pressure that is approximately 30 mm Hg above the systolic pressure. Once the electronic pressure sensor has detected the patient's blood pressure reading and pulse rate, the cuff automatically deflates. As the cuff deflates, decreasing numbers appear on the display screen.

10. Procedural Step. Following deflation of the cuff, the systolic and diastolic pressures and the pulse rate appear on the display screen. The systolic BP reading on this monitor is 121 and the diastolic BP reading is 76. The pulse rate is 72. Make a mental note of the readings and press the START/STOP button to turn off the monitor.

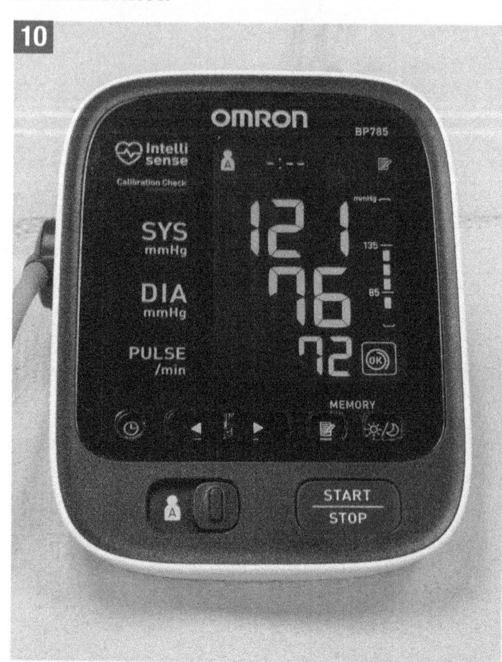

The readings appear on the display screen.

11. Procedural Step. Sanitize your hands.

12. Procedural Step. Document the results in the patient's medical record.

a. *Electronic health record:* In SimChart for the Medical Office, enter the systolic and diastolic readings, which arm was used, and what position the patient was in when the blood pressure was taken using textboxes, drop-down menus, and/or radio buttons.

b. *Paper-based patient record:* Document the date, the time, and the blood pressure reading. Make a notation in the patient's medical record if the lying or standing position was used to take blood pressure. Abbreviations that can be used are *L* (lying) and *St* (standing).

PPR Documentation Example

Date	
10/20/XX	2:30 p.m. BP: 121/76___S. Martinez, RMA

The Physical Examination

Check out the Evolve site at http://evolve.elsevier.com/Bonewit/today/ to access additional interactive activities and exercises to help you study and prepare for success.

LEARNING OUTCOMES	PROCEDURES
Preparation for the Physical Examination	
1. Identify the three components of a complete patient examination.	Prepare the examining room.
2. List the guidelines that should be followed in preparing the examining room.	Operate and care for items used during the physical examination, according to the manufacturers' instructions.
3. Identify equipment and instruments used during the physical examination.	Prepare a patient for a physical examination.
Measuring Weight and Height	
4. Explain the purpose of measuring weight and height.	Measure weight and height.
5. List the guidelines that should be followed when measuring weight and height.	
Body Mechanics	
6. Explain the benefits of proper body mechanics.	Demonstrate proper body mechanics when standing, sitting, and lifting an object.
7. Identify the basic principles that should be followed related to body mechanics.	
Positioning and Draping	
8. Explain the purposes of positioning and draping.	Position and drape a patient in each of the following positions: • Sitting • Supine • Prone • Dorsal recumbent • Lithotomy • Modified left lateral recumbent • Knee-chest • Fowler
9. List one use of each patient position.	
Wheelchair Transfer	
10. Explain the purpose of a wheelchair.	Transfer a patient from a wheelchair to the examining table and back again.
11. Describe the purpose of a transfer belt.	
Assessment of the Patient	
12. List and define the four techniques of examining the patient.	
13. State an example of the use of each examination technique.	
Assisting the Provider	
14. Describe the responsibilities of the medical assistant during the physical examination.	Assist the provider during a physical examination

CHAPTER OUTLINE

KEY TERMS

auscultation (os-kul-TAY-shun)
bariatrics (BAR-ee-AT-riks)
body mechanics
clinical diagnosis
diagnosis
differential (diff-er-EN-shul) diagnosis
inspection
mensuration (men-soo-RAY-shun)
palpation (pal-PAY-shun)
percussion (per-KUSH-un)
prognosis
symptom

INTRODUCTION TO THE PHYSICAL EXAMINATION

A complete patient examination consists of three parts: the *health history,* the *physical examination* of each body system, and *laboratory and diagnostic tests.* The provider uses the results to determine the patient's general state of health, to arrive at a diagnosis and prescribe treatment, and to observe any change in a patient's illness after treatment has been instituted.

An important and frequent responsibility of the medical assistant is to assist with a physical examination. Because health-promotion and disease-prevention activities have become an important focus of health care, individuals are becoming more aware of the need for a yearly physical examination to detect early signs of d and to prevent serious health problems. In addition, a physical examination may be a prerequisite for employment, participation in sports, attendance at summer camp, and admission to school. The physical examination is explained in detail in this chapter. Taking the health history, collecting specimens, and performing laboratory and diagnostic tests are discussed in other chapters.

DEFINITIONS OF TERMS

The medical assistant should know and understand the following terms related to the patient examination.

Final diagnosis. Often simply called the **diagnosis,** this term refers to the scientific method of determining and identifying a patient's condition through evaluation of the health history, the physical examination, laboratory tests, and diagnostic procedures. A final diagnosis is crucial because it provides a logical basis for treatment and prognosis.

Clinical diagnosis. The clinical diagnosis is an intermediate step in the determination of a final diagnosis. The clinical diagnosis of a patient's condition is obtained through evaluation of the health history and the physical examination without the benefit of laboratory or diagnostic tests. Laboratory and diagnostic imaging facilities usually require that the clinical diagnosis be entered on request forms; this information assists the facility in correlating data from their test results with the provider's needs. When the provider has analyzed the test results, a final diagnosis can often be established.

Differential diagnosis. Two or more diseases may have similar symptoms. A **symptom** is any change in the body or its functioning that indicates a disease might be present. The differential diagnosis involves determining which of these diseases is producing the patient's symptoms so that a final diagnosis can be established. For example, streptococcal sore throat and pharyngitis have similar symptoms. A differential diagnosis is made by collecting a throat specimen and performing a strep test.

Prognosis. The prognosis consists of the probable course and outcome of a patient's condition and the patient's prospects for recovery.

Risk factor. A risk factor is a physical or behavioral condition that increases the probability that an individual will develop a particular condition; examples are genetic factors, habits, environmental conditions, and physiologic conditions. The presence of a risk factor for a certain disease does not mean that the disease will develop; it means only that a person's chances of developing that disease are greater than those of a person without the risk factor. For example, cigarette smoking is a risk factor for developing lung cancer and heart disease. A person who smokes has a higher risk of developing lung cancer than a person who does not smoke or who has stopped smoking.

Screening test. A test performed on a large number of individuals (apparently in good health) for the early detection of a condition before it causes symptoms. Refer to *Highlight on Health Screening* for an outline of screening guidelines for common tests and procedures.

Acute illness. An acute illness is characterized by symptoms that have a rapid onset, are usually severe and intense, and subside after a relatively short time. In some cases, the acute episode progresses into a chronic illness. Examples of acute illness include colds, influenza, strep throat, and pneumonia.

Chronic illness. A chronic illness is characterized by symptoms that persist for longer than 3 months and show little change over a long time. Examples of chronic illness include diabetes mellitus, hypertension, and emphysema.

Therapeutic procedure. A therapeutic procedure is performed to treat a patient's condition with the goal of eliminating it or promoting as much recovery as possible. Examples of therapeutic procedures include administration of medication, ear and eye irrigations, and application of heat and cold.

Laboratory test. A laboratory test is the clinical analysis and study of a body substance to obtain objective data for the diagnosis, treatment, and management of a patient's condition. Examples of laboratory tests include the hemoglobin test, glucose test, urinalysis, and strep test.

Diagnostic procedure. A diagnostic procedure is a procedure performed to assist in the diagnosis of a patient's condition; examples include electrocardiography, colonoscopy, and mammography.

PREPARATION OF THE EXAMINING ROOM

Proper preparation of the examining room provides a comfortable and healthy environment for the patient and facilitates the physical examination. The following guidelines should be followed in preparing the examining room:

1. Ensure that the examining room is free of clutter and well lit.
2. Check the examining rooms daily to ensure there are ample supplies. Restock supplies that are getting low.
3. Empty waste receptacles frequently.
4. Replace biohazard containers as necessary. When removing biohazard containers from the examining room (see Chapter 2), follow the Occupational Safety and Health Administration (OSHA) Bloodborne Pathogens Standard.
5. Make sure the room is well ventilated, and install an air freshener to eliminate odors.
6. Maintain room temperatures that are comfortable not only for a fully clothed individual but also for an individual who has disrobed.
7. Clean and disinfect examining tables, countertops, and faucets daily.
8. Remove dust and dirt from furniture.
9. Change the examining table paper after each patient by unrolling a fresh length. Check to ensure there is an ample supply of gowns and drapes ready for use.
10. Ensure that the examining room door is closed during the examination to protect patient privacy.
11. Properly clean and prepare equipment, instruments, and supplies used for patient examination. Table 5.1 lists the equipment and supplies, along with their uses, that may be used during a physical examination.

HIGHLIGHT on Health Screening for Adults

The chance of developing certain diseases is greater at different ages. Periodic health screening is recommended for the detection and early treatment of disease.

Test or Procedure	Gender	Recommended Frequency (for Individuals of Average Risk)
Blood pressure	M and F	Every year beginning at age 20.
Cholesterol levels	M and F	Every 4–6 years beginning at age 20.
Cervical cancer screening	F	Every 3 years with a Pap test beginning at age 21 until age 29. Beginning at age 30, preferred screening includes a Pap test and an HPV test every 5 years until age 65.
Blood glucose level	M and F	Every 3 years beginning at age 45.
Testicular self-examination	M	Every month beginning at age 15.
Fecal occult blood test	M and F	Every year beginning at age 45.
Colonoscopy	M and F	Every 10 years beginning at age 45.
Prostate cancer screening	M	Should be offered by a health provider every year beginning at age 50 to men with a life expectancy of at least 10 years.
Chlamydia and gonorrhea	F	Every year for all sexually active woman age 25 and younger.
Mammography	F	Women between 40 and 44 years of age should have the choice to start annual breast cancer screening with mammograms if they wish to do so. Women between 45 and 54 years of age should undergo a mammogram every year. Women 55 years of age and older should switch to a mammogram every 2 years, or choose to continue yearly screening.
Electrocardiogram	M and F	One baseline recording starting at age 40. ■

F, Female; *HPV*, human papillomavirus; *M*, male; *Pap*, Papanicolaou.

Table 5.1 Equipment and Supplies for the Physical Examination

Item	Description and Purpose
Patient examination gown	Gown made of disposable paper or cloth that provides patient modesty, comfort, and warmth.
Drape	A length of disposable paper or cloth to cover a patient or parts of a patient to provide comfort and warmth and reduce exposure.
Sphygmomanometer	Instrument used to measure blood pressure.
Stethoscope	Instrument used to auscultate body sounds, such as blood pressure and lung and bowel sounds.
Thermometer	Instrument used to measure body temperature.
Upright balance scale	Device used to measure weight and height.
Otoscope	Lighted instrument with lens, used to examine external ear canal and tympanic membrane.
Tuning fork	Small metal instrument consisting of stem and two prongs, used to test hearing acuity.
Ophthalmoscope	Lighted instrument with lens, used for examining interior of eye.
Tongue depressor	Flat wooden blade used to depress patient's tongue during examination of mouth and pharynx.
Antiseptic wipe	Disposable pad saturated with antiseptic, such as alcohol, that is used to cleanse skin.
Tape measure	Flexible device calibrated in inches on one side and centimeters on the other side, used to measure patient (e.g., diameter of limb, head circumference).
Percussion hammer	Instrument with rubber head, used for testing neurologic reflexes.
Speculum	Instrument for opening body orifice or cavity for viewing (e.g., ear speculum, nasal speculum, vaginal speculum).
Disposable gloves	Gloves, usually latex, that are worn only once to provide protection from bloodborne pathogens and other potentially infectious materials.
Lubricant	Agent that is applied to provider's gloved hand or to speculum that reduces friction between parts to make insertion easier.
Specimen container	Container in which body specimen is placed for transport to laboratory (after it has been labeled).
Tissues	Used for wiping body secretions.
Cotton-tipped applicator	Small piece of cotton wrapped around the end of a slender wooden stick, used for collection of specimen from the body.
Overhead examination light	Light mounted on flexible movable stand to focus light on area for good visibility.
Basin	Container in which used instruments are deposited.
Biohazard container	Specially made container used for receiving items that contain infectious waste.
Waste receptacle	Container for used disposable articles that do not contain infectious waste.

12. Check equipment and instruments regularly to verify that they are in proper working condition to protect the patient from harm caused by faulty equipment.
13. Make sure equipment and supplies are ready for the examination and arranged for easy access by the provider. Equipment and supplies needed for the physical examination vary according to the type of examination and the provider's preference (Fig. 5.1).
14. Properly operate and care for each piece of equipment and each instrument. The manufacturer provides an operating manual, which should be read carefully and kept available for reference.

PREPARATION OF THE PATIENT

It is the medical assistant's responsibility to prepare the patient for the physical examination. After greeting and escorting the patient to the examining room, the medical assistant should identify the patient by asking the patient to state his or her full name and date of birth. This information should be compared with the demographic data indicated in the patient's medical record. The patient should *not* be asked whether he or she is a certain patient. For example, the patient should not be asked: "Are you Mary Williams?" The patient may not hear the medical assistant correctly or may not be paying attention and may answer in the affirmative even if he or she is not that patient. Proper identification is essential to avoid mistaking one patient for another. If the medical assistant performs a procedure on the wrong patient by mistake, he or she could be held liable. The medical assistant then takes vital signs and measures the weight and height of the patient. The results of these procedures are documented in the patient's medical record.

The medical assistant can reduce a patient's apprehension by addressing the patient by his or her name of choice, by adopting a friendly and supportive attitude, and by speaking clearly, distinctly, and slowly. The medical assistant should explain the purpose of the examination and offer to answer any questions.

The patient should be asked whether he or she needs to void before the examination. An empty bladder makes the examination easier and is more comfortable for the patient. If a urine specimen is needed, the patient is asked to void.

Instructions on disrobing for the examination should be specific so that the patient understands what items of clothing to remove and where to place the clothing. The disrobing area should be comfortable and should provide privacy. It is helpful to have a place for the patient to sit to make it easier to remove clothing and shoes. The area also should be equipped with hooks for hanging clothing. Instructions for putting on the examination gown and for locating the gown opening reduce patient confusion. If the medical assistant senses that the patient will have trouble undressing, assistance should be offered. Elderly and disabled patients sometimes have difficulty removing clothing.

The physical examination is performed with the patient positioned on an examining table, which is specially constructed to facilitate the examination. For safety, it is advisable to help the patient onto and off of the examining table.

HIGHLIGHT on Patient Coaching

The purpose of patient coaching is to help the patient develop habits, attitudes, and skills that enable the individual to maintain and improve his or her own health.

Fact: Patients who are active, informed participants in their health care are more apt to follow the provider's instructions than patients who are passive recipients of medical services.

Action: Provide patients with information on health care. Every patient interaction is an opportunity for teaching.

Fact: Adult learners are goal oriented and performance centered. They need and want information that would assist them in managing and improving their health.

Action: Review the information that you provide to patients, and determine whether it is nice to know or necessary to know. Select subject matter that is practical and useful and relates directly to the patient's needs.

Fact: The more information that is presented, the more the patient is likely to forget. Approximately one half of information presented to the patient is forgotten in the first 5 minutes after the patient receives it.

Action: When teaching, use the following pointers to help patients learn and retain information:

- Keep it short and be specific.
- Speak in terms the patient can understand.
- Focus on "how" rather than "why."
- Repeat and reinforce important information.
- Give practical examples, and provide ample time for patient practice.
- Ask for feedback from the patient to determine whether he or she understands the information.
- Provide the patient with written information.

Fact: Each individual has a distinct style of learning and learns best when using his or her preferred learning style. The three main learning styles are reading, listening, and doing. People often use more than one style for learning.

Action: Use a variety of teaching strategies to engage the various learning styles of patients. Examples of teaching strategies include explanations, printed handouts, audiovisual aids, demonstrations, and discussions.

Fact: Only two thirds of patients comply with health care instructions prescribed by the provider. Factors that influence compliance include the patient's adaptation to illness, motivation to change, physical capability, and support system.

Action: The following help to increase patient compliance with prescribed treatment:

- Address the patient by his or her name of choice. (Keep in mind that many patients object to being called by their first name by strangers.)
- Encourage the patient to take an active role in personal health care.
- Help the patient to set goals and objectives for change.
- Encourage care and support from family members.
- Make the patient aware of outside resources.
- Give positive reinforcement when the patient makes healthy changes. ■

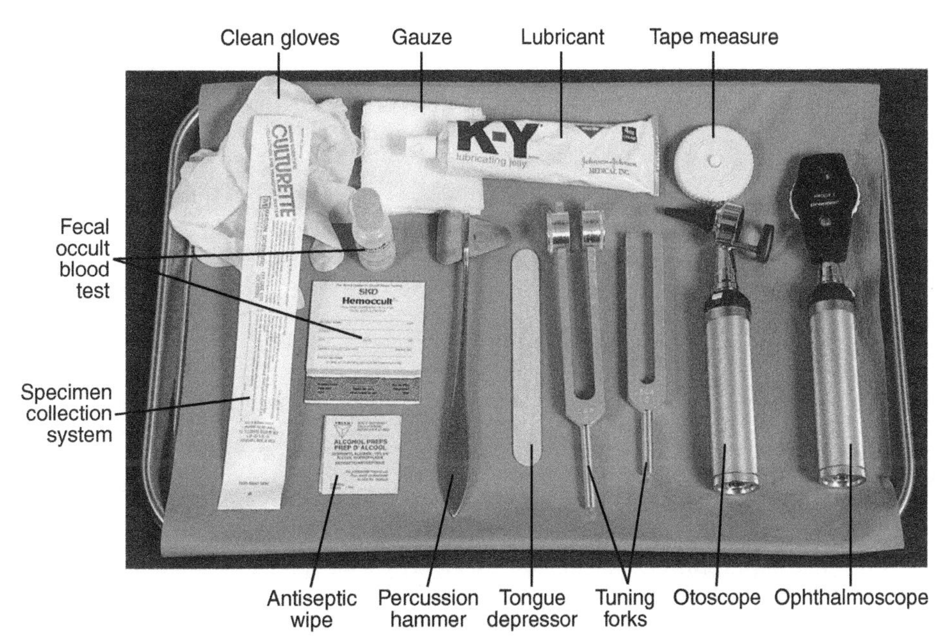

Fig. 5.1 Instruments and supplies used during the physical examination.

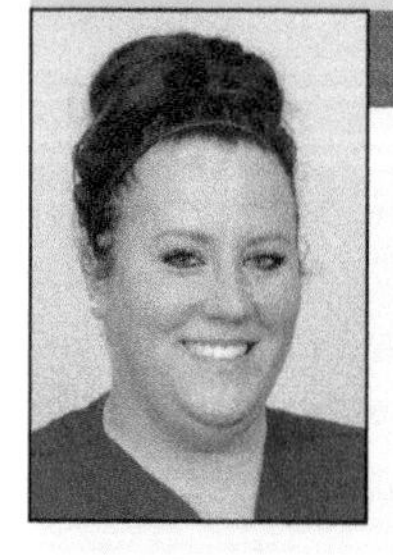

Putting It All Into Practice

My Name is Abby, and I am a certified medical assistant. I work in a medical clinic with a family medicine department of 10 physicians and 10 residents and interns. My duties cover a broad spectrum, from pediatrics to geriatrics, and include prenatal care, allergy injections, minor office surgery, electrocardiograms, colposcopies, immunizations, and wound care.

At our clinic, many of the patients are elderly. I occasionally come across geriatric patients who are not very cooperative and are "set in their ways." One 90-year-old woman, in particular, had a reputation in the office for being cantankerous and difficult to work with. One day when the physician ordered laboratory work on her, I prepared to draw blood from her tiny, frail body, praying that everything would go smoothly. As I helped her up after a successful "stick," she, of all people, reached to give me a hug and said to me, "I like you. That didn't even hurt!" She continued to hold my hand and talk to me as I walked her out of the office. This turned out to be the last time I would see her because she moved out of town, but not out of my heart, leaving a lasting impression on my life. ■

What Would You Do? What Would You *Not* Do?

Case Study 1

Abbey Auden, 35 years old, is at the medical office. Her husband got a backyard trampoline for their two school-aged children, and she decided to try it out. Abbey landed wrong on the trampoline and hurt her back and neck. For the past 5 days, she has been having headaches and back pain. Abbey refuses to have her weight taken because she has gained weight over the past several years and does not want to know how much she has gained. She does not understand why weight has to be taken at an office visit in the first place. Abbey says that many times when she should go to the doctor, she does not, just to avoid being weighed. She says she would not even be here now except that her husband insisted that she come. ■

MEASURING WEIGHT AND HEIGHT

The medical assistant routinely measures the weight and height of many types of patients. The process of measuring the patient is mensuration. A change in weight may be significant in the diagnosis of a patient's condition and in prescribing the course of treatment. Underweight and overweight patients who follow a diet therapy program should be weighed at regular intervals to determine their progress. Prenatal patients are weighed during each prenatal visit to assist in the assessment of fetal development and of the mother's health.

An adult's weight usually is measured during each office visit; an adult's height is typically measured only during the first visit or when a complete physical examination of the patient is requested. Children are weighed and their height (or length) is measured during each office visit to observe their pattern of growth and to calculate medication dosage.

TYPES OF SCALES

There are two types of scales commonly used in the medical office. These include the upright balance beam scale and the upright electronic digital scale. A balance beam scale uses sliding weights that are manually moved on horizontal calibration bars to measure the patient's weight. The patient's height is measured using a sliding vertical calibration rod with a measuring (headpiece) bar. Balance beam scales are quite accurate and do not require a power source. However, it is important that the medical assistant interpret the calibration markings correctly when measuring weight and height to prevent an error in the measurements. Specific guidelines for using a balance beam scale are presented in Box 5.1. Procedure 5.1 outlines the procedure for measuring height and weight using a balance beam scale.

An electronic scale (Fig. 5.5A) automatically measures a patient's weight and height and displays the results digitally on a display screen (see Fig. 5.5B). It is also able to determine a patient's body mass index (BMI) and display it on the screen of the scale. It takes less time to measure weight and height with an electronic scale as compared with a balance beam scale. The weight and height measurements are considered accurate; however, they can sometimes be affected by temperature and humidity. An electronic scale requires a power supply (e.g., battery and AC adapter).

BODY MASS INDEX

The patient's weight and height are used to determine BMI. The BMI strongly correlates with total body fat and therefore is used as a screening tool to identify patients who may be at risk for health problems associated with underweight, overweight and obesity (see the box Highlight on Body Mass Index). When using a balance beam scale, the BMI is determined by comparing a patient's weight and height against a BMI table (Fig. 5.6). The BMI can also be determined through the use of a BMI calculator available as part of an electronic health record (EHR) program or an internet BMI-calculator website. For adults 20 years and older, BMI is then interpreted using weight status categories. Adult patients with a BMI between 18.5 and 24.9 are considered to be within normal weight. Table 5.2 outlines each of the BMI ranges and the corresponding weight status categories.

BOX 5.1 Guidelines for Using a Balance Beam Scale

When using an upright balance scale to measure weight and height, use the following guidelines.

Weight

1. *Locate the scale to provide privacy for the patient.* Place the scale on a hard, level surface in a private location. Many patients are self-conscious about having their weight measured and prefer that it be done in privacy. Do not make weight-sensitive comments during the procedure. This is especially important for patients with eating disorders such as compulsive overeating and anorexia.
2. *Balance the scale before measuring weight.* If the scale is not balanced, the weight measurement will be inaccurate. The scale is balanced when the upper and lower weights are on zero and the indicator point comes to a rest in the center of the balance area.
3. *Assist the patient.* Assist the patient onto and off of the scale platform. The scale platform moves slightly and may cause the patient to become unsteady.
4. *Obtain an accurate weight.* Always ask the patient to remove his or her shoes. Measure weight with the patient in normal clothing. Ask the patient to remove heavy outer clothing, such as a sweater or a jacket.
5. *Interpret the calibration markings accurately.* The lower calibration bar is divided into 50-lb increments (Fig. 5.2A). The upper calibration bar is divided into pounds and quarter pounds. The longer calibration lines indicate pound increments, and the shorter calibration lines indicate quarter-pound and half-pound increments (see Fig. 5.2B).
6. *Determine the patient's weight correctly.* Add the measurement on the lower scale to the measurement on the upper scale. The result should be rounded to the nearest quarter pound. Occasionally the patient's weight may need to be converted to kilograms, which is the metric unit of measurement for weight. This may be required when determining medication dosage. The following formulas are used to convert weight measurements from one system to another.

Weight Conversion

Pounds to kilograms: Divide the number of pounds by 2.2:
 136 lb ÷ 2.2 = 61.8 kg

Kilograms to pounds: Multiply the number of kilograms by 2.2:
 75 kg × 2.2 = 165 lb

Height

1. *Provide for the patient's safety.* Follow the proper procedure when measuring the patient's height. An error in technique could result in injury. If a patient is placed on the scale in a forward position, the measuring bar could fall into the patient's face when he or she steps off of the scale, causing a facial injury.
2. *Interpret the calibration markings accurately.* Depending on the brand of scale, the calibration markings are divided into inches or feet and inches. (Fig. 5.3 is an example of a scale divided into feet and inches.) The calibration rod also is calibrated into centimeters, which is the metric unit of measurement for height. This unit of measurement is not typically used to measure height in the United States.
3. *Read the measurement correctly.* The height measurement is read from the top of the bar down and should be read to the nearest quarter inch. For most patients, you can read the height measurement at the junction of the stationary calibration rod and the movable calibration rod (Fig. 5.4A). However, if the patient's height is less than the top value of the stationary calibration rod, you must read the measurement from the bottom of the bar up directly on the stationary rod. (*Note*: The measuring bar must first be released (see Fig. 5.4B) and moved down to the stationary bar.) The highest calibration on the stationary rod of most scales is 50 inches; therefore patients with a height of 50 inches or less would have their height read directly from the stationary rod (see Fig. 5.4C).
4. *Document the height measurement correctly.* Document the height measurement in feet and inches. If the scale is calibrated in inches, convert the reading to feet and inches by dividing the number of inches by 12. A height measurement of 60 inches is documented as 5 feet (60 inches ÷ 12 = 5). If the patient's height measurement is 64 inches, the results would be documented as 5 feet, 4 inches.

What Would You Do? What Would You *Not* Do?

Case Study 2

Karen Steiner drops her 17-year-old daughter, Mikayla, off at the medical office for her sports physical examination. Mikayla is captain of the varsity cheerleading squad and is getting ready to start her senior year in high school. Mikayla's vital signs are normal, and she measures 5 feet, 6 inches tall and weighs 105 pounds. With some reluctance, Mikayla admits that she has been having problems with heartburn, and she is pretty sure she knows what is causing it. She says that she has to keep her weight down for cheerleading, and after eating dinner with her family, she makes herself vomit to get rid of the food in her stomach. Mikayla is not too concerned about doing this because a lot of the popular girls at school are doing the same thing. She says it is the easy way to stay slim, and she would like to lose another 10 pounds before football season starts. Mikayla wants some prescription drug samples to help with the heartburn because the over-the-counter pills that she has been taking are not working anymore. She does not want her parents to know about any of this because she is afraid that they would not understand and might make her drop out of cheerleading. ■

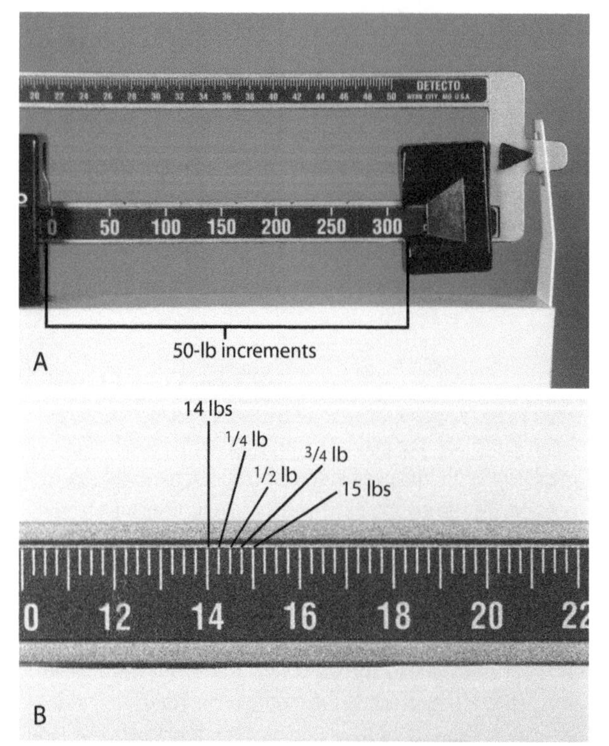

Fig. 5.2 Calibration markings for measuring weight. (A) Lower calibration bar. (B) Upper calibration bar.

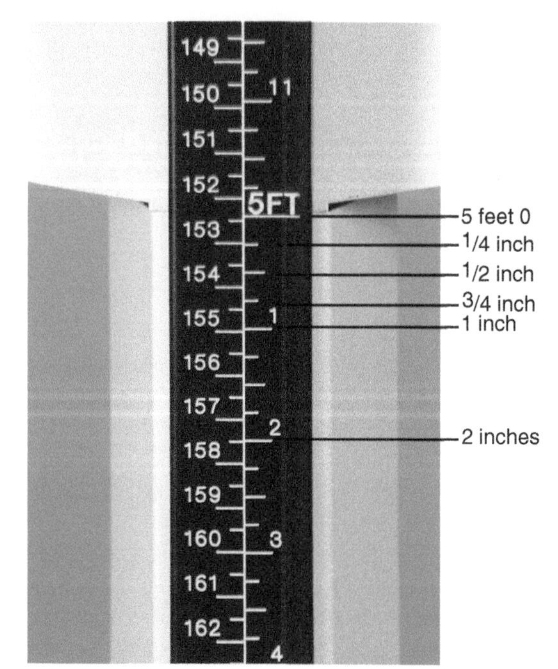

Fig. 5.3 Calibration markings for height.

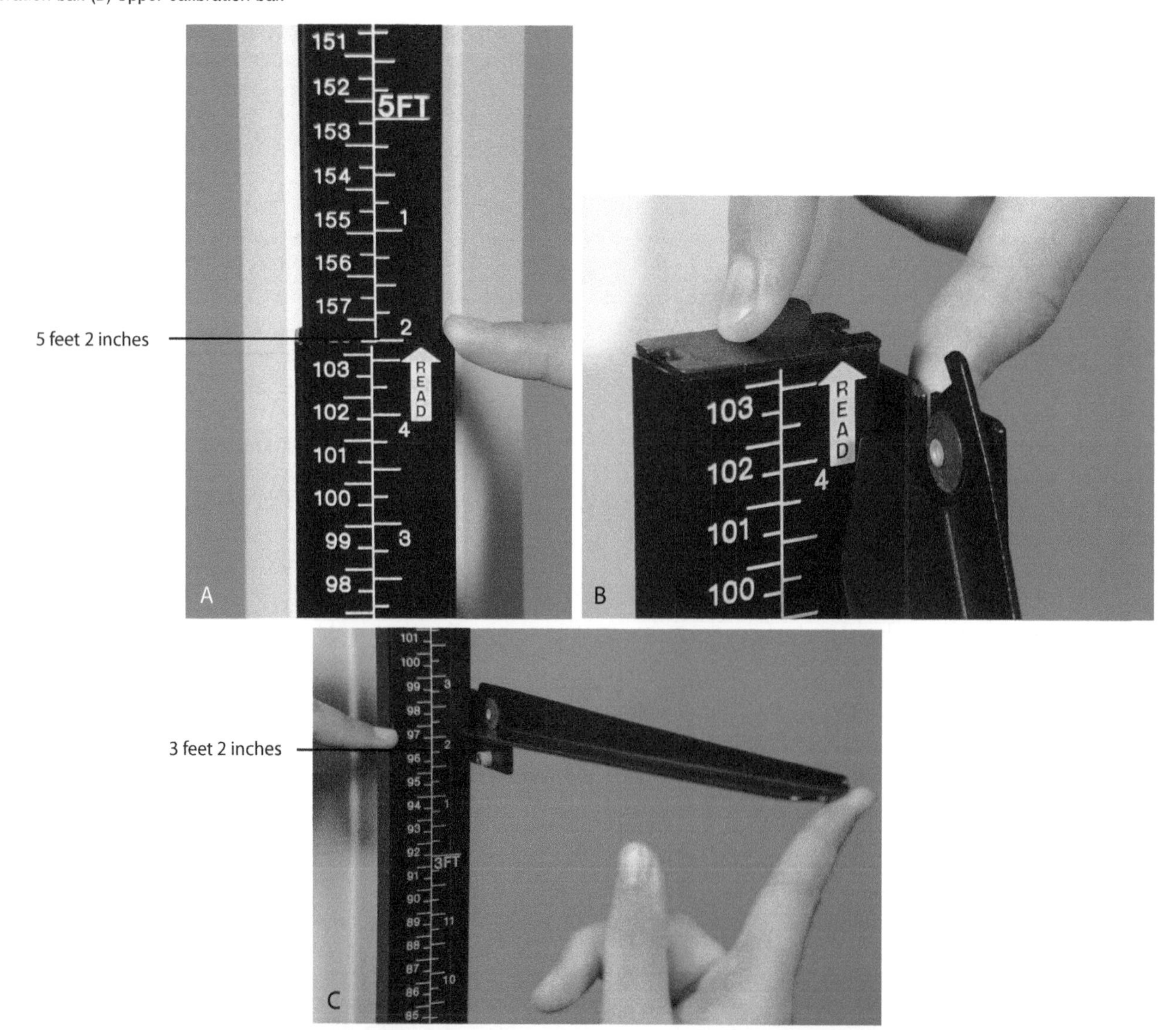

Fig. 5.4 (A) Reading a height measurement. The height measurement in this illustration is 6 feet, 1 inch. (B) Moving the measuring bar. (C) Reading a height measurement on the stationary calibration rod. The height measurement in this illustration is 3 feet, 2 inches.

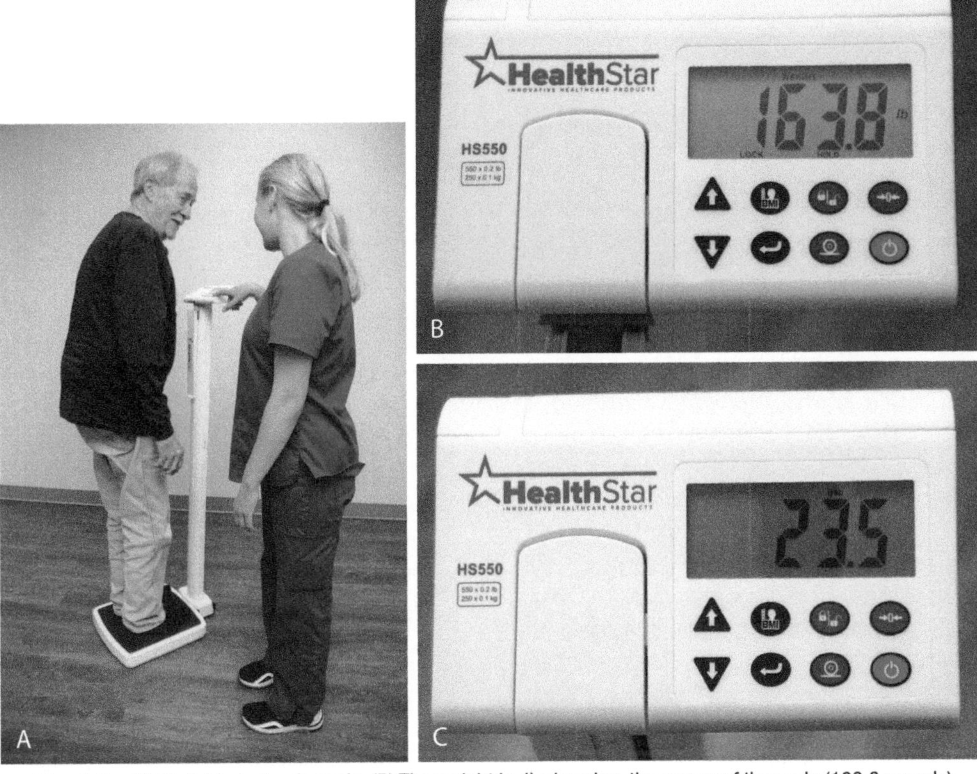

Fig. 5.5 (A) Upright electronic scale. (B) The weight is displayed on the screen of the scale (163.8 pounds). (C) The body mass index (BMI) is calculated using the weight and height measurements and displayed on the screen of the scale (BMI of 23.5).

BMI	19	20	21	22	23	24	25	26	27	28	29	30	31	32	33	34	35
Height (inches)	**Body Weight (pounds)**																
58	91	96	100	105	110	115	119	124	129	134	138	143	148	153	158	162	167
59	94	99	104	109	114	119	124	128	133	138	146	147	153	158	163	168	173
60	97	102	107	112	118	123	128	133	138	143	148	153	158	163	168	174	179
61	100	106	111	116	122	127	132	137	143	148	153	158	164	169	174	180	185
62	104	109	115	120	126	131	136	142	147	153	158	164	169	175	180	186	191
63	107	113	118	124	130	135	141	146	152	158	163	169	175	180	186	191	197
64	110	116	122	128	134	140	154	151	157	163	169	174	180	186	192	197	204
65	114	120	126	132	138	144	150	156	162	168	174	180	186	192	198	204	210
66	118	124	130	136	142	148	155	161	167	173	179	186	192	198	204	210	216
67	121	127	134	140	146	153	159	166	172	178	185	191	198	204	211	217	223
68	125	131	138	144	151	158	164	171	177	184	190	197	203	210	216	223	230
69	128	135	142	149	155	162	169	176	182	189	196	203	209	216	223	230	236
70	132	139	143	153	160	167	174	181	188	195	202	209	216	222	229	236	243
71	136	143	150	157	165	172	179	186	193	200	208	215	222	229	236	243	250
72	140	147	154	162	169	177	184	191	199	206	213	221	228	235	242	250	258
73	144	151	159	166	174	182	189	197	204	212	219	227	235	242	250	257	265
74	148	155	163	171	179	186	194	202	210	218	225	233	241	249	256	264	272
75	152	160	168	176	184	192	200	208	216	224	232	240	248	256	264	272	279
76	156	164	172	170	189	197	205	213	221	230	238	246	254	263	271	279	287

Fig. 5.6 Body mass index (BMI) table. To use the table, find the appropriate height in the left-hand column labeled Height. Move across to a given weight (in pounds). The number at the top of the column is the BMI at that height and weight. Pounds have been rounded off. (From National Heart, Lung, and Blood Institute, US Department of Health and Human Services.)

HIGHLIGHT on Cultural Diversity

Culture consists of the values, beliefs, and practices of a particular group of people. Culture is deeply rooted and is passed on from one generation to the next through communication. It includes areas such as religion, dietary practices, family lines of authority, family life patterns, beliefs, and health practices.

As the demographics of the United States continue to change, the medical assistant is faced with the challenge of providing care to an increasing number of cultural groups. It is important for the medical assistant to learn as much as possible about the cultural values of patients coming to the medical office. This is known as *cultural awareness* and can be accomplished by carefully observing and listening to patients to acquire knowledge of their cultural values.

Cultural sensitivity is respect and appreciation for cultural diversity, whereas *cultural competence* is understanding and using the cultural background of a patient to assist with the resolution of a problem. Because health practices are part of a patient's culture, changing them may have a negative impact on the patient. Whenever possible, the medical assistant should incorporate factors from a patient's cultural background into his or her health care.

Guidelines for achieving cultural competence

The following guidelines help the medical assistant in developing cultural awareness and sensitivity and in achieving cultural competence:

1. *Respect the patient's values, beliefs, and practices.* Even if you do not agree with them, it is important to respect the patient's right to hold these values and to not dismiss them as strange or odd. Cultural values play an important role in a patient's lifestyle. Patients from some cultures believe that losing blood depletes the body's strength and provides a route for the soul to leave the body. If a blood specimen is needed, these patients may become highly distressed or refuse to have their blood drawn. Members of some cultural groups believe that illness results when the body's natural balance or harmony is disturbed. To restore the balance, alternative forms of medicine, such as herbal remedies and aromatherapy, are used.
2. *Refrain from cultural stereotypes.* Not all people of a cultural group have the same beliefs, practices, and values. Assuming that all members of a cultural group are alike is known as *stereotyping* and should be avoided. Just as one would never assume that all people in the United States like hamburgers and baseball, every individual must be approached according to his or her specific beliefs and practices.
3. *Always address patients by their last names (and Mr., Mrs., Miss, Ms.) unless they give you permission to use other names.* In many cultures, using a first name to address anyone other than family or friends is considered disrespectful. Most older people in the United States dislike being called by their first name and feel it shows a lack of respect.
4. *Speak slowly and clearly.* Communicating with a patient may be difficult if the patient has a limited knowledge of English. With these patients, you should speak slowly and clearly in a normal tone and volume of voice. Speaking loudly does not help the patient to understand any better and may be offensive to the patient.
5. *Show respect for cultural lines of authority.* In many cultures, respect is given based on age and gender. In certain cultures, elders are considered the holders of the culture's wisdom and are highly respected. In other cultures, youth is valued over age. In certain cultures, men dominate and women have very little status. Because of this, a female patient from this type of culture may not be permitted to give her own health history or to answer questions. In addition, a male patient from this culture may not accept instructions from a female medical assistant.
6. *Use appropriate eye contact.* In most cultures, direct eye contact is important and generally shows that the other is attentive and listening. It conveys self-confidence, openness, interest, and honesty, whereas the lack of eye contact may be interpreted as secretiveness, shyness, guilt, or lack of interest. Other cultures consider eye contact impolite or an invasion of privacy; these patients show respect by avoiding direct eye contact.
7. *Be aware of cultural responses to illness.* The conditions under which an individual assumes the role of a (sick) patient and the way he or she performs in that role vary with culture. Individuals of some cultures resist the sick role and blame sickness on external forces as a means of punishment. These individuals may deny their illness and fail to provide much information when the medical assistant takes their symptoms. In other cultures, individuals take an optimistic view of the outcome of health care and, because of this, are more likely to offer information and to follow the provider's instructions.
8. Learn to appreciate the richness of diversity as an asset, rather than a hindrance, to communication and effective interaction with patients. ■

HIGHLIGHT on Body Mass Index

Body mass index

The body mass index (BMI) is an indirect measurement of body fat based on a patient's height and weight. Except for trained athletes, the BMI strongly correlates with the total body fat content in adults. This provides an indication of the risk of developing chronic health conditions associated with obesity. The National Heart, Lung, and Blood Institute (NHLBI), a federal agency, recommends that the BMI be determined in all adults. People of normal weight should have their BMI reassessed every 2 years.

Determining body mass index

BMI can be determined by using one of the following methods:

1. Use the BMI table (see Fig. 5.6).

HIGHLIGHT on Body Mass Index

2. Use the following website to have your BMI calculated automatically: https://www.nhlbi.nih.gov/health/educational/lose_wt/BMI/bmi-m.htm.
3. Use the following steps to calculate your BMI:
   a. Multiply your weight in pounds (without clothes or shoes) by 703. For an individual who weighs 135 lb:135 × 703 = 94,905.
   b. Divide this number by your height in inches. If this individual is 66 inches tall: 94,905 ÷ 66 = 1438.
   c. Divide this amount again by your height in inches, and round off to the nearest whole number: 1438 ÷ 66 = 21.79, or 22.

The BMI of this individual is 22.

Adult Obesity

The incidence of obesity in the United States has increased markedly, and obesity is now one of the most common problems encountered by primary care providers. Almost 69% of adults in the United States are either overweight or obese. That means that two out of every three Americans are overweight or obese. Obesity is associated with premature death and, after smoking, is currently the second leading cause of preventable death in the United States. According to the CDC, approximately 112,000 deaths in the United States each year are associated with obesity.

It has been determined that as the BMI increases to greater than 25, there is an increased risk of developing certain conditions associated with overweight and obesity, including the following:

- Hypertension
- Coronary heart disease
- Stroke
- Dyslipidemia (high blood cholesterol levels, high blood triglyceride levels, or both)
- Type 2 diabetes
- Colon cancer
- Gallbladder disease
- Gout
- Fatty liver disease
- Breast and endometrial cancers
- Infertility and polycystic ovary syndrome
- Sleep apnea and respiratory problems
- Osteoarthritis

Obesity is considered a chronic condition that requires a multiple treatment approach, including a behavioral therapy program, a low-calorie diet, and a suitable aerobic exercise program. Primary care providers often manage individuals with mild and moderate obesity, but morbidly obese patients are usually referred to a bariatric specialist. **Bariatrics** is the branch of medicine that deals with the treatment and control of obesity and diseases associated with obesity. Treatment of obesity may include one or more of the following:

- Dietary modification: based on medical evidence
- Physical activity: adjusted to the person's needs and abilities
- Behavioral modification: to help overcome unhealthy habits
- Medication: if appropriate, as a tool to help with the urge to eat
- Weight loss surgery: if appropriate, for those with severe obesity
- Prevention of weight regain: help with maintaining healthy habits
- Understanding, compassion, and respect. ■

Table 5.2 Interpretation of Body Mass Index

BMI	Weight Status Category
Less than 15	Very severely underweight
15–15.9	Severely underweight
16–18.49	Underweight
18.5–24.9	Healthy weight
25–29.9	Overweight
30–34.9	Obese Class I (Moderately obese)
35.0–39.9	Obese Class II (Severely obese)
40 or more	Obese Class III (Very severely obese)

BMI, Body mass index.

BODY MECHANICS

Daily activities in a medical office sometimes carry the risk of acute or chronic musculoskeletal injury. Because of this, the medical assistant should have a thorough knowledge of the principles of proper body mechanics and know when to use them. **Body mechanics** is the use of the correct muscles to maintain proper balance, posture, and body alignment to accomplish a task safely and efficiently without undue strain on muscles or joints. Proper body mechanics should be used when the medical assistant performs the following: standing, walking, sitting, lifting, positioning a patient on the examining table, and transferring a patient. The medical assistant should also use proper body mechanics at home in his or her activities of daily living. Using proper body mechanics prevents musculoskeletal strains to the back and other body structures such as the knees, neck, shoulders, and wrists.

The primary benefits of proper body mechanics include the following:

1. Allows an individual to conserve energy, which makes it easier to perform a task
2. Protects the body from injury by reducing stress and strain on muscles, nerves, joints, tendons, ligaments, and soft tissues
3. Helps to maintain proper body control and balance
4. Promotes effective, efficient, and safe movement

Studies show that health care workers sustain a significantly higher incidence of back injuries compared with workers in other professions. To help prevent an injury to the back, a primary focus of proper body mechanics is to keep the natural curves of the spine or vertebral column in proper alignment. The vertebral column has four curvatures. These curvatures increase the strength and resilience of the vertebral column and include the cervical curvature, thoracic curvature, lumbar curvature, and sacral curvature (Fig. 5.7). The vertebral column extends from the skull to the pelvis and consists of a series of bones known as *vertebrae.* The vertebrae are separated by shock-absorbing *intervertebral discs* (see Fig. 5.7). These discs allow an individual to bend and twist. Over time, with improper and repeated bending and twisting (especially while carrying an object), the discs can deteriorate, which causes them to narrow, to harden, and even to crack and tear. This condition is known as *degenerative disc disease.* With degenerative disc disease, the discs lose their shock-absorbing ability and cause the patient to experience localized pain and stiffness in the area of disc deterioration. In addition, once a disc is weakened, it can bulge out or rupture; this is known as a *herniated disc.*

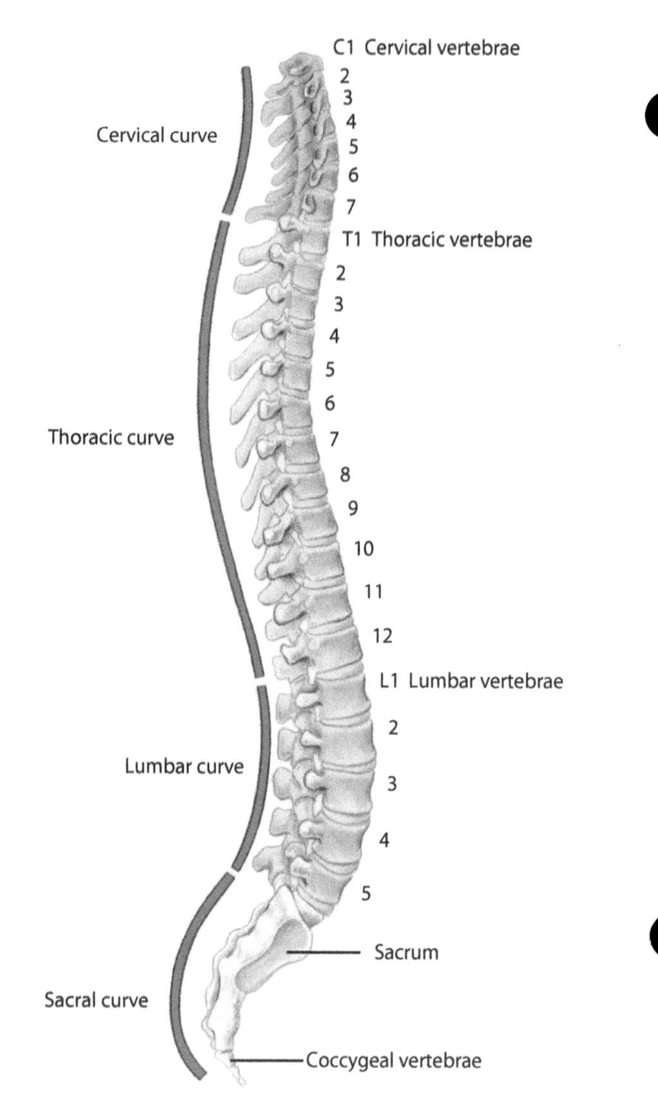

Fig. 5.7 Vertebral column. (From Applegate E: *The anatomy and physiology learning system,* ed 4, St. Louis, 2011, Elsevier.)

PRINCIPLES

There are some basic principles related to proper body mechanics that should be followed:

1. Movements should be smooth and coordinated rather than jerky.
2. Keeping the body in good physical condition through exercising, stretching, and weight training helps to prevent musculoskeletal injury.
3. To avoid straining the back, do not reach for something that is farther than 14 to 18 inches away.
4. Work at a comfortable height that avoids having to bend the neck or back forward to perform the task. People are usually most comfortable working at a height that is between the waist and elbow levels.
5. If possible, push, pull, or slide an object rather than lifting it. This conserves energy and places less strain on the back.
6. Lighter items should be stored on higher shelves or cabinets, and heavier items should be stored at or below waist level.
7. When an object from an overhead shelf or cabinet needs to be retrieved, use a step stool or chair to come up to the level of the object. Reaching for a stored overhead item can produce strain on the back.
8. When lifting an object or transferring a patient, the large muscles of the arms and legs should be used as much as possible and the back muscles as little as possible. The more muscle groups that are used, the more evenly the weight is distributed over the medical assistant's body, which puts less strain on the back.
9. When transferring a patient, encourage the patient to assist as much as possible.
10. If a patient becomes dizzy or faint or starts to fall, do not try to hold the patient in an upright position. Instead, balance yourself with your legs apart to form a wide base of support, and gently and gradually lower the patient to a chair or to the floor.
11. Always ask for assistance if you do not think you can lift a heavy object or transfer a patient.

APPLICATION OF BODY MECHANICS

The medical assistant should practice proper body mechanics when standing, sitting, lifting an object, positioning a patient on the examining table, and transferring a patient from a wheelchair to an examining table and back again, as outlined on the following pages.

Standing

It is important to maintain good posture by positioning the body in the correct standing position as outlined here. This provides the medical assistant with good balance and stability and reduces strain on the back by keeping the vertebral column at its natural alignment.

1. Wear comfortable low-heeled shoes that provide good support.

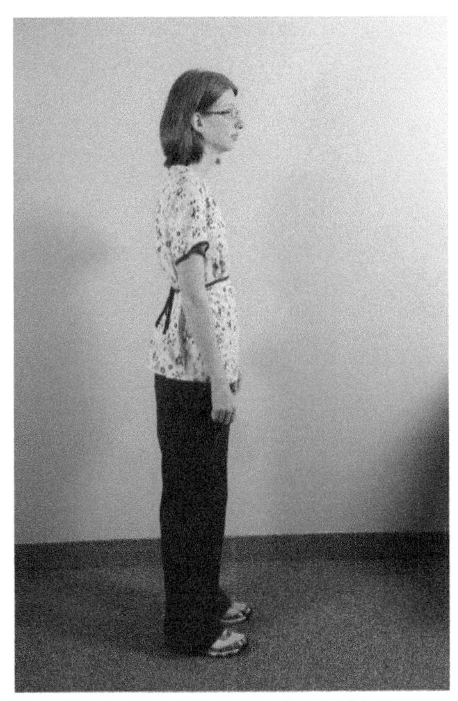

Fig. 5.8 Proper standing position.

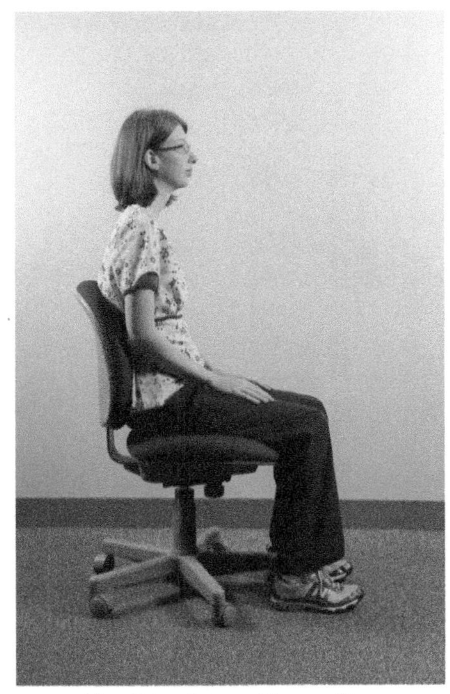

Fig. 5.9 Proper sitting position.

2. Hold the head erect at the midline of the body, the back as straight as possible with the pelvis tucked inward, the chest forward with the shoulders back, and the abdomen drawn in and kept flat. This helps to maintain appropriate alignment of the vertebral column (Fig. 5.8).
3. The knees should be slightly flexed with the feet pointing forward and parallel to each other approximately 3 inches apart. This provides a broad base of support and improves balance.
4. The arms should be positioned comfortably at the side, and the weight of the body should be evenly distributed over both feet.

Sitting

The medical assistant should use proper body mechanics when in a sitting position (Fig. 5.9), as follows:

1. Sit in a chair with a firm back.
2. Sit firmly with the back and buttocks supported against the back of the chair; avoid slumping. The body weight should be evenly distributed over the buttocks and thighs.
3. Use a small pillow or a rolled towel to support the lower back.
4. The feet should be flat on the floor, and the knees should be level with the hips.
5. If you need to sit for a prolonged period of time, use a footstool to raise one knee to reduce strain on the back.
6. Take frequent stretch breaks.

Lifting

The following steps outline the procedure for lifting an object while using proper body mechanics:

1. First determine the weight of the object to determine if you can safely lift it. Pushing the object with one foot can help you determine if you can lift it without assistance. Never lift anything heavier than you can easily manage.
2. Stand in front of the object, and balance yourself with the feet approximately 6 to 8 inches apart, toes pointed outward, and one foot slightly forward to provide a wide base of support. Tighten the stomach and gluteal muscles in preparation for lifting the object.
3. To lift the object, always bend the body at the knees and hips (Fig. 5.10A). This helps to maintain your center of gravity and allows the strong muscles of the legs to do the lifting. Never bend from the waist (see Fig. 5.10C).
4. Grasp the object firmly with both hands.
5. Keeping the back straight, lift the object smoothly with the leg muscles, not the back muscles (see Fig. 5.10B). The muscles of the back are not as strong and are more easily injured than the leg muscles.
6. Hold the object as close to the body as possible and at waist level. This allows the weight of the object to be lifted by the arm and leg muscles rather than the back muscles. To prevent strain on the back, never lift anything higher than the level of the chest.
7. If you need to turn after lifting the object, do not twist. Turn by pivoting your whole body. Twisting the spine can cause a serious back injury.
8. If you need to carry the object to another location, make sure the area of transport is dry and free of clutter.
9. Lower the object slowly, making sure to bend from the knees to allow the leg muscles to do the work.

POSITIONING AND DRAPING

Correct positioning of the patient facilitates the examination by permitting better access to the part being examined

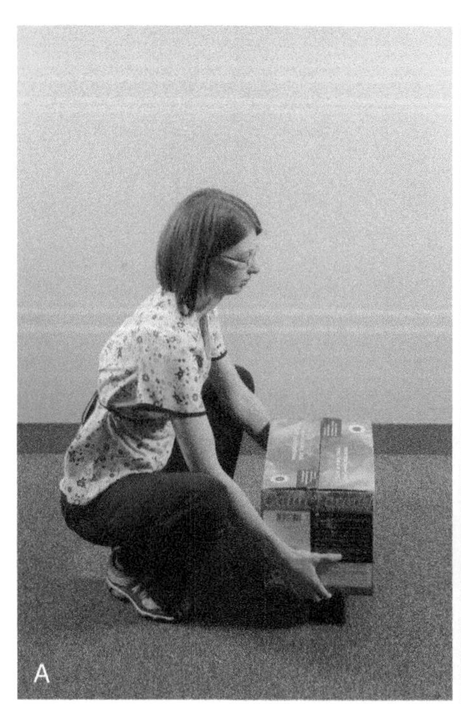

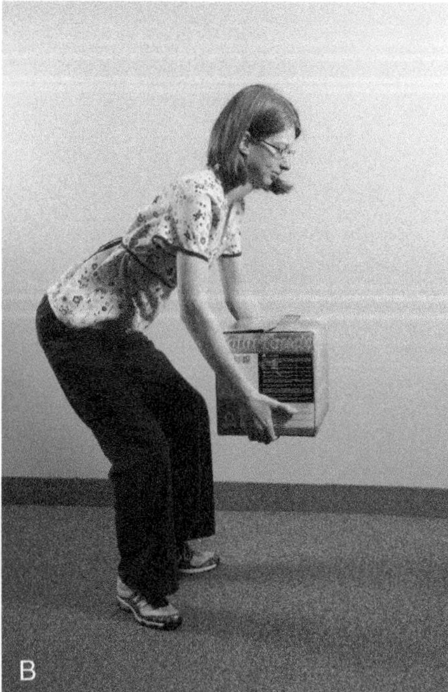

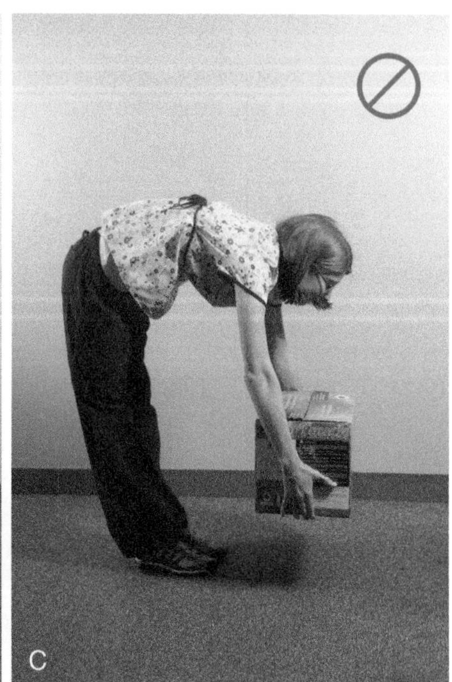

Fig. 5.10 (A) To lift the object, always bend the body at the knees and hips. (B) Lift with the leg muscles, while keeping the back straight. (C) Never bend from the waist.

or treated. The basic positions used in the medical office are sitting, supine, prone, dorsal recumbent, lithotomy, modified left lateral recumbent, knee-chest, and Fowler.

The position used depends on the type of examination or procedure to be performed. More than one position may be used to examine the same body part during the physical examination. The sitting and supine positions are both used to examine the chest. It is important to know the correct position for each examination or treatment. When positioning a patient, the medical assistant should explain the position to the patient and assist the patient in attaining it. The medical assistant should make sure to use proper body mechanics when positioning a patient to avoid musculoskeletal injuries.

It is important to take the patient's endurance and degree of wellness into consideration when positioning him or her. Patients who are weak or ill may be unable to assume a position or may require special assistance in attaining it. Some positions, such as the lithotomy and knee-chest positions, are embarrassing and uncomfortable. A patient should not be kept in these positions any longer than necessary. Some patients (especially the elderly) become dizzy after a time in certain positions, such as the knee-chest position. These patients should be allowed to rest before they get off the examining table. The medical assistant also should assist patients off the examining table to prevent falls.

The patient is draped during positioning to provide for modesty, comfort, and warmth. Only the part to be examined should be exposed. Patient gowns and drapes used in the medical office are usually made of paper but also may be made of cloth. Procedures 5.2–5.9 present proper positioning and draping of the patient.

WHEELCHAIR TRANSFER

A wheelchair is a chair mounted on wheels designed to make mobility easier for individuals who cannot walk or who are having difficulty walking because of illness or disability. Although some patients who come to the medical office in a wheelchair are able to transfer themselves from a wheelchair to an examining table, others may need assistance. The medical assistant plays an important role in the safe and efficient transfer of a patient from a wheelchair to an examining table and back again.

The OSHA recommends that assistive devices be used whenever possible to transfer patients. A transfer belt (also known as a *gait belt*) is a safety device that is approximately 1.5 to 2 inches wide and 48 or 60 inches long and is made of a durable fiber, such as canvas, nylon, or leather (Fig. 5.11). It can be used to assist in the safe transfer of a patient from a wheelchair to an examining table and back again. The transfer belt is wrapped around the patient's waist over his or her clothing and is securely fastened. The belt provides the medical assistant with a secure grip for holding onto the patient and controlling the patient's movement. This makes the transfer more comfortable for the patient because the medical assistant will not have to grasp the patient around the rib cage or under the axillae to make the transfer. Using a transfer belt also reduces the chance of the medical assistant hurting his or her musculoskeletal system while transferring a patient. Procedure 5.10 outlines the procedure for transferring a patient from a wheelchair to an examining table and back again using a transfer belt.

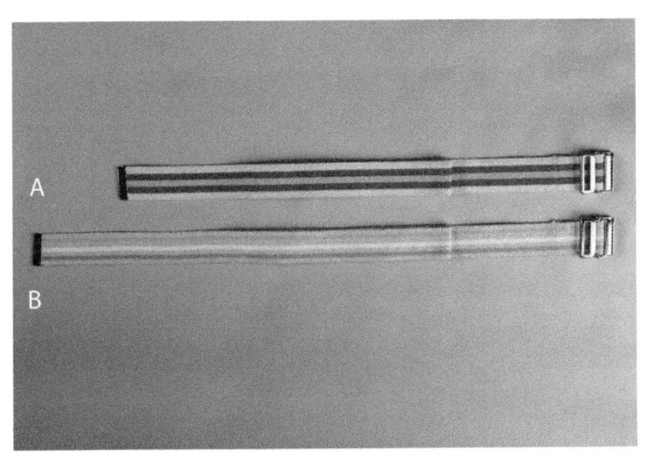

Fig. 5.11 Transfer belts. (A) Transfer belt that is 48 inches in length. (B) Transfer belt that is 60 inches in length.

It is important for the medical assistant to realize that it may not always be possible to transfer a patient from a wheelchair to the examining table, even with the use of a transfer belt. Before transferring a patient, the medical assistant should carefully assess his or her ability to make the transfer. There are certain factors that may place undue strain on the medical assistant's musculoskeletal system. These factors include patients who are overweight or patients who have conditions that limit their mobility (e.g., leg paralysis), making it impossible for the patient to assist with the transfer. If factors exist that might cause strain to the medical assistant's musculoskeletal system, the medical assistant should ask for assistance or notify the provider that it is not possible to transfer the patient to the examining table.

ASSESSMENT OF THE PATIENT

The extent of patient assessment during the physical examination depends on the purpose of the examination and the patient's condition. A complete physical examination involves a thorough assessment of all body systems. Table 5.3 outlines the specific assessments included in a complete physical examination. The provider uses an organized and systematic approach in performing a physical examination, starting with the patient's head and proceeding toward the feet. Using this type of approach facilitates the examination process and requires the fewest position changes by the patient.

With an EHR, the provider uses free-text entry, drop-down lists, and check-boxes to document findings on the screen of a computer monitor. The EHR program uses this information to generate the physical examination report. This means that by the end of the examination, the physical examination report is complete, and the provider does not need to dictate his or her findings at a later time. This alleviates the need for transcribing the provider's dictation into a written report. With a paper-based patient record (PPR), the provider documents the results of the physical examination in the patient's medical record, typically on a preprinted form.

Patients who exhibit symptoms of illness usually require only select portions of the physical examination. A patient who comes to the medical office with symptoms of bronchitis usually does not require a complete physical examination; rather, the provider examines the body system that is most likely to be associated with the symptoms. Four assessment techniques are used to obtain information during the physical examination: inspection, palpation, percussion, and auscultation.

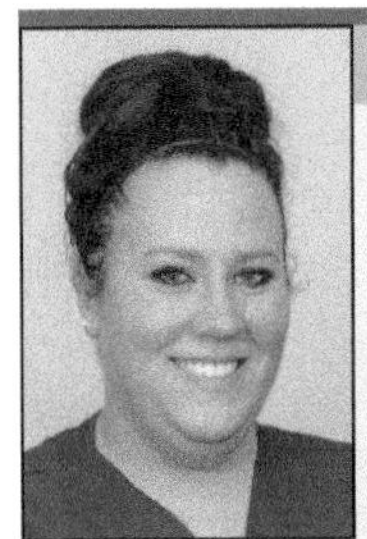

Memories *from* Practicum

Abby: During my practicum at a student health center at a 4-year college, I was responsible for working up patients for gynecologic examinations. The two-piece drapes had the top opening in the front and the bottom opening in the back. After explaining this to an Asian student who spoke very little English, I noticed that she had the openings opposite of what I had explained. I explained again, with words and gestures, that she needed to reverse the openings. To my surprise, she stood up, turned around in a circle, and sat down!

INSPECTION

Inspection involves observation of the patient for any signs of disease, and of the four assessment techniques, it is the one most frequently used. Good lighting is important for effective observation. The patient's color, speech, deformities, skin condition (e.g., rashes, scars, warts), body contour and symmetry, orientation to the surroundings, body movements, and anxiety level are assessed through inspection. The medical assistant should develop a high level of detailed observational skills to assist the provider in assessing physical characteristics.

PALPATION

Palpation is the examination of the body using the sense of touch (Fig. 5.12). The provider uses palpation to determine the placement and size of organs; the presence of lumps; and the existence of pain, swelling, or tenderness. Examining the breasts and taking the pulse are performed by palpation. Palpation often helps verify data obtained by inspection. The patient's verbal and facial expressions also are observed during palpation to assist in the detection of abnormalities.

The two types of palpation—light and deep—are categorized by the amount of pressure applied. *Light palpation* of structures is performed to determine areas of tenderness. The fingertips are placed on the part to be examined and are gently depressed approximately ½ inch. *Deep palpation* is used to examine the condition of organs such as those in the abdomen. Two hands are used for deep palpation. One hand is used to support the body from below, and the other hand is used to press over the area to be palpated. Deep palpation is used by the provider to perform a bimanual pelvic examination.

Table 5.3 Physician Assessment During the Physical Examination

Body Structure	Assessment	Normal Findings	Abnormal Findings
General appearance	Observation of body build, posture, gait	Good posture and balance Steady gait	Poor posture or balance Unsteady, irregular, or staggering gait
	Determination of weight and height	Weight within ideal range	Patient is overweight or underweight
	Observation of hygiene and grooming	Good hygiene and grooming	Poor hygiene and grooming
	Observation for signs of illness	No signs of illness	Obvious signs of illness
	Observation of attitude, emotional state, mood	Patient speaks clearly and is cooperative	Patient is uncooperative, withdrawn, incoherent, negative, or hostile
Skin	Inspection of skin for color, vascularity, lesions	Smooth, supple, free of blemishes	Blisters, wounds, lesions, rashes, swelling
		No unusual color	Unusual skin color (e.g., flushing, cyanosis, jaundice, pallor)
	Palpation of temperature, moisture, turgor, texture	Warm to touch	Rough, dry, flaky skin Poor skin turgor
Head and neck	Inspection of size, shape, contour of head	Round head with prominences in front and back	Head is asymmetric or of unusual size
	Inspection of hair and scalp	Hair is resilient, evenly distributed, and not excessively dry or oily	Loss of hair Scaliness or dryness of scalp Presence of lice or other parasites
	Palpation of head and neck	No lumps, swelling, tenderness, or lesions of head or neck	Lumps, swelling, tenderness, or lesions of head or neck
Eyes	Evaluation of visual acuity and color vision	Good visual ability with or without glasses or contact lenses	Poor visual acuity or blindness
		Appropriate color perception	Color blindness
	Evaluation of visual field	No visual field loss	Gaps in field of vision
	Inspection of eyelids and eyeballs	Eyes are bright	Dull or glossy eyes
	Inspection of conjunctiva	Pink mucous membranes	Inflamed mucous membranes Excessive tearing Drainage from eyes
	Inspection of eye movements	Eyes move equally in all directions	Drooping eyelids Uncoordinated eye movements
	Tests for pupillary reaction using penlight	Pupils are black, equal in size, react appropriately to light	Dilated, constricted, or unequal pupils
	Inspection of internal eye structures using ophthalmoscope	Reddish-pink retina, even caliber, intact retinal blood vessels	Cloudy lens or narrowed blood vessels
Ears	Test for hearing using tuning fork or audiometer	Good hearing ability	Limited hearing or deafness
	Inspection of size, shape, symmetry of ears	Ears are symmetric and proportionate to head	Ears are asymmetric and not proportionate to the head
	Inspection of external ear canal and tympanic membrane using an otoscope	Cerumen is soft and easily removed	Lesions, redness, or swelling of external ear canal
		No drainage or discomfort Skin of ear canal is intact, pink, warm, and slightly moist	Drainage from ear Pain when ear is moved Impacted cerumen
		Tympanic membrane is pearly gray and semitransparent	Tympanic membrane is red, bulging, or perforated
Nose	Inspection of size, shape, symmetry of nose	Nose is symmetric, straight, not tender	Nose is asymmetric, deformed, flaring, or tender
	Inspection of nostrils using nasal speculum	Septum is intact and midline	Deviation or perforation of septum
		Nasal mucosa is moist and pink	Redness, swelling, polyps, or discharge Nostrils are obstructed
	Test for sense of smell	Correct or very few incorrect responses to odors	Absent, decreased, exaggerated, or unequal responses to test substances

TABLE 5.3 Physician Assessment During the Physical Examination—cont'd

Body Structure	Assessment	Normal Findings	Abnormal Findings
Mouth and pharynx	Inspection of lips for contour, color, texture	Pink, moist, soft, smooth lips	Pallor, cyanosis, blisters, swelling, cracking, excessive dryness of lips
	Inspection of mucosa	Pink, moist mucous membranes	Pale or dry mucosa with ulcers or abrasions
	Inspection of gums and palate	Smooth, pink, moist, firm gums Hard palate is firm and white Soft palate is pink and cushiony	Gums are red, bleeding, swollen, tender, spongy, or receding
	Inspection of teeth	Smooth, white enamel; regularly spaced teeth or well-fitting dentures	Missing or loose teeth, dental caries, poor-fitting dentures
	Inspection of tongue	Moist, pink, slightly rough-surfaced tongue	Tongue is dry, furry, smooth, red, or ulcerated
	Inspection of pharynx	Pink and smooth pharynx	Pharynx is red, swollen, or ulcerated
		Tonsils are pink and normal in size	Tonsils are red or swollen
		Gag reflex is present	Absent gag reflex
Arms and hands	Inspection of hands and arms for general appearance	Firm, strong muscles	Muscle weakness, lack of control or coordination
		Normal range of motion in joints	Restricted range of motion
	Palpation of arm muscles	Good muscle control and coordination	
	Palpation for tenderness or lumps	No tenderness or lumps	Tenderness or lumps in hands or arms
	Inspection of fingernails	Colorless nail plate with a convex curve Smooth nail texture	Indentation, infection, brittleness, thickening, or angulation of nails Cyanosis or pallor of nails
Chest and lungs	Inspection of size and shape of chest	Chest is symmetric	Abnormal chest contour
	Assessment of respiratory rate, rhythm, depth	Normal respiratory rate, rhythm, depth	Labored, slow, rapid, or irregular respirations
	Percussion of chest		
	Auscultation of breath sounds	Normal breath sounds	Flat or dull lung sounds Noisy breath sounds
		No cough	Productive or nonproductive cough
	Palpation of ribs	No tenderness of ribs	Tenderness of ribs
Heart	Auscultation of heart sounds	Normal heart sounds	Irregular heartbeats or murmur
	Auscultation of apical pulse, rate, rhythm, volume	Regular, strong heartbeats	Rates slower or more rapid than normal
	Palpation of peripheral pulses	Palpable peripheral pulses	Weak or absent peripheral pulses
	Auscultation of blood pressure	Blood pressure within normal range for age	Low or high blood pressure
	Assessment of peripheral vascular perfusion	Skin is pink, resilient, moist	Cyanosis, pallor, edema
		Immediate return of color to nail beds	Poor capillary filling in nail beds
	Electrocardiogram to assess heart function	Normal heart function	Abnormal electrocardiogram
Breasts	Inspection of size, symmetry, contour	Breasts are round, smooth, symmetric	Retraction, dimpling, redness, or swelling of breasts
	Inspection of nipple	Nipples are round and equal in size, similar in color, appear soft and smooth Areola is round and pink	Bleeding, cracking, discharge, or inversion of nipples
	Palpation of breasts and axillary lymph nodes	No lumps in or tenderness of breasts or axillary lymph nodes	Lumps in or tenderness of breasts or axillary lymph nodes
Abdomen	Inspection of contour, symmetry, skin condition, integrity	Symmetric contour	Asymmetric contour
		Unblemished skin	Rash or other skin lesions
		Soft abdomen	Abdominal distention
	Auscultation of bowel sounds	Active bowel sounds	Increased, diminished, or absent bowel sounds
	Percussion to assess underlying organs Palpation of underlying organs, tenderness, lumps	Normal position and size of liver and spleen	Tenderness or lumps Enlarged liver or spleen

Continued

TABLE 5.3 Physician Assessment During the Physical Examination—cont'd

Body Structure	Assessment	Normal Findings	Abnormal Findings
Genitalia and rectum	Male		
	Inspection of penis and urethra	Penis is smooth	Ulceration or discharge from penis
	Inspection of scrotum and palpation of testes	Testicles are smooth, firm, and movable within scrotal sac Scrotum is symmetric	Lumps or tenderness of scrotum, testes, or prostate gland
	Palpation of rectum and prostate gland	Increased pigmentation in anal area Good anal sphincter tone	Enlarged prostate gland Hemorrhoids or relaxed anal sphincter
	Stool specimen to test for occult blood	Absence of occult blood in stool	Occult blood in stool
	Female		
	Inspection of external genitalia	External genitalia are smooth and without lesions	Ulceration or redness or swelling of external genitalia
	Inspection of vagina and cervix using vaginal speculum	Vaginal mucosa is pink and moist Cervix is pink and smooth	Lacerations, tenderness, redness, or discharge from vagina or cervix
	Specimen collection from vagina and cervix for Pap test	Pap test is normal	Pap test is abnormal
	Bimanual pelvic examination	No tenderness or lumps in uterus and ovaries	Tenderness in or lumps of uterus and ovaries
	Palpation of rectum	Good anal sphincter tone	Hemorrhoids or relaxed anal sphincter
	Stool specimen to test for occult blood	Increased pigmentation in anal area	Occult blood in stool
Legs and feet	Inspection of legs for general appearance and palpation of legs	Firm, strong muscles	Muscle weakness, lack of control or coordination
		Normal range of motion in joints	Restricted range of motion Tenderness or lumps Limp or foot dragging during walking
	Inspection of toenails	Smooth nail texture	Indentation, infection, brittleness, thickening, or angulation of nails
Neurologic	Determination of mental status and level of consciousness	Alert and responds appropriately	Responds inappropriately
		Oriented to person, place, and time	Disoriented
	Determination of sense of pain and touch	Normal responses to pain and touch	Diminished or absent response to stimuli
	Use of percussion hammer to test reflexes	Normal reflexes	Abnormal or absent reflexes

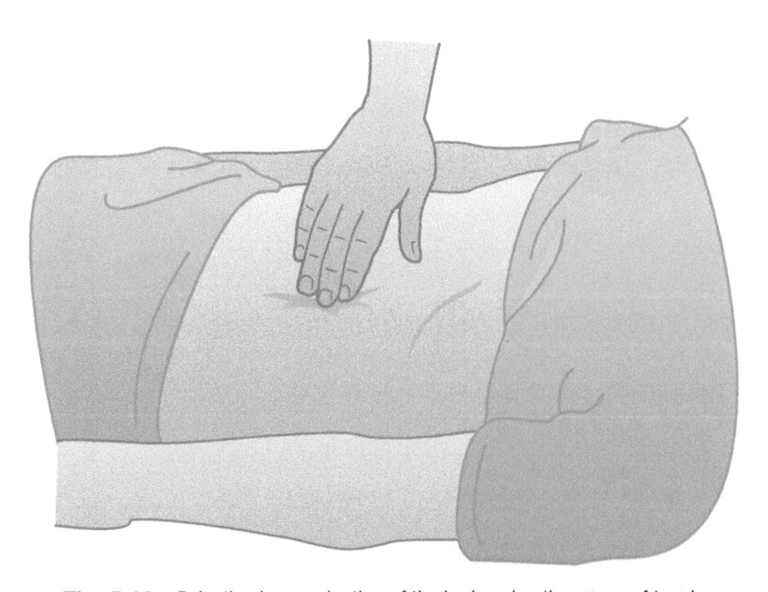

Fig. 5.12 Palpation is examination of the body using the sense of touch.

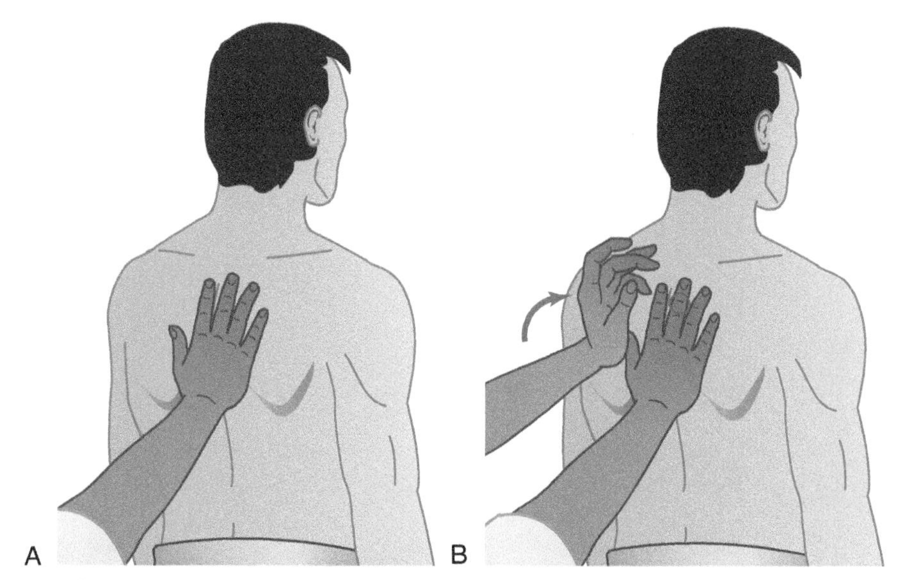

Fig. 5.13 Percussion involves tapping the patient with the fingers. (A) The nondominant hand is placed directly on the area to be assessed, with the fingers slightly separated. (B) The fingers of the dominant hand are used to strike the joint of the middle finger to produce a sound vibration.

PERCUSSION

Percussion involves tapping the patient with the fingers and listening to the sounds produced to determine the size, density, and locations of organs. This technique is often used to examine the lungs and abdomen.

The fingertips are used to produce a sound vibration similar to that of tapping a drumstick on a drum. The nondominant hand is placed directly on the area to be assessed, with the fingers slightly separated. The dominant hand is used to strike the joint of the middle finger placed on the patient to produce the sound vibration (Fig. 5.13). Structures that are dense, such as the liver, spleen, and heart, produce a dull sound. Empty or air-filled structures, such as the lungs, produce a hollow sound. Any condition that changes the density of an organ or tissue, such as fluid in the lungs, would change the quality of the sound.

AUSCULTATION

Auscultation is an examination technique that involves listening with a stethoscope to the sounds produced within the body. This technique is used to listen to the heart and lungs or to measure blood pressure (manual method). Environmental noise interferes with effective auscultation of body sounds and should be minimized. The diaphragm of the stethoscope chest piece is used to assess high-pitched sounds, such as lung and bowel sounds; the bell of the stethoscope chest piece is used to assess low-pitched sounds, such as those produced by the heart and vascular system. The chest piece should be cleaned with an antiseptic wipe and warmed with the hands before being placed on the patient.

What Would You Do? What Would You *Not* Do?

Case Study 3

Ben-Yi Sun has brought his father, Chang-Yi Sun, to the medical office. Chang-Yi Sun is 76 years old and lives with Ben-Yi and his family. Because there is a large Asian population in the community, the medical office personnel have learned two things about the Asian culture: (1) They are brought up to respect elders, and elders are always considered first, and (2) Asians have a great respect for harmony. If they do not understand something, they may not admit it to avoid disrupting harmony. Ben-Yi Sun speaks very good English, but his father understands only a few words of English. Chang-Yi Sun has been diagnosed with hypertension, and he needs education about going on a low-sodium diet. He also needs instructions on taking his blood pressure at home and documenting the results. ■

ASSISTING THE PROVIDER

During the patient assessment, the medical assistant should assist the provider as required. This includes helping the patient to change positions for the provider's examination of different parts of the body, handing the provider instruments and supplies, and reassuring the patient to reduce apprehension. When the examination is completed, the medical assistant should assist the patient off the examining table and provide additional information if needed, such as scheduling a return visit or patient education to promote wellness. Procedure 5.11 describes the procedure for assisting with the physical examination.

What Would You Do? What Would You *Not* Do? RESPONSES

Case Study 1
Page 148

What Did Abby Do?
- ❑ Empathized with Abbey and told her that a lot of patients feel just like she does about having their weight taken. Explained that the information in her medical record is strictly confidential.
- ❑ Told Abbey that weight is important so that the physician can properly diagnose and treat her condition and that medication dosage is often based on a person's weight.
- ❑ Told Abbey that she could stand on the scale backward while her weight is being measured so that she would not see the reading on the scale.
- ❑ Returned the weights to zero before Abbey got off the scale.
- ❑ Documented Abbey's weight in her medical record without telling her the results.
- ❑ Encouraged Abbey to see the physician when she needs to so that she stays as healthy as possible.

What Did Abby Not Do?
- ❑ Did not make any comments about Abbey's body or weight after weighing her.
- ❑ Did not criticize Abbey for letting her weight stand in the way of coming in when she needed health care.

Case Study 2
Page 149

What Did Abby Do?
- ❑ Listened carefully to Mikayla and showed concern verbally and nonverbally.
- ❑ Carefully documented the information relayed by Mikayla so that the physician would be aware of all aspects of Mikayla's problem.
- ❑ Told Mikayla that she needs to talk to the physician about wanting some medicine for heartburn.
- ❑ Encouraged Mikayla to talk to her parents about what's been going on with her.

What Did Abby Not Do?
- ❑ Did not agree with Mikayla that she needs to lose more weight.
- ❑ Did not make comments about Mikayla being too thin.

Case Study 3
Page 161

What Did Abby Do?
- ❑ Greeted Chang-Yi first before greeting his son.
- ❑ Spoke clearly and slowly to Ben-Yi in a normal tone of voice.
- ❑ Gave them a brochure on low-sodium diets and went over the foods that are low in sodium.
- ❑ Asked Chang-Yi (via Ben-Yi's translating) to indicate the foods he likes that he thinks would be low in sodium. Determined whether these foods are low in sodium.
- ❑ Showed Ben-Yi how to take his father's blood pressure.
- ❑ Had Ben-Yi practice taking his father's blood pressure.
- ❑ Made sure that Chang-Yi and Ben-Yi understood all of the information before they left the office.

What Did Abby Not Do?
- ❑ Be careful not to ignore Chang-Yi. ■

TERMINOLOGY REVIEW

Key Term	Word Parts	Definition
Audiometer	*audi/o:* hearing *-meter:* instrument used to measure	An instrument used to measure hearing.
Auscultation		The process of listening to the sounds produced within the body to detect signs of disease.
Bariatrics	*bar/o:* weight *-iatrics:* a branch of medicine	The branch of medicine that deals with the treatment and control of obesity and diseases associated with obesity.
Body mechanics		Use of the correct muscles to maintain proper balance, posture, and body alignment to accomplish a task safely and efficiently without undue strain on any muscle or joint.
Clinical diagnosis		A tentative diagnosis of a patient's condition obtained through evaluation of the health history and the physical examination, without the benefit of laboratory or diagnostic tests.
Diagnosis	*dia-:* through, complete *-gnosis:* knowledge	The scientific method of determining and identifying a patient's condition.

TERMINOLOGY REVIEW—cont'd

Key Term	Word Parts	Definition
Differential diagnosis		A determination of which of two or more diseases with similar symptoms is producing a patient's symptoms.
Inspection		The process of observing a patient to detect signs of disease.
Mensuration		The process of measuring a patient.
Palpation		The process of feeling with the hands to detect signs of disease.
Percussion		The process of tapping the body to detect signs of disease.
Prognosis	*pro-:* before *-gnosis:* knowledge	The probable course and outcome of a patient's condition and the patient's prospects for recovery.
Symptom		Any change in the body or its functioning that indicates a disease might be present.

PROCEDURE 5.1 Measuring Weight and Height

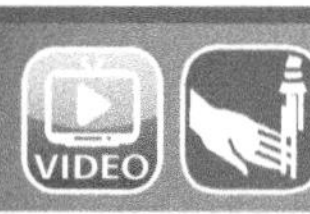

Outcome Measure weight and height.

Equipment/Supplies

- Upright balance scale
- Paper towel

Weight

1. **Procedural Step.** Sanitize your hands.
2. **Procedural Step.** Check the scale to ensure it is balanced as follows:
   a. Make sure the upper and lower weights are on zero. When the weights are on zero, they are all the way to the left of the calibration bars.

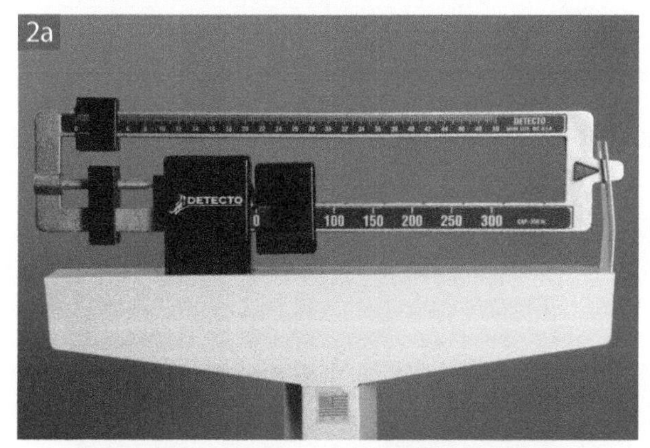

Ensure that the upper and lower weights are on zero.

   b. Look at the indicator point. If the scale is balanced, the indicator point is resting in the center of the balance area.
   c. If the indicator point rests below the center, adjust the screw on the balance knob by turning it clockwise (to the right) until the indicator point rests in the center of the balance area.

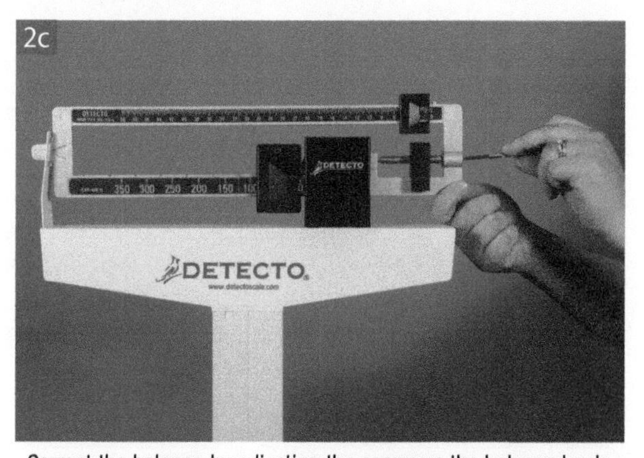

Correct the balance by adjusting the screw on the balance knob.

   d. If the indicator point rests above the center, adjust the screw on the balance knob by turning it counterclockwise (to the left) until the indicator point rests in the center of the balance area.

   Principle. If the scale is not balanced, the weight measurement will be inaccurate.
3. **Procedural Step.** Greet the patient, and introduce yourself.
4. **Procedural Step.** Identify the patient, and explain to the patient that you will be measuring his or her height and weight.

Continued

5. **Procedural Step.** Instruct the patient to remove shoes and outer clothing such as a jacket or sweater. A good medical aseptic practice is to place a paper towel on the platform of the scale to protect the patient's feet.
   Principle. Removing heavy clothing and shoes allows a more accurate measurement of the patient's weight.
6. **Procedural Step.** Assist the patient onto the scale, and instruct the patient not to move.
   Principle. It is not possible to balance the scale if the patient is moving.
7. **Procedural Step.** Balance the scale as follows:
   a. Move the lower weight to the notched groove that does not cause the indicator point to drop to the bottom of the balance area. Ensure that the lower weight is seated firmly in its groove.
   b. Slide the upper weight slowly along its calibration bar by tapping it gently until the indicator point comes to rest at the center of the balance area.
   Principle. Not seating the lower weight firmly in its groove results in an inaccurate reading.

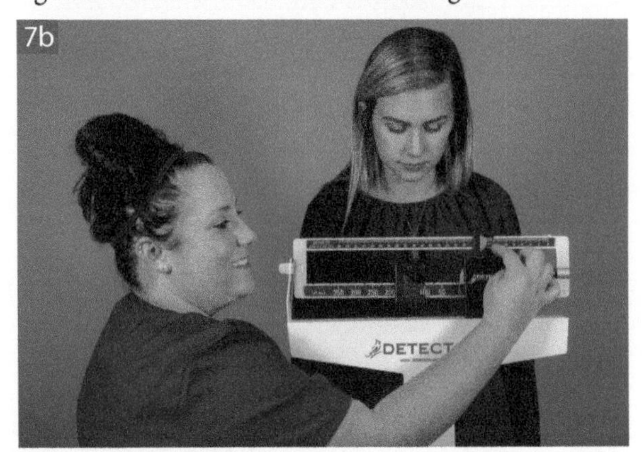

Slide the upper weight by tapping it gently.

8. **Procedural Step.** Read the results to the nearest quarter pound by adding the measurement on the lower scale to the measurement on the upper scale. Jot down this value, or make a mental note of it.
9. **Procedural Step.** Ask the patient to step off of the scale platform. Provide assistance if needed.

Height

1. **Procedural Step.** Slide the movable calibration rod upward until the measuring bar is well above the patient's apparent height. Open the measuring bar to its horizontal position.

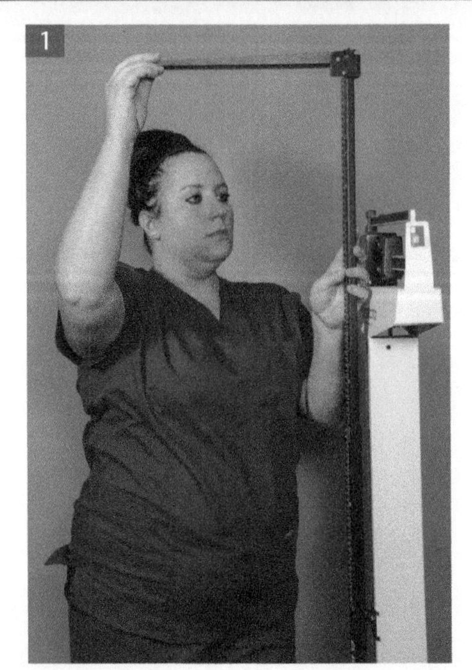

Slide the bar upward until it is well above the patient's height.

2. **Procedural Step.** Instruct the patient to step onto the scale platform with his or her back to the scale. Provide assistance if needed. Instruct the patient to stand erect and to look straight ahead.
   Principle. Looking straight ahead helps the patient to stand erect and balanced, which ensures an accurate measurement.
3. **Procedural Step.** Carefully lower the measuring bar (keeping it horizontal) until it rests gently on top of the patient's head with the hair compressed. The measuring bar should form a 90-degree angle with the calibration rod.
   Principle. The measuring bar must be at a 90-degree angle to ensure an accurate height measurement.

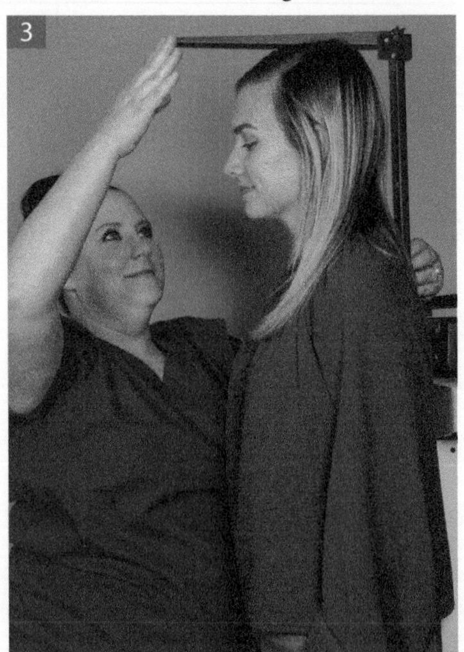

Lower the bar until it rests on top of the patient's head.

PROCEDURE 5.1 Measuring Weight and Height—cont'd

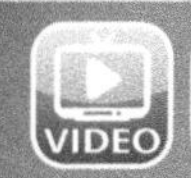

4. **Procedural Step.** Keeping the measuring bar in a horizontal position, instruct the patient to step down and put on his or her shoes. Hold the bar in a horizontal position until the patient has stepped off the scale.
5. **Procedural Step.** Read the height measurement from the top down to the nearest quarter-inch marking at the junction of the stationary calibration rod and the movable calibration rod. (*Note:* If the patient's height is less than the top value of the stationary rod, read the measurement from the bottom up directly on the stationary calibration rod.) Jot down this value, or make a mental note of it.

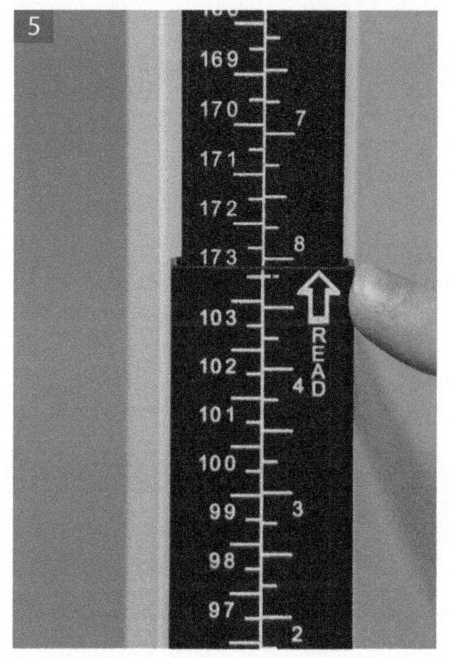

Read the measurement to the nearest quarter-inch marking.

6. **Procedural Step.** Return the measuring bar to its vertical (resting) position, and slide the movable calibration rod to its lowest position. Return the weights to zero.
7. **Procedural Step.** Sanitize your hands.
8. **Procedural Step.** Document the results in the patient's medical record.
   a. *Electronic health record:* In SimChart for the Medical Office, document the patient's weight and height measurements. You will be using textboxes, drop-down menus, and/or radio buttons to enter this information. (*Note:* The EHR automatically calculates and documents the patient's BMI from the weight and height measurements that are entered into the computer).
   b. *Paper-based medical record:* Document the date and time and the patient's weight and height measurements. The weight should be documented in pounds to the nearest quarter pound, and the height should be documented in feet and inches to the nearest quarter inch. If required by the medical office policy, determine the patient's BMI and document this number following the weight and height measurements (refer to the PPR documentation example).

PPR Documentation Example

Date	
11/5/XX	10:15 a.m. Wt: 126 1/2 lbs. Ht: 5' 8" BMI: 19.2
	——————————A. Erdy, CMA (AAMA)

Procedure 5.2

PROCEDURE 5.2 Sitting Position

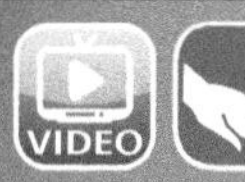

Outcome Position and drape a patient in the sitting position. The sitting position is used to examine the head, neck, chest, and upper extremities and to measure vital signs.

Equipment/Supplies

- Examining table
- Disposable patient gown
- Disposable patient drape

1. **Procedural Step.** Sanitize your hands. Greet the patient, and introduce yourself.
2. **Procedural Step.** Identify the patient, and explain the type of examination or procedure that will be performed.
3. **Procedural Step.** Provide the patient with a patient gown. Instruct the patient to remove clothing as appropriate for the type of examination being performed and to put on the patient gown with the opening in front.
4. **Procedural Step.** Pull out the footrest of the examining table, and assist the patient into a sitting position. The patient's buttocks and thighs should be firmly supported on the edge of the table.

Continued

PROCEDURE 5.2 Sitting Position—cont'd

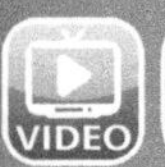

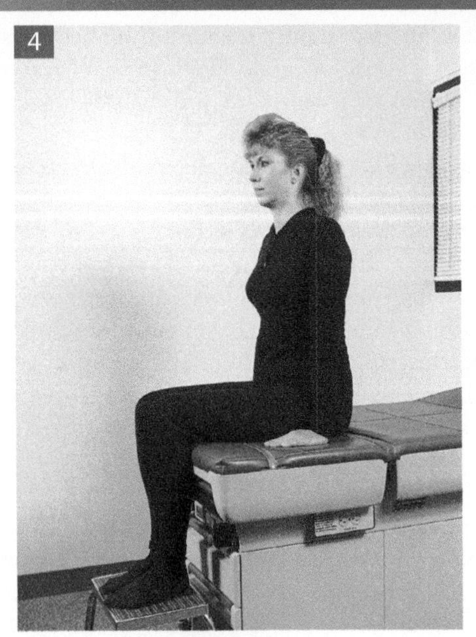

Sitting position.

5. Procedural Step. Place a drape over the patient's thighs and legs to provide warmth and modesty.

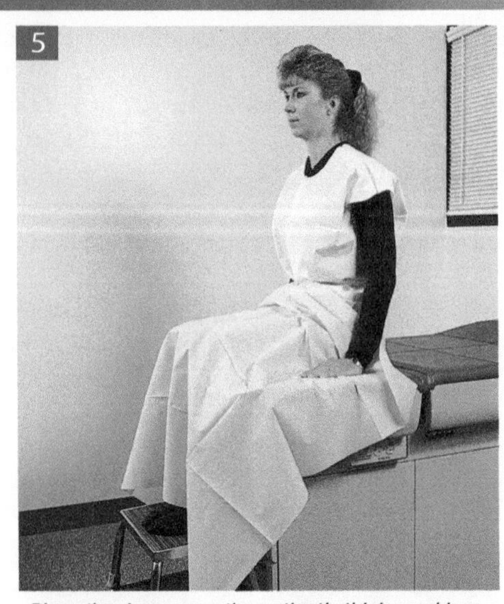

Place the drape over the patient's thighs and legs.

6. Procedural Step. After completion of the examination, assist the patient down from the table. Return the footrest to its normal position. Instruct the patient to get dressed. Discard the gown and drape in a waste container.

PROCEDURE 5.3 Supine Position

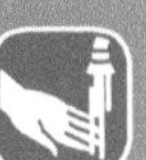

Outcome Position and drape a patient in the supine position. The supine position is used to examine the head, chest, abdomen, and extremities.

Equipment/Supplies

- Examining table
- Disposable patient gown
- Disposable patient drape

1. **Procedural Step.** Sanitize your hands. Greet the patient, and introduce yourself.
2. **Procedural Step.** Identify the patient, and explain the type of examination or procedure that will be performed.
3. **Procedural Step.** Provide the patient with a patient gown. Instruct the patient to remove clothing as appropriate for the type of examination being performed and to put on the patient gown with the opening in front.
4. **Procedural Step.** Pull out the footrest of the examining table, and assist the patient into a sitting position. Place a drape over the patient's thighs and legs.
5. **Procedural Step.** Ask the patient to move back on the table. As the patient is doing this, pull out the table extension while supporting the patient's lower legs.

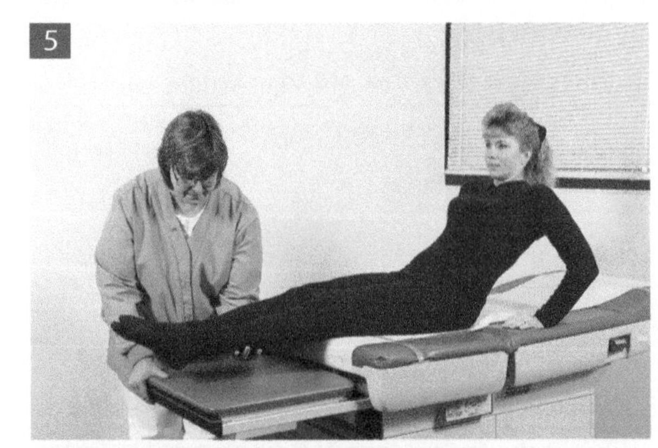

Pull out the table extension while supporting the patient's legs.

6. **Procedural Step.** Ask the patient to lie on his or her back with the legs together. Provide assistance if needed.

PROCEDURE 5.3 Supine Position—cont'd

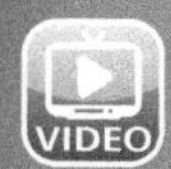

The patient's arms may be placed above the head or alongside the body.

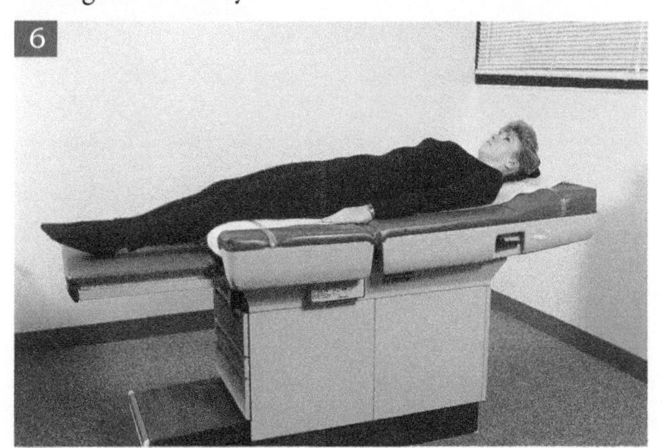

6 Position the patient on the back with the legs together.

7. **Procedural Step.** Position the drape lengthwise over the patient to provide warmth and modesty. As the provider examines the patient, move the drape according to the body parts being examined.

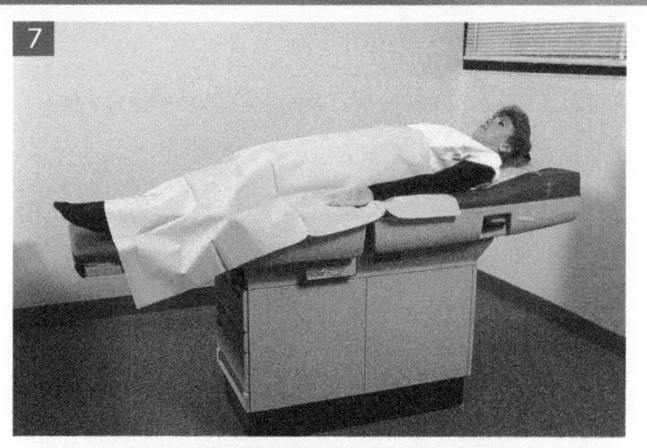

7 Place a drape lengthwise over the patient.

8. **Procedural Step.** After completion of the examination, assist the patient into a sitting position. Slide the table extension back into place while supporting the patient's lower legs.
9. **Procedural Step.** Assist the patient down from the table. Instruct the patient to get dressed. Return the footrest to its normal position. Discard the gown and drape in a waste container.

PROCEDURE 5.4 Prone Position

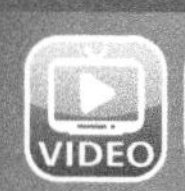

Outcome Position and drape a patient in the prone position. The prone position is used to examine the back and to assess extension of the hip joint.

Equipment/Supplies

- Examining table
- Disposable patient gown
- Disposable patient drape

1. **Procedural Step.** Sanitize your hands. Greet the patient, and introduce yourself.
2. **Procedural Step.** Identify the patient, and explain the type of examination or procedure that will be performed.
3. **Procedural Step.** Provide the patient with a patient gown. Instruct the patient to remove clothing as appropriate for the type of examination being performed and to put on the patient gown with the opening in back.
4. **Procedural Step.** Pull out the footrest of the examining table, and assist the patient into a sitting position. Place a drape over the patient's thighs and legs.
5. **Procedural Step.** Ask the patient to move back on the table. As the patient is doing this, pull out the table extension while supporting the patient's lower legs.
6. **Procedural Step.** Ask the patient to lie on his or her back. Provide assistance if needed. Position the drape lengthwise over the patient.
7. **Procedural Step.** Ask the patient to turn onto his or her stomach by rolling toward you. Provide assistance for this step by helping him or her turn and adjusting the drape to provide modesty.
Principle. This step prevents the patient from accidentally rolling off the table.

Continued

PROCEDURE 5.4 Prone Position—cont'd

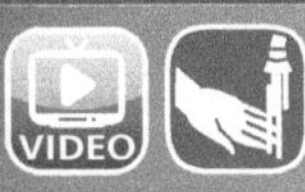

8. **Procedural Step.** Position the patient with the legs together and the head turned to one side. The arms can be placed above the head or alongside the body.

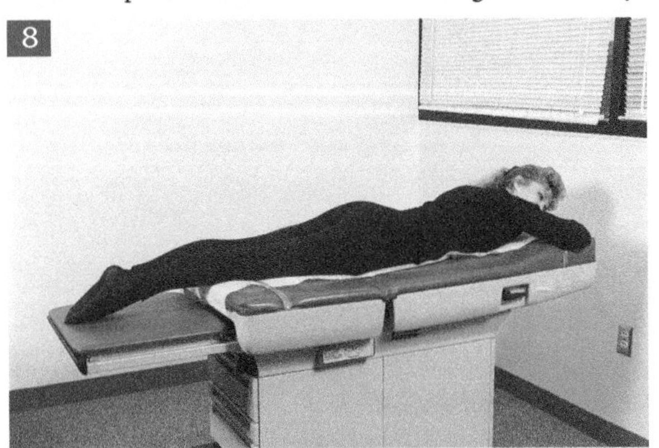
Position the patient's legs together with the head turned to one side.

9. **Procedural Step.** Adjust the drape as needed so that it is positioned lengthwise over the patient to provide warmth and modesty. As the provider examines the patient, move the drape according to the body parts being examined.

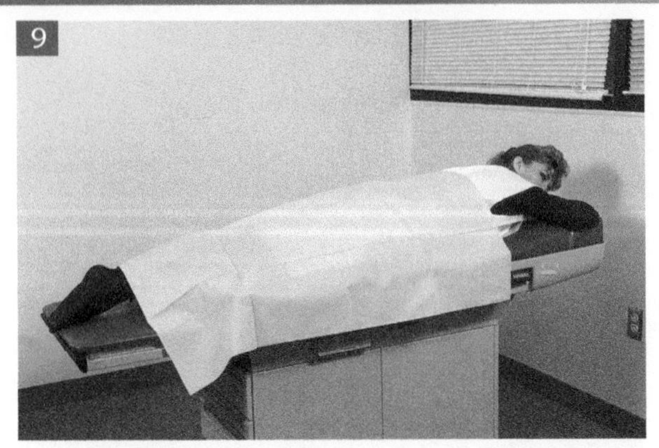
Place a drape lengthwise over the patient.

10. **Procedural Step.** After completion of the examination, ask the patient to turn back over by rolling toward you. Assist the patient into a supine position and then into a sitting position. Slide the table extension back into place while supporting the patient's lower legs.
11. **Procedural Step.** Assist the patient down from the table. Return the footrest to its normal position. Instruct the patient to get dressed. Discard the gown and drape in a waste container.

PROCEDURE 5.5 Dorsal Recumbent Position

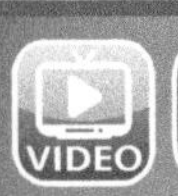

Outcome Position and drape a patient in the dorsal recumbent position. The dorsal recumbent position is used to perform vaginal and rectal examinations; to insert a urinary catheter; and to examine the head, neck, chest, and extremities of patients who have difficulty maintaining the supine position. The supine position is an uncomfortable position for patients with respiratory problems, back injury, or lower back pain. Bending the legs (rather than lying flat) is more comfortable for these patients and is easier to maintain.

Equipment/Supplies

- Examining table
- Disposable patient gown
- Disposable patient drape

1. **Procedural Step.** Sanitize your hands. Greet the patient, and introduce yourself.
2. **Procedural Step.** Identify the patient, and explain the type of examination or procedure that will be performed.
3. **Procedural Step.** Provide the patient with a patient gown. Instruct the patient to remove clothing as appropriate for the type of examination being performed and to put on the patient gown with the opening in front.
4. **Procedural Step.** Pull out the footrest of the examining table, and assist the patient into a sitting position. Place a drape over the patient's thighs and legs.
5. **Procedural Step.** Ask the patient to move back on the table. As the patient is doing this, pull out the table extension while supporting the patient's lower legs.
6. **Procedural Step.** Ask the patient to lie on his or her back. Provide assistance if needed. The arms can be placed above the head or alongside the body. Position the drape diagonally over the patient.

PROCEDURE 5.5 Dorsal Recumbent Position—cont'd

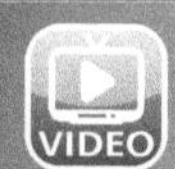

7. Procedural Step. Ask the patient to bend the knees and place each foot at the edge of the examining table with the soles of the feet flat on the table. Provide assistance during this step. Push in the table extension and the footrest.

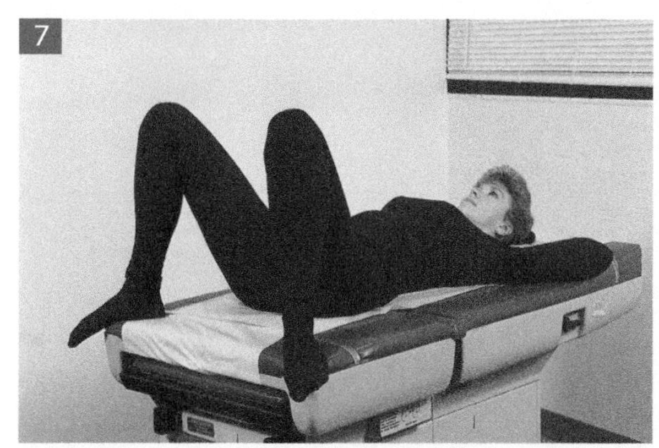

Ask the patient to bend the knees and place each foot at the edge of the examining table.

8. Procedural Step. Adjust the drape as needed to provide the patient with warmth and modesty. The drape should be positioned diagonally, with one corner over the patient's chest; the opposite corner falls between the patient's legs and completely covers the pubic area.

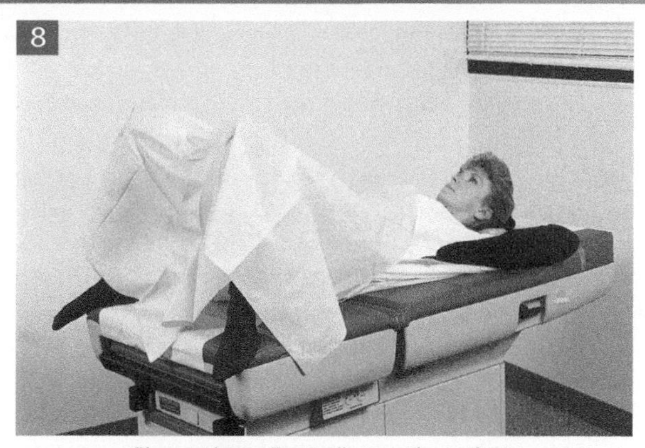

Place a drape diagonally over the patient.

9. **Procedural Step.** When the provider is ready to examine the genital area, the center corner of the drape is folded back over the abdomen.
10. **Procedural Step.** After completion of the examination, pull out the footrest and the table extension. Assist the patient into a supine position and then into a sitting position. Slide the table extension back into place while supporting the patient's lower legs.
11. **Procedural Step.** Assist the patient down from the table. Return the footrest to its normal position. Instruct the patient to get dressed. Discard the gown and drape in a waste container.

PROCEDURE 5.6 Lithotomy Position

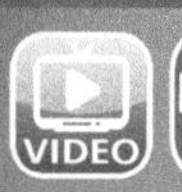
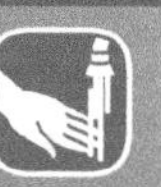

Outcome Position and drape a patient in the lithotomy position. The lithotomy position is used for vaginal, pelvic, and rectal examinations. The lithotomy position is the same as the dorsal recumbent position except that the patient's feet are placed in stirrups. The lithotomy position provides maximal exposure to the genital area and facilitates insertion of a vaginal speculum. Because this is an uncomfortable position for the patient to maintain, the patient should not be put into this position until just before the examination.

Equipment/Supplies

- Examining table
- Disposable patient gown
- Disposable patient drape

1. **Procedural Step.** Sanitize your hands. Greet the patient, and introduce yourself.
2. **Procedural Step.** Identify the patient, and explain the type of examination or procedure that will be performed.
3. **Procedural Step.** Provide the patient with a patient gown. Instruct the patient to remove clothing as appropriate for the type of examination being performed and to put on the patient gown with the opening in front. If the patient is wearing socks, tell her that she may keep them on during the procedure. ***Principle.*** Socks help to keep the patient's feet warm after they are placed in the metal stirrups.
4. **Procedural Step.** Some medical offices use disposable stirrup covers. If this is the case, apply a cover to each stirrup. Pull out the footrest of the examining table, and assist the patient into a sitting position. Place a drape over the patient's thighs and legs.

Continued

PROCEDURE 5.6 Lithotomy Position—cont'd

Principle. Stirrup covers provide a soft, warm, nonslip surface for the patient's feet.

5. **Procedural Step.** When the provider is ready to examine the patient, ask the patient to move back on the table. As the patient is doing this, pull out the table extension while supporting the patient's lower legs.
6. **Procedural Step.** Ask the patient to lie on the back. Provide assistance if needed. The arms can be placed above the head or alongside the body.
7. **Procedural Step.** Position the drape over the patient to provide warmth and modesty. The drape should be positioned diagonally with one corner over the patient's chest and the opposite corner between the patient's feet.
8. **Procedural Step.** Pull out the stirrups, and position them at an angle. Position the stirrups so that they are level with the examining table and pulled out approximately 1 foot from the edge of the table. Check to make sure the stirrups are not too far apart or too close together. Lock the stirrups into place.
   Principle. If the stirrups are too far apart, it is uncomfortable for the patient. If the stirrups are too close together, the patient will be unable to move her buttocks to the edge of the table as needed for the examination.
9. **Procedural Step.** Ask the patient to bend the knees and place each foot, one at a time, into a stirrup. Provide assistance during this step. Push in the table extension and the footrest.
10. **Procedural Step.** Instruct the patient to slide the buttocks all the way down to the edge of the examining table and to let her legs fall apart as far as is comfortable.

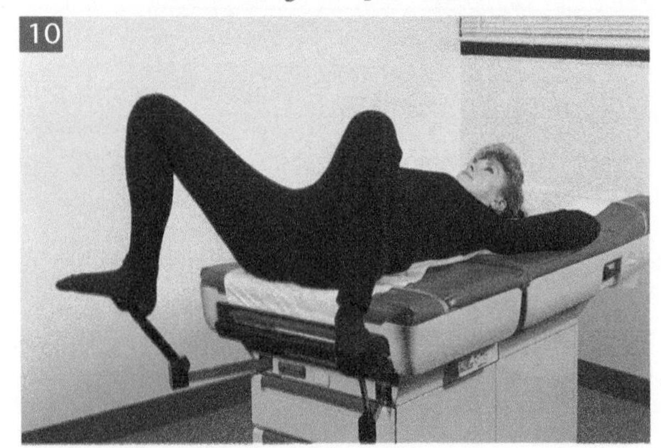

Ask the patient to slide the buttocks to the edge of the table and to rotate the thighs outward.

11. **Procedural Step.** Reposition the drape as needed so that one corner is over the patient's chest and the opposite corner falls between the patient's legs and completely covers the perineal area. When the provider is ready to examine the genital area, the center corner of the drape is pulled up and folded back over the knees.

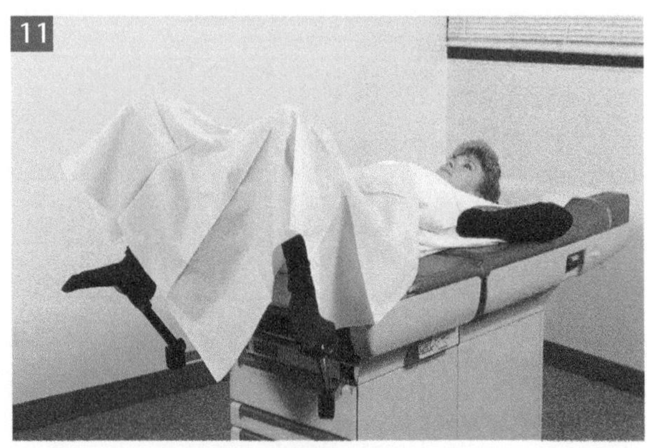

Position the drape diagonally.

12. **Procedural Step.** After completion of the examination, pull out the footrest and table extension. Ask the patient to slide the buttocks back from the end of the table. Lift the patient's legs out of the stirrups at the same time, and place them on the table extension (supine position). Remove the stirrup covers, and discard them in a waste container. Return the stirrups to their normal position. Assist the patient into a sitting position. Slide the table extension back into place while supporting the patient's lower legs.
    Principle. Lifting both the patient's legs out of the stirrups at the same time avoids strain on the back and abdominal muscles.
13. **Procedural Step.** Assist the patient down from the table. Return the footrest to its normal position. Instruct the patient to get dressed. Discard the gown and drape in a waste container.

PROCEDURE 5.7 Modified Left Lateral Recumbent Position

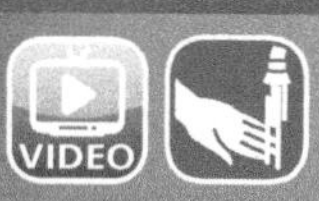

Outcome Position and drape a patient in the modified left lateral recumbent position. The modified left lateral recumbent position, (also known as Sims position) is used to examine the vagina and rectum, to measure rectal temperature, to perform a flexible sigmoidoscopy, and to administer an enema.

Equipment/Supplies

- Examining table
- Disposable patient gown
- Disposable patient drape

1. **Procedural Step.** Sanitize your hands. Greet the patient, and introduce yourself.
2. **Procedural Step.** Identify the patient, and explain the type of examination or procedure that will be performed.
3. **Procedural Step.** Provide the patient with a patient gown. Instruct the patient to remove clothing from the waist down and to put on the patient gown with the opening in back.
4. **Procedural Step.** Pull out the footrest of the examining table, and assist the patient into a sitting position. Place a drape over the patient's thighs and legs.
5. **Procedural Step.** Ask the patient to move back on the table. As the patient is doing this, pull out the table extension while supporting the patient's lower legs.
6. **Procedural Step.** Ask the patient to lie on his or her back. Provide assistance if needed.
7. **Procedural Step.** Position the drape lengthwise over the patient to provide warmth and modesty.
8. **Procedural Step.** Ask the patient to turn onto the left side. Provide assistance during this step to prevent the patient from accidentally rolling off the table and to adjust the drape to provide modesty. The patient's left arm should be positioned behind the body and the right arm forward with the elbow bent. Assist the patient in flexing the legs. The right leg is flexed sharply, and the left leg is flexed slightly.

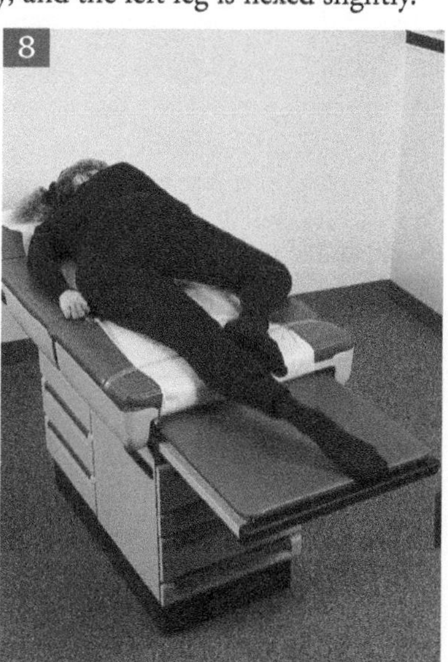

The right leg is flexed sharply, and the left leg is flexed slightly.

9. **Procedural Step.** Adjust the drape as needed. When the provider is ready to examine the patient, a small portion of the drape is folded back to expose the anal area.

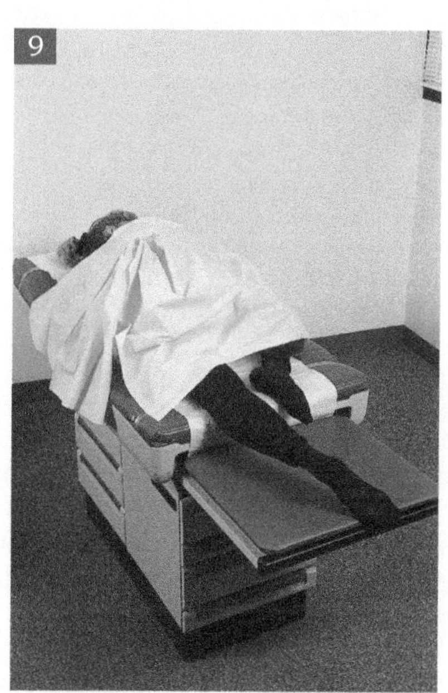

Adjust the drape as needed.

10. **Procedural Step.** After completion of the examination, assist the patient into a supine position and into a sitting position. Slide the table extension back into place while supporting the patient's lower legs.
11. **Procedural Step.** Assist the patient down from the table. Return the footrest to its normal position. Instruct the patient to get dressed. Discard the gown and drape in a waste container.

PROCEDURE 5.8 Knee-Chest Position

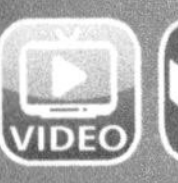

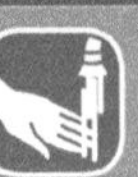

Outcome Position and drape a patient in the knee-chest position. The knee-chest position is used to examine the rectum and to perform a proctoscopic examination because it provides maximal exposure to the rectal area. This is a difficult position to maintain; the patient should not be put into this position until just before the examination.

Equipment/Supplies

- Examining table
- Disposable patient gown
- Disposable patient drape
- Pillow

1. **Procedural Step.** Sanitize your hands. Greet the patient, and introduce yourself.
2. **Procedural Step.** Identify the patient, and explain the type of examination or procedure that will be performed.
3. **Procedural Step.** Provide the patient with a patient gown. Instruct the patient to remove clothing from the waist down and to put on the gown with the opening in back.
4. **Procedural Step.** Pull out the footrest of the examining table, and assist the patient into a sitting position. Place a drape over the patient's thighs and legs.
5. **Procedural Step.** Ask the patient to move back on the table. As the patient is doing this, pull out the table extension while supporting the patient's lower legs.
6. **Procedural Step.** Assist the patient into the supine position and then into the prone position, making sure to have the patient roll toward you. Position the drape diagonally over the patient to provide warmth and modesty.
7. **Procedural Step.** Ask the patient to bend the arms at the elbows and rest them alongside the head. Ask the patient to elevate the buttocks while keeping the back straight. The patient's head should be turned to one side, and the weight of the body should be supported by the chest. A pillow under the chest can give additional support and aid in relaxation. The knees and lower legs are separated approximately 12 inches.

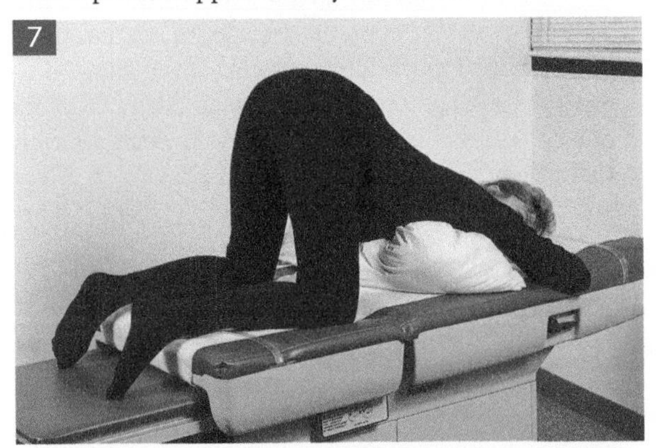

The buttocks are elevated, and the head is turned to one side.

8. **Procedural Step.** Adjust the drape diagonally as needed with one corner over the patient's back and the opposite corner over the buttocks and falling between the patient's legs. When the provider is ready to examine the patient, a small portion of the drape is folded back to expose the anal area.

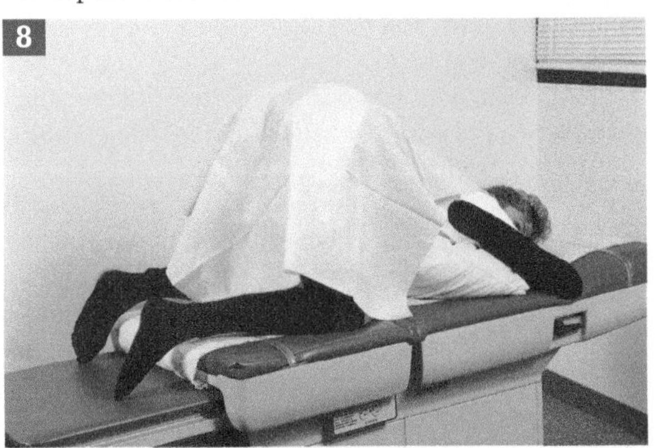

Position the drape diagonally.

9. **Procedural Step.** After completion of the examination, assist the patient into a prone position and then into a supine position. Allow the patient to rest in the supine position before he or she sits up.
   Principle. Patients (especially elderly ones) frequently become dizzy after being in the knee-chest position and should be allowed to rest before they sit up.
10. **Procedural Step.** Assist the patient into a sitting position. Slide the table extension back into place while supporting the patient's lower legs.
11. **Procedural Step.** Assist the patient down from the table. Return the footrest to its normal position. Instruct the patient to get dressed. Discard the gown and drape in a waste container.

PROCEDURE 5.9 Fowler Position

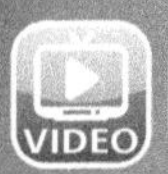

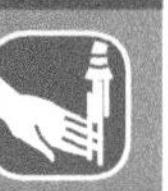

Outcome Position and drape a patient in the Fowler position. The Fowler position is used to examine the upper body of patients with cardiovascular and respiratory problems, such as congestive heart failure, emphysema, and asthma. These patients find it easier to breathe in this position than in a sitting or supine position. This position also is used to draw blood from patients who are likely to faint.

Equipment/Supplies

- Examining table
- Disposable patient gown
- Disposable patient drape

1. **Procedural Step.** Sanitize your hands. Greet the patient, and introduce yourself.
2. **Procedural Step.** Identify the patient, and explain the type of examination or procedure that will be performed.
3. **Procedural Step.** Provide the patient with a patient gown. Instruct the patient to remove clothing as appropriate for the type of examination being performed and to put on the patient gown with the opening in front.
4. **Procedural Step.** Position the head of the table as follows:
   a. For the semi-Fowler position, the table should be positioned at a 45-degree angle.
   b. For the full Fowler position, the table should be positioned at a 90-degree angle.
5. **Procedural Step.** Pull out the footrest of the examining table, and assist the patient into a sitting position. Place a drape over the patient's thighs and legs.
6. **Procedural Step.** Pull out the table extension while supporting the patient's lower legs. Ask the patient to lean back against the table head. Provide assistance during this step.

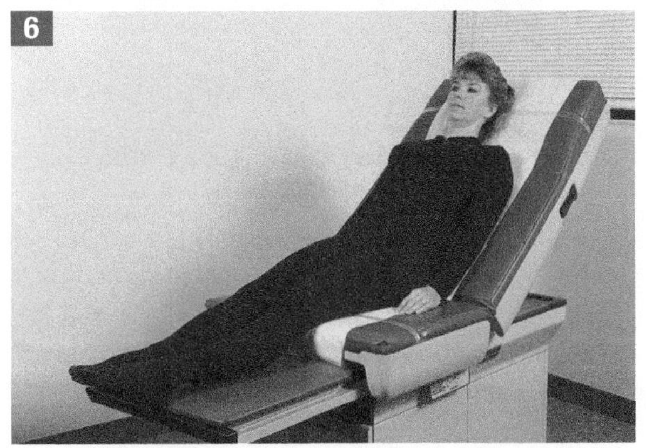

Ask the patient to lean back against the table head.

7. **Procedural Step.** Position the drape lengthwise over the patient to provide warmth and modesty. As the provider examines the patient, move the drape according to the body parts being examined.

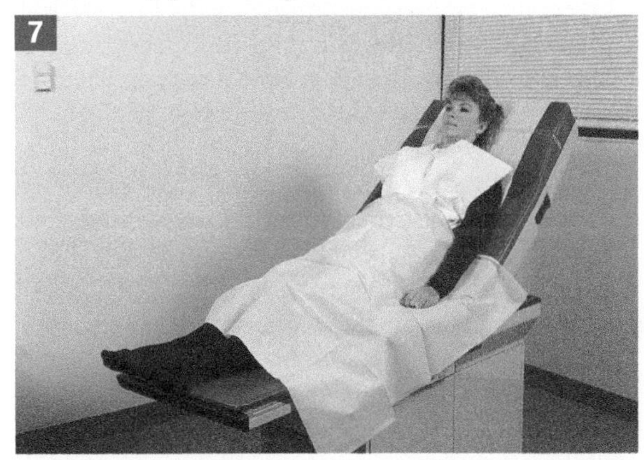

Position the table at a 45-degree angle for the semi-Fowler position.

8. **Procedural Step.** After completion of the examination, assist the patient into a sitting position. Slide the table extension back into place while supporting the patient's lower legs.
9. **Procedural Step.** Assist the patient down from the table. Instruct the patient to get dressed. Return the head of the table and the footrest to their normal positions. Discard the gown and drape in a waste container.

PROCEDURE 5.10 Wheelchair Transfer

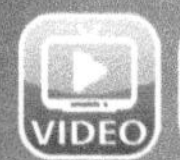

Outcome Transfer a patient from a wheelchair to the examining table and from an examining table to a wheelchair.

Equipment/Supplies

- Examining table
- Transfer belt

Transferring the Patient to the Examining Table

1. **Procedural Step.** Sanitize your hands.
2. **Procedural Step.** Greet the patient, and introduce yourself. Identify the patient, and explain the procedure.
3. **Procedural Step.** Evaluate the patient to determine his or her mental and physical capabilities to perform the transfer. Determine how heavy the patient is and if he or she is able to assist in the transfer. Assess whether or not you are able to perform the transfer safely. Do not perform the transfer if you think you may incur a musculoskeletal injury.
4. **Procedural Step.** Wrap the transfer belt snugly around the patient's waist over the patient's clothing with the buckle in front. Securely fasten the belt by threading it through the teeth of the buckle. Put the belt through the other two openings to lock it. The belt should be snug with just enough space between the belt and the patient's clothing to allow your fingers to be inserted comfortably between the belt and the patient's waist.
   Principle. Placing the transfer belt over the patient's clothing prevents abrasions to the patient's skin. The belt must be snug to prevent it from sliding upward on the patient's body.
5. **Procedural Step.** With the patient's stronger side next to the examining table, position the wheelchair at a 45-degree angle to the end of the examining table.

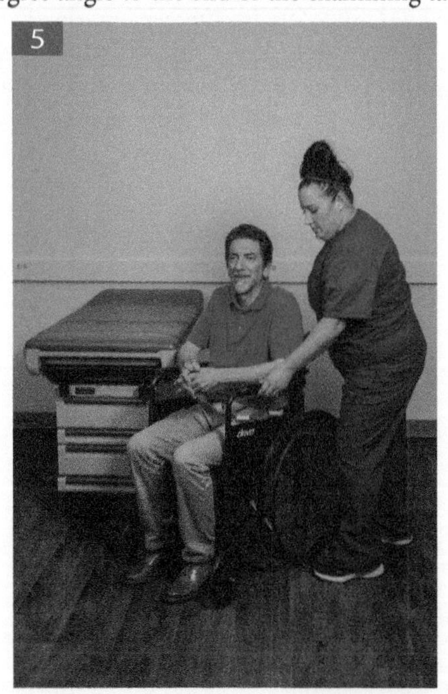

Position the wheelchair at a 45-degree angle.

6. **Procedural Step.** If the examining table is height adjustable, lower it to the same height as the wheelchair or slightly lower. If it is not height adjustable, pull out the footrest of the examining table.
7. **Procedural Step.** Lock the brakes of the wheelchair and fold back the wheelchair footrests.
   Principle. The wheels must be locked to prevent the chair from moving during the transfer. The wheelchair footrests must be out of the way to provide an unobstructed path for making the transfer.

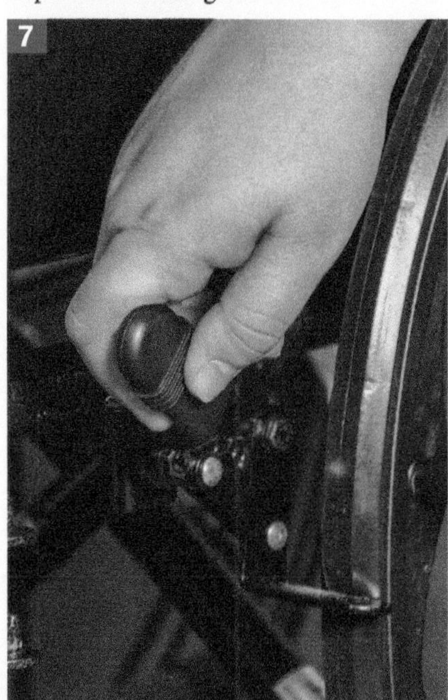

Lock the brakes.

8. **Procedural Step.** Inform the patient of what he or she will be required to do during the transfer. During the transfer, clearly state in a step-by-step manner what the patient should do. Encourage the patient to help as much as possible during the transfer by using the muscles of his or her arms and legs.
9. **Procedural Step.** Make sure the patient's feet are positioned flat on the floor.
   Principle. Making sure the patient's feet are flat on the floor provides the patient with balance and stability when he or she stands.
10. **Procedural Step.** Stand in front of the patient, with the feet apart approximately 6 to 8 inches, the toes pointed outward, one foot slightly forward, and the knees bent.
    Principle. This position conserves energy and provides a wide base of support for the transfer.

PROCEDURE 5.10 Wheelchair Transfer—cont'd

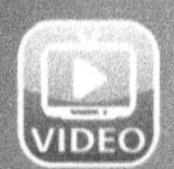

11. **Procedural Step.** Ask the patient to place his or her hands on the armrests of the wheelchair and to lean forward.

12. **Procedural Step.** Grasp the transfer belt on either side of the patient's waist using an underhand grasp.
Principle. The transfer belt provides a secure handle for holding onto the patient and controlling the patient's movement.

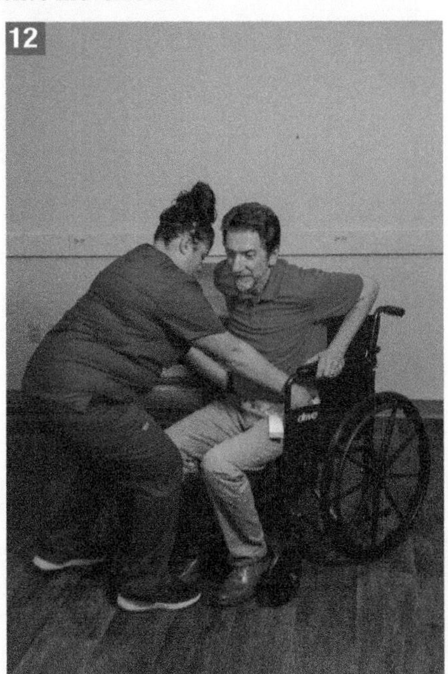

Grasp the transfer belt on either side of the patient's waist.

13. **Procedural Step.** Tighten your abdominal gluteal muscles in preparation for the transfer. Ask the patient to push off the armrests and into a standing position on the count of 3. At the same time, straighten your knees and assist the patient to a standing position by pulling upward on the transfer belt, making sure to keep your back straight.
Principle. The patient pushing upward with his or her arm and leg muscles provides an additional lifting force and reduces the chance of straining your back muscles. Lifting the patient using your knees and the transfer belt allows the strong muscles of the legs and arms to do the lifting, rather than the back muscles.

14. **Procedural Step.** Pivot the patient toward the examining table. Position the patient's buttocks and backs of the knees toward the examining table. Instruct the patient to step onto the footrest (backward) one foot at a time.
Principle. Pivoting prevents twisting of the spine, which can result in a serious back injury.

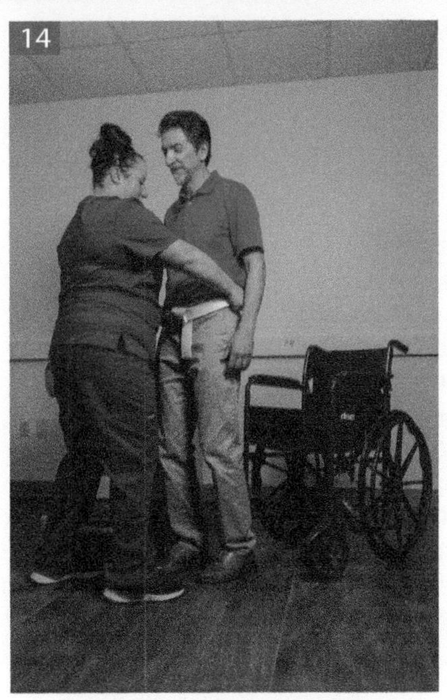

Position the patient toward the table.

15. **Procedural Step.** Gradually lower the patient into a sitting position on the examining table. Make sure the patient's buttocks and thighs are firmly supported on the table. Remove the transfer belt.

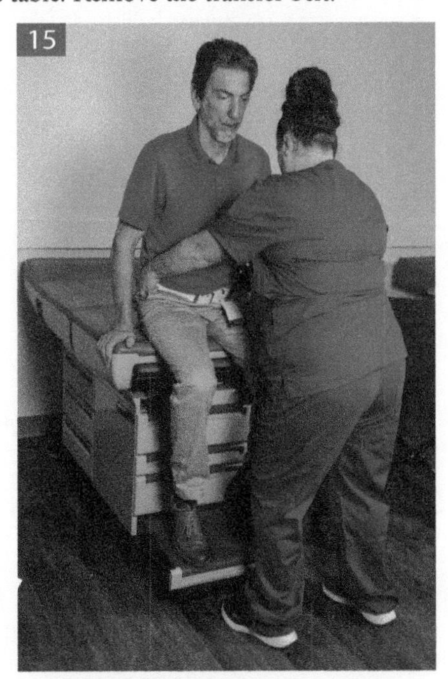

Gradually lower the patient onto the table.

16. **Procedural Step.** Unlock the wheelchair, and move it out of the way of the examining table. Push in the footrest of the examining table.

Continued

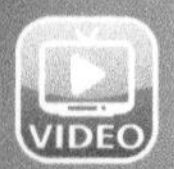

17. **Procedural Step.** Stay with the patient to prevent falls.

Transferring the Patient to the Wheelchair

1. **Procedural Step.** Wrap the transfer belt snugly around the patient's waist, and securely fasten it.
2. **Procedural Step.** Position the wheelchair at a 45-degree angle to the end of the examining table.
3. **Procedural Step.** If the examining table is height adjustable, lower it to the same height as the wheelchair or slightly lower. If it is not height adjustable, pull out the footrest of the examining table.
4. **Procedural Step.** Lock the wheelchair into place, and fold back the footrests.
5. **Procedural Step.** Inform the patient of what he or she will be required to do during the transfer.
6. **Procedural Step.** Stand in front of the patient, with the feet apart approximately 6–8 inches, the toes pointed outward, one foot slightly forward, and the knees bent.
7. **Procedural Step.** Ask the patient to place his or her arms on your shoulders. To prevent a neck injury, do not allow the patient to place his or her arms around your neck.

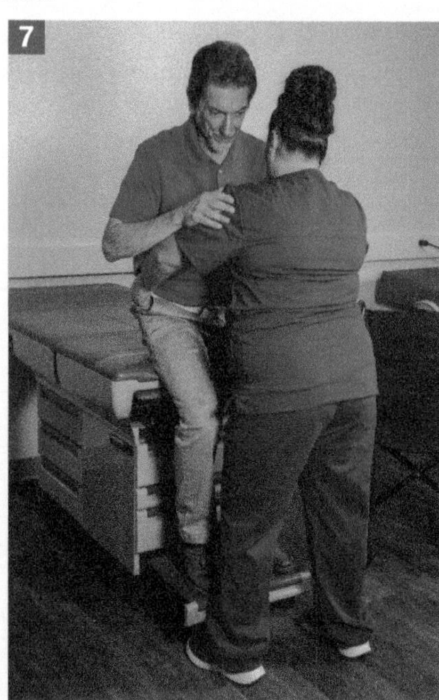

Ask the patient to put his or her arms on your shoulders.

8. **Procedural Step.** Grasp the transfer belt on either side of the patient's waist using an underhand grasp.
9. **Procedural Step.** Ask the patient to push to a standing position using his or her thigh and leg muscles on the count of 3. At the same time, straighten your knees and assist the patient to a standing position by pulling upward on the transfer belt.

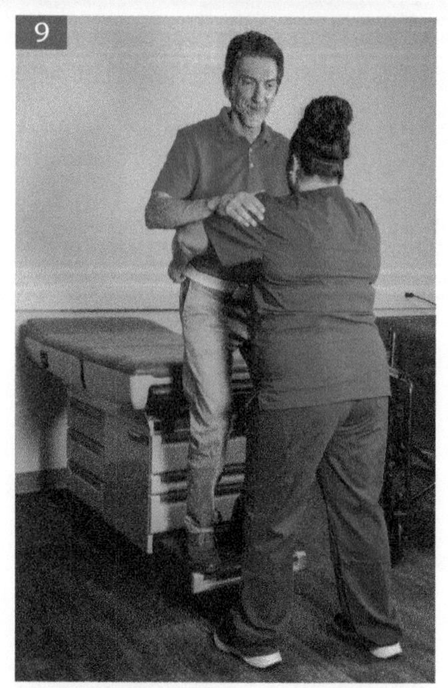

Assist the patient to a standing position.

10. **Procedural Step.** Instruct the patient to step down from the footrest, one foot at a time.
11. **Procedural Step.** Pivot the patient toward the wheelchair. Position the backs of the patient's legs against the seat of the wheelchair.
12. **Procedural Step.** Asked the patient to grasp the arm rests of the wheelchair. Bend at your knees, and gradually lower the patient into a sitting position in the wheelchair with the patient's buttocks at the back of the chair. Remove the transfer belt, and make sure the patient is comfortable.

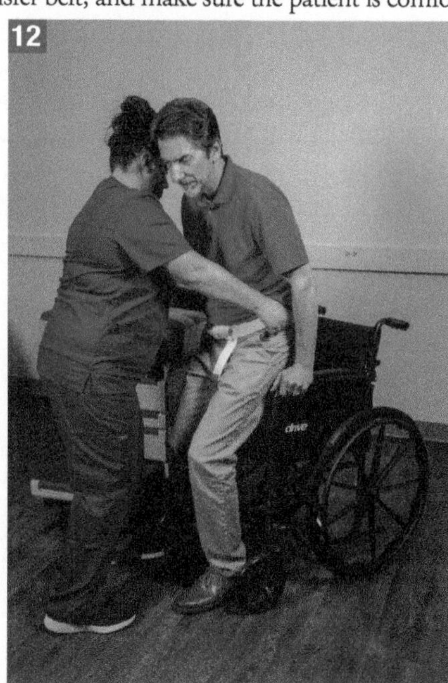

Gradually lower the patient into the wheelchair.

13. **Procedural Step.** Reposition the wheelchair footrests, and place the patient's feet in the footrests. Unlock the wheelchair.
14. **Procedural Step.** Push in the footrest of the examining table.

PROCEDURE 5.11 Assisting With the Physical Examination

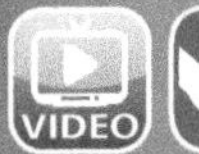

Outcome Prepare the patient, and assist with a physical examination.

Equipment/Supplies

- Examining table
- Equipment for the type of examination to be performed

1. **Procedural Step.** Prepare the examining room. Ensure that the room is clean, free of clutter, and well lit and that the room temperature is comfortable for the patient.
2. **Procedural Step.** Sanitize your hands.
3. **Procedural Step.** Assemble the equipment according to the type of examination to be performed and the provider's preference. Arrange the instruments and supplies in a neat and orderly manner on a table or tray. Do not allow one item to be placed on top of another.

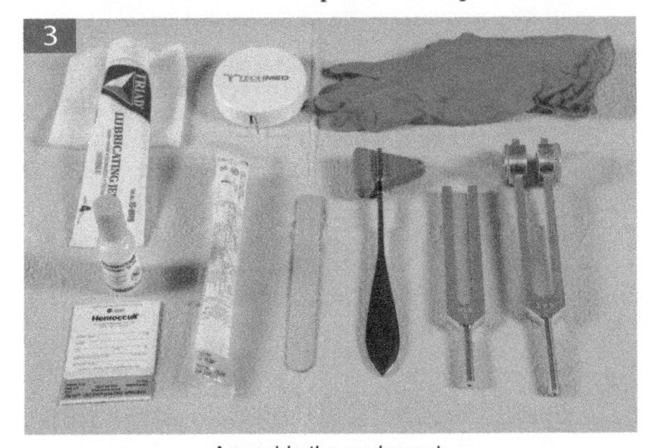

Assemble the equipment.

4. **Procedural Step.** Obtain the patient's medical record. (If an electronic health record [EHR] is being used, access the computer record for the appropriate patient.) Go to the waiting room, and ask the patient to come back to the examining room.
5. **Procedural Step.** Escort the patient to the examining room.
6. **Procedural Step.** Ask the patient to be seated. Greet the patient, and introduce yourself using a calm and friendly manner. Identify the patient by his or her full name and date of birth.
   Principle. Identifying the patient correctly avoids mistaking one patient for another. Using a calm and friendly manner helps to put the patient at ease.

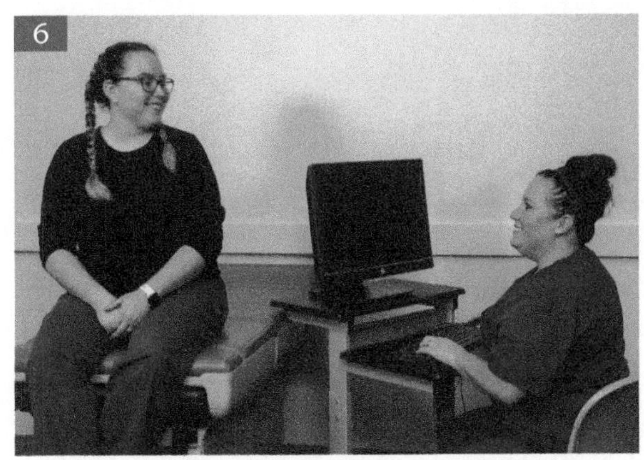

Greet and identify the patient by name and date of birth.

7. **Procedural Step.** Seat yourself so that you face the patient at a distance of 3–4 feet.
8. **Procedural Step.** Obtain essential information from the patient on allergies, current medications, and symptoms and document this information in the patient's medical record.
9. **Procedural Step.** Measure the patient's vital signs, and document the results.
10. **Procedural Step.** Measure the weight and height of the patient, and document the results. If required by the medical office policy, determine the patient's body mass index (BMI) and document this number following the weight and height measurements. (*Note:* The EHR automatically calculates and documents the patient's BMI from the weight and height measurements that are entered into the computer.)
11. **Procedural Step.** Instruct and prepare the patient for the examination as follows:
    a. Ask the patient whether he or she needs to empty the bladder before the examination. If a urine specimen is needed, the patient will be required to void into a urine container.
    b. Provide the patient with a patient gown. Instruct the patient to remove all clothing and to put on the patient gown. Offer assistance if you sense the patient may have trouble undressing.
    c. Tell the patient to have a seat on the examining table after putting on the patient gown. Leave the room to provide the patient with privacy.

Continued

PROCEDURE 5.11 Assisting With the Physical Examination—cont'd

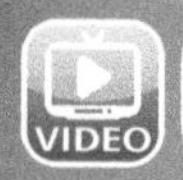

Principle. An empty bladder makes the examination easier and is more comfortable for the patient.

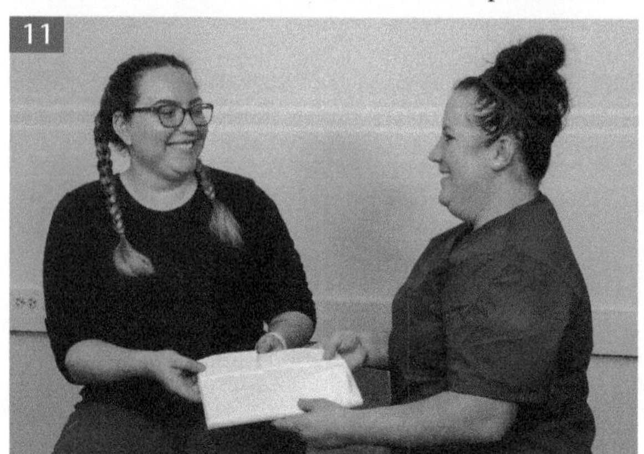

11 Instruct and prepare the patient for the examination.

12. **Procedural Step.** Make the medical record available to the provider. The medical office has a designated location where the record is placed, such as on a small shelf mounted on the wall next to the outside of the examining room door or in a chart holder on the outside of the examining room door. Position the medical record so that patient-identifiable information is not visible. If your office uses an EHR, you do not need to perform this step. With an EHR, the provider accesses the patient's record on the computer.
13. **Procedural Step.** Check to make sure that the patient is ready to be seen by the provider. Before entering a patient's room, knock lightly on the door to let the patient know that you are getting ready to enter the room. If a patient is ready to be seen, inform the provider. This may be done using a color-coded flagging system mounted on the wall next to the examining room.

    Principle. The Health Insurance Portability and Accountability Act (HIPAA) requires protection of a patient's health information.
14. **Procedural Step.** Assist the provider with examination of the body systems as follows:
    a. Ensure that the patient is positioned correctly in a sitting position on the examining table. This allows the provider to examine the patient's head, eyes, ears, nose, mouth and pharynx, neck, chest, lungs, and heart.
    b. Hand the provider the ophthalmoscope, otoscope, and tongue depressor.
    c. Dim the light when the provider is ready to use the ophthalmoscope. The dim light helps dilate the patient's pupils, providing the provider better visualization of the interior of the eye.
    d. After use, the tongue depressor should be transferred by holding it at the center to prevent contact with the patient's secretions, which may contain pathogens. Dispose of the tongue depressor in a regular waste container.

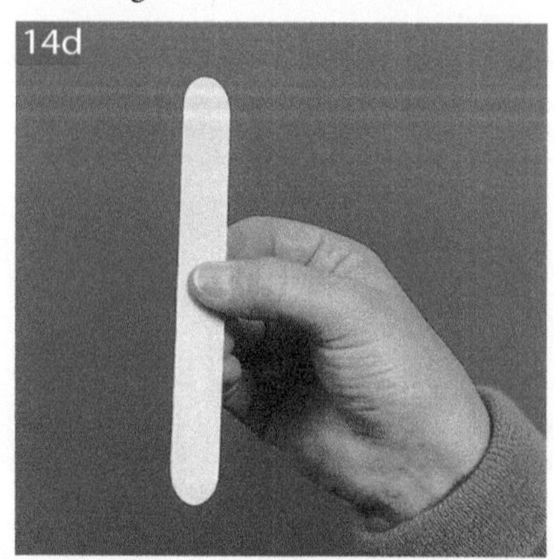

14d Transfer the tongue depressor by holding it at the center.

    e. Offer reassurance to the patient to reduce apprehension.
15. **Procedural Step.** Position the patient as required for examination of the remaining body systems. Place and drape the patient in the proper position for examination of a particular part of the body using proper body mechanics.
16. **Procedural Step.** Assist and instruct the patient as follows:
    a. Allow the patient to rest in a sitting position on the examining table before he or she gets off of it. Some patients become dizzy after being positioned on the examining table.
    b. Assist the patient off the examining table to prevent falls.
    c. Instruct the patient to get dressed. Provide assistance if needed.
    d. Provide the patient with any necessary instructions, such as patient education and scheduling a return visit. Give instructions involving medical care in terms the patient can understand; do not use medical terms.
    e. Sanitize the hands, and document in his or her medical record any instructions given to the patient.
    f. Escort the patient to the reception area.
17. **Procedural Step.** Clean the examining room in preparation for the next patient as follows:
    a. Discard the paper on the examining table. Then, apply gloves, and clean and disinfect the table. Unroll a fresh length of paper on the table.
    b. Discard all disposable supplies into an appropriate waste container.
    c. Ensure that there are ample numbers of clean gowns and drapes and other supplies.

PROCEDURE 5.11 Assisting With the Physical Examination—cont'd

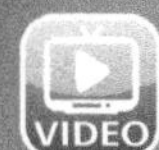

d. Remove reusable equipment to a work area for sanitization, sterilization, or disinfection as required by the medical office policy.

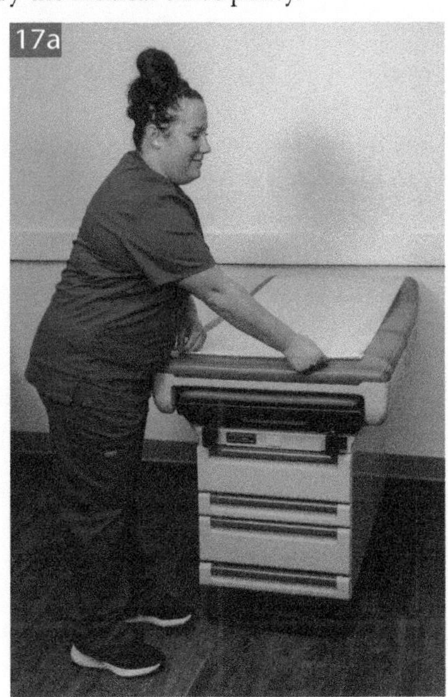

Unroll a fresh length of paper.

PPR Documentation Example

Date	
11/20/XX	11:30 a.m. CC. Shortness of breath x 2 days.
	T: 98.8° F (TA) P: 78 reg and strong, R: 20
	even and reg, BP: 110/68, Wt: 158, Ht: 5' 6"
	BMI: 25.5 ——— A. Erdy, CMA (AAMA)

Eye and Ear Assessment and Procedures

 Check out the Evolve site at http://evolve.elsevier.com/Bonewit/today/ to access additional interactive activities and exercises to help you study and prepare for success.

LEARNING OUTCOMES

The Eye

1. List and describe the structures that make up the eye.
2. Define visual acuity.
3. State the cause and visual difficulty of each of the following:
   - Myopia
   - Hyperopia
   - Astigmatism
   - Presbyopia
4. Explain the differences between an ophthalmologist, an optometrist, and an optician.
5. Explain the significance of the top and bottom numbers next to each line of letters on the Snellen eye chart.
6. Explain the difference between congenital and acquired color vision defects.
7. List the reasons to perform an eye irrigation and an eye instillation.

The Ear

8. List and describe the structures that make up the ear.
9. Identify conditions that may cause conductive and sensorineural hearing loss.
10. List and describe the ways in which hearing acuity can be tested.
11. List the reasons to perform an ear irrigation and an ear instillation.

PROCEDURES

Assess distance visual acuity.
Assess near visual acuity.
Assess color vision.
Perform an eye irrigation.
Perform an eye instillation.

Perform an ear irrigation.
Perform an ear instillation.

CHAPTER OUTLINE

INTRODUCTION TO THE EYE
Structure of the Eye
VISUAL ACUITY
Eye Specialists
Assessment of Distance Visual Acuity
- Conducting a Snellen Test
- Assessing Distance Visual Acuity in Preschool Children

Assessment of Near Visual Acuity
ASSESSMENT OF COLOR VISION
Ishihara Test
EYE IRRIGATION
EYE INSTILLATION
INTRODUCTION TO THE EAR
Structure of the Ear
ASSESSMENT OF HEARING ACUITY
Types of Hearing Loss
Hearing Acuity Tests
- Tuning Fork Tests
- Audiometry
- Tympanometry

EAR IRRIGATION
EAR INSTILLATION

KEY TERMS

astigmatism (uh-STIG-muh-tiz-em)
audiometer (aw-dee-OM-eh-ter)
canthus (KAN-thus)
cerumen
hyperopia (HYE-per-OP-ee-uh)
impacted cerumen
instillation (IN-still-AY-shun)
irrigation (EAR-ih-GAY-shun)
myopia (mye-OH-pee-uh)
otoscope (AH-toe-skope)
presbyopia (PRESS-bee-OH-pee-uh)
refraction (ree-FRAK-shun)
tympanic membrane (tim-PAN-ik MEM-brane)
visual acuity

Introduction to the Eye

The medical assistant is responsible for performing a variety of assessments and procedures that involve the eye. A visual acuity test is usually part of the routine physical examination. This test is a screening test to detect deficiencies in vision. The medical assistant may also be responsible for assessing color vision with the use of specially prepared colored plates. As a result of this testing, color blindness can be detected. Color blindness is an inability to distinguish certain colors; the most common problem is with the colors red and green. Color blindness is particularly significant if the patient is involved in an activity that relies on the ability to distinguish colors, such as electronics or interior decorating.

The medical assistant is responsible for performing or teaching the patient to perform eye irrigations and instillations. **Irrigation** is washing a body canal with a flowing solution. **Instillation** is dropping a liquid into a body cavity. Eye irrigations and instillations should be performed using the important principles of medical asepsis outlined in Chapter 2.

STRUCTURE OF THE EYE

The eye has three layers (Fig. 6.1). The outer layer is the *sclera,* which is composed of tough, white fibrous connective tissue. The front part of the sclera is modified to form a transparent covering over the colored part of the eye; this covering is the *cornea.*

The middle layer of the eye is the *choroid,* which is composed of many blood vessels and is highly pigmented. The blood vessels nourish the other layers of the eye, and the pigment works to absorb stray light rays. The front part of the choroid is specialized into the ciliary body, the suspensory ligaments, and the iris. The *ciliary body* contains muscles that control the shape of the lens. The function of the *suspensory ligaments* is to suspend the lens in place. The *lens* is responsible for focusing the light rays on the retina. The colored part of the eye is the *iris,* which controls the size of the pupil. The *pupil* is the opening in the eye that permits the entrance of light rays.

The third and innermost layer of the eye is the *retina.* Light rays come to a focus on the retina and subsequently are transmitted to the brain, by way of the optic nerve, to be interpreted.

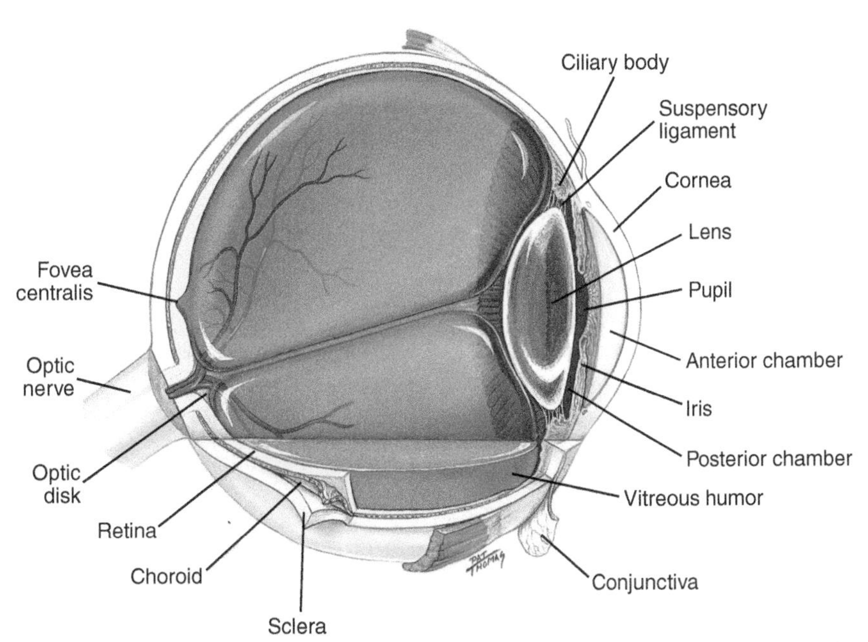

Fig. 6.1 The internal structure of the eye. (From Applegate EJ: *The anatomy and physiology learning system*, ed 4, St Louis: Elsevier; 2011.)

The *anterior chamber* is the area between the cornea and the iris, and the *posterior chamber* is the area between the iris and the lens. Both chambers are filled with a substance known as the *aqueous humor.* A transparent jelly-like material, known as *vitreous humor,* fills the eyeball between the lens and the retina. Its function is to help maintain the shape of the eyeball.

The *conjunctiva* is a membrane that lines the eyelids and covers the front of the eye except the cornea. The conjunctiva covering the sclera is transparent except for some capillaries, which allows the white sclera to show through.

Visual Acuity

Visual acuity refers to acuteness or sharpness of vision. A person with normal visual acuity can see clearly and is able to distinguish fine details close up and at some distance.

Errors of refraction are the most common causes of defects in visual acuity (Fig. 6.2). **Refraction** refers to the ability of the eye to bend the parallel light rays coming into it so that they can be focused on the retina. An *error of refraction* means that the light rays are not being refracted or bent properly and are not adequately focused on the retina. A defect in the shape of the eyeball can cause a refractive error. Errors of refraction can be improved with corrective lenses.

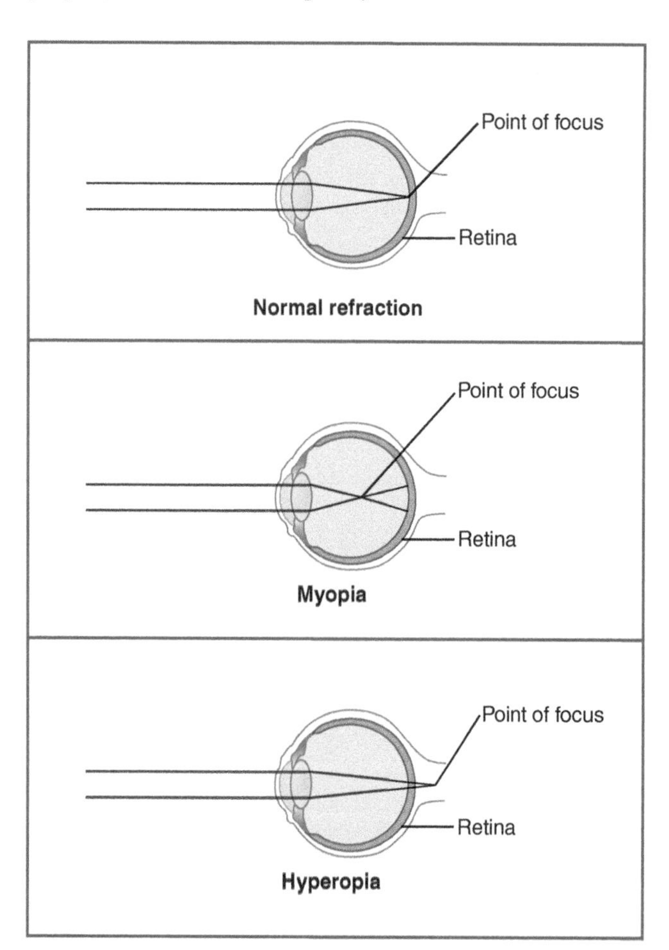

Fig. 6.2 Diagram of normal refraction compared with myopia (nearsightedness) and hyperopia (farsightedness), which are errors of refraction that cause visual defects.

A person who is nearsighted has a condition termed **myopia.** The eyeball is too long from front to back, causing the light rays to be brought to a focus in front of the retina. A myopic person has difficulty seeing objects at a distance and may squint and have headaches as a result of eyestrain. Corrective lenses (e.g., eyeglasses, contact lenses) or laser eye surgery can correct this condition, which then allows the light rays to come to a focus on the retina.

A person who is farsighted has a condition known as **hyperopia.** The eyeball is too short from front to back, resulting in a different type of refractive error, in which the light rays are brought to a focus behind the retina. The individual has difficulty viewing objects at a reading or working distance. An individual with hyperopia may experience blurring, headaches, and eyestrain while performing up-close tasks. Corrective lenses can correct this condition by causing the light rays to come to a focus on the retina.

Astigmatism is a refractive error that causes distorted and blurred vision for both near and far objects. A normal cornea has a round or spherical shape and is smooth. With astigmatism, the cornea is curved into an oval shape. This causes the light rays to focus on two different points on the retina, instead of just one, resulting in distorted and blurred vision. Astigmatism often occurs in combination with myopia or hyperopia and can be corrected with corrective lenses.

In most people, a decrease in the elasticity of the lens of the eye begins to occur after age 40 years. This condition, **presbyopia,** results in a decreased ability to focus clearly on close objects.

EYE SPECIALISTS

If a defect in visual acuity is detected, the patient is referred to an eye specialist for further evaluation. Several types of specialists are involved in the care of the eyes. An *ophthalmologist* is a physician who specializes in diagnosing and treating diseases and disorders of the eye. An ophthalmologist is qualified to prescribe ophthalmic and systemic medications and to perform eye surgery. An *optometrist* is a licensed primary health care provider who has expertise in measuring visual acuity and prescribing corrective lenses for the treatment of refractive errors. An optometrist also is qualified to diagnose and treat disorders and diseases of the eye and to prescribe ophthalmic medications. An optometrist is not a physician and is not permitted to prescribe systemic medications or to perform eye surgery. An *optician* is a professional who interprets and fills prescriptions for eyeglasses and contact lenses.

ASSESSMENT OF DISTANCE VISUAL ACUITY

Myopia can be diagnosed (in combination with other tests) by a distance visual acuity (DVA) test. In the medical office,

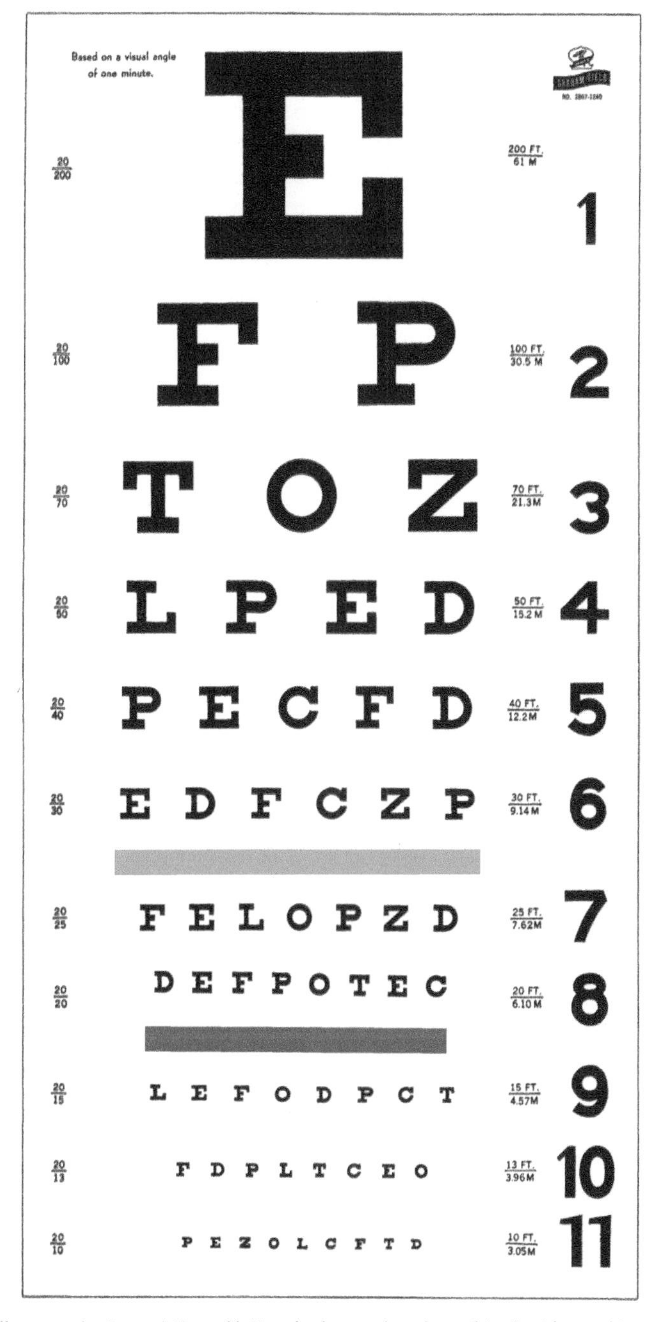

Fig. 6.3 Snellen eye chart consisting of letters in decreasing sizes; this chart is used to measure distance visual acuity.

the Snellen eye chart is most often used. Two types of charts are available. One type is used for school-age children and adults and consists of a chart of letters in decreasing sizes (Fig. 6.3). Another type is used for preschool children, non-English-speaking people, and nonreaders; it is composed of the capital letter *E* in decreasing sizes and arranged in different directions (Fig. 6.4). Visual acuity charts with pictures of familiar objects also are available for use with preschool children. Testing with these charts tends to be less accurate than with the Snellen charts. Some children are unable to identify the objects because of a lack of recognition, not because of a defect in visual acuity. It is suggested that the Snellen Big E chart be used with preschool children.

CONDUCTING A SNELLEN TEST

The visual acuity test should be performed in a well-lit room that is free of distractions. The test is usually performed at a distance of 20 feet; this can be conveniently marked off in the medical office with paint or a piece of tape so that it does not have to be remeasured every time the test is performed.

Two numbers, separated by a line, appear at the side of each row of letters on the chart. The number above the line represents the distance (in feet) at which the test is conducted. It is usually 20 feet because most eye tests are conducted at this distance. The number below the line represents the distance from which a person with normal visual acuity can read the

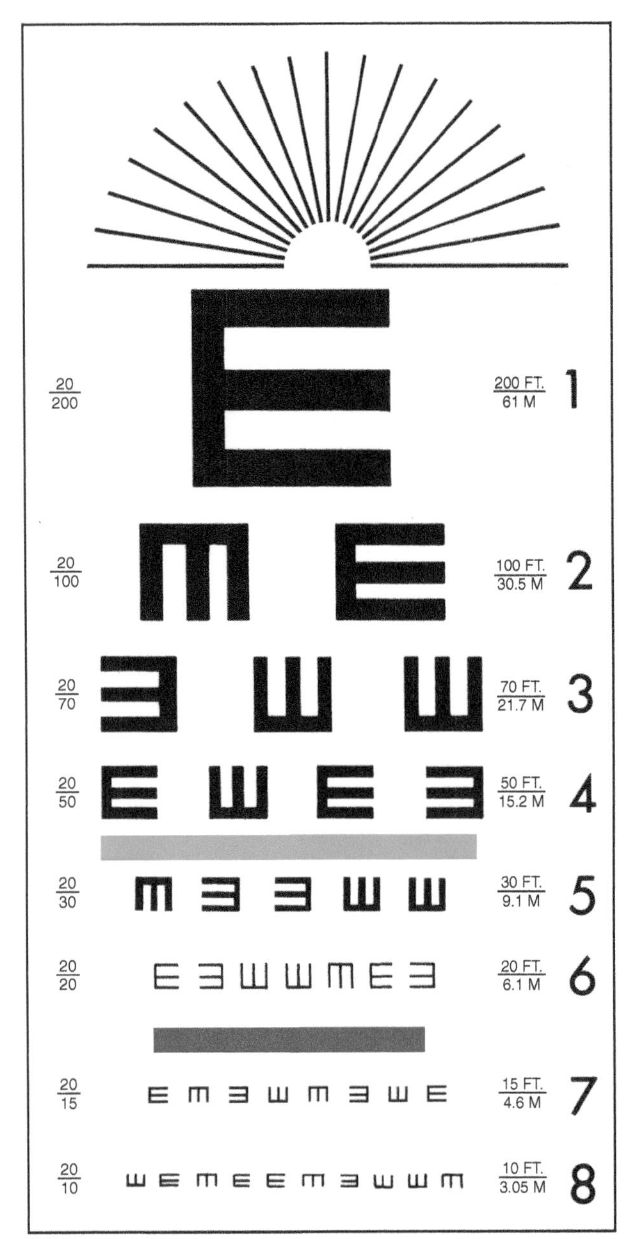

Fig. 6.4 Snellen Big E eye chart consisting of the capital letter *E* in decreasing sizes and arranged in different directions; this chart is used to measure distance visual acuity.

row of letters. The line marked 20/20 indicates normal DVA, or 20/20 vision. This means a person can read what he or she is supposed to read at a distance of 20 feet.

A visual acuity reading of 20/30 means this is the smallest line that the individual can read at a distance of 20 feet. People with normal acuity would be able to read this line at a distance of 30 feet.

A visual acuity reading of 20/15 means this is the smallest line that the individual can read at a distance of 20 feet. It indicates above-average acuity for distance vision. People with normal acuity would be able to read this line at 15 feet.

The acuity of each eye should be measured separately, traditionally beginning with the right eye. Most providers prefer that the patient wear his or her contact lenses or glasses (except reading). The medical assistant should document in the patient's medical record if corrective lenses were worn by the patient during the test. An eye occluder should be held over the eye not being tested. The patient's hand should not be used to cover the eye because this may encourage peeking through the fingers, especially in the case of children. The patient should be instructed to leave open the eye not being tested because closing it causes squinting of the eye that is being tested. The procedure for measuring DVA is outlined in Procedure 6.1.

ASSESSING DISTANCE VISUAL ACUITY IN PRESCHOOL CHILDREN

With minor variations, Procedure 6.1 can be used to test DVA in preschool children. The Snellen Big E chart is used for this purpose.

A child needs a complete and thorough explanation of what is expected of him or her before beginning the test. Tell the child you will be playing a pointing game. Do not force the child to play the game because the results then tend to be inaccurate. Draw the capital letter *E* on an index card, and teach the child to point in the direction of the open part of the *E* by turning the card in different directions (up, down, to the right, and to the left). Using such phrases as "fingers" or "the legs of the table" to describe the open part of the *E* helps the child understand what is expected (Fig. 6.5). Allow the child to practice the pointing game with the index card until you are sure this level of skill has been mastered. Be sure to praise the child when the correct response is given.

The child might need help holding the eye occluder in place. The aid of another person such as the parent would then be required.

ASSESSMENT OF NEAR VISUAL ACUITY

Near visual acuity (NVA) testing assesses the patient's ability to read close objects (i.e., at a reading or working distance); the test results are used to detect hyperopia and presbyopia.

The test is conducted with a card similar to the Snellen eye chart; however, the size of the type ranges from the size of newspaper headlines down to considerably smaller print such as would be found in a telephone directory (Fig. 6.6). The test card is available in a variety of forms, such as printed paragraphs, printed words, and pictures.

The test should be performed in a well-lit room free of distractions. It is conducted with the patient holding the test card at a distance between 14 and 16 inches. If the patient wears reading glasses, they should be worn during the test. The acuity should be measured in each eye separately, traditionally beginning with the right eye. An eye occluder should be held over the eye not being tested. The patient should be instructed to keep the covered eye open because closing it may cause squinting of the eye that is being tested. The patient is asked to read or identify orally each line or paragraph of type. During the test, the patient should be

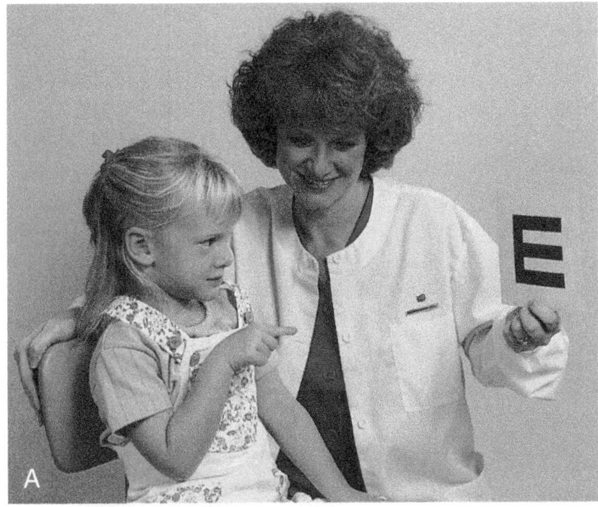

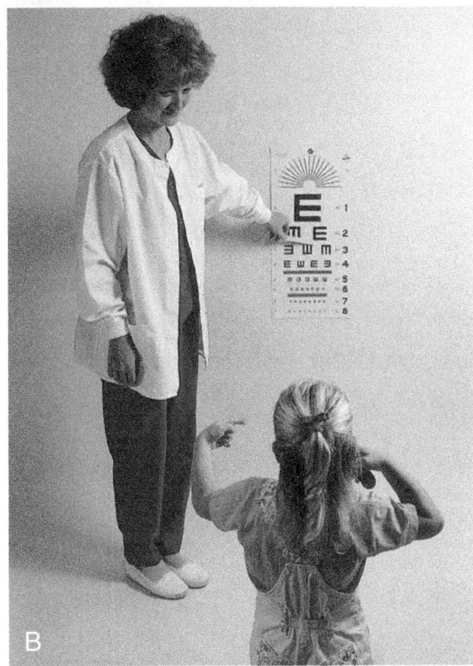

Fig. 6.5 (A) Cammie teaches a preschool child to point in the direction of the open part of the capital letter *E*. (B) Cammie performs the Snellen Big E visual acuity test.

observed for unusual symptoms, such as squinting, tilting the head, or watering of the eyes, which may indicate that the patient is having difficulty reading the card. The patient continues until reaching the smallest type that can be read.

The results are documented as the smallest type that the patient could comfortably read with each eye at the distance at which the card was held (i.e., 14 to 16 inches). The documentation is based on the type of test card used to conduct the test. One type of card uses a documentation method similar to that used with the Snellen eye test. For this type of NVA card, the results would be documented as 14/14 for a patient with normal NVA. This means the patient read what was supposed to be read at a distance of 14 inches. Also included in the documentation should be the date and time, corrective lenses worn, and any unusual symptoms exhibited by the patient.

Assessment of Color Vision

Defects in color vision may be classified as congenital or acquired. *Congenital defects* are more common and refer to a color vision deficiency that is inherited and is present at birth. Congenital color vision deficiencies most often affect males. *Acquired defects* refer to a color vision deficiency that is acquired after birth, resulting from such factors as an eye or brain injury, disease, and certain drugs. Color vision tests, such as the Ishihara test (Fig. 6.7), detect congenital color vision disturbances and are commonly performed in the medical office. A basic screening for color vision can be performed by asking the patient to identify the red and green lines on the Snellen eye chart.

What Would You Do? What Would You *Not* Do?

Case Study 1

Nicole Neason brings her daughter, Haley, to the office for a camp physical. Haley has just completed the fourth grade and is going to summer camp for 2 weeks with Tess, her best friend. Tess wears glasses, and Haley thinks they are really cool. She often asks to try on Tess's glasses and wishes she could wear glasses just like her best friend. When Haley is measured for visual acuity, she misses a few letters on the 20/70 line, the 20/50 line, the 20/40 line, and the 20/20 line. She is unable to read any of the letters on the 20/15 line. After the examination, Haley wants to know if she has missed enough letters to be able to get glasses. ■

ISHIHARA TEST

The Ishihara test for color blindness is a convenient and accurate method to detect total congenital color blindness and red-green color blindness by assessing an individual's ability to perceive primary colors and shades of color. The Ishihara book contains a series of polychromatic plates of primary-colored dots arranged to form a numeral against a background of similar dots of contrasting colors (see Fig. 6.7). Patients with normal color vision are able to read the appropriate numeral; however, patients with color vision defects read the dots either as not forming a number at all or as forming a number different from the one identified by the individual with normal color vision. The first plate in the Ishihara book is designed to be read correctly by all individuals (with normal vision and exhibiting color vision deficiencies) and should be used to explain the procedure to the patient.

The book includes plates with winding colored lines for patients who are unable to identify the numbers by name, such as preschool children and non–English-speaking people. The patient should be asked to trace the line formed by the colored dots using a cotton swab or the eraser end of a pencil. The patient's finger should not be used to do the tracing because over time soiled fingers can degrade the polychromatic plates.

No. 1.
.37M

In the second century of the Christian era, the empire of Rome comprehended the fairest part of the earth, and the most civilized portion of mankind. The frontiers of that extensive monarchy were guarded by ancient renown and disciplined valor. The gentle but powerful influence of laws and manners had gradually cemented the union of the provinces. Their peaceful inhabitants enjoyed and abused the advantages of wealth.

No. 2.
.50M

fourscore years, the public administration was conducted by the virtue and abilities of Nerva, Trajan, Hadrian, and the two Antonines. It is the design of this, and of the two succeeding chapters, to describe the prosperous condition of their empire; and afterwards, from the death of Marcus Antoninus, to deduce the most important circumstances of its decline and fall; a revolution which will ever be remembered, and is still felt by

No. 3.
.62M

the nations of the earth. The principal conquests of the Romans were achieved under the republic; and the emperors, for the most part, were satisfied with preserving those dominions which had been acquired by the policy of the senate, the active emulations of the consuls, and the martial enthusiasm of the people. The seven first centuries were filled with a rapid succession of triumphs; but it was

No. 4.
.75M

reserved for Augustus to relinquish the ambitious design of subduing the whole earth, and to introduce a spirit of moderation into the public councils. Inclined to peace by his temper and situation, it was very easy for him to discover that Rome, in her present exalted situation, had much less to hope than to fear from the chance of arms; and that, in the prosecution of

No. 5.
1.00M

the undertaking became every day more difficult, the event more doubtful, and the possession more precarious, and less beneficial. The experience of Augustus added weight to these salutary reflections, and effectually convinced him that, by the prudent vigor of

No. 6.
1.25M

his counsels, it would be easy to secure every concession which the safety or the dignity of Rome might require from the most formidable barbarians. Instead of exposing his person or his legions to the arrows of the Parthinians, he obtained, by an honor-

No. 7.
1.50M

able treaty, the restitution of the standards and prisoners which had been taken in the defeat of Crassus. His generals, in the early part of his reign, attempted the reduction of Ethiopia and Arabia Felix. They marched near a thou-

No. 8.
1.75M

sand miles to the south of the tropic; but the heat of the climate soon repelled the invaders, and protected the unwarlike natives of those sequestered regions

No. 9.
2.00M

The northern countries of Europe scarcely deserved the expense and labor of conquest. The forests and morasses of Germany were

No. 10.
2.25M

filled with a hardy race of barbarians who despised life when it was separated from freedom; and though, on the first

No. 11.
2.50M

attack, they seemed to yield to the weight of the Roman power, they soon, by a signal

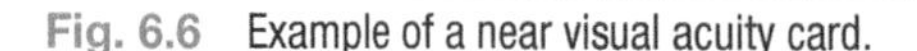

Fig. 6.6 Example of a near visual acuity card.

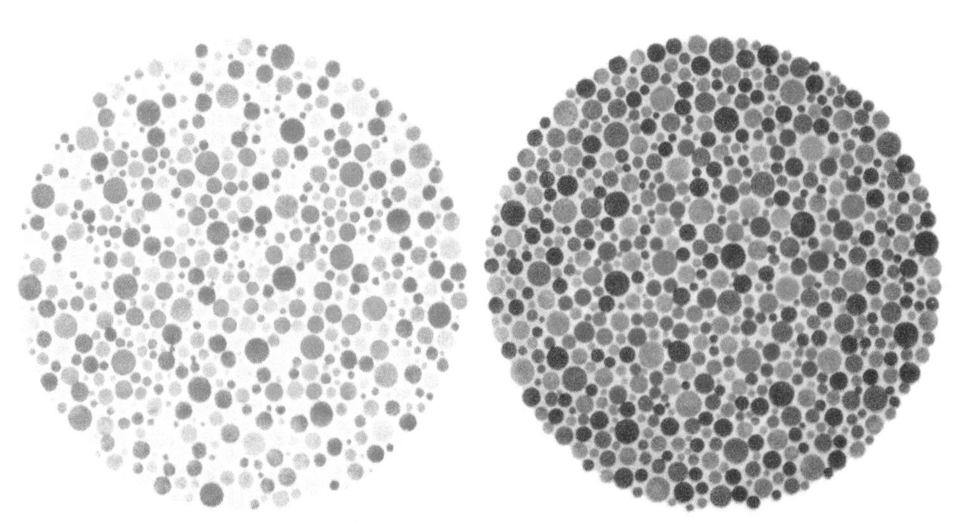

Fig. 6.7 Ishihara color plates. Polychromatic plates. In the left figure, a person with normal color vision reads 74, but a person with red-green color blindness reads 6. In the right figure, a red-blind person (protanope) reads 2, but a green-blind person (deuteranope) reads 4. A normal-vision person reads 42. Reproduced plates are not good for testing for color deficiency. (From Isihara J: *Tests for color blindness.* Tokyo; Kanehara; 1920.)

The Ishihara test should be conducted in a quiet room illuminated by natural daylight. If this is not feasible, a room lit with electric light may be used; however, the light should be adjusted to resemble the effect of natural daylight as much as possible. Using light other than just described, such as bright sunlight, may change the appearance of shades of color on the plates, leading to inaccurate test results.

The medical assistant is responsible for performing the color vision test and for documenting results in the patient's medical record. The provider assesses the results to determine whether the patient has a deficiency in color vision.

The Ishihara test consists of 14 color plates. Plates 1 through 11 are used to conduct the basic test, and plates 12, 13, and 14 are used to further assess patients who exhibit a red-green color deficiency. It is unnecessary to include these plates (12, 13, and 14) in the test of patients who exhibit normal color vision. In interpreting the results, if 10 or more plates are read correctly, the patient's color vision is considered normal. If 7 or fewer of the 11 Ishihara plates are read correctly, the patient is identified as having a color vision deficiency. It would be unusual for the medical assistant to obtain results in which the patient has read eight or nine plates correctly. The test is structured so that a patient with a color vision defect typically does not read eight or nine plates correctly and the rest incorrectly.

If a defect in color vision is detected, the patient is referred for additional assessment of color vision to an ophthalmologist or optometrist, who would use more precise color vision tests. The procedure for assessing color vision using the Ishihara color plates is outlined in Procedure 6.2.

Eye Irrigation

An eye irrigation involves washing the eye with a flowing solution. Eye irrigations are performed for the following purposes: to cleanse the eye by washing away foreign particles, ocular discharges, or harmful chemicals; to relieve inflammation through the application of heat; and to apply an antiseptic solution. Procedure 6.3 shows how to perform an eye irrigation.

Eye Instillation

An eye instillation involves the dropping of a liquid into the lower conjunctival sac of the eye. Eye instillations are performed to treat eye infections (with medication), to soothe an irritated eye, to dilate the pupil, and to anesthetize the eye during an eye examination or treatment. Medication to be instilled in the eye may come in the form of a liquid, as ophthalmic drops, or as an ophthalmic ointment. Eye drops are usually dispensed in a flexible plastic container with an attached dropper. Eye ointment is dispensed in a small metal tube with a small tip for applying the medication. Procedure 6.4 shows how to perform an eye instillation.

Putting It All Into Practice

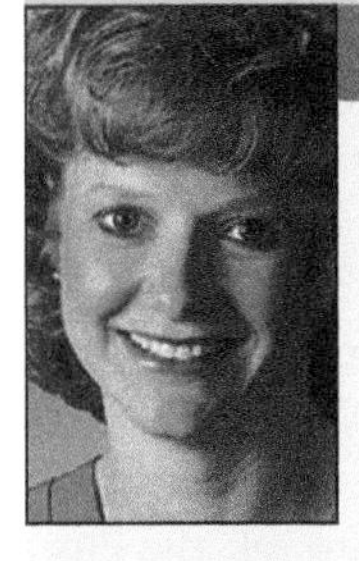

My name is Cammie Lindner, and I work for an ear, nose, and throat (ENT) surgeon. There are administrative responsibilities in my job; however, the focus is on the clinical aspects, including vital signs measurements, allergy testing, immunotherapy, and assisting with minor office surgeries, such as excision of skin lesions and tympanostomy tube insertions. Over past years in an ENT practice, there have been many challenging and rewarding situations. A recent incident was one that certainly falls into the rewards category.

A young girl came into the office from the emergency department for repair of a facial laceration. It had been quite a day for her, so it was understandable that she was a bit nervous and upset. As the suturing was being performed, she grasped her mother's hand as I tried to discuss interests and school with her. She did fine and was very relieved when the last suture was done.

On her return visit for suture removal, her mother could not accompany her. As I was showing her to the examination room, she quietly asked if I would be in the room. I said, "If you would like, I certainly will." She anxiously nodded yes. As the sutures were removed, she squeezed my hand tighter and tighter. After all of them were out, she first checked her appearance in the mirror and then turned before going out the door and gave me a big hug and a "thank you." Days like this one are truly great rewards and make you feel you really can make a difference in someone's care. ■

What Would You Do? What Would You *Not* Do?

Case Study 2

Peter Mitchell comes in with his 5-year-old son, Clive. Clive is diagnosed with conjunctivitis (pink eye), and the provider prescribes Polytrim ophthalmic suspension. Mr. Mitchell says that Clive does not cooperate very well when having drops put in his eyes and asks for any ideas that might make it less of an ordeal. Mr. Mitchell has 7-year-old twin girls at home and wants to know what can be done so they do not get pink eye. He asks if it would be all right to instill the drops in the twins' eyes as a preventive measure. ■

PATIENT COACHING Conjunctivitis

Answer questions that patients have about conjunctivitis.

What is conjunctivitis?

Conjunctivitis, often referred to as *pink eye,* is an inflammation of the conjunctiva (see illustration). The conjunctiva is a thin transparent membrane that covers the white of the eye. Conjunctivitis occurs when the conjunctiva becomes infected with a bacterium or virus. Other causes of conjunctivitis include allergies, prolonged wearing of contact lenses, and irritation from wind, dust, and smoke. Conjunctivitis is almost always harmless and clears up by itself within 2 weeks. If it is caused by a bacterium, the provider may prescribe antibiotic eye drops or ointment.

PATIENT COACHING Conjunctivitis—cont'd

What are the symptoms?
Most types of conjunctivitis are relatively painless. The eye is red or pink because of irritation, and there is a feeling of sandiness or grittiness in the eye. A discharge is usually present, which dries at night when the eyes are closed. This may cause the eyelids to be stuck together in the morning. Other symptoms include tearing, itching, and sensitivity to light.

Is it contagious?
Conjunctivitis caused by a virus or bacterium is highly contagious. It can be spread easily from one eye to another and throughout a family or classroom in a matter of days.

How can its spread be prevented?
The following measures help prevent the spread of conjunctivitis:
- Avoid touching or rubbing the infected eye, which can spread the infection to the other eye or to other people.
- Sanitize your hands frequently with soap, particularly after touching the eyes or face.
- Do not share washcloths, towels, or pillows with anyone.
- Do not wear contact lenses or eye makeup until the conjunctivitis is completely gone.
- Discard eye makeup that was used while you were infected to prevent reinfection.
- Encourage the patient to practice techniques that prevent the spread of conjunctivitis.
- If the provider has prescribed eye medication, teach the patient (or parent) the proper procedure for performing an eye instillation.
- Give the patient educational materials on conjunctivitis. ■

Introduction to the Ear

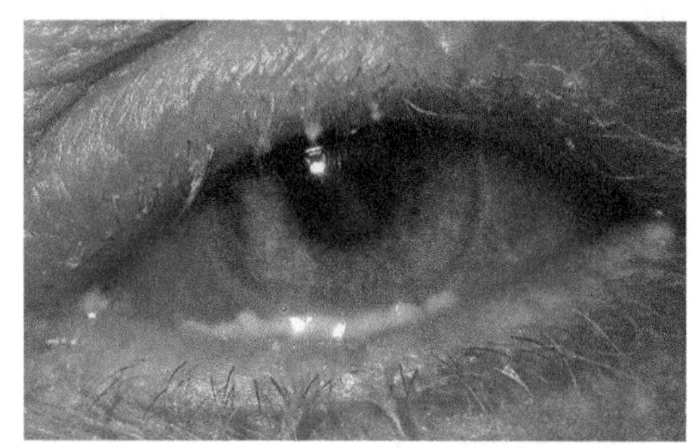
Bacterial conjunctivitis. (From Cuppett M, Walsh KM: *General medical conditions in the athlete*. St. Louis: Elsevier; 2005.)

The medical assistant is responsible for performing a variety of procedures that involve the ear. Hearing tests also may be part of the routine physical examination. During contact with the patient, the medical assistant should be alert to signs that indicate the patient might be having difficulty hearing what is being said. The medical assistant is responsible for assisting with hearing acuity tests such as tuning fork tests and audiometry. The medical assistant is also responsible for performing or teaching the patient to perform ear irrigations and instillations. Ear irrigations and instillations should be performed using the important principles of medical asepsis outlined in Chapter 2.

STRUCTURE OF THE EAR

The ear functions in hearing and in maintaining equilibrium. It consists of three divisions: the *external ear,* the *middle ear,* and the *inner ear.* The structures in the ear are illustrated in Fig. 6.8 and are described next.

The external ear is composed of the auricle (or pinna) and the external auditory canal, also known as the *external ear canal.* The opening into this canal is the *external auditory meatus.*

The *auricle* is a flap of cartilage covered with skin that projects from the side of the head. Its function is to receive and collect sound waves and to direct them toward the external auditory canal.

The *external auditory canal* is approximately 1 inch long in an adult and extends from the auricle to the tympanic membrane. It is lined with skin that contains fine hairs, nerve endings, and glands. The glands secrete earwax, or **cerumen,** a yellowish, waxy substance that lubricates and protects the ear canal. The canal has an S-shaped curve as it leads inward. The canal must be straightened during examination with an otoscope, ear instillation or irrigation, or aural temperature measurement.

The **tympanic membrane** is at the end of the external auditory canal. It is a pearly gray, semitransparent membrane that receives sound waves.

The middle ear is an air-filled cavity that contains three small bones, or *ossicles:* the malleus, the incus, and the stapes. The *eustachian tube* connects the middle ear to the nasopharynx. Air pressure between the external atmosphere and the middle ear is stabilized through the eustachian tube.

The inner ear contains the *cochlea,* which is the essential organ of hearing. The *semicircular canals* also are located in the inner ear and help to maintain equilibrium.

Assessment of Hearing Acuity

The assessment of hearing acuity is an integral part of a complete physical examination. It is possible for an individual to have hearing loss and not be aware of it. Early detection and treatment of hearing problems help prevent permanent hearing loss.

An individual with normal hearing should be able to hear the frequencies of normal speech, which range from 300 to 4000 Hz (hertz, or cycles per second) at a normal sound intensity. Patients who exhibit hearing loss are referred to an otolaryngologist or an audiologist for further evaluation.

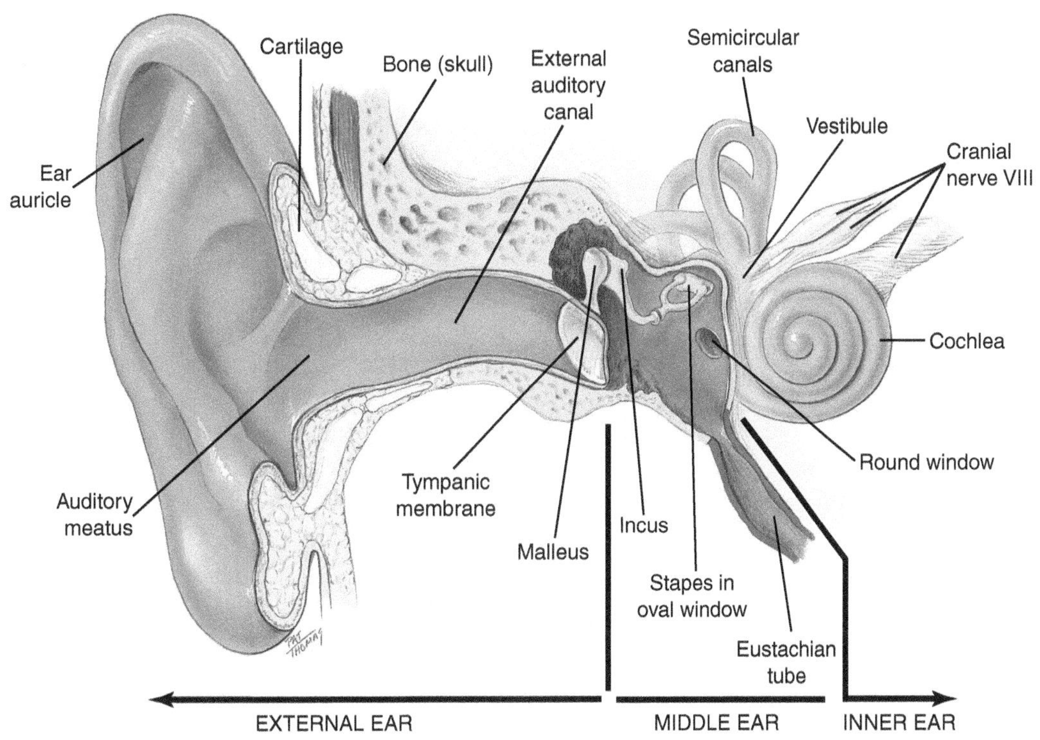

Fig. 6.8 Structure of the ear. (From Applegate EJ: *The anatomy and physiology learning system*, ed 3, St Louis: Elsevier; 2006.)

What Would You Do? What Would You *Not* Do?

Case Study 3

Willow Basil brings in her 6-year-old daughter, Jade. For the past 3 days, Jade has been running a fever and has had persistent pain and hearing loss in her left ear. Mrs. Basil practices alternative medicine and uses prescription medications as little as possible. She says that she has been trying herbal therapy and aromatherapy to make Jade better, but it does not seem to be helping. Jade is diagnosed with acute otitis media, and the physician prescribes amoxicillin for 10 days. Mrs. Basil wants to know if she has to give Jade the amoxicillin for the entire 10 days. She asks if she can stop using it when Jade starts feeling better. Mrs. Basil also wants to know if the ear infection will cause a permanent problem with Jade's hearing. ■

TYPES OF HEARING LOSS

There are three types of hearing loss: conductive, sensorineural, and mixed. *Conductive hearing loss* results when there is a physical interference with the normal conduction of sound waves through the external and middle ear. Because of the interference, the amount of sound reaching the inner ear is less than normal, resulting in hearing impairment. Conductive loss in the external ear may be caused by an obstruction in the external ear canal, such as swelling from external otitis (swimmer's ear), foreign bodies, benign growths such as polyps, and impacted cerumen. **Impacted cerumen** refers to cerumen that is wedged firmly together in the ear canal so as to be immovable. Conductive loss in the middle ear may be caused by serous otitis media (fluid in the middle ear) or acute otitis media (infection in the middle ear), a perforated **tympanic membrane** (eardrum), or otosclerosis. The cause of conductive hearing loss often can be detected by examining the external ear canal with an otoscope. An **otoscope** is an instrument used to examine the external ear canal and tympanic membrane. Hearing is frequently restored by removing the obstruction (e.g., impacted cerumen) or treating the disorder (e.g., serous otitis media).

Sensorineural hearing loss results from damage to the inner ear or auditory nerve. With this type of hearing loss, sound is conducted normally through the outer and middle ear structures, but because of a problem with the perception of sound waves, a hearing deficit occurs. Specific causes of sensorineural loss include hereditary factors, degenerative changes from the normal aging process known as *presbycusis,* intense noise exposure over time, tumors, ototoxicity caused by certain medications, and infectious diseases, such as measles, mumps, and meningitis. The most common cause of sensorineural hearing loss in an adult is presbycusis. As an individual ages, nerves and sensory receptor cells in the inner ear deteriorate, leading to a gradual loss of hearing. *Mixed hearing loss* is a combination of conductive and sensorineural loss.

HEARING ACUITY TESTS

Numerous tests can be used to assess hearing acuity. Tests range from qualitative tests using a tuning fork to highly specific quantitative tests using an audiometer. It is important to test only one ear at a time because a hearing deficit

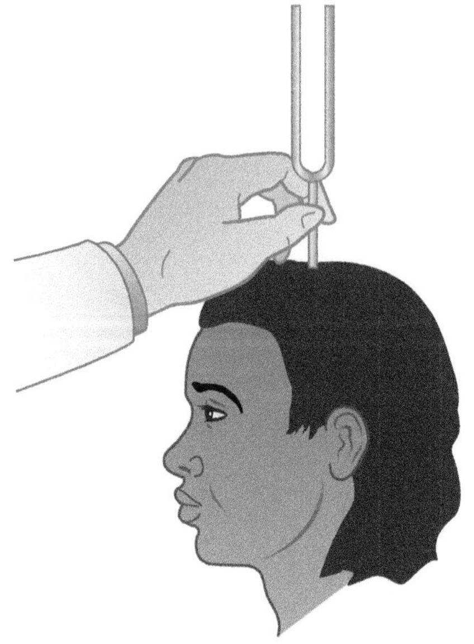

Fig. 6.9 Weber test.

can exist in one ear only. The ear not being tested should be blocked by an earplug or masked. *Masking* involves the presentation of sound (usually noise) to the ear not being tested so that the patient's response is based only on hearing in the ear being tested.

TUNING FORK TESTS

Tuning fork tests provide a general assessment of hearing acuity and may be part of the physical examination. A tuning fork with a frequency of 512 or 1024 Hz is usually used because these frequencies fall within the range of normal speech. The Weber and Rinne tests are the tuning fork tests most commonly performed by the provider; they are used to identify conductive and sensorineural hearing loss.

The *Weber test* is a useful assessment of hearing loss when one ear hears better than the other. The tuning fork is set in vibration, and the base of the fork is placed on the center of the patient's head. The patient is asked to indicate where the sound is heard best. A patient with normal hearing would hear the sound equally in both ears or in the center of the head. Fig. 6.9 illustrates the Weber test and describes the interpretation of the results.

The *Rinne test* compares the duration of sound perception by air conduction with that of bone conduction. The tuning fork is set in vibration, and the base of the fork is placed against the bone of the mastoid process. The patient is instructed to indicate when the sound is no longer heard. The prongs of the fork (still vibrating) are placed in the air about 1 inch from the opening of the patient's ear canal, and the patient indicates when the sound is no longer heard. An individual with normal hearing is able to hear the sound at least twice as long through air conduction as through bone conduction. Fig. 6.10 illustrates the Rinne test and describes the interpretation of results.

Memories *from* Practicum

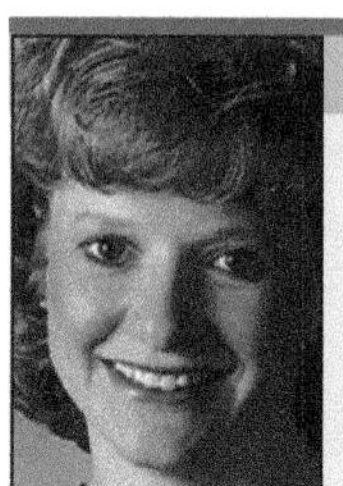

Cammie Lindner: There is one characteristic that is shared by all patients. I first noticed this during my practicum, and it does not seem to matter what type of practice it is. Patients like to feel special and to be treated that way. They like consistency in their provider and in the office staff and seeing familiar faces. This is especially hard during practicum. The time spent is too short to truly get to know the patients, but it is a great learning experience.

It is important to observe the staff and patient communication and interaction skills. By doing this, you can decide which ones you admire and those that you do not wish to copy. The following are just a few of the guidelines that have helped me: (1) Call patients by name, and be sure that they know your name. (2) Follow through with what you have told patients you will do, and keep them updated if circumstances change. (3) Smile, and do not let one patient's negative attitude interfere with your care of others. (4) Take time to listen.

When you do begin your career, it does not take long to get into a routine and to start knowing your patients. When patients see a familiar face, they are more willing to share information that can contribute to improved communication and good health care. ■

AUDIOMETRY

Audiometry is the measurement of hearing acuity using a special instrument called an **audiometer** (Fig. 6.11A). An audiometer quantitatively measures hearing for the various frequencies of sound waves. Audiometry is a more specific hearing acuity test because it provides information on how extensive a hearing loss is and which frequencies are involved. It is important that the test be conducted in a quiet room because outside noise may affect the results,

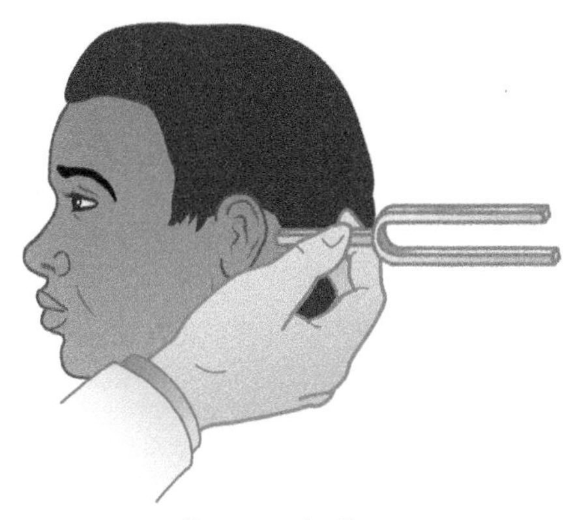

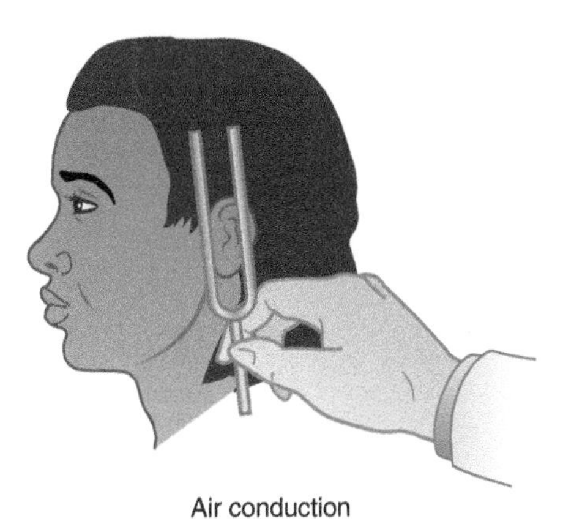

Normal Hearing
The patient hears the sound at least twice as long through air conduction as through bone conduction.

Conductive Hearing Loss
The patient hears the sound longer by bone conduction than by air conduction.

Sensorineural Hearing Loss
The sound is reduced. The patient will also hear the sound longer through air conduction than through bone conduction but not twice as long.

Fig. 6.10 Rinne test.

especially in the lower frequencies. The patient wears headphones placed snugly over the ears (see Fig. 6.11B). The audiometer delivers a single frequency at a time at specific intensities, starting with low-frequency tones of 250 to 500 Hz and going to very high frequencies of 6000 to 8000 Hz. The patient is asked to signal when he or she hears a sound so that the patient's hearing threshold for each frequency can be determined. The hearing acuity in each ear is assessed separately, and the results are plotted on a graph known as an *audiogram*. The medical assistant may be responsible for performing audiometry in the medical office. Before operating an audiometer, however, the medical assistant must receive extensive on-site training from an audiologist to ensure that proper technique is used to conduct the test.

TYMPANOMETRY

Tympanometry is not a hearing test, but it does help determine the cause of hearing loss, so it is presented in this section. The tympanometer consists of an earpiece attached to an electronic device (Fig. 6.12A). The earpiece is placed snugly in the patient's ear, and low-frequency sound waves are directed against the eardrum while pressure is applied in the ear canal (see Fig. 6.12B). With a normal ear, the eardrum exhibits mobility in response to the pressure, as indicated on a graphic readout known as a *tympanogram*. If there is fluid in the middle ear, the eardrum does not move but remains stiff, as indicated on the tympanogram. Tympanometry is useful in diagnosing serous otitis media (fluid in the middle ear), which is a common cause of temporary hearing loss in children.

Ear Irrigation

Ear irrigation is the washing of the external auditory canal with a flowing solution. Ear irrigations are performed for the following purposes: to cleanse the external auditory canal to remove cerumen, discharge, or a foreign body; to relieve inflammation by applying an antiseptic solution; and to apply heat to the ear. Before irrigating, impacted cerumen must be softened by instilling warm mineral oil or hydrogen peroxide for 10 to 15 minutes. An ear irrigation should not be performed if the tympanic membrane is perforated because this could result in severe irritation or infection of the middle ear.

Ear irrigations are most commonly performed in the medical office using either an ear irrigating syringe or an Elephant Ear Wash System. Procedure 6.5 shows how to perform an ear irrigation using both of these methods.

Ear Instillation

An ear instillation involves dropping a liquid into the external auditory canal. Ear instillations are performed to

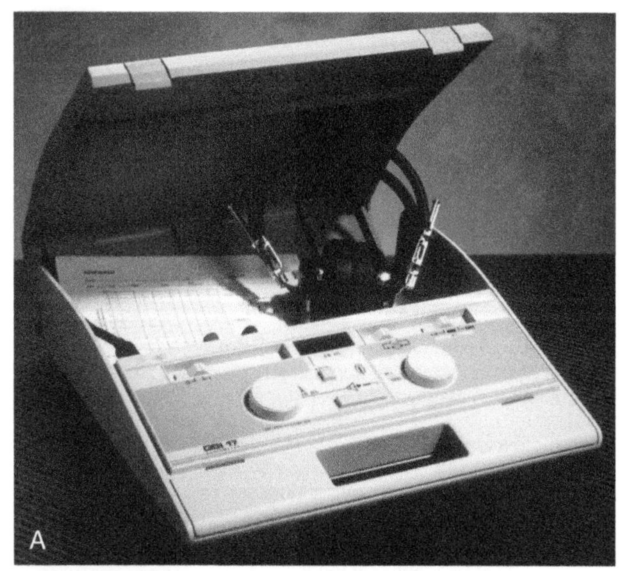

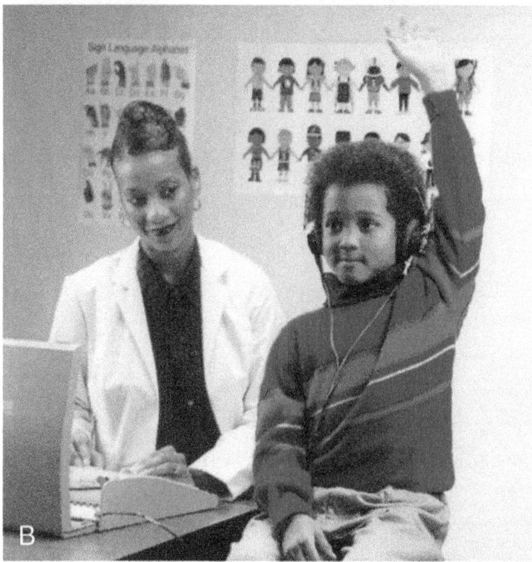

Fig. 6.11 (A) Audiometer. (B) The patient signals when he hears a sound. (Courtesy GSI [Grayson-Stadler], Milford, NH.)

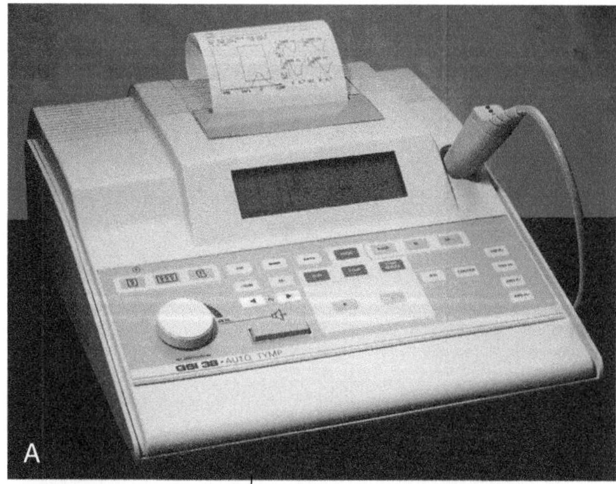

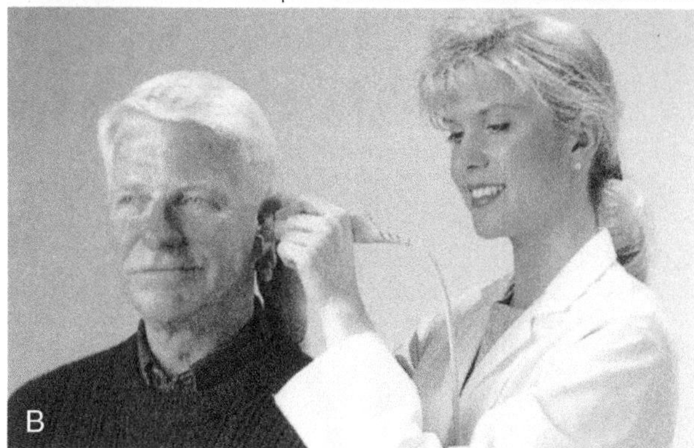

Fig. 6.12 (A) Tympanometer. (B) The earpiece is placed snugly in the patient's ear. (Courtesy GSI [Grayson-Stadler], Milford, NH.)

soften impacted cerumen, to combat infection with the use of antibiotic ear drops, and to relieve pain. The ear drops are usually dispensed in a flexible plastic container with an attached dropper. Procedure 6.6 shows how to perform an ear instillation.

PATIENT COACHING Acute Otitis Media

Answer questions that patients have about otitis media.

What is otitis media?

An infection of the middle ear is medically referred to as *acute otitis media.* It is an inflammation of the middle ear caused by an infection and can occur in one or both ears. It is common in young children 3 months to 3 years old but is unusual in adults. Otitis media is not serious if treated promptly and effectively. If not treated, however, otitis media can lead to serious complications, such as acute mastoiditis, meningitis, and permanent hearing loss.

What causes otitis media?

Otitis media is often the result of an upper respiratory infection or allergy that causes the eustachian tube to swell and become blocked. The blockage causes fluid to build up in the middle ear. This fluid is an ideal place for bacteria to grow. If this occurs, the result is acute otitis media.

What are the symptoms of otitis media and how is it diagnosed?

The most common symptoms are intense pain, fever, and temporary hearing loss. Other symptoms may include dizziness, nausea and vomiting, and (if the eardrum ruptures) drainage from the ear. To diagnose otitis media, the provider examines the ears with an otoscope. If otitis media is present, the eardrum is red and swollen (see illustration) as a result of irritation from the infection, and pus and mucus can be seen behind the eardrum.

PATIENT COACHING Conjunctivitis—cont'd

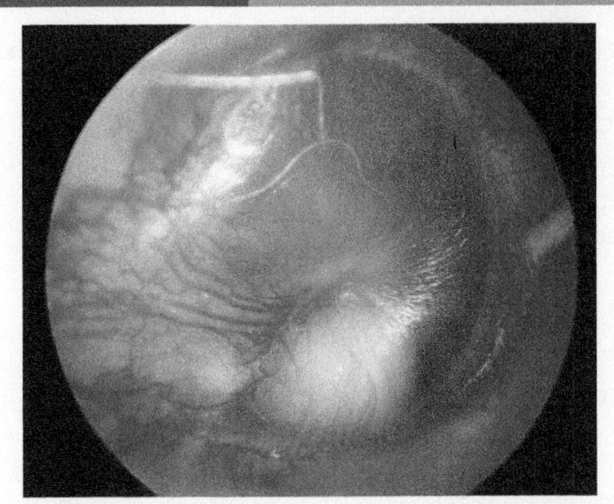

Chronic otitis media. (From Damjanov I, Linder J: *Pathology: a color atlas.* St Louis: Mosby; 1999.)

How is otitis media treated?

Otitis media is usually treated with an oral antibiotic for 10 to 14 days. It is important to complete the entire prescribed course of antibiotics; otherwise, the infection may recur. The provider also may recommend a decongestant to help open the blocked eustachian tube. After the acute infection is over, fluid may remain trapped in the middle ear. This condition is known as *serous otitis media* (see illustration) and, if not treated, may last for days, weeks, months, or even a year. Although fluid in the middle ear is painless, it may result in a feeling of fullness or pressure in the ears and temporary hearing loss.

Why is otitis media so common in children?

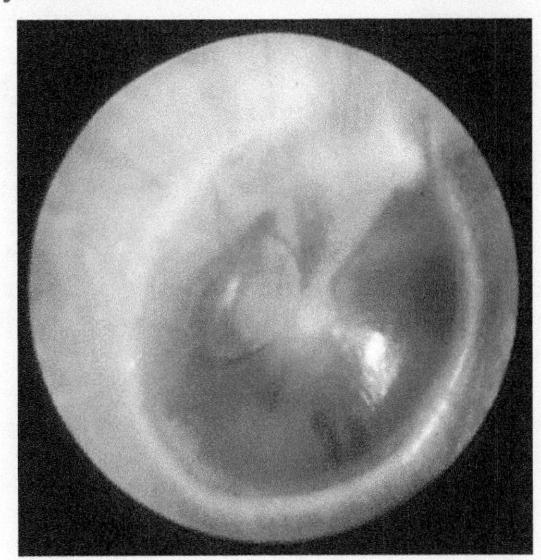

Serous otitis media. (From Swartz MH: *Textbook of physical diagnosis,* ed 5. Philadelphia: Elsevier; 2006.)

In children, the eustachian tube is positioned horizontally and is shorter and narrower than in adults. When a child has an upper respiratory infection, bacteria can travel easily to the middle ear resulting in otitis media. In addition, swelling from the respiratory infection can block this narrow tube, causing fluid to build up in the middle ear.

- Encourage the patient to complete the entire prescribed course of antibiotics.
- If the provider has prescribed ear drops, teach the patient (or parent) the proper procedure for performing an ear instillation.
- Encourage early treatment of upper respiratory infections.
- Give the patient educational materials on otitis media. ■

HIGHLIGHT on Hearing Impairment

Prevalence

The number of individuals with a hearing impairment has gradually increased over the past 20 years. Factors that contribute to this increase include an aging population and a noisier environment. It is estimated that approximately 35 million people in the United States have a hearing loss severe enough to interfere with their daily activities, and another 1 million individuals are profoundly deaf.

Hearing loss in children

Precise screening of preschool children for hearing loss is difficult. This is because tuning fork tests and audiometry require the ability to signal in response to sound, and children up to age 4 or 5 years have trouble mastering this skill. Most state, county, and local school systems require hearing screening as a prerequisite for entrance to school and again at periodic intervals, usually during the first, third, fifth, and seventh grades. Risk factors for hearing impairment in children include family history of deafness, premature birth, low birth weight, measles, mumps, high fevers, meningitis, recurrent or chronic ear infections, and the maternal rubella infection during pregnancy.

Signs of hearing impairment

Signs of hearing impairment in children are poor attentiveness, delayed speech development, and persistent problems with articulation. Signs of hearing impairment in adults include frequent requests for words or statements to be repeated, leaning toward the speaker, turning the head, cupping the ears, and speaking in a loud or unvaried tone of voice.

Common causes of hearing loss

The most common cause of conductive hearing loss in children is fluid in the middle ear, preventing the tympanic membrane from vibrating freely. In adults, the most common cause of conductive loss is otosclerosis, a condition in which the stapes becomes fixed because of calcium deposits and less able to pass on vibrations when sound enters the ear.

The loudness of sound is measured in units called *decibels* (dB). Sounds of less than 75 dB, even after long exposure, are unlikely to cause hearing loss. Normal conversation is approximately 60 dB, and a whisper in a quiet library is 30 to 40 dB. Permanent sensorineural hearing loss can result when the ear is repeatedly

Continued

HIGHLIGHT on Hearing Impairment—cont'd

bombarded with loud sounds over time. Standards set by the Occupational Safety and Health Administration (OSHA) indicate that continued exposure to noise louder than 85 dB eventually harms an individual's hearing by damaging the tiny hair cells in the organ of Corti. The organ of Corti is a structure in the cochlea (inner ear) that converts sound waves into nerve impulses for transmission to the brain. This type of sensorineural hearing loss is known as *noise-induced hearing loss.* It is most often seen in individuals who frequently listen to loud music, fire guns without wearing ear protection, or are exposed to loud noise as part of their jobs. The following are examples of common noises and the decibel level of each:

Noise	Decibels
Normal breathing	10
Humming of a refrigerator	40
Television	70
Vacuum cleaner	60–85
Motorcycle	95–100
Personal stereo system with earphones (on high)	115
Rock concert	120
Chain saw	120
Auto stereo on high	125
Jet taking off	140
Firecracker	150
Firearms	140–170

Hearing aids

Many hearing impairments can be helped with the use of a hearing aid. Individuals who benefit most from a hearing aid have mild to moderate conductive hearing loss. Individuals with sensorineural or mixed hearing loss have more trouble finding a suitable hearing aid and often get less satisfactory results. ■

What Would You Do? What Would You *Not* Do? RESPONSES

Case Study 1

Page 185

What Did Cammie Do?

- ❑ Talked with Haley (on her level) about why someone needs to wear glasses.
- ❑ Retested Haley with the Snellen chart to see if she missed the same letters.
- ❑ Tested Haley with the Big E chart to give the physician an additional measurement to make an interpretation of Haley's visual acuity.

What Did Cammie Not Do?

- ❑ Did not tell Haley that she needs glasses.
- ❑ Did not scold Haley for trying to miss letters on the test.

Case Study 2

Page 187

What Did Cammie Do?

- ❑ Gave Mr. Mitchell some suggestions on how to put drops in Clive's eyes so it is less scary. One idea is to have Clive lie down flat and close his eyes. Place the drops in the inner corner of his eye next to the bridge of his nose, letting them make a little lake there. When Clive relaxes and opens his eye, the drops will gently flow into his eye.
- ❑ Talked with Clive (on his level) about why he needs eye drops.
- ❑ Told Mr. Mitchell that the eye drops were prescribed for Clive and that they should be used only for Clive. Told him that if the twins developed conjunctivitis, he should call the office.
- ❑ Gave Mr. Mitchell suggestions for preventing the twins from getting conjunctivitis (not touching the infected eye, frequent handwashing, not sharing toys or towels).

What Did Cammie Not Do?

- ❑ Did not tell Mr. Mitchell to hold Clive down or force drops in his eyes.
- ❑ Did not tell Mr. Mitchell that he should know better than to think about giving the twins a medication not prescribed for them.

Case Study 3

Page 189

What Did Cammie Do?

- ❑ Explained to Mrs. Basil that Jade may begin to feel better after several days of antibiotics, but not all of the germs causing her ear infection will have been killed by then. If she does not give Jade the full course of antibiotics, the infection could come back.
- ❑ Documented all the medications that Mrs. Basil has administered to Jade.
- ❑ Gave Mrs. Basil a patient information brochure on acute otitis media.
- ❑ Told Mrs. Basil that she needs to talk to the physician about her concern regarding hearing loss because the physician is most qualified to answer that question.
- ❑ Encouraged Mrs. Basil to bring Jade in sooner when she develops fever and ear pain.

What Did Cammie Not Do?

- ❑ Did not criticize Mrs. Basil for waiting so long to bring Jade in.
- ❑ Did not offer a personal opinion about alternative medicine. ■

TERMINOLOGY REVIEW

Key Term	Word Parts	Definition
Astigmatism	*a-:* without *stigma/a:* point *-ism:* state of	A refractive error that causes distorted and blurred vision for both near and far objects due to a cornea that is oval-shaped.
Audiometer	*audi/o:* hearing *-meter:* instrument used to measure	An instrument used to measure hearing acuity quantitatively for the various frequencies of sound waves.
Canthus		The junction of the eyelids at either corner of the eye.
Cerumen		A yellowish waxy substance secreted by glands in the ear canal which functions to lubricate and protect the ear canal. Earwax.
Hyperopia	*hyper-:* above, excessive *-opia:* vision	A refractive error in which the light rays are brought to a focus behind the retina, resulting in difficulty viewing objects at a reading or working distance. Farsightedness.
Impacted cerumen		Cerumen that is wedged firmly together in the ear canal so as to be immovable.
Instillation		The dropping of a liquid into a body cavity.
Irrigation		The washing of a body canal with a flowing solution.
Myopia	*-opia:* vision	A refractive error in which the light rays are brought to a focus in front of the retina, resulting in difficulty viewing objects at a distance. Nearsightedness.
Otoscope	*ot/o:* ear *-scope:* to view	An instrument used to examine the external ear canal and tympanic membrane.
Presbyopia	*-opia:* vision	A decrease in the elasticity of the lens that occurs with aging, resulting in a decreased ability to focus on close objects.
Refraction		The deflection or bending of light rays by a lens.
Tympanic membrane	*tympan/o:* eardrum *-ic:* pertaining to	A thin, semitransparent membrane between the external ear canal and the middle ear that receives and transmits sound waves. Also known as the *eardrum.*
Visual acuity		Acuteness or sharpness of vision. A person with normal visual acuity can see clearly and is able to distinguish fine details close up and at some distance.

PROCEDURE 6.1 Assessing Distance Visual Acuity—Snellen Chart

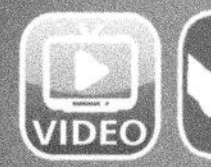

Outcome Assess distance visual acuity.

Equipment/Supplies

- Snellen eye chart
- Eye occluder
- Antiseptic wipe

1. **Procedural Step.** Sanitize your hands.
2. **Procedural Step.** Assemble the equipment. Perform the test in a well-lit room that is free of distractions. Wipe the eye occluder with an antiseptic wipe and allow it to dry completely.
   Principle. The eye occluder should be disinfected before use.
3. **Procedural Step.** Greet the patient and introduce yourself. Identify the patient and explain the procedure. Tell the patient that he or she will be asked to read several lines of letters. The patient should not have an opportunity to study or memorize the letters before beginning the test.
4. **Procedural Step.** Determine whether the patient wears contact lenses or glasses (other than reading glasses). If the patient wears such aids, he or she should be told to keep them on during the test.
5. **Procedural Step.** Ask the patient to stand on the marked line located 20 feet from the chart.
6. **Procedural Step.** Position the center of the Snellen chart at the patient's eye level. Stand next to the chart

PROCEDURE 6.1 Assessing Distance Visual Acuity—Snellen Chart—cont'd

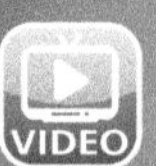

during the test to indicate to the patient the line to be identified.

Principle. Ensure that the chart is at the patient's eye level rather than at your eye level, to provide the most accurate results.

7. **Procedural Step.** Test the acuity of each eye separately. Measure the visual acuity of the right eye first.

   Principle. The medical assistant should establish a pattern of beginning with the same eye (traditionally the right eye) every time the test is performed. This helps to reduce errors during the documentation of results.

8. **Procedural Step.** Ask the patient to cover the left eye with the eye occluder. If the patient wears eyeglasses, tell him or her to place the occluder in front of the glasses gently to prevent the glasses from being moved out of their normal position. Instruct the patient to keep the left eye open. During the test, the medical assistant should check to make sure the patient is keeping the left eye open.

   Principle. Eyeglasses moved out of normal position may lead to inaccurate test results. Keeping the left eye open prevents squinting of the right eye, which temporarily improves vision, leading to inaccurate test results.

9. **Procedural Step.** Instruct the patient not to squint during the test because squinting temporarily improves vision. Ask the patient to identify orally one line at a time on the Snellen chart, starting with the 20/70 line (or a line that is several lines above the 20/20 line).

   Principle. It is best to start at a line above the 20/20 line to give the patient a chance to gain confidence and to become familiar with the test procedure.

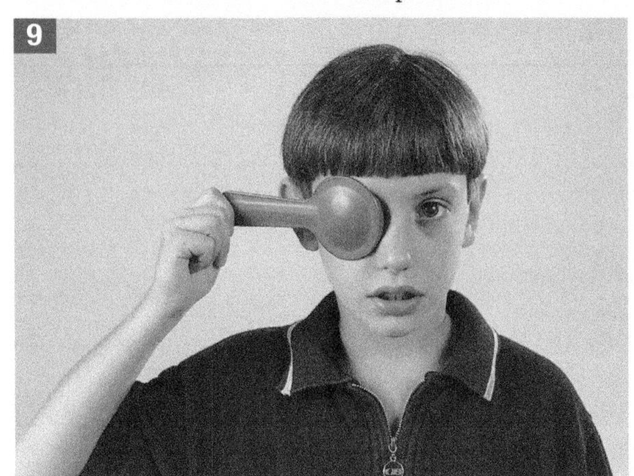

Ask the patient to identify one line at a time.

10. **Procedural Step.** If the patient is able to read the 20/70 line, proceed down the chart until reaching the smallest line of letters the patient can read. If the patient is unable to read the 20/70 line, proceed up the chart until the smallest line of letters the patient can read is reached.

11. **Procedural Step.** While the patient is reading the letters, observe him or her for unusual symptoms, such as squinting, tilting of the head, or watering of the eyes.

    Principle. These symptoms may indicate that the patient is having difficulty identifying the letters.

12. **Procedural Step.** On a small piece of paper, jot down the numbers that are displayed next to the smallest line of letters that the patient is able to read. If one or two letters are missed, document the visual acuity with a minus sign next to the bottom number, along with the number of letters missed. If more than two letters are missed, the previous line is documented.

13. **Procedural Step.** Ask the patient to cover the right eye with the eye occluder and to keep the right eye open. Measure the visual acuity in the left eye as described in steps 9 through 12. During the test, check to make sure the patient is keeping the right eye open.

    Principle. Keeping the right eye open prevents squinting of the left eye.

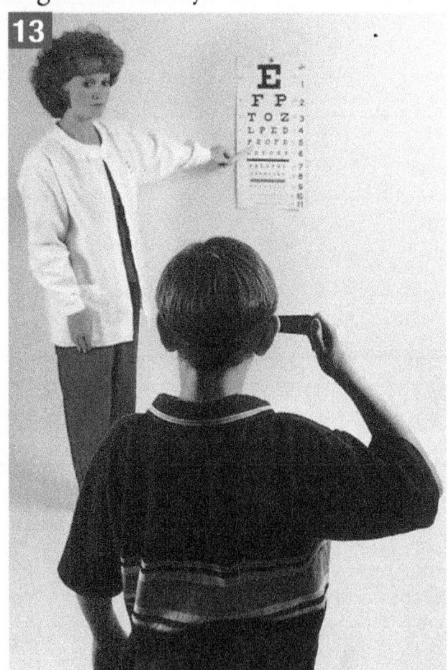

Ask the patient to cover the right eye and to keep the left eye open.

14. **Procedural Step.** Document the procedure in the patient's medical record.
    a. *Electronic health record:* In SimChart for the Medical Office, document the visual acuity results and any unusual symptoms the patient exhibited during the test using the correct radio buttons, drop-down menus, and free text fields. It should also be documented if the patient was wearing corrective lenses during the test and what type of corrective lenses were used (glasses or contact lenses).
    b. *Paper-based patient record:* Document the date and time, the name of the test (Snellen test), the

PROCEDURE 6.1 Assessing Distance Visual Acuity—Snellen Chart—cont'd

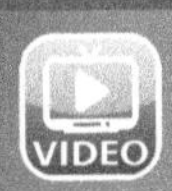

visual acuity results, and any unusual symptoms the patient exhibited during the test (refer to the PPR documentation). Also document whether the patient was wearing corrective lenses during the test. Use the following abbreviations: s̄c for "without correction" or c̄c for "with correction."

15. **Procedural Step.** Disinfect the eye occluder with an antiseptic wipe, and sanitize your hands.

PPR Documentation Example

Date	
11/5/XX	3:30 p.m. Snellen test, s̄c: Ⓡ eye 20/20-1.
	Ⓛ eye 20/25. Exhibited squinting, Ⓡ eye.——
	———————— C. Lindner, CMA (AAMA)

PROCEDURE 6.2 Assessing Color Vision—Ishihara Test

Procedure 6.2

Outcome Assess color vision.

Equipment/Supplies

- Ishihara book
- Cotton swab

1. **Procedural Step.** Sanitize your hands. Assemble the equipment.
2. **Procedural Step.** Conduct the test in a quiet room illuminated by natural daylight.
   Principle. Using unnatural light may change the appearance of the shades of color on the plates, leading to inaccurate test results.
3. **Procedural Step.** Greet the patient and introduce yourself. Identify the patient and explain the procedure. Using the first (practice) plate as an example, instruct the patient to orally identify numbers formed by colored dots. Tell the patient that 3 seconds will be given to identify each plate.
   Principle. The first plate is designed to be read correctly by all individuals and is used to explain the procedure to the patient.
4. **Procedural Step.** Hold the first color plate 30 inches (75 cm) from the patient, at a right angle to the patient's line of vision. The patient should keep both eyes open during the test.

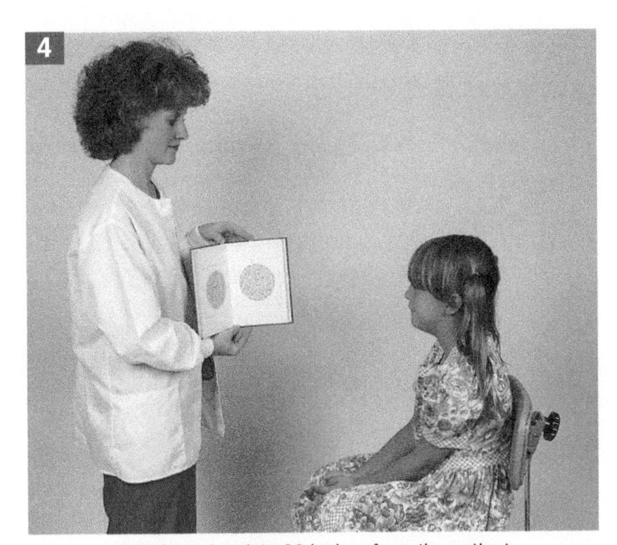

Hold the color plate 30 inches from the patient.

5. **Procedural Step.** Ask the patient to identify the number on the plate. If the plate consists of a traceable winding colored line, ask the patient to trace the line using a cotton swab or the eraser end of a pencil. The patient's finger should not be used to make the tracing.
   Principle. The patient's finger should not be used to trace the line because soiled fingers can degrade the plate over time.
6. **Procedural Step.** Document results after each plate. Continue until the patient has viewed all the plates.
   a. *Paper-based patient record:* To document color vision results, use the plate identification number and the

Continued

PROCEDURE 6.2 Assessing Color Vision—Ishihara Test—cont'd

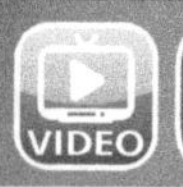

number given by the patient. If the patient is unable to identify a number, the mark X should be documented to indicate that the patient could not read the plate. Examples:

Plate 5: 6. This means the patient read the number 6 on plate 5 (instead of 74).

Plate 6: X. This means the patient could not identify a number on plate 6.

Plate 11: Traceable. This means that the patient correctly traced a winding line on plate 11.

As you can see from the results of this patient's color vision test, the patient correctly identified all 11 plates, which indicates normal color vision. Because the patient has normal color vision, the medical assistant did not need to include plates 12, 13, and 14 in the color vision test.

b. *Electronic health record:* In SimChart for the Medical Office, document the color vision results using the correct radio buttons, drop-down menus, and free text fields to indicate the plate identification number and the number given by the patient or to indicate that the patient is unable to identify a number.
Principle. Reading 10 or more plates correctly indicates normal color vision. If 7 or fewer plates are read correctly, the patient is identified as having a color vision deficiency.

7. **Procedural Step.** Complete the documentation entry.
   a. *Electronic health record:* In SimChart for the Medical Office, document any unusual symptoms the patient exhibited during the test, such as squinting or rubbing the eyes.
   b. *Paper-based patient record:* Document the date and time, the name of the test (Ishihara test), and any unusual symptoms the patient exhibited during the test, such as squinting or rubbing the eyes.
8. **Procedural Step.** Return the Ishihara book to its proper place. The book of color plates must be stored in a closed position to protect it from light.
Principle. Exposing the plates to excessive and unnecessary light results in fading of the color.

PPR Documentation Example

Plate No.	Normal Person	Results
1	12	12
2	8	8
3	5	5
4	29	29
5	74	74
6	7	7
7	45	45
8	2	2
9	X	X
10	16	16
11	Traceable	Traceable
11/6/XX	10:00 a.m.	
	C. Lindner, CMA (AAMA)	

PROCEDURE 6.3 Performing an Eye Irrigation

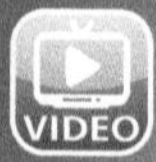
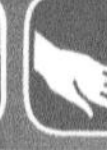

Outcome Perform an eye irrigation.

Equipment/Supplies

- Disposable gloves
- Irrigating solution
- Solution basin
- Bath thermometer
- Disposable rubber bulb syringe
- Basin
- Moisture-resistant towel
- Gauze pads

1. **Procedural Step.** Sanitize your hands.
2. **Procedural Step.** Assemble the equipment. If both eyes are to be irrigated, two sets of equipment must be used to prevent cross-infection from one eye to the other. Normal saline is usually used to irrigate the eye. Perform the following:
   a. Carefully check the label of the irrigating solution three times to make sure you have the correct solution. The first time is after you remove the solution container from the shelf. Compare the label of the solution container with the provider's instructions.
   b. Check the expiration date of the solution.

PROCEDURE 6.3 Performing an Eye Irrigation—cont'd

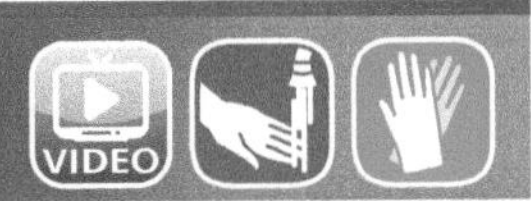

c. Warm the irrigating solution to body temperature (98.6°F [37°C]) by placing the solution container in a basin of warm water. Use a bath thermometer to make sure the temperature of the water used to warm the solution does not exceed body temperature.
d. Check the solution label a second time before pouring the solution.
e. Pour the solution as follows:
f. Palm the label of the container and remove the cap. Place the cap on a flat surface with the open end up. Pour the solution into the basin and replace the cap without contaminating it. Cover the basin to keep the solution warm.
g. Check the solution label a third time before returning the container to its storage area.

Principle. The solution label should be carefully checked three times to prevent an error. Outdated solutions may produce undesirable effects and should be discarded. If the solution is too cold or too warm, it will be uncomfortable for the patient. Palming the label prevents the solution from dripping on the label and obscuring it or loosening the label. Placing the cap open end up prevents contamination.

3. **Procedural Step.** Greet the patient and introduce yourself. Identify the patient and explain the procedure and the irrigation. If the patient wears glasses or contact lenses, ask him or her to remove them.
4. **Procedural Step.** Position the patient. The patient may be placed in a sitting or lying position. Place a moisture-resistant towel on the patient's shoulder to protect the patient's clothing. Position a basin tightly against the patient's cheek under the affected eye to catch the irrigating solution, and ask the patient to hold it in place. Ask the patient to tilt the head in the direction of the affected eye.

Principle. The patient is positioned so that the solution flows away from the unaffected eye to prevent cross-infection.

5. **Procedural Step.** Apply disposable gloves. Cleanse the eyelids from inner to outer **canthus** with a moistened gauze pad to remove any discharge or debris on the lids. The inner canthus is the inner junction of the eyelids next to the nose. The outer canthus is the junction of the eyelids farthest from the nose. Normal saline or the solution ordered for the irrigation may be used. Discard the gauze pad after each wipe.

Principle. The eyelids should be clean to prevent foreign particles from entering the eye during the irrigation. Cleansing from inner to outer canthus prevents cross-infection.

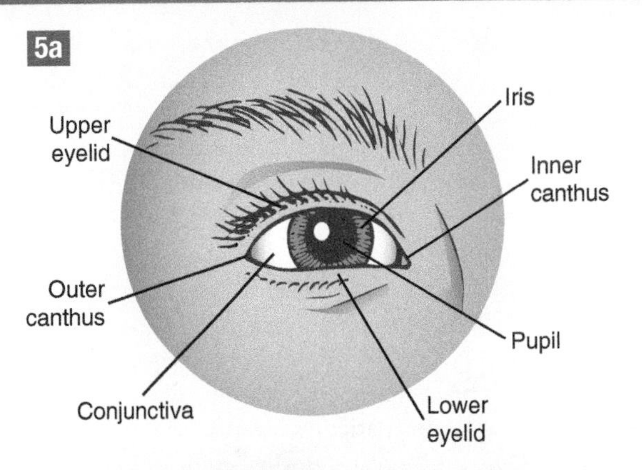

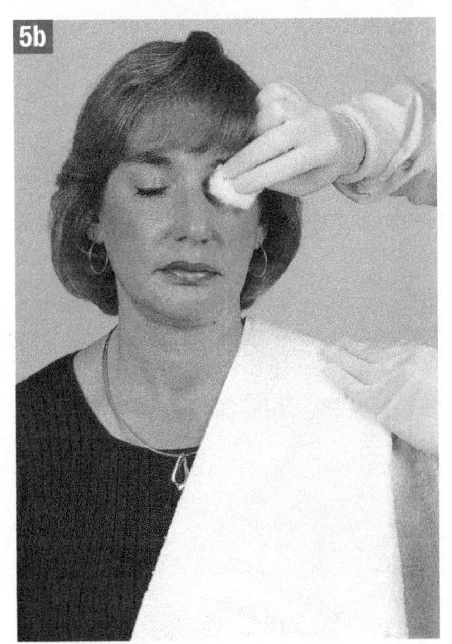

Cleanse the eyelids from inner to outer canthus.

6. **Procedural Step.** Fill the irrigating syringe with the solution by squeezing the bulb and slowly releasing it until the desired amount of solution enters the bulb. Instruct the patient to keep both eyes open and to find a focal point in the room and focus on it.

Principle. Looking at a focal point helps the patient keep the irrigated eye open during the procedure.

7. **Procedural Step.** Separate the eyelids with the index finger and thumb to expose the lower conjunctiva and to hold the upper eyelid open.

Principle. The medical assistant must hold the eye open during the procedure because the patient has a tendency to close it.

Continued

Procedure 6.3

PROCEDURE 6.3 Performing an Eye Irrigation—cont'd

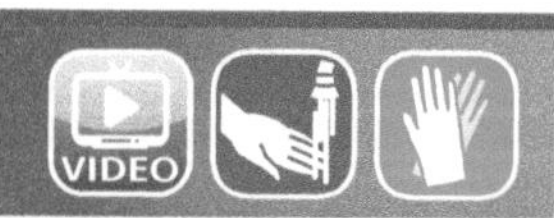

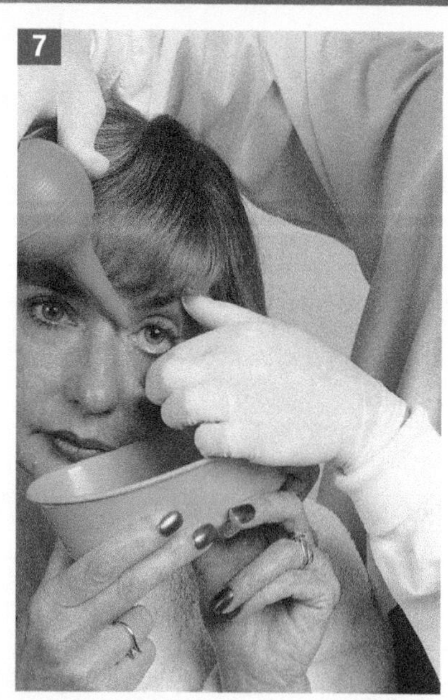

Separate the eyelids, and hold the tip of the syringe 1 inch above the eye.

8. **Procedural Step.** Hold the tip of the syringe approximately 1 inch above the eye. Gently release the solution onto the eye at the inner canthus. This allows the solution to flow over the eye at a moderate rate from the inner to the outer canthus. Direct the solution to the lower conjunctiva. To prevent injury, do not allow the tip of the syringe to touch the eye.
   Principle. The solution flows away from the unaffected eye to prevent cross-infection. The cornea is sensitive and can be harmed easily. The irrigating solution must be directed to the lower conjunctiva to prevent injury to the cornea.
9. **Procedural Step.** Refill the syringe, and continue irrigating until the desired results have been obtained or all the solution is used, depending on the purpose of the irrigation.
10. **Procedural Step.** Dry the eyelids from inner to outer canthus with a gauze pad.
11. **Procedural Step.** Remove the gloves, and sanitize your hands.
12. **Procedural Step.** Document the procedure in the patient's medical record.
    a. *Electronic health record:* In SimChart for the Medical Office, document, using the correct radio buttons, drop-down menus, and free text fields, which eye was irrigated; the type, strength, and amount of solution used; and any significant observations and patient reactions.
    b. *Paper-based patient record:* Document the following: the date and time; which eye was irrigated; the type, strength, and amount of solution used; and any significant observations and patient reactions (refer to the PPR documentation example).
13. **Procedural Step.** Remove reusable equipment to a work area for sanitization, sterilization, or disinfection as required by the medical office policy.

PPR Documentation Example

Date	
11/5/XX	10:30 a.m. Irrigated Ⓛ eye c̄ sterile saline at
	98.6° F. No complaints of discomfort.
	———————— C. Lindner, CMA (AAMA)

PROCEDURE 6.4 Performing an Eye Instillation

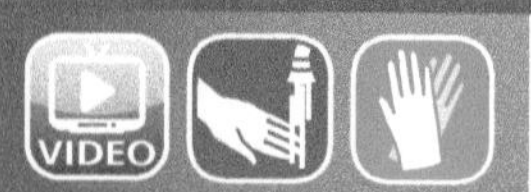

Outcome Perform an eye instillation.

Equipment/Supplies

- Disposable gloves
- Ophthalmic drops or ophthalmic ointment as ordered by the provider
- Tissues
- Gauze pads

1. **Procedural Step.** Sanitize your hands.
2. **Procedural Step.** Assemble the equipment, and perform the following:
   a. Check the drug label three times to make sure you have the correct medication. The first time should be when you remove the medication from the shelf. The medication label must bear the word *ophthalmic.*
   b. Check the medication label a second time against the provider's instructions. Also, check the dose ordered by the provider.
   c. Check the expiration date.

PROCEDURE 6.4 Performing an Eye Instillation—cont'd

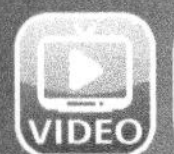  

d. Check the medication label a third time before the cap is removed to instill the medication (as indicated in Procedural Step 5).

Principle. The drug label should be carefully checked three times to prevent a medication error. Medication not bearing the word *ophthalmic* must never be placed in the eye because it could injure the eye. An outdated medication may produce undesirable effects and should be discarded.

3. **Procedural Step.** Greet the patient and introduce yourself. Identify the patient and explain the procedure and the purpose of the instillation. If the patient wears glasses or contact lenses, ask him or her to remove them.
4. **Procedural Step.** Help the patient into a sitting or supine position.
5. **Procedural Step.** Apply disposable gloves. Prepare the medication.

   Eye drops: If the medication requires mixing, shake the container well. Check the medication label for the third time, and remove the cap from the container.

   Eye ointment: Check the medication label for the third time, and remove the cap from the tip of the tube.
6. **Procedural Step.** Ask the patient to look up at the ceiling, and expose the lower conjunctival sac by using the fingers of the nondominant hand placed over a tissue. The fingers should be placed on the patient's cheekbone just below the eye, and the skin of the cheek should be drawn gently downward.

   Principle. Looking up helps keep the patient from blinking when the drops are instilled.
7. **Procedural Step.** Insert the medication.

   Eye drops: Invert the container and hold the tip of the dropper approximately ½ inch above the eye sac. Do not allow the dropper to touch the eye or any other surface. Gently squeeze the container and place the correct number of eye drops in the center of the lower conjunctival sac. Never place the drops directly on the eyeball. Replace the cap on the container.

   Eye ointment: Gently squeeze the tube and place a thin ribbon of ointment along the length of the lower conjunctival sac from the inner to outer canthus. Be careful not to touch the tip of the ointment tube to the eye or any other surface. Discontinue the ribbon by twisting the tube. Replace the cap on the tube.

   Principle. Touching the dropper or tip of the tube to the eye (or other surfaces) could injure the eye and contaminate the medication. Placing the medication in the conjunctival sac, rather than directly on the eyeball, is more comfortable for the patient.

7

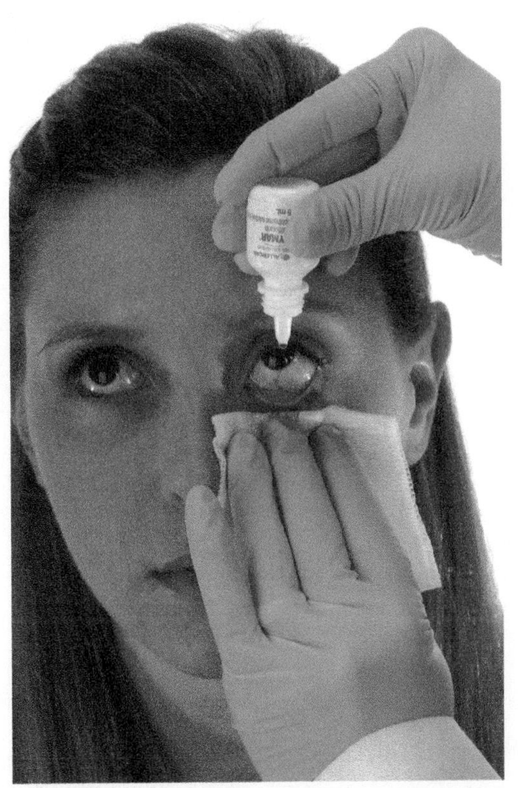

Ask the patient to look up, and insert the medication.

8. **Procedural Step.** Ask the patient to close his or her eyes gently and move the eyeballs. Instruct the patient not to shut the eyes tight or to blink and to keep the eyes closed for 1 to 2 minutes. Tell the patient that the instillation may blur the vision temporarily.

   Principle. Moving the eyeballs helps distribute the medication over the entire eye. Keeping the eyes closed allows the medication to be absorbed. If the eyes are shut tightly or if the patient blinks, the drops or ointment may be pushed out of the eye.
9. **Procedural Step.** Dry the eyelid from inner to outer canthus with a gauze pad to remove excess medication.
10. **Procedural Step.** Remove the gloves, and sanitize your hands.
11. **Procedural Step.** Document the procedure in the patient's medical record.

    a. *Electronic health record:* In SimChart for the Medical Office, document, using the correct radio buttons, drop-down menus, and free text fields, the name and strength of the medication, the number of drops or amount of ointment, which eye received the instillation, your observations, and the patient's reaction.

    b. *Paper-based patient record:* The medication dosage for eye drops is documented in the number of

Continued

PROCEDURE 6.4 Performing an Eye Instillation—cont'd

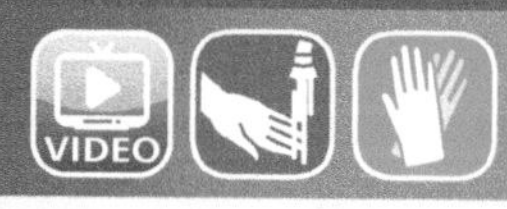

drops instilled. The documentation should include the date and time, the name and strength of the medication, the number of drops or amount of ointment, which eye received the instillation, your observations, and the patient's reaction (refer to the PPR documentation example).

12. Procedural Step. Return the medication to its proper storage area.

PPR Documentation Example

Date	
11/5/XX	2:30 p.m. Atropine sulfate 1%, 2 drops in each eye.
	Pt states a temporary blurring of vision. ——
	———————— C. Lindner, CMA (AAMA)

PROCEDURE 6.5 Performing an Ear Irrigation

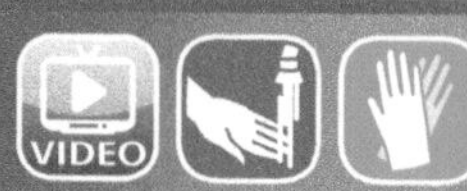

Outcome Perform an ear irrigation.

Equipment/Supplies

- Disposable gloves
- Irrigating solution
- Solution basin
- Bath thermometer
- Ear irrigating syringe or Elephant Ear Wash System
- Ear basin
- Moisture-resistant towel
- Gauze pads
- Ear wick

1. **Procedural Step.** Sanitize your hands.
2. **Procedural Step.** Assemble the equipment. If both ears are to be irrigated, two sets of equipment must be used to prevent cross-infection from one ear to the other.

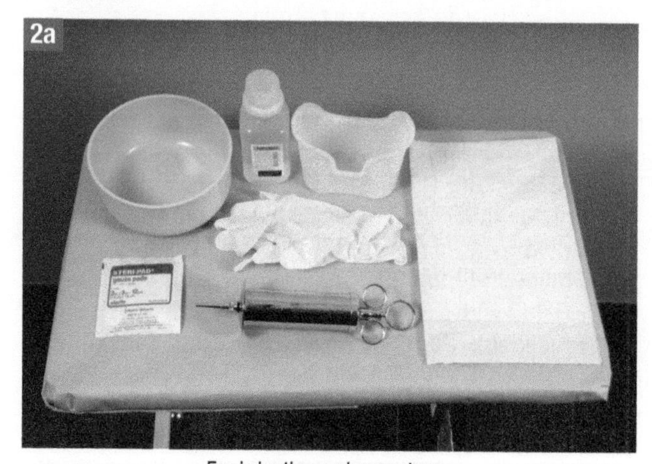

2a Ear irrigation syringe setup.

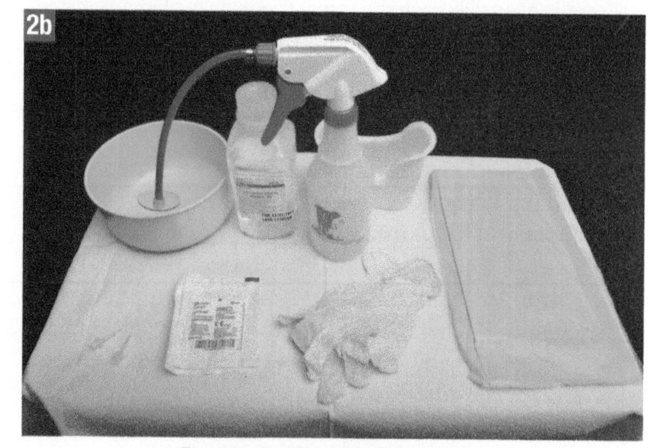

2b Elephant Ear Wash System setup.

3. **Procedural Step.** Prepare the irrigating solution:
   a. Carefully check the label of the irrigating solution three times to make sure you have the correct solution. The first time is after you remove the solution container from the shelf. Compare the label of the solution container with the provider's instructions.
   b. Check the expiration date of the solution.
   c. Warm the irrigating solution to body temperature (98.6°F [37°C]) by placing the solution container in a basin of warm water. Use a bath thermometer to make sure the temperature of the water used to warm the solution does not exceed body temperature.

PROCEDURE 6.5 Performing an Ear Irrigation—cont'd

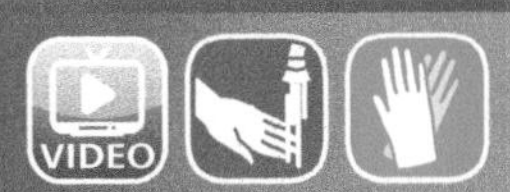

d. Check the solution label a second time before pouring the solution.
e. Pour the solution as follows:
Palm the label of the container and remove the cap. Place the cap on a flat surface with the open end up.
Ear irrigating syringe: Pour the solution into the basin and replace the cap without contaminating it. Cover the basin to keep the solution warm.
Elephant Ear Wash System: Remove the top of the spray bottle and pour the solution into the bottle. Replace the top of the spray bottle.
f. Check the solution label a third time before returning the container to its storage area.

Principle. The solution label should be carefully checked three times to prevent an error. An outdated solution may produce undesirable effects. If the solution is too cold or too warm, it might stimulate the inner ear and the patient may become dizzy. Palming the label prevents the solution from dripping on the label and obscuring it or loosening the label. Placing the cap open end up prevents contamination.

4. **Procedural Step.** Greet the patient and introduce yourself. Identify the patient and explain the procedure. Explain the purpose of performing the irrigation—for example, to remove cerumen. Tell the patient the procedure is not painful; however, he or she may feel a minimal amount of discomfort and occasional dizziness, fullness, and warmth as the ear solution comes in contact with the tympanic membrane.
5. **Procedural Step.** Position the patient in a sitting position. Place a moisture-resistant towel on the patient's shoulder under the ear to be irrigated to protect clothing and to prevent water from running down the neck. Position a basin tightly against the patient's neck under the affected ear to catch the irrigating solution, and ask the patient to hold it in place. Ask the patient to tilt the head in the direction of the affected ear.
Principle. The patient is positioned so that gravity aids the flow of the solution out of the ear and into the basin.
6. **Procedural Step.** Apply gloves. Cleanse the outer ear with a moistened gauze pad to remove any discharge or debris present. Normal saline or the solution ordered for the irrigation may be used.
Principle. The outer ear should be clean to prevent foreign particles from entering the ear canal during the irrigation.
7. **Procedural Step.** Prepare the irrigating device.
a. *Ear irrigating syringe:* Fill the syringe with the irrigating solution (approximately 50 mL). Expel air from the syringe.
Principle. Air forced into the ear is uncomfortable for the patient.
b. *Elephant Ear Wash System:* Twist a disposable tip onto the nozzle of the tubing, making sure to screw it firmly into place.

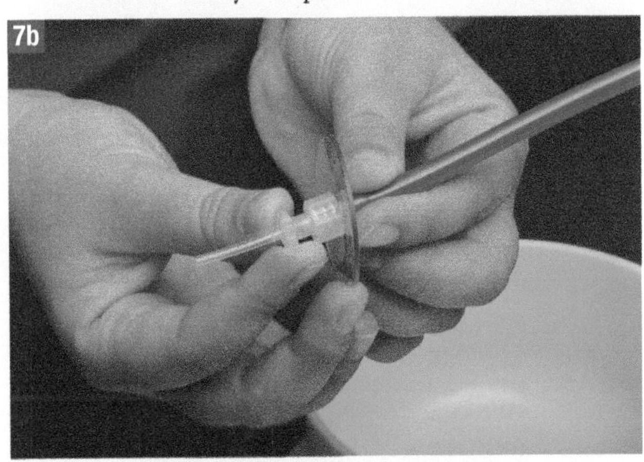

Twist a disposable tip onto the nozzle.

8. **Procedural Step.** Straighten the external ear canal. The canal is straightened by gently pulling the ear upward and backward for adults and children older than 3 years and downward and backward for children 3 years old or younger.
Principle. Straightening the canal permits the irrigating solution to reach all areas of the canal.
9. **Procedural Step.** Insert the tip of the irrigating device into the ear, but not too deeply. (*Note:* With regard to the ear irrigating syringe, make sure that the tip of the ear irrigating syringe does not obstruct the canal opening so that the solution can flow freely out of the canal. Obstruction of the canal causes pressure to build up in the canal, resulting in patient discomfort and possible injury to the tympanic membrane).
Principle. Inserting the tip of the syringe too deeply causes discomfort for the patient and possible injury to the tympanic membrane.
10. **Procedural Step.** Perform the irrigation.
a. *Ear irrigating syringe:* Inject the irrigating solution toward the roof of the ear canal by slowly depressing the plunger of the irrigating syringe.

Procedure 6.5

Continued

PROCEDURE 6.5 Performing an Ear Irrigation—cont'd

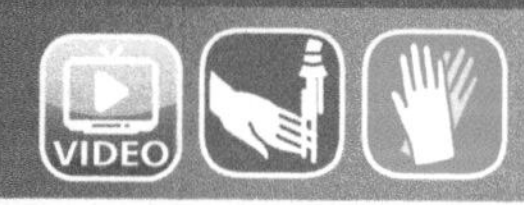

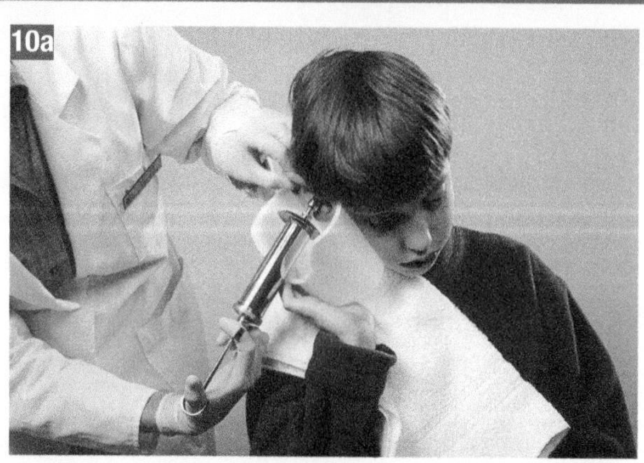

Inject the irrigating solution toward the roof of the ear canal.

b. *Elephant Ear Wash System:* Spray the irrigating solution toward the roof of the ear canal by depressing the trigger handle of the ear wash system. Make sure to keep the tubing fairly straight to prevent bending of the tubing. This ensures a good flow of solution into the ear.

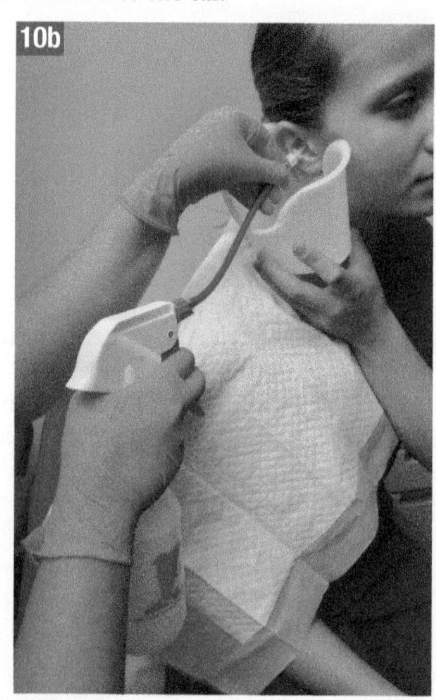

Spray the irrigating solution toward the roof of the ear canal.

Principle. The tip of the irrigating device should be directed at the roof of the canal to prevent injury to the tympanic membrane and to aid in the removal of foreign particles by allowing the solution to flow down the length of the canal and out the bottom. In addition, severe patient discomfort and dizziness may occur if the solution is injected directly onto the tympanic membrane.

11. **Procedural Step.** Continue irrigating until the desired results have been obtained or all the solution is used, depending on the purpose of the irrigation. Observe the returning solution to note the material present (e.g., cerumen, discharge, a foreign object) and the amount (small, moderate, or large).
12. **Procedural Step.** Dry the outside of the ear with a gauze pad. Have the patient lie on the affected side on the treatment table. Tell the patient that the ear will feel sensitive for a short time. Place a cotton wick loosely in the ear canal for 15 minutes if instructed to do so by the provider.
    Principle. Having the patient lie on the affected side allows any solution remaining in the ear canal to drain out. to drain out. A cotton wick makes the patient's ear feel less sensitive after the irrigation.
13. **Procedural Step.** Remove the gloves and sanitize your hands.
14. **Procedural Step.** Document the procedure in the patient's medical record.
    a. *Electronic health record:* In SimChart for the Medical Office, document, using the correct radio buttons, drop-down menus, and free text fields, which ear was irrigated; the type, strength, and amount of solution used; the amount and type of material returned in the irrigation solution; any significant observations, and patient reactions.
    b. *Paper-based patient record:* Document the following: the date and time; which ear was irrigated; the type, strength, and amount of solution used; the amount and type of material returned in the irrigating solution; any significant observations; and patient reactions (refer to the PPR documentation example).
15. **Procedural Step.** Remove equipment to a work area for sanitization, sterilization, disinfection, or disposal as required by the medical office policy.

PPR Documentation Example

Date	
11/15/XX	2:15 p.m. Irrigated (R) ear c̄ saline, 200 mL
	at 98.6° F. Mod amt of cerumen present in
	returned solution. Cotton wick placed in ear
	canal × 15 min. No complaints of discomfort.
	———————— C. Lindner, CMA (AAMA)

PROCEDURE 6.6 Performing an Ear Instillation

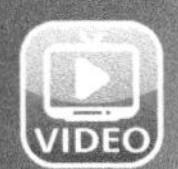

Outcome Perform an ear instillation.

Equipment/Supplies

- Disposable gloves
- Otic drops
- Gauze pad

1. **Procedural Step.** Sanitize your hands.
2. **Procedural Step.** Assemble the equipment, and perform the following:
   a. Check the drug label three times to make sure you have the correct medication. The first time should be when you remove the medication from the shelf. The medication label must bear the word *otic.*
   b. Check the medication label a second time against the provider's instructions. Also, check the dose ordered by the provider.
   c. Check the expiration date.
   d. Check the medication label a third time before the cap is removed to instill the medication (as indicated in Procedural Step 6).

   Principle. The drug label should be carefully checked three times to prevent a medication error. Medication not bearing the word *otic* must never be placed in the ear because it could injure the ear. An outdated medication may produce undesirable effects and should be discarded.
3. **Procedural Step.** Greet the patient and introduce yourself. Identify the patient and explain the procedure and the purpose of the instillation.
4. **Procedural Step.** Position the patient in a sitting position.
5. **Procedural Step.** Warm the drops to body temperature by holding the medication container in the palms of your hands for a few minutes. Do not warm the drops by placing them in hot water.

   Principle. If the drops are too cold or too warm, they might stimulate the inner ear, causing the patient to become dizzy.
6. **Procedural Step.** Apply gloves. If the medication requires mixing, shake the container well. Check the medication label for the third time, and remove the cap from the container.
7. **Procedural Step.** Ask the patient to tilt his or her head in the direction of the unaffected ear. Straighten the external auditory canal. The canal is straightened by pulling the ear upward and backward for adults and children older than 3 years and downward and backward for children 3 years old and younger. Gravity aids in the flow of medication into the ear canal.

   Principle. Straightening the canal permits the medication to reach all areas of the canal.
8. **Procedural Step.** Invert the container and place the tip of the dropper at the opening of the ear canal. Be careful not to touch the tip of the dropper to the ear. Gently squeeze the container and instill the correct number of drops along the side of the canal. Replace the cap on the container.

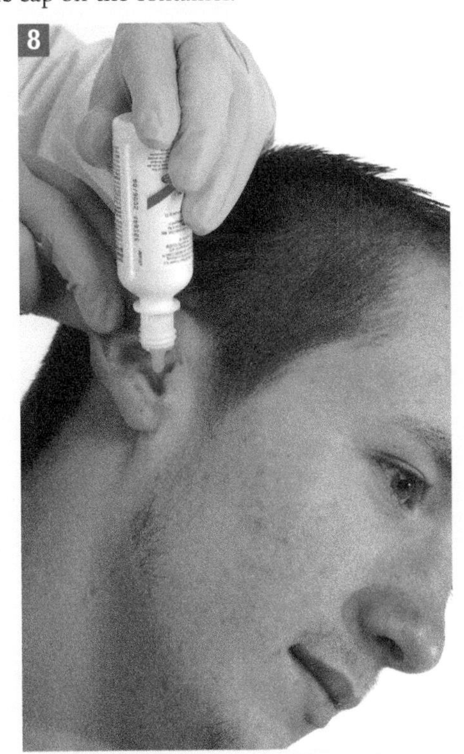

Instill the medication along the side of the ear canal.

9. **Procedural Step.** Instruct the patient to lie on the unaffected side for 2 to 3 minutes.

   Principle. Lying on the unaffected side prevents the medication from running out and allows complete distribution of the medication.
10. **Procedural Step.** Place a moistened cotton wick loosely in the ear canal for 15 minutes if instructed to do so by the provider.

    Principle. The cotton wick prevents the medication from running out when the patient is upright. Moistening the wick prevents the medication from being absorbed by the cotton.
11. **Procedural Step.** Remove the gloves, and sanitize your hands.

PROCEDURE 6.6 Performing an Ear Instillation—cont'd

12. **Procedural Step.** Document the procedure in the patient's medical record.
    a. *Electronic health record:* In SimChart for the Medical Office, document, using the correct radio buttons, drop-down menus, and free text fields, the strengths of the medication, the number of drops, which ear received the instillation, and any significant observations, as well as the patient's reaction.
    b. *Paper-based patient record:* Document the date and time, the name and strength of the medication, the number of drops, which ear received the instillation, any significant observations, and the patient's reaction (refer to the PPR documentation example).
13. **Procedural Step.** Return the medication to its storage area.

PPR Documentation Example

Date	
11/20/XX	9:30 a.m. Auralgan, 2 drops, (R) ear. No
	discharge present. Pt states a relief of pain.
	————————C. Lindner, CMA (AAMA)

Physical Agents to Promote Tissue Healing

 Check out the Evolve site at http://evolve.elsevier.com/Bonewit to access additional interactive activities and exercises to help you study and prepare for success.

LEARNING OUTCOMES

Local Application of Heat and Cold

1. State examples of moist and dry applications of heat and cold.
2. State the factors to consider when applying heat and cold.
3. List the effects of local application of heat, and state reasons for applying heat.
4. List the effects of local application of cold, and state reasons for applying cold.

Casts

5. List reasons for applying a cast.
6. Explain the purpose of each step in the cast application procedure.
7. List the guidelines that should be followed for proper cast care.

Splints and Braces

8. Describe a splint and explain its use.
9. Explain the purpose of a brace.

Ambulatory Aids

10. List factors that are taken into consideration when ambulatory aids are prescribed.
11. Explain the difference between an axillary crutch and a forearm crutch.
12. State conditions that may result when axillary crutches are not fitted properly.
13. List the guidelines that should be followed by the patient to ensure the safe use of crutches.
14. State the use of each of the following crutch gaits: four-point gait, two-point gait, three-point gait, swing-to gait, and swing-through gait.
15. List and describe the three types of canes.
16. Identify the patient conditions that warrant the use of a cane or walker.

PROCEDURES

Apply each of the following heat treatments:
- Heating pad
- Hot soak
- Hot compress
- Chemical hot pack
- Gel pack

Apply each of the following cold treatments:
- Ice bag
- Cold compress
- Chemical cold pack
- Gel pack

Assist with the application of a cast.
Assist with the removal of a cast.
Instruct a patient in proper cast care.

Apply a splint following the manufacturer's instructions.
Apply a brace following the manufacturer's instructions.

Measure a patient for axillary crutches.
Instruct a patient in the proper use of crutches.
Instruct a patient in the proper procedure for each of the following crutch gaits:
- Four-point
- Two-point
- Three-point
- Swing-to
- Swing-through

Instruct a patient in the use of a cane.
Instruct a patient in the proper use of a walker.

CHAPTER OUTLINE

KEY TERMS

ambulation (AM-byoo-LAY-shun)
ambulatory
brace
cast
compress (KOM-press)
edema (uh-DEE-muh)
erythema (err-uh-THEE-muh)
exudate (EKS-oo-date)
long arm cast
long leg cast
maceration (mass-er-AY-shun)
orthopedist (OR-thoe-PEE-dist)
short arm cast
short leg cast
soak
splint
sprain
strain
suppuration (SUP-er-AY-shun)

Introduction to Tissue Healing

Physical agents are often employed in the medical office to promote tissue healing for individuals who experience a disability as a result of injury, disease, or loss of a body part. Physical agents are used therapeutically to improve circulation, provide support, and promote the return of motion so that the individual can perform the activities of daily living. Physical agents frequently used in the medical office include heat and cold applied locally and ambulatory aids, such as crutches, canes, and walkers.

Local Application of Heat and Cold

The application of heat and cold is used therapeutically to treat conditions such as infection and trauma. The medical assistant is responsible for applying heat and cold therapy and for instructing patients in the procedure for applying heat or cold therapy at home. The medical assistant should have a basic understanding of the physiologic effects of heat and cold on the body and of possible adverse reactions if they are not administered correctly.

Heat and cold can be applied in moist or dry forms. Common applications of dry and moist heat and cold are as follows:

1. *Dry heat:* heating pad, chemical hot pack, gel pack
2. *Moist heat:* hot soak, hot compress
3. *Dry cold:* ice bag, chemical cold pack, gel pack
4. *Moist cold:* cold compress

Heat and cold are applied for short periods (typically 15 to 30 minutes) to produce the desired therapeutic results. The application may be repeated at time intervals specified by the provider. Prolonged application of heat or cold is not recommended because it can result in adverse secondary effects. The type of heat or cold application depends on the purpose of the application, the location and condition of the affected area, and the age and general health of the patient. The provider instructs the medical assistant to apply a heat or cold treatment based on these factors.

Heat and cold receptors in the skin readily adapt to changes in temperature, eventually resulting in diminished heat or cold sensations. The temperature remains the same and provides the intended therapeutic effects. The patient, not perceiving the same degree of temperature, may want to increase the intensity of the application, however, without realizing the inherent dangers. Excessive heat or cold could result in tissue damage. A common example of this situation is a patient who turns up the setting of a heating pad from medium to high when the heating pad no longer feels warm. The medical assistant should fully explain to the patient the necessity of maintaining a safe temperature range during the application.

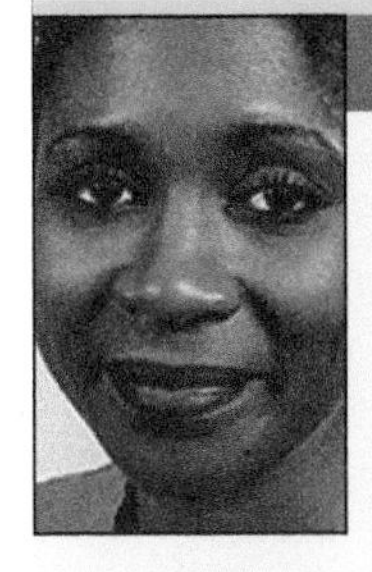

Putting It All into Practice

My name is Marlyne, and I am a Certified Medical Assistant. I work in a community health center. My primary responsibilities are to take patients back to the examination rooms and to prepare them for procedures and treatments. I take the patient's chief complaint and health history. I greet each patient in a kind and calm way. This helps put the patient at ease before the physician goes into the examining room.

I once worked in a private office with a small waiting room and a narrow hall. One of my regular patients was a healthy 20-year-old man who was confined to a wheelchair by a spinal injury from an automobile accident. He had great difficulty maneuvering his motorized chair in tight spaces, and he felt embarrassed and conspicuous sitting in the middle of the waiting room. I began bringing him through the larger back door into the physician's office, directly into an examination room. Talking about things we had in common, such as interests in sports and movies, made him feel more at ease. By making the situation as easy as possible for him, I was able to help him keep his dignity while not drawing attention to his special needs.

FACTORS AFFECTING THE APPLICATION OF HEAT AND COLD

Before applying heat or cold, certain factors must be taken into consideration to prevent unfavorable reactions, such as tissue damage. The temperature may need to be adjusted based on the following conditions:

1. *The age of the patient.* Young children and elderly patients tend to be more sensitive to the application of heat or cold.
2. *Location of the application.* Certain areas of the body are more sensitive to the application of heat or cold, especially thin areas of the skin and areas that are usually covered by clothing, such as the chest, back, and abdomen. The skin on the hands and face is not as sensitive and is better able to tolerate temperature change. Broken skin, such as is found with an open wound, is more sensitive to heat and cold and is more prone to tissue damage.
3. *Impaired circulation.* Patients with impaired circulation tend to be more sensitive to heat and cold. This impairment may be at the site of the application or may be a systemic problem involving the entire body that is a result of certain conditions (e.g., peripheral vascular disease, diabetes mellitus, congestive heart failure).
4. *Impaired sensation.* Patients with impaired sensation, such as diabetic patients, must be watched carefully because tissue damage may occur from the application of heat or cold without the patient's awareness.
5. *Individual tolerance to change in temperature.* Some individuals cannot tolerate temperature change as easily as others.

The medical assistant should observe the area to which the heat or cold has been applied before, during, and after treatment for signs indicating that a modification of temperature is needed. The patient should also be asked whether the application feels comfortable or is too hot or too cold. Prolonged erythema or paleness, pain, swelling, and blisters should be reported to the provider.

HEAT

LOCAL EFFECTS OF HEAT

The application of moderate heat to a localized area of the body for a short time (approximately 15 to 30 minutes) produces *dilation,* or an increase in diameter, of the blood vessels in the area as the body tries to rid itself of excess heat (Fig. 7.1). This results in an increased blood supply to the area, and tissue metabolism increases. Nutrients and oxygen are provided to the cells at a faster rate, and wastes and toxins are carried away faster. The skin in the area becomes warm and exhibits erythema. **Erythema** is a reddening of the skin caused by dilation of superficial blood vessels in the skin.

These physiologic effects of moderate heat applied to a localized area promote healing. Prolonged application of heat (longer than 1 hour) produces secondary effects, however, that reverses this healing process. Blood vessels constrict, and blood supply to the area decreases. The medical assistant must be careful to apply heat for the length of time specified by the provider.

PURPOSE OF APPLYING HEAT

Heat functions in relieving pain, congestion, muscle spasms, and inflammation. Conditions for which the local application of heat is often prescribed are low back pain, arthritis, menstrual cramping, and localized abscesses.

Heat promotes muscle relaxation and is often used for the relief of pain caused by excessive contraction of muscle fibers. **Edema**, or swelling, in the tissues can be reduced through the application of heat because the increased blood supply functions to increase the absorption of fluid from the tissues through the lymphatic system.

Heat (usually in the form of a hot compress) can be used to soften exudates. A **compress** is a soft, moist, absorbent cloth that is folded in several layers and applied to a part of the body in the local application of heat or cold. An **exudate** is a discharge produced by the body's tissues. Exudates may sometimes form a hard crust over an area and require removal. Heat also increases **suppuration**, or the process of pus formation, to help in the relief of inflammation by breaking down infected tissues. Heat is not recommended,

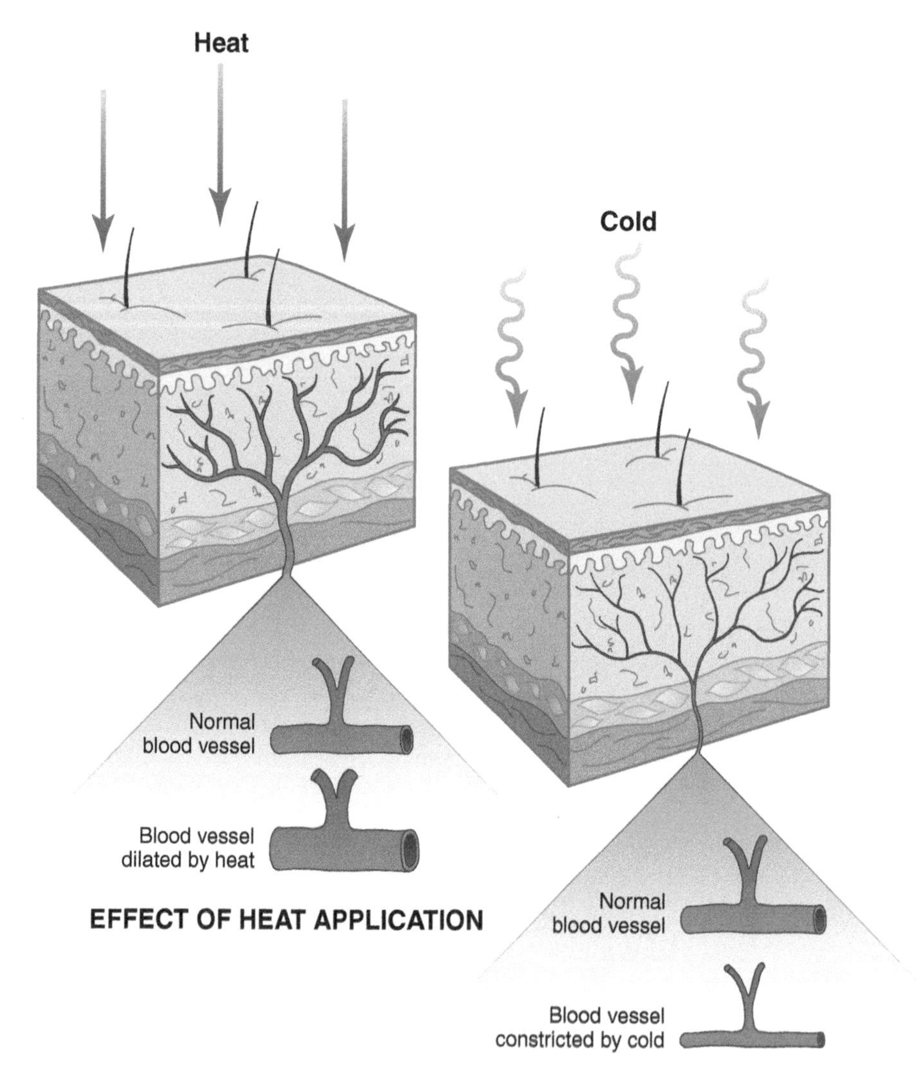

Fig. 7.1 Effects of the local application of heat and cold. (From Wood LA, Rambo BJ: *Nursing skills for allied health services*, vol 2, Philadelphi; WB Saunders; 1980.)

however, for the initial treatment of acute inflammation or trauma.

TYPES OF HEAT APPLICATIONS

The most common types of heat applications are described next, along with the conditions they are often used to treat.

Heating Pad

Heating pads are often used to relieve pain and muscle spasms. A heating pad consists of a network of wires that converts electrical energy into heat to provide a constant and even heat application. The wires must not be bent or crushed. This could damage the pad, resulting in overheating of parts of the pad and leading to burns or fire. Pins must not be inserted into the pad as a means of securing it; if a pin comes in contact with a wire, an electric shock could result. To prevent electric hazards, heating pads should not be used over areas that contain moisture, such as wet dressings.

Hot Soak

A **soak** is the direct immersion of a body part in water or a medicated solution. A soak can be applied to an extremity or a part of the torso. Hot soaks are often prepared using a ratio (e.g., two parts water to one part medication), and are used to cleanse open wounds, increase suppuration, increase the blood supply to an area to hasten the healing process, and apply a medicated solution to an area.

Hot Compress

A hot compress is a soft, moist, absorbent cloth, such as a washcloth, that is immersed in a warm solution and applied to a body part. Hot compresses are used to increase suppuration, improve circulation to a body part to aid in healing, promote drainage from infection, and soften exudates.

Applying a hot compress to an open wound requires the use of a sterile technique.

Chemical Hot Pack

Chemical hot packs are available in a variety of sizes and shapes. When activated, they provide a specific degree of heat for a specific period of time (usually 30 to 60 minutes), as indicated on the package label. A chemical hot pack consists of a vinyl bag containing calcium chloride crystals and a smaller bag (encased in the vinyl bag) containing water. Pressure is applied with the hands to break the inner bag. The water in the inner bag combines with the calcium chloride crystals to produce heat. After using the pack, it should be discarded in an appropriate receptacle. Chemical hot packs should be stored at room temperature and are used as an alternative to a heating pad to relieve pain and muscle spasms.

Procedures 7.1–7.3, and 7.6 (see later) present the proper application of heat with a heating pad, a hot soak, a hot compress, and a chemical hot pack.

What Would You Do? What Would You *Not* Do?

Case Study 1

Aaron Collins is at the office. Aaron recently helped a friend move, and the next day he developed intense pain in his lower back. To alleviate the pain, he slept on a heating pad, but when he woke up, his back was red and blistered. Aaron says he turned the setting on the heating pad to high because his back was hurting so much and he thought that it would help his back feel better sooner. Aaron wants to know the best way to apply heat using a heating pad. He also wants to know what he can do to prevent low back pain in the future.

COLD

LOCAL EFFECTS OF COLD

The application of moderate cold to a localized area produces constriction, or a decrease in diameter, of blood vessels in the area as the body attempts to prevent heat loss (see Fig. 7.1). This constriction leads to a decreased blood supply to the area. Tissue metabolism decreases, less oxygen is used, and fewer wastes accumulate. The skin becomes cool and pale. Prolonged application of cold (longer than 1 hour) has a reverse secondary effect. Blood vessels dilate, and tissue metabolism is increased. To prevent secondary effects, the medical assistant must only apply cold for the recommended length of time.

PURPOSE OF APPLYING COLD

The application of moderate cold for a short time is used to prevent edema. Cold may be applied immediately after an individual has sustained direct trauma, such as a bruise, minor burn, sprain, strain, joint injury, or fracture. A **sprain** involves trauma to a joint that causes injury to the ligaments, while a **strain** is the overstretching of a muscle caused by trauma. The cold limits the accumulation of fluid in the body tissues by constricting blood vessels and reducing the leakage of fluid into the tissues. Through constriction of peripheral blood vessels, cold can be used to control bleeding. Cold temporarily relieves pain through its anesthetic, or numbing, effect, which reduces stimulation of the pain receptors. Cold also slows the movement of blood and tissue fluids in the affected area, resulting in less pressure against pain receptors and therefore less pain. In the early stages of an infection, the local application of cold inhibits the activity of microorganisms. In this way, suppuration is decreased, and inflammation is reduced. Cold applications should always be placed in a protective covering because applying cold directly to the skin could result in a skin burn.

TYPES OF COLD APPLICATIONS

Ice Bag

An ice bag consists of a waterproof bag with a screw-on cap. Before use, it must be filled with small pieces of ice and placed in a protective covering. Ice bags are used to prevent swelling, control bleeding, and relieve pain and inflammation.

Cold Compress

A cold compress is a soft, moist, absorbent cloth, such as a washcloth, that is immersed in a cold solution and applied to a body part. Cold compresses are used to relieve pain and inflammation and to treat conditions such as headache, injury to the eye, and pain after tooth extraction.

Chemical Cold Pack

Chemical cold packs are available in a variety of sizes and shapes. When activated, they provide a specific degree of coldness for a specific period of time (usually 30 to 60 minutes), as indicated on the package label. Most cold packs consist of a vinyl bag of ammonium nitrate crystals. Enclosed in this bag is a smaller vinyl bag of water. The cold pack is activated by applying pressure until the inner bag ruptures. This releases the water into the larger bag, and a chemical reaction occurs between the crystals and the water, producing coldness. These packs are disposable, and when the coldness diminishes, they should be discarded in an appropriate receptacle. Chemical cold packs should be stored at room temperature. They are used as an alternative to ice bags for the local application of cold to prevent swelling, control bleeding, and relieve pain and inflammation.

Procedures 7.4–7.6 present proper application of cold with an ice bag, a cold compress, and a chemical cold pack.

Gel Pack

A gel pack consists of a reusable vinyl or nylon bag containing a water-based gel that can be heated or cooled (Fig. 7.2). A gel pack is flexible and molds well to a body area.

Gel packs can be used for the local application of heat as an alternative to a heating pad, or the local application of cold as an alternative to an ice bag. Before using a gel pack, it is important to check it for damage. If the bag is ruptured or leaking, it must be discarded. Depending on the type of application required, the pack should be heated or cooled by carefully following the specific instructions accompanying the pack. General guidelines for the application of a gel pack are outlined in Box 7.1.

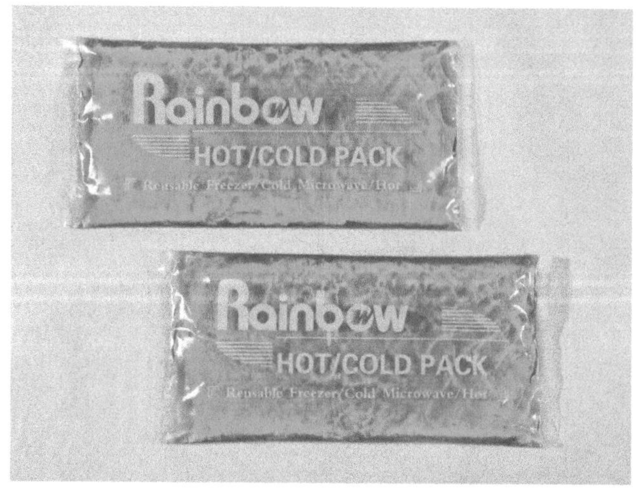

Fig. 7.2 Gel packs.

PATIENT COACHING Low Back Pain

Answer questions patients have about low back pain.

What causes low back pain?

Low back pain is one of the most common health problems in the United States. Approximately 80% of Americans are affected by low back pain at some time during their life. The most frequent cause of low back pain is poor posture and poor body mechanics, which strain the muscles and ligaments that support the back. Most cases of low back pain can be prevented by practicing good body mechanics. Other causes of low back pain include physical inactivity, excessive body weight, disc damage, osteoarthritis, spondylitis, and congenital deformities.

What is the treatment for low back pain?

To treat low back pain caused by strain, the provider may prescribe a combination of one or more of the following: bed rest, local application of heat or cold, massage, medications, back manipulation, use of back-supporting devices, deep-heating treatments such as ultrasound, and exercises to strengthen the supporting structures of the back and prevent the back pain from recurring or becoming chronic.

How can low back pain be prevented?

- Wear comfortable low-heeled shoes that offer good support.
- Maintain correct posture while sitting, standing, and sleeping.
- Never lift anything heavier than you can easily manage. To lift an object, always bend the body at the knees and hips. Never bend from the waist. List the object with the leg muscles and hold it close to the body at waist level. Never lift anything higher than chest level.
- Sit in a chair with a firm back.
- The car seat should be positioned so that the driver's back is straight, and the knees are raised.
- Maintain a healthy body weight.

BOX 7.1 Gel Pack Application Guidelines

Gel Pack Heat Therapy

1. A gel pack used for heat therapy should be stored at room temperature.
2. Before heating the pack, the gel should be evenly distributed in the pack and the pack laid flat in a microwave.
3. Microwave the gel pack on high power for the length of time specified in the instructions accompanying the pack (usually 1 min).
4. Use heat resistant gloves to remove the gel pack from the microwave.
5. Knead the gel pack using heat-resistant gloves to evenly distribute the heat in the pack.
6. If the pack is too hot, allow it to cool before applying it to the treatment area.
7. If the pack is not hot enough, return it to the microwave and heat the pack in 10-s intervals until it reaches the desired temperature.
8. Make sure to avoid overheating the gel pack to prevent it from swelling up and bursting.
9. Before application to the treatment area, wrap the gel pack in a protective covering such as a dry towel to provide for patient comfort.

Gel Pack Cold Therapy

1. Place the gel pack in the freezer for the length of time specified in the instructions accompanying the pack (usually 1–2 h).
2. The gel pack can be permanently stored in the freezer.
3. Before application to the treatment area, wrap the gel pack in a protective covering such as a dry towel to provide for patient comfort.

Casts

A **cast** is a stiff cylindrical casing that is used to immobilize a body part until healing occurs. Casts are applied most often when an individual sustains a fracture (Fig. 7.3). The cast keeps the fractured bones aligned until proper healing occurs. Casts also are used to support and stabilize weak or dislocated joints; to promote healing after a surgical correction, such as knee surgery; and to aid in the nonsurgical correction of deformities, such as congenital dislocation of the hip.

Casts are applied by an orthopedist, also known as an *orthopedic surgeon*. An **orthopedist** is a physician who specializes in the diagnosis and treatment of disorders of the musculoskeletal system. An orthopedist treats patients with deformities, injuries, and diseases of the bones, joints, ligaments, tendons, muscles, nerves, and skin. The role of the medical assistant in cast application is to assemble the equipment and supplies, prepare the patient for the procedure, assist the provider during the application, provide or reinforce cast care instructions, and clean the examining room after the application.

An important goal of cast management is the prevention of pressure areas, which are most apt to occur over bony prominences. A *pressure area* occurs when the cast presses or rubs against the patient's skin and prevents adequate circulation to the area. When this occurs, the patient usually feels a painful rubbing, burning, or stinging sensation under the cast. If permitted to continue, the pressure can cause the skin to break down, leading to the development of a *pressure ulcer* (Fig. 7.4). If not treated, a pressure ulcer progresses from a simple red patch of skin to erosion into the subcutaneous tissue and eventually erosion into the muscle and bone. Deep pressure ulcers often become infected by invading organisms and develop gangrene. It is important to detect the occurrence of a pressure area early so that prompt treatment can be instituted to prevent serious complications.

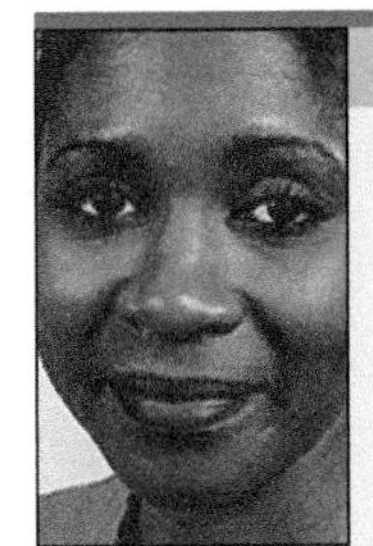

Memories *from* Practicum

Marlyne: At my first practicum site, I was scared to death about having to give injections to small children. I did not want to hurt them. A 6-month-old infant was brought to the office for her immunizations. My practicum supervisor wanted me to give the injections. The infant was so small, and she was crying before I even gave her the first injection. I knew that when I gave the injection, she was going to cry even more and that made me feel bad. My supervisor was there with me, and she talked me through it. It turned out that it was not as bad as I had thought it would be. My supervisor was very helpful in keeping me calm. After that first experience, I felt much more comfortable when I had to give an injection to a small child.

SYNTHETIC CASTS

Synthetic casts are the most common type of cast used to immobilize a body part. A synthetic cast consists of knitted fabric tape made of fiberglass, polyester and cotton, or plastic. The tape is impregnated with polyurethane resin that is activated when soaked in water. Of the three kinds of synthetic material, fiberglass is used most often. Synthetic tape comes in different colors and is packaged as an individual roll in an airtight pouch (Fig. 7.5). Synthetic tape is available in widths ranging from 2 to 8 inches.

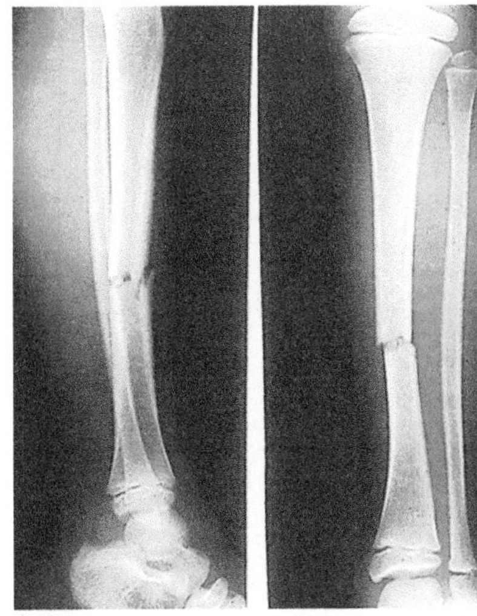

Fig. 7.3 A fracture of the tibia in the left lower leg. (From McRae R, Esser M: *Practical fracture treatment*, ed 4, Philadelphia: Churchill Livingstone; 2002.)

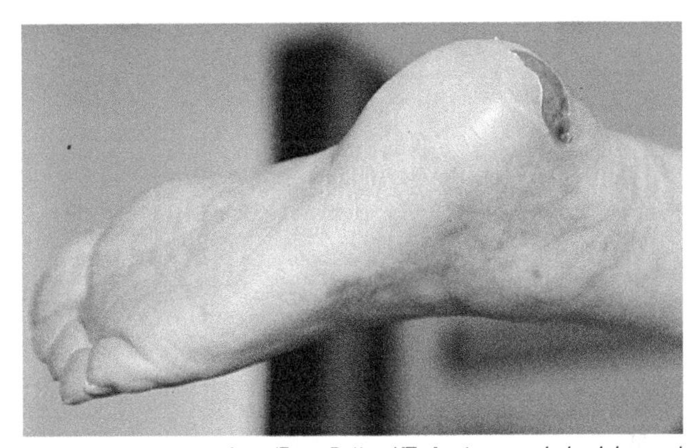

Fig. 7.4 Pressure ulcer. (From Patton KT: *Anatomy and physiology*, ed 9, St Louis: Elsevier; 2016.)

CAST APPLICATION

The provider applies the cast so that it fits snugly but still allows adequate circulation necessary for proper healing. Four to 6 weeks are usually required for the complete healing of a fracture.

Casts are classified according to the body part they cover. The types of casts most frequently applied in the medical office and common uses of each are illustrated and described in Fig. 7.6. The type of cast applied depends on the nature of the patient's injury or condition. A **short arm cast** is used for a dislocated wrist, and a **long arm cast** is used for a fracture of the humerus.

The following steps are performed in applying a cast:

1. **Inspect the skin.** The area to which the cast is to be applied must be clean and dry. The patient's skin should be inspected for redness, bruises, and open areas. This information should be documented in the patient's medical record because it may assist in evaluating patient complaints after the cast has been applied.

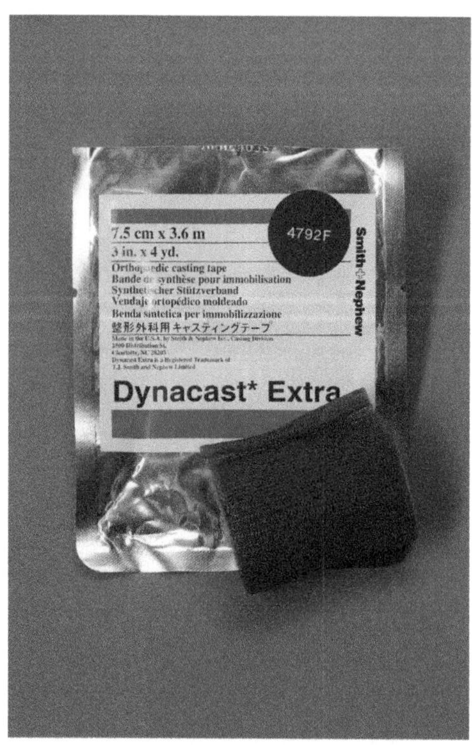

Fig. 7.5 A roll of synthetic tape comes packaged in an airtight pouch.

Short arm cast

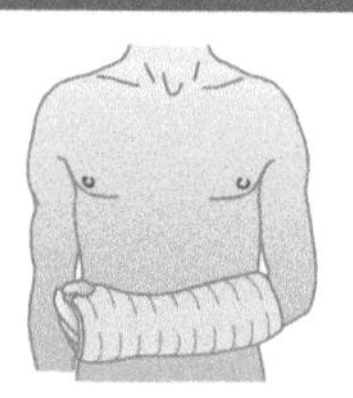

Extends from below the elbow to the fingers.

Use:
- Fracture of the hand or wrist
- Postoperative immobilization

Long arm cast

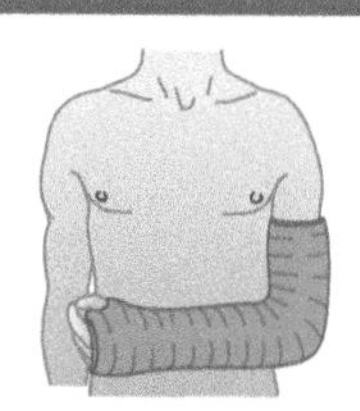

Extends from the upper arm to the fingers, usually with a bend in the elbow.

Use:
- Fracture of the humerus, forearm, or elbow
- Postoperative immobilization

Short leg cast

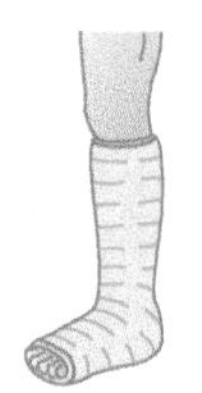

Begins just below the knee and extends to the toes.

Use:
- Fracture of the foot, ankle, or distal tibia or fibula
- Severe sprain or strain
- Postoperative immobilization
- Correction of a deformity

Long leg cast

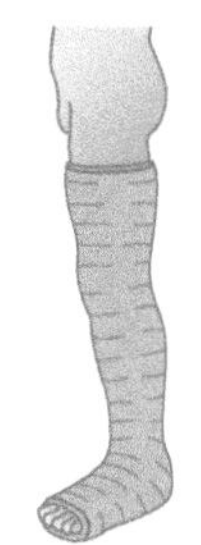

Extends from the midthigh to the toes.

Use:
- Fracture of the distal femur, knee, or lower leg
- Soft tissue injury to the knee or knee dislocation
- Postoperative immobilization

Fig. 7.6 Types of casts.

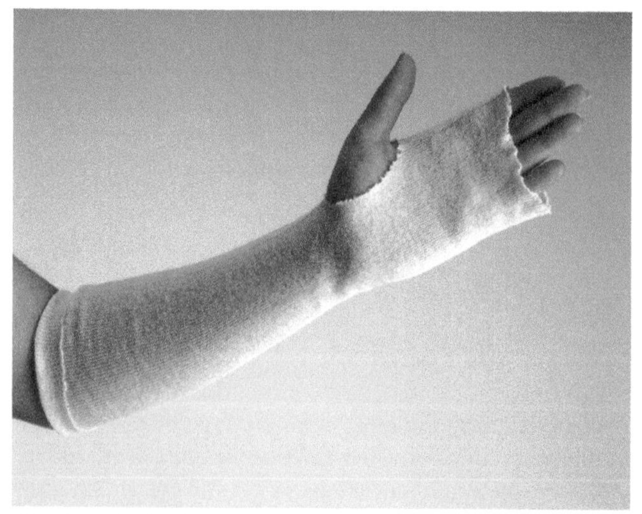

Fig. 7.7 Application of a stockinette.

2. **Apply the stockinette.** Before applying the cast, the provider covers the body part with a stockinette (Fig. 7.7). A stockinette consists of a soft, tubular, knitted cotton material that stretches up to three times its original width to accommodate the diameter of the body part. It is put on like a stocking. The purpose of the stockinette is to provide patient comfort and to cover the rough edges at the ends of the cast. Stockinettes come in widths ranging from 2 to 12 inches; the width used depends on the diameter of the part to be covered. Typically, a 3-inch width is used for arm casts, a 4-inch width is used for leg casts, and a 10- to 12-inch width is used for body casts.
3. **Apply the cast padding.** Cast padding consists of a soft cotton material that comes in a roll in widths ranging from 2 to 6 inches. The purpose of cast padding is to prevent pressure areas and to shield the patient's skin when the cast is removed. Two or three layers are applied directly over the stockinette, using a spiral turn. Each turn overlaps the preceding one by one-half the width of the roll. Extra layers of padding are applied over bony prominences to prevent pressure areas (Fig. 7.8).
4. **Prepare the synthetic tape.** The roll of synthetic tape is fully immersed in cool, room-temperature water (68°F to 75°F [20°C to 24°C]) for a period of time recommended by the manufacturer. Fiberglass tape is immersed for 5 to 15 seconds. The airtight pouch containing a roll of synthetic tape should remain sealed until just before it is time to immerse the roll in the water. This is because air causes the resin in the tape to harden and become rigid, making it unacceptable for use.
5. **Apply the cast tape.** The synthetic tape is applied over the cast padding. The provider wears rubber gloves during the procedure to protect the hands from the casting material. The tape is wrapped over the body part, using a spiral turn, until the desired number of layers have been applied (Fig. 7.9). Generally, three or four layers are applied for a non–weight-bearing cast (e.g., short

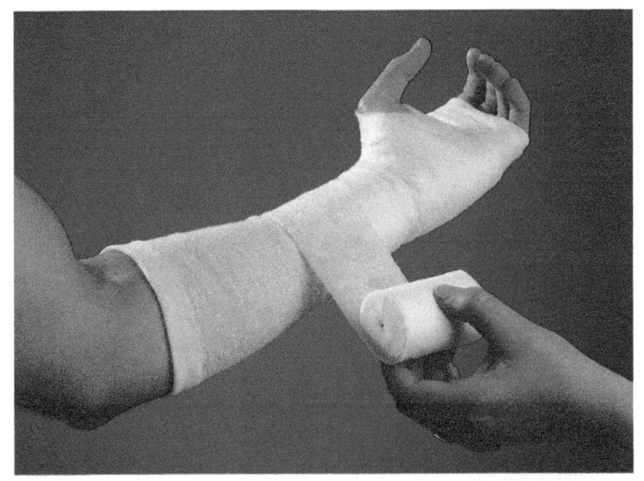

Fig. 7.8 Application of cast padding. (Courtesy 3M Health Care, St Paul, MN.)

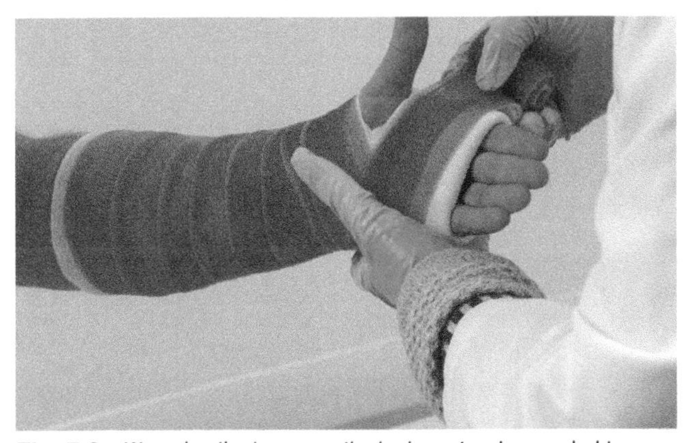

Fig. 7.9 Wrapping the tape over the body part, using a spiral turn.

arm cast or long arm cast), and five to eight layers are applied for a weight-bearing cast (e.g., **short leg cast** or **long leg cast**).

6. **Allow the cast to dry.** The cast is allowed to dry for a period of time specified by the manufacturer. A fiberglass cast usually dries within 30 minutes. Only when a cast is completely dry does it become hard and inflexible and able to bear weight. The provider usually prescribes a supportive device, such as a sling or crutches, to prevent unnecessary strain and to minimize swelling during the healing process.

PRECAUTIONS

The following precautions should be observed during and after cast application.

- Remove excess casting particles. Remove synthetic casting material with a swab moistened with alcohol or acetone. If cast particles are not removed, they may work their way under the cast, resulting in irritation and infection.
- Before the patient leaves the medical office, the provider checks the circulation, sensation, and movement of the exposed extremity to ensure that the cast is not too tight. The provider also ensures that all joints excluded from the cast are free to move.

GUIDELINES FOR CAST CARE

The medical assistant is often responsible for explaining or reinforcing the guidelines that should be followed by a patient with a cast to promote the healing process. These guidelines are often presented on an instruction sheet that is signed by the patient, with a copy filed in the patient's medical record. Guidelines for cast care include the following:

- Allow the cast to dry before putting any pressure or weight on the cast. Synthetic casts can bear weight approximately 30 minutes to 1 hour after application.
- Elevate the cast above heart level for the first 24 to 48 hours to decrease swelling and pain. This can be accomplished by propping the casted extremity on pillows or some other type of support.
- Gently move the toes or fingers frequently to prevent swelling and joint stiffness and to increase circulation.
- Apply ice to the casted extremity to reduce swelling. Place small pieces of ice in an ice bag, and loosely wrap it around the cast at the level of the injury.
- Take precautions to prevent dirt, sand, powder, and other foreign particles from becoming trapped under the cast. They can cause irritation to the skin, leading to infection.
- Do not apply powder for itching under the cast. Do not use any object to scratch the skin under the cast. Inserting anything under the cast, such as a pencil, coat hanger, or knitting needle, may cause a break in the skin, which could become infected. Also, the object may become lost in the cast.
- Do not engage in activities that could cause injury because of impairment of your physical abilities (e.g., driving a car).
- Keep the cast dry. When taking a bath or shower, cover the cast with a plastic bag and secure the bag to the skin with waterproof tape. If possible, hang the casted limb over the side of the tub or outside of the shower. Although the material making up a synthetic cast is moisture-resistant, the cast padding is not. If a synthetic cast becomes wet, it must be dried as soon as possible to prevent maceration. **Maceration** is the softening and breaking down of the skin, which can lead to infection.
- To dry a wet cast, first, blot the outside of the cast with an absorbent towel. This should be followed by the application of a blow dryer on a cool or the lowest heat setting using a sweeping motion over the entire cast until it is completely dry. The patient should be instructed not to use the high setting on the blow dryer because this amount of heat could burn the skin.
- Inspect the skin around the cast at regular intervals to check for redness, sores, or swelling.
- Do not trim the cast or break off any rough edges because this may weaken or break the cast. If the surface of the cast has a rough edge, a metal nail file or emery board

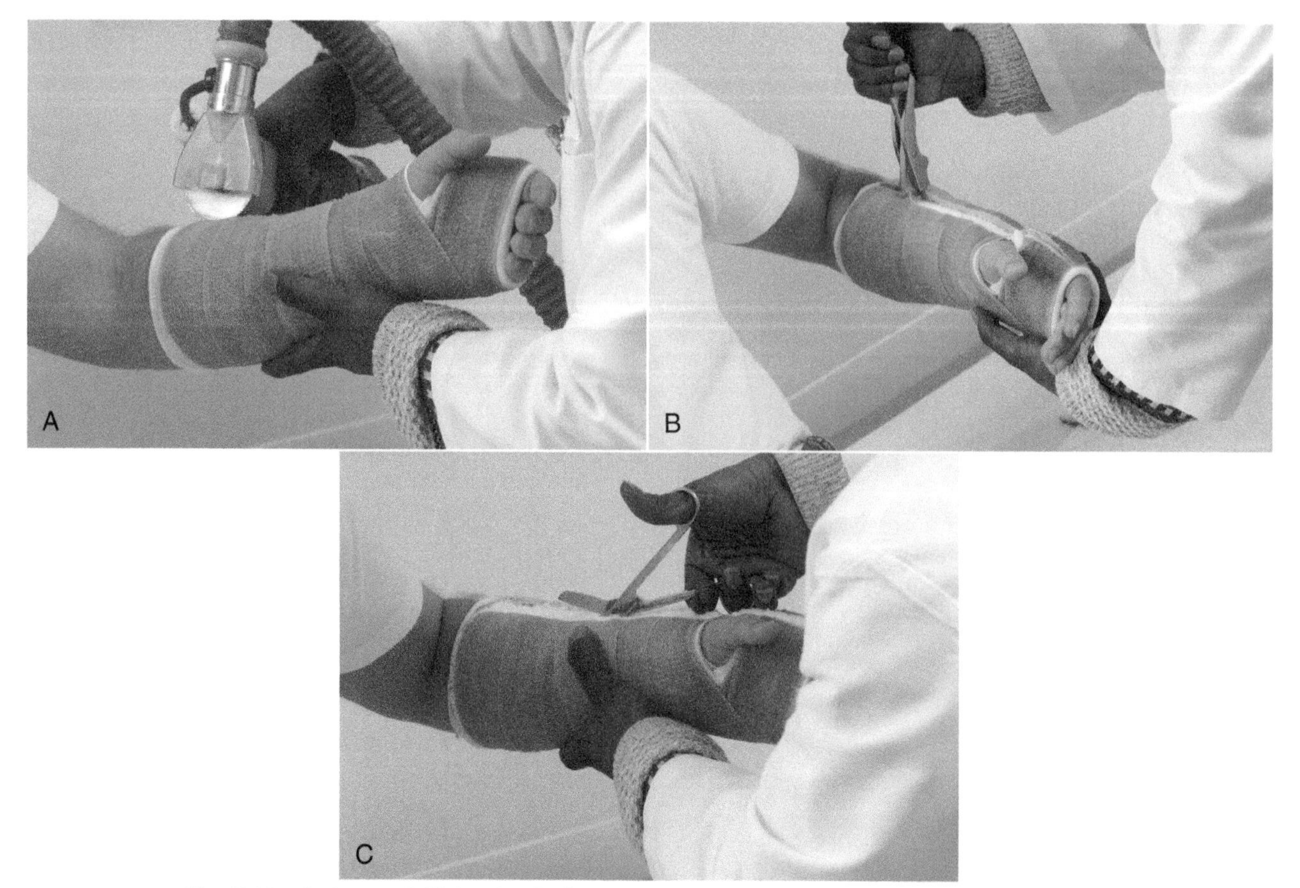

Fig. 7.10 Cast removal. (A) A cast cutter is used to cut the entire length of the cast. (B) The cast is pried open with a cast spreader. (C) Bandage scissors are used to cut through the cast padding and stockinette.

can be used to smooth it. Notify the provider if the cast becomes loose, broken, dented, or cracked, because the cast may need to be replaced.

SYMPTOMS TO REPORT

The patient should report the following symptoms *immediately* to the provider; they may indicate that the cast is too tight, or an infection is developing:

- Increased pain or swelling that does not go away with the application of an ice bag, medication, elevation, or rest
- A feeling that the cast is too tight. Slight pressure applied with the thumbnail to the fingernail or toenail should cause it to blanch white, and then when the pressure is released, the nail should immediately return to its normal color. If this does not occur, it could indicate insufficient blood flow to the extremity from a cast that is too tight.
- Tingling, numbness, or loss of movement of the fingers or toes
- Coldness, paleness, or blueness of the fingers or toes
- Painful rubbing, burning, or stinging under the cast
- Foul odor or drainage coming from the cast
- Sore areas around the edge of the cast
- Chills, fever, nausea, or vomiting

CAST REMOVAL

The easiest and safest way to remove a cast is to bivalve it—this means cutting the cast into two halves, resulting in an anterior shell and a posterior shell. To bivalve a cast, the provider cuts the entire length of the cast on two opposite sides down to the level of the cast padding. The cuts are made with a cast cutter. A cast cutter is a handheld electric saw with a circular blade that oscillates, which means that the saw vibrates but does not rotate (Fig. 7.10A). The medical assistant should reassure the patient that, although the saw is noisy, only a tickling sensation and some heat are felt from the saw's vibration. After cutting the cast, the provider pries it apart with a cast spreader (see Fig. 7.10B). Next, the provider uses bandage scissors to cut through the cast padding and stockinette (see Fig. 7.10C). The cast is carefully removed from the patient's extremity.

The skin of the affected extremity typically appears yellow and scaly. The extremity also appears thinner, and the muscles are flabby. The medical assistant should explain to the patient that this is normal and results from a lack of use of the extremity. The provider may recommend exercises or physical therapy or both to help the patient regain strength and function of the body part.

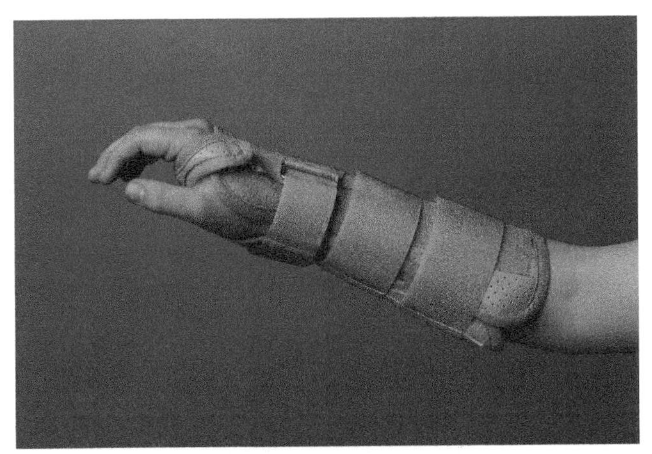

Fig. 7.11 Arm splint.

What Would You Do? What Would You *Not* Do?

Case Study 2

Christina Themes calls the office. Two days ago, Christina fell while she was inline skating and broke the radius and ulna of her right arm. The physician applied a long arm fiberglass cast. While at the medical office, Christina received oral and written instructions on how to care for her cast. Christina says that in all the confusion, she misplaced the instructions. She said she didn't want to bother anyone at the office, so she did what she could to make her arm feel better. She says that it didn't work because now her arm is swollen and hurts. She took a bath, and the cast got wet, so she wants to know how to dry it. Christina asks if it would be possible to have one of those removable casts, so she can take it off when she takes a bath.

SPLINTS AND BRACES

Along with casts, splints and braces are used to assist in the treatment of fractures. A **splint** is a rigid removable device used to support and immobilize a displaced or fractured part of the body. Splints also are commonly used to protect areas that are sprained or strained. Splints are molded to fit specific parts of the body and are well padded to provide patient comfort and to prevent pressure areas. A splint can be custom made by an orthopedist using plaster or fiberglass casting materials. Splints also are commercially available and consist of two parts: a rigid material such as plastic or fiberglass, and straps with Velcro that hold the splint in place (Fig. 7.11).

A splint may be applied initially to a fractured limb because it can be adjusted to accommodate swelling from injuries more easily than a cast. After the swelling subsides, a cast is usually applied. When the fracture is almost healed, the cast may be removed, and another splint applied. This allows for bathing of the extremity and easy removal for therapy until the fracture heals completely and the splint is no longer needed.

A **brace** is designed to support a part of the body and hold it in its correct position to allow for the functioning of the body part while healing takes place. An example of a brace is a *short leg walker,* which consists of a rigid lightweight frame with a removable padded liner (Fig. 7.12). A short leg walker is often used, instead of a cast, to heal a stable fracture (e.g., stress fracture) of the lower leg. A short leg walker is available in different sizes so it can be properly fitted to extend from just below the patient's knee to the toes. Special fasteners or straps with Velcro are used to hold the walker in place and allow for adjustment of it (see Fig. 7.12). A short leg walker permits walking and standing, which encourage healing. It also can be removed to permit bathing of the leg.

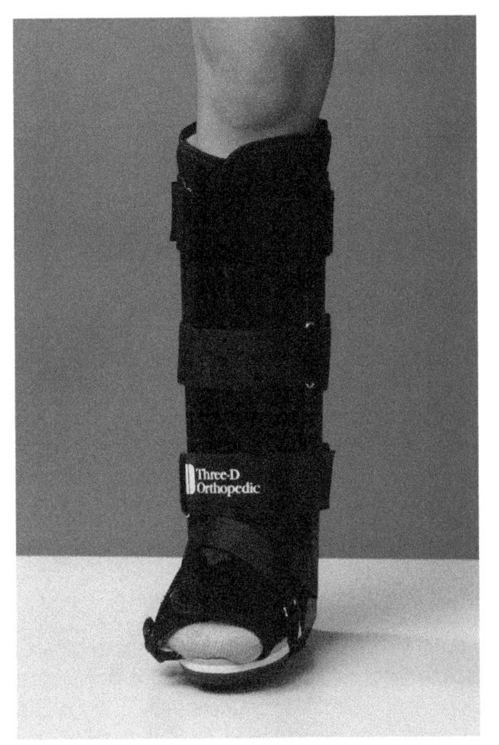

Fig. 7.12 Short leg walker, which is an example of a leg brace.

PATIENT COACHING Cast Care

- Teach the patient the important guidelines of cast care.
- Emphasize the importance of contacting the provider immediately if any signs of circulatory impairment or infection occur.
- If the provider has prescribed cold to reduce swelling, teach the patient the procedure for applying an ice bag to the casted extremity.
- Emphasize the importance of returning to have the cast checked by the provider.
- If the provider prescribes isometric exercises to maintain the muscle tone of the affected extremity, provide the patient with a sheet that illustrates the exercises.
- Provide the patient with printed materials on cast care.

Ambulatory Aids

Mechanical assistive devices are used by individuals who require aid in ambulation. The word **ambulation** means walking; patients who are **ambulatory** are able to walk as opposed to being confined to a wheelchair or a bed. Ambulatory aids

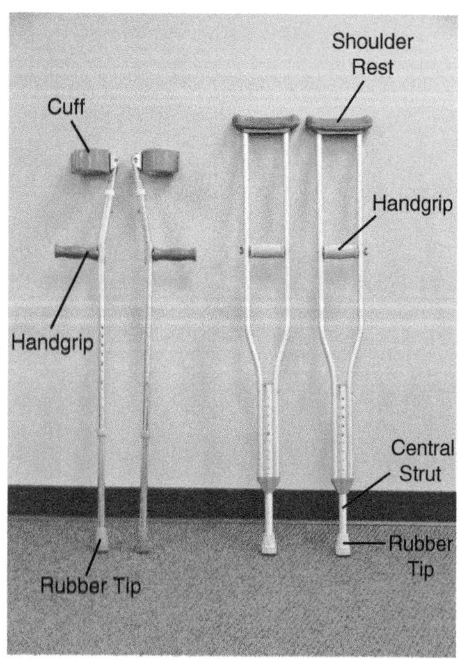

Fig. 7.13 Types of crutches. Forearm crutch is on the left and axillary crutch is on the right. (Modified from Niedzwiecki B, Pepper J, Weaver PA: *Kinn's the medical assistant*, ed 14, St. Louis: Elsevier; 2020.)

include crutches, canes, and walkers. The device used depends on factors such as the type and severity of the disability, the amount of support required, and the patient's age and degree of muscular coordination. The ambulatory aid may be prescribed for a temporary condition, such as a fracture, a sprain to a lower extremity, and disability after orthopedic surgery. It also may be prescribed for a long-term condition, such as paralysis, deformity, and permanent weakness of the lower extremities.

CRUTCHES

Crutches are artificial supports that are used by patients requiring assistance in walking as a result of disease, injury, or birth defects of the lower extremities. Crutches function by removing weight from the legs and transferring it to the arms. The two main crutch types are the axillary crutch and the forearm crutch (Fig. 7.13). The axillary crutch and the forearm crutch require rubber tips, which increase surface tension, to prevent the crutches from slipping on the floor.

The *axillary crutch* is used most frequently and is made of tubular aluminum or wood. This type of crutch has a shoulder rest and handgrips and extends from the ground almost to the patient's axilla.

The *forearm crutch* (also known as an *elbow crutch)* consists of a single adjustable tube of aluminum that extends to the forearm. A metal or plastic cuff attached to the crutch fits securely around the patient's forearm, and a handgrip covered with rubber extends from the crutch for weight-bearing. The cuff and the handgrip stabilize the patient's wrists to make walking safer and easier. One advantage of the forearm crutch is that the individual can release the handgrip, enabling use of the hand, while the cuff holds the crutch in place. Forearm crutches are used most often by individuals with long term disabilities such as paraplegia or cerebral palsy.

AXILLARY CRUTCH MEASUREMENT

The patient must be measured for axillary crutches to ensure the correct crutch length and proper placement of the handgrip. Incorrectly fitted crutches increase the patient's risk of developing back pain, nerve damage, and injuries to the axillae and palms of the hands. Procedure 7.7 presents the correct way to measure a patient for axillary crutches.

If the crutches are too long, the shoulder rests exert pressure on the patient's axillae. This can injure the radial nerve in the brachial plexus, which eventually may lead to *crutch palsy*, a condition of muscular weakness in the forearm, wrist, and hand. In addition, crutches that are too long force the patient's shoulders forward, preventing the patient from pushing his or her body off the ground. Crutches that are too short force the patient to be bent over and uncomfortable, also making them awkward to use. If the handgrips are too low, pressure is put on the patient's axillae, whereas handgrips that are too high are awkward.

Aluminum crutches consist of aluminum tubes. Spring-loaded pushbuttons on an inner tube "pop out" into holes on an outer tube to allow proper adjustment of the crutch length.

Wooden crutches are made with bolts and wing nuts, which allow proper adjustment of the length and handgrip level.

PATIENT COACHING Crutches

- Teach patients the guidelines for the proper use of crutches.
- Provide the patient with an exercise sheet that illustrates exercises to strengthen arm muscles before beginning crutch walking.
- Teach the patient the crutch gaits prescribed by the provider, and have the patient demonstrate the gaits before leaving the office.
- Provide the patient with a list of local vendors who provide crutch services, such as repairs and supplies (e.g., rubber tips, crutch pads).
- Provide the patient with printed educational materials on the use of crutches and crutch gaits.

CRUTCH GUIDELINES

It is important that the patient receive specific guidelines to ensure safety while using crutches, to prevent injuries and falls. The medical assistant is responsible for instructing the patient in the following guidelines:

1. Wear well-fitting flat shoes with firm, nonskid soles to provide good traction and stability.
2. Use good posture to prevent strain on muscles and joints and to maintain proper body balance.
3. Support your weight with your hands on the handgrips and the axillary pads pressing against the sides of the rib cage.

The body weight should not be supported by the axillae because the pressure on the axillae may cause crutch palsy.

4. Look ahead when walking, rather than down at your feet.
5. Be aware of the surface on which you are walking. It should be clean, flat, dry, and well-lit. Throw rugs and objects serving as obstacles should temporarily be removed from your environment to prevent falls.
6. Keep the crutches about 4 to 6 inches out from the sides of your feet when walking to prevent obstruction of the pathway for the feet.
7. Take steps by moving the crutches forward a safe and comfortable distance, preferably 6 inches. When first learning to use the crutches, take small steps rather than large ones. Do not move forward more than 12 to 15 inches with each step. A greater distance might cause the crutches to slide forward and make you lose your balance.
8. Report tingling or numbness in the upper body to the provider. You might be using the crutches incorrectly, or they might be the wrong size for you.
9. Extra padding can be added to the shoulder rests of your crutches to make them more comfortable. If you do this, ensure that the extra padding does not press against your axillae, but rather against your lateral rib cage. The handgrips also can be padded for increased comfort.
10. To prevent slipping, keep the crutch tips dry to maintain their surface friction. If they become wet, dry them completely before use.
11. Inspect the crutch tips regularly. They should be securely attached. If the crutch tips are worn down, they should be replaced with tips of the proper size.
12. For wooden crutches, periodically check the wing nuts holding the central strut and handgrips in place to ensure that they are tight.

CRUTCH GAITS

The type of crutch gait used depends on the amount of weight the patient is able to support with one or both legs and the patient's physical condition and muscular coordination. The patient should learn both a fast and slow gait. The faster gait is used for making speed in open areas, and the slower one is used in crowded places. In addition, learning more than one gait reduces patient fatigue because a different combination of muscles is used for each gait. Procedure 7.8 provides guidelines and charts for use in instructing the patient on how to walk with crutches.

CANES

A cane is a lightweight, easily movable device made of aluminum or wood with a rubber tip and is used to help provide balance and support. Canes are generally used by patients who have weakness on one side of the body, such as patients with hemiparesis, joint disabilities, or defects of the neuromuscular system. The three main types of canes are: the *standard cane,* the *tripod cane,* and the *quad cane* (Fig. 7.14). The standard cane provides the least amount of support and is used by patients who require only slight assistance in walking. The tripod and quad canes have three and four legs, respectively, a bent shaft, and a T-shaped handle with grips. They are easier to hold and provide greater stability than a standard cane because of the wider base of support. In addition, multilegged canes are able to stand alone, which frees the arms when the patient is getting up from a chair. The disadvantage of a multilegged cane is that it is bulkier and more difficult to move.

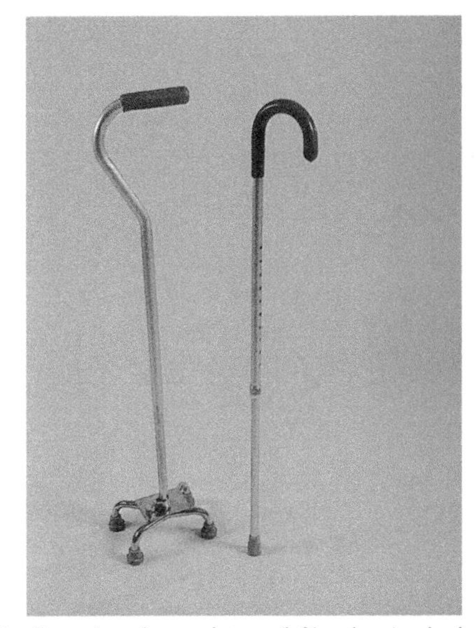

Fig. 7.14 Examples of a quad cane *(left)* and a standard cane *(right)*. (Courtesy 3M Health Care, St Paul, MN.)

A cane is held on the side of the body opposite the side that needs support. The cane length must be properly adjusted to ensure optimal stability. The cane handle should be approximately level with the greater trochanter, and the elbow should be flexed at a 25- to 30-degree angle. The patient should be instructed to stand erect and not lean on the cane to ensure good balance. Procedure 7.9 presents guidelines instructing the patient on how to walk with a cane.

WALKERS

A walker is an ambulatory aid consisting of an aluminum frame with handgrips and four widely placed legs with rubber suction tips and one open side (Fig. 7.15). A walker is light and easily movable. Walkers are available with wheels that facilitate the movement of the walker. They are also available with a fold-up feature that allows them to be easily transported in a vehicle. For proper ambulation, the walker should extend from the ground to approximately the level of the patient's hip joint. Procedure 7.10 presents guidelines on instructing the patient on how to walk with a walker.

Walkers are used most often by geriatric patients with weakness or balance problems. Walkers are also used during the healing process for patients who have had knee or hip joint replacement surgery. These patients need more help with balance and walking than can be provided by crutches or a cane. Because of its wide base, a walker provides the patient with a great amount of stability and security. Disadvantages of a walker include a slow pace and difficulty in maneuvering the walker in a small room.

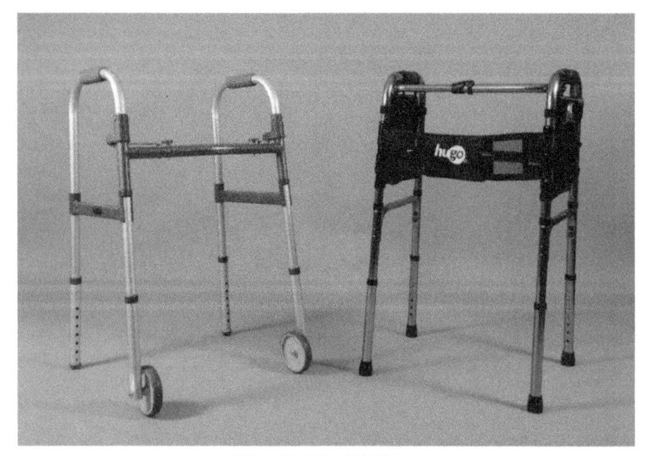

Fig. 7.15 Walkers.

What Would You Do? What Would You *Not* Do?

Case Study 3

Thaddeus Bernard calls the office. Thaddeus fractured the femur of his left leg 2 weeks ago in a skiing accident. The physician applied a long leg fiberglass cast, and Thaddeus was properly fitted with aluminum crutches. Thaddeus says that he is having some problems with his crutches. He is complaining of weakness in his forearms and hands and some tingling and numbness in his fingers. He also says that he has bruises under his arms. Thaddeus says that after he got home, his crutches did not seem to fit right, so he readjusted them. Thaddeus is getting ready to return to college and wants to know the best way to carry his books while using crutches.

What Would You Do? What Would You *Not* Do? RESPONSES

Case Study 1

Page 211

What Did Marlyne Do?

- ❑ Empathized with Aaron for being in so much pain.
- ❑ Explained to Aaron that he should never sleep on a heating pad because the heat builds up and causes the type of burn he experienced.
- ❑ Explained to Aaron that it is best to apply heat for 15 to 30 minutes at a time with the pad set no higher than the medium setting. Told him that the pad may not feel warm after his body gets used to it, but that it is still helping him. Told Aaron that the high setting could burn his skin.
- ❑ Told Aaron how to prevent low back pain by using good body mechanics, especially during lifting.

What Did Marlyne Not Do?

- ❑ Did not criticize Aaron for sleeping on the heating pad or turning the pad to the high setting.

Case Study 2

Page 217

What Did Marlyne Do?

- ❑ Reassured Christina that the medical staff is there to help her, and she should never hesitate to call when she needs information or is having a problem.
- ❑ Asked Christina what she did to try to make her arm feel better and documented this information in her medical record. Checked with the physician to determine whether he wanted to see Christina.
- ❑ Reeducated Christina on proper cast care instructions over the phone and mailed her another cast care instruction sheet.
- ❑ Explained to Christina how to dry her cast properly by first blotting it and then using a hairdryer. Told her that if she is unable to dry her cast completely, she will need to come in to have it replaced.
- ❑ Explained to Christina that the physician applied the type of cast that would best treat her injury and help her to heal.

What Did Marlyne Not Do?

- ❑ Did not criticize Christina for waiting so long to call the office.
- ❑ Did not tell Christina it would be a good idea for her to have a "removable cast."

Case Study 3

Page 220

What Did Marlyne Do?

- ❑ Listened carefully and empathetically to Thaddeus' problems with and concerns about his crutches.
- ❑ Explained to Thaddeus that the crutches were adjusted to fit him properly at the office and that some problems may have developed after he readjusted them.
- ❑ Scheduled an appointment for Thaddeus to come in that day so the physician could examine him, and his crutches could be checked for proper length.
- ❑ Went over crutch guidelines and crutch gaits with Thaddeus again when he came to the office for his appointment.
- ❑ Told Thaddeus that he should use a backpack to carry his books to keep his hands free to move on his crutches. Stressed that he should keep his backpack as light as possible and keep the weight evenly distributed on his back (i.e., use both straps).

What Did Marlyne Not Do?

- ❑ Did not tell Thaddeus to readjust the crutches himself.
- ❑ Did not tell Thaddeus that he should have paid more attention when he was being instructed in crutch guidelines.

Terminology Review

Medical Term	Word Parts	Definition
Ambulation		Walking or moving from one place to another.
Ambulatory		Able to walk as opposed to being confined to bed or a wheelchair.
Brace		An orthopedic device used to support and hold a part of the body in the correct position to allow functioning and healing.
Cast		A stiff cylindrical casing used to immobilize a body part until healing occurs.
Compress		A soft, moist, absorbent cloth that is folded in several layers and applied to a part of the body in the local application of heat or cold.
Edema		The retention of fluid in the tissues, resulting in swelling.
Erythema	*hem/o:* blood	Reddening of the skin caused by dilation of superficial blood vessels in the skin.
Exudate		A discharge produced by the body's tissues.
Long arm cast		A cast that extends from the axilla to the fingers of the hand, usually with a bend in the elbow.
Long leg cast		A cast that extends from the midthigh to the toes.
Maceration		The softening and breaking down of the skin as a result of prolonged exposure to moisture.
Orthopedist	*orth/o:* straight *-ist:* specialist	A physician who specializes in the diagnosis and treatment of disorders of the musculoskeletal system, which includes the bones, joints, ligaments, tendons, muscles, and nerves.
Short arm cast		A cast that extends from below the elbow to the fingers.
Short leg cast		A cast that begins just below the knee and extends to the toes.
Soak		The direct immersion of a body part in water or a medicated solution.
Splint		An orthopedic device used to support and immobilize a part of the body.
Sprain		Trauma to a joint that causes injury to the ligaments.
Strain		An overstretching of a muscle caused by trauma.
Suppuration		The process of pus formation.

PROCEDURE 7.1 Applying a Heating Pad

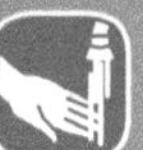

Outcome Apply a heating pad.

Equipment/Supplies

- Heating pad with a protective covering

1. **Procedural Step.** Sanitize your hands.
2. **Procedural Step.** Assemble the equipment.
3. **Procedural Step.** Greet the patient and introduce yourself. Identify the patient and explain the procedure. Explain the purpose of the application (e.g., to relieve pain).
4. **Procedural Step.** Place the heating pad in the protective covering.
   Principle. The protective covering provides more comfort for the patient and absorbs perspiration.

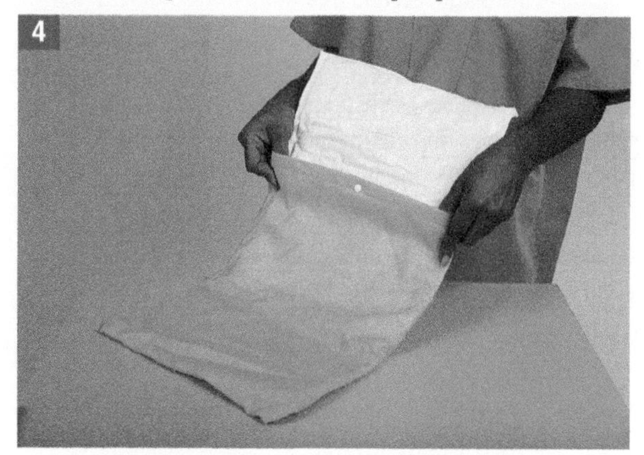

Place the heating pad in a protective covering.

5. **Procedural Step.** Connect the plug to an electric outlet. Set the selector switch at the proper setting, as designated by the provider (usually low or medium).
6. **Procedural Step.** Place the heating pad on the patient's affected body area. Ask the patient how the temperature feels. The heating pad should feel warm but not uncomfortable.
7. **Procedural Step.** Instruct the patient not to lie on the pad or turn the control higher to prevent burns.
   Principle. Lying on the pad causes heat to accumulate and burn the patient. The patient's heat receptors eventually become adjusted to the temperature change, resulting in a decreased heat sensation, and the patient may be tempted to increase the temperature. Turning the control higher results in excessive heat on the patient's skin, which could burn the patient.
8. **Procedural Step.** Check the patient periodically for signs of an increase or decrease in redness or swelling and ask the patient whether the site is painful. Administer the treatment for the proper length of time as designated by the provider.
9. **Procedural Step.** Sanitize your hands.
10. **Procedural Step.** Document the procedure in the patient's medical record.
    a. *Electronic health record (EHR):* Using an EHR such as SimChart for the Medical Office, use the correct radio buttons, drop-down menus, and free text fields to document the method of heat application, the location and duration of the application, the appearance of the application site, and the patient's reaction. Also, document any instructions provided to the patient on applying a heating pad at home.
    b. *Paper-based patient record:* Document the date and time, method of heat application (heating pad), temperature setting of the pad, location and duration of the application, appearance of the application site, and the patient's reaction. Also, document any instructions provided to the patient on applying a heating pad at home (refer to the PPR documentation example).
11. **Procedural Step.** Properly care for the equipment and return it to its storage location. Also, if the protective covering is disposable, throw it away; if it is reusable, either wash it in the washing machine or sanitize it before reusing it.

PPR Documentation Example

Date	
12/10/XX	10:15 a.m. Heating pad on medium setting
	applied to lower back x 20 min. Area appears
	pink following application. Pt states a relief
	of pain and better mobility. Provided
	instructions on the application of a heating
	pad at home. ——— M. Cooper, CMA (AAMA)

PROCEDURE 7.1

PROCEDURE 7.2 Applying a Hot Soak

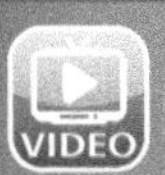

Outcome Apply a hot soak.

Equipment/Supplies

- Soaking solution ordered by the provider
- Bath thermometer
- Basin
- Bath towels

1. **Procedural Step.** Sanitize your hands.
2. **Procedural Step.** Assemble the equipment. Check the label on the solution container to make sure you have the correct solution as ordered by the provider. Place the solution container in a basin of warm water. Warm the soaking solution to a temperature between 105°F and 110°F (41°C and 44°C).
3. **Procedural Step.** Greet the patient and introduce yourself. Identify the patient and explain the procedure. Explain the purpose of the application (e.g., to apply a medicated solution).
4. **Procedural Step.** Fill the basin one-third to two-thirds full with the warmed soaking solution.
5. **Procedural Step.** Check the temperature of the solution with a bath thermometer. The temperature for an adult should be 105°F–110°F (41°C–44°C).
6. **Procedural Step.** Assist the patient into a comfortable position to avoid fatigue and muscle strain. Pad the side of the basin with a towel for the patient's comfort.
7. **Procedural Step.** Slowly and gradually immerse the patient's affected body part in the solution. Ask the patient how the temperature feels.
   Principle. The affected body part should gradually become accustomed to the change in temperature.
8. **Procedural Step.** Test the temperature of the solution frequently. To keep the solution at a constant temperature, remove cooler fluid every 5 min and replace it with the hot solution. Pour the hot solution near the edge of the basin by placing your hand between the patient and the solution. Stir the solution as you pour.
   Principle. The solution should be added away from the patient's body part to prevent splashing hot fluid on the patient. Stirring in the solution helps distribute the heat and keep the temperature constant.

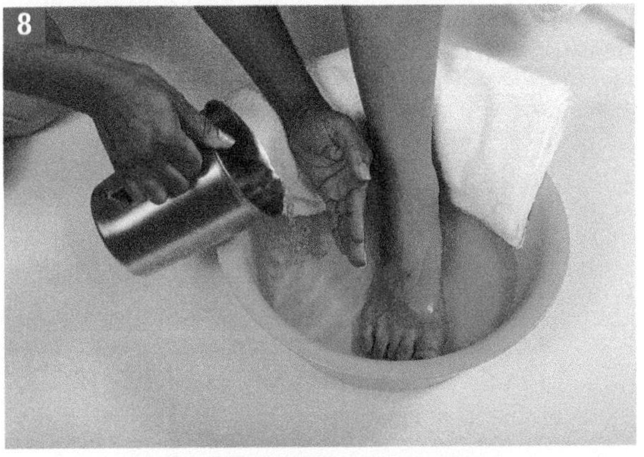

Replace cooler solution with hot solution.

9. **Procedural Step.** Check the patient's skin periodically for signs of an increase or decrease in redness or swelling and ask the patient whether the site is painful. Apply the hot soak for the proper length of time as designated by the provider (usually 15 min).
10. **Procedural Step.** Dry the affected part completely and gently.
11. **Procedural Step.** Sanitize your hands.
12. **Procedural Step.** Document the procedure in the patient's medical record.
    a. *Electronic health record (EHR):* Using an EHR such as SimChart for the Medical Office, use the correct radio buttons, drop-down menus, and free text fields to document the method of heat application, name and strength of the solution, the temperature of the soak, the location and duration of the application, the appearance of the application site, and the patient's reaction.
    b. *Paper-based patient record:* Document the date and time, method of heat application (hot soak), name and strength of the solution, the temperature of the soak, location and duration of the application, the appearance of the application site, and the patient's reaction (refer to the PPR documentation example).
13. **Procedural Step.** Properly care for equipment and return it to its storage location.

PPR Documentation Example

Date	
12/12/XX	1:15 p.m. Normal saline hot soak at 105° F
	applied to (R) ankle x 20 min. Area appears
	pink following application. Pt states less
	stiffness in ankle. ————————
	———————— M. Cooper, CMA (AAMA)

PROCEDURE 7.3 Applying a Hot Compress

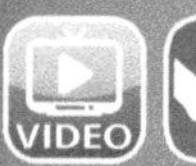

Outcome Apply a hot compress.

Equipment/Supplies

- Solution ordered by the provider
- Bath thermometer
- Basin
- Washcloths
- Waterproof covering
- Towel

1. **Procedural Step.** Sanitize your hands.
2. **Procedural Step.** Assemble the equipment. Check the label on the solution container to make sure you have the correct solution as ordered by the provider. Place the solution container in a basin of warm water. Warm the soaking solution to a temperature between 105°F and 110°F (41°C and 44°C).
3. **Procedural Step.** Greet the patient and introduce yourself. Identify the patient and explain the procedure. Explain the purpose of the application (e.g., to soften an exudate).
4. **Procedural Step.** Fill the basin half full with the warmed solution. Check the temperature of the solution with the bath thermometer. The temperature for an adult should be 105°F–110°F (41°C–44°C).
5. **Procedural Step.** Completely immerse the compress in the solution. Wring the compress to remove excess moisture. The compress should be wet but not dripping. Apply it lightly at first to the affected site to allow the patient to become used to the heat gradually. You may want to cover the compress with a waterproof cover to help hold in the heat. Ask the patient how the temperature feels. The compress should be as hot as the patient can comfortably tolerate.
   Principle. The waterproof cover prevents cool air currents from coming into contact with the compress and reduces the number of times the compress needs to be changed.

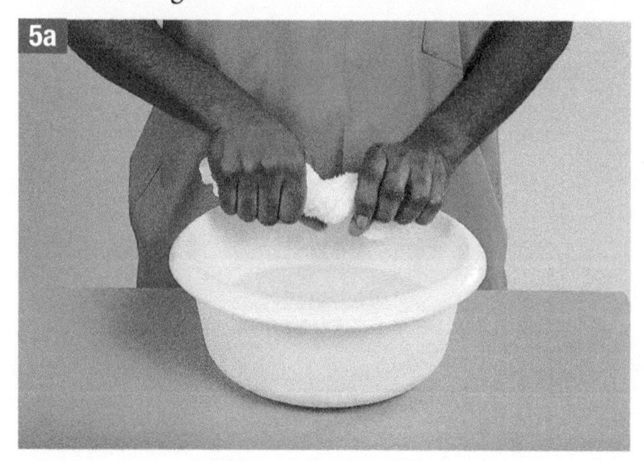

5a Wring out the compress.

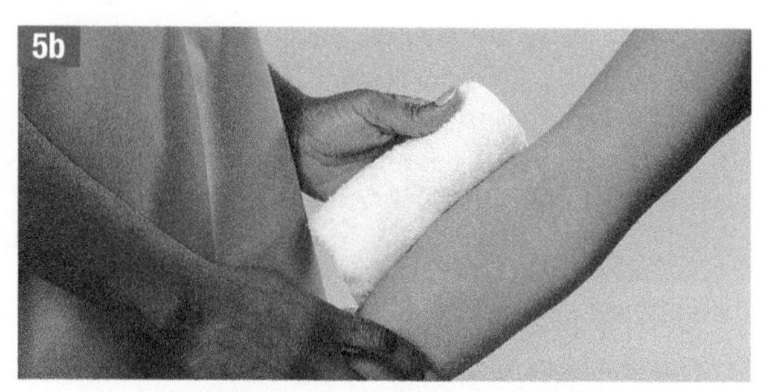

5b Apply the compress to the affected site.

6. **Procedural Step.** Place additional compresses in the solution so that they are ready for use.
7. **Procedural Step.** Repeat the application of the compress every 2–3 min for the duration of time specified by the provider (usually 15–20 min). Check the patient's skin periodically for signs of an increase or decrease in redness or swelling and ask the patient whether the site is painful.
8. **Procedural Step.** Check the temperature of the solution periodically. Remove cooler fluid and replace it with the hot solution if needed. Administer the treatment for the proper length of time as designated by the provider.
9. **Procedural Step.** Dry the affected part thoroughly and gently.
10. **Procedural Step.** Sanitize your hands.
11. **Procedural Step.** Document the procedure in the patient's medical record.
    a. *Electronic health record (EHR):* Using an EHR such as SimChart for the Medical Office, use the correct radio buttons, drop-down menus, and free text fields to document the method of heat application, name and strength of the solution, the temperature of the solution, location and duration of the application, the appearance of the application site, and the patient's reaction.
    b. *Paper-based patient record:* Document the date and time, method of heat application (hot compress), name and strength of the solution, the temperature of the solution, location and duration of the application, the appearance of the application site, and the patient's reaction (refer to the PPR documentation example).

PROCEDURE 7.3 Applying a Hot Compress—cont'd

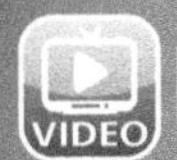
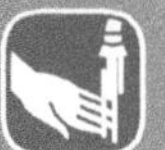

12. **Procedural Step.** Properly care for equipment and return it to its storage location.

PPR Documentation Example

Date	
12/20/XX	10:30 a.m. Normal saline hot compress at
	110° F applied to (R) forearm x 20 min.
	No complaints of discomfort. ————
	———————— M. Cooper, CMA (AAMA)

PROCEDURE 7.4 Applying an Ice Bag

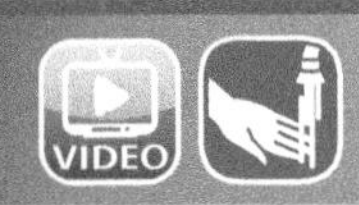

Outcome Apply an ice bag.

Equipment/Supplies

- Ice bag with a protective covering
- Small pieces of ice (ice chips or crushed ice)

1. **Procedural Step.** Sanitize your hands.
2. **Procedural Step.** Assemble the equipment.
3. **Procedural Step.** Greet the patient and introduce yourself. Identify the patient and explain the procedure. Explain the purpose of applying the ice bag (e.g., to prevent swelling).
4. **Procedural Step.** Check the ice bag for leakage.
   Principle. A leaking bag would get the patient wet and cause chilling.
5. **Procedural Step.** Fill the bag one-half to two-thirds full with small pieces of ice.
   Principle. Small pieces of ice work better than large pieces because they reduce the air spaces in the bag, resulting in better conduction of cold. In addition, small pieces of ice allow the bag to mold better to the body area.
6. **Procedural Step.** Expel air from the bag by squeezing the empty top half of the bag together and screwing on the stopper.
   Principle. Air is a poor conductor of cold and makes it difficult to mold the ice bag to the body area.

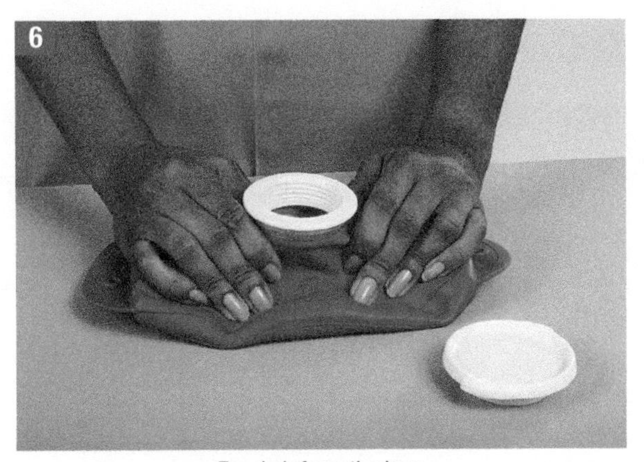

6 Expel air from the bag.

7. **Procedural Step.** Place the bag in the protective covering.
   Principle. The protective covering provides for patient comfort and absorbs the moisture that condenses on the outside of the bag.
8. **Procedural Step.** Place the bag on the patient's affected body area. Ask the patient how the temperature feels. The application of ice is usually uncomfortable, but most patients tolerate it when they know how much benefit may be derived from it.
   Principle. Individuals vary in their ability to tolerate cold.
9. **Procedural Step.** Check the patient's skin periodically for signs of an increase or decrease in redness or swelling and ask the patient whether the site is painful.

Continued

PROCEDURE 7.4 Applying an Ice Bag—cont'd

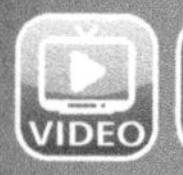

If extreme paleness and numbness or a mottled blue appearance occur at the application site, remove the bag and notify the provider.

10. **Procedural Step.** Refill the bag with ice as necessary and change the protective covering if needed. Administer the treatment for the proper length of time, as designated by the provider (usually, until the area feels numb, approximately 15–30 min).
11. **Procedural Step.** Sanitize your hands.
12. **Procedural Step.** Document the procedure in the patient's medical record.
    a. *Electronic health record (EHR):* Using an EHR such as SimChart for the Medical Office, use the correct radio buttons, drop-down menus, and free text fields to document the method of cold application, location and duration of the application, the appearance of the application site, and the patient's reaction. Also, document any instructions provided to the patient on applying an ice bag at home.
    b. *Paper-based patient record:* Document the date and time, method of cold application (ice bag), location and duration of the application, the appearance of the application site, and the patient's reaction. Also, document any instructions provided to the patient on applying an ice bag at home (refer to the PPR documentation example).
13. **Procedural Step.** Properly care for the ice bag. Dispose of or launder the protective covering as required. Cleanse the ice bag with a warm detergent solution, rinse thoroughly, and dry by hanging the bag upside down with the top removed. Store the bag by screwing on the stopper, leaving air inside to prevent the sides from sticking together.

PPR Documentation Example

Date	
12/22/XX	11:30 a.m. Ice bag applied to Ⓡ knee x 20
	min. Pt complained of slight discomfort
	during the application. Area appears less
	swollen following application. Provided
	instructions on the application of an ice
	bag at home._____M. Cooper, CMA (AAMA)

PROCEDURE 7.5 Applying a Cold Compress

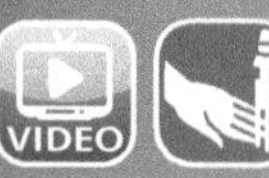

Outcome Apply a cold compress.

Equipment/Supplies

- Ice cubes
- Basin
- Washcloths
- Towel
- Ice bag

1. **Procedural Step.** Sanitize your hands.
2. **Procedural Step.** Assemble the equipment. Check the label on the solution container to make sure you have the correct solution as ordered by the provider.
3. **Procedural Step.** Greet the patient and introduce yourself. Identify the patient and explain the procedure. Explain the purpose of the application (e.g., to treat an eye injury).
4. **Procedural Step.** Place large ice cubes in the basin. Add the solution until the basin is half full.
   Principle. Using larger pieces of ice prevents them from sticking to the compress and slows the rate at which they melt in the solution.

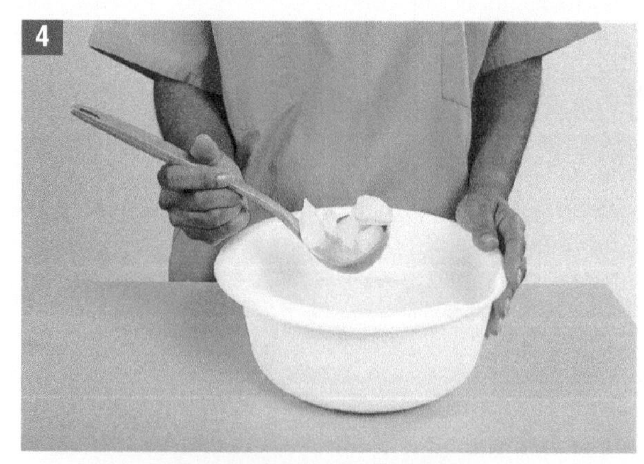

Place large ice cubes in the basin.

5. **Procedural Step.** Completely immerse the compress in the solution. Wring the compress to rid it of excess

PROCEDURE 7.5

PROCEDURE 7.5 Applying a Cold Compress—cont'd

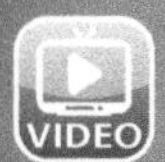

moisture. The compress should be wet but not dripping. Apply it lightly at first to the affected site to allow the patient to become used to the cold gradually. The compress can be covered with an ice bag to help keep it cold and to reduce the number of times it needs to be changed. Ask the patient how the temperature feels.

6. **Procedural Step.** Place additional compresses in the solution to be ready for use.
7. **Procedural Step.** Repeat the application of the compress every 2–3 min for the duration of time specified by the provider (usually 15–20 min). Check the patient's skin periodically for signs of an increase or decrease in redness or swelling and ask the patient whether the site is painful.
8. **Procedural Step.** Add ice if needed to keep the solution cold. Administer the treatment for the proper length of time designated by the provider.
9. **Procedural Step.** Thoroughly dry the affected part.
10. **Procedural Step.** Sanitize your hands.
11. **Procedural Step.** Document the procedure in the patient's medical record.
    a. *Electronic health record (EHR):* Using an EHR such as SimChart for the Medical Office, use the correct radio buttons, drop-down menus, and free text fields to document the method of cold application, location and duration of the application, the appearance of the application site, and patient's reaction.
    b. *Paper-based patient record:* Document the date and time, method of cold application (cold compress), location and duration of the application, the appearance of the application site, and patient's reaction (refer to the PPR documentation example).
12. **Procedural Step.** Properly care for equipment and return it to its storage location.

PPR Documentation Example

Date	
12/27/XX	9:15 a.m. Normal saline cold compress applied
	to bridge of nose x 15 min. Nose appears less
	swollen following application. Tolerated
	application well —— M. Cooper, CMA (AAMA)

PROCEDURE 7.6 Applying a Chemical Pack

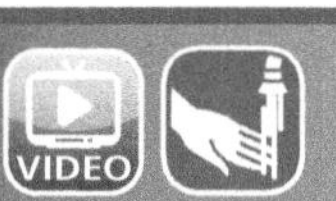

Outcome Apply a chemical cold pack and a chemical hot pack.

Equipment/Supplies

- Chemical cold pack
- Chemical hot pack

The procedure for applying a chemical cold or hot pack is as follows:

1. **Procedural Step.** Shake the crystals to the bottom of the bag.
2. **Procedural Step.** Squeeze the bag firmly with your hands to break the inner water bag.
3. **Procedural Step.** Shake the bag vigorously to mix the contents.
4. **Procedural Step.** Cover the bag with a protective covering.
5. **Procedural Step.** Apply the bag to the affected area. Check the patient's skin periodically.
6. **Procedural Step.** Administer the treatment for the proper length of time.
7. **Procedural Step.** Discard the bag in an appropriate receptacle.
8. **Procedural Step.** Sanitize your hands.
9. **Procedural Step.** Document the procedure in the patient's medical record.
    a. *Electronic health record (EHR):* Using an EHR such as SimChart for the Medical Office, use the correct radio buttons, drop-down menus, and free text fields to document the method of application (chemical cold or hot pack), location and duration of the application, the appearance of the application site, and patient's reaction.
    b. *Paper-based patient record:* Document the date and time, method of application (chemical cold or hot

Continued

PROCEDURE 7.6 Applying a Chemical Pack—cont'd

pack), location and duration of the application, the appearance of the application site, and patient's reaction (refer to the PPR documentation example).

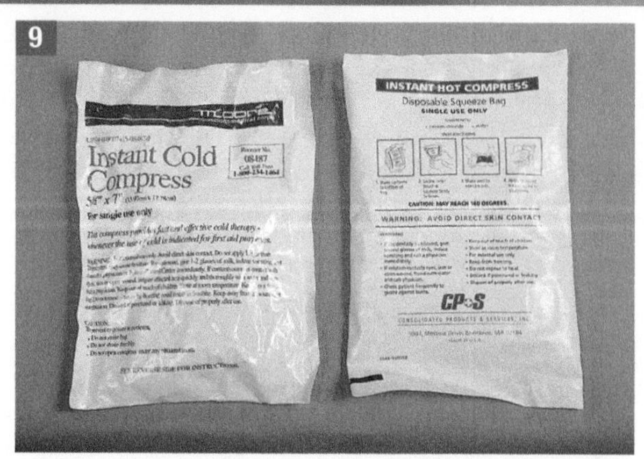

Chemical packs. (A) Chemical cold pack. (B) Chemical hot pack.

PROCEDURE 7.7 Measuring for Axillary Crutches

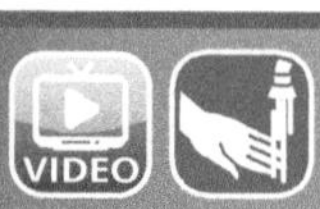

Outcome Measure an individual for axillary crutches.

Equipment/Supplies

- Axillary crutches
- Goniometer

1. **Procedural Step.** Greet the patient and introduce yourself. Identify the patient and inform the patient that you will be measuring him or her for axillary crutches. Discuss the importance of properly fitted crutches with the patient.

Determining Crutch Length

For you to determine crutch length correctly, the patient must wear shoes while being measured. The measurement can be taken while the patient is standing.

2. **Procedural Step.** Ask the patient to stand erect.
3. **Procedural Step.** Position the crutches with the crutch tips at a distance of 2 inches (5 cm) in front of and 4–6 inches (15 cm) to the side of each foot. (The large dots in the figure represent crutch tips.)

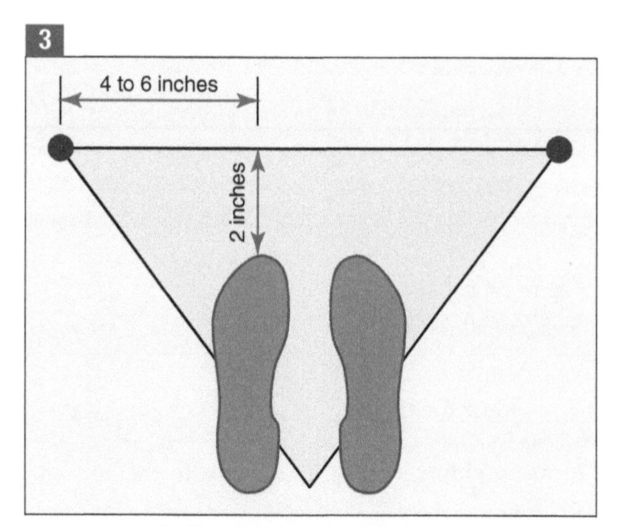

Position for measuring for crutches.

4. **Procedural Step.** Adjust the crutch length so that the shoulder rests are approximately 1½ –2 inches (about two finger widths) below the axillae.
   - *Aluminum crutches.* The length of the crutch is adjusted by pressing the spring-loaded push button with your thumb and sliding the outer tube upward or downward as necessary to attain the proper length. The spring-loaded button on the inner tube should be allowed to "pop out" into the appropriate hole on the outer tube.

PROCEDURE 7.7 Measuring for Axillary Crutches—cont'd

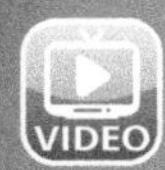

- *Wooden crutches.* The length of the crutch is adjusted by removing the bolt and wing nut and sliding the central strut (support piece) at the bottom upward or downward as necessary to attain the proper length. The strut is secured by replacing the bolt and securely fastening the wing nut.

Handgrip Positioning

When the crutch length has been adjusted, the correct placement of the handgrips must be determined.

5. **Procedural Step.** Ask the patient to stand erect with a crutch under each arm and to support his or her weight by the handgrips.
6. **Procedural Step.** Adjust the handgrips on the crutches so that the patient's elbow is flexed to an angle of approximately 30 degrees. The handgrip level is adjusted by removing the bolt and wing nut and sliding the handgrip upward or downward, as required. The handgrip is secured by replacing the bolt and tightly fastening the wing nut. The angle of elbow flexion can be verified by using a measuring device known as a goniometer. A goniometer is an instrument that measures the angle of a joint.
7. **Procedural Step.** Check the fit of the crutches. If the crutches are measured correctly, the medical assistant should be able to insert two fingers between the top of the crutches and the axillae when the patient is standing erect with the crutches under the arms.

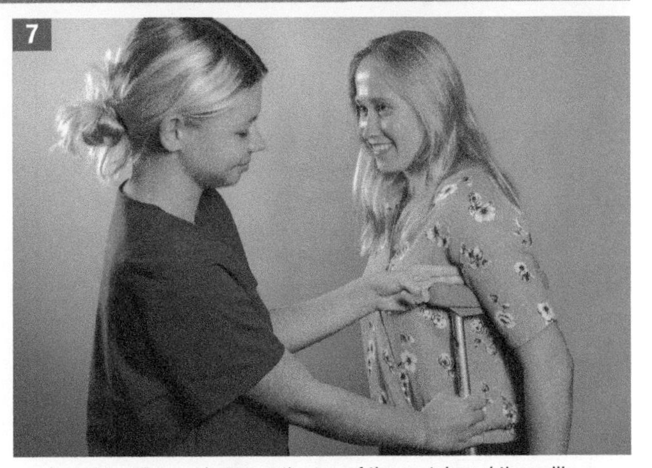

Insert two fingers between the top of the crutch and the axilla.

8. **Procedural Step.** Document the procedure in the patient's medical record.
   a. *Electronic health record (EHR):* Using an EHR such as SimChart for the Medical Office, use the appropriate radio buttons, drop-down menus, and free text fields to document the axillary crutch measurement procedure.
   b. *Paper-based patient record:* Document the date and time and the axillary crutch measurement procedure.

PROCEDURE 7.8 Instructing a Patient in Crutch Gaits

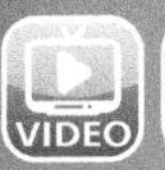

Outcome Instruct a patient in the following crutch gaits: four-point, two-point, three-point, swing-to, and swing-through.

Equipment/Supplies

- Axillary crutches

1. **Procedural Step.** Greet the patient and introduce yourself. Identify the patient and inform the patient that you will be instructing him or her in crutch gaits. Discuss the importance of the proper use of crutches with the patient.
2. **Procedural Step.** Instruct the patient in the tripod position as follows:
   a. Stand erect and face straight ahead.
   b. Place the tips of the crutches 4–6 inches (15 cm) in front of the feet and 4–6 inches (10–15 cm) to the side of each foot. (The large dots in the figure represent crutch tips.)

Principle. The tripod position is the basic crutch stance used before crutch walking. It provides a wide base of support and enhances stability and balance.

Continued

PROCEDURE 7.8

PROCEDURE 7.8 Instructing a Patient in Crutch Gaits —cont'd

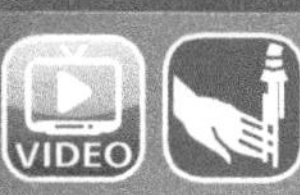

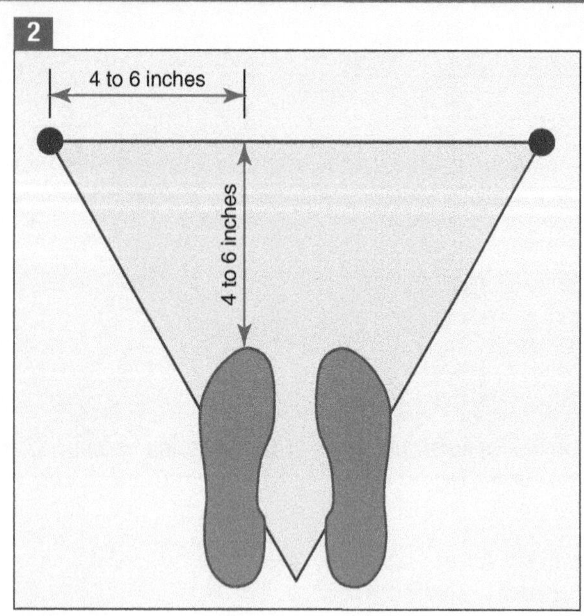

Tripod position.

3. Procedural Step. Instruct the patient in the following crutch gaits.

a. Four-Point Gait: The four-point gait is a basic and slow gait. To use this gait, the patient must be able to bear considerable weight on both legs. The four-point gait is the most stable and the safest of the crutch gaits because it provides at least three points of support at all times. It is used most often by patients who have leg muscle weakness or spasticity, poor muscular coordination or balance, or degenerative leg joint disease. Instruct the patient in the procedure for the four-point gait, following the steps in the accompanying figure.

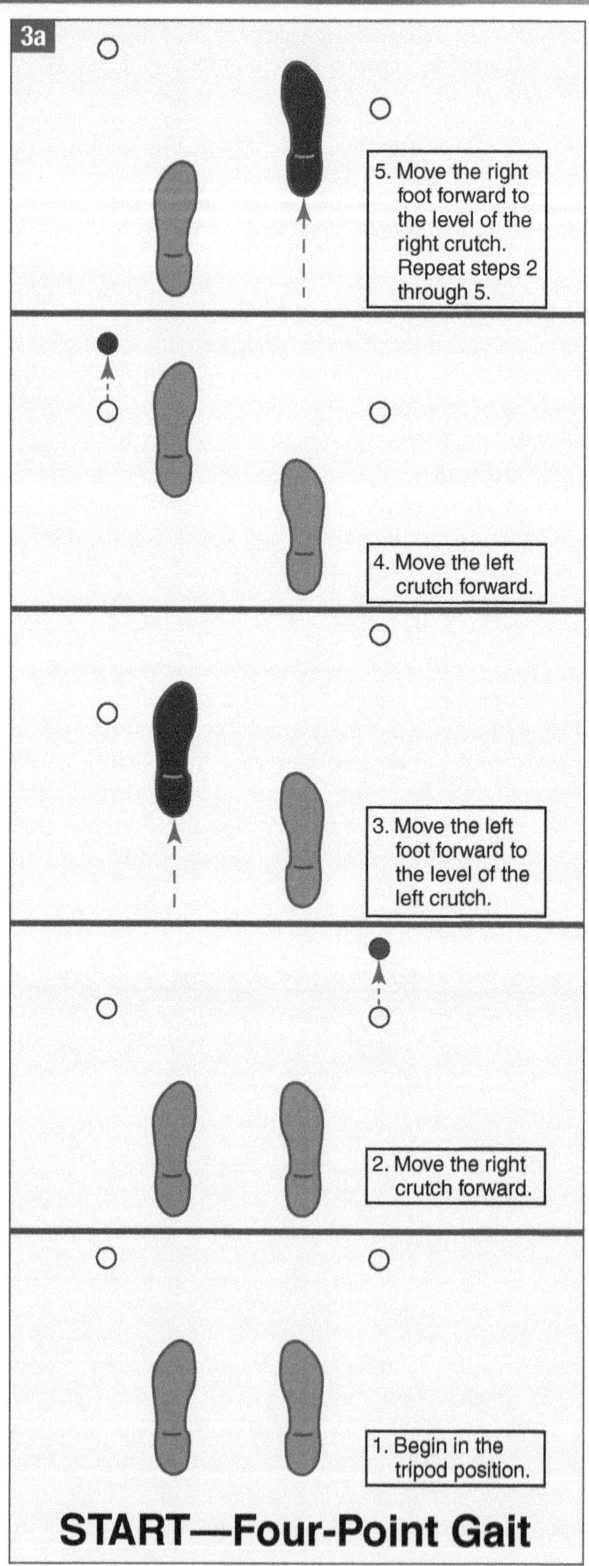

PROCEDURE 7.8 Instructing a Patient in Crutch Gaits—cont'd

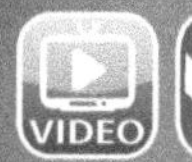

PPR Documentation Example

Date	
12/15/XX	1:30 p.m. Instructed pt in four-point gait. Pt was able to demonstrate four-point gait. ———————— M. Cooper, CMA (AAMA)

PPR Documentation Example

Date	
12/16/XX	2:30 p.m. Instructed pt in two-point gait. Pt was able to demonstrate two-point gait. ———————— M. Cooper, CMA (AAMA)

b. Two-Point Gait: The two-point gait is similar to, but faster than, the four-point gait. This gait requires better balance because only two points support the body at one time. The two-point gait is used when the patient is capable of partial weight-bearing on each foot and has good muscular coordination. Instruct the patient in the procedure for the two-point gait, following the steps in the accompanying figure.

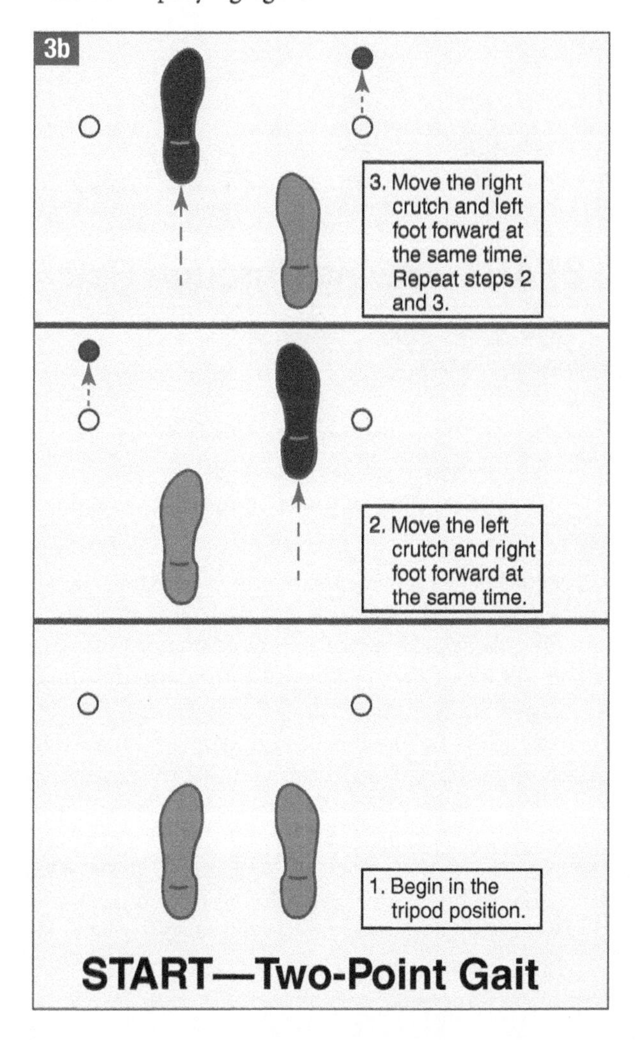

c. Three-Point Gait: The three-point gait is used by patients who cannot bear weight on one leg. The patient must be able to support his or her full weight on the unaffected leg. With this gait, the crutches and the unaffected leg alternately bear the patient's weight. This gait is used most often by amputees without a prosthesis, patients with musculoskeletal or soft tissue trauma to a lower extremity (e.g., fracture, sprain), patients with acute leg inflammation, and patients who have had recent leg surgery. To use this gait, the patient must have good muscular coordination and arm strength. Instruct the patient in the procedure for the three-point gait, following the steps in the accompanying figure.

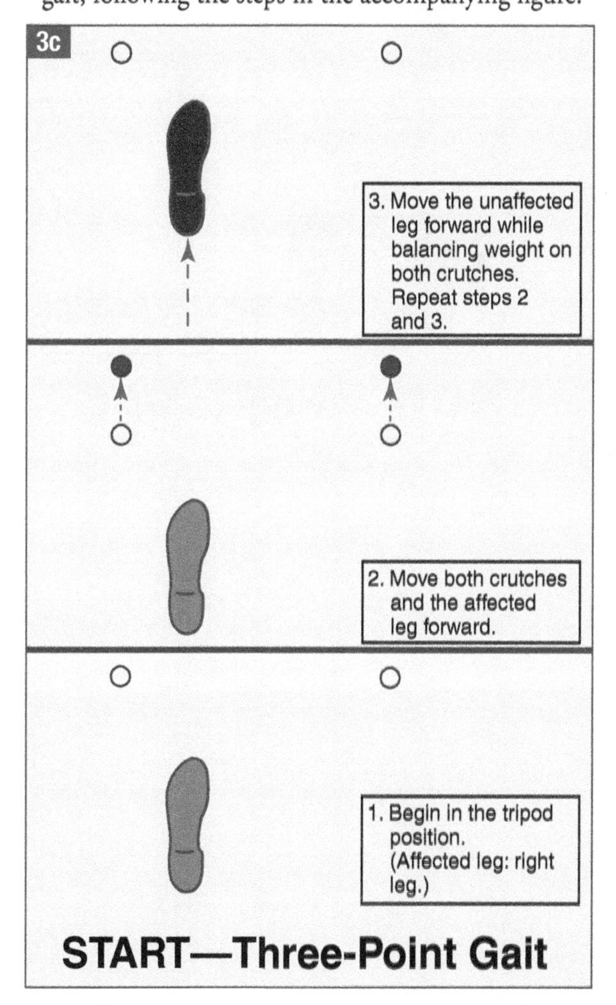

Continued

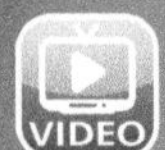

d. Swing Gaits: The swing gaits include the swing-to gait and the swing-through gait and are used by patients with severe lower extremity disabilities, such as paralysis, and by patients who wear supporting braces on their legs.Instruct the patient in the procedures for the swing-to and the swing-through crutch gaits, following the steps in the accompanying figures.

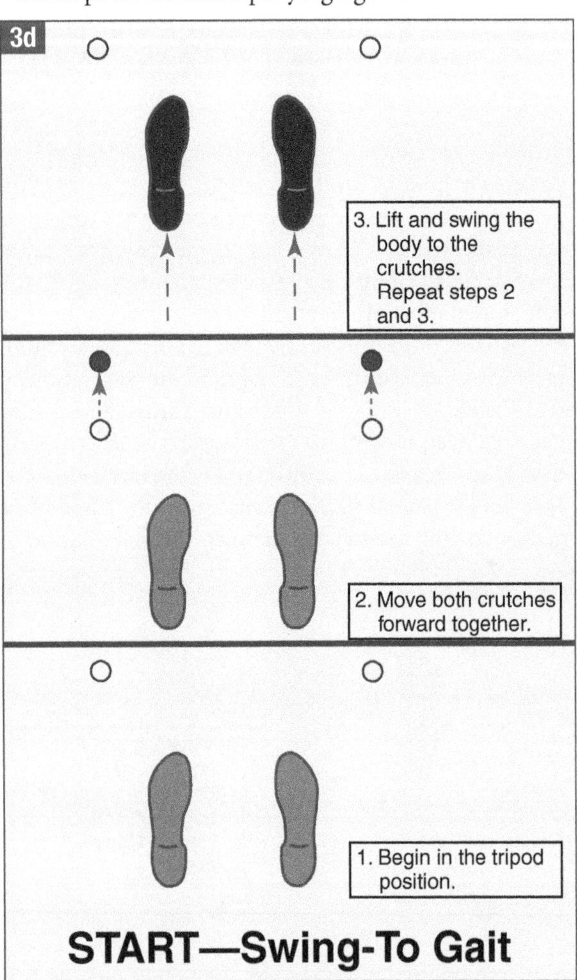

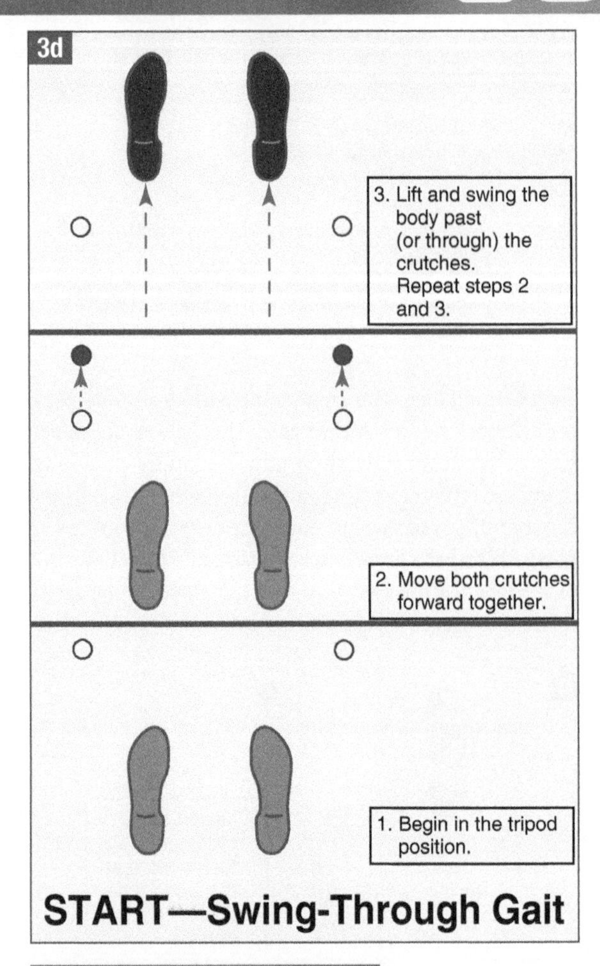

PPR Documentation Example

Date	
12/18/XX	3:30 p.m. Instructed pt in swing-to and
	swing-through gaits. Pt was able to demon-
	strate swing gaits.— M. Cooper, CMA (AAMA)

4. **Procedural Step.** Document the procedure in the patient's medical record.
   a. *Electronic health record (EHR):* Using an EHR such as SimChart for the Medical Office, use the appropriate radio buttons, drop-down menus, and free text fields to document the type of instructions given to the patient. Document that the patient was able to properly demonstrate the crutch gaits.
   b. *Paper-based patient record:* Document the date and time and the type of instructions given to the patient. Document that the patient was able to properly demonstrate the crutch gaits (refer to the PPR documentation example).

PPR Documentation Example

Date	
12/17/XX	2:30 p.m. Instructed pt in three-point gait. Pt
	was able to demonstrate three-point gait. —
	———————— M. Cooper, CMA (AAMA)

PROCEDURE 7.9 Instructing a Patient in Use of a Cane

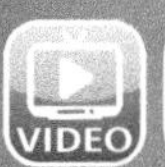

Outcome Instruct the patient in the use of a cane.

Equipment/Supplies

- Cane

1. **Procedural Step.** Greet the patient and introduce yourself. Identify the patient and inform the patient that you will be showing him or her how to use a cane. Discuss the importance of proper cane use with the patient.

Instruct the patient as follows:

2. **Procedural Step.** Hold the cane on the strong side of the body (i.e., in the hand opposite the affected extremity).
3. **Procedural Step.** Place the tip of the cane 4–6 inches to the side of the foot.
4. **Procedural Step.** Move the cane forward approximately 12 inches (1 foot).
5. **Procedural Step.** Move the affected leg forward to the level of the cane.
6. **Procedural Step.** Move the strong leg forward and ahead of the cane and weak leg.
7. **Procedural Step.** Repeat steps 3 through 5.

Note: The cane and the affected leg can be moved forward simultaneously (steps 3 and 4); however, the patient has less support with this method.

8. **Procedural Step.** Document the procedure in the patient's medical record.
   a. *Electronic health record (EHR):* Using an EHR such as SimChart for the Medical Office, use the appropriate radio buttons, drop-down menus, and free text fields to document the type of instructions given to the patient. Document that the patient was able to demonstrate the proper use of a cane.
   b. *Paper-based patient record:* Document the date and time and the type of instructions given to the patient. Document that the patient was able to demonstrate the proper use of a cane (refer to the PPR documentation example).

PPR Documentation Example

Date	
12/20/XX	2:30 p.m. Instructed pt in the procedure for
	using a cane. Pt was able to demonstrate
	proper use of a cane. ————————
	M. Cooper, CMA (AAMA)

PROCEDURE 7.10 Instructing a Patient in Use of a Walker

Outcome Instruct the patient in the use of a walker.

Equipment/Supplies

- Walker

1. **Procedural Step.** Greet the patient and introduce yourself. Identify the patient and inform the patient that you will be showing him or her how to use a walker. Discuss the importance of proper walker use with the patient.

Instruct the patient as follows:

2. **Procedural Step.** Pick up the walker and move it forward approximately 6 inches.
3. **Procedural Step.** Move the right foot and then the left foot up to the walker.
4. **Procedural Step.** Repeat steps 1 and 2.
5. **Procedural Step.** Document the procedure in the patient's medical record.
   a. *Electronic health record (EHR):* Using an EHR such as SimChart for the Medical Office, use the appropriate radio buttons, drop-down menus, and free text fields to document the type of instructions given to the patient. Document that the patient was able to demonstrate the proper use of a walker.
   b. *Paper-based patient record:* Document the date and time and the type of instructions given to the patient. Document that the patient was able to demonstrate the proper use of a walker (refer to the PPR documentation example).

PPR Documentation Example

Date	
12/21/XX	9:30 a.m. Instructed pt in the procedure for
	using a walker. Pt was able to demonstrate
	proper use of a walker. ————————
	M. Cooper, CMA (AAMA)

8 The Gynecologic Examination and Prenatal Care

 Check out the Evolve site at http://evolve.elsevier.com/Bonewit to access additional interactive activities and exercises to help you study and prepare for success.

LEARNING OUTCOMES

Gynecologic Examination

Introduction

1. State the purpose of the gynecologic examination.
2. Identify the components of the gynecologic examination.

Breast Examination

3. Explain the purpose of a breast examination.
4. Identify the breast cancer screening guidelines recommended by the American Cancer Society.

Pelvic Examination

5. Explain the purpose of a pelvic examination.
6. List and describe the four parts of the pelvic examination.
7. State the purpose of cervical cancer screening.
8. Identify the cervical cancer screening guidelines recommended by the American College of Obstetricians and Gynecologists.
9. Explain the purpose of the Pap test and the human papillomavirus test.
10. List and describe the patient preparation recommended for cervical cancer screening.
11. List and describe each category on a cytology request for a Pap test.
12. List and describe the procedures that may be performed as a result of an abnormal Pap test result.

Gynecologic Infections

13. Identify the symptoms, diagnosis, and treatment of each of the following gynecologic infections:
    - Bacterial vaginosis
    - Vulvovaginal candidiasis
    - Trichomoniasis
    - Chlamydia
    - Gonorrhea
    - Genital herpes
    - Human papillomavirus infection

Prenatal Care

Prenatal Visits

14. Explain the purpose of each part of the prenatal record.
15. List and explain each part of the initial prenatal examination.
16. List and explain the purpose of each prenatal laboratory test.
17. Explain the purpose of return prenatal visits.

PROCEDURES

Instruct a patient in the procedure for a breast self-examination.

Prepare a patient for a gynecologic examination.

Assist the provider with a gynecologic examination.

Complete a cytology requisition form.

Assist in the collection of a gynecologic specimen for the detection of a vaginal infection or sexually transmitted infection.

Calculate the expected date of delivery (EDD).

Complete a prenatal health history.

Assist the provider with an initial prenatal examination.

5. Explain the purpose of each of the following:
    - Carrier screening
    - First trimester prenatal screening test
    - Noninvasive prenatal test
    - Multiple marker test
    - Obstetric ultrasound scan
    - Amniocentesis
    - Fetal heart rate monitoring

Assist the provider with a return prenatal examination.

Six-Week Postpartum Visit

6. Explain the purpose of the 6-week postpartum visit.
7. List and explain the purpose of each of the procedures included in the postpartum examination.

Assist the provider with a 6-week postpartum examination.

CHAPTER OUTLINE

INTRODUCTION TO THE GYNECOLOGIC EXAMINATION AND PRENATAL CARE

GYNECOLOGIC EXAMINATION

Terms Related to Gynecology

Breast Examination

Breast Cancer Screening Guidelines

Pelvic Examination

- Inspection of External Genitalia, Vagina, and Cervix
- Cervical Cancer Screening
- Bimanual Pelvic Examination
- Rectal-Vaginal Examination

GYNCOLOGIC INFECTIONS

Vaginal Infections

- Bacterial Vaginosis
- Vulvovaginal Candidiasis
- Trichomoniasis

Sexually Transmitted Infections

- Chlamydia
- Gonorrhea
- Genital Herpes
- Human Papillomavirus Infection

PRENATAL CARE

Obstetric Terminology

Prenatal Visits

- Initial Prenatal Visit
- Return Prenatal Visits
- Six Weeks Postpartum Visit

KEY TERMS

Gynecology

amenorrhea (AY-men-ah-REE-ah)
cervix (SER-viks)
colposcopy (kol-POS-koe-pee)
cytology (sy-TOL-oh-jee)
dysmenorrhea (DIS-men-ah-REE-ah)
dyspareunia (DIS-pah-ROO-nee-ah)
dysplasia (dis-PLAY-shah)
ectocervix (EK-toe-SER-viks)
endocervix (EN-doe-SER-viks)
external os (eks-TER-nal AHS)
gynecology (gie-nuh-KOL-oh-jee)
menopause (MEN-oh-paws)
menorrhagia (men-uh-RAY-jee-ah)
metrorrhagia (met-ro-RAY-jee-ah)
parity (PEAR-ih-tee)
perimenopause (PEAR-ee-MEN-oh-paws)
perineum (pear-ih-NEE-um)
preterm birth
risk factor
vulva (VUL-va)

Obstetrics

abortion (ah-BOR-shun)
Braxton Hicks contractions (BRAK-stun HIKS con-TRAK-shuns)
dilation (of the cervix) (die-LAY-shun)
effacement (eh-FAYS-ment)
embryo (EM-bree-oh)
engagement
expected date of delivery (EDD)
fetal heart rate
fetal heart tones
fetus (FEE-tus)
fundus (FUN-dus)
gestation (jess-TAY-shun)
gestational age (jess-TAY-shun-al)
gravidity (gra-VID-ih-teed)
infant
lochia
multigravida (MUL-tee-GRAV-ih-duh)
multipara (mul-TIH-pear-uh)
nullipara (nul-IH-pear-uh)
obstetrics (ob-STEH-triks)
parity
position
postpartum (poest-PAR-tum)
preeclampsia (PREE-ih-KLAMP-see-ah)
prenatal (pree-NAY-tul)
presentation
preterm birth
primigravida (PRIH-mih-GRAV-ih-duh)
primipara (prih-MIH-pear-uh)
puerperium (PYOO-ur-PEER-ee-um)
quickening
term birth
toxemia (tok-SEE-mee-uh)
trimester (try-MES-ter)

Introduction to the Gynecologic Examination and Prenatal Care

The medical assistant should have knowledge of gynecology and obstetrics to assist in examinations and treatments in these specialties. Gynecologic examinations are frequently and routinely performed in the medical office. Prenatal care consists of a series of scheduled medical office visits for the promotion of the health of the mother and fetus during the pregnancy. Obtaining the patient's cooperation makes the gynecologic or prenatal examination proceed more smoothly and, as a result, makes the patient feel more comfortable. The medical assistant can help by explaining the purpose of the procedure to the patient. If the patient understands the beneficial results to be derived from the examination, she is more likely to participate as required. For means of convenience, this chapter is divided into the following two sections: the gynecologic examination and prenatal care.

Gynecologic Examination

Gynecology is the branch of medicine that deals with health maintenance and diseases of the female reproductive system. The gynecologic examination is frequently and routinely performed in the medical office and generally includes a *breast examination* and a *pelvic examination.*

The purpose of the gynecologic examination is to assess the health of the female reproductive organs to detect early signs of disease, leading to early diagnosis and treatment. This examination may be included as a part of a general physical examination, or it may be performed by itself. Although assisting with a gynecologic examination is a routine procedure for the medical assistant, the patient may not consider it a routine examination. To reduce apprehension or embarrassment, the medical assistant should fully explain the procedure to the patient and offer to answer any questions.

TERMS RELATED TO GYNECOLOGY

The medical assistant should have a thorough knowledge of the female reproductive system (Fig. 8.1) and the following terms associated with the female reproductive system:

Amenorrhea. Absence or cessation of the menstrual period. Amenorrhea occurs normally before puberty, during pregnancy, and after menopause.

Cervix. The lower narrow end of the uterus that opens into the vagina.

Colposcopy. Examination of the cervix using a colposcope (a lighted instrument with a magnifying lens).

Dysmenorrhea. Pain that is associated with the menstrual period.

Dyspareunia. Pain in the vagina or pelvis experienced by a woman during sexual intercourse.

Dysplasia. The growth of abnormal cells. Dysplasia is a precancerous condition that may or may not develop into cancer.

Menopause The permanent cessation of menstruation, which usually occurs between the ages of 45 and 55 with an average age of 51.

Menorrhagia. Excessive bleeding during a menstrual period, in the number of days, the amount of blood, or both. Also called *dysfunctional uterine bleeding* (DUB).

Metrorrhagia. Bleeding between menstrual periods.

Perimenopause. Before the onset of menopause, the phase during which a woman with regular periods changes to irregular cycles and increased periods of amenorrhea.

Perineum. The external region between the vaginal orifice and the anus in a female and between the scrotum and the anus in a male.

Risk factor. Anything that increases an individual's chance of developing a disease. Some risk factors (e.g., smoking) can be avoided, but others cannot (e.g., age and family history).

BREAST EXAMINATION

The provider usually begins the gynecologic examination with the breast examination. The medical assistant is responsible for assisting the patient into the supine position. The provider inspects the breasts and nipples for swelling, dimpling, puckering, and change in skin texture. The nipples are checked for abnormalities such as bleeding and discharge. The breasts and axillary lymph nodes are palpated for lumps, hard knots, and thickening.

The patient should know how to examine her breasts at home for the presence of lumps and other changes with a breast self-examination (BSE). Most breast cancers are first discovered by women themselves. The American College of Obstetricians and Gynecologists (AGOG) recommends that women 20 years of age and older examine their breasts once every month. The American Cancer Society (ACS) states that a BSE is an option for women starting in their 20s. The ACS recommends that women become familiar with how their breasts normally look and feel and report any changes to a health care provider.

The medical assistant may be responsible for instructing the patient in the BSE procedure at the medical office (Procedure 8.1). If a lump or other change is discovered, the woman should schedule an appointment with her provider as soon as possible. Most breast lumps are not cancerous, but the provider must make that diagnosis.

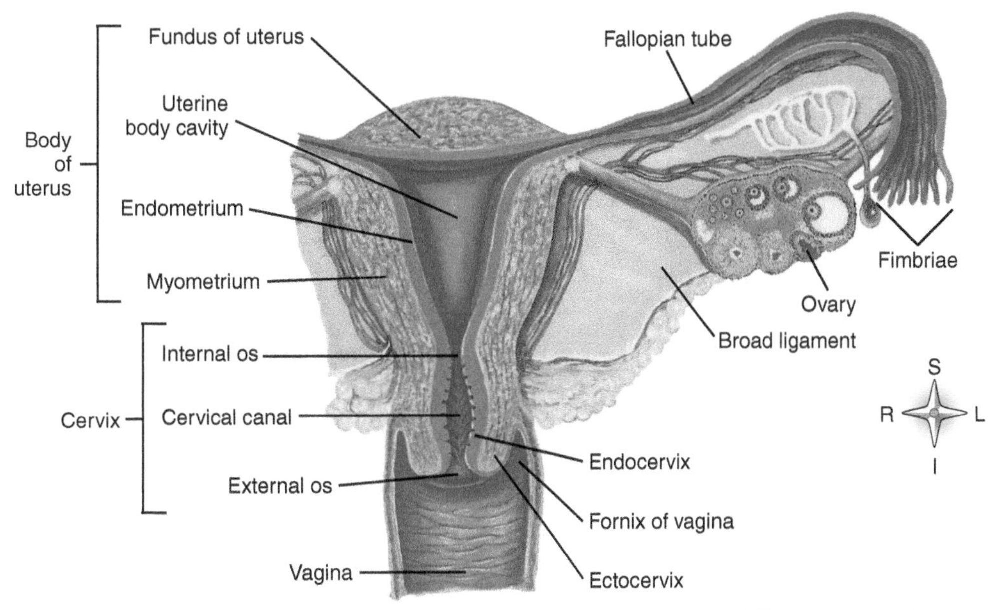

Fig. 8.1 The female reproductive system. (Modified from Thibodeau GA, Patton KT: *Anatomy and physiology,* ed 5, St Louis: Elsevier; 2003.)

BREAST CANCER SCREENING GUIDELINES

The ACS publishes breast cancer screening recommendations for women at average risk for breast cancer. A woman at *average risk* does not have a personal history of breast cancer, a family history of breast cancer, a genetic mutation known to increase risk of breast cancer (such as BRCA) and has not had chest radiation therapy before the age of 30. The ACS breast cancer screening recommendations are outlined in Box 8.1.

PELVIC EXAMINATION

The purpose of the pelvic examination is to assess the size, shape, and location of the reproductive organs and to detect the presence of disease. The pelvic examination consists of the following components:

- Inspection of the external genitalia, vagina, and cervix
- Collection of a specimen for cervical cancer screening
- Bimanual pelvic examination
- Rectal-vaginal examination

For the pelvic examination, the patient is positioned in the lithotomy position. The patient lies on the table on her back, with her feet in the stirrups and her buttocks at the bottom edge of the table. The stirrups should be level with the examining table and pulled out approximately 1 foot from the edge of the table. The patient's knees should be bent and relaxed, and her thighs should be rotated outward as far as is comfortable. This position helps relax the vulva and perineum and facilitates insertion of the vaginal speculum. The patient should be properly draped to reduce exposure and to provide warmth. The lithotomy position is difficult to maintain, and the patient should not be placed in this position until the provider is ready to begin the examination.

Putting It All Into Practice

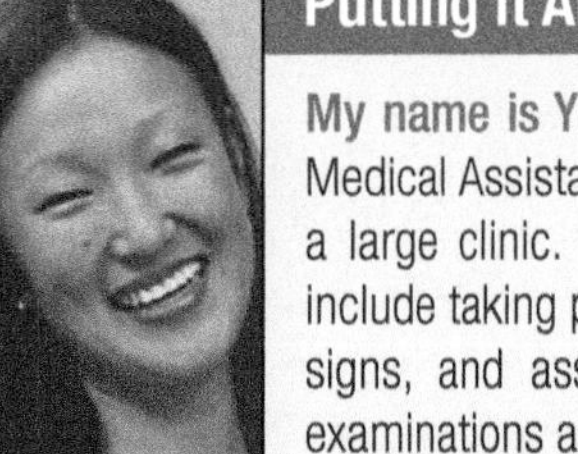

My name is Yin-Ling, and I am a Registered Medical Assistant. I work with 10 physicians in a large clinic. My primary job responsibilities include taking patient histories, measuring vital signs, and assisting physicians with patient examinations and procedures.

One experience that has probably affected me more than any other occurred while I was working in obstetrics and gynecology. A full-term prenatal patient came in for a routine weekly appointment late one afternoon. By this stage of the pregnancy, you have seen the patients often enough to develop a more personal relationship. I was taking her vital signs and asking the routine questions when she said, "I haven't felt the baby move for 2 days." This immediately sent up a red flag, but I was careful to hide my concern until I was out of her room. The physician was unable to pick up any fetal heart tones, so she immediately did an ultrasound. It showed that the fetus had died. The patient was alone and extremely upset. I stayed with her until her family arrived.

Although little medical treatment was given during this time, I do believe that my medical assisting training and experience made a difference in my knowing what to do and say to help comfort the patient during this difficult time. ■

BOX 8.1 American Cancer Society Breast Cancer Screening Recommendations for Women at Average Breast Cancer Risk

- Women between 40 and 44 should have the choice to start annual breast cancer screening with mammograms if they wish to do so.
- Women 45–54 should get mammograms every year.
- Women 55 and older should switch to a mammogram every other year, or they can choose to continue yearly mammograms.
- Screening should continue as long as a woman is in good health and is expected to live 10 more years or longer.
- All women should be familiar with how their breasts normally look and feel and report any changes to a health care provider right away.

PATIENT COACHING Breast Self-Examination

Answer questions patients have about breast self-examination.

Why is it important to examine my breasts?

The purpose of a breast self-examination is not just to find lumps, but also to notice when there are changes in your breasts. The best way to do this is to become as familiar as possible with how your breasts normally look and feel. By examining your breasts, you will learn what is normal for you, and it will be easier to notice changes.

What is considered normal?

Breast tissue normally feels a little lumpy and uneven. The left and right breasts may not be the same size; most women's breasts are slightly different in size. Many women have a normal thickening or ridge of firm tissue under the lower curve of the breast where it attaches to the chest wall. Throughout your life, changes also can occur in the size, shape, and feel of your breasts because of aging, weight changes, the menstrual cycle, pregnancy, breastfeeding, and use of birth control pills or other hormones.

What should be reported to the provider?

Early breast cancer does not usually cause pain. When breast cancer first develops, there may be no symptoms at all. As the cancer grows, it can cause changes that should be reported to the provider. Contact your provider immediately if any of the following changes occurs:

- Any new lump, hard knot, or thickening in the breast or underarm area
- A change in the size or shape of the breast
- A puckering or dimpling of the skin of the breast or nipple
- A change in skin texture of the breast or nipple
- A nipple that becomes retracted (pulled in)
- A discharge or bleeding from the nipple ■

What Would You Do? What Would You *Not* Do?

Case Study 1

Carol Wooster, 47 years old, has come to the office for a gynecologic examination. She has not had a gynecologic examination in 10 years. Mrs. Wooster picked up a breast self-examination (BSE) brochure at a local health fair and performed a BSE at home. She is now concerned because she found some unusual things. Her right breast is slightly larger than her left breast, her left nipple is pulled in, and she found some freckles on her right breast. Mrs. Wooster explains that she has not had a gynecologic examination in such a long time because her periods have been normal and regular. Mrs. Wooster is afraid that the physician will be annoyed with her for not having had the examination sooner. ■

The medical assistant can help the patient relax during the examination by telling her to breathe deeply, slowly, and evenly through the mouth. If the patient is relaxed, it is easier for the provider to insert the vaginal speculum and to perform the bimanual pelvic examination; it also is more comfortable for the patient. Procedure 8.2 outlines the medical assistant's role in assisting the provider with a gynecologic examination.

INSPECTION OF EXTERNAL GENITALIA, VAGINA, AND CERVIX

The provider begins the pelvic examination with inspection of the external genitalia. The **vulva** is inspected for swelling, ulceration, and redness.

Next, the provider inserts a vaginal speculum into the vagina. Specula are available in two forms–plastic and metal. *Plastic specula* are used most commonly in the medical office; they are disposable and are designed to be used only once and then discarded. A plastic speculum permits a light source to be directly attached to it and the plastic blades facilitate visualization of the vagina. *Metal specula* are reusable and must be sanitized and sterilized after each use. Vaginal specula come in three sizes–small, medium, and large. The provider determines the size required based on the physical and sexual maturity of the patient. The function of the speculum is to hold the walls of the vagina apart to allow visual inspection of the vagina and cervix (Fig. 8.2).

A metal vaginal speculum is cold and should be warmed before use by placing it on a heating pad or by storing it in a warming drawer. A warmed speculum is more comfortable for the patient. It is important not to overheat the speculum, however; one that is too hot is just as uncomfortable as one that is too cold. A disposable plastic speculum does not hold the cold and does not need to be warmed.

The provider inspects the vagina and cervix for color, lacerations, ulcerations, redness, nodules, and discharge.

If an abnormal discharge is present, the provider obtains a specimen for laboratory evaluation. Examples of pathologic conditions that may produce a discharge include vaginal infections such as *bacterial vaginosis (BV), vulvovaginal candidiasis (VVC), trichomoniasis, chlamydia,* and *gonorrhea,* which are discussed in detail later.

CERVICAL CANCER SCREENING

Cervical cancer screening is used for the early detection of cancer of the cervix. Almost all cervical cancers are caused by the human papillomavirus (HPV). HPV is a common virus that can be transmitted from one individual to another during sexual intercourse. There are many types of HPV, but most of these do not pose a health risk. Certain types of HPV are called *high-risk* because they can cause abnormal changes to the cervical cells (known as **dysplasia**) that can lead to cervical cancer over time. Although infection with a high-risk HPV is the most important risk factor for

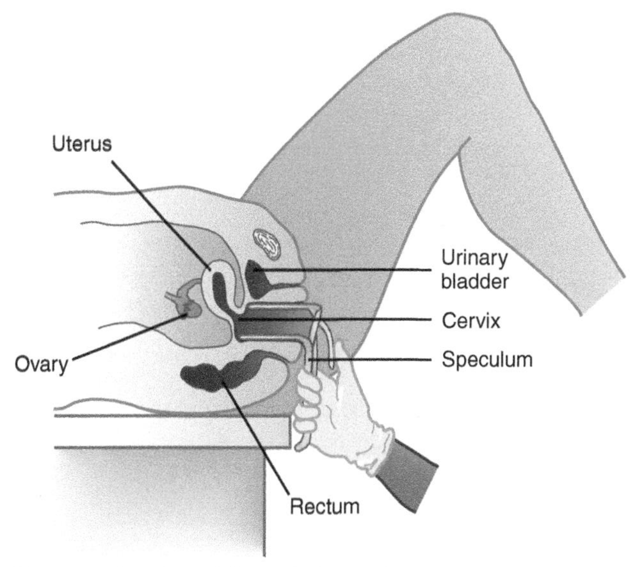

Fig. 8.2 Insertion of the vaginal speculum for visualization of the vagina and cervix.

HIGHLIGHT on Breast Cancer

Breast cancer is one of the most common types of cancer among American women. The American Cancer Society estimates that one of every eight women in the United States develops breast cancer at some point in her lifetime. Every year, more than 200,000 women learn they have breast cancer, and about 40,000 of them die from the disease. Most women (82%) diagnosed with breast cancer are older than 50 years old, but breast cancer does occur in younger women.

Survival rate

The 5-year survival rate for breast cancer that has spread to a distant site in the body (metastasized) is only 21%. The 5-year survival rate for small, localized tumors is 94%. If the cancer has spread to lymph nodes in the region of the breast, the 5-year survival rate is 73%. These encouraging statistics are the result of advances in the early detection of breast cancer and better treatment, including improved surgical procedures, radiation therapy, chemotherapy, hormonal therapy, and biologic therapy.

Risk factors

Breast cancer results from the abnormal growth of cells in breast tissue. It occurs more often in the left breast than in the right, and more often in the upper outer quadrant of the breast. The cause of abnormal growths in the breasts is unknown; therefore, every woman should consider herself at risk for breast cancer. Certain factors seem to place a woman at higher-than-normal risk for breast cancer, however, including the following:

- **Gender.** Women are much more likely than men to develop breast cancer.
- **Age.** The risk of breast cancer increases as women get older. Most women diagnosed with breast cancer are older than age 50.
- **Personal history.** Women with cancer in one breast have a greater chance of developing a new cancer in the other breast or in another part of the same breast.
- **Family history.** A woman's risk of developing breast cancer increases if her mother, sister, or daughter had breast cancer, especially at a young age.
- **Dense breast tissue.** Women with dense breast tissue (meaning they have more glandular tissue than fat tissue as seen on a mammogram) have a higher risk of developing breast cancer.
- **Breast biopsy.** Women who have had a breast biopsy that indicated certain types of benign breast disease (characterized by atypical hyperplasia) have an increased risk of developing breast cancer.
- **Breast cancer genes.** A woman who has inherited mutations in breast cancer genes (mutations of the *BRCA1* and *BRCA2* genes) from either parent is more likely to develop breast cancer.
- **Reproductive history.** Women who began menstruating at an early age (younger than age 12) or who went through menopause at a late age (after age 55) have a slightly increased risk of breast cancer.
- **Childbearing.** Women who have never had a child or women who had their first child late (after age 30) have a slightly increased risk of developing breast cancer.

Continued

HIGHLIGHT on Breast Cancer—cont'd

- **Hormone replacement therapy (HRT).** Studies indicate that the long-term use of estrogen and progesterone combination HRT for relief of menopausal symptoms increases the risk of breast cancer.
- **Radiation treatment.** Women who have had radiation of the chest before age 30 as treatment for another type of cancer (e.g., Hodgkin disease) have a significantly increased risk of developing breast cancer.
- **Race.** Caucasian women are diagnosed more frequently than Hispanic, Asian, or African American women.
- **Lifestyle factors.** Studies suggest that the use of alcohol (more than two drinks per day) increases the risk of breast cancer. Obesity, especially for women after menopause, also may increase the risk of breast cancer.

Warning signs

The warning signs of possible breast cancer include a lump, hard knot, or thickening in the breast or armpit; a change in breast color or texture; dimpling or puckering; nipple discharge; changes in the size or shape of the breast; and an enlargement of the lymph nodes.

Diagnosis

A biopsy is the only conclusive method of determining whether a breast lump or suspicious area seen on a mammogram is benign or malignant. A biopsy involves the surgical removal and analysis of all or part of the lump. Biopsy methods include fine needle aspiration biopsy (collection of a sample of fluid from the lump), core needle biopsy (removal of a core of tissue from the lump), and surgical excisional biopsy (removal of all or part of the lump). The provider may recommend one or more of these procedures to evaluate a lump or other change in the breast.

Approximately 80% of breast lumps are benign. A lump or suspicious area is often the result of a benign breast condition, such as normal hormonal changes, fibrocystic breast disease, or a fibroadenoma.■

the development of cervical cancer, there are other factors that place a woman at higher risk for cervical cancer. These include:

- Cigarette smoking
- Weakened immune system due to human immunodeficiency virus (HIV) infection, organ transplantation, chemotherapy, or long-term steroid use
- Having given birth to three or more children
- Use of oral contraceptives for more than 5 years
- Diethylstilbestrol (DES) exposure before birth

Nearly all cancers of the cervix can be cured if detected early enough. The American College of Obstetricians and Gynecologists (ACOG) publishes recommendations for cervical cancer screening which are outlined in Box 8.2. Cervical cancer screening consists of two types of tests: the Pap test and the HPV test which are described in more detail as follows.

BOX 8.2 American College of Obstetricians and Gynecologists Cervical Cancer Screening Recommendations

- Cervical cancer screening should start at age 21. Women under age 21 should not be tested.
- Women between the ages of 21 and 29 should have a Pap test performed every 3 years. HPV testing should not be used in this age group unless it is needed after an abnormal Pap test result.
- Women between the ages of 30 and 65 have three options for screening. They can have a Pap test plus an HPV test (known as *cotesting*) performed every 5 years. They can have a Pap test alone every 3 years, or they can have a primary HPV test every 5 years. A primary HPV test is an HPV test that is done by itself for screening. The FDA has approved certain tests to be primary HPV tests.
- Women who are at high risk for cervical cancer or who have had abnormal Pap test results should be screened more often. Women who have been vaccinated against HPV should still follow these guidelines for their age group.
- Women over the age of 65 who have had regular cervical cancer screenings in the past 10 years with normal results should not be screened for cervical cancer. Once screening is stopped, it should not be started again. Women with a history of a serious cervical pre-cancer should continue to be screened for at least 20 years after that diagnosis, even if it goes past age 65.
- A woman who has had her uterus and cervix removed (total hysterectomy) for reasons not related to cervical cancer and who has no history of cervical cancer or serious pre-cancer should not be screened.

Pap Test

The Pap test is a simple and painless **cytology** evaluation named after its developer, Dr. George Papanicolaou (1883–1962). To perform the evaluation, a sampling of cells is collected from the cervix and examined under the microscope for the presence of abnormal cells.

The primary purpose of the Pap test is to detect abnormal cells (dysplasia) that may develop into cervical cancer if not treated. It usually takes years or even decades for abnormal cervical cells to develop into cancer. The Pap test can also determine the presence of noncancerous conditions such as infection and inflammation. The Pap test detects the presence of cancer cells, however in regularly screened individuals, most abnormal cells are discovered before they become cancerous. In some cases, the Pap test can detect cancer of the endometrium; however, it is less reliable in doing so.

Human Papillomavirus Test

The HPV test is a DNA test that detects the genetic material of high-risk types of HPV that have infected the cervical cells. Approximately 70% of all cervical cancers are caused by HPV types 16 and 18. The HPV test can be performed on the same liquid-based cytology specimen that is collected for a Pap test. Essentially, the Pap test looks for the presence of abnormal cells of the cervix while the HPV test looks for high-risk HPVs that may cause the cervical cells to become abnormal. Performing an HPV test is not necessary under the age of 30 (unless it is needed following an abnormal Pap test result). This is because cervical HPV infections in younger women usually go away on their own without causing problems.

Patient Instructions

The medical assistant should provide the patient with patient preparation instructions for cervical cancer screening which help to ensure accurate test results. It is recommended that the specimen not be collected during the patient's menstrual period. The patient should be instructed to schedule cervical cancer screening approximately 10 to 20 days after the first day of her last menstrual period (LMP). The patient should be told not to douche or insert tampons, vaginal medications, lubricants, or contraceptive spermicides into the vagina for 2 days before having cervical cancer screening. Douching and tampon insertion reduce the number of cells available for analysis, and vaginal medications, lubricants, and spermicides change the pH of the vagina, making the specimen nonrepresentative or invalid. The patient also should be told to abstain from sexual intercourse for 2 days before undergoing cervical cancer screening. Recent sexual intercourse can produce inflammatory changes that can interfere with visualization of abnormal cells that may be present.

Specimen Collection Techniques

With a vaginal speculum in place, the provider collects a sampling of epithelial cells from the cervix for evaluation by the laboratory. A scraping of cells must be collected from both the ectocervix and the endocervix (refer to Fig. 8.1).

The **ectocervix** is the outermost layer of the cervix that projects into the vagina and consists of a thin, flat layer of cells, approximately 10 layers thick, known as *stratified squamous epithelial cells.* The **endocervix** is the inner part of the cervix that forms a narrow canal that connects the vagina to the uterus; it is lined with a mucous membrane made up of *simple columnar epithelial cells* that produce mucus. A scraping of epithelial cells may also be collected from the vagina; however, this is not usually done unless the provider has observed a lesion on the vaginal wall, or the maturation index is to be determined. The collection devices and techniques used by the provider to obtain the epithelial cells is described next.

Vaginal Specimen

If a vaginal specimen is needed, it is collected first, before the ectocervical and endocervical specimens are obtained. The rounded end of a plastic cytospatula is used to collect the specimen. If a routine vaginal specimen is being obtained, it is collected from the vaginal pool in the posterior fornix of the vagina, which is located just below the cervix (Fig. 8.3A). If the provider is collecting a specimen from a lesion on the vaginal wall, a scraping of cells is taken from the area of the lesion. To obtain a specimen for determination of the maturation index (discussed later), the provider obtains the vaginal specimen from the upper one-third of the lateral vaginal wall.

Ectocervical Specimen

The provider collects the ectocervical specimen by placing the S-shaped end of a plastic cytospatula just inside the cervical canal at the **external os**. The external os is the opening of the cervical canal of the uterus into the vagina. The physician next rotates the blade of the cytospatula 360 degrees over the surface of the ectocervix at the squamocolumnar junction, where cervical cancer is most often found (see Fig. 8.3B).

Endocervical Specimen

The provider collects the endocervical specimen by inserting a cytobrush into the endocervical canal and rotating the cytobrush (see Fig. 8.3C). The cytobrush is made up of soft bristles designed to be inserted into the canal without causing damage to it.

Ectocervical and Endocervical Combined Specimen

A scraping of cells from the ectocervix and endocervix can be collected at the same time using a flexible plastic collection device known as a *cytobroom*. The provider inserts the central bristles of the cytobroom into the endocervical canal deep enough to allow the shorter bristles to contact the outside of the cervix fully. The cytobroom is gently pushed and rotated in a clockwise direction to collect an ectocervical and endocervical combined specimen (see Fig. 8.3D).

Preparation of the Specimen

The most commonly used method to prepare a cytology specimen for evaluation is the liquid-based method; brand names of liquid-based systems include *ThinPrep* and *SurePath*. Following collection, the specimen is placed in a plastic collection vial containing a liquid preservative. The preservative maintains the specimen and prevents it from drying out during transport to the laboratory. Use of the liquid-based method provides a high-quality specimen which

Vaginal Specimen

Vaginal speculum

Posterior fornix

The rounded end of the spatula is used to obtain the vaginal specimen from the posterior fornix of the vagina.

A

Ectocervical Specimen

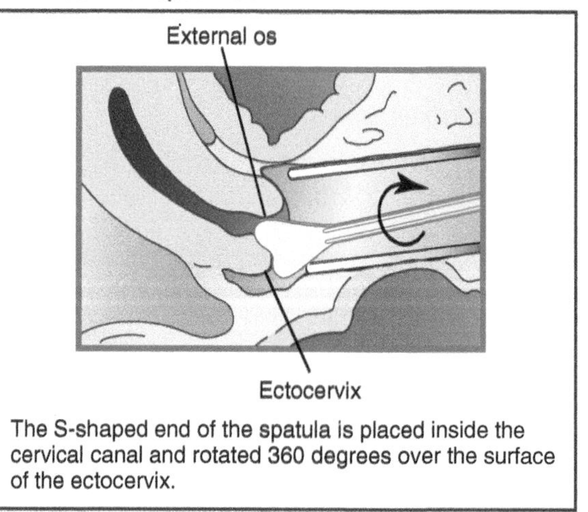

The S-shaped end of the spatula is placed inside the cervical canal and rotated 360 degrees over the surface of the ectocervix.

B

Endocervical Specimen

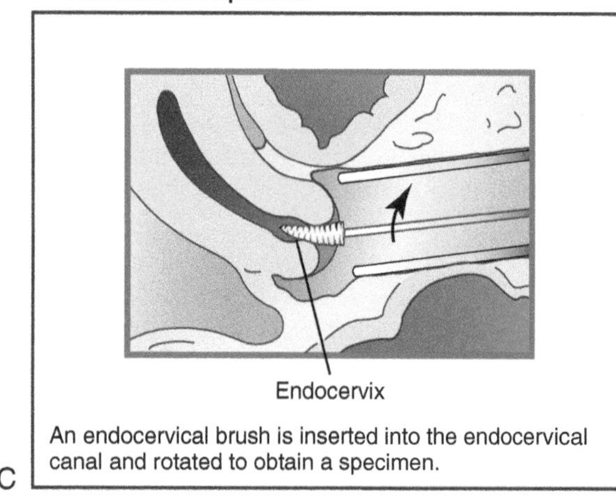

An endocervical brush is inserted into the endocervical canal and rotated to obtain a specimen.

C

Ectocervical and Endocervical Combined Specimen

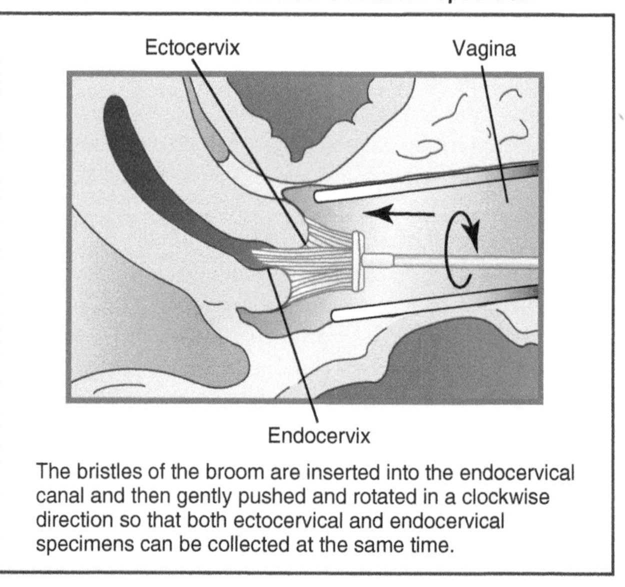

The bristles of the broom are inserted into the endocervical canal and then gently pushed and rotated in a clockwise direction so that both ectocervical and endocervical specimens can be collected at the same time.

D

Fig. 8.3 Obtaining the Pap specimen. (A) Vaginal specimen. (B) Ectocervical specimen. (C) Endocervical specimen. (D) Ectocervical and endocervical combined specimen.

results in fewer slides that are unsatisfactory for evaluation. A high-quality specimen also reduces the occurrence of false-negative test results.

The specimen for a liquid-based preparation is obtained using one or more of the specimen collection techniques previously described; the technique employed is based on physician preference. A plastic cytospatula (S-shaped end) may be used to collect the ectocervical specimen and a cytobrush may be used to collect an endoectocervical specimen. Alternatively, a cytobroom can be used to collect an ectocervical and endocervical combined specimen. If a vaginal specimen is needed, it is collected first using the rounded end of a cytospatula.

Once the specimen has been collected, the medical assistant is responsible for performing one of the following steps depending on the brand of liquid-based preparation being used:

1. Rinse the collection device in the vial of liquid preservative and discard the collection device (performed with ThinPrep).
2. Remove the tip of the collection device, deposit it in the vial of preservative, and discard the handle (performed with SurePath).

Cytology Request

A cytology request must accompany all Pap specimens. Fig. 8.4 is an example of a cytology request form. The medical assistant is responsible for completing the request, which includes the following categories.

General Information

General information includes the provider's name, address, and phone number and the patient's name, address, identification number, date of birth, and date of LMP. Insurance

GYN CYTOLOGY REQUISITION

THOMAS WOODSIDE, MD
501 MAIN ST
ST. LOUIS, MO 63146
(314) 555–0093

PATIENT INFO

Patient's Name (Last) | (First) | (MI) | Date of Birth MO DAY YR | Collection Time : AM PM | Collection Date MO DAY YR | Patient's ID #

Patient's Address | Phone

City | State | ZIP

RESP. PARTY

Name of Responsible Party (if different from patient)

Address of Responsible Party | APT #

City | State | ZIP

INSURANCE

Patient's Relationship to Responsible Party ☐ 1. Self ☐ 2. Spouse ☐ 3. Child ☐ 4. Other

Insurance Company Name | Plan | Carrier Code

Subscriber/Member # | Location | Group #

Insurance Address | Physician's Provider #

City | State | ZIP

Employer's Name or Number | Insured SSN

Diagnosis/Signs/Symptoms in ICD-9 Format (Highest Specificity)

REQUIRED

ICD-9 codes are the internationally accepted method of describing the clinical picture of the patient. All diagnoses should be provided by the ordering physician or his or her authorized designee. The following is a partial list of common diagnoses in ICD-9 format. Most third party payers require an ICD-9 code to indicate the medical necessity of the test(s) and/or profile(s) ordered. For a complete list of all ICD-9 codes, please refer to a current ICD-9 manual.

V76.2 Routine Cervical Pap Smear	616.0 Cervicitis	626.8 Abnormal Bleeding
V15.89 High Risk Cervical Screening	616.10 Vaginitis	627.1 Postmenopausal Bleeding
V22.2 Pregnancy	617.0 Endometriosis, Uterus	627.3 Atrophic Vaginitis
079.4 Human Papillomavirus	622.1 Dysplasia, Cervix	795.0 Abnormal Cervical Pap Smear
180.0 Malignant Neoplasm, Cervix	623.0 Dysplasia, Vagina	

COLLECTION METHOD

Liquid-Based Prep
192055 ☐ ThinPrep Pap Test
192039 ☐ ThinPrep Pap Test w/reflex to HPV Hybrid Capture when ASC-US or SIL
192047 ☐ ThinPrep Pap Test w/reflex to high-risk only HPV Hybrid Capture when ASC-US

Pap Smear
009100 ☐ 1 Slide **009191** ☐ 2 Slides

Pap Smear and Maturation Index
009209 ☐ 1 Slide **190074** ☐ 2 Slides

SOURCE OF SPECIMEN

☐ **Ectocervical**
☐ **Endocervical**
☐ **Vaginal**

Date LMP
___/___/___
Mo Day Year

COLLECTION TECHNIQUE

☐ **Spatula**
☐ **Brush**
☐ **Broom**
☐ **Other** ____________

PATIENT HISTORY

☐ **Pregnant**
☐ **Lactating**
☐ **Oral Contraceptives**
☐ **Postmenopausal**
☐ **Hormone Replacement Therapy**
☐ **PMP Bleeding**
☐ **Postpartum**
☐ **IUD**
☐ **Postcoital Bleeding**
☐ **DES Exposure**
☐ **Previous Abnormal Pap Test**
☐ **Other** ____________

PREVIOUS TREATMENT | **Date/Results**

☐ **None**
☐ **Colposcopy and Bx** ____________
☐ **Cervical Cryotherapy** ____________
☐ **LEEP** ____________
☐ **Laser Treatment** ____________
☐ **Conization** ____________
☐ **Hysterectomy** ____________
☐ **Radiation** ____________
☐ **Chemotherapy** ____________

Fig. 8.4 Cytology request form.

information also is required in this section for third-party billing.

Date and Time of Collection

The date and time of collection indicate to the laboratory the number of days that have passed since the collection, providing the laboratory with information regarding the freshness of the specimen.

Test(s) Requested

The test(s) desired by the provider are indicated by selecting the appropriate box adjacent to the test(s).

Source of the Specimen

The purpose of this category is to identify the origin of the specimen because it is impossible for the laboratory to obtain this information by looking at the specimen. The medical assistant selects one or more of the following boxes on the form: ectocervical, endocervical, or vaginal.

Collection Technique

The collection device or devices used to obtain the specimen must be indicated. The medical assistant selects one or more of the following boxes on the form: spatula, brush, or broom.

Patient History

Information on the present and past health status of the patient is specified under the patient history category. The medical assistant must check the following boxes that apply to the patient: pregnant, lactating, oral contraceptives, postmenopausal (PMP), hormone replacement therapy, PMP bleeding, postpartum, intrauterine device (IUD), postcoital bleeding, diethylstilbestrol (DES) exposure, and previous abnormal Pap test. This information assists the laboratory in evaluating the specimen.

Previous Treatment

Any previous treatment for a precancerous or cancerous condition of the cervix is indicated under this category. The medical assistant checks the appropriate box on the form if any of the following procedures have been performed on the patient: colposcopy and biopsy, cryotherapy, loop electrocautery excision procedure (LEEP), laser treatment, conization, hysterectomy, radiation, and chemotherapy.

Evaluation of the Specimen

Following collection, the liquid-based cytology specimen is transported to an outside laboratory for further processing and evaluation. Before a Pap evaluation can be performed, the specimen must undergo a processing procedure. The specimen is placed in an automated slide preparation processor which performs several important functions. First, it separates the cells from debris present in the specimen, and then it disperses a representative cell sample onto a slide in a thin, uniform layer. The slide is next immersed in a fixative to maintain the normal appearance of the cells.

Before the Pap slide can be evaluated, it must be stained by a laboratory technician. The purpose of staining is to allow better viewing of the morphology of the epithelial cells. The slide is studied under a microscope for evidence of abnormalities by a specially trained technician, known as a *cytotechnologist.* When an abnormality is detected, it is reviewed by a *cytopathologist* (a provider specializing in pathology), who makes a final evaluation.

A more recent development in the evaluation of Pap slides is the use of automated cytology computer-imaging devices. An abnormal slide may contain only a few abnormal cells among thousands of normal cells. Because of this, these abnormal cells may be missed during the evaluation by the cytotechnologist. A cytology computer-imaging device is able to examine every cell on the slide and select and display cells that appear "most abnormal." The cytotechnologist can evaluate these cells further under a microscope. In this way, the cytotechnologist can focus his or her expertise and decision making on preselected areas of the slide.

Maturation Index

The maturation index must be performed on a sampling of cells taken from the upper third of the lateral vaginal wall. The *maturation index* refers to the percentage of parabasal, intermediate, and superficial cells present in the specimen. The maturation index provides an endocrine evaluation of the patient, which can assist the provider in evaluating the cause of infertility, menopausal or PMP bleeding, or amenorrhea and can help assess the results of treatment with hormones. Numerous factors affect the results of the maturation index; it is important to indicate on the cytology request the presence of abnormal bleeding; hormone treatment; or treatment with digitalis, corticosteroids, or thyroid medication.

Cytology Report

The Bethesda System (TBS) is the standard for reporting the results of a Pap test on the cytology report (Fig. 8.5). The National Cancer Institute in Bethesda, Maryland, developed this system. It provides a detailed cytologic description, rather than a numerical result (as with the previous class I through V system). For this reason, TBS is a more effective means of communicating the results of the Pap test to the provider. TBS separates the cytology report into the following categories:

1. **Specimen Adequacy.** This category refers to the quality of the specimen collected by the provider. The specimen is described using one of the following classifications:
   - **Satisfactory for Evaluation.** This indicates that the specimen was of sufficient sampling and quality for a comprehensive assessment of the cells.
   - **Unsatisfactory for Evaluation.** This indicates that the overall sampling or quality of the specimen was inadequate. A reason is given for the inability to evaluate the Pap specimen, such as too few cells were collected or the presence of blood or inflammation is obscuring the cells.
2. **General Categorization.** This category provides the medical office with a quick review of the report. The following classifications are used to categorize the specimen:
   - **Negative for Intraepithelial Lesion or Malignancy.** This indicates that the epithelial cells were normal and that there were no precancerous or cancerous findings. This classification also is assigned to a specimen that exhibits certain benign (noncancerous) changes. Benign changes can be caused by vaginal infections, such as bacterial vaginosis chlamydia, trichomoniasis, candidiasis, and herpes. Benign changes also can be caused by inflammation resulting from the normal cell repair process, radiation, and chemotherapy. Any benign findings of importance (e.g., vaginal infections) are described in detail in the Interpretation/Result section of the cytology report.

GYN CYTOLOGY REPORT

RIVERVIEW MEDICAL LABORATORY DEPARTMENT OF PATHOLOGY 2501 GRANT AVENUE ST. LOUIS, MO 63146 (314) 555–3443	PATIENT: Heather Jones PATIENT NO: 45876 DOB: 10/20/65 SUBMITTING: T. Woodside, MD

	SPECIMEN TYPE
Date of Specimen: 7/01/XX	
Date Received: 7/02/XX	[X] ThinPrep [ ] Conventional Pap Smear
Date Reported: 7/06/XX	
Performed By: Richard McVay, Cytotechnologist	**Checked By:** Melissa Wagner, Pathologist

SPECIMEN ADEQUACY	GENERAL CATEGORIZATION
[X] **Satisfactory for Evaluation** [ ] **Unsatisfactory for Evaluation**	[ ] **Negative for Intraepithelial Lesion or Malignancy (*see Interpretation/Result*)** [X] **Epithelial Cell Abnormality (*see Interpretation/Result*)** [ ] **Other (*see Interpretation/Result*)**

INTERPRETATION/RESULT

A. BENIGN CELLULAR CHANGES

- [ ] Infection:
  - [ ] Trichomonas vaginalis
  - [ ] Fungal organisms morphologically compatible w/Candida species
  - [ ] Cellular changes associated with herpes simplex virus
  - [ ] Bacterial infection morphologically compatible with gardnerella
  - [ ] Cytoplasmic inclusions suggestive of chlamydia
- [ ] Reactive changes
  - [ ] Without inflammation
  - [ ] With inflammation
  - [ ] Atrophy with inflammation (atrophic vaginitis)
  - [ ] Radiation effect
  - [ ] Repair
  - [ ] Hyperkeratosis
  - [ ] Parakeratosis

B. EPITHELIAL CELL ABNORMALITIES

- [X] Squamous Cell
  - [X] Atypical Squamous Cells of Undetermined Significance (ASC-US)
  - [ ] Atypical Squamous Cells of Higher Risk (ASC-H)
  - [ ] Low-Grade Squamous Intraepithelial Lesion (LSIL)
  - [ ] High-Grade Squamous Intraepithelial Lesion (HSIL)
  - [ ] Squamous Cell Carcinoma
- [ ] Glandular Cell
  - [ ] Atypical Glandular Cells of Undetermined Significance (AGUS)
  - [ ] Adenocarcinoma

Fig. 8.5 Cytology report form (The Bethesda System).

- **Epithelial Cell Abnormality.** This classification indicates abnormal cell changes. The abnormality is described in detail in the Interpretation/Result section of the report.
- **Other.** This classification is used to indicate that no abnormality was found in the cells, but the findings indicate some increased risk. The presence of normal-appearing endometrial cells in a PMP woman may indicate an abnormality of the endometrium. These findings are described in detail in the Interpretation/Result section of the report.

3. **Interpretation/Result.** This part of the report provides the provider with a detailed description of findings. This includes any significant benign changes (e.g., vaginal infections) and any abnormal changes in the epithelial cells. Table 8.1 lists and describes the findings most frequently reported.
4. **Automated Review.** This category indicates whether the specimen was evaluated using an automated computer-imaging device. The name of the device and the results are specified in this section.
5. **Ancillary Testing.** This category is used if an additional test method is used to evaluate the specimen. If abnormal cells are detected on the Pap slide, a HPV test may be performed. The name of the test method and the results would be reported under this category.

TABLE 8.1 Pap Test Results

Test Result	Interpretation
Normal: Negative for intraepithelial lesion or malignancy	Epithelial cells were normal, and there were no precancerous or cancerous findings.
ASC-US: Atypical squamous cells of undetermined significance	Cells are only slightly abnormal. Nature and cause of abnormality cannot be determined. These slightly altered cells usually return to normal on their own, resulting in negative results on subsequent Pap tests.
ASC-H: Atypical squamous cells of higher risk	Minor abnormal changes in cells with unknown causes, but at risk of progressing to high-grade lesion (HSIL). Further testing is required to determine whether this is a minor condition or one that may progress to HSIL.
LSIL: Low-grade squamous intraepithelial lesion	Abnormal cells that show definite minor changes but are unlikely to progress to cancer (general term for this is *mild dysplasia*). LSIL may be caused by HPV infection, but of a type that is not likely to lead to cervical cancer.
HSIL: High-grade squamous intraepithelial lesion	Abnormal cell changes that have a higher likelihood of progressing to cancer. Although not cancerous yet, abnormal cells may become cancerous if treatment is not obtained (general term for this is *moderate-to-severe dysplasia*). HSIL is often caused by HPV infection of a type associated with cervical cancer.
Carcinoma	Usually means patient has cervical cancer. Most women with cervical cancer also test positive for HPV infection.

HPV, Human papillomavirus.

TABLE 8.2 Procedures Performed Following Abnormal Pap Test Results

Procedure	Description
Colposcopy (Refer to Chapter 10: Minor Office Surgery)	Colposcopy is performed to examine the vagina and cervix using a magnifying device (colposcope) to detect areas of abnormal tissue growth that may not be visible with the naked eye.
Cervical Biopsy (Refer to Chapter 10: Minor Office Surgery)	A cervical biopsy is performed in combination with colposcopy to remove a cervical tissue specimen for examination by a pathologist to detect the presence of cervical dysplasia or cancer of the cervix.
LEEP (Loop electrosurgical excision procedure)	LEEP uses an electrical current which is passed through a thin wire loop which functions as a scalpel to remove abnormal cells from the cervix. The tissue is examined by a pathologist to detect the presence of cervical dysplasia or cancer of the cervix.
Cervical Cryotherapy (Refer to Chapter 10: Minor Office Surgery)	Cryotherapy involves the application of extreme cold to destroy abnormal cervical cells that show changes that may lead to cancer. It is performed only after a colposcopy confirms the presence of cervical dysplasia.
Laser Treatment	Laser therapy involves the use of heat from a laser beam to destroy abnormal cervical cells.
Conization	Conization involves the removal of a cone-shaped section of the cervix containing abnormal cells using a scalpel, a laser, or the LEEP technique.

Abnormal Pap Test Results

Abnormal Pap test results can be caused by infection and inflammation, precancerous lesions, and cancerous lesions. Although an abnormal Pap result is found in every 1 in 10 tests, most abnormal results are not due to cancer but rather are caused by infection or inflammation.

The Pap test is a screening test; therefore, an abnormal test result requires further evaluation before a final diagnosis can be made. The type of test or procedure performed depends on the age of the patient and the Pap test result category (see Table 8.1). For example, a 21-year-old patient with a result of atypical squamous cells of undetermined significance (ASC-US) may require a repeat Pap test in 12 months. On the other hand, a 35-year-old patient with a result of high-grade squamous intraepithelial lesion (HSIL) may require colposcopy and biopsy or a LEEP. Procedures that are commonly performed following an abnormal Pap test result are outlined in Table 8.2.

BIMANUAL PELVIC EXAMINATION

After obtaining the smear for the Pap test, the provider withdraws the speculum and performs a bimanual pelvic examination. The provider inserts the index and middle fingers of a lubricated gloved hand into the vagina. The fingers of the other hand are placed on the woman's lower abdomen. Between the two hands, the provider can palpate the size, shape, and position of the uterus and ovaries and can detect tenderness or lumps (Fig. 8.6).

RECTAL-VAGINAL EXAMINATION

The last part of the pelvic examination is a rectal-vaginal examination. The provider inserts one gloved finger into the vagina and another gloved finger into the rectum to obtain information about the tone and alignment of the pelvic organs and the adjacent region (ovaries, fallopian tubes, and ligaments of the uterus). The presence of hemorrhoids, fistulas, and fissures also can be noted. During this examination, the provider may want to obtain a fecal specimen from the rectum to test for occult blood in the stool (e.g., Hemoccult). This is typically performed on women beginning at 40 years of age. The medical assistant is responsible for assisting with the collection and testing of the specimen for occult blood. This procedure (fecal occult blood testing) is presented in detail in Chapter 13.

Gynecologic Infections

Gynecologic infections are commonly seen in the medical office and can be classified into the following categories: *vaginal infections* and *sexually transmitted infections (STIs).* Vaginal infections are caused by the overgrowth of an organism normally present in the vagina, while STIs are caused by the transmission of a pathogen through sexual contact with an infected partner. In most areas, vaginal infections are much more common than STIs.

The medical assistant is responsible for assembling the appropriate supplies for the collection of a suspected pathogen. The medical assistant must label the specimen with the patient's name and date of birth, the date, and the source of the specimen. If the specimen is to be transported to an outside medical laboratory for evaluation, a laboratory request form must be completed. The request form indicates the source of the specimen, the physician's clinical diagnosis, and the laboratory test requested. The physician's clinical assessment of the patient's signs and symptoms, along with the results of the laboratory evaluation of the specimen, are used to diagnose the presence of a gynecologic infection.

Medical assistants should protect themselves from infection with a pathogen while assisting with the collection of the specimen by practicing good techniques of medical asepsis. A thorough discussion of common vaginal infections and STIs is presented next.

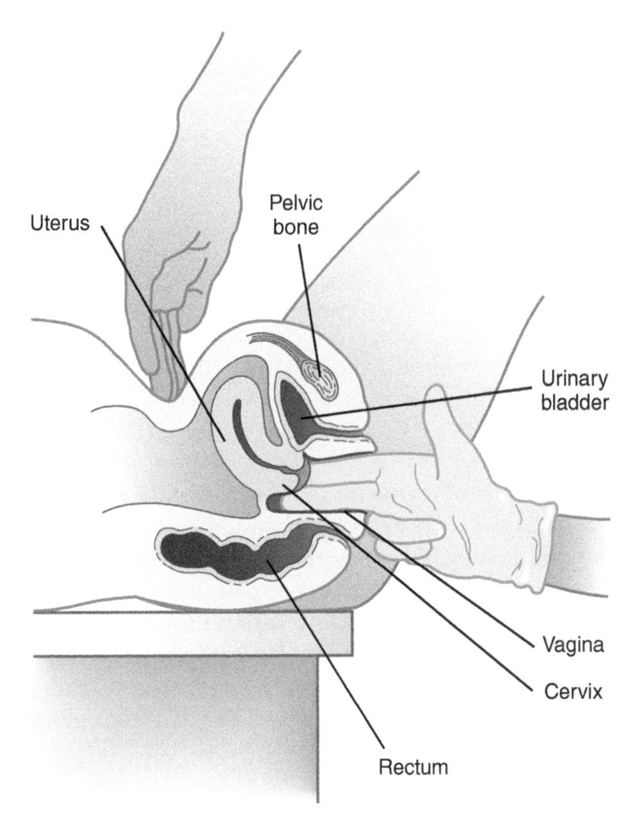

Fig. 8.6 The bimanual pelvic examination.

VAGINAL INFECTIONS

The vagina provides a warm, moist environment, which tends to encourage the growth of various organisms that can result in a vaginal infection, or *vaginitis*. If an unusual vaginal discharge is present, suggesting a vaginal infection, a specimen is obtained to identify the invading organism. A specimen of the vaginal discharge is collected at the medical office and is evaluated there or placed in an appropriate specimen container that is picked up by a laboratory courier and transported to an outside medical laboratory for evaluation. The patient should be instructed not to douche or use a feminine hygiene product before coming to the medical office because the physician may not be able to observe the discharge or to obtain a specimen for analysis.

The most common vaginal infections include bacterial vaginosis, vulvovaginal candidiasis, and trichomoniasis which are discussed in more detail as follows.

BACTERIAL VAGINOSIS

Description

Bacterial vaginosis (BV) is the most common cause of abnormal vaginal discharge in women of childbearing age (14 to 49). In the United States, as many as 30% of women of childbearing age are infected with BV. In the past, BV has been known by different names such as *Gardnerella vaginitis* and *nonspecific vaginitis.*

BV is caused by an imbalance in the normal flora of the vagina, known as the *vaginal flora*. The factors that upset the normal balance of the vaginal flora are not yet completely understood. The majority of the vaginal flora (95%) consists of lactobacilli which are beneficial to the body. When the vaginal flora is altered, anaerobic bacteria normally present in the vagina in small numbers (such as Gardnerella vaginalis) begin to grow and multiply. This results in the replacement of the beneficial lactobacilli with these harmful anaerobic bacteria along with a decrease in the acidity of the vagina.

The normal pH of the vagina ranges from 3.8 to 4.5, which is considered mildly acidic; this works to repress the growth of the harmful anaerobic bacteria.

A patient with BV will have a vaginal pH of 4.5 or higher; this means that there is a decrease in the acidity of the vagina which promotes the growth of the harmful anaerobic bacteria.

Many women with BV have no symptoms and are not aware of having the condition. When symptoms are present, they commonly include an abnormal amount of a thin, grayish-white vaginal discharge which has a foul-smelling or "fishy" odor. Any woman can develop BV, but some behaviors or activities have been found to increase the risk of developing this condition. They include vaginal douching, new or multiple sexual partners, IUDs, recent antibiotic use, and cigarette smoking.

If left untreated, BV can lead to significant health complications. Having BV increases the risk of infection by a number of STIs such as chlamydia, gonorrhea, genital herpes, and HIV. BV also increases the risk of pelvic inflammatory disease (PID), pregnancy complications, and postsurgical complications following gynecologic procedures such as a hysterectomy.

Diagnosis and Treatment

BV can be identified in the medical office. This involves using a sterile swab to place a small amount of the vaginal discharge on a microscope slide, adding a drop of isotonic saline to it and placing a coverslip over the mixture to protect it. The provider examines the slide under the microscope to observe for the presence of vaginal epithelial cells that are coated with bacteria known as *clue cells*. Clue cells are a good indication that BV is present. The provider may also check the pH of the vagina to determine if the pH is higher than 4.5 (also suggestive of BV). In addition to determining the presence of clue cells and checking the vaginal pH, the provider may perform a *whiff test*. This involves placing a small amount of vaginal discharge on a microscope slide and adding a drop of 10 percent potassium hydroxide (KOH) to it and then checking the odor of the specimen. A characteristic fishy odor is considered a positive whiff test and is also suggestive of BV.

If the provider prefers to have an outside laboratory evaluate the specimen, it must be placed in the appropriate specimen container and transported to the laboratory for evaluation. A nucleic acid hybridization test (NAT) known as a *DNA-probe test* is used to detect BV. The brand name of this test is Affirm VP III (Becton Dickinson, San Jose, CA). The probe test uses DNA technology to detect the presence of BV. The DNA-probe test can also simultaneously determine the presence of VVC and trichomoniasis. The provider collects a vaginal specimen using a sterile swab. After collection, the specimen is placed in a tube containing a transport medium to preserve the specimen until it reaches the laboratory.

Several antibiotics are effective in the treatment of BV. These include metronidazole (Flagyl) taken either orally or as a vaginal gel (Metrogel). A vaginal clindamycin cream (Cleocin) is also effective in treating BV. Tinidazole (Tindamax) can be used to treat BV and tends to have fewer side effects than the other antibiotics. Once the natural balance of the vaginal flora has been disrupted, the body sometimes has difficulty in getting back to normal. Because of this, BV has a tendency to recur following treatment, requiring a second round of antibiotic therapy.

VULVOVAGINAL CANDIDIASIS

Description

Candida albicans is a yeastlike fungus normally found in the intestinal tract and is a frequent contaminant of the vagina; however, it usually does not produce symptoms indicating a vaginal infection. Conditions such as pregnancy, diabetes mellitus, a weakened immune system, and prolonged antibiotic therapy may cause changes in the vagina that may precipitate vulvovaginal candidiasis (VVC), commonly referred to as a "yeast infection." The vaginal changes result in the overgrowth of *C. albicans* in the vagina. Symptoms of VVC include white patches on the mucous membrane of the vagina; a thick, odorless, cottage cheese–like discharge; vulval irritation; and dysuria. The discharge is extremely irritating and usually results in burning and intense itching.

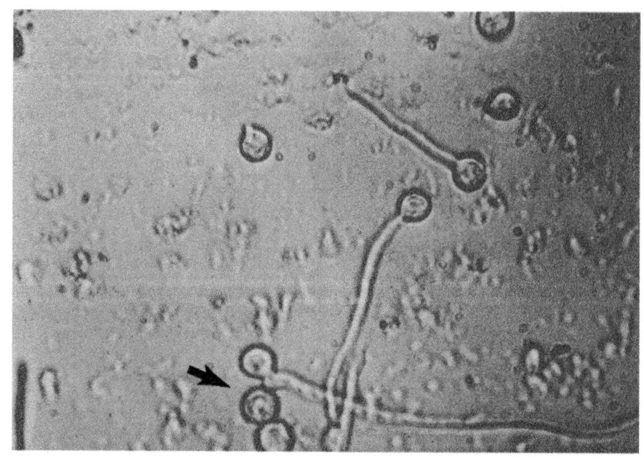

Fig. 8.7 *Candida albicans (arrow)* under a microscope. (Modified from Mahon C, Manuselis G: *Textbook of diagnostic microbiology,* ed 5, St Louis: Elsevier; 2015.)

Diagnosis and Treatment

VVC may be identified microscopically in the medical office by placing a specimen of the vaginal discharge on a slide using a sterile swab and adding a drop of a 10% solution of KOH. The KOH dissolves cellular debris present in the smear and allows better visualization of yeast buds, spores, or hyphae (fungus filaments) indicating the presence of *C. albicans* (Fig. 8.7). If the physician prefers to have an outside laboratory evaluate the specimen, it must be placed in the appropriate specimen container and transported to the laboratory. The recommended testing method for VVC is the DNA-probe test (Affirm VP III).

VVC is treated with the application of vaginal ointments or suppositories, such as miconazole (Monistat), clotrimazole (Gyne-Lotrimin), and nystatin (Mycostatin), or the oral administration of fluconazole (Diflucan). VVC has a tendency to recur; the patient should be instructed to contact the medical office if symptoms of the yeast infection reappear.

TRICHOMONIASIS

Description

Trichomonas vaginalis, the causative agent of trichomoniasis (trich), is a one-celled pear-shaped protozoan with flagella, which allow for the motility of the organism (Fig. 8.8). Because trichomoniasis is spread through sexual intercourse, it is also classified as an STI. It is included in this section because the symptoms are similar to those of a vaginal infection. Women between the ages of 40 and 49 years are more likely than adolescents or young adults to be infected with trichomoniasis.

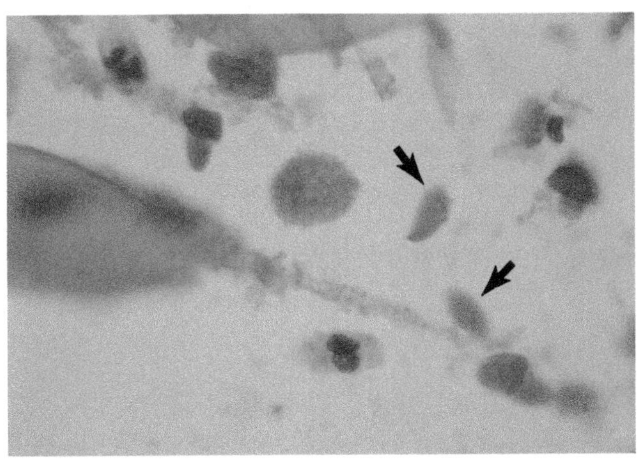

Fig. 8.8 *Trichomonas vaginalis (arrow)* under a microscope. (Modified from Mahon C, Manuselis G: *Textbook of diagnostic microbiology,* ed 3, St Louis: Elsevier; 2007.)

Women infected with trichomoniasis may not have any symptoms. When symptoms do occur they include a profuse, frothy vaginal discharge that is usually yellowish green and has an unpleasant odor; itching and irritation of the vulva and vagina; dyspareunia; and dysuria. The cervix may exhibit small red spots, a condition known as "strawberry cervix."

Diagnosis and Treatment

Trichomonas may be identified at the medical office by a wet preparation, which involves placing a small amount of the discharge on a microscope slide using a sterile swab, adding a drop of isotonic saline to it, and placing a coverslip over the mixture to protect it (Fig. 8.9). The slide is examined under the microscope by the provider and observed for the presence of the lashing movements of the flagella and the motility of the organism. If the physician prefers to have an outside laboratory evaluate the specimen, it must be placed in the appropriate specimen container and transported to the laboratory for evaluation. The recommended testing method for trichomonas is the DNA-probe test (Affirm VP III).

Trichomoniasis is treated with the oral administration of metronidazole (Flagyl) or tinidazole (Tindamax). The woman and her sexual partner must be treated at the same time to prevent reinfection because her partner may harbor the organism without displaying noticeable symptoms.

Wet Preparation

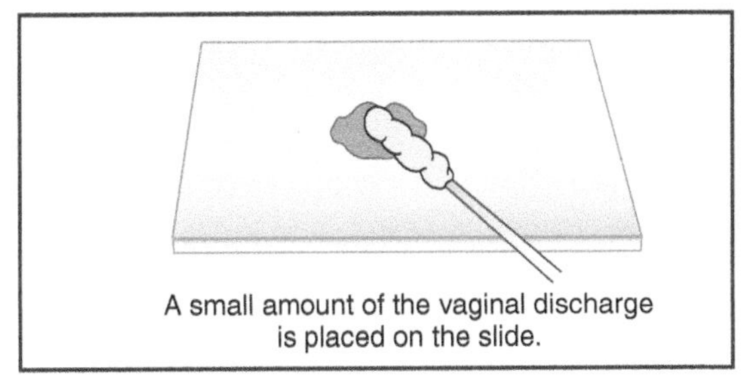

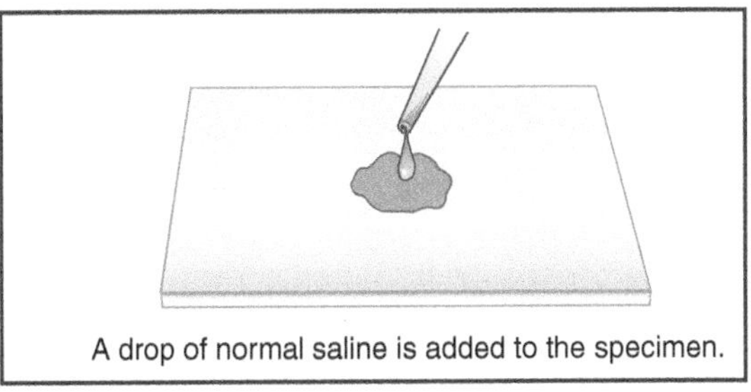

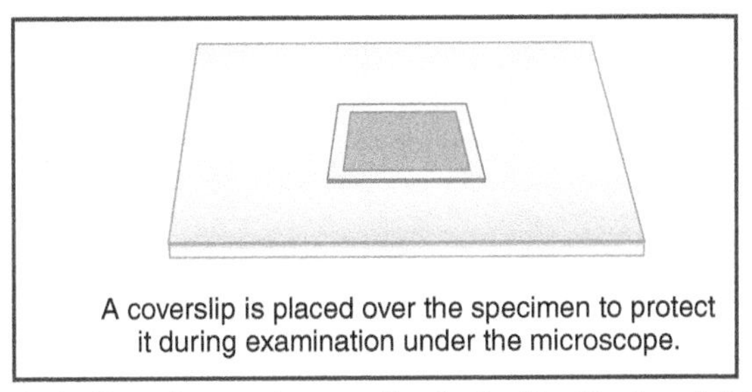

Fig. 8.9 Preparing a wet preparation for the identification of *Trichomonas vaginalis.*

SEXUALLY TRANSMITTED INFECTIONS

STIs are infections that are commonly spread through sexual contact with an infected individual and are among the most common infectious diseases in the United States (Refer to *Highlight on Sexually Transmitted Infections*). Most STIs initially do not cause symptoms. This results in a greater risk of transmitting the infection to others. Because of this, the CDC has set forth screening recommendations for the detection of STIs in asymptomatic individuals. These recommendations are discussed in this section.

More than twenty STIs have been identified and are most often caused by bacteria and viruses. The most common STIs are chlamydia, gonorrhea, genital herpes, and HPV, which are discussed in this section. Other STIs include hepatitis B, syphilis, and HIV, which are discussed in other chapters within this text. Of these, chlamydia, gonorrhea, and syphilis are curable with antibiotics, while genital herpes, HPV, hepatitis B, and HIV are treatable but not curable.

CHLAMYDIA

Description

Chlamydia is caused by the bacterium *Chlamydia trachomatis.* It is a gram-negative intracellular bacterium that grows and multiplies in the cytoplasm of the host cell. Chlamydia is the most frequently reported and fastest spreading sexually transmitted disease in the United States, particularly among adolescent girls and young women. Because of this, the CDC recommends annual routine screening for chlamydia of all sexually active females 25 years of age or younger. The CDC also recommends annual screening for women older than 25 with risk factors such as new or multiple sex partners, or a sex partner who has an STI.

Most women with chlamydia have no symptoms and are not aware of having the condition. Because of this, many women do not seek medical care until serious complications have occurred. After infection, chlamydia first attacks the cervix, resulting in cervicitis. If symptoms do occur, they may include one or more of the following: dysuria, itching and irritation of the genital area, and a yellowish, odorless vaginal discharge. These symptoms usually appear 1 to 3 weeks after the patient has been infected.

If not treated, chlamydia can spread further into the female reproductive tract and cause PID. The symptoms of PID include lower abdominal pain, fever, nausea and vomiting, dyspareunia, vaginal discharge, and bleeding between periods. Complications of PID are serious and include chronic pelvic pain, scarring of the fallopian tubes, ectopic pregnancy, and infertility.

Symptoms of a chlamydial infection in men include mild dysuria and a thin, watery discharge from the penis. Men are more likely to have symptoms than women; however, the symptoms may appear only early in the day and be so mild that they are ignored. If the infection is not treated, it can cause *epididymitis,* a painful condition of the testicles that could result in infertility.

Diagnosis and Treatment

The recommended test method for chlamydia is a nucleic acid amplification (NAA) test. NAA testing became available within the last decade and is considered the most sensitive and promising test for the identification of chlamydia (and gonorrhea). NAA tests are able to detect the presence of the genetic material (DNA) of chlamydia bacteria.

The following types of specimens can be used with a NAA test:

- Endocervical specimen
- Vaginal specimen (provider-collected or patient-collected)
- Urethral specimen (male)

After collection, the specimen is placed in a tube containing a transport medium to preserve the specimen until it reaches the laboratory. See Box 8.3, *Chlamydia and Gonorrhea Specimen Collection* for instructions on how to assist with the collection of an endocervical and urethral specimen. NAA testing can also be performed on a liquid-based cytology specimen for a Pap test.

Women who do not need a pelvic exam as part of their clinical evaluation can be screened for chlamydia and gonorrhea by providing a *patient-collected* vaginal specimen. Many women prefer this method of collection over a provider-collected specimen. Studies show that the results from a patient-collected specimen are just as accurate as a provider-collected specimen. Refer to Box 8.4 which outlines the procedure for instructing a patient in obtaining a patient-collected vaginal specimen.

Many NAA tests on the market can also use a *first-catch* urine specimen to perform the test. A first-catch urine specimen involves the collection of urine that has remained in the bladder for 1 hour. A first-catch urine specimen is the preferred specimen to test for chlamydia in a male. The procedure for obtaining a first-catch urine specimen is presented in Chapter 16 (Urinalysis).

When diagnosed early, chlamydia can be treated successfully with antibiotics. The antibiotics most often used are azithromycin (Zithromax) and doxycycline taken orally. The patient's partner(s) also should be tested for chlamydia so that if treatment is needed, it can be administered as soon as possible.

GONORRHEA

Description

Gonorrhea is caused by the bacterium *Neisseria gonorrhoeae,* which is a gram-negative diplococcus. Gonorrhea is an infection of the genitourinary tract that is transmitted through sexual intercourse. Chlamydia often occurs in association with gonorrhea; approximately 25% to 40% of patients infected with gonorrhea also have chlamydia. The CDC recommends annual routine screening for gonorrhea of all sexually active females 25 years of age or younger. The CDC also recommends annual screening for women older than 25 with risk factors such as new or multiple sex partners, or a sex partner who has an STI.

Women who have contracted gonorrhea may have no symptoms or may exhibit dysuria and an increased vaginal discharge that is yellow in color. The symptoms of gonorrhea (if they occur) appear 2 to 10 days after infection and may be so mild that they are ignored. As the disease progresses, it can spread farther into the reproductive tract, resulting in PID. As mentioned previously, PID can lead to serious complications such as infertility.

Men who have contracted gonorrhea tend to exhibit more symptoms than women, including dysuria and a whitish discharge from the penis, which may progress to a thick and creamy discharge. The burning and pain experienced during urination are often severe, which usually prompts an infected man to seek early treatment. If not treated, gonorrhea may cause epididymitis, which could lead to infertility.

Diagnosis and Treatment

The recommended method for diagnosing gonorrhea is a NAA test which detects the presence of the genetic material (DNA) of gonorrhea bacteria. The type of specimens that can be used for the NAA gonorrhea test are the same as those previously described for the NAA test for chlamydia.

Gonorrhea can be treated with antibiotics, however in recent years, gonorrhea bacteria have become resistant to the antibiotics typically used to treat the disease. Because of this, the CDC now recommends dual therapy (using two drugs) to treat gonorrhea. This includes the administration of ceftriaxone by injection and an oral dose of azithromycin. The patient's partner(s) also should be tested for gonorrhea so that if treatment is needed, it can be administered as soon as possible.

BOX 8.3 Chlamydia and Gonorrhea Specimen Collection

Nucleic Acid Amplification Test

The procedure for collecting an endocervical and urethral specimen for a nucleic acid amplification test is outlined below. Chlamydia and gonorrhea tests can be performed on the same specimen.

1. The medical assistant assembles supplies needed to collect the specimen, including a vaginal speculum, clean disposable gloves, and the specimen collection kit. The medical assistant should check the expiration date on the collection kit to make sure it has not expired. The collection kit includes cotton-tipped swabs and a tube of transport medium.
2. The transport tube must be labeled with the following information: patient's name, date of birth, and identification number, date and time of collection, and physician's name and telephone number.

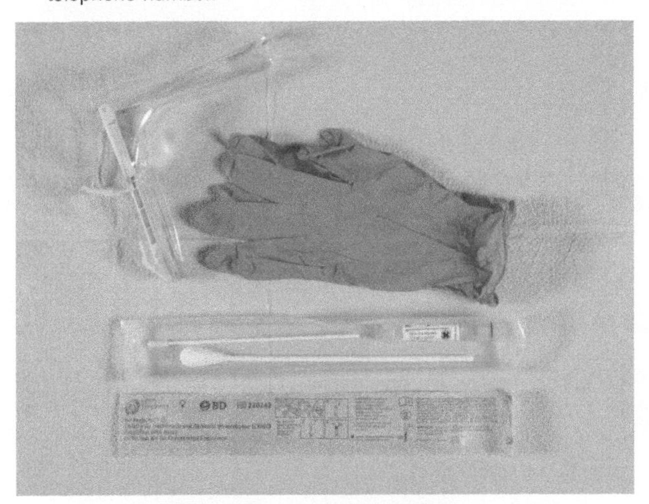

DNA probe setup (female patient).

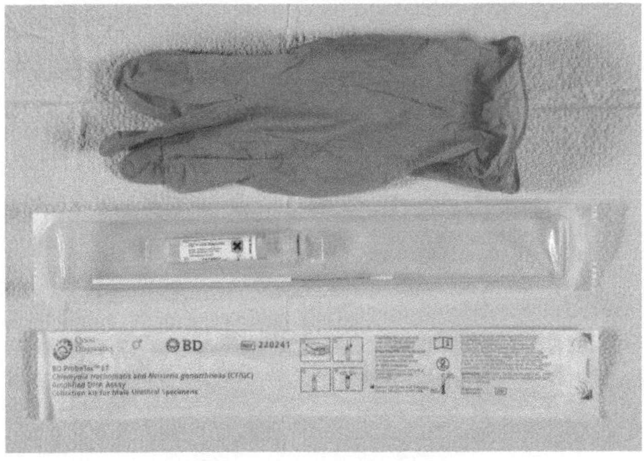

DNA probe setup (male patient).

3. The physician collects the specimen as follows:
   - **Female Patient:** The physician inserts a vaginal speculum into the vagina. Using a cotton-tipped swab, the physician first removes excess mucus or discharge from the cervix, and discards the swab. Next, the physician collects the specimen by inserting another cotton-tipped swab into the endocervical canal and rotating it for 15–30 s. This ensures a good sampling of the specimen.
   - **Male Patient:** The patient must not urinate for 1 h before the collection to prevent any urethral discharge from being washed away. The physician inserts a small-tipped cotton swab 2–4 cm into the penis. The swab is gently rotated for 2–3 s to dislodge cells and to ensure contact with all urethral surfaces.
4. The provider carefully withdraws the swab.
5. The medical assistant should ensure that the transport medium is at the bottom of the tube. The medical assistant unscrews the cap and holds the tube for the physician.
6. The physician inserts the swab into the transport tube, breaks off the shaft of the swab at the score line, and discards the top of the shaft.

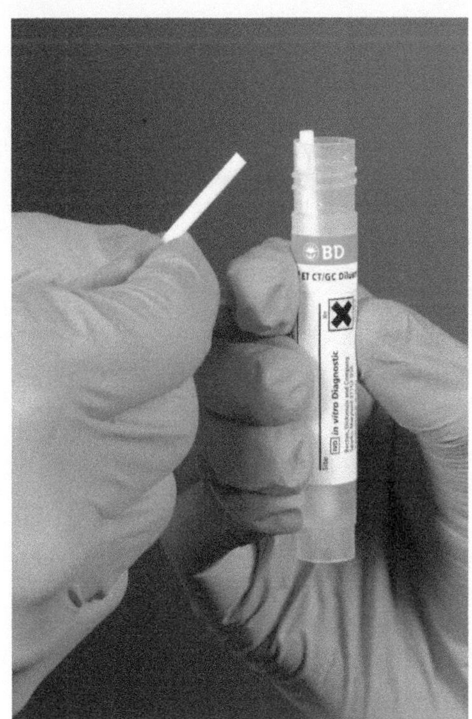

Breaking off shaft of swab.

7. The medical assistant places the cap on the tube and twists it until it clicks into place. The tube is placed in a biohazard specimen transport bag along with the laboratory requisition for pickup by the laboratory.

BOX 8.4 Patient-Collected Vaginal Specimen

Patient-collected specimens for chlamydia and gonorrhea are becoming more commonplace especially among younger individuals. The specimen can be collected in the privacy of a rest room at the medical office. The medical assistant should provide the patient with an instruction sheet for the collection of the specimen and go over the instructions with the patient and offer to answer any questions.

The medical assistant should perform the following:

1. Sanitize the hands.
2. Obtain a nucleic acid amplification (NAA) collection kit and check the expiration date. The kit includes a NAA transport tube and a sterile collection swab.
3. Open the collection kit package and label the transport tube with the patient's name, the date, the type of specimen (vaginal), and your initials.
4. Greet the patient and introduce yourself. Identify the patient and explain the procedure.
5. Escort the patient to the rest room and place the transport tube on a flat surface.
6. Partially open the swab package to expose the shaft of the swab and place the package on a flat surface within easy reach of the patient.

The medical assistant should instruct the patient in the collection of the specimen as follows:

1. Thoroughly wash your hands and dry them. Do not cleanse or wipe the genital area.
2. Remove all clothing from the waist down. Comfortably position yourself to maintain balance in a sitting or standing position by sitting on the toilet or standing with the legs spread apart.
3. Carefully remove the sterile swab from the package with your dominant hand taking care not to touch the tip, drop it, or lay it down. If the swab is contaminated request a new collection kit.
4. Hold the collection swab by placing your thumb and forefinger in the middle of the shaft covering the black score line.
5. Expose the vaginal opening by spreading apart the folds of skin around the vaginal opening (labia) with your nondominant hand.

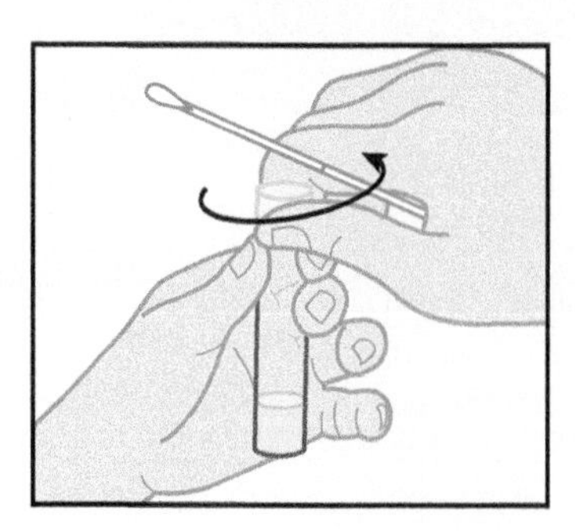

6. Carefully insert the soft tip of the swab into your vagina about 2 inches past the opening of the vagina (approximately the length of your little finger).
7. Gently rotate the swab for 10–30 s making sure the swab touches the walls of the vagina.

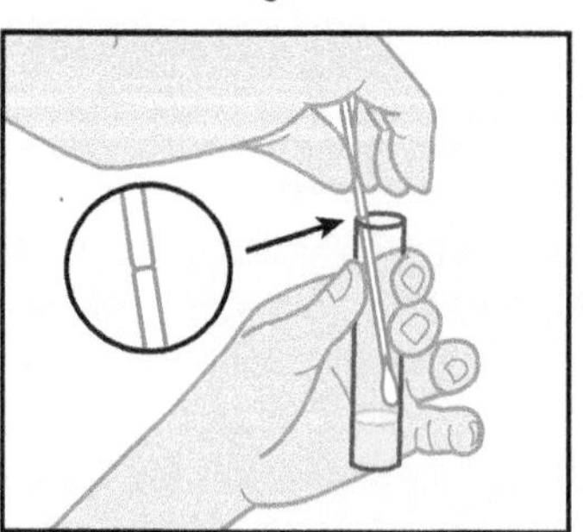

8. Withdraw the swab without touching the skin outside the vagina. Contamination of the swab may lead to inaccurate test results.
9. While still holding the swab in your dominant hand, carefully unscrew the cap from the transport tube.

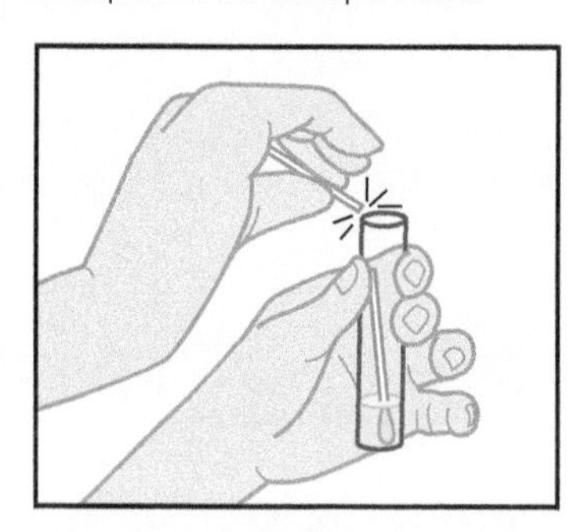

10. Immediately lower the swab in the transport tube until the visible black score line on the shaft is lined up with the rim of the tube. Be careful not to touch the swab to any surface prior to placing it in the tube. The tip of the swab will be just above the liquid in the tube.

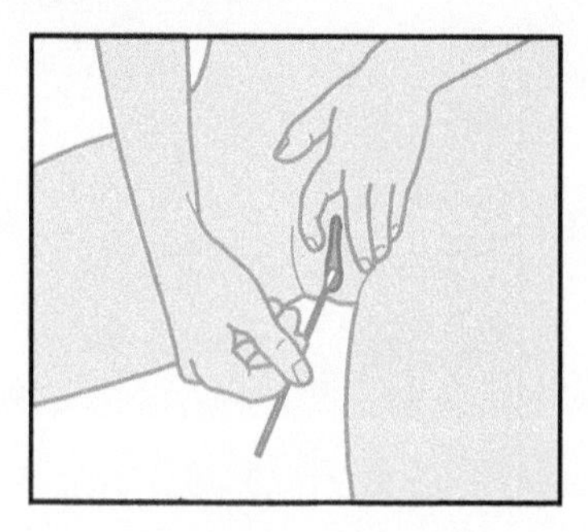

11. Carefully break the swab shaft at the black score line by leaning the shaft against the tube rim and applying gentle pressure. Be careful not to spill the liquid. Dispose of the broken-off end of the shaft in a biohazard waste container.

BOX 8.4 Patient-Collected Vaginal Specimen—cont'd

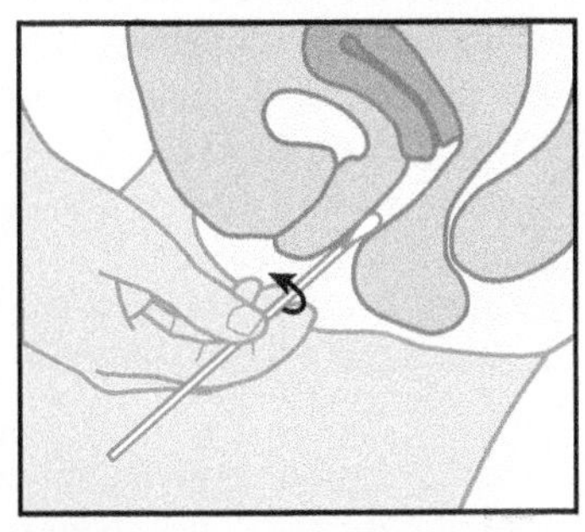

12. Tightly screw the cap onto the transport tube.
13. Thoroughly wash hands.
14. Return the transport tube to the medical assistant.

The medical assistant should perform the following:

1. Apply gloves before accepting the transport tube from the patient.
2. Place the NAA transport tube in a biohazard specimen transport bag and seal the bag. Insert the laboratory requisition into the outside pocket of the bag.
3. Remove gloves and sanitize the hands.
4. Place the specimen bag in the appropriate location for pickup by the laboratory.

GENITAL HERPES

Description

Genital herpes is one of the most common STIs in the United States. Approximately 50 million individuals in the United States are infected with genital herpes, which translates to about one in six adults. Genital herpes occurs most often in individuals aged 14 to 49 and is more common in women than in men because it is more easily transmitted from men to women than from women to men during sexual intercourse.

Genital herpes is caused by the herpes simplex virus (HSV). There are two types of HSV; these include HSV type 1 (HSV-1) and HSV type 2 (HSV-2). The most common cause of genital herpes is HSV-2. HSV-1 is more often the cause of cold sores, however HSV-1 can be transmitted to the genital area during oral sex resulting in genital herpes.

Most individuals infected with HSV do not have symptoms or only have very mild symptoms which go unnoticed or are mistaken for another condition. Because of this, most individuals with genital herpes are not aware of having this condition. If symptoms do occur, they typically include small fluid-filled blisters on or around the genitals, anus, or lips. These blisters break open resulting in painful sores or ulcers. The ulcers eventually scab over and heal within 2 to 4 weeks following an initial herpes infection. Systemic symptoms that may occur, especially during the first outbreak, include fever, muscle aches, swollen lymph nodes, and headaches. There is no cure for herpes; once an individual is infected with HSV, the virus stays in the body for life causing recurrent outbreaks. Recurrent outbreaks are generally shorter in duration and less severe than the initial outbreak of genital herpes. Outbreaks are usually most frequent in the first year following infection and usually decrease in number over time.

Diagnosis and Treatment

The recommended test method for diagnosing genital herpes is a NAA test which detects the genetic material (DNA) of the herpes virus. Antiviral medications can be taken during an outbreak to shorten the length and severity of an outbreak. These antiviral medications include acyclovir, valacyclovir, and famciclovir. Taking a daily dose of an antiviral medication (known as *suppressive therapy*) can help to prevent or decrease the number of outbreaks and reduce the likelihood of transmitting the virus to a partner.

HUMAN PAPILLOMAVIRUS INFECTION

Description

HPV infection is the most common STI in the United States. More than 79 million Americans are currently infected with HPV and approximately 14 million individuals become newly infected each year. There are 100 different types of HPV; approximately 40 of these types can affect the genitals and are transmitted through skin-to-skin contact during vaginal, anal, or oral sex. Genital HPV infections are so common that nearly all sexually active individuals will contract at least one type of HPV infection in their lifetime. Individuals who are not sexually active almost never develop HPV infections.

Most individuals with genital HPV infections do not exhibit symptoms and therefore do not know that they are infected. Because of this, they may unknowingly transmit the HPV infection to a partner. Most sexually transmitted HPV infections (90%) are cleared from the body by the immune system within 1 to 2 years following infection and the patient does not experience any health problems. In some instances, HPV infections persist and eventually cause genital warts or precancerous lesions.

Sexually transmitted HPVs are divided into the following two categories:

- *Low-Risk HPVs:* A low-risk HPV has a low risk of causing cancer. Infection with a low-risk HPV can result in the development of genital warts. Genital warts rarely cause discomfort and pain and usually appear as flat lesions, cauliflower-like bumps, or tiny stem-like protrusions. Genital warts can affect the vulva, vagina, cervix, and anus in women and the penis, scrotum, and anus in men. The diagnosis of genital warts is usually made through visual inspection. Treatment of genital warts may include topical medications, cryosurgery, electrocautery, laser treatments, or surgical excision.
- *High-Risk HPVs:* A high-risk HPV has a high risk of causing cancer. Infection with persistent high-risk HPVs cause abnormal cellular changes which may lead to precancerous lesions. These precancerous lesions may eventually result in cancer of the cervix, vulva, vagina, penis, anus, mouth, or pharynx. It usually takes years or even decades for cancer to develop following infection with a high-risk HPV.

Diagnosis and Treatment

The only HPV-related cancer for which routine screening is recommended is cervical cancer. As previously discussed, cervical cancer screening tests include the Pap test and the HPV test. The Pap test detects the presence of abnormal cervical cells that may develop into cancer if not treated while the HPV test detects the presence of high-risk HPV infections of the cervix which may cause the cervical cells to become abnormal. The ACOG guidelines (presented in Box 8.2) recommend that women ages 21 to 29 have a Pap test every three years. Women between the ages of 30 and 65 should have a Pap test combined with an HPV test every 5 years. This is known as *co-testing*. As alternatives, a woman in this age group can have a Pap test every 3 years or a primary HPV test every 5 years.

There are no screening tests available to detect high-risk HPV infections or abnormal cellular changes that may lead to HPV-related cancer of the vulva, vagina, penis, anus, mouth, or pharynx. The diagnosis of these conditions is usually made through visual inspection which is then confirmed through a biopsy.

There is currently no treatment available which will eliminate HPV from the body. There are treatments, however, for the health problems that may result from persistent HPV infections such as HPV-related cancers and genital warts. Although there is no cure for HPV infections, a vaccine is available to prevent sexually-transmitted HPV infections that may lead to HPV-related cancers and genital warts. The HPV vaccine (Gardasil 9) does not protect against sexually-transmitted HPV infections already contracted by an individual, therefore the HPV vaccine should be administered before an individual becomes sexually active (refer to the Patient Coaching box on HPV Vaccine).

PATIENT COACHING Human Papillomavirus Vaccine

Answer questions that patients have regarding the HPV vaccine.

What HPV vaccine is approved for use in the United States?

The HPV vaccine approved by the FDA for use in the United States is Gardasil 9 (Merck).

Gardasil 9 protects against infection with nine types of HPV that are most likely to result in genital warts and HPV-related cancers. Gardasil 9 does not protect against all the HPV types that may lead to cervical cancer; therefore it is important for women to continue routine cervical cancer screening.

What protection is provided by the HPV vaccine?

The HPV vaccine prevents HPV infections associated with the following HPV-related conditions:

Female

- Cervical, vulvar, and vaginal cancer
- Anal cancer
- Genital warts

Male

- Anal cancer
- Genital warts

Who should get the HPV vaccine?

The CDC recommends routine vaccination of both girls and boys starting at 11 or 12 years of age, but it can be administered as early as 9 years of age through 26 years of age.

What is the immunization schedule for the HPV vaccine?

- *Ages 9 to 14:* Pre-adolescents and adolescents between the ages of 9 and 14 years of age should receive the HPV vaccine as a two-dose series with the second dose being administered 6 to 12 months following the first dose.
- *Ages 15 to 26:* Individuals between the ages of 15 and 26 years of age should receive the HPV vaccine as a three-dose series with the second dose administered 1 to 2 months after the first dose, and the third dose administered 6 months after the first dose.

What are the side effects of the vaccine?

Many individuals who receive the HPV vaccine have no side effects at all or have very mild side effects. If side effects occur, they commonly include soreness, redness or swelling at the injection site, fever, and headache.

HIGHLIGHT on Sexually Transmitted Infections

Sexually transmitted infections (STIs) are among the most common infectious diseases in the United States today. The CDC estimates that there are 20 million new infections each year in the United States. If this trend continues, at least one in four Americans will contract an STI at some time in his or her life. STIs are most prevalent among teenagers and young adults; more than half of all new STI cases are contracted by individuals 15–24 years old.

Transmission

STIs are spread most often by sexual contact with the penis, vagina, mouth, or anus of an infected person. They are less commonly spread by skin-to-skin contact and through the use of contaminated needles among drug users.

Symptoms

An STI sometimes causes no symptoms at all, particularly in women. If symptoms do occur, they include one or more of the following: an unusual discharge from the penis or vagina; itching, redness, or soreness of the genitals; sores or blisters on or around the genitals, anus, or both; and pain or burning during urination. With or without symptoms, an STI can be spread to someone else. If symptoms develop, they may be so mild that they go unnoticed, or they may be confused with symptoms of other diseases. Because of this, STIs may go undetected and untreated. If not treated, many STIs result in serious complications, such as infertility. In addition, some STIs can be passed from an infected mother to her infant before or during birth. An individual diagnosed with an STI should inform his or her sex partner immediately so that the partner can also be treated. This reduces the risk that the sex partner will develop serious complications from the STI.

Treatment

When diagnosed early, most STIs can be treated effectively, and many can be cured. Antibiotics can cure STIs caused by bacteria which include chlamydia, gonorrhea, and syphilis. Antiviral medications have been developed to control the symptoms of certain STIs caused by viruses (e.g., genital herpes, HIV), however these medications cannot eliminate the virus from the body. Currently, a preventive vaccine is available for hepatitis B and HPV.

Risk Factors

Sexually active individuals who are at increased risk for contracting an STI should have regular health checkups to be tested for STIs. Factors that increase the risk of contracting an STI include the following:

- Unprotected sex
- Multiple sexual partners
- Having a history of one or more STIs
- Alcohol use
- Illicit drug use
- Injecting drugs
- Being under 25 years of age
- Living in a community with a high prevalence of STIs

Individuals at increased risk should learn to recognize the symptoms of STIs and check themselves for signs of STI infection once a month. If an individual thinks he or she has an STI, a physician should be consulted as soon as possible. If an individual has been treated for an STI and still has symptoms, he or she should return to the physician for further evaluation. It is possible to have more than one STI at a time and to become reinfected with the same STI.

Prevention and Control Measures

All STIs can be prevented. The best way to prevent STIs is to practice abstinence or to have a mutually monogamous sexual relationship with an uninfected partner. If an individual's lifestyle does not follow one of these patterns, the following can be done to reduce the risk of contracting an STI:

- Get vaccinated for Hepatitis B and HPV.
- Before having a sexual relationship, partners should discuss their sexual histories with each other and get tested for STIs.
- Use a condom during sexual intercourse. If the condom is not used correctly, however, an individual still could contract an STI. Make sure to use a water-based lubricant with condoms to keep the condom from breaking.
- Limit the number of sexual partners. The risk of an STI increases with each new partner, particularly if it is unknown how many previous partners that person has had.
- Do not have sex with anyone who exhibits the symptoms of an STI.
- Obtain annual STI testing if you have risk factors for contracting an STI.
- If you have an STI, take all prescribed medication and abstain from intercourse until a physician has determined that you are no longer contagious.

What Would You Do? What Would You *Not* Do?

Case Study 2

Brooke Fairchild comes to the office. She is 16 years old, and her father is a lawyer and her mother is a chemical engineer. Her boyfriend was diagnosed 2 weeks ago with chlamydia. Brooke was hesitant to come in because she does not have any symptoms and her boyfriend always uses a condom. She is worried about her parents finding out that she is sexually active and what they will think if she has an STI. Brooke also is afraid and extremely embarrassed about what will be "done to her" to determine whether she has chlamydia. She tells Yin-Ling that she is thinking of leaving the office and not seeing the physician at all. (*Note:* Brooke lives in a state that allows minors to receive health care services without parental consent.) ■

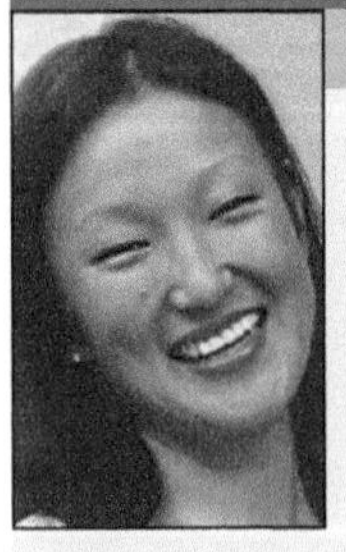

Memories *from* Practicum

Yin-Ling: During my practicum, I was assigned to an OB/GYN clinic. They had an ultrasound technician working there who ran all the scans on prenatal patients. The ultrasound scans I observed always looked like a big blob to me—I could never see anything.

One day, a patient that the ultrasound technician knew really well came into the office. The patient agreed to let me come in for her ultrasound. It was her first time getting an ultrasound. When the technician put the ultrasound probe on her abdomen, we could see the outline of the whole baby. You could even see a tiny arm and fingers, and it looked like the baby was waving. The look of joy and amazement on the mom's face was unforgettable. After that, I knew I was in the right profession. ■

Prenatal Care

Obstetrics is the branch of medicine that deals with the supervision of women's health during pregnancy, childbirth, and the puerperium. **Prenatal** care refers to the care of a pregnant woman before delivery of the infant. Prenatal care consists of a series of scheduled medical office visits for promotion of the health of the mother and fetus through prevention of disease and early detection, diagnosis, and treatment of problems common to pregnancy (e.g., anemia, urinary tract infection, and preeclampsia). Early detection of medical problems helps prevent serious complications in the mother and the fetus.

OBSTETRIC TERMINOLOGY

The medical assistant should know the common terms related to obstetrics, as follows:

Braxton Hicks contractions. Intermittent and irregular painless uterine contractions that occur throughout pregnancy. They occur more frequently toward the end of pregnancy and are sometimes mistaken for true labor pains.

Dilation (of the cervix). Stretching of the external os (of the cervix) from an opening of a few millimeters to an opening large enough to allow the passage of an infant (approximately 10 cm).

Effacement. Thinning and shortening of the cervical canal from its normal length of 1 to 2 cm to a structure with paper-thin edges in which there is no canal at all. Effacement occurs late in pregnancy, during labor, or both. The purpose of effacement, along with dilation, is to permit the passage of the infant into the birth canal.

Embryo. The child in utero from the time of conception through the first 8 weeks of development (i.e., the first 2 months of development).

Engagement. The entrance of the fetal head or the presenting part into the pelvic inlet.

Fetus. The child in utero, from the third month after conception to birth; during the first 2 months of development, it is called an *embryo.*

Fundus. The dome-shaped upper portion of the uterus between the fallopian tubes.

Gestation. The period of intrauterine development from conception to birth; the period of pregnancy. The average pregnancy lasts about 280 days, or 40 weeks, from the date of conception to childbirth.

Gestational age. The age of the fetus between conception and birth.

Infant. A child from birth to 12 months old.

Multigravida. A woman who has been pregnant more than once.

Multipara. A woman who has completed two or more pregnancies to the age of viability regardless of whether they ended in live infants or stillbirths.

Nullipara. A woman who has not carried a pregnancy to the point of fetal viability (20 weeks of gestation).

Position. The relation of the presenting part of the fetus to the maternal pelvis.

Postpartum. Occurring after childbirth.

Preeclampsia. A major complication of pregnancy, the cause of which is unknown, characterized by increasing hypertension, albuminuria, and edema. If the condition is neglected or is not treated properly, preeclampsia may develop into eclampsia, which could cause maternal convulsions and coma. Preeclampsia generally occurs between the 20th week of pregnancy and the end of the first week postpartum.

Presentation. Indication of the part of the fetus that is closest to the cervix and is delivered first. A cephalic presentation is a delivery in which the fetal head is presenting against the cervix. A breech presentation is a delivery in which the buttocks or feet are presented instead of the head.

Primigravida. A woman who is pregnant for the first time.

Primipara. A woman who has carried a pregnancy to fetal viability (20 weeks of gestation) for the first time regardless of whether the infant was stillborn or alive at birth.

Puerperium. The period of time (usually 4 to 6 weeks) after delivery in which the uterus and the body systems are returning to normal.

Quickening. The first movements of the fetus in utero as felt by the mother, which usually occurs between 16 and 20 weeks of gestation and is felt consistently thereafter.

Toxemia. A condition that can occur in pregnant women that includes preeclampsia and eclampsia. If preeclampsia goes undiagnosed or is not satisfactorily controlled, it could develop into eclampsia, which is characterized by convulsions and coma.

Trimester. Three months, or one third, of the gestational period. The 9 months of pregnancy are divided into three trimesters, each consisting of 3 months. From conception to 3 months is the first trimester, from 4 to 6 months is the second trimester, and from 7 to 9 months is the third trimester.

PRENATAL VISITS

Medical office visits for prenatal and postpartum care of the pregnant woman can be grouped into three major categories as follows:

1. First prenatal visit
2. Return prenatal visits
3. Six weeks postpartum visit

INITIAL PRENATAL VISIT

The first prenatal visit generally occurs after the woman has missed her second menstrual period; if problems exist, the woman is seen after missing her first menstrual period. Regardless of whether or not the patient is happy and excited about the pregnancy, the first visit is often a stressful experience for the patient. The medical assistant plays an important role in relaxing the patient and relieving her anxiety.

The first prenatal visit requires more time than subsequent prenatal visits; sufficient time should be scheduled to allow a complete and accurate initial assessment of the pregnant woman. The components of the first prenatal visit vary depending on the medical office, but they generally include the following:

- Completion of a prenatal record form.
- Initial prenatal examination, consisting of a complete physical examination. Of particular importance are breast, abdominal, and pelvic examinations.
- Prenatal patient education.
- Laboratory tests.

Prenatal Record

The prenatal record provides information regarding the past and present health of the patient and serves as a database and flow sheet for subsequent prenatal visits. The prenatal record is essential in helping identify high-risk patients. The medical assistant is usually responsible for collecting a portion of the information required for the prenatal record. Many types of prenatal record forms are available (Fig. 8.10). The specific form used in the medical office is based on the provider's preference and the method used for conducting the prenatal examination.

Obtaining and documenting information in the prenatal record from one visit to the next provides an opportunity for the medical assistant to develop a rapport with the patient. It is also an excellent time to relay information to her regarding various aspects of the prenatal and postnatal periods, such as an explanation of the changes occurring in her body, the signs and symptoms of labor, nutrition of the infant (breastfeeding and bottle feeding), and care of the newborn infant. The prenatal record form should be completed in a quiet setting that is free from distractions. This gives the patient the confidence to discuss areas of concern openly, which helps ensure a complete and accurate prenatal history.

During the first prenatal visit, the medical assistant should relay his or her name and position to the patient to help build a supportive relationship with her and to allow her to ask for the medical assistant by name when contacting the medical office. The prenatal record is similar to and contains much of the same information as the health history described in Chapter 5. Particular attention is given to factors that may influence the course of pregnancy, as described in the following paragraphs.

Past Medical History

The past medical history focuses on conditions that could affect the health of the mother and fetus, such as diabetes, hypertension, heart disease, autoimmune disorders, kidney disease, liver disease, varicosities or phlebitis, alcohol and tobacco intake, drug addiction, Rh sensitization, pulmonary disease (e.g., tuberculosis, asthma), bleeding tendencies, surgeries, anesthetic complications, previous abnormal Pap tests, infertility problems, STIs, and drug allergies. In addition, the medical assistant solicits information from the patient regarding immunizations and childhood diseases to provide the provider with the information needed to assess her antibody protection against such diseases.

Rubella, if contracted during pregnancy, can be dangerous to the developing fetus; the earlier in pregnancy the infection occurs, the greater is the chance of birth defects. The infant may be born with heart defects, cataracts, intellectual disabilities, and deafness. Patients who do not have antibody protection against rubella are given a rubella immunization within 6 weeks of delivery. Fortunately, rubella has become quite rare in the United States due to the routine rubella vaccination of children. The rubella vaccination cannot be given to a pregnant woman because it may be harmful to the fetus. These patients should be told to avoid exposure to children with rubella during their pregnancy.

Menstrual History

A menstrual history is obtained from the patient. It includes the date of onset of menstruation, the menstrual interval cycle, the duration, the amount of flow (documented as small, moderate, or large), and any gynecologic disorders. The form also includes a space for the patient to indicate whether or not she was using a method of contraception when she became pregnant.

Obstetric History

A thorough obstetric history is a component of the prenatal record and provides the opportunity to obtain information from the patient related to previous pregnancies. Information that is obtained and explored includes gravidity, parity, and other information related to previous pregnancies.

Gravidity and parity provide data with respect to the pregnancy, and the medical assistant should develop skill in recording this information. **Gravidity (G)** is recorded using one digit, which indicates the number of times a woman has been pregnant regardless of the duration of the pregnancy and including the current pregnancy. A woman who is pregnant for the second time but had a spontaneous abortion during the first pregnancy would be recorded as *G: 2.* A woman who is pregnant for the second time (and did not have a spontaneous abortion) also would be recorded as *G: 2.*

Parity refers to the condition of having borne offspring regardless of the outcome. It is recorded using four abbreviations and digits, which represent the following pregnancy outcomes:

1. **Term birth (T).** Delivery after 37 weeks regardless of whether the child was born alive or stillborn.
2. **Preterm birth (P).** Delivery between 20 and 37 weeks regardless of whether the child was born alive or stillborn.
3. **Abortion (A).** Termination of the pregnancy before the fetus reaches the age of viability (20 weeks). An abortion can be spontaneous or elective.
4. **Living children (L).** Number of living children.

Example: A woman has been pregnant four times with the following outcomes: a spontaneous abortion, a full-term stillbirth, a preterm birth of a healthy child, and a full-term birth of a healthy child. The recording would be as follows:**G: 4** *(pregnancies);* **T: 2** *(term);* **P: 1** *(preterm);* **A: 1** *(abortion);* **L: 2** *(living children).*

Multiple births (twins, triplets) count as one pregnancy and one delivery. If a woman had been pregnant two times and had a set of full-term healthy twins and a set of preterm

PRENATAL HEALTH HISTORY

PATIENT INFORMATION

Date: ____ EDD: ____ Referred By: ____

Name: ____ (LAST FIRST MIDDLE) Phone (home): ____

Phone (work): ____

Address: ____ Emergency Contact: ____

____ (CITY STATE ZIP) Phone: ____

Date of Birth: ___/___/___ Age: ___ Marital Status: ____

Occupation: ____

Education: ☐ High School ☐ College ☐ Post-graduate

PAST MEDICAL HISTORY

	O Neg + Pos	DETAIL POSITIVE REMARKS INCLUDE DATE AND TREATMENT		O Neg + Pos	DETAIL POSITIVE REMARKS INCLUDE DATE AND TREATMENT
1. DIABETES			16. D (Rh) SENSITIZED		
2. HYPERTENSION			17. PULMONARY (TB, ASTHMA)		
3. HEART DISEASE			18. RHEUMATIC FEVER		
4. AUTOIMMUNE DISORDER			19. BLEEDING TENDENCY		
5. KIDNEY DISEASE/UTI			20. GYN SURGERY		
6. NEUROLOGIC/EPILEPSY					
7. PSYCHIATRIC			21. OPERATIONS/HOSPITALIZATIONS (YEAR AND REASON)		
8. HEPATITIS/LIVER DISEASE					
9. VARICOSITIES/PHLEBITIS					
10. THYROID DYSFUNCTION			22. ANESTHETIC COMPLICATIONS		
11. TRAUMA/DOMESTIC VIOLENCE			23. HISTORY OF ABNORMAL PAP		
12. BLOOD TRANSFUSION			24. UTERINE ANOMALY/DES		

	AMT/DAY PREPREG.	AMT/DAY PREG.	# YEARS USE		O Neg + Pos	DETAIL POSITIVE REMARKS
				25. INFERTILITY		
13. TOBACCO				26. SEXUALLY TRANSMITTED DISEASE		
14. ALCOHOL						
15. STREET DRUGS				27. OTHER		

IMMUNIZATIONS:

Mark an X next to those you have had.

☐ Influenza ☐ Chickenpox
☐ Hepatitis B ☐ Pneumococcal
☐ Hib ☐ Tuberculin Test
☐ Polio ☐ Tetanus Booster
☐ MMR

ALLERGIES:

List all allergies (foods, drugs, environment). ☐ None

____

MENSTRUAL HISTORY

Menarche: Age at Onset ____ GYN Disorders (List): ____

Frequency: Q ____ Days

Duration: ____ Days

Amount of Flow: ☐ Small ☐ Moderate ☐ Large

On contraceptive at conception? ☐ Yes ☐ No

Fig. 8.10 Example of a prenatal record form.

OBSTETRIC HISTORY

G ____________ (Total Pregnancies) T ____________ (Term) P ____________ (Preterm) A ____________ (Abortions) L ____________ (Living Children)

PREVIOUS PREGNANCIES:

DATE MONTH/ YEAR	WEEKS GEST.	LENGTH OF LABOR	BIRTH WEIGHT	SEX M/F	TYPE DELIVERY	ANES.	MATERNAL COMPLICATIONS	INFANT COMPLICATIONS

PRESENT PREGNANCY HISTORY

NAUSEA			ABDOMINAL PAIN		
VOMITING			URINARY COMPLAINTS		
FATIGUE			VAGINAL BLEEDING		
BREAST CHANGES			VAGINAL DISCHARGE		
INDIGESTION			PRURITUS		
CONSTIPATION			ACCIDENTS		
PERSISTENT HEADACHES			SURGERY		
DIZZINESS			X-RAYS		
VISUAL DISTURBANCE			RUBELLA EXPOSURE		
EDEMA (SPECIFY AREA)			OTHER VIRAL INFECTIONS		

LMP _____/_____/_____ (Mo Day Year) **Amount of Flow:** ☐ **Small** ☐ **Moderate** ☐ **Large**

CURRENT MEDICATIONS: (Include prescription, OTC, herbal, and vitamins). ☐ **None**

Medication **Frequency**

____

____

____

INITIAL PHYSICAL EXAMINATION

DATE ____/____/____

1. HEENT	☐ NORMAL	☐ ABNORMAL	12. VULVA	☐ NORMAL	☐ CONDYLOMA	☐ LESIONS
2. FUNDI	☐ NORMAL	☐ ABNORMAL	13. VAGINA	☐ NORMAL	☐ INFLAMMATION	☐ DISCHARGE
3. TEETH	☐ NORMAL	☐ ABNORMAL	14. CERVIX	☐ NORMAL	☐ INFLAMMATION	☐ LESIONS
4. THYROID	☐ NORMAL	☐ ABNORMAL	15. UTERUS SIZE	______ WEEKS		☐ FIBROIDS
5. BREASTS	☐ NORMAL	☐ ABNORMAL	16. ADNEXA	☐ NORMAL	☐ MASS	
6. LUNGS	☐ NORMAL	☐ ABNORMAL	17. RECTUM	☐ NORMAL	☐ ABNORMAL	
7. HEART	☐ NORMAL	☐ ABNORMAL	18. DIAGONAL CONJUGATE	☐ REACHED	☐ NO	_____CM
8. ABDOMEN	☐ NORMAL	☐ ABNORMAL	19. SPINES	☐ AVERAGE	☐ PROMINENT	☐ BLUNT
9. EXTREMITIES	☐ NORMAL	☐ ABNORMAL	20. SACRUM	☐ CONCAVE	☐ STRAIGHT	☐ ANTERIOR
10. SKIN	☐ NORMAL	☐ ABNORMAL	21. SUBPUBIC ARCH	☐ NORMAL	☐ WIDE	☐ NARROW
11. LYMPH NODES	☐ NORMAL	☐ ABNORMAL	22. GYNECOID PELVIC TYPE	☐ YES	☐ NO	

COMMENTS (Number and explain abnormals): ____

____

____

______________________________ **EXAM BY** ______________________________

Fig. 8.10, cont'd

Continued

PATIENT'S NAME ____

INTERVAL PRENATAL HISTORY

Date 20___	Weeks Gestation	Height of Fundus (cm)	Weight	B/P	Urine Glucose	Urine Protein	FHT	Vaginal Examination	Presentation	Edema	Discharge	Bleeding	Contractions	Fetal Activity	NST	Next Appt.	Initials
				/													
				/													
				/													
				/													
				/													
				/													
				/													
				/													
				/													
				/													
				/													
				/													
				/													
				/													

PLANS/EDUCATION **(COUNSELED ☑)**

- ☐ ANESTHESIA PLANS ____________________
- ☐ TOXOPLASMOSIS PRECAUTIONS (CATS/RAW MEAT) ____________________
- ☐ CHILDBIRTH CLASSES ____________________
- ☐ PHYSICAL/SEXUAL ACTIVITY ____________________
- ☐ LABOR SIGNS ____________________
- ☐ NUTRITION COUNSELING ____________________
- ☐ BREAST OR BOTTLE FEEDING ____________________
- ☐ NEWBORN CAR SEAT ____________________
- ☐ POSTPARTUM BIRTH CONTROL ____________________
- ☐ ENVIRONMENTAL/WORK HAZARDS ____________________
- ☐ TUBAL STERILIZATION ____________________
- ☐ VBAC COUNSELING ____________________
- ☐ CIRCUMCISION ____________________
- ☐ TRAVEL ____________________
- ☐ LIFESTYLE, TOBACCO, ALCOHOL ____________________

REQUESTS ____________________

TUBAL STERILIZATION CONSENT SIGNED — **DATE** ___/___/___ — **INITIALS** ____________

Fig. 8.10, cont'd

LABORATORY		PATIENT'S NAME ______		
INITIAL LABS	**DATE**	**RESULTS**	**REVIEWED**	**COMMENTS**
BLOOD TYPE	/ /	A B AB O		
Rh FACTOR	/ /	☐ Pos ☐ Neg		
Rh ANTIBODY SCREEN	/ /	☐ Pos ☐ Neg		
HCT/HGB	/ /	____% ____ g/dL		
RUBELLA ANTIBODY TITER	/ /	Immune Nonimmune		
VDRL	/ /	☐ NR ☐ R		
HBsAg (HEPATITIS B)	/ /	☐ Pos ☐ Neg		
HIV	/ /	☐ Pos ☐ Neg ☐ Declined		
URINE CULTURE/SCREEN	/ /			
PAP TEST	/ /	☐ Normal ☐ Abnormal		
CHLAMYDIA	/ /	☐ Pos ☐ Neg		
GONORRHEA	/ /	☐ Pos ☐ Neg		
7–20 WEEK LABS (WHEN INDICATED/ELECTED)	**DATE**	**RESULTS**	**REVIEWED**	**COMMENTS**
ULTRASOUND #1 (7–12 WEEKS)	/ /	EDD:		
ULTRASOUND #2 (18–20 WEEKS)	/ /	EFW:		
Multiple Marker Test (15–20 WEEKS)	/ /			
CVS	/ /			
AMNIOCENTESIS	/ /			
24–28 WEEK LABS (WHEN INDICATED)	**DATE**	**RESULTS**	**REVIEWED**	**COMMENTS**
HCT/HGB	/ /	____ % ____ g/dL		
GCT (24–28 WKS)	/ /	1 Hour ________		
GTT (IF SCREEN ABNORMAL)	/ /	____ FBS ____ 1 Hour ____ 2 Hour ____ 3 Hour		
D (Rh) ANTIBODY SCREEN	/ /			
D IMMUNE GLOBULIN (RhIG) GIVEN (28 WKS)	/ /	SIGNATURE		
32–36 WEEK LABS	**DATE**	**RESULTS**	**REVIEWED**	**COMMENTS**
HCT/HGB (32 WKS)	/ /	____ % ____ g/dL		
ULTRASOUND #3 (34 WKS)	/ /	EFW:		
GROUP B STREP (35–37 WKS)	/ /	☐ Pos ☐ Neg		
ADDITIONAL LAB TESTS	**DATE**	**RESULTS**	**REVIEWED**	**COMMENTS**
	/ /			
	/ /			
	/ /			
	/ /			
	/ /			

Fig. 8.10, cont'd

healthy triplets, the recording would be: **G: 2 T: 1 P: 1 A: 0 L: 5.**

If a woman is a multigravida, information about each pregnancy is obtained, including the date of delivery, gestation in weeks, length of labor in hours, birth weight and sex of the newborn, type of delivery (vaginal or cesarean section), type of anesthesia, and any maternal or infant complications. The obstetric history assists in identifying areas that may need to be investigated further or monitored during the prenatal period. Women with previous complications, such as premature labor, gestational diabetes, or postpartum hemorrhaging, are at risk for having these problems again.

Present Pregnancy History

The present pregnancy history establishes a baseline for the present health status of the prenatal patient. In addition, the patient is queried regarding any warning signs that may be present and that may place the mother or fetus in jeopardy, such as persistent headaches, visual disturbances, abdominal pain, vaginal bleeding, or discharge. The patient also is asked whether she has experienced any of the early signs of pregnancy, such as nausea, vomiting, fatigue, spotting, and swollen/tender breasts.

All prescribed or over-the-counter medications (including vitamin supplements and herbal products) the patient is taking must be documented. Certain medications cross the placental barrier and could be harmful to the developing fetus. The patient should be instructed not to take any medications without first checking with the provider.

In the space provided under the present pregnancy history, the medical assistant needs to document the date of the first day of the patient's LMP. The LMP is used to calculate the due date or **expected date of delivery (EDD)**.

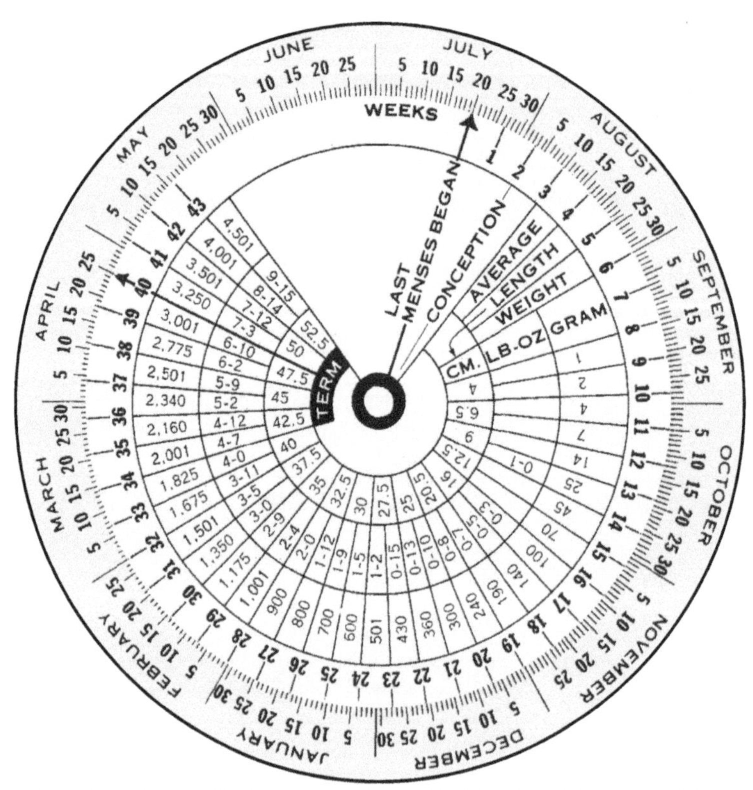

Fig. 8.11 Gestation calculator. The last menstrual period is July 20, and the expected date of delivery is April 25.

Gestation calculators are commercially available that can be used to determine the EDD by lining up an arrow and the date of the LMP, using a movable inner cardboard wheel (Fig. 8.11). There are also many online gestation calculators available as well as a variety of gestation calculator applications designed for mobile devices. In addition, electronic health record software automatically calculates the EDD after the LMP has been entered into the computer. If the patient is unsure of the date of her LMP, the provider estimates the length of gestation by other methods, such as fundal height measurement and sonography.

Interval Prenatal History

The interval prenatal history also is included in the prenatal record form; its purpose is to update the record. During every return visit, essential data, including weight, blood pressure, urine testing results, fundal height measurement, and fetal heart rate (FHR), are collected and documented in this section. A general inquiry is made regarding the occurrence of additional signs of pregnancy, such as fetal movement or Braxton Hicks contractions, and how the patient is feeling and any concerns or symptoms since the last prenatal visit. This information is documented in the prenatal record and assists the medical staff in planning, implementing, and evaluating individual needs. Particular attention is focused on risk factors, such as hypertension, thrombophlebitis, and uterine bleeding, which could influence the course of the pregnancy.

Initial Prenatal Examination

Purpose

The initial prenatal examination is of particular importance because it results in confirmation of the pregnancy and establishes a baseline for the woman's state of health. It includes a thorough gynecologic examination (breast and pelvic examinations) and a general physical examination of the other body systems, although the latter may be performed during a subsequent prenatal visit, depending on the medical office routine.

Women often have little or no medical supervision during their childbearing years; the physical examination is of particular importance in establishing a baseline for the woman's general state of health and in identifying high-risk prenatal patients. Conditions such as obesity, hypertension, severe varicosities, and uterine size inappropriate for the due date can be diagnosed by the provider, and necessary treatment or monitoring can be instituted to help prevent complications.

Preparation of the Patient

When the patient arrives at the medical office and the prenatal record form has been completed, the medical assistant is responsible for taking and documenting the patient's vital signs, height, and weight to provide a database for subsequent prenatal visits. The patient is asked to disrobe completely and put on an examining gown with the opening in front. The medical assistant must give complete and thorough instructions so that the patient knows exactly what is expected. The patient should be asked whether she needs to empty her bladder because an empty bladder facilitates the examination and is more comfortable for her. If the office policy is such that a specimen is needed for urine testing at the initial prenatal visit, the patient will be required to void.

Special precautions should be taken in assisting the prenatal patient. The medical assistant should support the patient as she gets onto and off the scale and examining table to ensure her safety and comfort. This is especially important as the pregnancy progresses and the patient becomes more awkward and off balance.

The medical assistant is responsible for setting up the tray required for the examination. The setup includes the equipment and supplies required for the procedures to be performed. During the prenatal examination, the medical assistant is responsible for positioning the patient as required for each aspect of the examination and assisting the provider as necessary.

Patient Education

At the conclusion of the initial prenatal examination and after the patient is dressed, the provider counsels the patient on health promotion and disease prevention. Topics that are often discussed include nutrition, weight gain, rest, sleep, employment, exercise, travel, sexual intercourse, dental care, smoking, alcohol, and drugs. Many offices have a prenatal guidebook designed especially for this purpose that is given to each patient to use as a reference. Some offices also use a series of teaching films that the patient views during the return prenatal visit while waiting to see the provider. The provider also prescribes a daily vitamin supplement to be taken during the prenatal period to ensure that the mother and fetus obtain an adequate supply of vitamins and minerals.

When the provider is finished talking with the patient, the medical assistant is responsible for scheduling the next prenatal visit and for ensuring that the patient understands the instructions for maintaining health and preventing disease during the pregnancy. The medical assistant should tell the patient to report the occurrence of any warning signs during the pregnancy (see Box 8.5, Warning Signs During Pregnancy) and not to take any medications without first checking with the provider. The patient also should be encouraged to contact the medical office should any questions or problems arise.

BOX 8.5 Warning Signs During Pregnancy

Signs of Infection
- Fever
- Vaginal discharge
- Dysuria
- Increased frequency of urination
- Marked decrease in urinary output

Signs of Spontaneous Abortion
- Vaginal bleeding
- Persistent low back pain
- Abdominal pain and cramping

Signs of Preeclampsia
- Severe, persistent headache
- Dizziness
- Blurred vision
- Sudden swelling of hands, feet, or face
- Sudden rapid weight gain
- Abdominal pain

Signs of Placental or Fetal Problems
- Vaginal spotting or bleeding
- Abdominal pain and cramping
- Back pain
- Noticeable decrease in fetal activity
- No fetal movement

Signs of Preterm Labor
- Regular or frequent contractions (more than four to six per hour)
- Recurring low, dull backache
- Menstrual-like cramping
- Unusual pressure in the pelvis, low back, abdomen, or thighs

Laboratory Tests

The provider orders many laboratory tests to assist in the assessment of the patient's state of health and to detect problems that may put the pregnancy at risk. Several tests, such as the Pap test and the chlamydia and gonorrhea tests, require the provider to collect the specimens at the medical office and have them transported by laboratory courier to an outside laboratory for evaluation. The specimen required for the prenatal blood tests (known as a prenatal profile) must be obtained through a venipuncture to provide a sufficient quantity of blood for the number of tests ordered. The blood specimen is collected at the medical office or at an outside laboratory.

It is important to have these initial tests completed as soon as possible to provide the provider with the test results by the time of the next scheduled prenatal visit. Based on the results of the prenatal examination and the laboratory tests, the provider may order additional tests to assess the patient's condition. Certain tests and procedures, such as the glucose challenge test (GCT) and the group B streptococcus (GBS) test, are scheduled later in the pregnancy. The prenatal laboratory tests that are usually performed on a pregnant woman are described next.

Urine Tests

Urinalysis

A complete urinalysis, including physical, chemical, and microscopic analyses of the urine, is performed;

a clean-catch midstream urine specimen is generally required for the test. If bacteria are found in the urine specimen, the provider usually requests a urine culture and sensitivity test to determine the possible presence of a urinary tract infection. A pregnancy test also may be performed on the urine specimen, if ordered by the provider.

Swab Tests

Pap Test

A Pap test is done for the detection of abnormalities of cell growth to diagnose precancerous or cancerous conditions of the cervix. This test also can be used for hormonal assessment (maturation index) and to assist in the detection of vaginal infections.

Chlamydia and Gonorrhea

Specimens are taken from the endocervical canal and sent to the laboratory to rule out chlamydia and gonorrhea. A patient who is diagnosed with chlamydia or gonorrhea requires immediate treatment with an appropriate antibiotic to prevent problems for herself and her child.

If a chlamydial or gonorrheal infection is present at the time of delivery, the bacteria causing these conditions could infect the infant's eyes during passage through the birth canal. This may result in a type of conjunctivitis known as *ophthalmia neonatorum*, which, if not treated, could lead to blindness. For this reason, most states require that pregnant women be tested for chlamydia and gonorrhea, and that the eyes of newborns be treated with an antibiotic ointment immediately after birth to kill any harmful bacteria that may be present.

Vaginal Infections

If an excessively irritating vaginal discharge is present, the provider obtains a specimen to rule out bacterial infections including BV, trichomoniasis, and VVC. If a vaginal infection is diagnosed, the prenatal patient will be treated with the appropriate medication. BV and trichomoniasis increase the risk of premature birth and low birth weight. It is important to control VVC before delivery to prevent the development of *thrush*, a yeast-like infection of the infant's mucous membranes of the mouth or throat.

Group B Streptococcus

GBS is a common bacterium often found in the vagina and rectum of healthy women. Normally, one in four pregnant women carries GBS. GBS is not harmful to a pregnant woman, but it can cause life-threatening infections in the newborn. While passing through the birth canal, a newborn can become infected with the bacteria carried by the mother. When infected, the infant may develop an infection of the blood (septicemia), pneumonia, or meningitis.

To prevent GBS infection of the newborn, a pregnant woman is tested for the bacteria between 35 and 37 weeks of gestation. Using two swabs, the provider collects specimens from the vagina and the rectum. The specimen swabs are placed in a transport tube and sent to the laboratory to be cultured for GBS. If GBS is found, intravenous antibiotics are administered to the woman every 4 hours during labor until delivery. In most cases, this antibiotic administration prevents the newborn from becoming infected with GBS. In situations in which the newborn does become infected with GBS, antibiotics are administered immediately, and the infant is closely monitored.

What Would You Do? What Would You *Not* Do?

Case Study 3

Johanna Kruger is 24 years old and pregnant with her first child. She is at the office for her first prenatal visit. She is quite upset. One of her neighbors had minimal prenatal care and just had a baby, and the baby died 24 hours later from a group B strep infection. Johanna is afraid that the same thing will happen to her baby. She wants to be tested for group B streptococcus as soon as possible. She has some antibiotics at home and is thinking of taking them. Johanna is worried because she has been experiencing some problems with her pregnancy. She feels nauseous all day, her breasts are swollen and tender, and yesterday she had some spotting. Johanna is hesitant to tell all of this to the physician because he might think she worries too much. ■

Blood Tests

Complete Blood Count

The complete blood count (CBC) is a basic screening test used to assist in assessing the patient's state of health. It includes a hemoglobin, hematocrit, white blood cell count, red blood cell count, differential white blood cell count, platelet count, and red blood cell indices. Of particular importance with respect to the prenatal patient are the hemoglobin and hematocrit evaluations, which are described here.

Hemoglobin and Hematocrit

Low hemoglobin or hematocrit values are seen in cases of anemia. Prenatal patients have a tendency to develop anemia because there is an increased demand for and correlating increased production of red blood cells during pregnancy; the provider carefully reviews the results of these tests. If the hemoglobin or hematocrit value is low, further hematologic evaluation is usually required. If necessary, therapy is instituted, which usually consists of an iron supplement and nutritional counseling. The hemoglobin and hematocrit values are checked again at approximately 32 weeks of gestation as a precaution against anemia before delivery.

Rh Factor and ABO Blood Type

Tests are performed to anticipate ABO blood type and Rh factor incompatibilities. If the patient is Rh-negative, the possibility of an Rh incompatibility exists. This situation warrants the performance of an Rh antibody titer test and repeat antibody titers throughout the pregnancy to determine whether the mother's antibody level is increasing.

An increased Rh antibody level could be dangerous to the developing fetus. It can result in severe anemia, jaundice, brain damage, heart failure, and sometimes death of the fetus.

Glucose Challenge Test

A glucose challenge test (GCT) is performed between 24 and 28 weeks of gestation to screen for gestational diabetes mellitus (GDM). This test works by assessing the body's response to a measured glucose solution. The patient does not need to fast for this test, and no preparation is required other than arriving at the laboratory at the scheduled time. To perform the GCT, the patient is asked to drink 50 g of a glucose solution, and her glucose level is measured 1 hour later. A woman with a glucose level of less than 140 mg/dL does not have GDM and requires no further testing. If the glucose level is greater than 140 mg/dL, the test is abnormal. Not all women with elevated results have diabetes, however, and further testing using the 3-hour oral glucose tolerance test (OGTT) must be performed before a final diagnosis can be made. (*Note:* Refer to Chapter 19 for information on the OGTT.)

HIGHLIGHT on Gestational Diabetes Mellitus

Definition of Gestational Diabetes Mellitus

Gestational diabetes mellitus (GDM) is a condition in which a pregnant woman who has never had diabetes mellitus develops an elevated glucose level (hyperglycemia). Every year, approximately 3% to 5% of pregnant women in the United States are diagnosed with GDM. Because most women with GDM have no symptoms, the American Diabetes Association recommends that all pregnant women be screened for GDM during the second trimester of the pregnancy.

Cause of Gestational Diabetes Mellitus

GDM develops from a physical interaction between the mother and the fetus. The placenta of the fetus produces hormones to preserve the pregnancy. These hormones are excreted into the mother's circulatory system in increasing amounts during the second trimester of pregnancy. These hormones counteract the effect of the mother's insulin, which results in a condition known as *insulin resistance.* In most cases, the mother's pancreas responds to insulin resistance by producing additional insulin to keep the blood glucose at a normal level. Some women are unable to produce enough extra insulin, however, which causes an elevation of their blood glucose level and results in GDM.

Problems for the Child

If GDM is not treated or if it is poorly controlled, problems can occur in the unborn child. The extra glucose crosses the placenta and enters the fetus' circulatory system. To decrease the elevated glucose level, the fetus' pancreas produces large amounts of insulin. The increased insulin converts the extra glucose into fat, resulting in the development of a large infant with a condition known as *macrosomia.* Infants with macrosomia may be too large to be born vaginally and may require a cesarean birth. Although the infant does not have diabetes, he or she is at risk for developing type 2 diabetes later in life. Other problems that can occur at birth include hypoglycemia, breathing difficulties, and jaundice.

Problems for the Mother

Problems that a mother with GDM can develop include an increased incidence of preeclampsia, infection, postpartum bleeding, and injury to the birth canal if the infant is delivered vaginally. Another problem is the development of polyhydramnios (excess amount of amniotic fluid), which causes the uterus to stretch and take up more space in the abdominal cavity. This can result in breathing difficulties for the mother during the pregnancy. GDM almost always resolves after delivery. This is because when the placenta is removed, the hormones causing the problem also are removed. The mother's insulin can work normally without resistance. Some women go on to develop type 2 diabetes later in life, however.

Risk Factors for Gestational Diabetes Mellitus

Certain factors put some women at greater risk for developing GDM. These women are usually screened earlier and more often for GDM during the pregnancy. Risk factors for GDM include the following:

- Obesity
- Family history of diabetes mellitus
- Previous birth of an infant weighing more than 9 lb
- Previous birth of an infant who was stillborn or had a birth defect
- Previous GDM diagnosis
- Age older than 25 years
- Polyhydramnios
- Belonging to an ethnic group known to have higher rates of GDM (Hispanic, African American, Native American, Asian, Pacific Islander)

Treatment

If a woman is diagnosed with GDM, the treatment is focused on keeping her glucose at a safe level. This includes special meal plans, exercise, daily blood glucose testing, and insulin injections, if needed. If the blood glucose is controlled during pregnancy, most women with GDM are able to prevent maternal or fetal complications.

Syphilis Test

The microorganism that causes syphilis, *Treponema pallidum,* is able to cross the placental barrier and infect the fetus; this could result in intrauterine death or could cause the fetus to be born with congenital syphilis. Infants with congenital syphilis are often born with deformities and may become blind, deaf, paralyzed, and develop intellectual disabilities. The tests most commonly employed to screen for the presence of syphilis are the Venereal Disease Research Laboratory (VDRL) test and the rapid plasma reagin (RPR) test. The test results are reported as nonreactive, weakly reactive, or reactive. Because these tests are screening tests, a weakly reactive or reactive test result warrants more specific testing to arrive at a diagnosis for syphilis. Examples of these tests are the fluorescent treponemal antibody absorption (FTA-ABS) test and the *Treponema pallidum* particle agglutination assay (TPPA) test.

A prenatal test for syphilis is mandated by most states and should be performed early in the pregnancy, before fetal damage occurs. A patient who has contracted syphilis requires treatment with an appropriate antibiotic.

Rubella Antibody Titer

The rubella antibody titer assesses the level of antibody against rubella (German measles) in the patient's blood and is used to determine whether the woman is immune to rubella. If the mother contracts rubella during pregnancy, serious congenital abnormalities can occur in the fetus. Patients who lack immunity should be immunized against rubella within 6 weeks of delivery.

Rh Antibody Titer (on Rh-Negative Blood Specimens)

An Rh antibody titer detects the quantity of circulating Rh antibodies against red blood cells. These antibodies can occur in a pregnant woman who is Rh-negative and is carrying an Rh-positive fetus; an Rh antibody titer is performed on all Rh-negative blood specimens. Repeat antibody titer levels also are performed during the pregnancy to determine whether the woman's antibody level is increasing. As was previously indicated, an increased Rh antibody level could be dangerous to the developing fetus. As a preventive measure, Rh-negative women with the potential of having an Rh-positive infant and who test negative for Rh antibodies are given two injections of Rh immune globulin (RhoGAM). The Rh immune globulin prevents the formation of Rh antibodies in the mother, which avoids Rh incompatibility complications during the next pregnancy. The first injection is given at 28 weeks of gestation, and the second injection is administered within 72 hours of delivery.

Hepatitis B and Human Immunodeficiency Virus

The Centers for Disease Control and Prevention (CDC) recommends that pregnant women have the hepatitis B surface antigen (HBsAg) test to screen for hepatitis B virus. Women who have positive HBsAg test results have an increased risk of spontaneous abortion or preterm labor. In addition, the mother may transmit hepatitis B to the infant, particularly during delivery or in the first few days of life. This risk can be greatly reduced by administering hepatitis B immune globulin (HBIG) and the hepatitis B vaccine within 12 hours of birth to the newborns of women who have tested positive for hepatitis B.

Infants born to women who are HIV positive are at risk of developing the disease. If antiretroviral drugs are taken during pregnancy and the infant is delivered by cesarean section, the chance of transmitting HIV to the infant is reduced significantly. Because of this, the CDC recommends that testing for HIV be included in the routine panel of prenatal screening tests for all pregnant women, and that separate written consent is not required. The CDC further recommends that the patient should be notified that HIV testing will be performed unless the patient declines the test. The CDC recommends that repeat HIV screening be performed in the third trimester in geographic areas that have elevated rates of HIV infection among pregnant women.

RETURN PRENATAL VISITS

Return prenatal visits provide the opportunity for a continuous assessment of the health of the mother and the fetus. During each visit, essential data are collected and documented in the prenatal record, resulting in an updated record at each visit, as is discussed in this section. If signs or symptoms of a pathologic condition are present, the provider performs select aspects of the physical examination as necessary to diagnose and treat the condition. In addition, diagnostic and laboratory tests may be ordered to assist in diagnosis and treatment. The usual schedule of visits for prenatal care is listed below. A patient who exhibits complications is seen more frequently for closer monitoring.

- 0 to 28 weeks of gestation: Every 4 weeks
- 29 to 35 weeks: Every 2 weeks
- 36 weeks until delivery: Every week

The return prenatal visit also provides the opportunity for the provider and the medical assistant to lend support to the mother, to provide her with ongoing prenatal education to reduce apprehension and anxiety, and to ensure that the mother is well informed and prepared during her pregnancy, childbirth, and the postpartum period. The medical assistant plays an important role in prenatal education and should take the necessary time with each patient to provide appropriate information and to allow the patient to ask questions. Procedure 8.3 outlines the medical assistant's role in the return prenatal visit.

The patient is asked to provide a urine specimen during each return prenatal visit. The medical assistant is responsible for testing the specimen for glucose and protein using a reagent strip and for documenting results in the prenatal record. A positive reaction to glucose may indicate the development of GDM or a prediabetic condition, and a positive reaction to protein may indicate a urinary tract infection or preeclampsia. Further testing usually is needed to arrive at a final diagnosis and to institute treatment. Hypertension is the most common medical disorder of pregnancy and

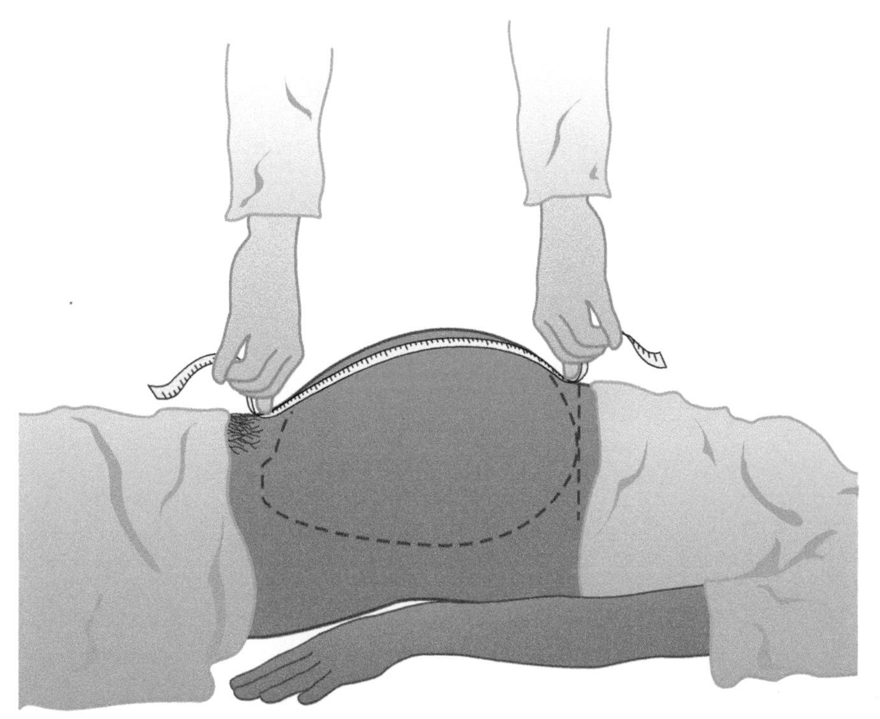

Fig. 8.12 Measurement of fundal height. The provider places one end of a centimeter tape measure on the superior aspect of the symphysis pubis and measures to the top of the uterine fundus.

occurs in 10% to 12% of all pregnancies. Because of this, the medical assistant must make sure to obtain an accurate blood pressure measurement.

During the return visit, the provider performs one or more of the following procedures, depending on the stage of the pregnancy: (1) palpation of the woman's abdomen to measure fundal height, (2) measurement of the FHR, and (3) a vaginal examination. These procedures are discussed in detail next.

Fundal Height Measurement

The pregnant uterus rises gradually into the abdominal cavity, and the fundus is palpable between 8 and 13 weeks of gestation. The first fundal height measurement, which is usually performed during the first prenatal visit, is used as a guideline for all subsequent measurements. The provider measures the fundal height by placing one end of a flexible, nonstretchable centimeter tape measure on the superior aspect of the symphysis pubis and measuring to the crest or top of the uterine fundus (Fig. 8.12). The measurement is documented on a flow chart in the patient's prenatal record. By 20 weeks, the fundus reaches the lower border of the umbilicus, and between 36 and 37 weeks, it reaches the tip of the sternum. During the first and second trimesters, measuring the fundal height provides a rough estimate of the duration of the pregnancy (Fig. 8.13). Because fetal weights vary considerably during the third trimester, it is difficult to use fundal height measurements as an estimate of the duration of the pregnancy in the last trimester.

In addition to assessing the duration of the pregnancy, the fundal height measurements permit variations from normal to become apparent and are used to assess whether fetal growth is progressing normally. Growth that is too rapid or too slow must be evaluated further by the provider as a possible indication of high-risk conditions, such as multiple pregnancies, polyhydramnios, ovarian tumor, intrauterine growth retardation, intrauterine death, or an error in estimating the fetal progress.

Fetal Heart Tones

Fetal heart tones refer to the heartbeat of the fetus as heard through the mother's abdominal wall and the **fetal heart rate** is the number of times per minute that the fetal heart beats. The normal FHR is between 120 and 160 beats per minute with a regular rhythm. A very slow or rapid FHR usually indicates fetal distress. The fetal heart tones can be heard with a Doppler fetal pulse detector between 10 and 12 weeks of gestation. The Doppler fetal pulse detector converts ultrasonic waves into audible sounds of the fetal pulse.

The Doppler device consists of a main control unit and a probe (Fig. 8.14A). The probe head contains a transducer and electronic components, which generate the sound waves. The probe head is delicate and must be handled carefully, making sure not to drop or knock the head to prevent damaging it.

Because air is a poor conductor of sound, an ultrasound coupling gel must first be spread on the mother's abdomen in the area to be examined. The gel is usually applied by the medical assistant, and its purpose is to increase conductivity of the sound waves between the abdomen and the transducer.

The provider places the head of the probe into the gel on the mother's abdomen and slowly moves it until the

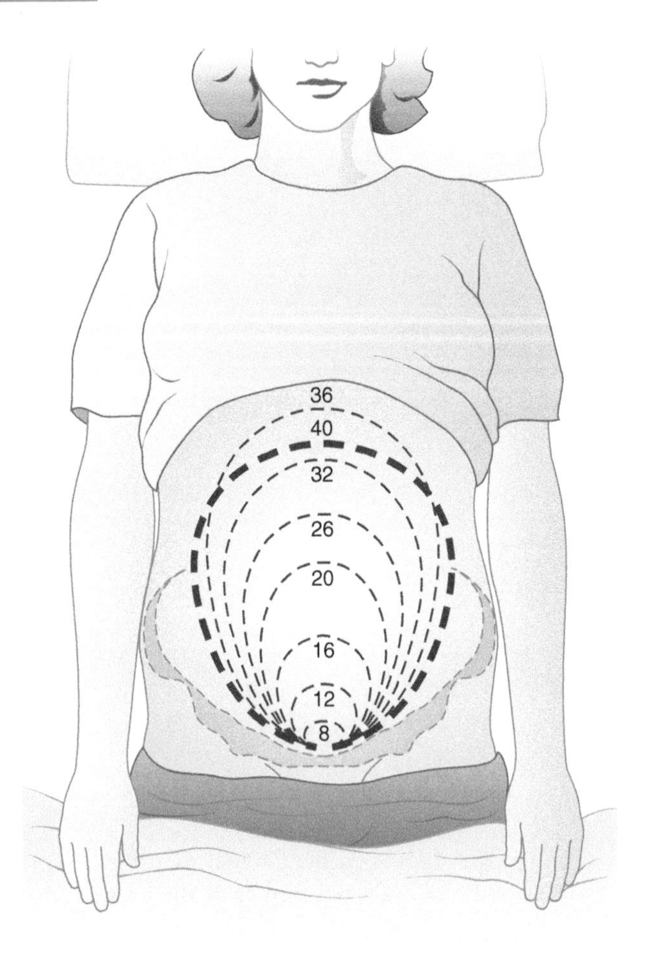

Fig. 8.13 Fundal height showing gestational age in weeks.

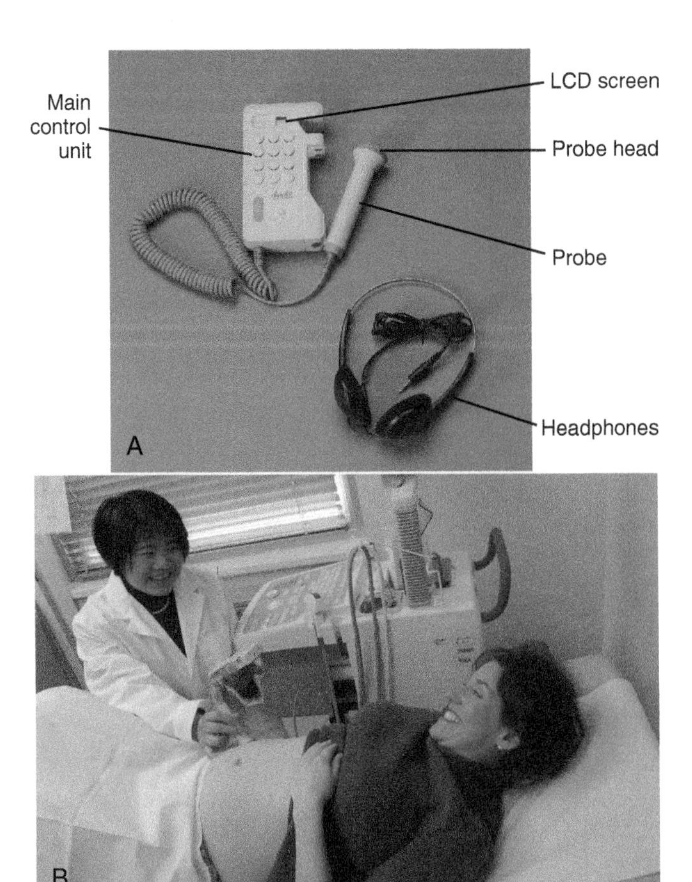

Fig. 8.14 (A) Parts of a Doppler device. (B) The probe of the Doppler device is moved across the abdomen to detect the fetal pulse.

fetal heart tones are located. The Doppler device amplifies the fetal heart tones, and they are broadcast through a built-in loudspeaker in the main unit. A volume control provides adjustment of the sound level as required. (Fetal heart tones sound like the hoofbeats of a galloping horse, and when the probe is over the placenta, a windlike sound is heard.) The Doppler device also may have an LCD screen, which provides a digital display of the fetal pulse rate. Stereo headphones come with the Doppler device to allow private listening. The loudspeaker is muted when the headphones are connected (see Fig. 8.14B).

After the procedure, the medical assistant should remove excess gel from the mother's abdomen with a paper towel. The probe head is cleaned using a damp cloth or a paper towel. The Doppler device should be properly stored in its carrying case to prevent it from becoming damaged.

Vaginal Examination

In the absence of vaginal bleeding, vaginal examinations may be performed at any time during the pregnancy; however, in a normal pregnancy, there is usually no need to perform a vaginal examination until the patient nears term. The vaginal examination is usually begun approximately 2 to 3 weeks from the EDD and is performed to confirm the presenting part and to determine the degree, if any, of cervical dilation and effacement. The purpose of dilation and effacement is to permit the passage of the infant from the uterus into the birth canal (Fig. 8.15).

What Would You Do? What Would You *Not* Do?

Case Study 4

Wynita Lopez is at the office with her husband. She is 36 years old and 14 weeks pregnant. It took Wynita a long time—almost 8 years—to get pregnant. She is excited and happy about being pregnant but, at the same time, upset and confused. Her test results on her first trimester prenatal screening test came back indicating an increased risk for Down syndrome. Wynita and her husband understand that the only way to know for sure is to have an amniocentesis. Wynita does not know what to do and cannot stop crying. She is afraid of having an amniocentesis because of the slight risk of miscarriage. Wynita and her husband are unsure what their decision would be if the baby did have Down syndrome. Her husband is visibly distressed and wants Wynita to decide whether or not to have an amniocentesis. Right now she wants as much information as she can get about all of this before she makes a decision. ■

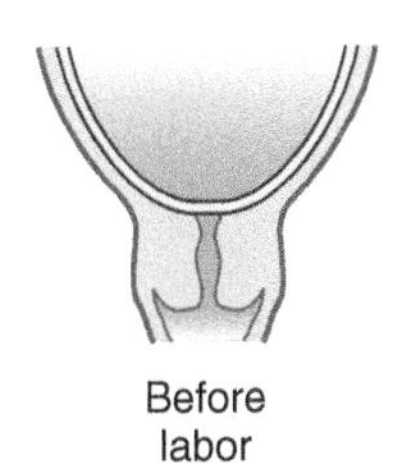

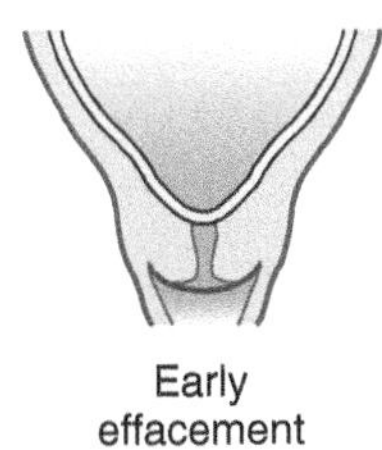

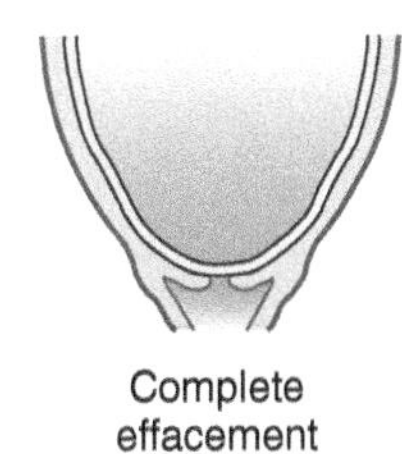

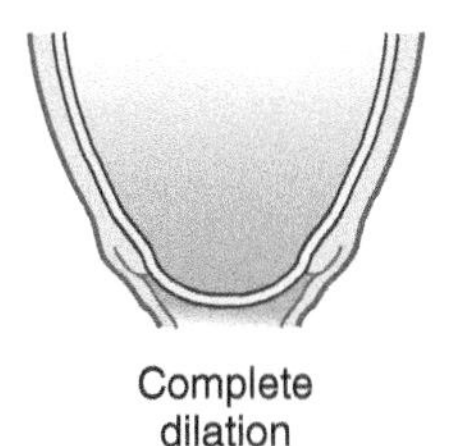

Fig. 8.15 Effacement and dilation occur to permit the passage of the infant into the birth canal. The cervical canal shortens from its normal length of 1–2 cm to a structure with paper-thin edges in which there is no canal at all. The cervix dilates from an opening a few millimeters wide to an opening large enough to allow the passage of the infant (approximately 10 cm).

Special Tests and Procedures

The pregnancy can be evaluated with one or more of the following special tests and procedures: carrier screening, first trimester prenatal screening (FTPS) test, noninvasive prenatal test (NIPT), multiple marker test, obstetric ultrasound scan, amniocentesis, and FHR monitoring. These are not considered routine tests and procedures; however, they involve a slight risk or no risk at all to the mother or the fetus. It is important for the medical assistant to have a general knowledge of these tests and procedures which are described next in more detail.

Carrier Screening

Carrier screening can determine if a woman or her partner carries a gene for specific genetic disorders such as cystic fibrosis and sickle cell disease. In many cases, both parents must carry the same gene to have a child affected with a genetic disorder. Carrier screening can be performed before or during the pregnancy. The test is performed using a blood specimen or tissue sample that is swabbed from inside the cheek. The provider often recommends carrier screening if the woman or her partner has a genetic disorder, has a child with a genetic disorder, has a family history of a genetic disorder, or belongs to an ethnic group that has an increased risk of a specific genetic disorder.

First Trimester Prenatal Screening Test

The FTPS test, also known as *Ultrascreen*, is a prenatal evaluation available to pregnant women between 11 and 14 weeks of gestation. The purpose of the FTPS is to assess the patient's risk of certain fetal genetic disorders which include Down syndrome, Trisomy 18, and other less common chromosomal abnormalities. The FTPS test cannot determine the risk of neural tube defects such as spina bifida.

The FTPS test consists of a combination of the following two tests: (a) A blood test to measure a protein (pregnancy-associated protein A) and a hormone (human chorionic gonadotropin) present in the blood of a pregnant woman and (b) an ultrasound to measure the fluid accumulation behind the neck of the fetus known as *nuchal translucency*. The FTPS is a screening test. Abnormal test results always necessitate further testing to determine whether a fetal abnormality actually exists such as amniocentesis.

Noninvasive Prenatal Test

The NIPT, also known as *cell-free DNA test*, is a laboratory test used to assess whether a patient is at increased risk of having a fetus affected by certain genetic disorders. During pregnancy some of the DNA from the baby crosses into the mother's bloodstream. This DNA carries the baby's genetic information. This fetal DNA is tested to check for certain genetic disorders that include Down syndrome, Trisomy 13, Trisomy 18, and problems with the number of sex chromosomes. This test can also determine the gender of the baby. This NIPT can be performed as early as 9 to 10 weeks of gestation and up until delivery. The NIPT is a screening test. Abnormal test results always necessitate further testing to determine whether a fetal abnormality actually exists such as amniocentesis.

Multiple Marker Test

The multiple marker (quad screen) test is a laboratory test available to pregnant women between 15 and 20 weeks of gestation. Its purpose is to screen for the presence of certain fetal abnormalities, which include neural tube defects, Down syndrome, trisomy 18, and ventral wall defect. Because the multiple marker test has a high incidence of false-positive test results, it is not a mandatory prenatal test; however, the AGOG believes that this test should be offered to all pregnant women regardless of maternal age. The multiple marker test is a screening test. Abnormal test results always require further testing, such as amniocentesis, to determine whether a fetal abnormality actually exists.

Obstetric Ultrasound Scan

An obstetric ultrasound scan is a diagnostic imaging technique, similar to sonar, used to view the fetus in utero. It allows continuous viewing of the fetus and shows fetal movement. An ultrasound technologist usually performs the procedure. The primary purpose of an ultrasound scan is to evaluate the health of the fetus and to determine gestational age. This is accomplished by viewing the image of the fetus and by taking various measurements of the image, such as crown-rump length; biparietal diameter, which is a side-to-side measurement of the fetal head; femur length; and abdominal circumference.

Obstetric ultrasound scanning uses high-frequency sound waves that are directed into the uterus through a transducer. When the sound waves reach the uterus, they "bounce" back to the transducer, similar to an echo. These reflected sound waves are converted into an image, or *sonogram* (Fig. 8.16), which is displayed on a monitor screen. The monitor is positioned so the mother can view the image on the screen. There are two methods for performing an ultrasound scan: the transabdominal method and the endovaginal method.

Although an obstetric ultrasound scan can be performed at any time during the pregnancy, it is often performed at between 7 and 12 weeks of gestation and again at between 18 and 20 weeks. A third scan is sometimes done around 34 weeks of gestation. Box 8.6 outlines this schedule and what can be assessed at these times.

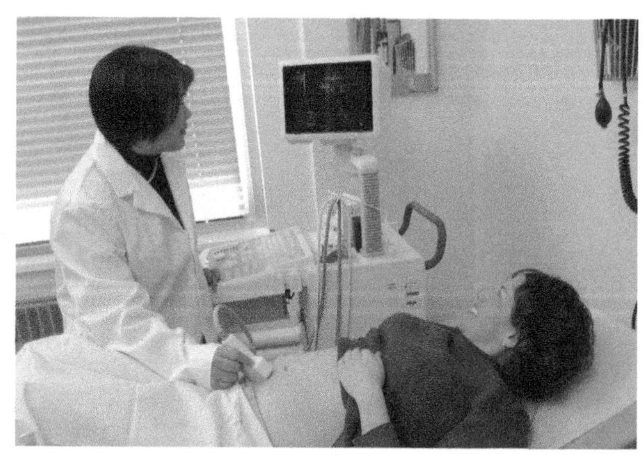

Fig. 8.16 Obstetric ultrasound scan.

Transabdominal Ultrasound Scan

Transabdominal ultrasound is the scanning method performed most often. The patient must have a full bladder for this examination. This is accomplished by instructing

BOX 8.6 Purpose of Obstetric Ultrasound Scanning

Between 7 and 12 Weeks

- To confirm pregnancy by detecting fetal heart motion
- To determine gestational age by taking measurements of the embryo and embryonic sac
- To measure nuchal translucency
- To detect an ectopic pregnancy

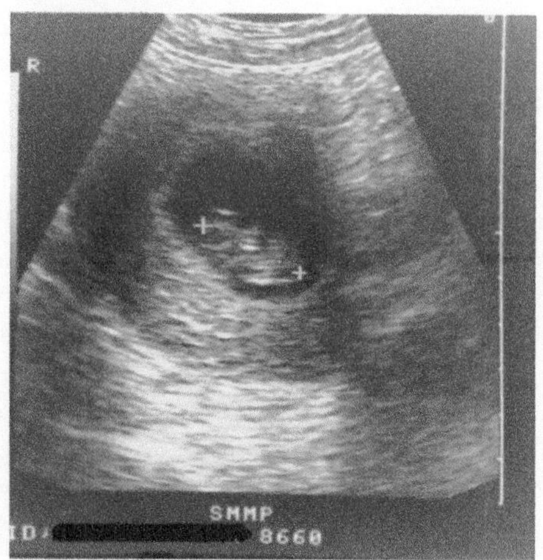

Embryo at approximately 9 weeks of gestation. (From Greer I, Cameron IT, Kitchener HC, Prentice A: *Mosby's color atlas and text of obstetrics and gynecology,* St Louis: Mosby; 2001.)

Between 18 and 20 Weeks

- To determine fetal growth, size, and weight by taking measurements of the fetus
- To detect the presence of multiple fetuses
- To examine the brain, spinal cord, heart, lungs, gastrointestinal tract, reproductive organs, kidneys, bladder, bowel, and extremities of the fetus
- To detect congenital abnormalities
- To determine the location of the placenta
- To determine the cause of bleeding or spotting

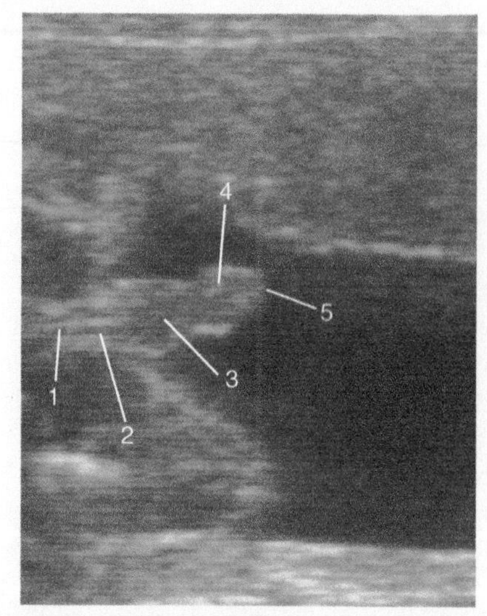

Erect fetal penis. *1,* urethra; *2,* corpus cavernosum; *3,* shaft; *4,* glans; *5,* foreskin. (From Callen P: *Ultrasonography in obstetrics and gynecology,* ed 4, Philadelphia: WB Saunders; 2000.)

BOX 8.6 Purpose of Obstetric Ultrasound Scanning—cont'd

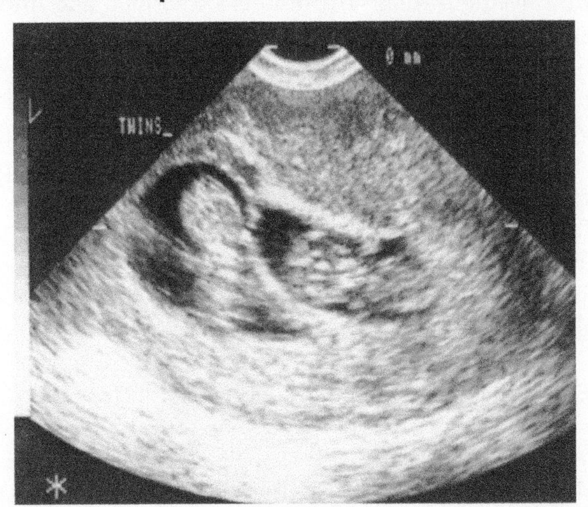

Sonogram of twins. (From Greer I, Cameron IT, Kitchener HC, Prentice A: *Mosby's color atlas and text of obstetrics and gynecology*, St Louis: Mosby; 2001.)

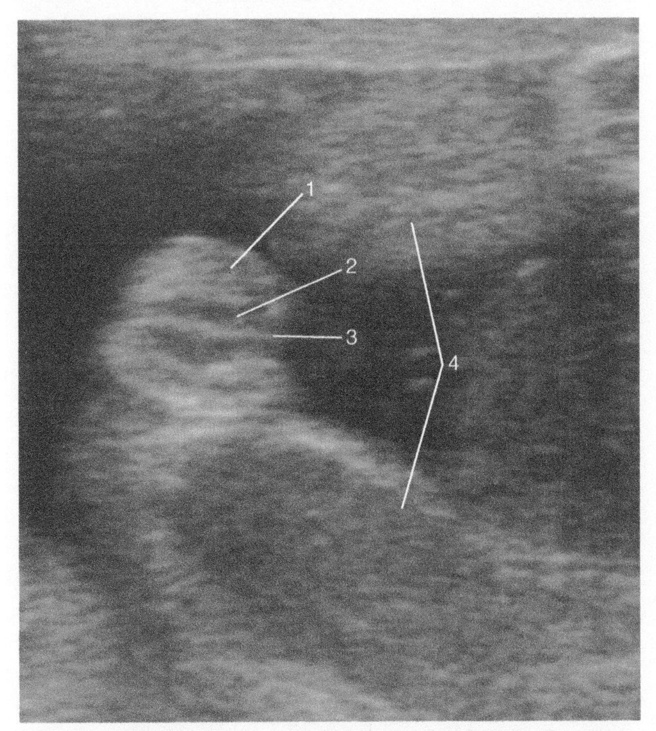

External female genitalia. *1,* major labium; *2,* minor labium; *3,* vaginal cleft; *4,* thighs. (From Callen P: *Ultrasonography in obstetrics and gynecology,* ed 4, Philadelphia: WB Saunders; 2000.)

At 34 Weeks

- To evaluate fetal growth, size, and weight by taking measurements of the fetus
- To verify the location of the placenta
- To confirm fetal presentation in uncertain cases

Other Purposes

- To diagnose uterine and pelvic abnormalities during pregnancy
- To view the fetus, placenta, and amniotic fluid during tests such as amniocentesis and chorionic villus sampling
- To confirm intrauterine death

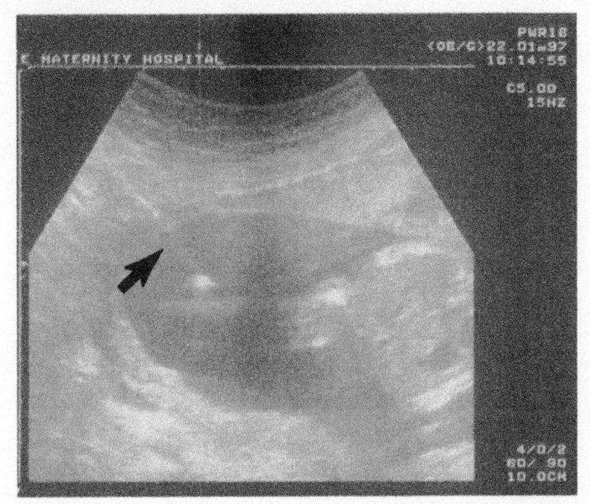

Amniocentesis being performed under ultrasound guidance. (From Greer I, Cameron IT, Kitchener HC, Prentice A: *Mosby's color atlas and text of obstetrics and gynecology,* St Louis: Mosby; 2001.)

the patient to consume 32 oz of fluid approximately 1 hour before the procedure. A full bladder acts as an "acoustic window" through which the sound waves can travel to provide a clear visualization of the uterus. In addition, a full bladder holds the uterus stable and pushes away any bowel that might interfere with the image. The patient lies on an examining table in a supine position and is draped with the abdomen exposed. A coupling agent, in the form of a liquid gel, is applied to the patient's abdomen to increase the transmission of the sound waves. An abdominal probe (containing

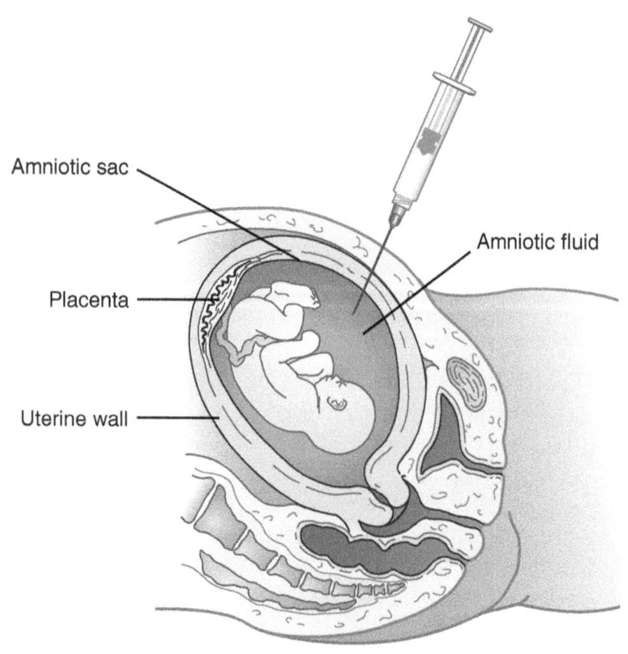

Fig. 8.17 Amniocentesis.

a transducer) is placed into the gel, and the probe is moved slowly over the patient's abdomen; the image of the fetus is displayed on the screen of the monitor (Fig. 8.17). Three-dimensional and four-dimensional (3-D and 4-D, respectively) ultrasound are types of transabdominal ultrasound. A 3-D ultrasound exam takes thousands of images at once. These images are formatted into a 3-D image which looks more lifelike. A 4-D image is similar to a 3-D image, but it also shows movement.

Endovaginal Ultrasound Scan

In the early stages of the pregnancy (up to 12 weeks), endovaginal scanning is preferred over transabdominal scanning. The patient must have an empty bladder for this scan, which makes the examination more comfortable. The patient is placed in the lithotomy position, and a vaginal probe is placed in the patient's vagina. The image of the embryo is displayed on the screen of the monitor. An endovaginal ultrasound scan provides clearer visualization of the uterus at the beginning of the pregnancy because the probe is situated in the vagina, which places it closer to the uterus.

Amniocentesis

Amniocentesis is a diagnostic procedure that can be performed between 15 and 18 weeks of gestation. Amniocentesis aids in prenatal diagnosis of certain genetically transmitted errors of metabolism, congenital abnormalities, and chromosomal disorders such as Down syndrome. It also is used to detect fetal jeopardy or distress and, later in the pregnancy, to assess fetal lung maturity. Amniocentesis also can determine whether the fetus is a boy or a girl.

To perform the procedure, the provider inserts a long, thin needle through the mother's abdomen and into the amniotic sac surrounding the fetus (see Fig. 8.17). An obstetric ultrasound scan is always performed in conjunction with amniocentesis so that the provider can view the position of the fetus, placenta, and amniotic fluid. This allows the provider to know the exact place to insert the needle. The provider withdraws a sample (about 1 tablespoon) of fluid, which contains fetal cells. The fluid is sent to a laboratory for study. It usually takes 1 to 3 weeks to evaluate the amniotic fluid and report the results.

Although the complication rate for an amniocentesis is extremely low, the procedure is not risk free. There is a slight risk of bleeding, leakage of fluid, and infection of the amniotic fluid. There also is a slight possibility of miscarriage. Because of these risks, amniocentesis is offered only to women whose pregnancies are at risk for fetal abnormalities. This includes women who are 35 years old or older, women who have a child with a genetic or neural tube defect, women who have abnormal multiple marker test results, women who have or whose partner has a chromosomal abnormality, and women who are or whose partner is a carrier for a metabolic disease.

Fetal Heart Rate Monitoring

FHR monitoring is performed later in the pregnancy to obtain information on the physical condition of the fetus. Specific conditions that may warrant this procedure are fetal growth that is not progressing well, decreased amniotic fluid, decreased fetal activity, elevation of the mother's blood pressure, gestational diabetes, and an overdue infant.

To perform the procedure, an electronic microphone is strapped to the mother's abdomen to amplify the fetal heartbeat. A gel is usually applied under the microphone to make the sounds clearer. The fetal heartbeat is heard and displayed on a screen and printed on special paper.

There are two kinds of FHR monitoring procedures: the nonstress test and the contraction stress test (CST). The *nonstress test* (NST) monitors changes in the FHR in response to the fetus' spontaneous movements. The mother is instructed to press a button when she feels the fetus move. In a normal test, the fetus' heart rate increases when the fetus moves. To prepare for the NST, the mother must be instructed to eat a light meal within 2 hours of the procedure to stimulate fetal movement.

If the results of the NST are abnormal, a *contraction stress test* (CST) may be performed. This test is similar to the NST except that mild contractions of the uterus are stimulated for a short period of time. The CST is used to evaluate the response of the fetus' heart rate to the contractions to determine whether the fetus would be able to withstand the stress of repeated contractions during labor. If the results of the test are abnormal, further evaluation is required to evaluate the well-being of the fetus and to determine how and when delivery of the fetus should be carried out.

SIX-WEEK POSTPARTUM VISIT

The **puerperium** includes the period of time in which the body systems are returning to their prepregnant or nearly prepregnant state, which usually is 4 to 6 weeks after delivery. During this time, numerous changes occur in the woman's body. The *involution of the uterus* (i.e., the process by which it returns to its normal size and state) occurs; this includes healing of any injuries sustained to the birth canal during delivery.

During the puerperium, the patient experiences a vaginal discharge shed from the lining of the uterus, known as **lochia**. Lochia consists of blood, tissue, white blood cells, mucus, and some bacteria. The color of the lochia is an indication of the progress of the healing of the uterus. For the first 3 days after delivery, the lochia consists almost entirely of blood and, because of its red color, is termed *lochia rubra.* By approximately 4 days postpartum, the amount of blood decreases, and the discharge becomes pink or brownish and is known as *lochia serosa.* By 10 days postpartum, the flow should decrease, and the lochia should become yellowish white; this is known as *lochia alba.* Lochia usually continues in consistently decreasing amounts (from moderate to scant to occasional spotting) and becomes paler in color until the third week after delivery, when it usually disappears altogether. It would not be considered unusual for the discharge to last the entire 6 weeks, however.

The patient should be instructed to contact the medical office under the following circumstances: if the amount of discharge increases rather than decreases; if the discharge is absent within the first 2 weeks after delivery; if it changes to red after having been yellowish white, which indicates bleeding; or if it takes on a foul odor, which indicates infection. Menstruation usually begins approximately 2 months after delivery in a nonnursing mother and 3 to 6 months after delivery in a nursing mother.

During the puerperium, the patient should be encouraged to avoid fatigue, to avoid lifting heavy objects, and to consume a nutritious, well-balanced diet that helps maintain health and promote healing. The physician will want to see the patient at the medical office at the end of the 6-week period. The purpose of the 6 weeks postpartum visit is to evaluate the general mental and physical condition of the patient, to ensure there are no residual problems from childbearing, and to provide the patient with education regarding postpartum depression and methods of contraception and infant care. During this visit, the patient is queried about problems or abnormalities related to postpartum depression, vaginal discharge, urinary or bowel function, and breastfeeding if she is nursing. This information is documented in the patient's medical record. The postpartum visit provides an excellent opportunity for the medical assistant to instruct the patient in the technique for performing a BSE and to educate her on the importance of returning to the medical office as needed for a Pap test.

During the postpartum examination, the physician evaluates the patient's general mental status and physical appearance, performs breast and pelvic examinations, and checks to determine whether the muscle tone has returned to the muscles of the abdominal wall. During the puerperium, atypical cells may be sloughed off into the cervical and vaginal mucus as part of the normal healing process. Because of this, the Pap test is not included in the postpartum visit. If the patient has problems with hemorrhoids or varicosities, the physician discusses any further treatment required. If the patient does not have antibody protection to rubella, as has been evidenced through the prenatal laboratory tests, she receives rubella immunization at this time (if it was not administered in the hospital). In addition, hemoglobin and hematocrit determinations usually are performed on the postpartum patient to screen for anemia caused by blood loss during delivery and the puerperium.

Responsibilities of the medical assistant during the postpartum visit include measuring and documenting the patient's vital signs and weight and preparing the patient for the examination. The patient is required to disrobe completely for this examination and to put on an examining gown with the opening in front. Table 8.3 lists the procedures commonly included in the 6-week postpartum visit and the purpose of each.

TABLE 8.3 Six-Week Postpartum Examination

Procedure	Purpose
Vital signs • Temperature • Pulse • Respiration • Blood pressure	To ensure vital signs fall within normal limits and that blood pressure has returned to normal prepregnant level.
Weight	To determine whether patient's weight has returned to prepregnant measurement. If not, nutritional counseling may be indicated.
Breast examination	To ensure breasts are not sore or tender and no cysts or lumps are present. In nonnursing mother, breasts are examined to determine whether they have returned to their prepregnant size. In nursing mother, nipples are examined for cracks, redness, soreness, and fissures.
Pelvic examination	To ensure that involution of uterus is complete and to determine whether the cervix has healed. To ensure that episiotomy (if performed) and any injuries sustained by the birth canal have healed. To ensure that no abnormal vaginal discharge is present.
Rectal-vaginal examination	To ensure pelvic floor has regained its muscle tone. To determine whether hemorrhoids are present.
Evaluation of patient's general mental and physical condition	To ensure body systems have returned to their prepregnant state. To discuss and evaluate signs and symptoms of postpartum depression.

What Would You Do? What Would You *Not* Do? RESPONSES

Case Study 1
Page 238

What Did Yin-Ling Do?

- ❑ Reassured Mrs. Wooster that the physician is there to help her and stressed that he will be pleased that she has come to the office for an examination.
- ❑ Commended Mrs. Wooster on performing a breast self-examination (BSE) at home to become familiar with her breast tissue. Asked her whether she had any questions on how to perform a BSE.
- ❑ Told Mrs. Wooster that some breast changes are normal and others are not normal, and the only way to know for sure is to be examined by the physician.
- ❑ Told Mrs. Wooster that it is important to have a periodic gynecologic examination even if her periods are normal. Explained to her that some conditions can be present without symptoms. Gave Mrs. Wooster a patient information brochure on gynecologic examinations.
- ❑ Took plenty of time with Mrs. Wooster so that she would feel comfortable coming back again in the future for a gynecologic examination.

What Did Yin-Ling Not Do?

- ❑ Did not criticize Mrs. Wooster for waiting so long to schedule a gynecologic examination.

Case Study 2
Page 255

What Did Yin-Ling Do?

- ❑ Stressed to Brooke how important it is that she be seen by the physician. Explained that she could be infected with chlamydia and not know it because chlamydia often has no symptoms, especially in women.
- ❑ Explained to Brooke that state law allows her to be treated for a sexually transmitted infection without permission from her parents. Told her the law was created to encourage minors to seek treatment for sexually transmitted infections.
- ❑ Commended Brooke on practicing safe sex. Relayed to her that if a condom is not used correctly, or if it tears, she might not be protected from getting a sexually transmitted infection. That is another reason she should be tested.
- ❑ Explained to Brooke what will occur during the examination and what the physician will be doing. Relayed techniques that Brooke could use to relax during the procedure.

What Did Yin-Ling Not Do?

- ❑ Did not tell Brooke everything would be all right and that she probably does not have chlamydia.
- ❑ Did not try to prevent Brooke from leaving if she still insists on doing so.

Case Study 3
Page 264

What Did Yin-Ling Do?

- ❑ Tried to calm Johanna by telling her that it is normal for her to be worried and concerned. Explained that the purpose of her prenatal visits is so that the physician can keep a close watch on her and detect any problems that might occur.
- ❑ Reassured Johanna that she does not need to be afraid to tell the physician any of her concerns because he is there to help her and her baby.
- ❑ Told Johanna that it is important not to take any medications during her pregnancy without first checking with the physician because some medications could be harmful to her baby.
- ❑ Told Johanna that her problems and concerns would be relayed to the physician and that he would want to talk to her about them. Explained that the physician also would talk with her about being tested for group B streptococcus.

What Did Yin-Ling Not Do?

- ❑ Did not tell Johanna that it was all right to take the antibiotics.
- ❑ Did not tell Joanna that her neighbor should have gotten better prenatal care.

Case Study 4
Page 268

What Did Yin-Ling Do?

- ❑ Escorted Mr. and Mrs. Lopez to a private room in the office. Tried to relax them and told them that whatever they choose to do will be the right decision for them.
- ❑ Gave Mrs. Lopez the information she requested that was available at the office and provided her with a list of resources approved by the physician that she could contact for further information.
- ❑ Asked Mr. and Mrs. Lopez whether they had any more questions they wanted to ask the physician.

What Did Yin-Ling Not Do?

- ❑ Did not give Mr. and Mrs. Lopez advice on what they should do. ■

TERMINOLOGY REVIEW

Medical Term	Word Parts	Definition
Abortion		The termination of the pregnancy before the fetus reaches the age of viability (20 weeks).
Amenorrhea	*a-:* without *men/o:* menstruation *-orrhea:* flow, excessive discharge	The absence or cessation of the menstrual period. Amenorrhea occurs normally before puberty, during pregnancy, and after menopause.

TERMINOLOGY REVIEW—cont'd

Medical Term	Word Parts	Definition
Braxton Hicks contractions		Intermittent and irregular painless uterine contractions that occur throughout pregnancy. They occur more frequently toward the end of pregnancy and are sometimes mistaken for true labor pains.
Cervix		The lower narrow end of the uterus that opens into the vagina.
Colposcopy	*colp/o:* vagina- *scopy:* visual examination	Examination of the cervix using a colposcope (a lighted instrument with a magnifying lens).
Cytology	*cyt/o:* cell- *ology:* study of	The science that deals with the study of cells, including their origin, structure, function, and pathology.
Dilation (of the cervix)		The stretching of the external os from an opening a few millimeters wide to an opening large enough to allow the passage of an infant (approximately 10 cm).
Dysmenorrhea	*dys-:* difficult, painful, abnormal *men/o:* menstruation *-orrhea:* flow, excessive discharge	Pain associated with the menstrual period.
Dyspareunia	*dys-:* difficult, painful, abnormal	Pain in the vagina or pelvis experienced by a woman during sexual intercourse.
Dysplasia	*dys-:* difficult, painful, abnormal *plasia:* a growth	The growth of abnormal cells. Dysplasia is a precancerous condition that may or may not develop into cancer.
Ectocervix	*ecto-:* outside, outer	The outermost layer of the cervix that projects into the vagina consisting of stratified squamous epithelial cells.
Effacement		The thinning and shortening of the cervical canal from its normal length of 1–2 cm to a structure with paper-thin edges in which there is no canal at all. Effacement occurs late in pregnancy, during labor, or both. The purpose of effacement along with dilation is to permit the passage of the infant into the birth canal.
Embryo		The child in utero from the time of conception through the first 8 weeks of development.
Endocervix	*endo-:* within	The inner part of the cervix that forms a narrow canal that connects the vagina to the uterus.
Engagement		The entrance of the fetal head or the presenting part into the pelvic inlet.
Expected date of delivery (EDD)		Projected birth date of the infant.
External os		The opening of the cervical canal of the uterus into the vagina.
Fetal heart rate		The number of times per minute the fetal heart beats.
Fetal heart tones		The sounds of the heartbeat of the fetus heard through the mother's abdominal wall.
Fetus		The child in utero from the third month after conception to birth; during the first 2 months of development, it is called an *embryo.*
Fundus		The dome-shaped upper portion of the uterus between the fallopian tubes.
Gestation		The period of intrauterine development from conception to birth; the period of pregnancy. The average pregnancy lasts about 280 days, or 40 weeks, from the date of conception to childbirth.
Gestational age		The age of the fetus between conception and birth.
Gravidity	*gravid/o:* pregnancy	The total number of pregnancies a woman has had regardless of duration, including a current pregnancy.
Gynecology	*gynec/o:* woman *-ology:* study of	The branch of medicine that deals with health maintenance and diseases of the female reproductive system.
Infant		A child from birth to 12 months of age.
Internal os		The internal opening of the cervical canal into the uterus.
Lochia		A discharge from the uterus after delivery that consists of blood, tissue, white blood cells, and some bacteria.
Menopause	*men/o:* menstruation	The permanent cessation of menstruation, which usually occurs between the ages of 45 and 55.

Continued

TERMINOLOGY REVIEW—cont'd

Medical Term	Word Parts	Definition
Menorrhagia	*men/o:* menstruation *-orrhagia:* rapid flow of blood	Excessive bleeding during a menstrual period, in the number of days or the amount of blood or both. Also called *dysfunctional uterine bleeding* (DUB).
Metrorrhagia	*metr/o:* uterus *-orrhagia:* rapid flow of blood	Bleeding between menstrual periods.
Multigravida	*multi-:* many *gravid/o:* pregnancy	A woman who has been pregnant more than once.
Multipara	*multi-:* many *par/o:* bear, give birth to	A woman who has completed two or more pregnancies to the age of fetal viability regardless of whether they ended in live infants or stillbirths.
Nullipara	*nulli-:* none *par/o:* bear, give birth to	A woman who has not carried a pregnancy to the point of fetal viability (20 weeks of gestation).
Obstetrics		The branch of medicine concerned with the care of the woman during pregnancy, childbirth, and the postpartal period.
Parity	*par/o:* bear, give birth to	The condition of having born offspring regardless of the outcome.
Perimenopause	*peri-:* surrounding *men/o:* menstruation	Before the onset of menopause, the phase during which the woman with regular periods changes to irregular cycles and increased periods of amenorrhea.
Perineum		The external region between the vaginal orifice and the anus in a female and between the scrotum and the anus in a male.
Position		The relation of the presenting part of the fetus to the maternal pelvis.
Postpartum	*post-:* after *par/o:* bear, give birth to	Occurring after childbirth.
Preeclampsia		A major complication of pregnancy, the cause of which is unknown, characterized by increasing hypertension, albuminuria, and edema. If this condition is neglected or is not treated properly, it may develop into eclampsia, which could cause maternal convulsions and coma. Preeclampsia generally occurs between the 20th week of pregnancy and the end of the first week postpartum.
Prenatal	*pre-:* in front of, before *nat/o:* birth *-al:* pertaining to	Before birth.
Presentation		Indication of the part of the fetus that is closest to the cervix and is delivered first. A cephalic presentation is a delivery in which the fetal head is presenting against the cervix. A breech presentation is a delivery in which the buttocks or feet are presented instead of the head.
Preterm birth	*pre:* in front of, before	Delivery occurring between 20 and 37 weeks of gestation regardless of whether the child was born alive or stillborn.
Primigravida	*prim/i:* first *gravid/o:* pregnancy	A woman who is pregnant for the first time.
Primipara	*prim/i:* first *par/o:* bear, give birth to	A woman who has carried a pregnancy to fetal viability (20 weeks of gestation) for the first time regardless of whether the infant was stillborn or alive at birth.
Puerperium		The period of time, usually 4 to 6 weeks after delivery, in which the uterus and the body systems are returning to normal.
Quickening		The first movements of the fetus in utero as felt by the mother, which usually occur between 16 and 20 weeks of gestation and are felt consistently thereafter.
Risk factor		Anything that increases an individual's chance of developing a disease. Some risk factors (e.g., smoking) can be avoided, but others cannot (e.g., age and family history).
Term birth		Delivery occurring after 37 weeks of gestation regardless of whether the infant was born alive or stillborn.
Toxemia		A condition that can occur in pregnant women that includes preeclampsia and eclampsia. If preeclampsia goes undiagnosed or is not satisfactorily controlled, it could develop into eclampsia, characterized by convulsions and coma.
Trimester	*tri-:* three	Three months, or one third, of the gestational period of pregnancy.
Vulva		The region of the external female genital organs.

PROCEDURE 8.1 Breast Self-Examination Instructions

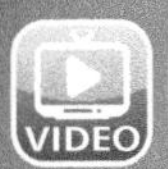

Outcome Instruct a patient in the procedure for performing a breast self-examination.

Equipment/Supplies

- Small pillow

1. **Procedural Step.** Greet the patient and introduce yourself. Identify the patient and inform the patient that you will be showing her how to perform a breast self-examination. Discuss with her the purpose of a breast self-examination (see the *Patient Coaching* box on Breast Self-Examination).
2. **Procedural Step.** Explain to the patient that a complete breast self-examination should be performed in three ways—before a mirror, lying down, and in the shower.
   Principle. Using three methods results in a thorough examination, making it more likely that breast changes will be detected.

Instruct the patient in the procedure for performing a breast self-examination as follows:

Before a Mirror

3. **Procedural Step.** Remove clothing from the waist up. Stand in front of a large mirror with your arms relaxed at your sides. Observe each breast for the following and, if present, report them to your provider
   a. Change in size or shape
   b. Swelling, puckering, or dimpling of the skin
   c. Change in skin texture
   d. Retraction of the nipple
   e. Changes in size or position of one nipple compared with the other
   Principle. Puckering and dimpling of the skin or retraction of the nipple may mean that a tumor is pulling the skin inward.
4. **Procedural Step.** Slowly raise your arms over your head, and repeat the same inspection listed in step 3.
   Principle. When the arms are moved at the same time into the same positions, both breasts and nipples should react to the movement in the same way. A change in one breast (e.g., dimpling or puckering of the skin) and not the other should be reported to your provider.

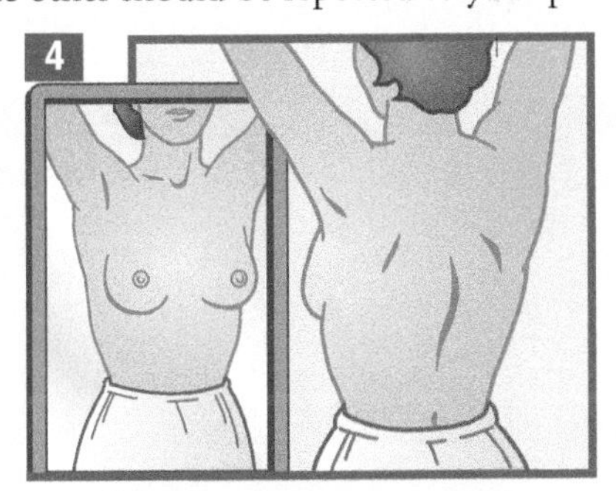

Raise your arms over your head.

5. **Procedural Step.** Rest your palms on your hips and press down firmly to flex your chest muscles. Repeat the inspection in step 3.
   Principle. Flexing the chest muscles allows abnormalities to become more apparent.

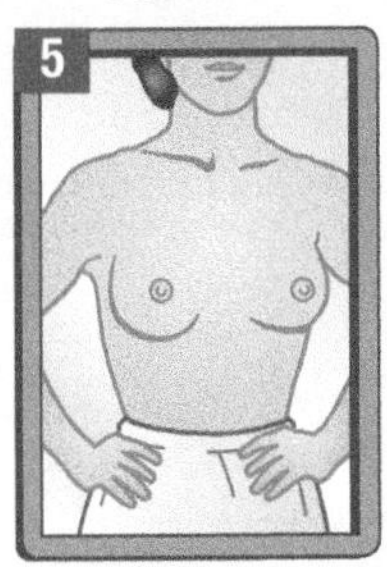

Press down firmly to flex the chest muscles.

6. **Procedural Step.** Gently squeeze the nipple of each breast with your fingertips and look for a discharge.

Lying Down

7. **Procedural Step.** To examine the right breast, lie on your back and place a small pillow (or folded towel) under your right shoulder. Place your right hand behind your head.
   Principle. The purpose of this step is to flatten the breast and distribute the breast tissue more evenly on the chest, making it easier to palpate the breast tissue.
8. **Procedural Step.** Extend your left hand with the fingers held flat. The pads of the middle three fingers of the left hand are used to perform the examination. The finger pads include the top third of each finger. Do not use the tips of the fingers. Use small rotating motions (about the size of a dime) and continuous firm pressure with the finger pads.
   Principle. The finger pads are more sensitive than the fingertips, making it easier to detect an abnormality.

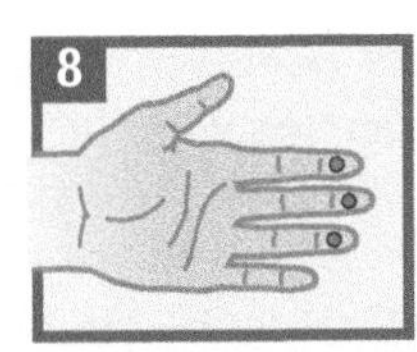

Use the pads of the middle three fingers.

9. **Procedural Step.** Use one of the following patterns to move around the breast: circular, vertical strip, or wedge. Choose the pattern that is easiest for you. When

Continued

PROCEDURE 8.1 Breast Self-Examination Instructions—cont'd

you have chosen a pattern, use the same pattern each time you examine your breasts.

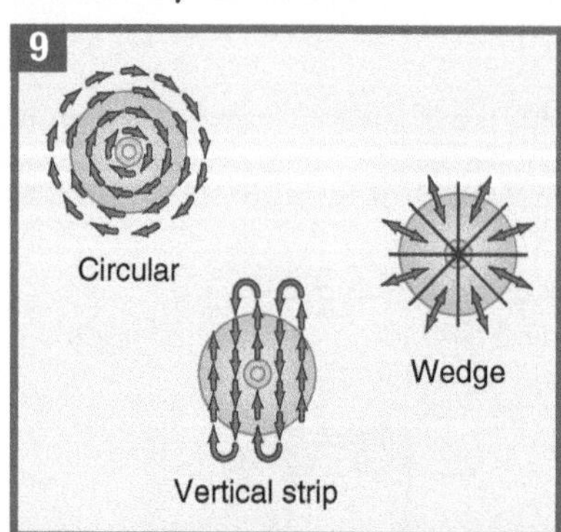

Use one of three patterns to examine the breasts.

Circular

a. Visualize the breast as a clock face.
b. Start at the outside top edge of the breast.
c. Proceed clockwise around the entire outer rim of the breast until your fingers return to the starting point.
d. Move in about 1 inch toward the nipple, and make the same circling motion again.
e. Move around the breast in smaller and smaller circles until you reach the nipple.

Vertical Strip

a. Mentally divide the breast into strips.
b. Start in the underarm area and slowly move your fingers downward until they are below the breast.
c. Move your fingers about 1 inch toward the middle, and slowly move back up.
d. Repeat until the entire breast has been examined.

Wedge

a. Mentally divide your breast into wedges, similar to the pieces of a pie.
b. Starting at the outer edge of the breast, move your fingers toward the nipple and back to the edge of the breast.
c. Check your entire breast, covering one small wedge-shaped section at a time.

Principle. Using a specific pattern ensures that the entire breast is examined.

10. Procedural Step. Holding the middle three fingers of your hand together with the thumb extended, use your finger pads and the pattern you selected to examine the right breast thoroughly. Press firmly enough to feel the different breast tissues. The breast should be palpated for lumps, hard knots, and thickening. Breast tissue normally feels a little lumpy and uneven.

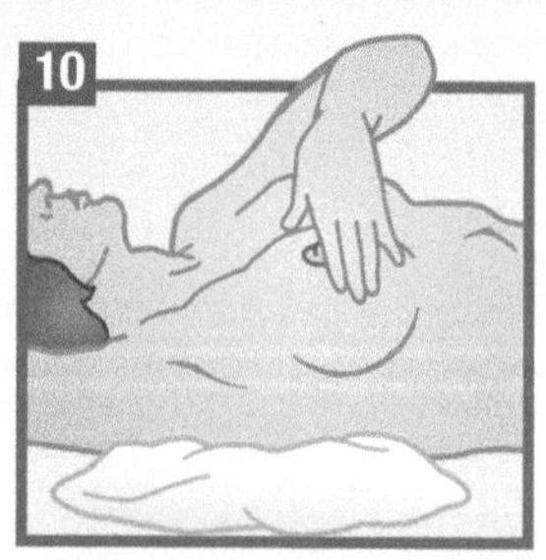

Examine the right breast.

11. Procedural Step. Examine the entire chest area from your collarbone to the base of a properly fitted bra and from the breastbone to the underarm. Pay special attention to the area between the breast and the underarm, including the underarm itself. A ridge of firm tissue in the lower curve of the breast is normal. Continue the examination until every part of the breast has been examined, including the nipple.

Principle. An enlarged node in the armpit also can be a sign of breast cancer even if nothing can be felt in the breast.

12. Procedural Step. Repeat this procedure on the left breast. Place a small pillow (or folded towel) under the left shoulder, and place your left hand behind your head. Use the finger pads of the right hand to examine the left breast.

In the Shower

13. Procedural Step. Gently lather each breast.

Principle. Fingers glide easily over wet, soapy skin, making it easier to detect changes in the breast.

14. Procedural Step. Place your right hand behind your head. Extend your left hand with the fingers held flat. With the finger pads of the middle three fingers, use small rotating motions (about the size of a dime) and continuous firm pressure with the finger pads to examine the right breast. Use your preferred pattern (circular, vertical strip, or wedge) to palpate for lumps, hard knots, and thickening. Examine the area between the breast and the underarm, including the underarm itself.

Principle. The upright position makes it easier to examine the upper and outer portions of the breast.

15. Procedural Step. Repeat the procedure on the left breast. Place the left arm behind the head, and use the right fingers to examine the left breast.

PROCEDURE 8.1 Breast Self-Examination Instructions—cont'd

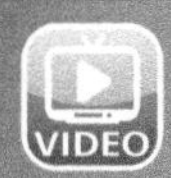

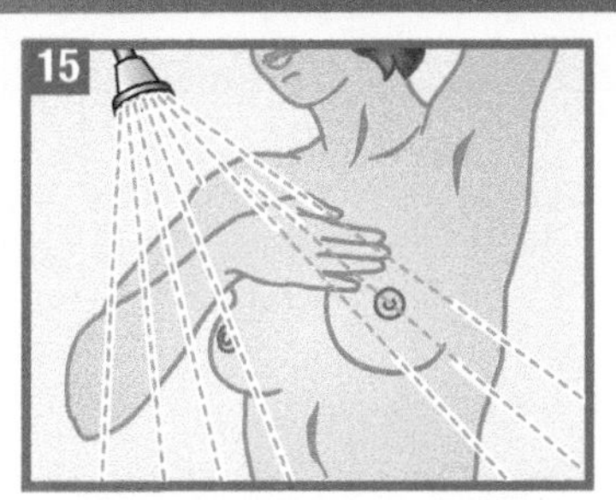
Examine the breasts in the shower.

16. **Procedural Step.** Instruct the patient to report lumps and other changes to the provider immediately. Reassure the patient that most breast lumps are not cancerous, but the only way to know for sure is to see the provider as soon as possible.
17. **Procedural Step.** Document the procedure in the patient's medical record.
    a. *Electronic health record (EHR):* Using an EHR such as SimChart for the Medical Office, document the type of instructions given to the patient using the appropriate radio buttons, drop-down menus, and free text fields. If you gave a printed instruction sheet or educational brochure to the patient, document this as well.
    b. *Paper-based patient record:* Document the date and time and the type of instructions given to the patient. If you gave a printed instruction sheet or educational brochure to the patient, document this as well (refer to the PPR documentation example).

PPR Documentation Example

Date	
9/7/XX	11:00 a.m. Instructions provided for a
	BSE. Pt given a BSE educational brochure.
	——————————— Y. Wu, RMA

Procedure 8.2

PROCEDURE 8.2 Assisting with a Gynecologic Examination

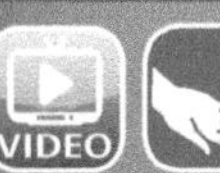
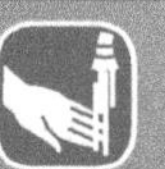

Outcome Assist with a gynecologic examination. The following procedure describes the medical assistant's role in assisting with a gynecologic examination consisting of breast and pelvic examinations, including a liquid-based Pap test and a fecal occult blood test.

Equipment/Supplies

- Disposable gloves
- Examining gown and drape
- Disposable vaginal speculum
- Vial with preservative (ThinPrep, SurePath)
- Plastic cytospatula and cytobrush or cytobroom
- Water-based lubricant
- Gauze pads
- Fecal occult blood test
- Tissues
- Cytology request form
- Biohazard specimen transport bag

1. **Procedural Step.** Sanitize your hands.
2. **Procedural Step.** Assemble the equipment. Complete as much of the cytology request form as possible. Some information on the form, such as the last menstrual period (LMP), requires input from the patient and must be completed later.

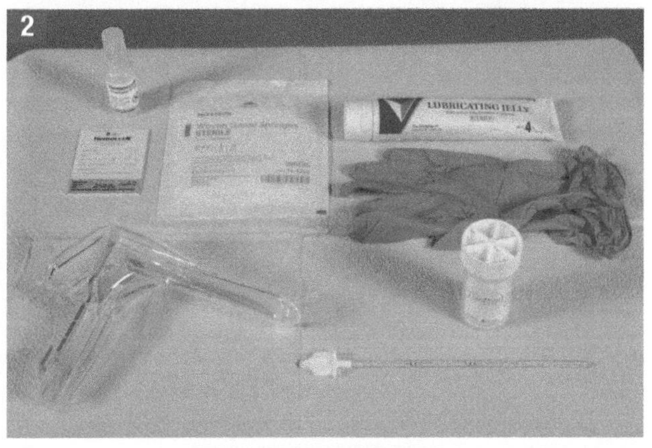

Assemble the equipment.

Continued

PROCEDURE 8.2 Assisting with a Gynecologic Examination—cont'd

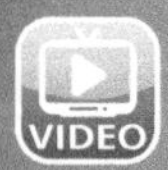

3. **Procedural Step.** Check the expiration date on the specimen vial. Label the vial with the date and the patient's name, date of birth, and identification number. The identification number is located on the cytology request form.
   Principle. If the vial is outdated, it should be discarded because it may lead to inaccurate test results.
4. **Procedural Step.** Greet the patient and introduce yourself.
5. **Procedural Step.** Escort the patient to the examining room and ask her to be seated. Identify the patient. Seat yourself so that you are facing the patient. Ask the patient whether she has any problems or concerns, and document this information in the patient's medical record. Ask the patient the necessary questions to complete the rest of the cytology request form.
6. **Procedural Step.** Measure the patient's vital signs, height, and weight, and document the results in the patient's medical record.
7. **Procedural Step.** Instruct and prepare the patient for the examination as follows:
   a. Ask the patient whether she needs to empty the bladder before the examination. If a urine specimen is needed, instruct the patient in the proper collection of the specimen.
   b. Provide the patient with a patient gown. Instruct the patient to remove all clothing and to put on the patient gown with the opening in front. If the patient is wearing socks, tell her she can keep them on. Offer assistance if you sense the patient may have trouble undressing.
   c. Tell the patient to have a seat on the examining table after she has put on the examining gown.
   d. Leave the room to give her privacy.

   Principle. An empty bladder makes the examination easier and is more comfortable for the patient. Wearing socks helps keep the patient's feet warm during the examination.

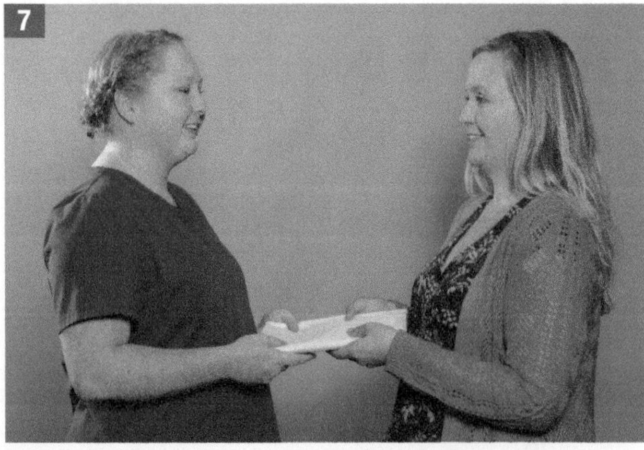

Instruct and prepare the patient for the examination.

8. **Procedural Step.** Make the medical record available for review by the provider. The medical office has a designated location where the record is placed, such as a small shelf mounted on the wall next to the outside of the examining room door or a chart holder on the outside of the examining room door. Position the medical record so that patient-identifiable information is not visible. If your office uses an electronic health record (EHR), you do not need to perform this step. With an EHR, the provider accesses the patient's record on the computer.
   Principle. The provider will want to review the patient's measurements and urine test results documented by the medical assistant. The Health Insurance Portability and Accountability Act (HIPAA) requires protection of a patient's health information.
9. **Procedural Step.** Check to make sure the patient is ready to be seen by the provider. Before entering the room, always knock lightly on the door to let the patient know you are getting ready to enter the room. Inform the provider that the patient is ready. This may be done using a color-coded flagging system mounted on the wall next to the examining room.
10. **Procedural Step.** Assist the patient into a supine position, and properly drape her for the breast examination.
11. **Procedural Step.** Assist the patient into the lithotomy position for the pelvic examination.
12. **Procedural Step.** Prepare the vaginal speculum by thinly lubricating the blades of the speculum with a water-based lubricant. Never apply lubricant to the tip of the speculum.
    Principle. Lubricating the vaginal speculum facilitates its insertion into the vagina.
13. **Procedural Step.** Prepare the light for the provider as follows:
    a. *Overhead examination lamp:* Adjust and focus the light for the provider.
    b. *Speculum-illumination system:* Snap the light source device into the light holder on the vaginal speculum and turn it on. The lighting system produces a beam of light that shines through the blades of the speculum for visualization of the vagina and cervix.

    Principle. Visualization of the vagina and cervix requires direct light.
14. **Procedural Step.** Hand the vaginal speculum to the provider. Reassure the patient, and help her relax the abdominal muscles during the examination by telling her to breathe deeply, slowly, and evenly through the mouth.

Continued

PROCEDURE 8.2 Assisting with a Gynecologic Examination—cont'd

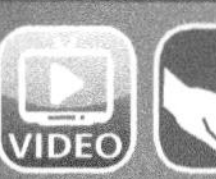

Principle. If the patient is relaxed, the examination proceeds more smoothly and is more comfortable for her.

15. Procedural Step. Apply gloves, and assist with the collection of the Pap specimen as follows:

ThinPrep

Cytospatula and Cytobrush Method

(1) Remove the cap from the ThinPrep vial, and hold it so that the provider can insert the cytospatula into the vial.

(2) Rinse the plastic cytospatula in the liquid preservative by vigorously swirling it around in the solution 10 times.

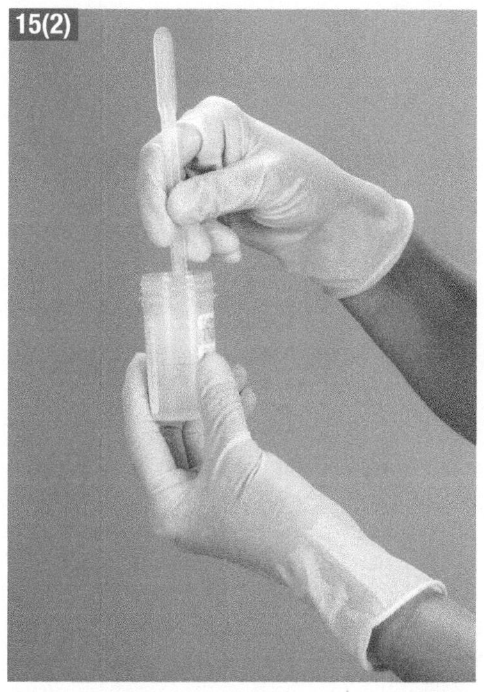

Vigorously swirl the cytospatula in the preservative.

(3) Discard the cytospatula in a biohazard waste container.

(4) Hold the vial so that the provider can insert the cytobrush into the vial.

(5) Rinse the cytobrush in the liquid preservative by vigorously rotating it in the solution 10 times while pushing the cytobrush against the vial wall. Swirl the cytobrush in the solution to further release cellular material.

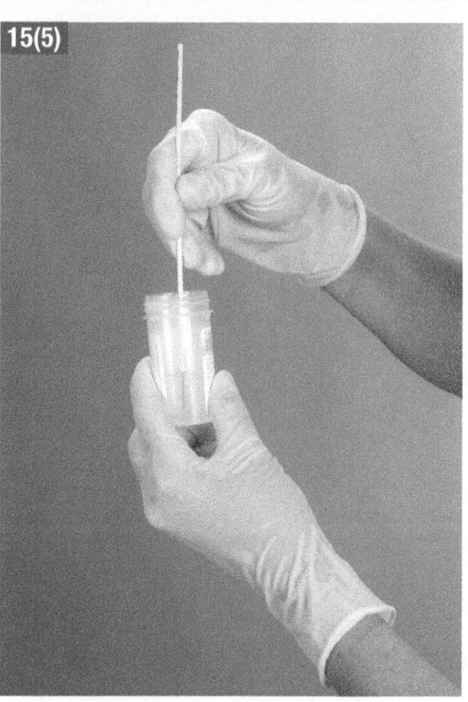

Rotate the cytobrush in the preservative.

(6) Discard the cytobrush in a biohazard waste container. Securely tighten the cap so that the torque line on the cap passes the torque line on the vial.

Cytobroom Method

(1) Remove the cap from the ThinPrep vial, and hold it so that the provider can insert the cytobroom into the vial.

(2) Rinse the cytobroom in the liquid preservative by pushing the cytobroom vigorously into the bottom of the vial 10 times. This motion forces the cytobroom bristles apart, releasing cervical cells into the solution. Swirl the cytobroom vigorously in the liquid preservative to further release cellular material.

Continued

PROCEDURE 8.2 Assisting with a Gynecologic Examination—cont'd

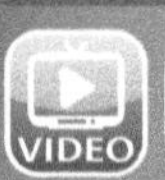

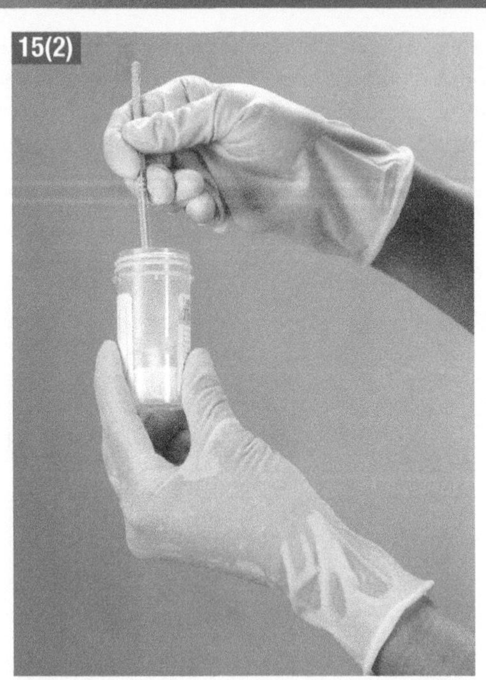

Push the cytobroom vigorously into the bottom of the vial.

(3) Discard the cytobroom in a biohazard waste container. Tighten the cap so that the torque line on the cap passes the torque line on the vial.

SurePath

(1) Remove the cap from the SurePath vial, and hold it so that the provider can insert the collection device into the vial.
(2) Break off (cytospatula and cytobrush method) or disconnect the tip (cytobroom method) of the collection device from the handle.
(3) Discard the handle of the collection device in a waste container.
(4) Repeat the above steps until the provider has collected all of the specimens needed for the Pap test.
(5) Securely tighten the cap on the vial.

16. **Procedural Step.** Turn off the examining lamp or disconnect the light source from the vaginal speculum. Discard the disposable vaginal speculum in a biohazard waste container. Apply lubricant to a gauze square. Hold it out so that the provider can apply lubricant to his or her gloves to perform the bimanual and rectal-vaginal examinations. Assist with the collection of the fecal specimen for the fecal occult blood test.

Principle. Applying lubricant to a gauze square (rather than directly to the provider's gloved fingers) prevents the opening of the tube of lubricant from touching the provider's gloves and contaminating the contents of the tube.

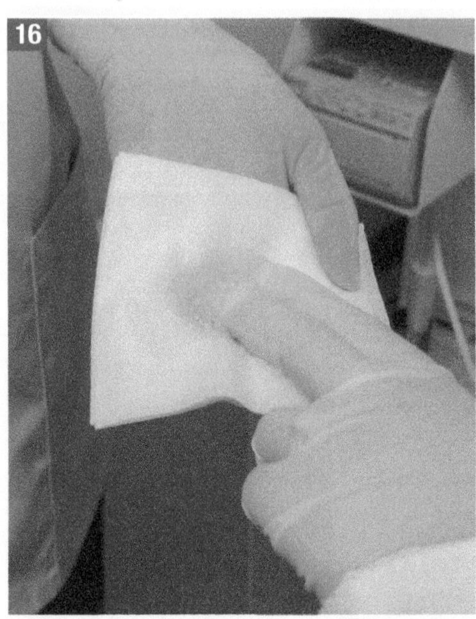

Hold the gauze with the lubricant for the provider.

17. **Procedural Step.** After the examination, assist the patient into a sitting position, and allow her the opportunity to rest for a moment. Offer the patient tissues to remove excess lubricant from the perineum. Assist the patient off the examining table.
Principle. Some patients (especially the elderly) become dizzy after lying on the examining table and should be allowed to rest after sitting up.
18. **Procedural Step.** Instruct the patient to get dressed. Tell the patient how and when she will be notified of the Pap test results.
19. **Procedural Step.** Test the fecal occult blood specimen, and document the results in the patient's medical record.
20. **Procedural Step.** Prepare the Pap specimen for transport to the laboratory. Place the vial in a biohazard specimen transport bag and seal the bag. Insert the cytology requisition into the outside pocket of the bag and tuck the top of the requisition under the flap. Place the bag in the appropriate location for pickup by the laboratory.

PROCEDURE 8.2 Assisting with a Gynecologic Examination—cont'd

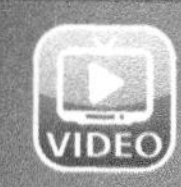
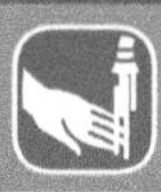

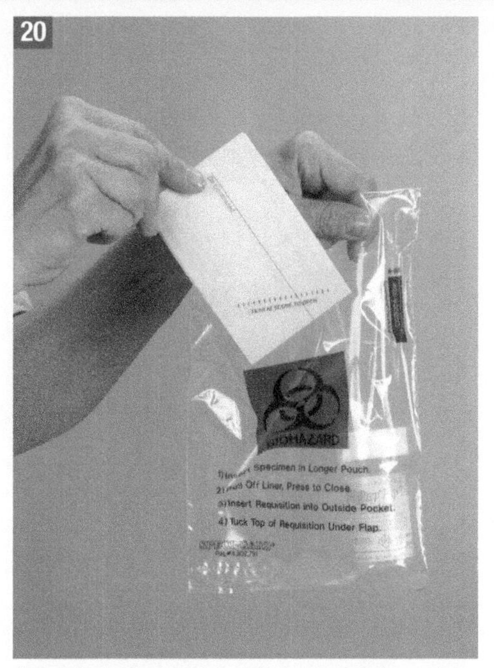

Insert the laboratory request into the outside pocket.

21. **Procedural Step.** Document the transport of the Pap specimen to an outside laboratory in the patient's medical record.
22. **Procedural Step.** Clean the examining room.

PPR Documentation Example

Date	
9/7/XX	10:00 a.m. Hemoccult: negative.
	Instructions provided for BSE. ThinPrep
	Pap specimen to Medical Center Laboratory
	for cytology. ———————Y. Wu, RMA

PROCEDURE 8.3 Assisting with a Return Prenatal Examination

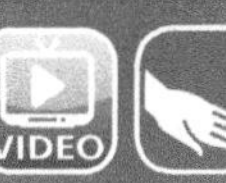

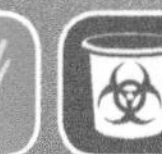
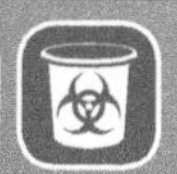

Outcome Assist with a return prenatal examination.

Equipment/Supplies

- Urine specimen container
- Centimeter tape measure
- Doppler fetal pulse detector
- Ultrasound coupling gel
- Paper towel
- Disposable vaginal speculum
- Disposable gloves
- Water-based lubricant
- Gauze pads
- Examining gown and drape

1. **Procedural Step.** Sanitize your hands.
2. **Procedural Step.** Set up the tray for the prenatal examination. The equipment and supplies depend on the procedures to be included in the examination, which may include one or more of the following:
   a. Fundal height measurement
   b. Measurement of fetal heart tones
   c. Examination of the legs, feet, and face for edema and development of varicosities
   d. Taking a specimen for the diagnosis of a vaginal infection
   e. Vaginal examination

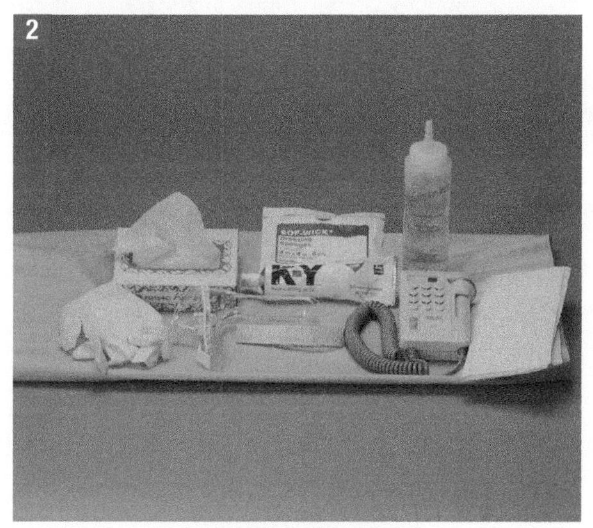

Set up the prenatal tray.

Continued

PROCEDURE 8.3 Assisting with a Return Prenatal Examination—cont'd

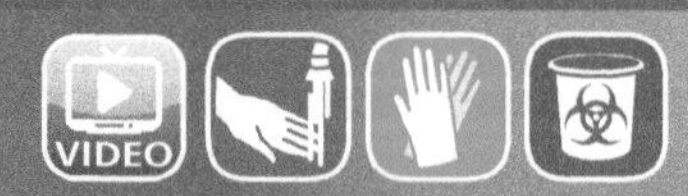

3. **Procedural Step.** Greet the patient and introduce yourself. Identify the patient and explain the procedure. Provide the patient with a urine specimen container, and ask her to obtain a urine specimen.
   Principle. A urine specimen is needed to test for glucose and protein at each prenatal visit. In addition, an empty bladder makes the examination easier and is more comfortable for the patient.
4. **Procedural Step.** Escort the patient to the examining room, and ask her to be seated. Seat yourself so that you are facing the patient. Ask the patient whether she has experienced any problems since the last prenatal visit, and document information in the appropriate section in her prenatal record.
   Principle. The provider investigates any unusual or abnormal signs or symptoms relayed by the patient.
5. **Procedural Step.** Measure the patient's blood pressure, and document the results in the prenatal record. If the blood pressure is elevated, allow the patient to relax, and then measure the blood pressure again.
   Principle. Taking the blood pressure again gives you the opportunity to determine whether the elevation was due to emotional excitement.

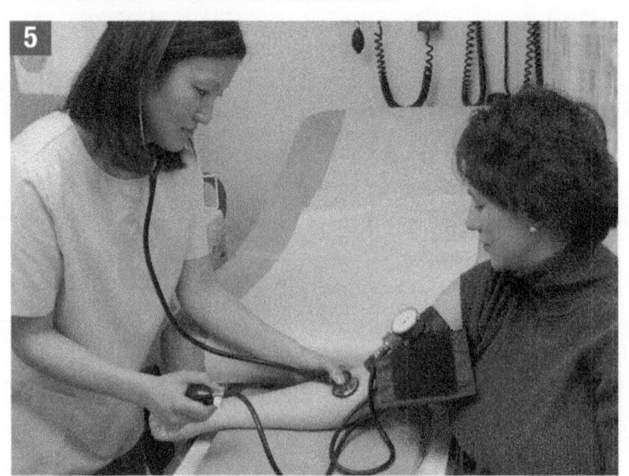

Measure the patient's blood pressure.

6. **Procedural Step.** Weigh the patient, and document the results in the prenatal record.
   Principle. Maternal weight gain or loss assists in assessing fetal development, as well as the mother's nutrition and state of health.

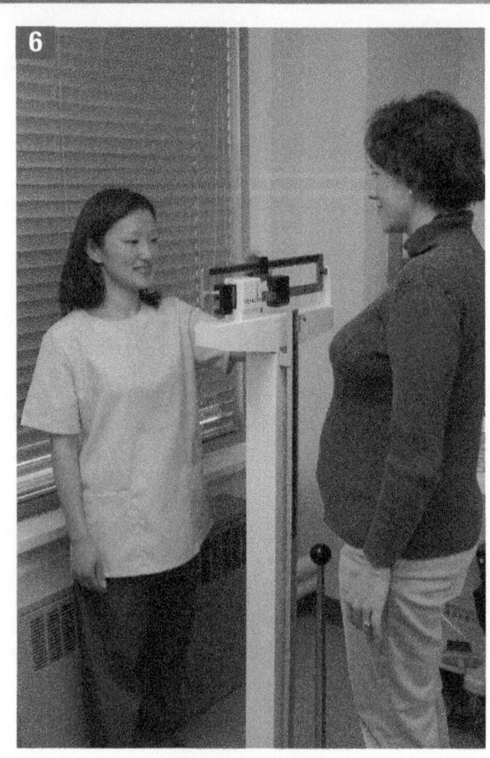

Weigh the patient.

7. **Procedural Step.** Instruct and prepare the patient for the examination. Have her remove or pull up her outer clothing to expose the abdominal area. If the provider will be performing a vaginal examination, the patient also must remove her panties; otherwise, she may leave them on. Tell the patient to have a seat on the examining table when she is finished getting ready for the examination. Leave the room to give her privacy.
8. **Procedural Step.** Using a reagent strip, test the urine specimen for glucose and protein, and document the results in the prenatal record. *Note:* The urine specimen may be tested at any time before the provider examines the patient; however, a convenient time to test the specimen is while the patient is disrobing.
   Principle. The prenatal patient's urine must be tested at every visit to assist in early detection and prevention of disease.
9. **Procedural Step.** Make the medical record available for review by the provider. The medical office has a designated location where the record is placed, such as a small shelf mounted on the wall next to the outside of the examining room door or in a chart holder on the outside of the examining room door. Position the medical record so that patient-identifiable information is not visible. If your office uses an EHR, you

Continued

PROCEDURE 8.3 Assisting with a Return Prenatal Examination—cont'd

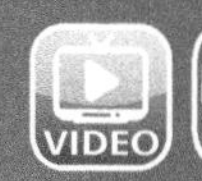
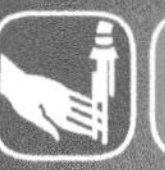
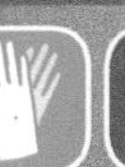

do not need to perform this step. With an EHR, the provider accesses the patient's record on the computer.

Principle. The provider will want to review the patient's medical record and information documented by the medical assistant. HIPAA requires protection of a patient's health information.

10. **Procedural Step.** Check to make sure the patient is ready to be seen by the provider. Before entering a patient's room, always knock lightly on the door to let the patient know you are getting ready to enter the room. Inform the provider. This may be done using a color-coded flagging system mounted on the wall next to the examining room.
11. **Procedural Step.** Assist the patient into a supine position, and properly drape her. Provide support and reassurance to the patient to help her relax during the examination.

    Principle. The patient should be properly draped so that she is warm and comfortable.
12. **Procedural Step.** Assist the provider as required for the prenatal examination, as follows:
    a. Fundal height measurement: Hand the provider the tape measure for determination of the fundal measurement.
    b. *Fetal heart tones:* Apply a liberal amount of coupling gel to the patient's abdomen. Turn on the Doppler fetal pulse detector and hand it to the provider. When the provider is finished, remove excess gel from the patient with a paper towel. Clean the probe head of the Doppler device with a damp cloth or a paper towel. Place the probe head back in its holder.

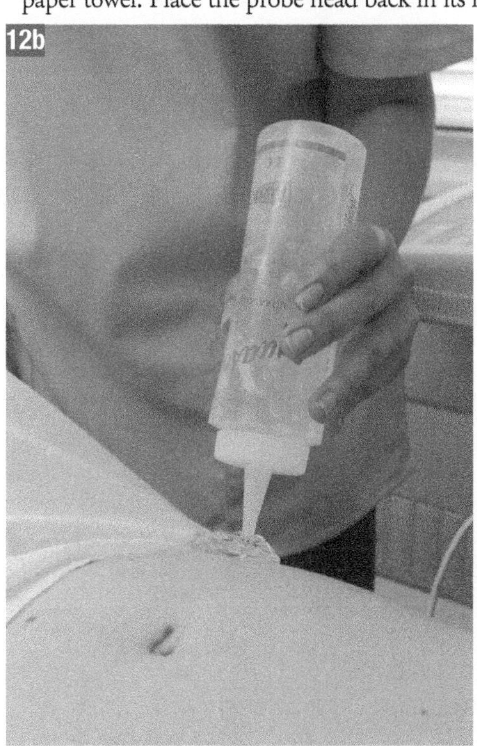

Apply a liberal amount of coupling gel.

    c. *Vaginal specimen:* Assist the patient into the lithotomy position if a specimen is to be taken for the detection of a vaginal infection. Assist with collection of the specimen as required.
    d. *Vaginal examination:* Assist the patient into the lithotomy position if a vaginal examination is to be performed.
13. **Procedural Step.** After the examination, assist the patient into a sitting position, and allow her the opportunity to rest for a moment. If a vaginal examination was performed, offer the patient tissues to remove excess lubricating jelly from the perineum. Assist her off the examining table to prevent falls. Instruct the patient to get dressed. Leave the room to provide the patient with privacy.

    Principle. The patient may become dizzy after being on the examining table and should be allowed to rest before getting off the table. The medical assistant must provide for the safety of the prenatal patient while she is getting off the examining table.

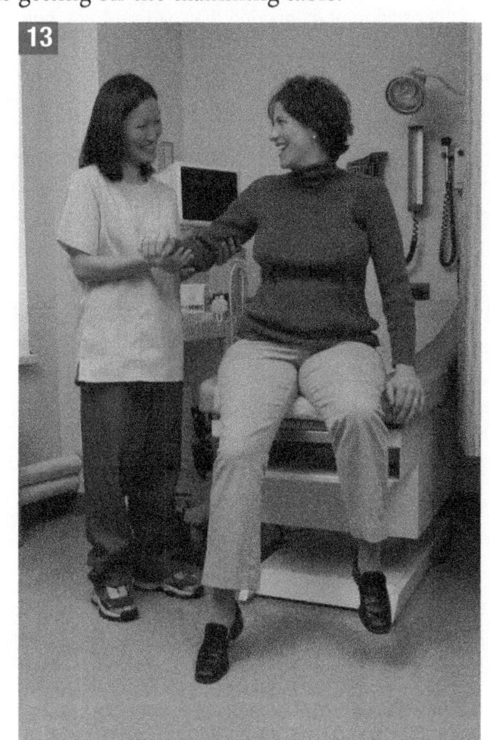

Assist the patient off the examining table.

14. **Procedural Step.** Provide the prenatal patient teaching and further explanation of the provider's instructions as required to meet individual patient needs. Escort the patient to the reception area.
15. **Procedural Step.** Clean the examining room in preparation for the next patient, and, if necessary, prepare specimens for transport to an outside medical laboratory.

The Pediatric Examination

 Check out the Evolve site at http://evolve.elsevier.com/Bonewit/today/ to access additional interactive activities and exercises to help you study and prepare for success.

LEARNING OUTCOMES

Pediatric Office Visits

1. List the components of the well-child visit.
2. State the usual schedule for well-child visits.
3. Explain the purpose of the sick-child visit.
4. List the procedures performed by the medical assistant during pediatric office visits.
5. Explain why it is important to develop a rapport with the pediatric patient.

Growth Measurements

6. State the importance of measuring the child's weight, height (or length), and head circumference during each office visit.
7. State the functions served by a growth chart.

Pediatric Blood Pressure Measurement

8. State the importance of measuring a child's blood pressure.
9. List the three factors that determine whether a child has hypertension.

Collection of a Urine Specimen

10. List the reasons for collecting a urine specimen from a child.

Pediatric Injections

11. State the range for the gauge and length of needles used for intramuscular and subcutaneous pediatric injections.
12. Explain the use of each of the following pediatric injection sites: vastus lateralis and deltoid.

Immunizations

13. Describe the schedule for immunization of infants and children recommended by the American Academy of Pediatrics.
14. State the information that must be provided to parents as required by the National Childhood Vaccine Injury Act.
15. List the information that must be documented in the medical record after administering an immunization.

Newborn Screening Test

16. Explain the purpose of a newborn screening test.
17. List the symptoms of phenylketonuria.
18. State what occurs if phenylketonuria is left untreated.

PROCEDURES

Carry an infant using the following positions:
1. Cradle
2. Upright

Measure the weight and length of an infant.
Measure the head and chest circumference of an infant.

Measure the blood pressure of a child.
Plot pediatric growth values on a growth chart.

Collect a urine specimen using a pediatric urine collector.

Locate the following pediatric intramuscular injection sites:
3. Vastus lateralis
4. Deltoid

Administer an intramuscular injection to an infant.
Administer a subcutaneous injection to an infant.

Read and interpret a vaccine information statement.
Document information on an immunization administration record.

Collect a specimen for a newborn screening test.

CHAPTER OUTLINE

KEY TERMS

adolescent
immunity (ih-MYOO-nih-tee)
immunization (IM-yoo-nih-ZAY-shun)
infant
length
pediatrician (PEE-dee-uh-TRIH-shun)
pediatrics (pee-dee-AT-riks)
preschool (PREE-skool) child
school-age child
toddler (TOD-ler)
toxoid (TOKS-oid)
vaccine (vak-SEEN)
vertex (VER-teks)

Introduction to the Pediatric Examination

Pediatrics is the branch of medicine that deals with the care and development of children, and the diagnosis and treatment of diseases in children. A **pediatrician** is a physician who specializes in pediatrics. Many physicians in general practice accept pediatric patients. It is essential that the medical assistant develop the skills needed to assist the physician in the care and treatment of children.

Pediatric Office Visits

There are two broad categories of pediatric patient office visits. The first is the *well-child visit* (also termed *health maintenance visit*), in which the physician progressively evaluates the growth and development of the child. A patient history update and physical examination are performed during each well-child visit, and are directed toward discovering any abnormal conditions commonly associated with the stage of development reached by the child. Table 9.1 provides an outline of normal development during infancy. The child also receives necessary immunizations during these visits.

The interval between well-child visits depends on the medical office, but it frequently follows this schedule after birth: 3 to 5 days, 1 month, 2 months, 4 months, 6 months, 9 months, 12 months, 15 months, 18 months, 24 months, 2½ years, 3 years, 4 years, and once a year thereafter.

The second category of pediatric patient office visits is the *sick-child visit.* The child is exhibiting the signs and symptoms of a disease, and the physician evaluates the patient's condition to arrive at a diagnosis and to prescribe a treatment.

During well-child and sick-child visits, the medical assistant performs many of the same procedures that have been presented in previous and subsequent chapters (e.g., measurement of temperature, pulse, respiration, and blood pressure; measurement of weight and height; measurement of visual and hearing acuity; assisting with the physical examination; administration of medication; collection of specimens). This chapter discusses procedures specifically related to the pediatric patient, and the variations of the procedures previously mentioned.

What Would You Do? What Would You *Not* Do?

Case Study 1

My-Lai Chang comes into the office with Christopher Chang, her 1-month-old son. Christopher is here for his 1-month well-child visit. Mrs. Chang is distraught and says that Christopher has episodes of nonstop crying every day that last 2 to 3 h at a time. She is breastfeeding Christopher and says that the crying is worse after he nurses. Mrs. Chang realizes that Christopher has colic and feels guilty because it seems "her milk" is making it worse. She is also having problems with sore nipples and engorgement. She really wanted to breastfeed Christopher, but she is thinking of stopping because it just seems too hard to do. Christopher measures in the 50th percentile for weight and length. Mrs. Chang is worried that he is not growing and thinks she may not be producing enough milk. ■

DEVELOPING A RAPPORT

The medical assistant must establish a rapport with the pediatric patient. If the medical assistant gains the child's trust and confidence, the child is likely to cooperate during an examination or procedure. Interacting with children requires special techniques. The techniques employed depend on the age of the child. **Toddlers** (1 to 3 years old) and **preschool children** (3 to 6 years old) often respond well to making a game of the procedure. Explaining the purpose of an instrument (e.g., the stethoscope) to a **school-age child** (6 to 12 years old) and allowing him or her to hold the instrument or even to help during the procedure may overcome fears in that age group (Fig. 9.1). **Adolescents** (12 to 18 years old) respond best by discussing the risks of a procedure and allowing them to have input in the decision-making process.

Table 9.1 Milestones of Gross and Fine Motor Development in Infancy

Average Age (Months)	Gross Motor	Fine Motor
1	Turns head from side to side	Grasping reflex present
2	Holds head at 45-degree angle when prone	Holds rattle briefly
3	Begins rolling over	Grasps rattle or dangling objects
4	Slight head lag when pulled to sitting position	Brings objects to mouth
5	No head wobble when held in sitting position	Transfers objects from hand to hand
6	Sits without support	Manipulates and examines large objects with hands
7	Stands while holding on	Reaches for, grabs, and retains object
8	Pulls self to stand	Grasps objects with thumb and finger
9	Crawls backward	Begins to show hand preference
10	Creeps on hands and knees	Hits cup with spoon
11	Walks using furniture for support	Picks up small objects with thumb and forefinger (pincer grasp)
12	Stands alone easily	Puts three or more objects into container
12–16	Walks alone easily	Turns two or three pages in large cardboard book

From Leahy JM, Kizilay PE: *Foundations of nursing practice,* Philadelphia: Saunders; 1998.

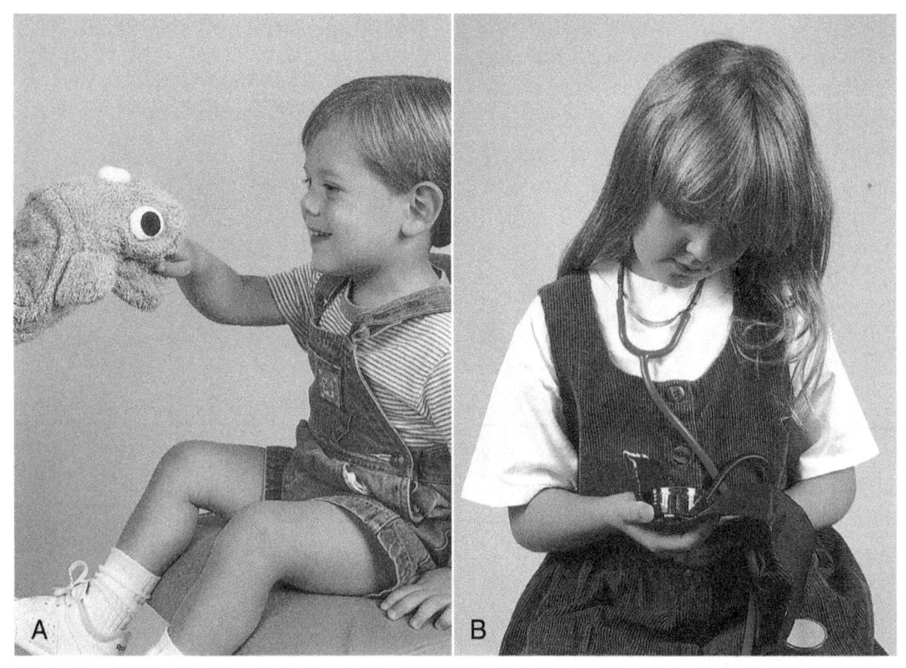

Fig. 9.1 The medical assistant should develop a rapport with children to gain their trust and cooperation. Making a game of the procedure (A) and explaining the purpose of the stethoscope and allowing the child to hold it (B) help the child overcome fears.

The medical assistant should always explain the procedure to children who are able to understand. Each child must be approached at his or her level of understanding. To do this, the medical assistant should know what to expect from a child at a particular age, in terms of motor and social development. Each child has his or her own individual rate of development; the descriptions of normal development based on age are meant to serve as a guide only, and may have to be modified to meet individual needs. In addition, it is normal for an ill child to regress to an earlier level of behavior. Table 9.2 outlines techniques that can be used with various age groups to gain their cooperation during an examination or procedure.

CARRYING THE INFANT

An **infant** is a child from birth to 12 months old. The medical assistant needs to lift and carry the infant to perform various procedures, such as measurement of length and weight. The infant should be lifted and carried in a manner that is safe and comfortable. Proper positions include the cradle and upright positions.

Table 9.2 Techniques for Interaction With Children

Technique	Infant (Birth–1 year)	Toddler (1–3 years)	Preschool (3–6 years)	School Age (6–12 years)	Adolescent (12–18 years)
Avoid sudden motion and loud or abrupt noises	•		•		
Limit number of strangers in room	•				
Use distractions, bright objects, rattles, and talking to gain cooperation	•				
Physically restrain child if necessary to ensure safety	•	•	•		
Allow physical contact with parent during procedure	•	•	•		
Encourage parent to comfort child after procedure	•	•	•		
Use play to explain procedure (e.g., dolls, puppets)		•	•		
Perform procedures quickly, if possible		•	•		
Use concrete terms, rather than abstract terms		•	•		
Avoid words that have more than one meaning (e.g., shot)		•	•		
Give child permission to cry, yell, or otherwise express pain verbally		•	•		
Praise child for cooperative behavior		•	•	•	
Allow child to handle equipment, if possible			•	•	
Make sure child understands body part to be involved			•	•	
Try to describe how procedure will feel			•	•	
Tell child about any discomfort that may be felt, but don't dwell on it			•	•	
Stress benefits of anything child may find pleasurable afterward (e.g., stickers, feeling better)			•	•	
Give child choices when possible (e.g., arm to use)			•	•	
Suggest ways to maintain control (e.g., counting, deep breathing, relaxation)			•	•	
Use drawing and diagrams to illustrate parts of body that will be involved			•	•	
Encourage participation such as holding instrument during procedure			•	•	
Include child in decision-making process				•	•
Discuss risks of procedure					•
Provide information about appearance changes that might result					•
Give child educational brochures or have him or her view videos about procedure					•
Ask parent to step out if child does not want parent in examining room					•

Cradle Position: To place an infant in a cradle position, the medical assistant slides one hand and forearm under the infant's back and grasps the infant's arm from behind. The thumb and fingers should encircle the infant's forearm. The infant's head, shoulders, and back are supported by the medical assistant's forearm. Next, the medical assistant slips the other hand and forearm up and under the infant's buttocks. The infant is cradled in the arm with his or her body resting against the medical assistant's chest (Fig. 9.2).

Upright Position: To place an infant in an upright position, the medical assistant slips one hand and forearm under the infant's head and shoulders. The fingers should be spread apart to support the infant's head and neck. The other

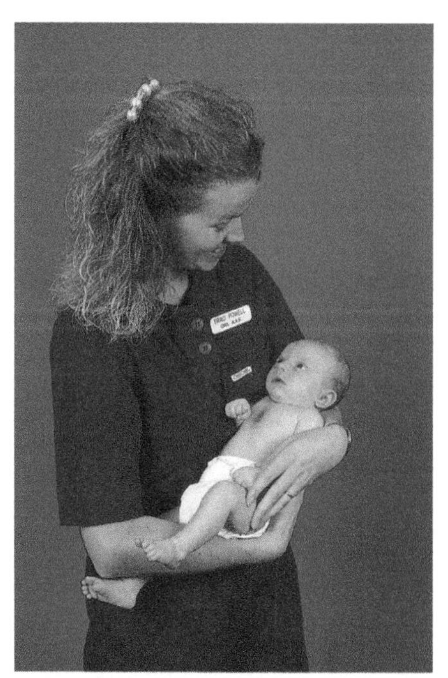

Fig. 9.2 Traci holds the infant in the cradle position.

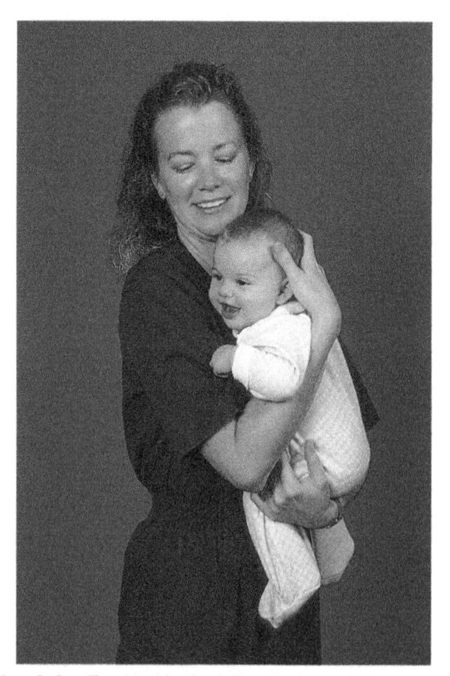

Fig. 9.3 Traci holds the infant in the upright position.

hand and forearm are slipped under the infant's buttocks to help support the infant's weight. The infant should be allowed to rest against the medical assistant's chest with the cheek resting on the medical assistant's shoulder (Fig. 9.3).

GROWTH MEASUREMENTS

One of the best methods to evaluate the progress of a child is to measure his or her growth. The weight, height (or length), and head circumference (up to age 3 years) of a child should be measured during each office visit and plotted on a growth chart.

WEIGHT

A child's weight is often used to determine nutritional needs and the proper dosage of medication to administer to the child. The medical assistant should exercise care in measuring weight. Infants are weighed in a recumbent position, as outlined in Procedure 9.1. Older children are weighed in a standing position, as presented in Chapter 5.

LENGTH AND HEIGHT

Another measure of a child's growth is **length**, or height (stature). Length is measured in children younger than 24 months. The recumbent length is a measurement from the **vertex** (top) of the head to the heel of the infant in a supine position, as outlined in Procedure 9.1. Two people are often needed to determine the length of an infant accurately. The parent's help can be requested; the medical assistant must provide the parent with thorough instructions on what needs to be done. Older children have their height measured in a standing position (Fig. 9.4), as presented in Chapter 5.

Putting It All Into Practice

My name is Traci, and I am a Certified Medical Assistant. I work in the pediatrics department of a large multispecialty clinic. My job responsibilities are mostly clinical; however, I do assist in the front office when needed. I love working with the children and have enjoyed watching them grow over the years.

A co-worker and I recently organized a local American Association of Medical Assistants (AAMA) chapter. Our chapter provides AAMA continuing education units (CEUs). Our members attend state and national conventions every year, and they hold state and national leadership positions. It is my goal to see the medical assisting profession continue to grow and advance in the health care field.

It is interesting how your education, training, and experience all come together, especially in a crisis. Early one morning when I arrived at work, a mother rushed in with a small child who was approximately 2 years old. The child was dusky in color, panicky, and having trouble breathing. Apparently, the child had gotten into some dry beans the previous night and had inhaled one into her lung. The physicians were not in the building yet, and this child was in respiratory distress. We immediately called a Code Blue, put her on oxygen, and made arrangements for an ambulance to take her to Children's Hospital, where a surgeon was waiting. All went well, and she is a healthy little girl today.

Looking back, I am grateful for a good, solid medical assisting education; a Pediatric Advance Life Support (PALS) certification; and experience in working with children so that I was able to help that child through a life-threatening experience. I firmly believe that no matter how long a person has been in the medical field or what his or her profession is, continuing education is essential to stay current in the ever-changing health care field. ■

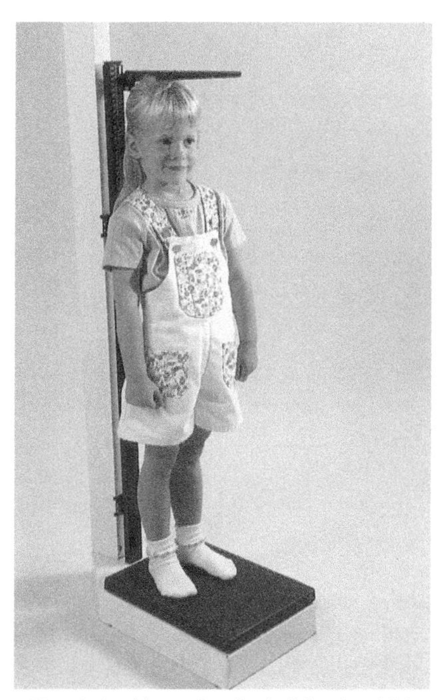

Fig. 9.4 Measuring the height of a child.

HEAD AND CHEST CIRCUMFERENCE

Infancy is a period of rapid brain growth. Because of this, the head circumference is an important measurement. The head circumference for a newborn ranges from 32 to 38 cm (12½ to 15 inches). A 10-cm (4-inch) increase in head circumference occurs within the first year of life.

The head circumference of children younger than 3 years should be routinely measured and plotted on a head circumference growth chart. Measurement of head circumference is an important screening measure for microencephaly and macroencephaly.

At birth, a newborn's head circumference is about 2 cm larger than his or her chest circumference. The chest grows at a faster rate than the cranium, and between 6 months and 2 years of age, the measurements are about the same. After age 2 years, the chest circumference is greater than the head circumference. The measurement of the chest circumference is valuable in a comparison with the head circumference, but not by itself. The chest circumference is not typically measured on a routine basis; this measurement is done only when a heart or lung abnormality is suspected. Procedure 9.2 outlines the procedure for measuring the head and chest circumference of an infant.

GROWTH CHARTS

Growth charts should be part of every child's permanent record. The National Center for Health Statistics developed growth charts to assist physicians in determining whether the growth of a child is normal. The charts can be used to identify children with growth or nutritional abnormalities. In offices with an electronic medical record, the growth percentiles are automatically calculated and plotted on a growth chart when the child's growth measurements are entered into the computer. This "electronic" growth chart is maintained in the child's electronic medical record and can be printed out if needed. In some offices, the medical assistant may be responsible for manually plotting the child's measurements on a preprinted growth chart (Procedure 9.3).

Growth charts provide a means of comparing a child's weight and length (or height) with those of other children of the same age. For example, the medical assistant calculates the growth percentile of an 18-month-old boy and finds that he is in the 25th percentile for weight and the 80th percentile for length. This means that 75% of 18-month-old boys weigh more than he does, and 25% weigh less than he does. It also means that 20% of 18-month-old boys are taller, and 80% are shorter. Although comparing a child with other children of the same age is one use of growth charts (particularly by parents), it is not the most important use.

The primary use of growth charts is to look at the child's growth pattern. If a child has always hovered around a certain percentile in height and weight, there is no need for concern. If a child is in the 20th percentile for weight but has always been in this percentile, he is likely growing normally. It would be more of a concern if the child had been in the 75th percentile and dropped to the 40th percentile. The physician investigates any significant change or rapid increase or decrease in a child's growth pattern.

HIGHLIGHT on Childhood Obesity

Statistics

An epidemic of childhood obesity is occurring in the United States and has become a serious public health problem. Childhood obesity occurs when a child consumes more calories than the body can burn. Approximately 31% of Americans under the age of 20 are overweight or obese. A child is considered overweight if his or her weight falls in the 85th to 95th percentile for age, gender, and height on the National Center for Health Statistics growth charts. When a child's weight exceeds the 95th percentile for age, gender, and height, he or she is considered obese.

Causes

The primary causes of childhood obesity are overeating and inadequate exercise. Other causes include the following:

1. Family history of obesity
2. Medical illnesses (e.g., endocrine or neurological problems)
3. Medications (e.g., steroids, certain psychiatric medications)
4. Stressful life events (e.g., divorce, moves, deaths, abuse)
5. Family and peer problems
6. Low self-esteem
7. Depression or other emotional problems

Continued

HIGHLIGHT on Childhood Obesity—cont'd

Related Problems

Problems associated with childhood obesity include high blood pressure, elevated blood cholesterol levels, type 2 diabetes, orthopedic problems caused by increased stress on weight-bearing joints, skin disorders (e.g., dermatitis), sleep apnea, low self-esteem, social isolation, and feelings of rejection and depression. Some authorities believe that the social and psychological problems are the most significant consequences of childhood obesity.

Prevention

The risk of obesity tends to be greater among children who have obese parents. After age 3, the likelihood that obesity will persist into adulthood increases as an obese child gets older. When an obese child reaches age 6, the probability is more than 50% that obesity will persist into adulthood. Among obese adolescents, 70% to 80% remain obese as adults.

It is much easier to prevent childhood obesity than to treat it after it has occurred. Authorities believe that the primary focus should be on educating parents about the problems associated with childhood obesity and helping them employ preventive measures. Preventing obesity in childhood is critical because habits formed during childhood frequently carry into adulthood. Guidelines for preventing childhood obesity include the following:

1. Provide a healthy diet with a focus on fruits and vegetables
2. Avoid oversized portions
3. Encourage active play
4. Promote healthy snacks
5. Do not use food for reward, comfort, or bribes
6. Limit television, video, and computer time
7. Limit the amount of "junk" food kept in the home
8. Do not make the child eat when he or she is not hungry
9. Do not offer dessert as a reward for finishing a meal
10. Encourage the child to drink water instead of sweet beverages
11. Do not frequently eat at fast-food restaurants

Treatment

The treatment of childhood obesity is difficult, and the success rate is not particularly high. Children seem to be most successful at losing weight and keeping it off when the entire family is involved. Parents should eat healthy meals and snacks with their children. The most successful diets are those that use ordinary foods in controlled portions, rather than diets that require the avoidance of specific foods. Parents also should spend time being active with their children. Activities should stress self-improvement rather than competition. ■

PEDIATRIC BLOOD PRESSURE MEASUREMENT

The American Academy of Pediatrics recommends that all children 3 years and older have their blood pressure measured annually. Measuring pediatric blood pressure helps to identify children at risk for developing hypertension as adults. High blood pressure in children can be caused by kidney disease, and, to a lesser degree, by heart disease. When the condition is treated, the blood pressure usually returns to normal. Overweight children usually have higher blood pressure than children of normal weight. Losing weight through a prescribed diet and regular physical activity often reduces blood pressure in these children.

SPECIAL GUIDELINES FOR CHILDREN

The procedure for measuring blood pressure in children is the same as that for adults and is presented in Chapter 4. Some special pediatric guidelines must be taken into consideration.

CORRECT CUFF SIZE

The most important criterion in obtaining an accurate pediatric blood pressure measurement is in the selection of the correct cuff size. If the cuff is too small, the reading may be falsely high. If the cuff is too large, the reading may be falsely low. Blood pressure cuffs come in a variety of sizes and are measured in centimeters. The size of a cuff refers to its inner inflatable bladder, rather than its fabric cover. Table 9.3 lists the range of cuff sizes commercially available. The name of the cuff (e.g., child, adult) does not imply that it is appropriate for that age. An 8-year-old obese child may need an adult-sized cuff.

Table 9.3 Acceptable Bladder Dimensions for Arms of Different Sizes

Cuff	Bladder Length (cm)	Arm Circumference Range at Midpoint
Newborn	6	Less than 6 cm
Infant	15	6–15 cm
Child	21	16–21 cm
Small adult	24	22–26 cm
Adult	30	27–34 cm
Large adult	38	35–44 cm
Adult thigh	42	45–52 cm

For an accurate blood pressure measurement, the bladder of the cuff should encircle 80% to 100% of the arm. The child's arm circumference should be assessed at the midpoint between the acromion process (shoulder) and the olecranon process (elbow). Fig. 9.5 shows how to determine the correct pediatric cuff size. Additional methods for determining correct cuff size are presented in Chapter 4.

DETERMINATION OF PROPER CUFF SIZE

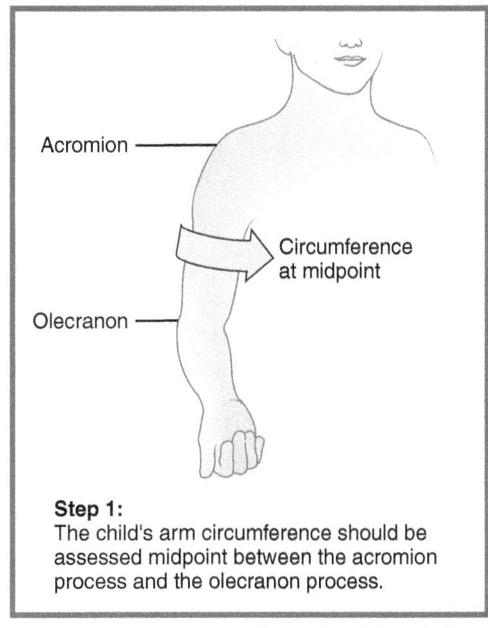

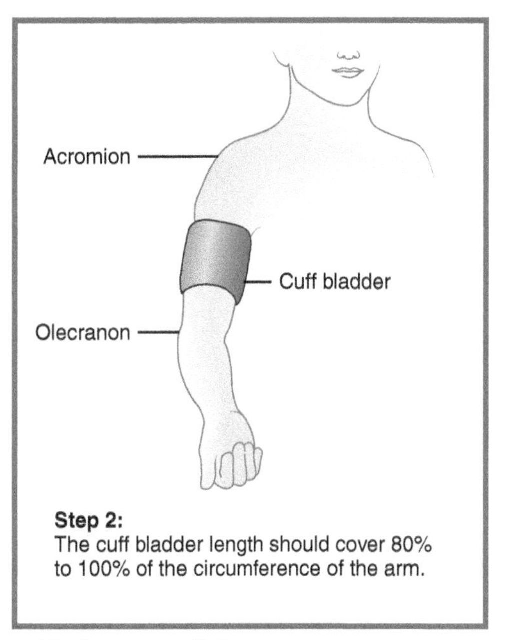

Fig. 9.5 Determination of proper blood pressure cuff size.

COOPERATION OF THE CHILD

Another important factor to consider when taking pediatric blood pressure is preparing the child for the procedure. It is important to gain the child's cooperation and to ensure that the child is relaxed. Apprehension can cause the blood pressure to be falsely high. To reduce a child's anxiety level, carefully explain the procedure to the child, and, if appropriate, allow him or her to handle the equipment before measurement of the blood pressure. The blood pressure should be measured after the child has been sitting quietly for 3 to 5 minutes (Fig. 9.6).

What Would You Do? What Would You *Not* Do?

Case Study 2

Wanda Tilley comes to the office with her 10-year-old daughter, Courtney. Courtney has a skin condition on her legs that needs to be evaluated by the physician. Courtney has been obese since she was 4 years old. Mrs. Tilley also is obese and is not too concerned about Courtney's weight. She says that Courtney must have inherited her "fat gene," and there's not much that can be done about it. Courtney's favorite activities are playing video games and reading. She would like to join the community swim team, but she's too embarrassed for anyone to see her in a swim suit. Courtney says the other kids are always making fun of her at school. She says that they call her "two-ton Tilley" and "double-roll," and they don't want to sit with her at lunch. Courtney wants her mom to home-school her because she's getting to the point where she can't take it anymore. She doesn't want the doctor to examine her because she thinks he will scold her for being so fat. ■

BLOOD PRESSURE CLASSIFICATIONS

Blood pressure varies depending on the age of the child and his or her height and gender. The National High Blood Pressure Education Program (NHBPEP) prepared a set of tables that physicians use to determine whether a child's blood pressure is higher than the average among children of the same age and height. If a child has a blood pressure that is higher than 90% to 95% of most other children of the same age, height, and gender, the child may have high blood pressure.

The NHBPEP tables (one for boys and one for girls) allow precise classification of blood pressure according to body size, which avoids misclassifying children at the extreme ends of normal growth. A very tall child would not be mistakenly diagnosed as having hypertension, and hypertension would not be missed in a very short child. The NHBPEP tables used by physicians to assist in the diagnosis of hypertension in children can be found at the National Heart, Lung, and Blood Institute website.

Blood pressure varies throughout the day in children as a result of normal fluctuations in physical activity and emotional stress. A single blood pressure reading taken on one occasion does not characterize the child's blood pressure accurately. If a child's blood pressure is elevated, an average of two or more blood pressure readings taken on two or more separate office visits must be taken before the physician can make a diagnosis of hypertension.

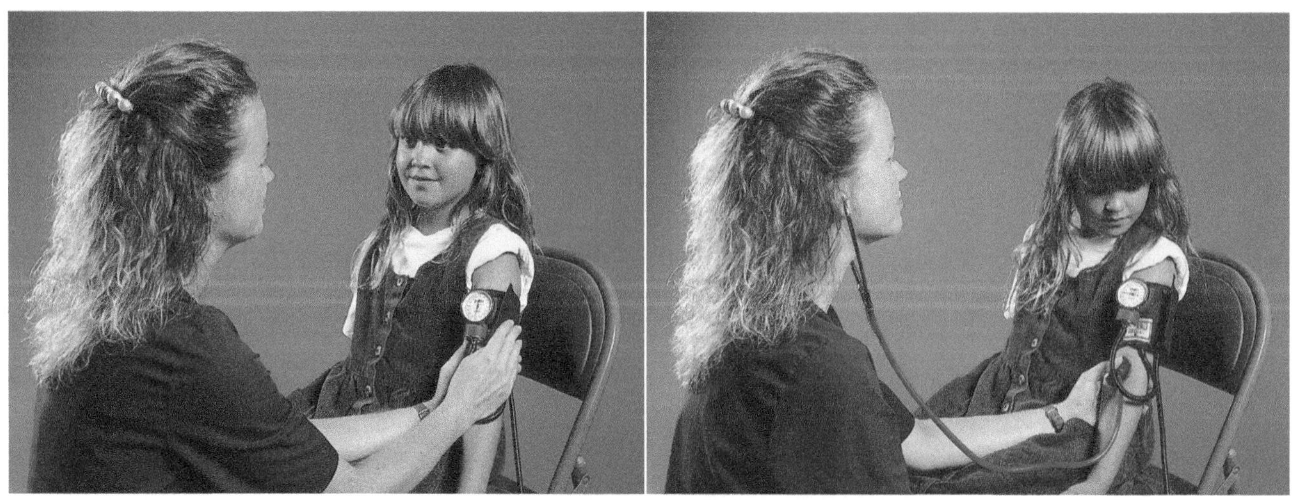

Fig. 9.6 Traci measures the blood pressure of a pediatric patient.

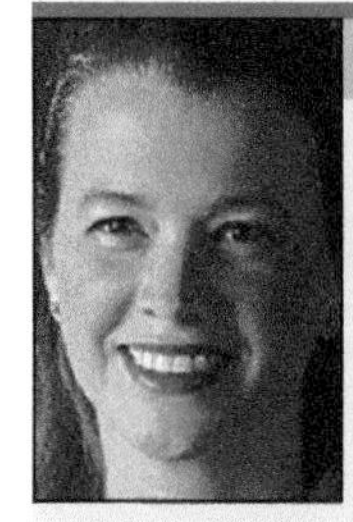

Memories *from* Practicum

Traci: I still remember how difficult it was at times as a student. I had been out of high school for more than a year, so I had to get back into the routine of studying. I worried about whether I would do well, whether I would be able to find a good job, and whether I would like medical assisting. Adding to these concerns was the financial burden of putting myself through 2 years of school. I took advantage of grants and student loans. Throughout the last 6 months of my education, I also worked full-time as an aide on the midnight shift at a nursing home while attending school full-time during the day. As if that were not enough, my first child was well on her way into this world as I was finishing up the last quarter of my degree. There were so many times that I was tired, frustrated, and broke, but I kept pushing myself to do my best because I knew this was going to be my lifetime career, and I wanted to excel in my profession. My determination paid off. Today I have a great medical assisting position that I love, with an institution that is one of the best employers in the area. ■

COLLECTION OF A URINE SPECIMEN

A urinalysis may be performed on a pediatric patient for the following reasons: to screen for the presence of disease as part of a general physical examination, to assist in the diagnosis of a pathologic condition (e.g., urinary tract infection), or to evaluate the effectiveness of therapy. The collection of a urine specimen from a child who exhibits bladder control is performed using the technique outlined in Chapter 16. Collecting a urine specimen from an infant or young child who cannot urinate voluntarily involves the use of a pediatric urine collector. Pediatric urine collectors are designed to be used with both genders. The urine collector consists of a clear plastic disposable bag containing a hypoallergenic pressure-sensitive adhesive around the opening of the bag. The adhesive firmly attaches the urine collector to the skin surrounding the genitalia. Procedure 9.4 outlines the procedure for applying a pediatric urine collector.

PEDIATRIC INJECTIONS

Administering an injection to a child is an important responsibility. The experience a child has with early injections influences the child's attitude toward later ones. If the child is old enough to understand, the procedure should be explained. The medical assistant should be honest and should attempt to gain the child's trust and cooperation. The child should be told the truth about the injection—that it will hurt, but only for a short time. It also is advisable to explain that the medicine is being given to help him or her. Another person (e.g., parent, health care worker) should be present to assist. The assistant can help position the child and can divert or restrain him or her if necessary. If the child struggles and fights excessively, the medical assistant should delay the injection and consult the physician. After the injection has been administered, the medical assistant or the child's parent should hold the infant, provide comfort, and show approval so that the child associates something other than pain with this procedure.

The administration of injections is presented in Chapter 11. Before undertaking the study of pediatric injections, the medical assistant should review this chapter thoroughly, concentrating on the locations of injection sites and the procedures for preparing and administering injections. The same basic technique is used to administer an injection to an adult and a child. Variations in procedure are explained in the following section.

INTRAMUSCULAR INJECTIONS

An intramuscular injection is administered directly into muscle tissue. The gauge and length of the needle used for intramuscular injections vary, depending on the consistency of the medication to be administered and the size of the child. Thick or oily preparations require a larger needle lumen, and the needle must be long enough to reach muscle tissue. A needle length ranging from ⅝ inch to 1 inch is typically used to administer an intramuscular injection to a child, and in general the gauge of the needle ranges from 22 to 25, depending on the viscosity (thickness) of the medication.

Intramuscular Injection Sites

The specific site for injection of the medication depends on the age of the child which is indicated in the package insert accompanying the medication. The two most commonly used pediatric injection sites are the vastus lateralis and the deltoid. The dorsogluteal site is not recommended for infants and children. This is because an injection into this site may come dangerously close to the sciatic nerve; an injection into the sciatic nerves results in pain, numbness and weakness of the leg and foot.

Vastus Lateralis Site

The vastus lateralis site is recommended for infants and young children under the age of 3 years. It is located on the anterior surface of the midlateral thigh, away from major nerves and blood vessels, and it is large enough to accommodate the injected medication (Fig. 9.7A). To locate the vastus lateralis site in an infant or young child, divide the mid–anterior thigh into thirds. The injection is administered into the middle third of the thigh (see Fig. 9.7B).

The length of the needle used depends on the overall size of the thigh. The needle should be long enough to penetrate the muscle belly for proper absorption to occur. A 1-inch needle is often used for a normal-sized infant or child; however, the length of the needle may need to be decreased (e.g., ⅝ inch) for a newborn or preterm infant and increased (e.g., 1¼ inches) for an obese child. For administration of the injection, the infant or toddler should be held on the assistant's lap in a "cuddle" or semi-recumbent position. The site should be clearly visible and the assistant should restrain the child to prevent as much movement as possible. The medical assistant must grasp the thigh to compress the muscle tissue and to stabilize the extremity (Fig. 9.8A). The injection is administered at a 90-degree angle as illustrated in Fig. 9.8B, by following the procedure outlined in Chapter 11.

Deltoid Site

The deltoid muscle is shallow and can accommodate only a small amount of medication (0.5 to 1 mL). In addition, repeated injections at this site are painful. Because the deltoid site is so small in an infant, it should not be used to administer an injection until a child is 3 years of age. The length of the needle should be adjusted according to the amount of subcutaneous tissue over the injection site. For example, a ⅝-inch needle is often used for a normal-sized 4-year-old, but a 1-inch needle may be required for an obese child of the same age. For administration of the injection, the deltoid muscle mass should be grasped at the injection site and compressed between the thumb and fingers. The needle should be inserted pointing slightly upward toward the shoulder (Fig. 9.9).

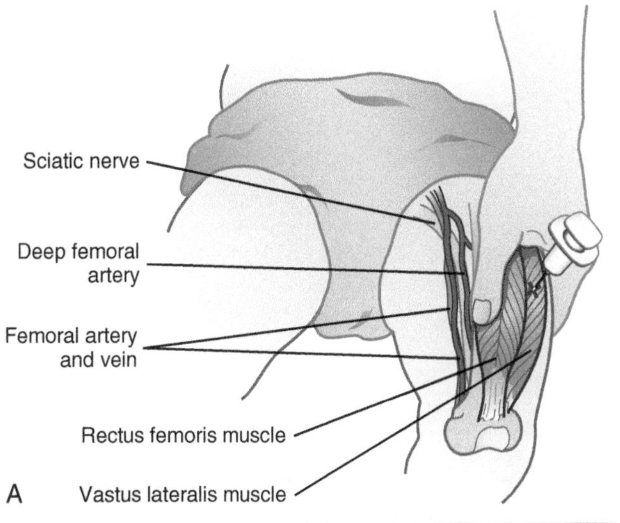

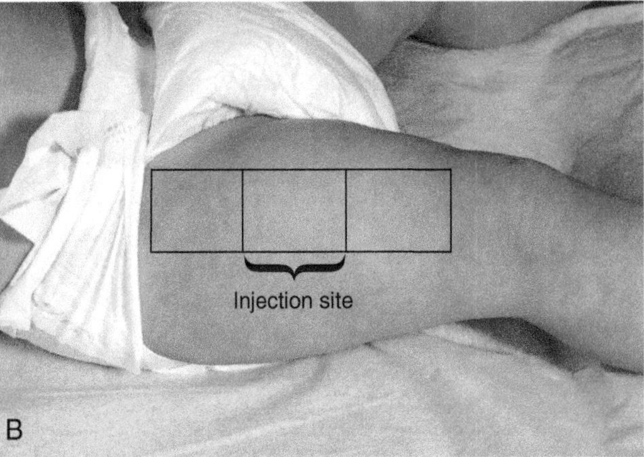

Fig. 9.7 (A) Vastus lateralis intramuscular injection site. (B) Location of the vastus lateralis injection site in an infant. Divide the mid-anterior thigh into thirds. The injection is administered into the middle third of the thigh. (A, Courtesy Wyeth Laboratories, Philadelphia, PA.)

SUBCUTANEOUS INJECTIONS

A subcutaneous injection is made into the subcutaneous tissue, which consists of adipose (fat) tissue located just under the skin. The length of the needle used to administer a pediatric subcutaneous injection ranges from ½ inch to ⅝ inch, and the gauge of the needle ranges from 23 to 25.

Subcutaneous tissue is located all over the body; however, certain sites are more commonly used because they are located where bones and blood vessels are not near the surface of the skin. The recommended subcutaneous site for an infant younger than 12 months of age is the anterior thigh. For a child 12 months of age or older, the recommended subcutaneous site is the lateral part of the upper arm or the anterior thigh.

For administration of the injection, the area surrounding the injection site should be grasped and held in a cushion fashion and the needle should be inserted at a 45-degree

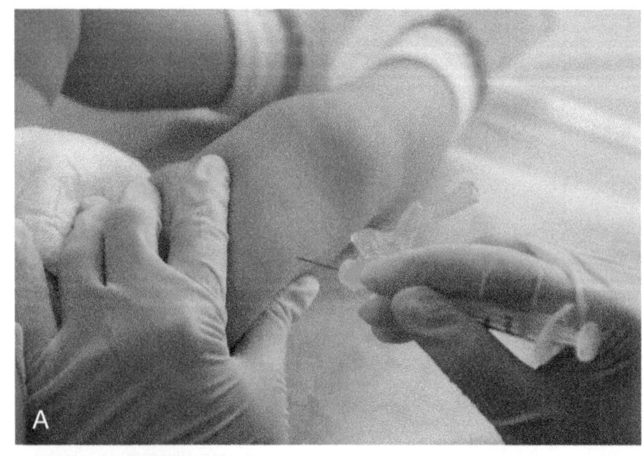

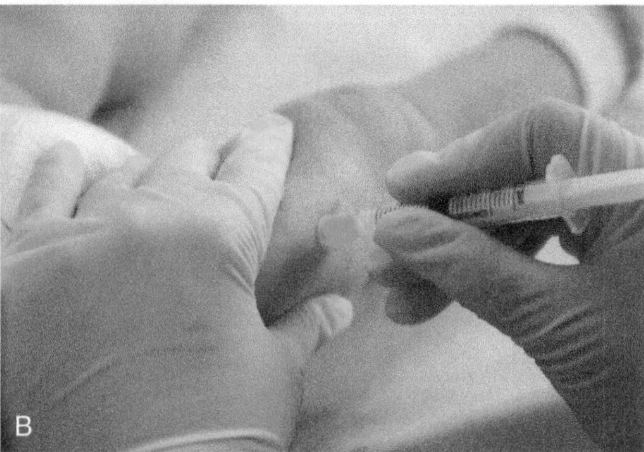

Fig. 9.8 (A) Compression of the vastus lateralis muscle. (B) Intramuscular injection into the vastus lateralis injection site.

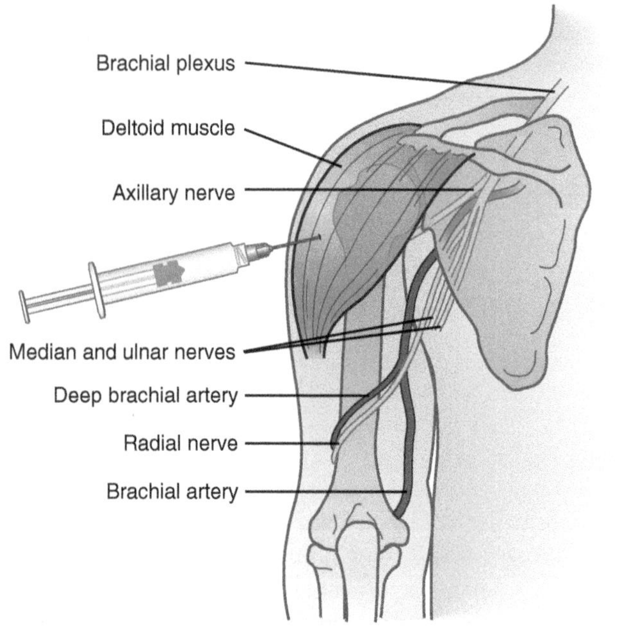

Fig. 9.9 Deltoid intramuscular injection site. (Courtesy Wyeth Laboratories, Philadelphia, PA.)

angle. This ensures that the subcutaneous tissue and not muscle tissue is entered. The designated pediatric subcutaneous injection sites do not contain any large blood vessels. Because of this, the Centers for Disease Control and Prevention (CDC) recommends that aspiration of the syringe is not necessary before administration of an immunization through the subcutaneous route. Studies show that not aspirating before administration of the immunization reduces pain at the injection site. It is extremely important, however, that the medical assistant always review and follow the medication administration policies set forth at her or his medical office.

IMMUNIZATIONS

Immunity is the resistance of the body to the effects of harmful agents, such as pathogenic microorganisms and their toxins. The process of becoming immune or rendering an individual immune through the use of a vaccine or toxoid is known as active, artificial **immunization**. A **vaccine** is a suspension of attenuated (weakened) or killed microorganisms administered to an individual to prevent an infectious disease by stimulating the production of antibodies in that individual (e.g., hepatitis B vaccine). A **toxoid** is a toxin (a poisonous substance produced by a bacterium) that has been treated by heat or chemicals to destroy its harmful properties (e.g., tetanus toxoid). It is administered to an individual to prevent an infectious disease by stimulating the production of antibodies in that individual. Immunizations build the body's defenses and protect an individual from attack by certain infectious diseases.

Immunizations should be administered to infants and young children during well-child visits according to an immunization schedule. The American Academy of Pediatrics recommends that the schedule outlined in Fig. 9.10 be followed. This schedule is intended as a guide to be used with any modifications needed to meet the requirements of an individual or group.

The medical assistant should be familiar with each immunization that is administered, including its use, common side effects, route of administration, dose, and method of storage. The drug manufacturer includes a package insert with each vaccine and toxoid that contains this information. Drug references, such as the *Prescribers' Digital Reference* (available online), also can be used to locate information on immunizations. Immunizations administered to infants and children, along with brand names, routes of administration, and common minor problems, are listed in Table 9.4. Certain immunizations can be administered together in the same injection. A combined immunization is just as effective as the individual immunization and results in fewer injections for the infant or child. For example, diphtheria, tetanus, and pertussis (DTaP), hepatitis B, and polio (DTaP-HepB-IPV) immunizations can be combined together in the same injection. Table 9.5 provides a list of combined immunizations administered to infants and children, along with brand names and the routes of administration.

Parents should be provided with an immunization record card (Fig. 9.11) at their infant's first well-child visit. They

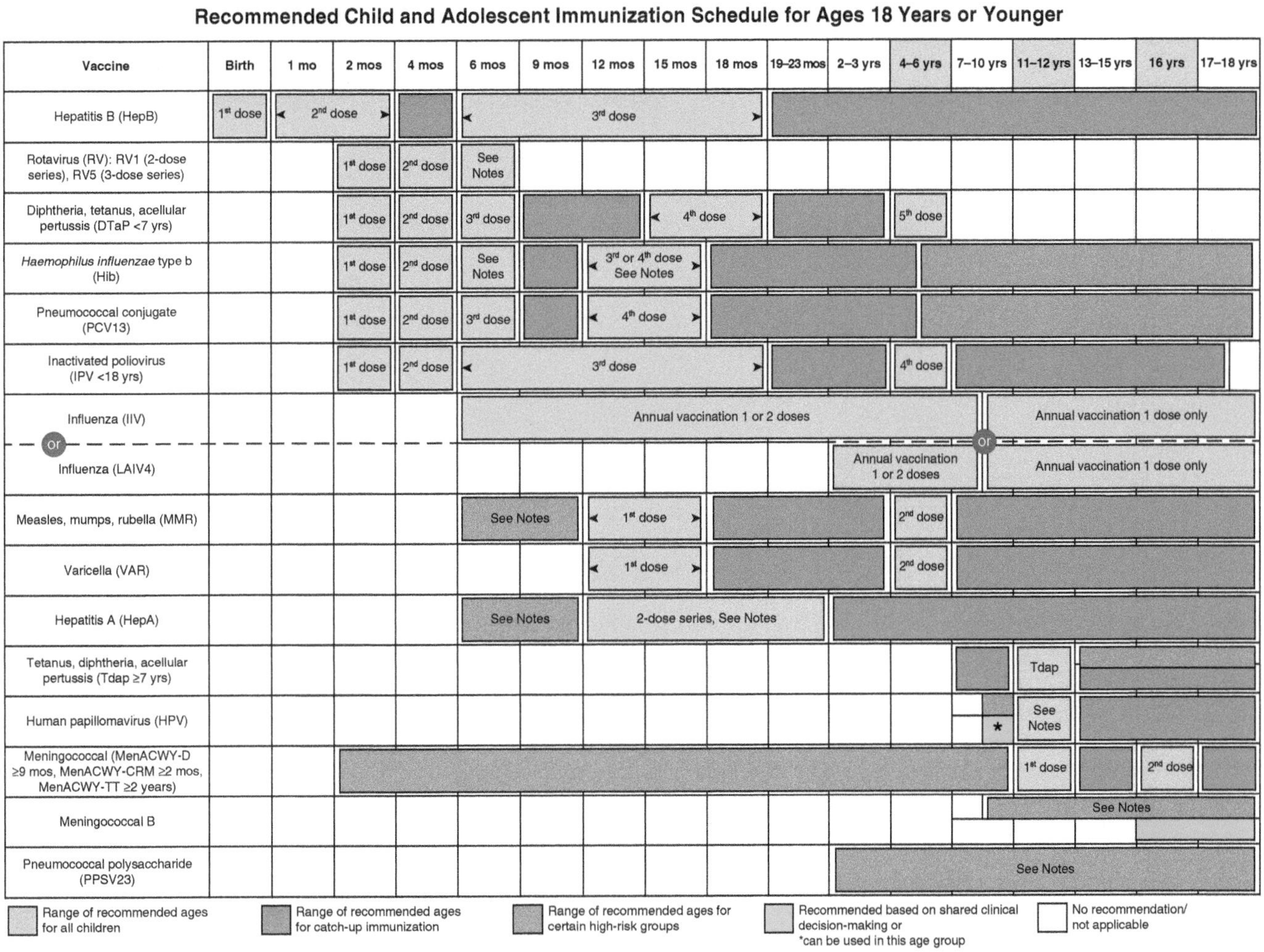

Recommended Child and Adolescent Immunization Schedule for Ages 18 Years or Younger

Vaccine	Birth	1 mo	2 mos	4 mos	6 mos	9 mos	12 mos	15 mos	18 mos	19–23 mos	2–3 yrs	4–6 yrs	7–10 yrs	11–12 yrs	13–15 yrs	16 yrs	17–18 yrs
Hepatitis B (HepB)	1st dose	2nd dose			3rd dose												
Rotavirus (RV): RV1 (2-dose series), RV5 (3-dose series)			1st dose	2nd dose	See Notes												
Diphtheria, tetanus, acellular pertussis (DTaP <7 yrs)			1st dose	2nd dose	3rd dose			4th dose				5th dose					
Haemophilus influenzae type b (Hib)			1st dose	2nd dose	See Notes		3rd or 4th dose See Notes										
Pneumococcal conjugate (PCV13)			1st dose	2nd dose	3rd dose		4th dose										
Inactivated poliovirus (IPV <18 yrs)			1st dose	2nd dose	3rd dose							4th dose					
Influenza (IIV)					Annual vaccination 1 or 2 doses								Annual vaccination 1 dose only				
or																	
Influenza (LAIV4)											Annual vaccination 1 or 2 doses		Annual vaccination 1 dose only				
Measles, mumps, rubella (MMR)					See Notes		1st dose					2nd dose					
Varicella (VAR)							1st dose					2nd dose					
Hepatitis A (HepA)					See Notes		2-dose series, See Notes										
Tetanus, diphtheria, acellular pertussis (Tdap ≥7 yrs)														Tdap			
Human papillomavirus (HPV)													*	See Notes			
Meningococcal (MenACWY-D ≥9 mos, MenACWY-CRM ≥2 mos, MenACWY-TT ≥2 years)														1st dose		2nd dose	
Meningococcal B														See Notes			
Pneumococcal polysaccharide (PPSV23)											See Notes						

Range of recommended ages for all children | Range of recommended ages for catch-up immunization | Range of recommended ages for certain high-risk groups | Recommended based on shared clinical decision-making or *can be used in this age group | No recommendation/not applicable

Fig. 9.10 Immunization schedule. (Modified from Department of Health and Human Services, Centers for Disease Control and Prevention, Atlanta, GA, 2021.)

Table 9.4 Infant and Childhood Immunizations

Immunization (and Abbreviation)	Brand Names	Route of Administration	Common Minor Problems after Administration
Hep B (hepatitis B vaccine)	Engerix-B Recombivax HB	IM	Mild fever Soreness at injection site
DTaP (diphtheria and tetanus toxoids and acellular pertussis vaccine)	Acel-Imune Certiva Daptacel Infanrix Tripedia	IM	Fever, irritability, tiredness, poor appetite, and vomiting Redness or swelling at injection site Soreness or tenderness at injection site (occurs 1–3 days after the injection and occurs more often after the fourth or fifth dose in the series than after earlier doses)
Hib (*Haemophilus influenzae* type b vaccine)	ActHIB HibTITER PedvaxHIB	IM	Redness, swelling, and warmth at injection site; fever greater than 101°F (38.3°C) (occurs within 1 day after injection; may last 2–3 days)
IPV (inactivated polio vaccine)	IPOL	IM or SC	Soreness at the injection site
PCV (pneumococcal conjugate vaccine)	Prevnar	IM	Redness, swelling, and tenderness at the injection site; fever Irritability and drowsiness Loss of appetite
RV (rotavirus vaccine)	Rotarix RotaTeq	PO	Irritability, temporary diarrhea, and vomiting
MMR (measles, mumps, and rubella vaccines)	M-M-R II	SC	Fever, mild rash, swelling of glands in the cheeks or neck (occur 7–12 days after administration)

Continued

TABLE 9.4 Infant and Childhood Immunizations—cont'd

Immunization (and Abbreviation)	Brand Names	Route of Administration	Common Minor Problems after Administration
Var (varicella) (chickenpox vaccine)	Varivax	SC	Fever, mild rash Soreness or swelling at injection site
Hep A (hepatitis A vaccine)	Havrix Vaqta	IM	Soreness at the injection site Headache, loss of appetite, and tiredness (usually last 1–2 days)
MCV4 (meningococcal vaccine)	Menactra	IM	Pain and redness at injection site Fever (usually lasts 1–2 days)
HPV (human papillomavirus vaccine)	Gardasil Cervarix	IM	Pain, redness, swelling, or itching at injection site Fever
Influenza vaccine (injection)	Afluria Fluarix FluLaval FluShield Fluvirin Fluzone Fluzone Intradermal	IM ID	Soreness, redness, or swelling at the injection site, fever and malaise Hoarseness; sore, red, or itchy eyes Cough, fever, aches (occur soon after injection and usually last 1–2 days)
Influenza vaccine (nasal spray)	FluMist	IN	Runny nose, nasal congestion or cough Headache, muscle aches, abdominal pain, or occasional vomiting or diarrhea Fever; wheezing

ID, Intradermal; *IM,* intramuscular; *IN,* intranasal; *PO,* oral; *SC,* subcutaneous.

Table 9.5 Infant and Childhood Combination Immunizations

Combined Immunization	Brand Name	Route of Administration
DTaP-HepB-IPV	Pediarix	IM
DTaP-Hib-IPV	Pentacel	IM
DTaP-IPV	Kinrix	IM
DTaP-Hib	TriHIBit	IM
Hib-HepB	Comvax	IM
MMRV	ProQuad	SC

See Table 9.4 for the common minor problems that may occur following administration of each individual immunization.

DTaP, Diphtheria, tetanus, and pertussis; *HepB,* hepatitis B; *Hib,* Haemophilus influenzae type b; *IM,* intramuscular; *IPV,* inactivated polio vaccine; *MMRV,* measles, mumps, rubella, varicella; *SC,* subcutaneous.

should be instructed to bring this card to every visit so that their child's immunizations can be recorded. Parents should be informed of the possible normal side effects of each immunization and given instructions on how to respond if they occur.

NATIONAL CHILDHOOD VACCINE INJURY ACT

The National Childhood Vaccine Injury Act (NCVIA) requires that parents be provided with information about the benefits and risks of childhood immunizations. To help medical offices comply with these regulations, the CDC developed a set of vaccine information statements (VISs). A VIS explains, in lay terminology, the benefits and risks of a vaccine or toxoid. It also contains information about reporting a moderate or severe reaction, the National Vaccine Injury Compensation Program, and how to obtain more information about the vaccine or toxoid. See Fig. 9.12 for a DTaP VIS.

The NCVIA requires that the appropriate and most current VIS be given to the child's parent or guardian each and every time before the child receives a dose of any immunization listed in Table 9.4. The medical assistant must give the parent or guardian enough time to read the VIS and an opportunity to ask questions before the immunization is administered. In addition, the medical assistant must document the following information in the patient's medical record: the name and publication date of each VIS provided to the parent, and the date the VIS was given to the parent. The publication date of the VIS is located at the bottom left or right corner of the VIS. Following the administration of the immunization, the NCVIA requires the following information be documented in the patient's medical record: the date of administration, the manufacturer and lot number, the signature and title of the health care provider who administered the immunization, and the name and address of the medical office where it was administered. Fig. 9.13 shows an example of an immunization administrative record that is included in a patient's medical record.

IMMUNIZATION RECORD					
Name ______					
Birthdate ______					
Immunization	DATE	DATE	DATE	DATE	DATE
Hep B (Hepatitis B)					
DTaP (Diphtheria, Tetanus, and Pertussis)					
Hib (*Haemophilus influenzae* Type b)					
IPV (Inactivated Polio Vaccine)					
PCV (Pneumococcal Conjugate Vaccine)					
RV (Rotavirus vaccine)					
MMR (Measles, Mumps, Rubella)					
Varicella (Chickenpox)					
Hep A (Hepatitis A)					
MCV4 (Meningococcal Vaccine)					
HPV (Human Papillomavirus)					
Influenza					
Tuberculin (Mantoux) RESULT					
Tetanus Booster					
Other					

Fig. 9.11 Immunization record card.

VACCINE INFORMATION STATEMENT

DTaP (Diphtheria, Tetanus, Pertussis) Vaccine: *What You Need to Know*

Many Vaccine Information Statements are available in Spanish and other languages. See www.immunize.org/vis

Hojas de información sobre vacunas están disponibles en español y en muchos otros idiomas. Visite www.immunize.org/vis

1 Why get vaccinated?

DTaP vaccine can prevent **diphtheria, tetanus**, and **pertussis**.

Diphtheria and pertussis spread from person to person. Tetanus enters the body through cuts or wounds.

- **DIPHTHERIA (D)** can lead to difficulty breathing, heart failure, paralysis, or death.
- **TETANUS (T)** causes painful stiffening of the muscles. Tetanus can lead to serious health problems, including being unable to open the mouth, having trouble swallowing and breathing, or death.
- **PERTUSSIS (aP)**, also known as "whooping cough," can cause uncontrollable, violent coughing which makes it hard to breathe, eat, or drink. Pertussis can be extremely serious in babies and young children, causing pneumonia, convulsions, brain damage, or death. In teens and adults, it can cause weight loss, loss of bladder control, passing out, and rib fractures from severe coughing.

2 DTaP vaccine

DTaP is only for children younger than 7 years old. Different vaccines against tetanus, diphtheria, and pertussis (Tdap and Td) are available for older children, adolescents, and adults.

It is recommended that children receive 5 doses of DTaP, usually at the following ages:

- 2 months
- 4 months
- 6 months
- 15–18 months
- 4–6 years

DTaP may be given as a stand-alone vaccine, or as part of a combination vaccine (a type of vaccine that combines more than one vaccine together into one shot).

DTaP may be given at the same time as other vaccines.

3 Talk with your health care provider

Tell your vaccine provider if the person getting the vaccine:

- Has had an **allergic reaction after a previous dose of any vaccine that protects against tetanus, diphtheria, or pertussis**, or has any **severe, life-threatening allergies**.
- Has had **a coma, decreased level of consciousness, or prolonged seizures within 7 days after a previous dose of any pertussis vaccine (DTP or DTaP)**.
- Has **seizures or another nervous system problem**.
- Has ever had **Guillain-Barré Syndrome** (also called GBS).
- Has had **severe pain or swelling after a previous dose of any vaccine that protects against tetanus or diphtheria**.

In some cases, your child's health care provider may decide to postpone DTaP vaccination to a future visit.

Children with minor illnesses, such as a cold, may be vaccinated. Children who are moderately or severely ill should usually wait until they recover before getting DTaP.

Your child's health care provider can give you more information.

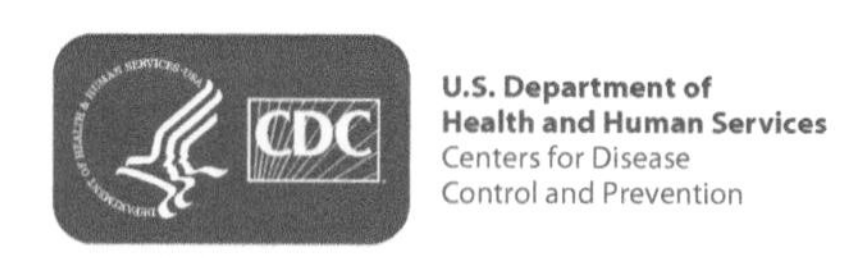

Fig. 9.12 Vaccine information statement for diphtheria, tetanus, and pertussis (DTaP). (Courtesy Centers for Disease Control and Prevention, Atlanta, GA, 2020.)

4 Risks of a vaccine reaction

- Soreness or swelling where the shot was given, fever, fussiness, feeling tired, loss of appetite, and vomiting sometimes happen after DTaP vaccination.
- More serious reactions, such as seizures, non-stop crying for 3 hours or more, or high fever (over 105°F) after DTaP vaccination happen much less often. Rarely, the vaccine is followed by swelling of the entire arm or leg, especially in older children when they receive their fourth or fifth dose.
- Very rarely, long-term seizures, coma, lowered consciousness, or permanent brain damage may happen after DTaP vaccination.

As with any medicine, there is a very remote chance of a vaccine causing a severe allergic reaction, other serious injury, or death.

5 What if there is a serious problem?

An allergic reaction could occur after the vaccinated person leaves the clinic. If you see signs of a severe allergic reaction (hives, swelling of the face and throat, difficulty breathing, a fast heartbeat, dizziness, or weakness), call **9-1-1** and get the person to the nearest hospital.

For other signs that concern you, call your health care provider.

Adverse reactions should be reported to the Vaccine Adverse Event Reporting System (VAERS). Your health care provider will usually file this report, or you can do it yourself. Visit the VAERS website at **www.vaers.hhs.gov** or call **1-800-822-7967**. *VAERS is only for reporting reactions, and VAERS staff do not give medical advice.*

6 The National Vaccine Injury Compensation Program

The National Vaccine Injury Compensation Program (VICP) is a federal program that was created to compensate people who may have been injured by certain vaccines. Visit the VICP website at **www.hrsa.gov/vaccinecompensation** or call **1-800-338-2382** to learn about the program and about filing a claim. There is a time limit to file a claim for compensation.

7 How can I learn more?

- Ask your health care provider.
- Call your local or state health department.
- Contact the Centers for Disease Control and Prevention (CDC):
  - Call **1-800-232-4636** (**1-800-CDC-INFO**) or
  - Visit CDC's website at **www.cdc.gov/vaccines**

Vaccine Information Statement (Interim)

DTaP (Diphtheria, Tetanus, Pertussis) Vaccine

Office use only

04/01/2020 | 42 U.S.C. § 300aa-26

Fig. 9.12, cont'd

IMMUNIZATION ADMINISTRATION RECORD

Name ______________________________
(first) (MI) (last)

DOB ______________________________

Physician ______________________________

Address ______________________________

____

SITE ABBREVIATIONS:

RVL: Right vastus lateralis
LVL: Left vastus lateralis
RD: Right deltoid
LD: Left deltoid
PO: By mouth
IN: Intranasal

Vaccine	Type of Vaccine[1] (generic abbreviation)	Date Given (mo/day/yr)	Dose	Site	Vaccine		Vaccine Information Statement		Signature and Title of Vaccinator
					Lot #	Mfr.	Date on VIS	Date Given	
Hepatitis B[2] (e.g., HepB, Hib-HepB, DTaP-HepB-IPV) Give IM.									
Diphtheria, Tetanus, Pertussis[2] (e.g., DTaP, DTaP-Hib, DTaP-HepB-IPV, DT, DTaP-Hib-IPV, Tdap, DTaP-IPV, Td) Give IM.									
***Haemophilus influenzae* type b**[2] (e.g., Hib, Hib-HepB, DTaP-Hib-IPV, DTaP-Hib) Give IM.									
Polio[2] (e.g., IPV, DTaP-HepB-IPV, DTaP-Hib-IPV, DTaP-IPV) Give IPV SC or IM. Give all others IM.									
Pneumococcal (e.g., PCV, conjugate; PPV, polysaccharide) Give PCV IM. Give PPV SC or IM.									
Rotovirus Give oral.									
Measles, Mumps, Rubella[5] (e.g., MMR, MMRV) Give SC.									
Varicella[5] (e.g., Var, MMRV) Give SC.									
Hepatitis A Give IM									
Meningococcal (e.g., MCV4, MPSV4) Give MCV4 IM and MPSV4 SC.									
Human papillomavirus (e.g., HPV) Give IM									
Influenza[5] (e.g., TIV, inactivated; LAIV, live attenuated) Give TIV IM. Give LAIV IN.									
Other									

1. Record the generic abbreviation for the type of vaccine given (e.g., DTaP-Hib, PCV), *not* the trade name.
2. For combination vaccines, fill in a row for each separate antigen in the combination.

Fig. 9.13 Immunization administration record included in a patient's medical record. (Modified from Immunization Action Coalition, St Paul, MN.)

What Would You Do? What Would You *Not* Do?

Case Study 3

Stacy Jones, a legal secretary, brings her 5-year-old son, Matthew, in for a kindergarten physical. Stacy has read the vaccine information statements for the diphtheria, tetanus, and pertussis (DTaP), inactivated polio vaccine (IPV), and measles-mumps-rubella (MMR) immunizations that Matthew will be getting at this visit and has some questions. She wants to know why polio is not given orally anymore. She also wants to know why children are immunized against chickenpox because it is such a harmless disease. She is annoyed because she thinks that children are receiving too many unnecessary injections these days. Matthew is extremely afraid of "shots" and says that no one with a needle is getting anywhere near him. Stacy is protective of Matthew and knows that he will be hard to handle. She wants to know whether this set of immunizations could just be skipped. She says that most of these diseases do not even exist anymore and that she noticed, from reading the vaccine sheets, that there are a lot of possible side effects. ■

NEWBORN SCREENING TEST

PURPOSE OF THE TEST

A newborn screening test is performed on an infant to screen for the presence of certain metabolic and endocrine diseases. The diseases that are screened for vary by state but typically include phenylketonuria (PKU), biotinidase deficiency, congenital adrenal hyperplasia, maple sugar urine disease, congenital hypothyroidism, galactosemia, homocystinuria, and sickle cell anemia. The most important of these is PKU, which is discussed in greater detail in the following paragraphs.

PHENYLKETONURIA

PKU is a congenital hereditary disease caused by a lack of the enzyme *phenylalanine hydroxylase.* This enzyme is needed to convert phenylalanine, an amino acid, into tyrosine, which is an amino acid needed for normal metabolic functioning. Without this enzyme, phenylalanine accumulates in the blood and, if the accumulation is left untreated, causes mental retardation and other abnormalities, such as tremors and poor muscle coordination. In most cases, on early detection, a special low-phenylalanine diet and close periodic monitoring can prevent adverse effects. Normal development usually occurs if treatment is started before the child reaches 3 to 4 weeks of age. To promote the best development of cognitive abilities, most authorities recommend lifelong dietary restriction of phenylalanine. Although PKU is not a common condition (affecting 1 in every 12,000 births), early diagnosis and treatment lead to a better prognosis.

Phenylalanine can be detected in the blood of an affected infant only after the infant has been receiving breast or formula milk. Infants taking formula can be tested earlier than breast-fed infants because formula contains phenylalanine, whereas the "first breast milk," or colostrum, does not. The test results of breastfed infants are usually invalid until the mother begins producing milk.

NEWBORN SCREENING REQUIREMENTS

All states require by law that infants undergo newborn screening. The best time to perform the test is between 1 and 7 days after birth. In most states, the newborn screening test is performed before the infant leaves the hospital. If the test has abnormal or invalid results, the infant needs to be retested. Most repeat tests are required because of invalid test results caused by the collection of an inadequate amount of the blood specimen. Newborn screening retesting is usually performed at a hospital laboratory but may sometimes be performed in the medical office.

The newborn screening test card (Fig. 9.14) includes an information section that must be completed before the test is performed. The newborn screening test is performed on capillary blood obtained from the fleshy part of the lateral or medial posterior curve of the plantar surface of the infant's heel (Procedure 9.5). The blood specimen is placed on a special filter paper attached to the newborn screening test card and is mailed to an outside laboratory for analysis. The results are ready in a few days. If one of the newborn screening test results is positive, further testing is performed.

PATIENT COACHING Childhood Immunizations

- Encourage parents to have their children immunized.
- Emphasize to parents the importance of maintaining an immunization record card that documents all of their child's immunizationss
- Provide parents with educational materials on the importance of immunizations.
- Answer questions patients have about childhood immunizations.

What is immunity?

Immunity is the resistance of the body to microorganisms that cause disease. When an individual has an infection, the body responds by producing disease-fighting substances known as *antibodies.* Antibodies usually remain in the body even after the individual has recovered from the disease. This protects the individual from getting that disease again.

Continued

PATIENT COACHING Childhood Immunizations—cont'd

How do immunizations prevent disease?

The pathogens that cause disease or their toxins are weakened or killed and made into vaccines. These vaccines are injected into the body, and the body reacts to them the same way that it responds to the disease itself—by producing antibodies. These antibodies last for a long time, often for life, to defend the body against disease.

What childhood diseases can be prevented through immunization?

The reduction of childhood disease by immunization during the past 50 years has been dramatic. Fourteen diseases can be prevented by routine immunization of children: hepatitis B, diphtheria, tetanus, pertussis (whooping cough), *Haemophilus influenzae* type b infections, polio, measles, mumps, rubella (German measles), chickenpox (varicella), pneumococcal infections (meningitis and blood infections), hepatitis A, rotavirus, and influenza (flu). Except for tetanus, all these diseases are contagious. They can be spread from child to child and from one community to another. When children are not protected against them, serious outbreaks of disease can still occur.

Haven't most of these diseases been eliminated in the United States?

Although most of the vaccine-preventable diseases have been reduced to very low levels in the United States, this is not true worldwide. Some of these diseases are quite prevalent in other countries. An infected traveler can bring these diseases into the United States without knowing it. If Americans were not immunized, these diseases could quickly spread throughout the population and cause an epidemic. Only when a disease has been eradicated worldwide is it safe to stop immunizing for that particular disease.

Do immunizations have side effects?

Immunizations are among the safest and most reliable medications available. Minor side effects may occur, however, after administration of an immunization. They do not last long and may include a slight fever and irritability; redness, swelling, and soreness at the injection site; and a mild rash. Rarely, the effects can be more serious; if any unusual symptoms occur after immunization, it is important to contact the physician immediately. Overall, the benefits of immunizations to prevent childhood diseases are greater than the possible risks for almost all children.

Are immunizations required by law?

Every state has laws requiring immunization against some or all of these diseases before children enter school. Children who get their immunizations benefit from the protection these immunizations provide. Immunizations also contribute to the well-being of everyone by reducing the chance for disease to spread. School immunization requirements for each state can be found at the following websites: www.nnii.org/vaccinelnfo/index.cfm#state and www.immunize.org/states. ■

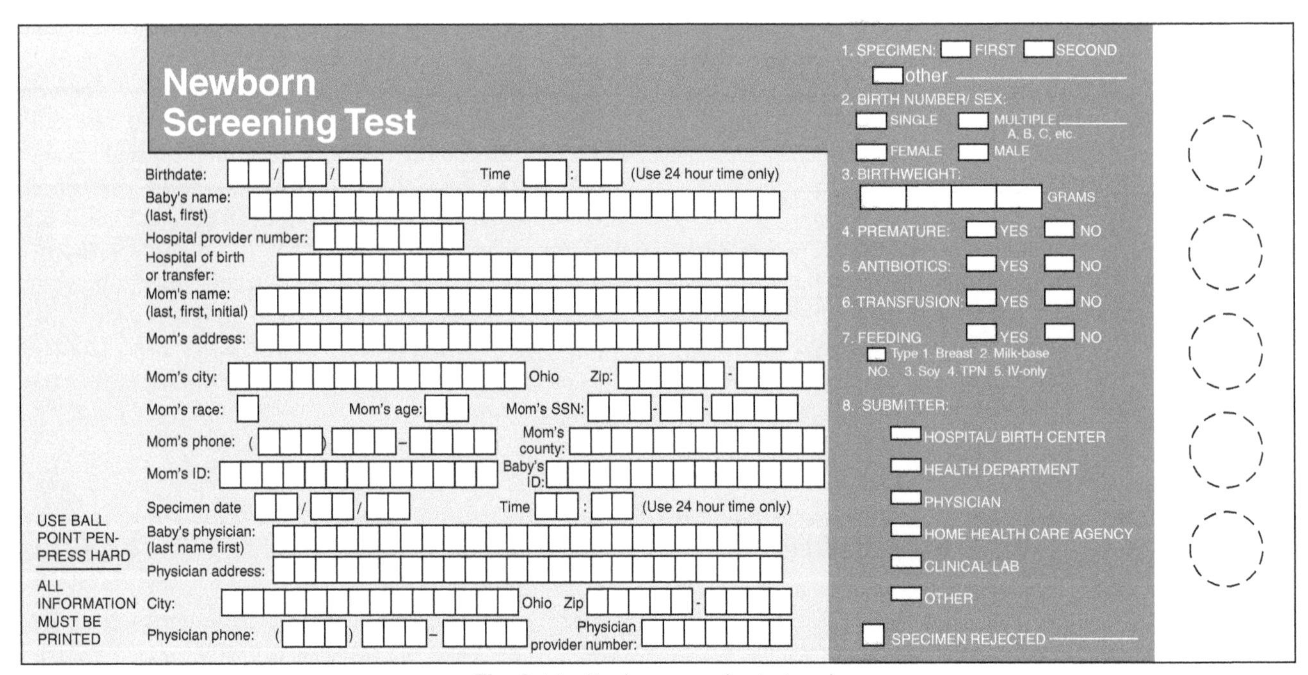

Newborn Screening Test

Birthdate: __/__/__ Time __:__ (Use 24 hour time only)
Baby's name: (last, first)
Hospital provider number:
Hospital of birth or transfer:
Mom's name: (last, first, initial)
Mom's address:
Mom's city: Ohio Zip: -
Mom's race: Mom's age: Mom's SSN: - -
Mom's phone: ( ) - Mom's county:
Mom's ID: Baby's ID:
Specimen date __/__/__ Time __:__ (Use 24 hour time only)
Baby's physician: (last name first)
Physician address:
City: Ohio Zip -
Physician phone: ( ) - Physician provider number:

USE BALL POINT PEN-PRESS HARD

ALL INFORMATION MUST BE PRINTED

1. SPECIMEN: FIRST SECOND other
2. BIRTH NUMBER/ SEX: SINGLE MULTIPLE A, B, C, etc. FEMALE MALE
3. BIRTHWEIGHT: GRAMS
4. PREMATURE: YES NO
5. ANTIBIOTICS: YES NO
6. TRANSFUSION: YES NO
7. FEEDING YES NO Type 1. Breast 2. Milk-base NO. 3. Soy 4. TPN 5. IV-only
8. SUBMITTER: HOSPITAL/ BIRTH CENTER; HEALTH DEPARTMENT; PHYSICIAN; HOME HEALTH CARE AGENCY; CLINICAL LAB; OTHER

SPECIMEN REJECTED

Fig. 9.14 Newborn screening test card.

What Would You Do? What Would You *Not* Do? RESPONSES

Case Study 1

Page 287.

What Did Traci Do?

- ❑ Listened patiently to Mrs. Chang and allowed her to vent her frustrations.
- ❑ Reassured Mrs. Chang that her milk is very nutritious for Christopher. Gave her a brochure on breastfeeding that included information on what to do for sore nipples and engorgement.
- ❑ Gave Mrs. Chang the names and phone numbers of community resources for nursing mothers.
- ❑ Told Mrs. Chang that Christopher's weight and length do not fall in the underweight category on his growth chart. Showed her Christopher's growth chart so that she could see that Christopher is progressing normally.

What Did Traci Not Do?

- ❑ Did not tell Mrs. Chang to cheer up because the colic would eventually go away on its own.
- ❑ Did not give a personal opinion on whether Mrs. Chang should breastfeed or bottle feed her infant.

Case Study 2

Page 293.

What Did Traci Do?

- ❑ Explained to Mrs. Tilley that childhood obesity has increased dramatically in the United States and has become a serious health concern.
- ❑ Told Mrs. Tilley that she could have a big impact on Courtney's life by preparing healthy meals, eating them with her, and by becoming involved in activities with Courtney, such as taking walks.
- ❑ Spent some time talking with Courtney about her interests and complimented Courtney on her achievements.
- ❑ Encouraged Courtney to join the swim team, told her that lots of people do not like to be seen in a swim suit, and encouraged her not to let that stand in her way of doing something she wants to do.
- ❑ Reassured Courtney that the doctor wants to help her and that he would never say anything bad about her weight.

What Did Traci Not Do?

- ❑ Did not agree with Mrs. Tilley that there is nothing that can be done about Courtney's weight problem.
- ❑ Did not tell Courtney that she needs to lose weight or she might develop serious health problems such as diabetes.

Case Study 3

Page 303.

What Did Traci Do?

- ❑ Explained to Stacy that it is rare, but sometimes a child develops polio from getting the oral polio vaccine. Told her that this does not occur with the injectable polio vaccine.
- ❑ Explained to Stacy that chickenpox is usually a mild disease, but it can be serious, especially in young infants and adults.
- ❑ Explained to Stacy that most side effects from immunizations are mild and that complications from the diseases far outweigh the possible side effects.
- ❑ Told Stacy that these diseases have been reduced to very low levels in the United States, but they still occur in other countries. Explained that infected travelers can bring these diseases to the United States and infect individuals who are not immunized.
- ❑ Reminded Stacy that these immunizations are required for Matthew to start kindergarten.
- ❑ Talked with Matthew on his level about why he needs to be immunized.
- ❑ Told Matthew that they would play a game so that it wouldn't hurt as much. Taught him to hold up his finger and pretend that it was a birthday candle; when the injection was given, told him to keep blowing out the candle until he was told to stop.
- ❑ Told Matthew that he could choose a prize from the treasure chest after he had his immunizations.

What Did Traci Not Do?

- ❑ Did not ignore or minimize Stacy's concerns.
- ❑ Did not tell Stacy it would be all right to skip Matthew's immunizations.
- ❑ Did not refer to the immunizations as "shots" when talking with Matthew.
- ❑ Did not tell Matthew that it would not hurt when he gets his immunizations.

TERMINOLOGY REVIEW

Key Term	Word Parts	Definition
Adolescent		An individual 12–18 years old.
Immunity		The resistance of the body to the effects of a harmful agent, such as a pathogenic microorganism and its toxins.
Immunization (active, artificial)		The process of becoming immune or of rendering an individual immune through the use of a vaccine or toxoid.
Infant		A child from birth to 12 months old.

Continued

TERMINOLOGY REVIEW—cont'd

Key Term	Word Parts	Definition
Length (recumbent)		The measurement from the vertex of the head to the heel of the foot of a patient in a supine position.
Pediatrician	*pedi/a:* child	A physician who specializes in the care and development of children and the diagnosis and treatment of children's diseases.
Pediatrics	*pedi/a:* child	The branch of medicine that deals with the care and development of children and the diagnosis and treatment of children's diseases.
Preschool child	*pre-:* in front of; before	A child 3–6 years old.
School-age child		A child 6–12 years old.
Toddler		A child 1–3 years old.
Toxoid		A toxin (a poisonous substance produced by a bacterium) that has been treated by heat or chemicals to destroy its harmful properties. It is administered to an individual to prevent an infectious disease by stimulating the production of antibodies in that individual.
Vaccine		A suspension of attenuated (weakened) or killed microorganisms administered to an individual to prevent an infectious disease by stimulating the production of antibodies in that individual.

PROCEDURE 9.1 Measuring the Weight and Length of an Infant

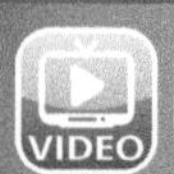

Outcome Measure the weight and length of an infant.

Equipment/Supplies

- Pediatric balance scale (table model)

1. **Procedural Step.** Sanitize your hands.
2. **Procedural Step.** Greet the infant's parent and introduce yourself. Identify the infant and explain the procedure to the parent. The weight of the infant is usually measured first. Depending on the medical office policy, ask the parent to perform one of the following:
   a. Remove the infant's clothing and put a dry diaper on the infant.
   b. Remove the infant's clothing, including the diaper.

   Principle. The infant should not be weighed with a wet diaper because it could increase the infant's weight considerably. Also, growth charts for infants and young children base their percentiles on the weight of the child without clothing.
3. **Procedural Step.** Unlock the pediatric scale, and place a clean paper protector on it. Check the balance scale for accuracy, making sure to compensate for the weight of the paper.

   Principle. The paper protector prevents cross-contamination and reduces the spread of disease from one patient to another.
4. **Procedural Step.** Gently place the infant on his or her back on the table of the scale. Place one hand slightly above the infant as a safety precaution.
5. **Procedural Step.** Balance the scale as follows:
   a. Move the lower weight to the notched groove that does not cause the indicator point to drop to the bottom of the calibration area. Ensure that the lower weight is seated firmly in its groove.
   b. Slowly slide the upper weight along its calibration bar by tapping it gently until the indicator point comes to rest at the center of the balance area.

   Principle. Not seating the lower weight firmly in its groove results in an inaccurate reading.

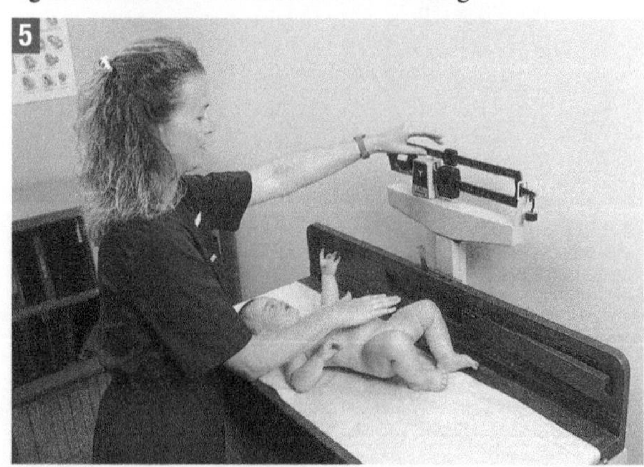

Balance the scale.

PROCEDURE 9.1 Measuring the Weight and Length of an Infant—cont'd

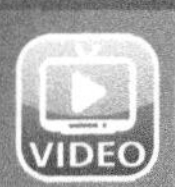

6. Procedural Step. Read the results while the infant is lying still. Jot down this value or make a mental note of it. (*Note:* The result on the pictured scale is 15 lb, 2 oz.)

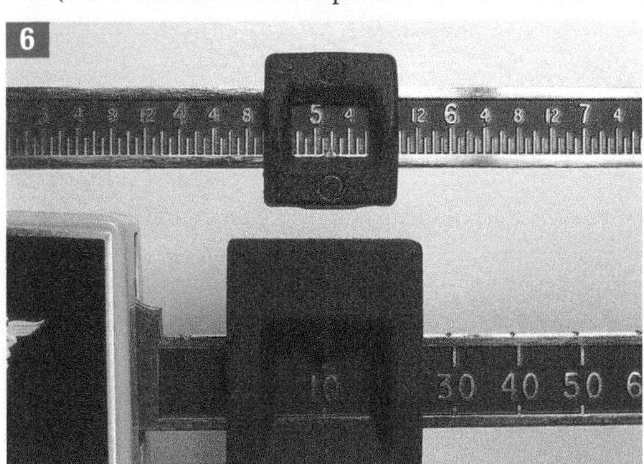

Read the results in pounds and ounces.

7. Procedural Step. Return the balance to its resting position, and lock the scale.

8. Procedural Step. Place the vertex (top) of the infant's head against the headboard at the zero mark. Ask the parent to hold the infant's head in this position.

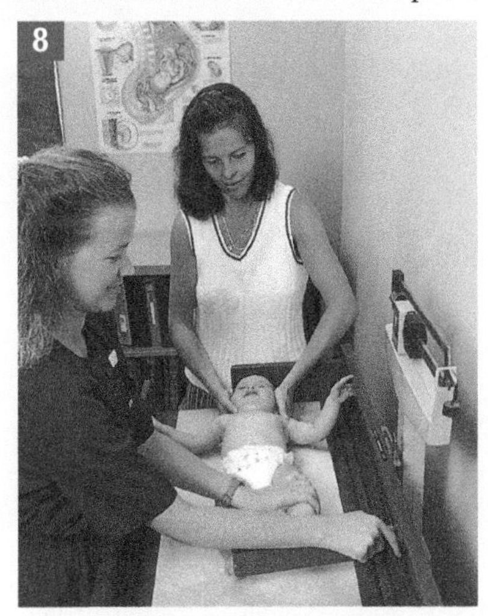

Properly position the infant.

9. Procedural Step. Straighten the infant's knees, and place the soles of his or her feet firmly against the upright footboard (to create a right angle).

10. Procedural Step. Read the infant's length in inches to the nearest ⅛-inch from the measure. Jot down this value or make a mental note of it. (*Note:* The result on this scale is 25½ inches.)

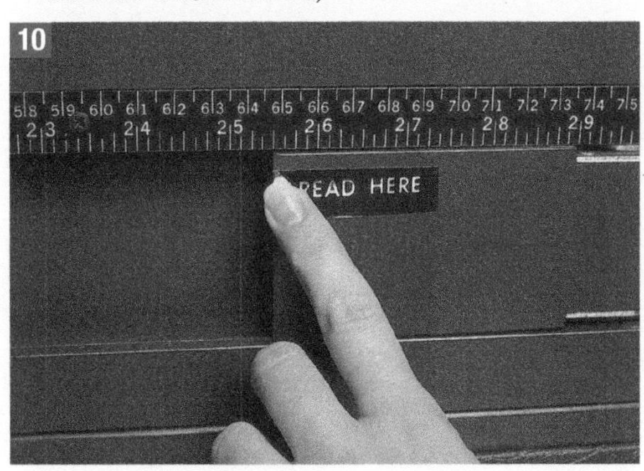

Read the length in inches.

11. Procedural Step. Gently remove the infant from the table, and hand him or her to the parent. Return the headboard and footboard to their resting positions.

12. Procedural Step. Sanitize your hands.

13. Procedural Step. Document the results in the patient's medical record.

a. *Electronic health record (EHR):* Document the infant's weight and length measurements using the appropriate radio buttons, drop-down menus, and free text fields. The electronic medical record will automatically calculate the child's growth percentiles and plot them on a growth chart once you enter the infant's weight and length measurements into the computer.

b. *Paper-based patient record (PPR):* Document the date and time and the infant's weight and length measurements (refer to the PPR documentation example).

PPR Documentation Example

Date	
8/10/XX	9:30 a.m. Wt. 15 lbs. 2 oz. Length 25 1/2 in.
	______________ T. Powell, CMA (AAMA)

PROCEDURE 9.1

PROCEDURE 9.2 Measuring Head and Chest Circumference of an Infant

Outcome Measure the head and chest circumference of an infant.

Equipment/Supplies

- Flexible nonstretch tape measure

Measurement of Head Circumference

1. **Procedural Step.** Sanitize your hands, and assemble the equipment.
2. **Procedural Step.** Greet the infant's parent and introduce yourself. Identify the infant and explain the procedure to the parent.
3. **Procedural Step.** Position the infant. The infant should be placed on his or her back on the examining table. An alternative position is to have the parent hold the infant.
4. **Procedural Step.** Position the tape measure around the infant's head at the greatest circumference. This is usually accomplished by placing the tape slightly above the eyebrows and pinna of the ears and around the occipital prominence at the back of the skull.

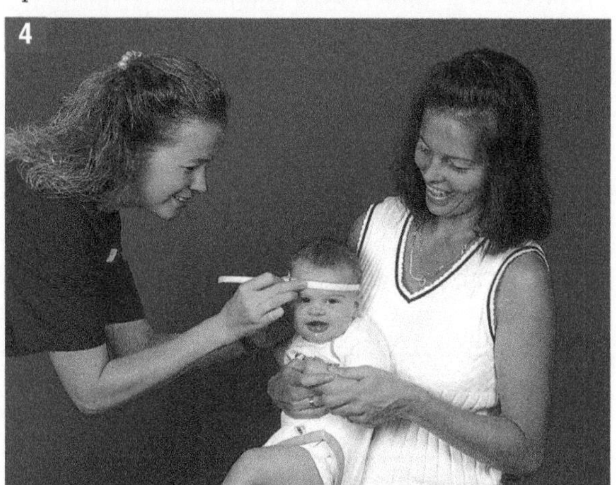

Position the tape measure around the infant's head.

5. **Procedural Step.** Read the results in centimeters (or inches) to the nearest 0.5 cm (or ¼ inch). Jot down this value or make a mental note of it. Sanitize your hands.
6. **Procedural Step.** Document the results in the patient's medical record.
   a. *Electronic health record (EHR):* Document the infant's head circumference measurement using the appropriate radio buttons, drop-down menus, and free text fields. The electronic medical record will automatically calculate the child's head circumference percentile and plot it on a growth chart once you enter the infant's head circumference measurement into the computer.
   b. *Paper-based patient record:* Document the date and time and the infant's head circumference measurement in centimeters (refer to the PPR documentation example).

PPR Documentation Example

Date	
8/10/XX	10:00 a.m. Head circumference: 42.5 cm. ___
	________________T. Powell, CMA (AAMA)

Measurement of Chest Circumference

1. **Procedural Step.** Sanitize your hands, and assemble the equipment.
2. **Procedural Step.** Greet the infant's parent and introduce yourself. Identify the infant and explain the procedure to the parent.
3. **Procedural Step.** Position the infant on his or her back on the examining table.
4. **Procedural Step.** Encircle the tape around the infant's chest at the nipple line. It should be snug, but not so tight that it leaves a mark.

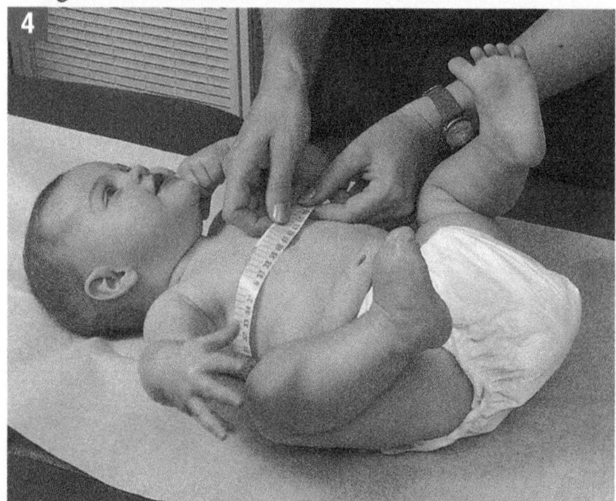

Encircle the tape around the infant's chest.

5. **Procedural Step.** Read the results in centimeters (or inches) to the nearest 0.5 cm (or ¼-inch). Jot down this value or make a mental note of it. Sanitize your hands.
6. **Procedural Step.** Document the results in the patient's medical record.
   a. *Electronic health record (EHR):* Document the infant's chest circumference measurement using the appropriate radio buttons, drop-down menus, and free text fields.
   b. *Paper-based patient record:* Document the date and time and the infant's chest circumference measurement in centimeters (refer to the PPR documentation example).

PPR Documentation Example

Date	
8/15/XX	10:00 a.m. Chest circumference: 42 cm. ___
	________________T. Powell, CMA (AAMA)

PROCEDURE 9.3 Calculating Growth Percentiles

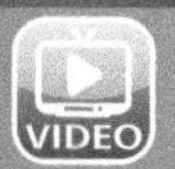

Outcome Plot a pediatric growth value on a growth chart.

Equipment/Supplies

- Pediatric growth chart

1. **Procedural Step.** Select the proper growth chart.
2. **Procedural Step.** Locate the child's age in the horizontal column at the bottom of the chart.
3. **Procedural Step.** Locate the growth value in the vertical column under the appropriate category (weight, length or stature, and head circumference).
4. **Procedural Step.** Draw an imaginary vertical line from the child's age mark and an imaginary horizontal line from the child's growth mark. Find the site at which the two lines intersect on the graph, and place a dot on this site.

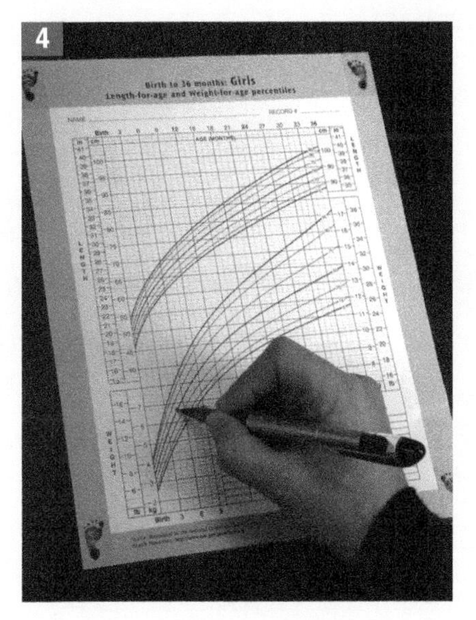

5. **Procedural Step.** To determine the percentile in which the child falls, follow the curved percentile line upward to read the value located on the right side of the chart. Interpolation is needed if the value does not fall exactly on a percentile line. (*Interpolation* means that you must estimate a percentile that falls between a larger and a smaller known percentile.)
6. **Procedural Step.** Document the results in the patient's medical record. Include the date and time and each growth percentile. (Refer to the PPR documentation example).

   In a medical office that uses an electronic health record, the growth percentiles are automatically calculated when you enter the child's weight, length, and head circumference measurements into the computer. The growth percentiles are plotted and displayed on an electronic growth chart that is maintained as part of the child's electronic record.

PPR Documentation Example

Date	
10/22/XX	10:30 a.m. Weight: 55%. Length: 70%.______
	Head Circum: 67% ——T. Powell, CMA (AAMA)

PROCEDURE 9.3 Calculating Growth Percentiles—cont'd

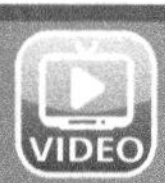

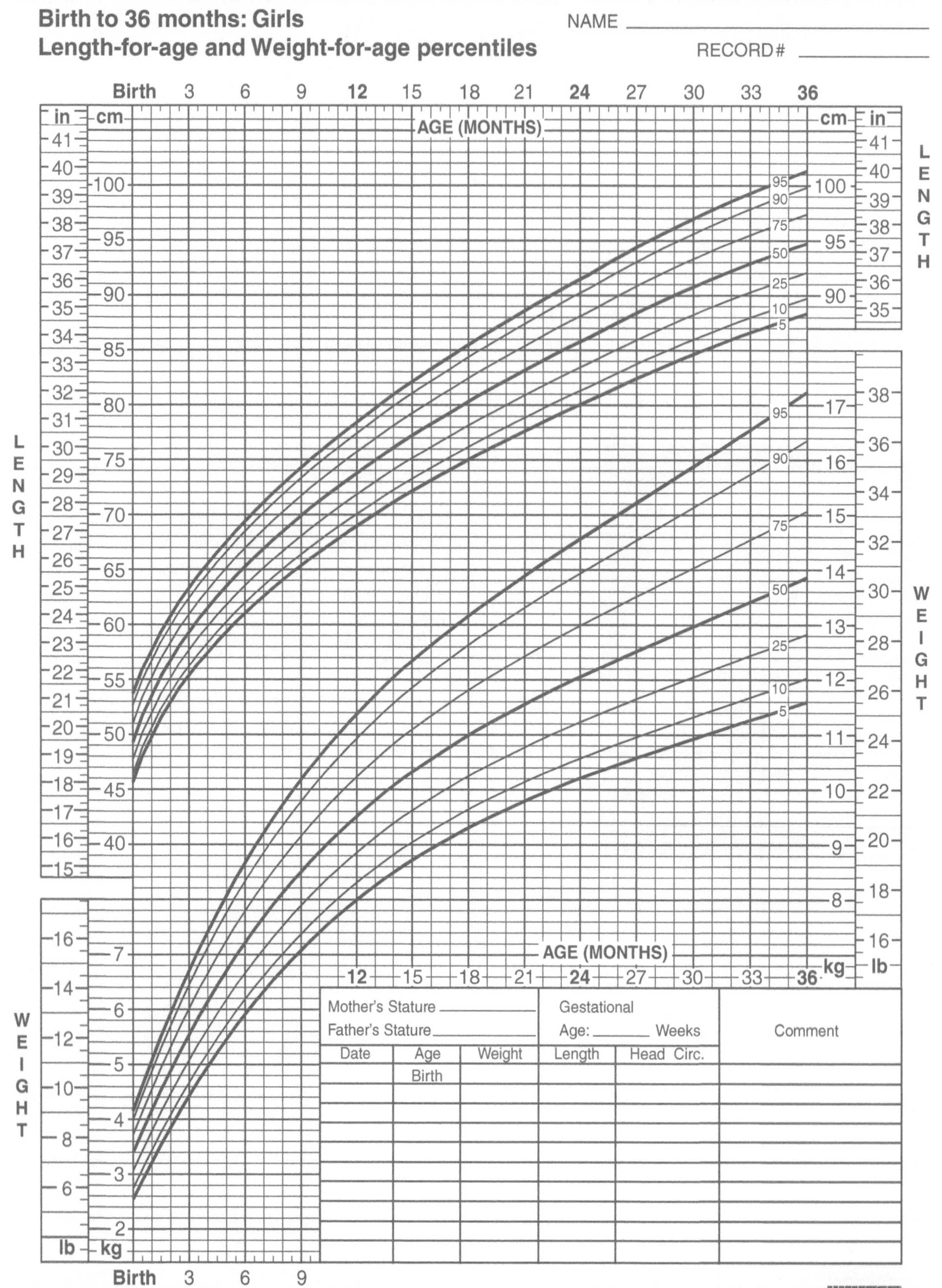

Published May 30, 2000 (modified 4/20/01).
SOURCE: Developed by the National Center for Health Statistics in collaboration with the National Center for Chronic Disease Prevention and Health Promotion (2000).
http://www.cdc.gov/growthcharts

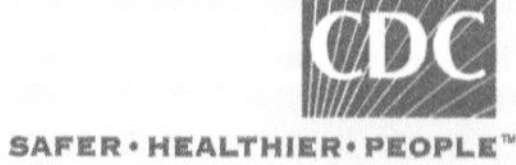

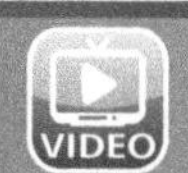

PROCEDURE 9.3 Calculating Growth Percentiles—cont'd

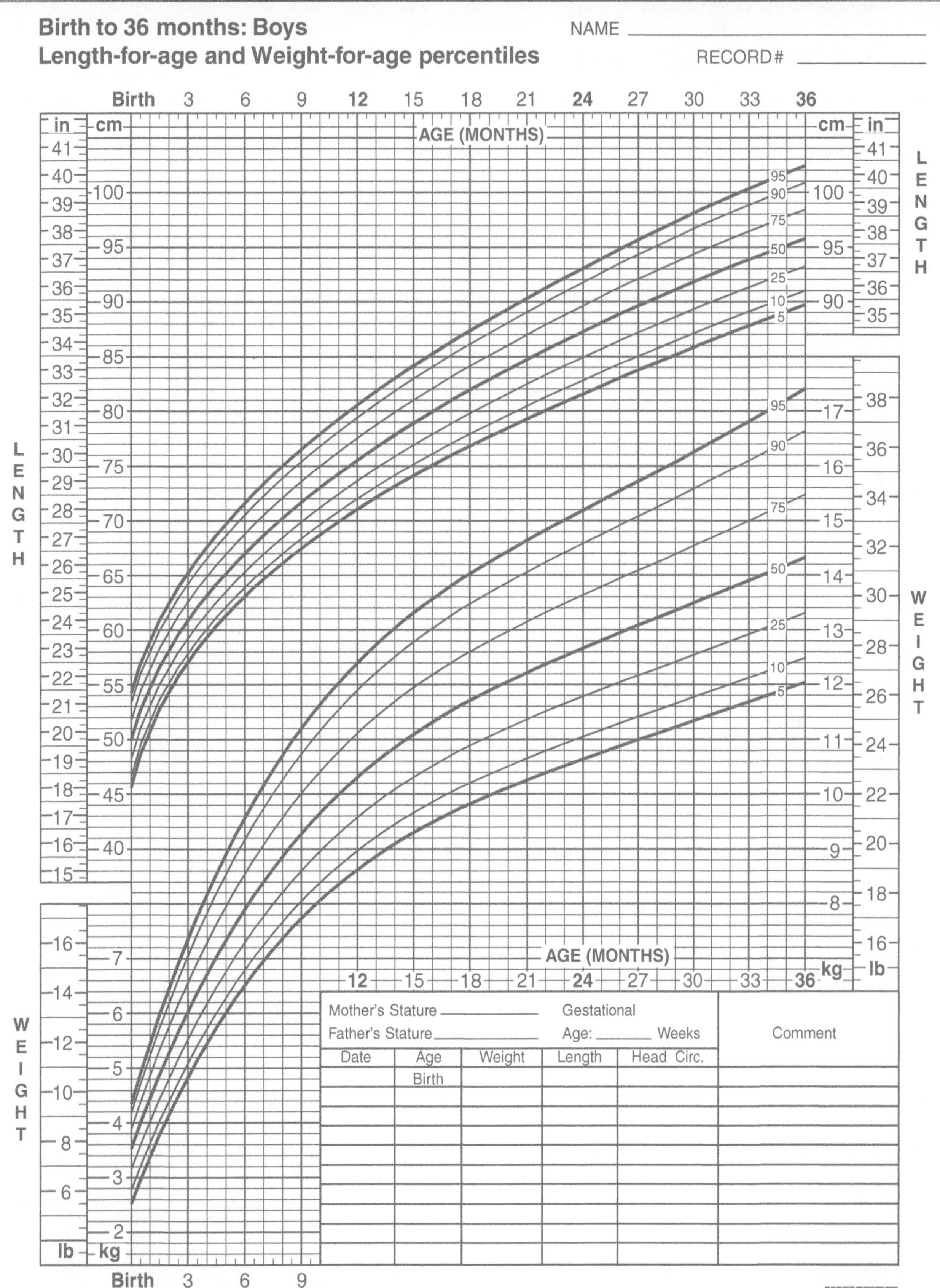

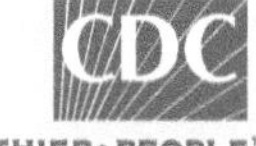

PROCEDURE 9.3

PROCEDURE 9.4 Applying a Pediatric Urine Collector

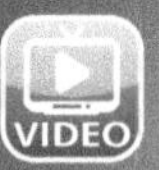

Outcome Apply a pediatric urine collector.

Equipment/Supplies

- Disposable gloves
- Personal antiseptic wipes
- Pediatric urine collector bag
- Urine specimen container and label
- Regular waste container

1. **Procedural Step.** Sanitize your hands.
2. **Procedural Step.** Assemble the equipment.
3. **Procedural Step.** Greet the infant's parent and introduce yourself. Identify the infant and explain the procedure to the parent.
4. **Procedural Step.** Apply gloves. Position the child. The child should be placed on his or her back with the legs spread apart. The medical assistant may need another individual to hold the child's legs apart.
   Principle. This position facilitates cleansing of the genitalia and permits proper application of the urine collector bag.
5. **Procedural Step.** Cleanse the child's genitalia.
   Female: Using a front-to-back motion (pubis to anus), cleanse each side of the meatus with a separate wipe. With a third wipe, cleanse directly down the middle (directly over the urinary meatus). Discard each wipe after cleansing. Allow the area to dry completely.
   Male: If the child is not circumcised, retract the foreskin of the penis. Cleanse the area around the meatus and the urethral opening (meatal orifice) in a manner similar to that used to cleanse the female patient. Use a separate wipe for each swipe. Cleanse the scrotum last, using a fresh wipe. Discard each wipe after cleansing. Allow the area to dry completely.
   Principle. The urinary meatus and surrounding area must be cleansed to prevent contaminants, such as baby powder, fecal material, and microorganisms, from entering the urine specimen, which could affect the test results. A front-to-back motion must be used to prevent drawing microorganisms from the anal area into the area being cleansed. The area must be completely dry to ensure an airtight adhesion of the collection bag to prevent leakage of urine.
6. **Procedural Step.** Remove the paper backing from the urine collector bag. This exposes the hypoallergenic adhesive surface around the opening of the bag. Firmly attach the bag in the following manner:
   Female: Stretch the perineum taut, and firmly place the bottom of the adhesive surface on the infant's perineum. Starting at the perineum and working upward, firmly press the adhesive surface to the skin surrounding the external genitalia, ensuring there is no puckering. The opening of the bag should be directly over the urinary meatus. The excess of the bag should be positioned toward the child's feet.
   Male: Position the bag so that the child's penis and scrotum are projected through the opening of the bag. Starting at the perineum and working upward, firmly press the adhesive surface to the skin surrounding the penis and scrotum, ensuring there is no puckering. The excess of the bag should be positioned toward the child's feet.
   Principle. The adhesive surface of the bag must be attached securely with no puckering to prevent leakage.

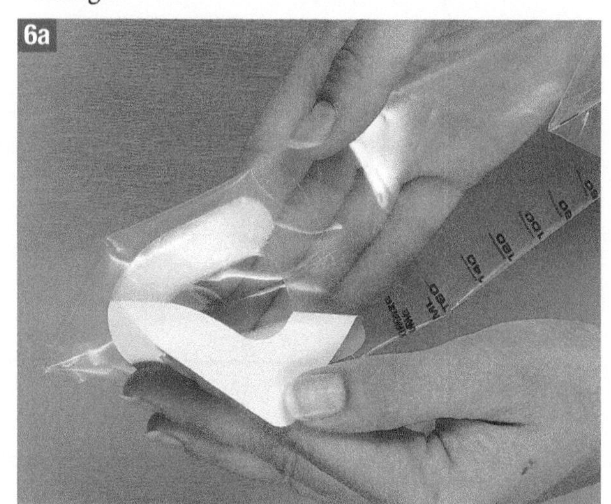

Remove paper backing from the urine collector bag.

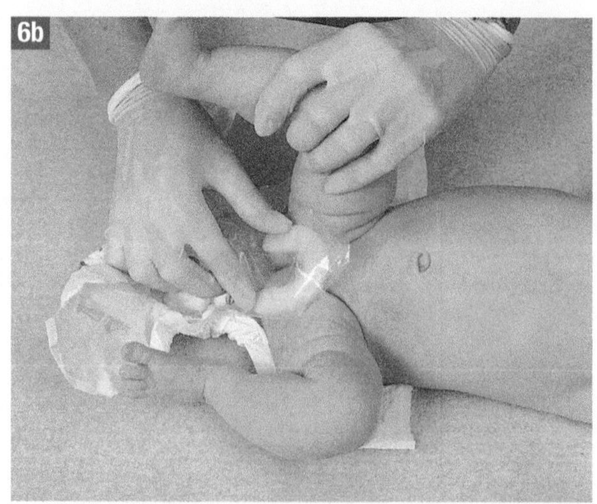

Firmly press the adhesive surface to the skin surrounding the external genitalia.

PROCEDURE 9.4 Applying a Pediatric Urine Collector—cont'd

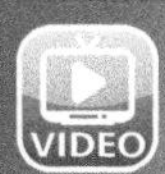

6c

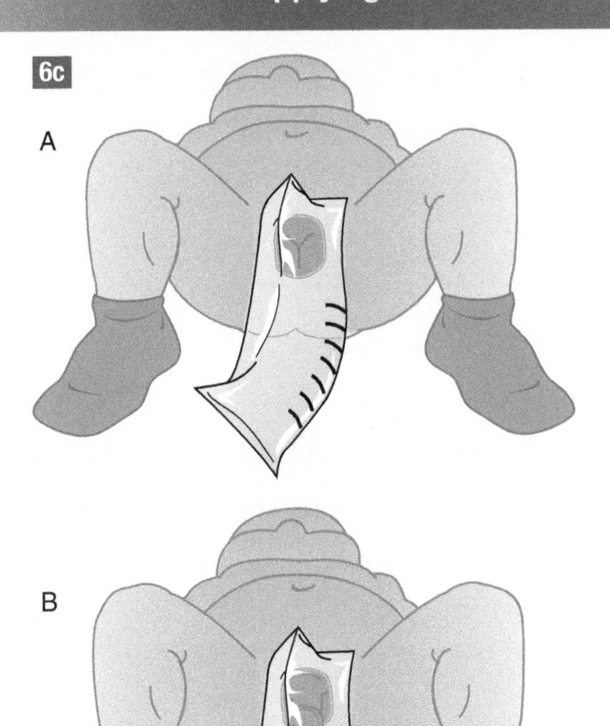

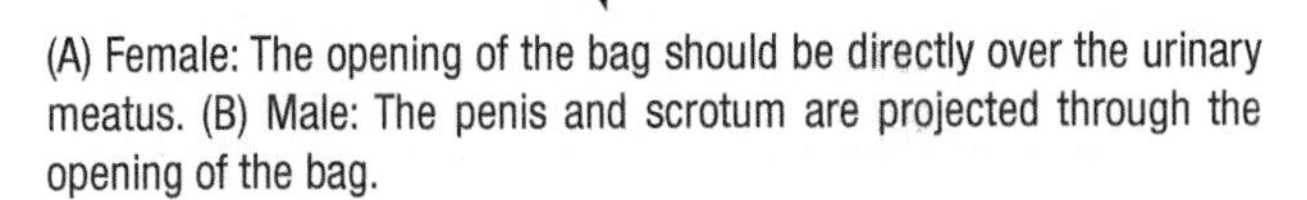

(A) Female: The opening of the bag should be directly over the urinary meatus. (B) Male: The penis and scrotum are projected through the opening of the bag.

7. **Procedural Step.** Loosely diaper the child. Check the urine collector bag every 15 minutes until a urine specimen is obtained.
   Principle. The diaper helps hold the urine collector bag in place. The bag must be checked frequently. Once the infant has urinated, moisture from the urine may cause the adhesive surface to become loose and leak, especially with an active infant.
8. **Procedural Step.** When the child has voided, gently remove the urine collector bag by holding the bottom of the adhesive surface against the infant's skin and carefully peeling the bag off from the top to the bottom.
   Principle. The bag must be removed gently because pulling the adhesive away too quickly may cause discomfort and irritation of the child's skin.
9. **Procedural Step.** Cleanse the genital area with a personal antiseptic wipe. Rediaper the child.
10. **Procedural Step.** Transfer the urine specimen into a urine specimen container, and tightly apply the lid. Label the container with the child's name and date of birth, the date, the time of collection, and the type of specimen (i.e., urine). Dispose of the collector bag in a regular waste container. (*Note:* The urine collector bag can be used as a urine container to transport the specimen to the laboratory. This is accomplished by folding the adhesive sponge ring in half along its vertical axis and pressing the adhesive surfaces firmly together to ensure a tight seal.)
11. **Procedural Step.** Based on the medical office routine, test the urine specimen or prepare it for transfer to an outside laboratory; be sure to include a completed laboratory request form. If the specimen cannot be tested or transferred immediately, preserve it by placing it in the refrigerator.
    Principle. Changes occur in a urine specimen that is left sitting out at room temperature, which can lead to inaccurate test results.
12. **Procedural Step.** Remove the gloves, and sanitize your hands.
13. **Procedural Step.** Document the procedure in the patient's medical record.
    a. *Electronic health record (EHR):* Document the type of specimen (i.e., urine) and the testing that was completed, using the appropriate radio buttons, drop-down menus, and free text fields. If the specimen is to be transported to an outside laboratory, document this information, including the laboratory tests ordered.
    b. *Paper-based patient record:* Document the date, the time of collection, and the type of specimen (i.e., urine). If the specimen is to be transported to an outside laboratory, document this information, including the laboratory tests ordered (refer to the PPR documentation example).

PPR Documentation Example

Date	
8/12/XX	10:15 a.m. Urine specimen collected for
	culture. Picked up by Medical Center Lab on
	8/12/XX.__________T. Powell, CMA (AAMA)

PROCEDURE 9.5 Newborn Screening Test

Outcome Collect a capillary blood specimen for a newborn screening test.

Equipment/Supplies:

- Disposable gloves
- Infant heel warmer or warm compress
- Antiseptic wipe
- Sterile 2 × 2 gauze pad
- Sterile lancet
- Adhesive bandage
- Newborn screening test card
- Mailing envelope
- Biohazard sharps container

1. **Procedural Step.** Sanitize your hands, and assemble the equipment.

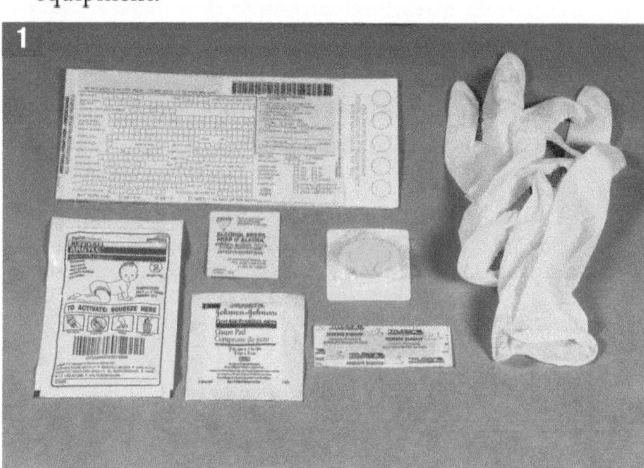

Assemble the equipment.

2. **Procedural Step.** Greet the infant's parent and introduce yourself. Identify the infant and explain the procedure to the parent.
3. **Procedural Step.** Complete the information section of the newborn screening card.
4. **Procedural Step.** Select an appropriate puncture site. The fleshy part of the lateral and medial posterior curves of the plantar surface of the heel can be used.
   Principle. The fleshy lateral and medial posterior curves of the heel are used to avoid calcaneal complications such as inflammation of the bone caused by penetrating the bone with the lancet.

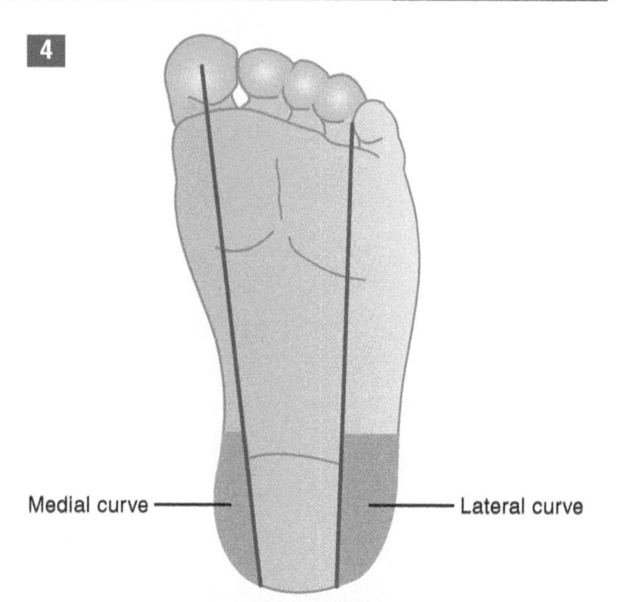

Plantar surface of the heel.

5. **Procedural Step.** Warm the puncture site with a commercially available infant heel warmer or a warm compress for approximately 5 minutes.
   Principle. Warming the puncture site increases capillary circulation and promotes bleeding.

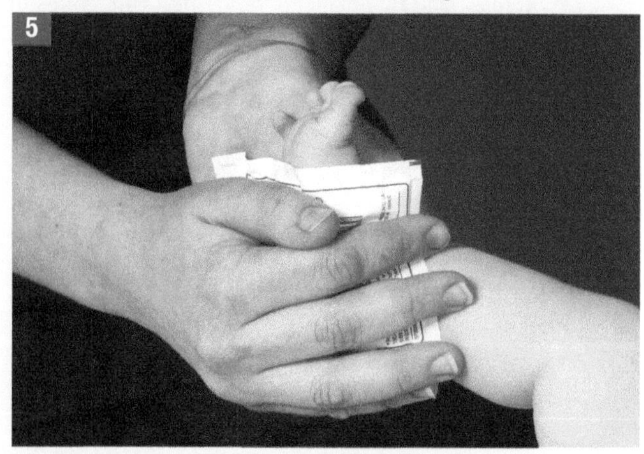

Warm the puncture site.

6. **Procedural Step.** Cleanse the puncture site with an antiseptic wipe, and allow it to air dry. Do not wipe the area with gauze to speed the drying process.

Principle. The site must be allowed to air dry to give the alcohol enough time to destroy microorganisms. If the site is wet, the patient will feel a stinging sensation when the puncture is made.

7. **Procedural Step.** Apply gloves. Grasp the infant's foot around the puncture site, and, without touching the cleansed site, make a puncture with the sterile lancet. The puncture should be made at a right angle to the lines of the skin. Dispose of the lancet in a biohazard sharps container.
Principle. Touching the site after cleansing would contaminate it, and the cleansing process would have to be repeated.

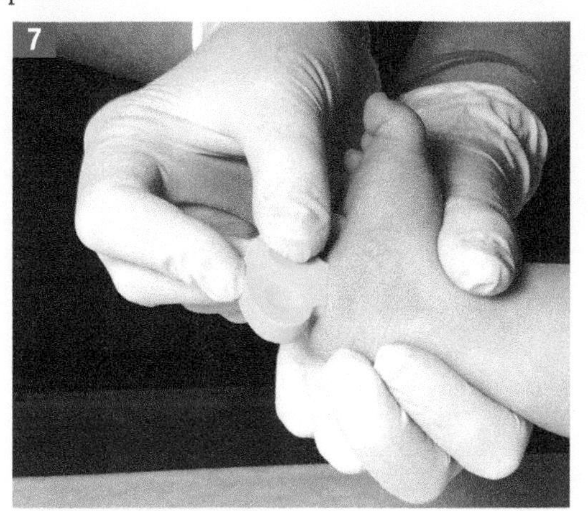

Grasp the infant's foot and make the puncture.

8. **Procedural Step.** Wipe away the first drop of blood with a gauze pad.
Principle. The first drop of blood is diluted with alcohol and tissue fluid and is not a suitable specimen.

9. **Procedural Step.** Encourage a large drop of blood to form by exerting gentle pressure without excessively squeezing the area. Place one side of the filter paper next to the infant's heel. Touch the drop of blood to the center of the first circle on the test card, and completely fill the first circle with the blood specimen. The proper amount of specimen is obtained when the blood can be observed soaking completely through the filter paper from one side to the other.
Principle. Excessive squeezing would cause dilution of the blood sample with tissue fluid, leading to inaccurate test results.

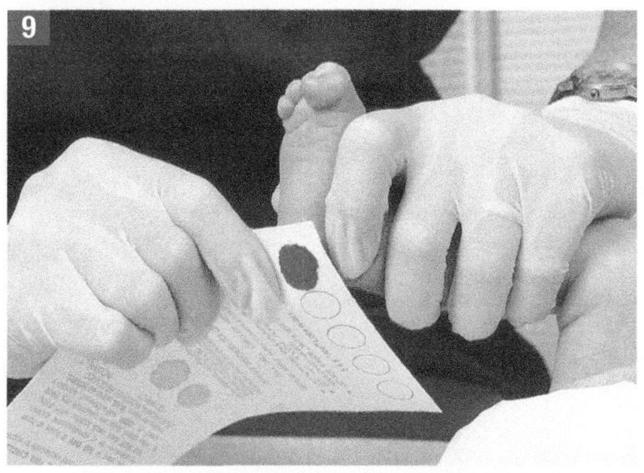

Completely fill the circle with the blood specimen.

10. **Procedural Step.** Repeat Procedure Step 9 until all the circles on the card are completely filled with blood. Be careful not to touch the blood specimens on the card with your gloved hand.
Principle. The circles must be completely filled to ensure enough of a blood sample to perform the test. Most repeat tests are required because of inadequate specimen collection. Touching the blood specimen could lead to inaccurate test results.

11. **Procedural Step.** Hold a piece of gauze over the puncture site, and apply pressure to control the bleeding. Remain with the infant until the bleeding stops. If needed, apply an adhesive bandage.

12. **Procedural Step.** Remove the gloves, and sanitize your hands.

13. **Procedural Step.** Allow the test card to air dry in a horizontal position for at least 3 h at room temperature on a nonabsorbent surface. Do not allow the wet blood specimen to come in contact with any other surface. Do not expose the test card to heat, moisture, or direct sunlight. Do not place the specimen in a biohazard specimen bag or any other type of plastic bag.
Principle. Placing the test card in a plastic bag interferes with proper drying of the specimen.

14. **Procedural Step.** After the blood is completely dry, place the test card in its protective envelope, and mail it to an outside laboratory for testing within 48 h.
Principle. The test card should be mailed within 48 h to ensure accurate test results.

15. **Procedural Step.** Document the procedure in the patient's medical record.
    a. *Electronic health record (EHR):* Document the date and time, the type of procedure, the puncture site location, and information regarding transfer to an outside laboratory, using the appropriate radio buttons, drop-down menus, and free text fields.
    b. *Paper-based patient record:* Document the date and time, the type of procedure, the puncture site location, and information regarding transfer to an outside laboratory (refer to the PPR documentation example).

PPR Documentation Example

Date	
8/15/XX	9:30 a.m. Blood specimen collected from
	(R) medial heel. Sent to Newborn Screening
	Lab on 8/15/XX for newborn screening test.
	________________T. Powell, CMA (AAMA)

Minor Office Surgery

 Check out the Evolve site at http://evolve.elsevier.com/Bonewit/today/ to access additional interactive activities and exercises to help you study and prepare for success.

LEARNING OUTCOMES

Surgical Asepsis
1. State the characteristics of a minor surgical procedure.
2. Identify procedures that require the use of surgical asepsis.
3. Describe the medical assistant's responsibilities during a minor surgical procedure.
4. List the guidelines to follow to maintain surgical asepsis during a sterile procedure.
5. Identify surgical instruments commonly used in the medical office and explain the use and care of each instrument.

Wound Healing
6. Explain the differences between a closed and an open wound and give examples.
7. List and explain the three phases of the healing process.
8. List and describe the different types of wound exudates.
9. List the functions of a dressing.

Methods of Wound Closure
10. Explain the method used to measure the diameter of suturing material.
11. Describe the two types of sutures (absorbable and nonabsorbable) and give examples of their uses.
12. Categorize suturing needles according to type of point and shape.
13. State the advantages and wound care instructions for each of the following wound closure methods: sutures, surgical skin staples, topical tissue adhesives, and skin closure tape.

Medical Office Surgical Procedures
14. Explain the purpose of and procedure for each of the following minor surgical operations: sebaceous cyst removal, incision and drainage of a localized infection, mole removal, needle biopsy, ingrown toenail removal, colposcopy, cervical punch biopsy, and cryosurgery.
15. Explain the principles underlying each step in the minor office surgery procedures.

Bandaging
16. State the functions of a bandage, and list the guidelines for applying a bandage.
17. Identify the common types of bandages used in the medical office.

PROCEDURES

Apply and remove sterile gloves.
Open a sterile package.
Add an article to a sterile field.
Pour a sterile solution.

Change a sterile dressing.

Set up a tray for suture insertion.
Remove sutures.
Remove surgical staples.
Assist the provider with the application of a topical tissue adhesive.
Apply and remove skin closure tape.

Assist the physician with minor office surgery.

Apply each of the following bandage turns:
- Circular
- Spiral
- Spiral-reverse
- Figure-eight
- Recurrent

CHAPTER OUTLINE

KEY TERMS

abrasion (ah-BRAY-shun)
abscess (AB-sess)
absorbable suture (ab-SOR-ba-bul SOO-chur)
approximation (ah-PROKS-ih-MAY-shun)
bandage
biopsy (BYE-op-see)
capillary action (KAP-ill-air-ee AK-shun)
colposcope (KOL-poh-skope)
colposcopy (kol-POS-koh-pee)
contaminate (kon-TAM-in-ate)
contusion (kon-TOO-shun)
cryosurgery (KRY-oh-SURJ-er-ee)
exudate (EKS-oo-date)
fibroblast (FYE-broh-blast)
forceps (FORE-seps)
furuncle (FYOOR-un-kul)
hemostasis (hee-moe-STAY-sis)
incision (in-SIH-shun)
infection (in-FEK-shun)
infiltration (in-fill-TRAY-shun)
inflammation (in-flah-MAY-shun)
laceration (lass-ur-AY-shun)
ligate (LIH-gate)
local anesthetic (LOE-kul an-es-STET-ik)
Mayo (MAY-oe) tray
needle biopsy (NEE-dul BYE-op-see)
nonabsorbable suture (non-ab-SOR-ba-bul SOO-chur)
postoperative (post-OP-er-uh-tiv)
preoperative (pree-OP-er-uh-tiv)
puncture (PUNK-shur)
scalpel (SKAL-pul)
scissors
sebaceous cyst (suh-BAY-shus SIST)
serum (SEER-um)
sterile (STARE-ul)
surgery
surgical asepsis (SUR-jih-kul ay-SEP-sis)
sutures (SOO-churz)
swaged (SWAYJD) needle
wound

Introduction to Minor Office Surgery

The term **surgery** is defined as the branch of medicine that deals with operative and manual procedures for correction of deformities and defects, repair of injuries, and diagnosis and treatment of certain diseases. *Minor office surgery* (also known as *minor surgery*) refers to a surgical procedure that is restricted to the management of minor conditions and injuries that does not require the use of general anesthesia. Minor surgical procedures have the following characteristics:

- Are performed in an ambulatory health care facility, such as a physician's office or clinic
- Can be performed in a short period of time, usually in less than 1 hour
- Require a local anesthetic, a topical anesthetic, or no anesthetic

- Can be performed safely with a minimum of discomfort to the patient
- Do not, under normal circumstances, pose a major risk to life or to the function of an organ or body parts.

Various types of minor surgical operations are performed in the medical office, such as insertion of sutures, sebaceous cyst removal, incision and drainage of infections, mole removal, needle biopsies, cervical biopsies, and ingrown toenail removal. The physician explains the nature of the surgical procedure and any risks to the patient and offers to answer questions. The medical assistant is responsible for **preoperative** instructions (e.g., explaining the patient preparation required for the procedure) and for obtaining the patient's signature on a written consent to treatment form, thus granting the physician permission to perform the surgery (Fig. 10.1).

Additional responsibilities of the medical assistant include preparing the treatment room, preparing the patient, preparing the minor surgery tray, assisting the physician during the procedure, administering **postoperative** care to the patient, and cleaning the treatment room after the procedure.

The treatment room must be spotlessly clean, and the medical assistant should ensure that the physician has adequate lighting for the procedure. The patient is positioned and draped according to the procedure to be performed. The skin is prepared as specified by the physician. Hair around the operative site is a contaminant and may need to be removed by shaving. The skin is cleansed, and an appropriate antiseptic is applied to the area to reduce the number of microorganisms present.

The medical assistant prepares the minor surgery tray using a **sterile** technique. The specific instruments and supplies included in each setup vary depending on the type of surgery to be performed and the physician's preference. The medical assistant must become familiar with the instruments and supplies required for each surgical procedure performed in the medical office.

During the minor surgery, the medical assistant is present to assist the physician as needed and to lend support to the patient. The medical assistant should become completely familiar with the assisting techniques (e.g., swabbing blood from the operative site) required for each surgical

(attach label or complete blanks)

First name: ____________ Last name: ____________

Date of Birth: ______ Month ______ Day ______ Year

Account Number: ____________

Procedure Consent Form

I, ______________________________, hereby consent to have

Dr. ____________ perform ______________________________

I have been fully informed of the following by my physician:

1. The nature of my condition.
2. The nature and purpose of the procedure.
3. An explanation of risks involved with the procedure.
4. Alternative treatments or procedures available.
5. The likely results of the procedure.
6. The risks involved with declining or delaying the procedure.

My physician has offered to answer all questions concerning the proposed procedure.

I am aware that the practice of medicine and surgery is not an exact science, and I acknowledge that no guarantees have been made to me about the results of the procedure.

Patient ______________________ Date ____________
(or guardian and relationship)

Witnessed ______________________ Date ____________

Fig. 10.1 Consent to treatment form.

procedure performed in the medical office and should learn to anticipate the physician's needs to help the procedure go quickly and smoothly.

After the minor surgery, the medical assistant should remain with the patient as a safety precaution to prevent accidental falls and other injuries and to make sure the patient understands the postoperative instructions. The medical assistant removes and properly cares for all used instruments and supplies and cleans the treatment room in preparation for the next patient.

SURGICAL ASEPSIS

Surgical asepsis, also known as *sterile technique,* refers to practices that keep objects and areas sterile, or free from all living microorganisms and spores. Surgical asepsis protects the patient from pathogenic microorganisms that may enter the body and cause disease. It is always employed under the following circumstances: when caring for broken skin, such as open wounds and suture punctures; when a skin surface is being penetrated, as by a surgical incision for a mole removal or the administration of an injection (the needle must remain sterile); and when a body cavity is entered that is normally sterile, such as during the insertion of a urinary catheter. Sterility of instruments and supplies is achieved through the use of disposable sterile items or by sterilizing reusable articles.

A sterile object that touches any unsterile object is automatically considered **contaminated** and must not be used. If the medical assistant is in doubt or has a question concerning the sterility of an article, he or she should consider it contaminated and replace it with a sterile article.

Sterility of the hands cannot be attained. Sanitizing the hands renders them medically aseptic and must be performed before and after every surgical procedure using proper technique (see Chapter 2). To prevent contamination of sterile articles, sterile gloves must be worn while picking up or transferring articles during a sterile procedure. Procedure 10.1 describes the procedure for applying and removing sterile gloves.

Specific guidelines must be observed during a sterile procedure to maintain the sterile field. See Box 10.1, *Guidelines for Maintaining a Sterile Field.*

BOX 10.1 Guidelines for Maintaining a Sterile Field

1. Take precautions to prevent sterile packages from becoming wet. Wet packages draw microorganisms into the package owing to the **capillary action** (the action that causes the liquid to rise along a wick, a tube, or a gauze dressing) of the liquid, resulting in contamination of the sterile package. If a sterile package that has been prepared at the medical office becomes wet, it must be rewrapped and resterilized; if a disposable sterile package becomes wet, it must be discarded.
2. A 1-inch border around the sterile field is considered contaminated or unsterile because this area may have become contaminated while the sterile field was being set up.
3. Always face the sterile field. If you must turn your back to it or leave the room, a sterile towel must be placed over the sterile field.
4. Hold all sterile articles above waist level. Anything out of sight might become contaminated. The sterile articles also should be held in front of you and should not touch your uniform.
5. To avoid contamination, place all sterile items in the center, not around the edges, of the sterile field.
6. Be careful not to spill water or solutions on the sterile field. The area beneath the field is contaminated, and microorganisms are drawn up onto the field by the capillary action of the liquid, resulting in contamination of the field.
7. Do not talk, cough, or sneeze over a sterile field. Water vapor from the nose, mouth, and lungs is carried outward by the air and contaminates the sterile field.
8. Do not reach over a sterile field. Dust or lint from your clothing may fall onto it, or your unsterile clothing may accidentally touch it.
9. Do not pass soiled dressings over the sterile field.
10. Always acknowledge if you have contaminated the sterile field so that proper steps can be taken to regain sterility.

INSTRUMENTS USED IN MINOR OFFICE SURGERY

A variety of surgical instruments are used for minor office surgery. Most instruments are made of stainless steel and have either a bright, highly polished finish or a dull finish. The medical assistant should become familiar with the name, use, and proper care of all instruments used in the medical office. Surgical instruments are named according to one or more of the following: (1) function (e.g., splinter forceps); (2) design (e.g., mosquito hemostatic forceps); and (3) the individual who developed the instrument (e.g., Kelly hemostatic forceps). The parts of an instrument are illustrated in Fig. 10.2; some common instruments are described here and are illustrated in Fig. 10.3.

SCALPELS

A **scalpel** is a small straight surgical knife consisting of a handle and a thin, sharp steel blade. A scalpel is used to make surgical incisions and can divide tissue with the least possible trauma to the surrounding structures. Both disposable and reusable scalpels are available. A disposable scalpel consists of a nonslip plastic handle and a permanently

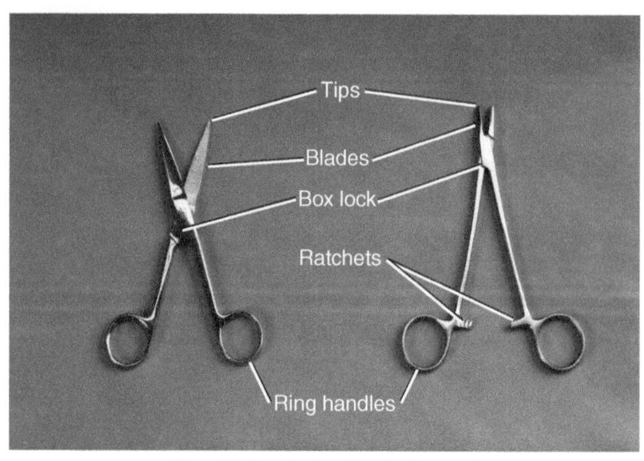

Fig. 10.2 Parts of an instrument.

attached steel blade that is individually packaged to maintain sterility. Scalpels that are reusable consist of a reusable stainless steel handle to which a disposable steel blade is attached. The blade comes individually packaged in a moisture-proof sterile package.

SCISSORS

Scissors are cutting instruments that have ring handles and straight (str) or curved (cvd) blades. Both blade tips may be sharp (s/s), both may be blunt (b/b), or one tip may be blunt and the other sharp (b/s). The two parts of a pair of scissors come together at a hinge joint known as a *box lock* (see Fig. 10.2). The type of scissors employed depends on the intended use. The various types of scissors are listed and described next.

- *Operating scissors* have straight delicate blades with sharp cutting edges and are used to cut through tissue. They are available with sharp/sharp, blunt/blunt, or blunt/sharp blade tips.
- *Suture scissors* are used to remove sutures. The hook on the tip aids in getting under a suture, and the blunt end prevents puncturing of the tissues.
- *Bandage scissors* are inserted beneath a dressing or bandage to cut it for removal. The flat blunt prow can be inserted beneath a dressing without puncturing the skin.
- *Dissecting scissors* have thick beveled blades with a fine cutting edge used to divide or separate tissue rather than cut it. Dissecting scissors are available with straight or curved blades. Both blade tips of dissecting scissors are blunt.

FORCEPS

Forceps are instruments for grasping, squeezing, or holding tissue or an item such as sterile gauze. Some forceps have two prongs and a spring handle (e.g., thumb, tissue, splinter, dressing forceps) that provides the proper tension for grasping an object such as tissue, a foreign object, or sterile gauze. Some forceps have serrations (e.g., thumb and hemostatic forceps), which are sawlike teeth that grasp tissue and prevent it from slipping out of the jaws of the instrument. As is shown in Fig. 10.3, some varieties have toothed clasps on the handle, known as *ratchets* (see Fig. 10.2), to hold the tips securely together and lock them in place (e.g., Allis tissue forceps, hemostatic forceps). The ratchets are designed to allow locked closure of the instrument at two or more positions. The various types of forceps are listed and described next.

- *Thumb forceps* have serrated tips and are used to pick up tissue or to hold tissue between adjacent surfaces.
- *Tissue forceps* have teeth that are used to grasp tissue and prevent it from slipping. Tissue forceps are identified by the number of opposing teeth on each jaw (e.g., 1 × 2, 2 × 3, 3 × 4). Tissue forceps are sometimes referred to as "rat-toothed" forceps because the pointed projections resemble the teeth of a rat. The teeth should approximate tightly when the instrument is closed.
- *Splinter forceps* have sharp points that are useful in removing foreign objects, such as splinters, from the tissues.
- *Dressing forceps* are used in the application and removal of dressings. They are also used to hold or grasp sterile gauze or sutures during a surgical procedure. Dressing forceps have blunt ends that contain coarse cross-striations used for grasping.
- *Hemostatic forceps* have serrated tips, ratchets, ring handles, and box locks and are available with straight or curved blades. Hemostats are used to clamp off blood vessels and to establish **hemostasis** until the vessels can be closed with sutures. The serrations on a hemostat prevent the blood vessel from slipping out of the jaws of the instrument. The ratchets keep the hemostat tightly shut and locked in place when it is closed. The ring handles allow for a secure grasp of the hemostat and also are used to select the desired ratchet position. The serrated blades should mesh together smoothly when the hemostat is closed; if they spring back open, the instrument is in need of repair. *Mosquito hemostatic forceps* have small, fine tips and are smaller and more delicate than standard Kelly hemostatic forceps. Mosquito hemostatic forceps are used to hold delicate tissue or to clamp off smaller blood vessels, whereas standard hemostatic forceps are used to grasp and compress larger blood vessels.
- *Sponge forceps* have ring handles, ratchets, box locks, and large serrated rings on the blade tips for holding sponges. A *sponge* is a porous, absorbent pad, such as a 4-inch gauze pad, used to absorb fluids, apply medication, or cleanse an area.

MISCELLANEOUS INSTRUMENTS

Various miscellaneous instruments used in the medical office are listed and described next.

- *Needle holders* have serrated tips, ring handles, ratchets, and box locks. A needle holder is used to firmly grasp a curved needle for insertion of the needle through the skin flaps of an incision. The serrated tips of a needle holder are designed to hold a curved needle securely without damaging it. A needle holder is sometimes referred to as a "driver" because it functions to "drive" the curved needle through the skin.
- *Retractors* are used to hold tissues aside to improve the exposure of the operative area.

CARE OF SURGICAL INSTRUMENTS

Surgical instruments are expensive, are delicate yet durable, and last for many years if handled and maintained properly. The care an instrument receives depends to a large degree on the parts making up the instrument (e.g., box lock, ratchet, cutting edge, serrations). The medical assistant works with instruments while setting up a sterile tray, performing certain procedures such as suture removal and sterile dressing change, and cleaning up after minor office surgery and during the sanitization and sterilization process. During each

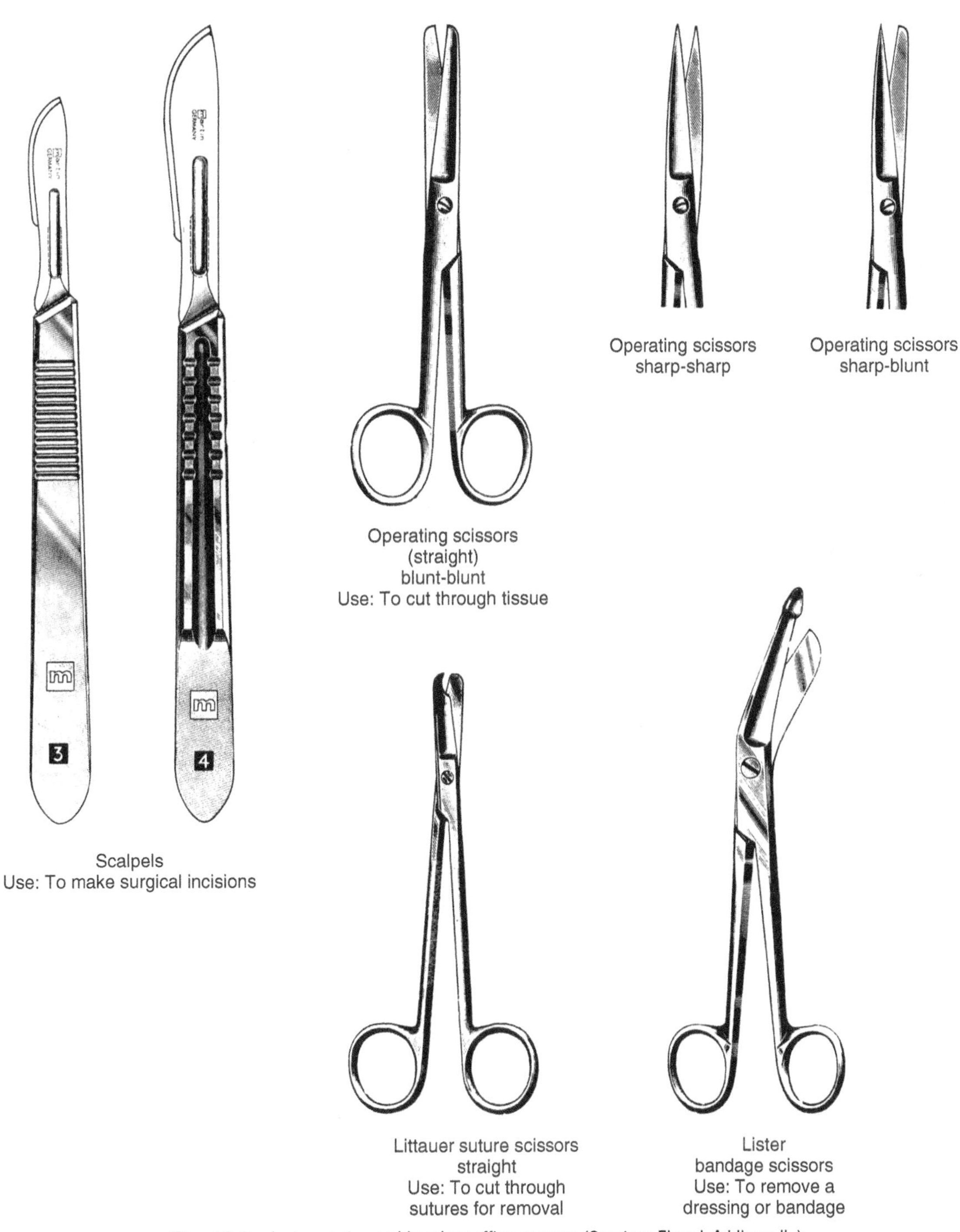

Fig. 10.3 Instruments used in minor office surgery. (Courtesy Elmed, Addison, IL.)

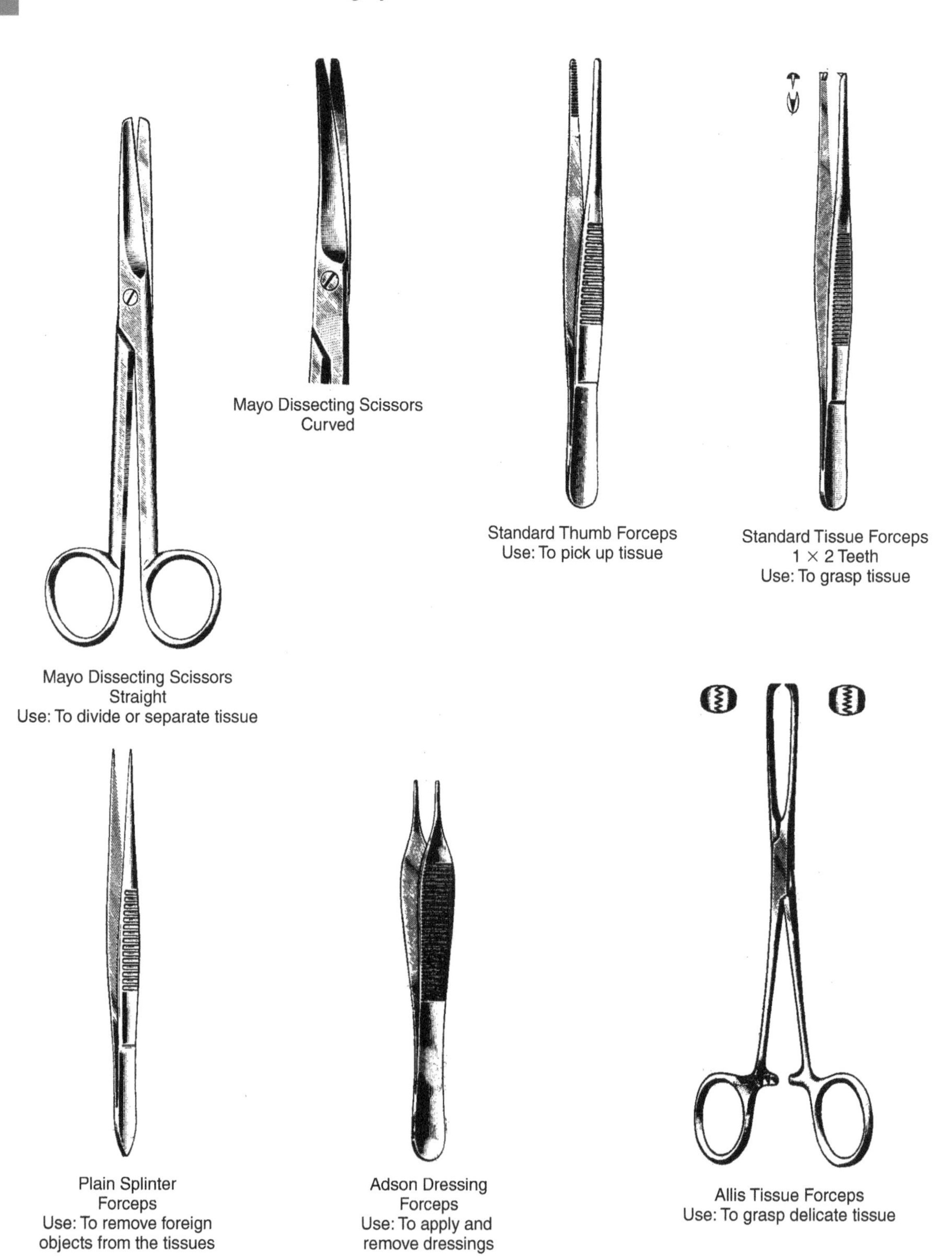

Fig. 10.3 cont'd

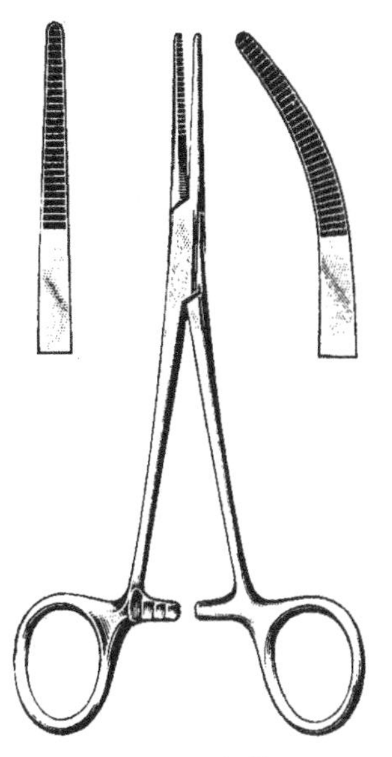

Kelly Hemostatic Forceps
Straight or Curved
Use: To clamp off blood vessels

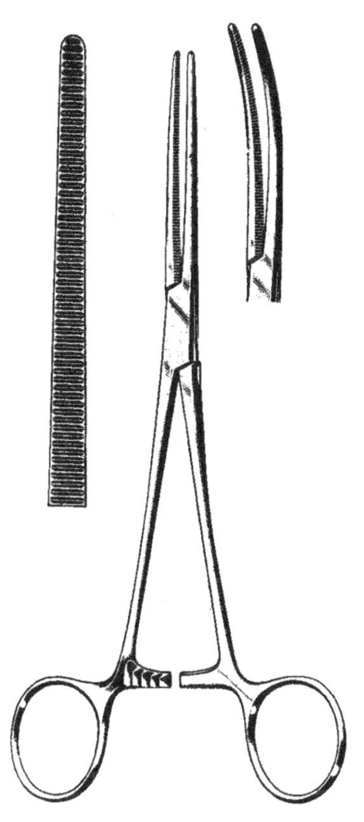

Rochester-Pean Hemostatic Forceps
Straight or Curved

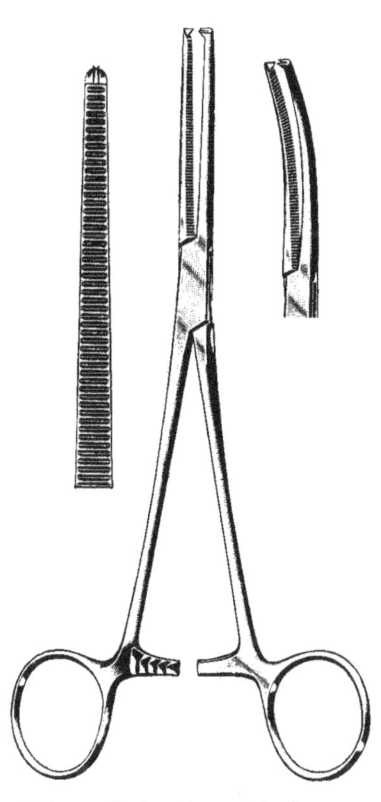

Ochsner-Kocher Hemostatic Forceps
Straight or Curved
1 × 2 Teeth

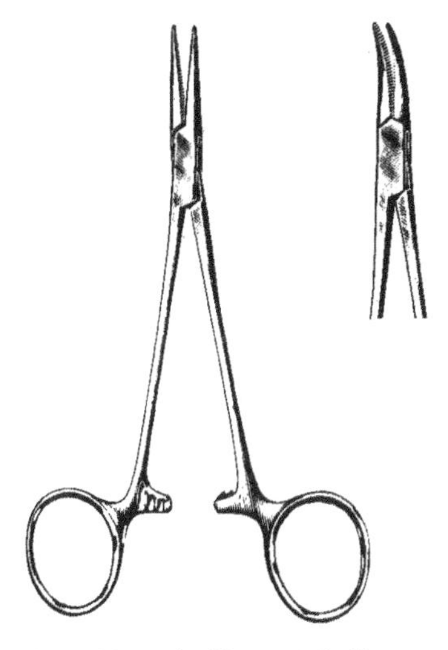

Halsted Mosquito Hemostatic Forceps
Straight and Curved
Use: To hold delicate tissue or to clamp off small blood vessels

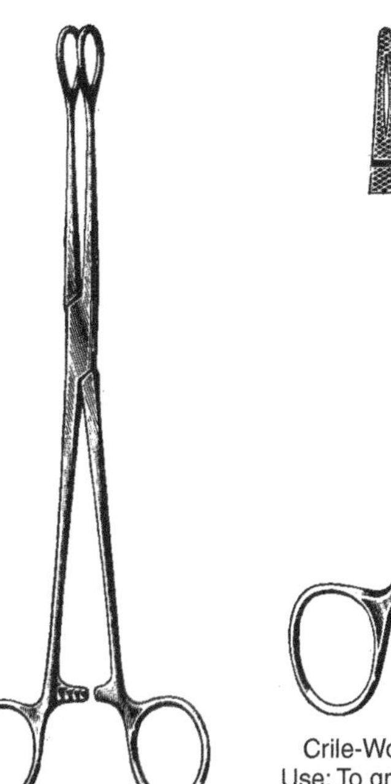

Foerster
Sponge Forceps
Use: To hold a sponge

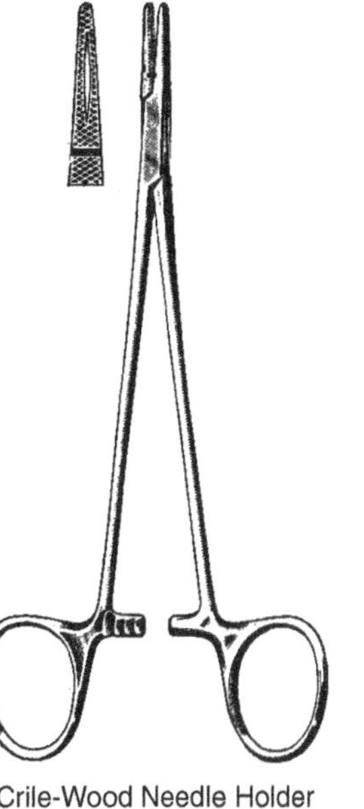

Crile-Wood Needle Holder
Use: To grasp a curved needle

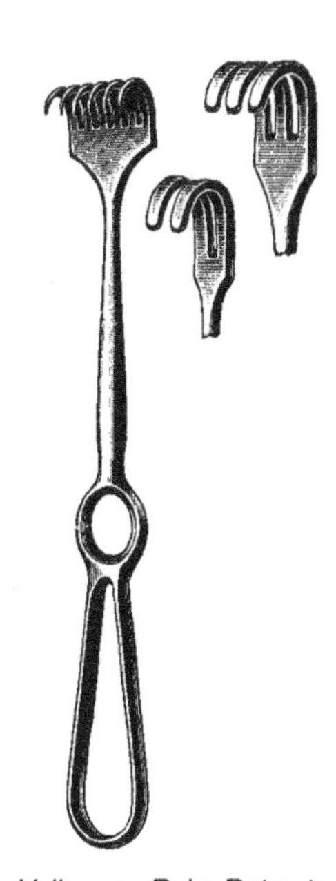

Volkmann Rake Retractor
Use: To hold tissue aside

Fig. 10.3 cont'd

GYNECOLOGIC INSTRUMENTS

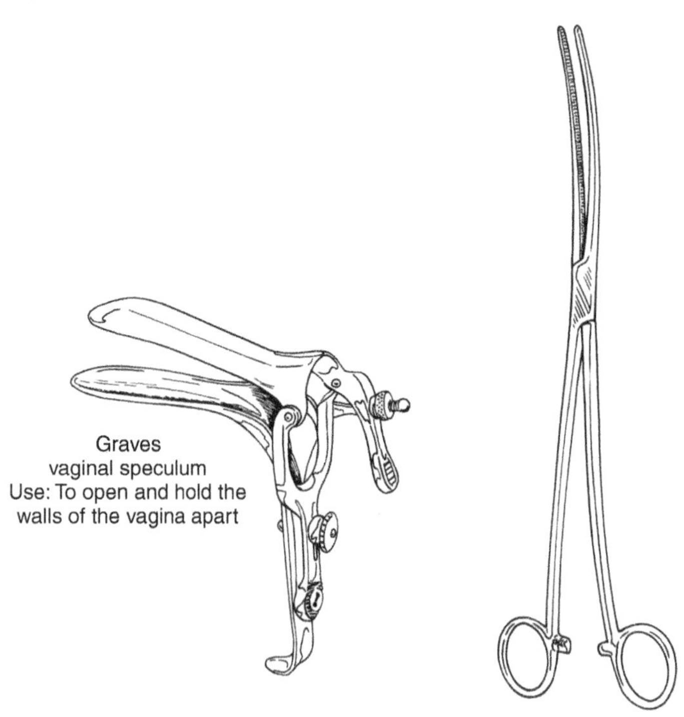

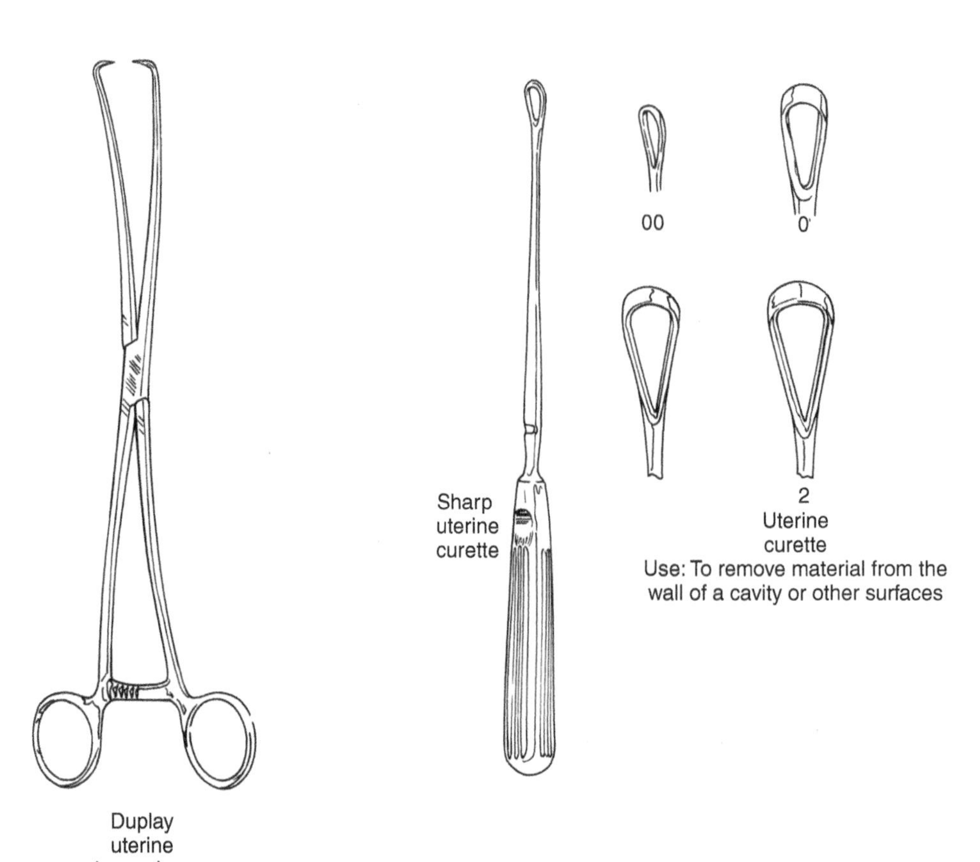

Fig. 10.3 cont'd

of these procedures, guidelines must be followed to prolong the life span of each instrument and to ensure its proper functioning:

1. Always handle instruments carefully. Dropping an instrument on the floor or throwing an instrument into a basin could damage it.
2. Do not pile instruments in a heap because they become entangled and might be damaged when separated.
3. Keep sharp instruments separate from the rest of the instruments to prevent damaging or dulling the cutting edge. Also, keep delicate instruments, such as lensed instruments, separate to protect them from damage.
4. To prolong the proper functioning of the ratchet, keep instruments with a ratchet in an open position when not in use.
5. Rinse blood and body secretions off an instrument as soon as possible to prevent them from drying and hardening on the instrument.
6. When performing procedures that require surgical instruments, always use the instrument for the purpose for which it was designed. Substituting one type of instrument for another could damage it.
7. Sanitize and sterilize instruments using proper technique.

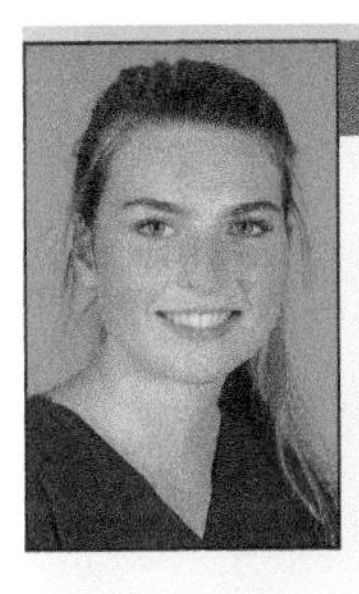

Putting It All Into Practice

My name is Heidi, and I have worked as the office manager of an internal medicine office for the past 7 years. My job includes front and back office duties, including scheduling appointments, transcription, patient calls, patient workups, injections, electrocardiograms, and venipuncture. The most interesting part of my job is dealing with the many different personalities of the patients I come in contact with daily.

A patient who had not been to the clinic for a while came in one day. His graduation from college had been delayed because he had developed a pilonidal cyst that needed to be surgically removed. At onset, these cysts can be very painful and usually require daily cleaning and packing. From my experience with pilonidal cyst care, I knew that 1–2 months of treatment are usually required before full recovery is achieved.

The physician and I prepared for the initial treatment and noticed that the surgical site was very large and deep. We knew this treatment would take much longer than usual. Treatment was provided daily for 3 months. Subsequent treatments continued every other day for 2 months. Through our continuous contact, we became good friends with the patient.

Our patient graduated at the end of the spring quarter and moved out of state. He stays in contact with us and is still undergoing treatment. He made a difference in our lives because he always maintained a positive attitude and was very pleasant, making our job easier. We made a difference in his life through the good health care we provided and our continuing friendship. ■

COMMERCIALLY PREPARED STERILE PACKAGES

Commercially prepared disposable packages are used frequently and may contain one particular article (e.g., sterile dressing) or a complete sterile setup (e.g., one for the removal of sutures). The directions for opening the package are stated on the outside of the package; they should be followed carefully to prevent contamination of the sterile contents. Procedure 10.2 describes opening a sterile package.

One type of commercially prepared package is the peel-apart package (commonly referred to as a *peel-pack*). This type of sterile package has an edge with two flaps that can be pulled apart in the following manner: Grasp each unsterile flap between your bent index finger and extended thumb, and, rolling your hands outward, pull the package apart (Fig. 10.4A). The inside of the wrapper and the contents are sterile, and to prevent contamination, they must not be touched with the bare hands. The medical assistant can place the contents of the peel-pack directly on the sterile field by stepping back slightly from the field and gently ejecting or "flipping" the contents onto the center of the sterile field (see Fig. 10.4B). Stepping back prevents the unsterile outer wrapper and the medical assistant's hands from crossing over the sterile field, which would result in contamination.

The contents of the package also can be removed with a sterile gloved hand. This technique is useful during minor office surgery, when the physician needs additional supplies, such as gauze pads and sutures. The medical assistant opens the sterile package, and the physician removes the sterile contents from the package using a gloved hand (see Fig. 10.4C). The inside of the package can be used as a sterile field by opening the peel-apart package completely and laying it flat on a clean dry surface (see Fig. 10.4D).

Once a sterile package has been opened and set up, the medical assistant may need to pour a sterile solution, such as an antiseptic, into a container located on the field. To do so, the steps of surgical asepsis outlined in Procedure 10.3 should be followed.

WOUNDS

A **wound** is a break in the continuity of an external or internal surface caused by physical means. Wounds can be accidental or intentional (as when the physician makes an incision during a surgical operation). There are two basic types of wounds: closed and open.

A *closed wound* involves an injury to the underlying tissues of the body without a break in the skin surface or mucous membrane; an example is a contusion, or bruise. A **contusion** results when the tissues under the skin are injured and is often caused by a blunt object. Blood vessels rupture, allowing blood to seep into the tissues, which

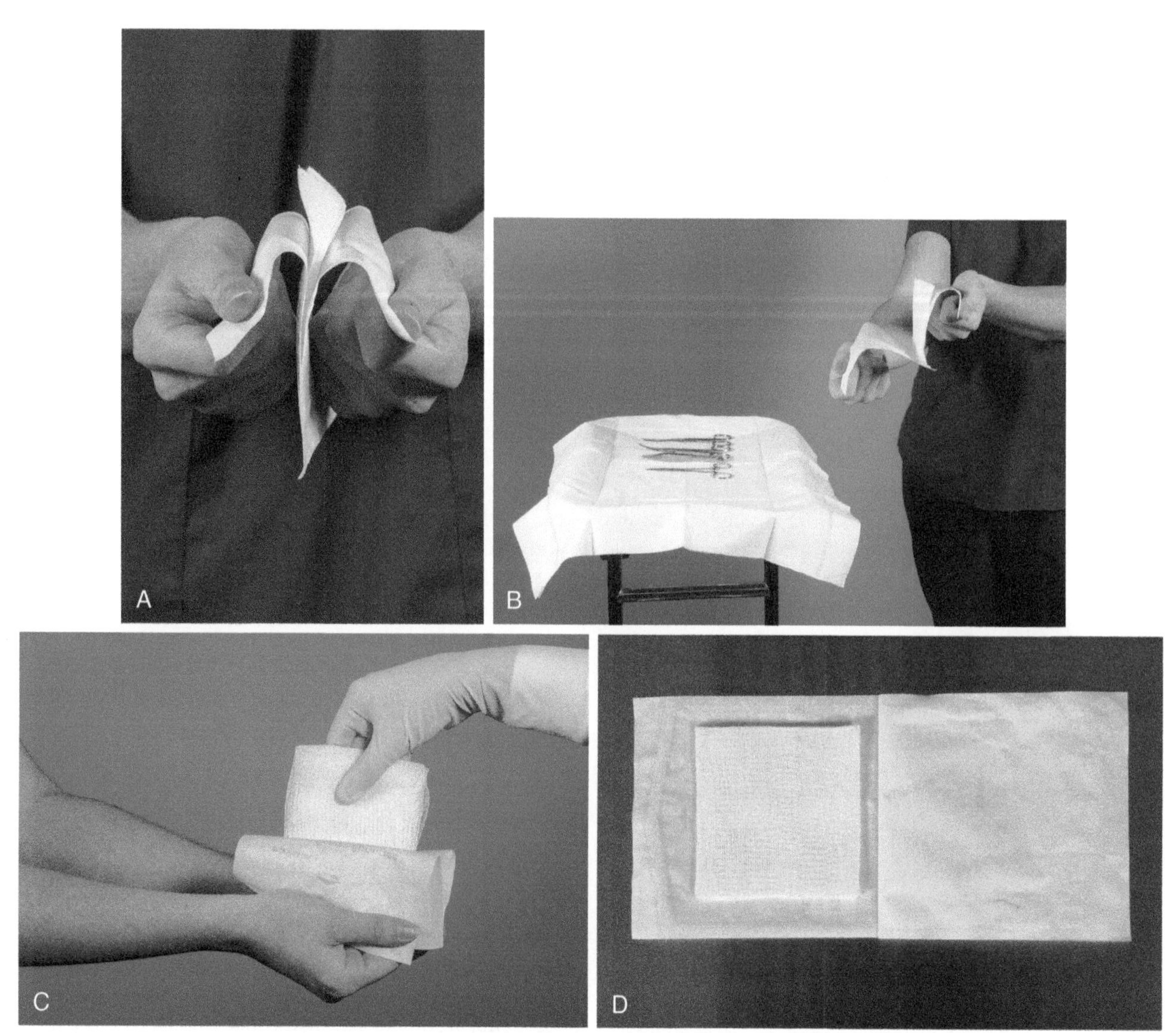

Fig. 10.4 Methods for removing the sterile contents of a peel-apart package so that sterility is maintained. (A) Grasp each flap between a bent index finger and an extended thumb, and roll hands outward to pull apart. (B) Step back and eject the contents onto the field. (C) The medical assistant opens the pack, and the physician removes the sterile contents with a gloved hand. (D) The inside of the peel-apart package can be used as a sterile field.

results in a bluish discoloration of the skin. After several days, the color of the contusion turns greenish yellow as a result of the oxidation of blood pigments. Bruising commonly occurs with injuries such as fractures, sprains, strains, and black eyes. *Open wounds* involve a break in the skin surface or mucous membrane that exposes the underlying tissues; examples include incisions, lacerations, punctures, and abrasions. Fig. 10.5 illustrates specific wounds.

- An **incision** is a clean, smooth cut caused by a sharp instrument, such as a knife, razor, or piece of glass. Deep incisions are accompanied by profuse bleeding; in addition, damage to muscles, tendons, and nerves may occur.
- A **laceration** is a wound in which the tissues are torn apart, rather than cut, leaving ragged and irregular edges. Lacerations are caused by dull knives, large objects that have been driven into the skin, and heavy machinery. Deep lacerations result in profuse bleeding, and a scar often results from the jagged tearing of the tissues.
- A **puncture** is a wound made by a sharp-pointed object piercing the skin layers—for example, a nail, splinter, needle, wire, knife, bullet, or animal bite. A puncture wound has a very small external skin opening, and for this reason, bleeding is usually minor. A tetanus booster may be administered with this type of wound because the tetanus bacteria grow best in a warm anaerobic environment, such as the one in a puncture.
- An **abrasion** or scrape is a wound in which the outer layers of the skin are scraped or rubbed off, resulting in the oozing of blood from ruptured capillaries. Abrasions are often caused by falling on gravel and floors (floor burn). These falls can result in skinned knees and elbows.

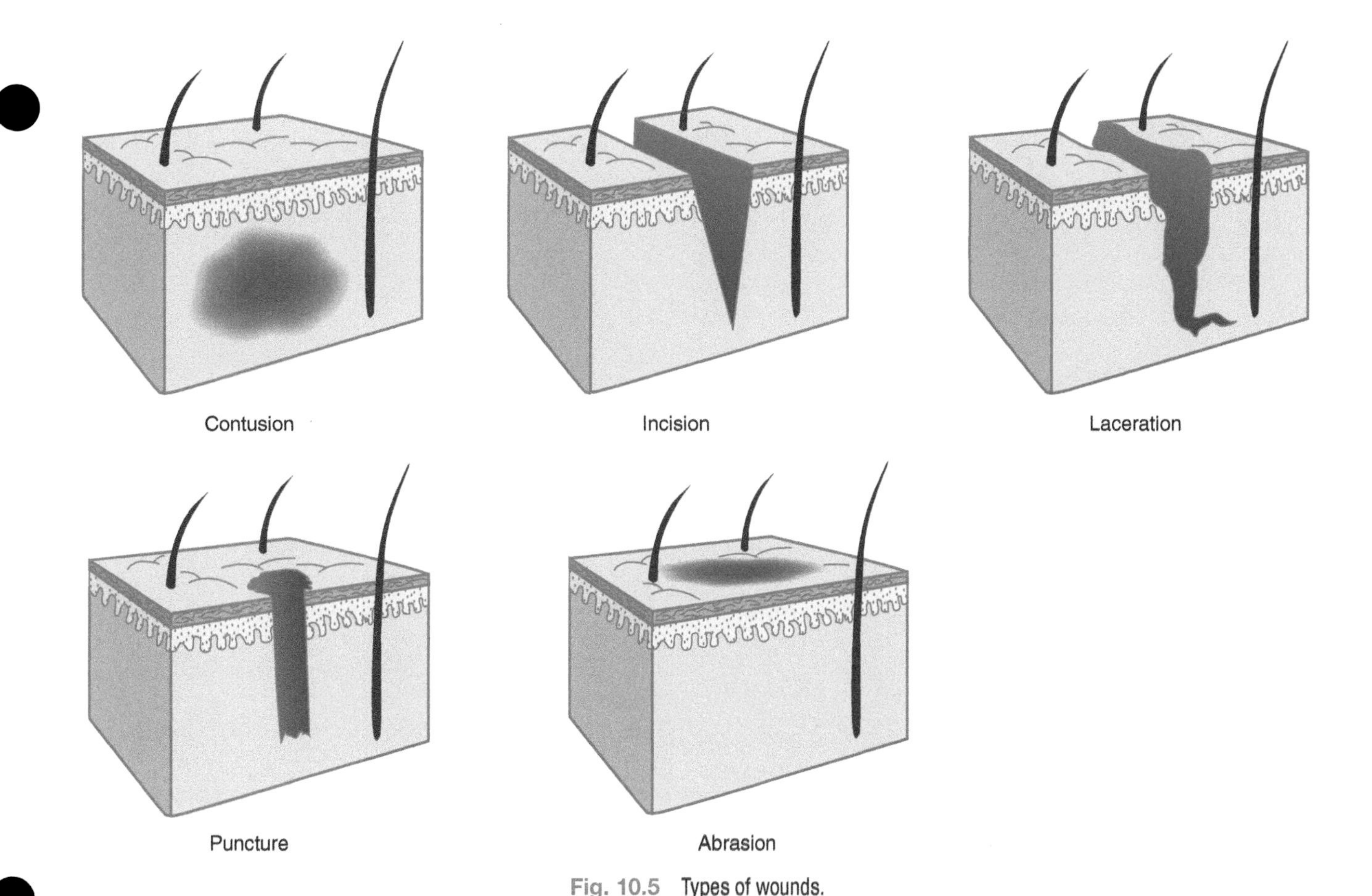

Fig. 10.5 Types of wounds.

WOUND HEALING

The skin is a protective barrier for the body and is considered its first line of defense. When the surface of the skin has been broken, it is easy for microorganisms to enter and cause **infection**. The body has a natural healing process that works to destroy invading microorganisms and to restore the structure and function of damaged tissues, as is described next.

Phases of Wound Healing

Wound healing occurs in three phases, which are described here and illustrated in Fig. 10.6.

Phase 1

Phase 1, also called the *inflammatory phase,* begins as soon as the body is injured. This phase lasts approximately 3 to 4 days. During this phase, a fibrin network forms, resulting in a blood clot that "plugs" up the opening of the wound and stops the flow of blood. The blood clot eventually becomes the scab. The inflammatory process also occurs during this phase. **Inflammation** is the protective response of the body to trauma, such as cuts and abrasions, and to the entrance of foreign matter, such as microorganisms. During inflammation, the blood supply to the wound increases, which brings white blood cells and nutrients to the site to assist in the healing process. The four local signs of inflammation are redness, swelling, pain, and warmth. The purpose of inflammation is to destroy invading microorganisms and to remove damaged tissue debris from the area so that proper healing can occur.

Phase 2

Phase 2 is also called the *proliferative phase* and typically lasts 4 to 20 days. During this phase, the wound is rebuilt with new connective tissue known as *granulation tissue.* The function of granulation tissue is to fill in the wound and protect the surface of the wound. Granulation tissue consists primarily of collagen and microscopic blood vessels and is formed in the following sequence. **Fibroblasts** migrate to the wound and begin to synthesize collagen. Collagen is a white protein that provides strength to the wound. As the amount of collagen increases, the wound becomes stronger, and the chance that the wound will open decreases. There also is a growth of new capillaries to provide an abundant blood supply to the granulation tissue. The presence of granulation tissue is part of the natural healing process and its presence indicates that wound healing is progressing normally. Granulation tissue exhibits the following characteristics:

- Translucent red or dark pink in color
- Soft and moist to the touch
- Bumpy or granular in appearance
- Painless

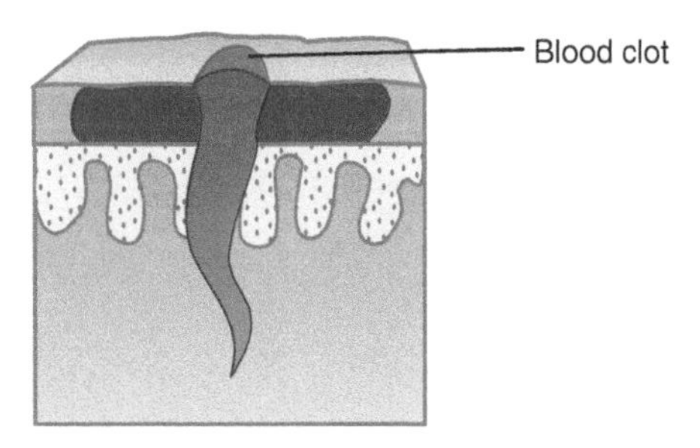

Phase 1: Inflammatory Phase

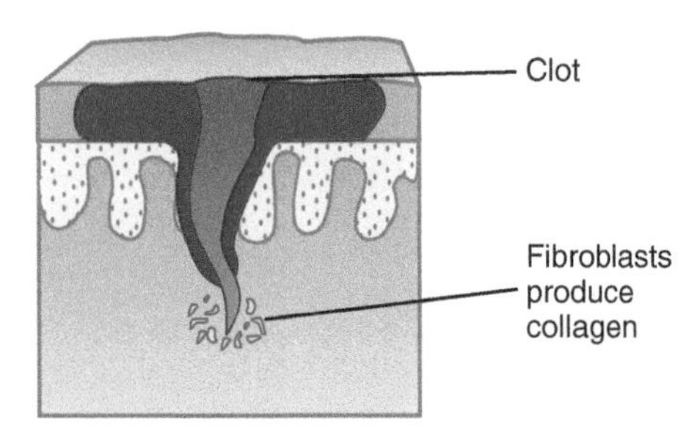

Phase 2: Proliferative Phase

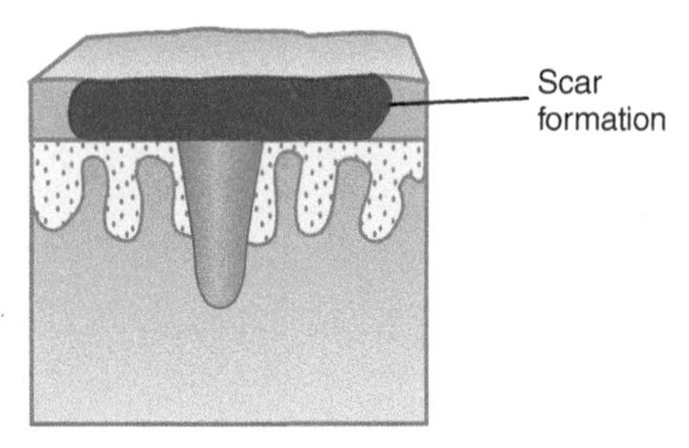

Phase 3: Maturation Phase

Fig. 10.6 Phases of wound healing.

Phase 3

Phase 3, also known as the *maturation phase,* begins as soon as granulation tissue forms and can last for 2 years. During this phase, collagen continues to be synthesized, and the granulation tissue eventually hardens to white scar tissue. Scar tissue is not true skin and does not contain nerves or have a blood supply.

The medical assistant should always inspect the wound when providing wound care. The wound should be observed for signs of inflammation and the amount of healing that has occurred. This information should be documented in the patient's record.

Wound Drainage

The medical term for drainage is **exudate** that is produced as a normal part of the healing process. An exudate consists of material, such as fluid and cells that have escaped from blood vessels during the inflammatory process and is deposited in tissue or on tissue surfaces. The function of an exudate is to flush foreign debris and dead tissue from the wound and to provide a moist environment to assist in wound healing. When providing wound care, the medical assistant should always inspect the wound for drainage and document this information in the patient's medical record. There are three major types of exudates: serous, sanguineous, and purulent.

- *Serous exudate.* A serous exudate consists chiefly of **serum**, which is the clear portion of the blood. Serous drainage is clear and watery. An example of a serous exudate is the fluid in a blister from a burn.
- *Sanguineous exudate.* A sanguineous exudate is red and consists of red blood cells. This type of drainage results when capillaries are damaged, allowing the escape of red blood cells, and is frequently seen in open wounds. A bright-red sanguineous exudate indicates fresh bleeding, and a dark exudate indicates older bleeding.
- *Purulent exudate.* A purulent exudate contains pus, which consists of leukocytes, dead liquefied tissue debris, and dead and living bacteria. Purulent drainage is usually thick and has an unpleasant odor. It is white in color but may acquire tinges of pink, green, or yellow depending on the type of infecting organism. The process of pus formation is *suppuration.*

In addition to the exudates just described, mixed types of exudates are often observed in a wound. A *serosanguineous exudate* consists of clear and blood-tinged drainage and is commonly seen in surgical incisions. A *purosanguineous exudate* consists of pus and blood and is often seen in a new wound that is infected.

STERILE DRESSING CHANGE

Surgical asepsis must be maintained when one is caring for and applying a dry sterile dressing (abbreviated as *DSD*) to an open wound. The medical assistant must take care to prevent infection in clean wounds and to decrease infection in wounds already infected. The function of a sterile dressing is to protect the wound from contamination and trauma, to absorb drainage, and to restrict motion, which may interfere with proper wound healing. The size, type, and amount of dressing material used during a sterile dressing change depend on the size and location of the wound and the amount of drainage.

Sterile folded *gauze pads* are used in the medical office for a sterile dressing change. This type of dressing absorbs drainage, but the gauze has a tendency to stick to the wound when the drainage dries. Gauze pads come in a variety of sizes, including 4 × 4, 3 × 3, and 2 × 2; the 4 × 4 size is used most frequently.

Nonadherent pads also are used as a sterile dressing; they have one surface impregnated with agents that prevent the dressing from sticking to the wound. One brand of this type of material is Telfa pads. The nonadherent side, which is shiny, is placed next to the wound. Telfa dressings are often used to cover burned skin. Procedure 10.4 presents the procedure for changing a sterile dressing.

METHODS OF WOUND CLOSURE

Wound closure may be required to close a surgical incision or to repair an accidental wound. It is typically required when tissue has been damaged to the extent that it cannot heal naturally on its own.

The most common methods of wound closure include sutures, surgical staples, topical skin adhesives (surgical glue), and skin closure tape. The purpose of wound closure is approximation, or the bringing together of the edges of the wound to hold them in place until enough healing has taken place so that the wound can withstand ordinary stress and no longer needs support from the wound closure material. It also protects the wound from further contamination and minimizes the amount of scar formation. The method of wound closure chosen by the physician depends on the characteristics of the wound and the location of the wound. These four methods are described next along with the advantages and disadvantages of each.

SUTURES

Sutures are most commonly used to close a wound. Suturing is a method of wound closure used to sew skin and other body tissues together to close a surgical incision or to close a wound caused by an injury. A **local anesthetic** is necessary to numb the area before the sutures are inserted. The suture is applied using a surgical needle and suturing material and secured with a surgical knot. Sutures minimize the risk of bleeding and infection that accompany surgical incisions and skin injuries. Closing a wound with sutures is one of the oldest known medical procedures. The ancient Egyptians are believed to have been the first to close wounds with a needle and thread nearly 4000 years ago.

Types of Sutures

Sutures are available in two types: absorbable and nonabsorbable. **Absorbable sutures** are made of a material that is gradually digested and absorbed by the body in a relatively short period of time. The amount of time can range from 7 days to several months depending on the type of tissue being sutured and the size and type of absorbable suture being used.

Absorbable sutures consist of surgical gut (Surgigut) or synthetic materials, such as polyglycolic acid (Dexon), polyglactin 910 (Vicryl), polydioxanone (PDS II), polyglyconate (Maxon), and poliglecaprone (Monocryl), lactomer (Polysorb), and Caprosyn (Fig. 10.7A). Surgical gut

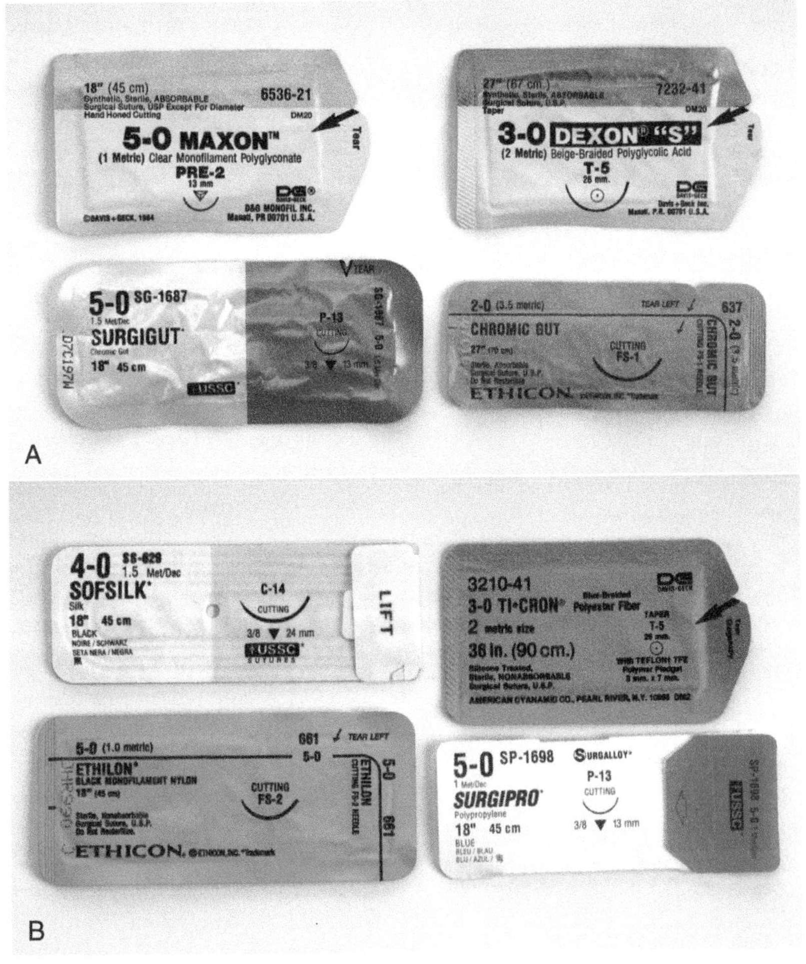

Fig. 10.7 Swaged suture packets. (A) Absorbable sutures. (B) Nonabsorbable sutures.

is made from sheep or cow intestine. This type of suturing material is gradually digested by tissue enzymes and is absorbed by the body's tissues 7 to 21 days after insertion depending on the kind of surgical gut employed. *Plain surgical gut* has a rapid absorption time, whereas *chromic surgical gut* is treated to slow down its rate of absorption in the tissues. Absorbable sutures frequently are used to suture subcutaneous tissue, fascia, intestines, bladder, and peritoneum and to **ligate**, or tie off, vessels. Because suturing of this type of tissue is typically done during surgery performed by the physician in the hospital with the patient under a general anesthetic, the medical office may not stock absorbable suture material.

Nonabsorbable sutures (see Fig. 10.7B) are not absorbed by the body and may remain permanently in the body tissues and become encapsulated by fibrous tissue or may be removed (e.g., skin sutures). Nonabsorbable sutures are used to suture skin; this type of suture is used frequently in the medical office. Nonabsorbable sutures are made from materials that are not affected by tissue enzymes. These materials include silk (Sofsilk), nylon (Ethilon), polyester (Ti-Cron, Surgidac), polypropylene (Prolene, Surgipro), polybutester (Novafil and Vascufil), stainless steel, and surgical skin staples.

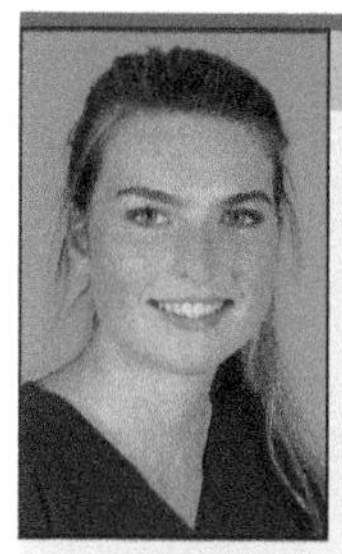

Memories *from* Practicum

Heidi: I remember observing my first minor office surgery during my practicum. It was a sebaceous cyst removal. The cyst was located on the calf of the patient's left leg. I helped in setting up the surgical tray and prepared and draped the site. I tried to explain to the patient what was going to occur to prepare her for the procedure. I think the patient was calmer than I was. The physician entered the room with a medical assistant on hand. Although I was in the room primarily to observe, I helped the physician with his surgical gloves and in numbing the site. I watched the physician make the incision and remove a large cyst.

Everything was going smoothly until the physician started to suture the wound. I felt like someone had turned the heat up really high; the room seemed to get really hot. I started to feel dizzy. I smiled at the physician and excused myself. He just smiled back at me, and I left the room. I went outside the room and caught my breath. I regained my composure and reentered the room. The physician was still suturing the wound. As I watched him insert the needle through the skin and pull the suture tight, it really got to me. I smiled and told the physician that I would wait outside until they were done. After the physician left the room, I went back to help clean up. I felt so stupid. Later that day, the physician looked at me and said, "Got a little warm in there, didn't it?" He just laughed and said that what I did was normal and not to worry about it. He made me feel better about myself. After that incident, I went in alone and helped him with cyst removals, and it did not bother me at all. ■

Suture Size and Packaging

Sutures are measured by their gauge, which refers to the diameter of the suturing material. The sizes range from numbers below 0 (pronounced "aught") to numbers above 0. The diameter of the suture material increases with each number above 0 and decreases with each number below 0. If the size of a particular suture material ranges from 7-0 to 5, available sizes include 7-0, 6-0, 5-0, 4-0, 3-0, 2-0, 0, 1, 2, 3, 4, and 5. Size 7-0 sutures are very fine sutures, and size 5 sutures are very heavy sutures. Size 2-0 (00) sutures have a smaller diameter than size 0 sutures.

Nonabsorbable sutures with a smaller gauge (5-0 to 6-0) are used for suturing incisions in delicate tissue, such as the face and neck, whereas nonabsorbable heavy sutures are used for firmer tissue, such as the chest and abdomen. Finer sutures leave less scar formation and are used when cosmetic results are desired.

Sutures come in a box of individually packaged sutures (Fig. 10.8A). The box of sutures is stamped with an expiration date that must be checked each time a suture package is removed from the box. Each individual suture package consists of an outer peel-apart envelope and a sterile inner packet (see Fig. 10.8B). Packages are labeled according to the type of suture material (e.g., surgical silk), the size (e.g., 4-0) and length of the suturing material (e.g., 18 inches), the date of manufacture, and the expiration date of the suture. The type and size of material used are based on the nature and location of the tissue being sutured and the physician's preference. To repair a laceration of the arm, the physician might use a 4-0 surgical silk suture. The physician informs the medical assistant of the type and size of sutures needed.

Suture Needles

Needles used for suturing are made from stainless steel alloys and are categorized according to their type of point and their shape. A needle with a sharp point is a *cutting needle,* and one with a round point is a *noncutting needle.* Cutting needles (Fig. 10.9A) are used for firm tissues such as skin; the sharp point helps push the needle through the tissue. Noncutting or blunt needles are used to penetrate tissues that offer a small amount of resistance, such as the fascia, intestine, liver, spleen, kidneys, subcutaneous tissue, and muscle.

A suture needle may be curved or straight (see Fig. 10.9A). *Curved needles* permit the physician to dip in and out of the tissue. A needle holder must be used with a curved needle. A *straight needle* is used when the tissue can be displaced sufficiently to permit the needle to be pushed and pulled through the tissue. Straight needles do not require the use of a needle holder.

Some needles have an eye through which the suture material is inserted; however, most needles are **swaged** (see Fig. 10.9B). *Swaged* means that the suture and needle are one continuous unit; the needle is permanently attached to the end of the suture. Swaged needles are used frequently

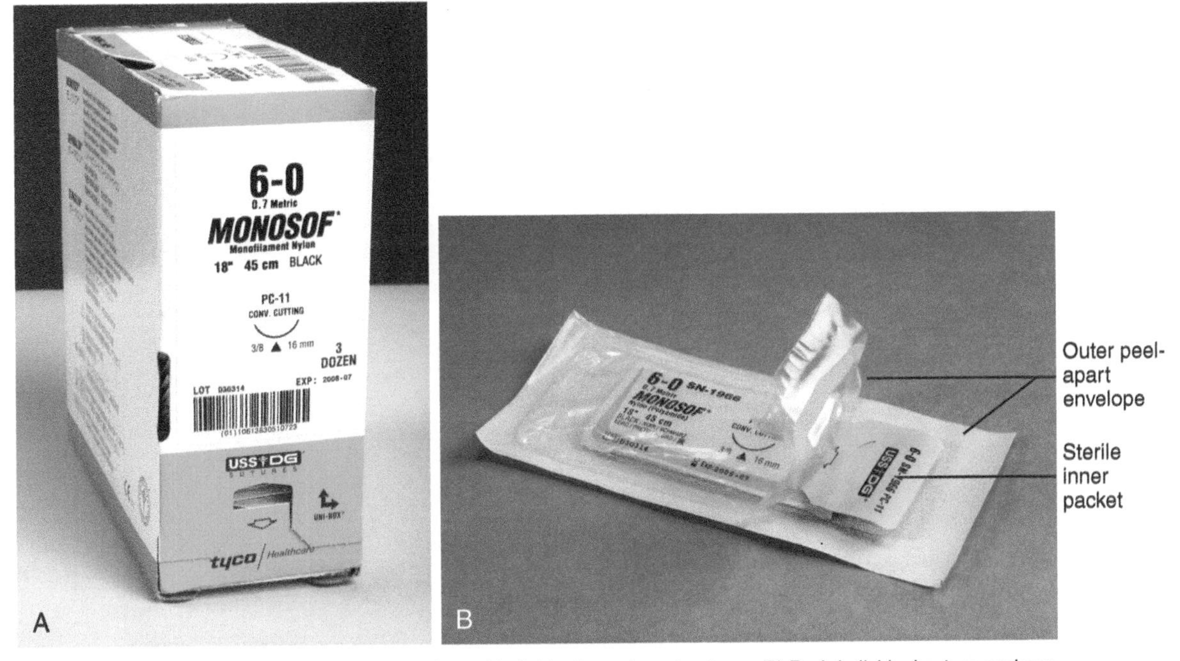

Fig. 10.8 (A) Sutures come in a box of individually packaged sutures. (B) Each individual suture package consists of an outer peel-apart envelope and a sterile inner packet.

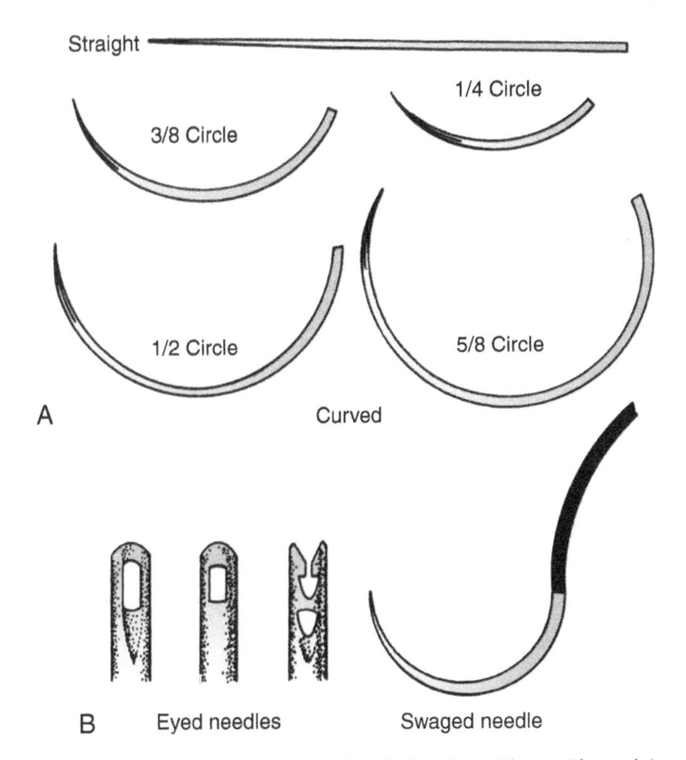

Fig. 10.9 Common suture needles. (A) Needles with a cutting point. (B) Eyed needles and a swaged needle. (B, Modified from Nealon TF, Jr.: *Fundamental skills in surgery,* ed 4, Philadelphia: WB Saunders; 1994.)

because they offer several advantages over eyed needles. One advantage is that the suture material does not slip off the needle, as might occur with suture material threaded through the eye of a needle. Another advantage is that tissue trauma is reduced because a swaged needle has only a single strand of suture that must be pulled through the tissue compared with a double strand in an eyed needle. The swaged needle can be pulled through the tissue with less resulting trauma. Swaged suture packets are labeled to specify the type, size and length of suture material, the type of needle point (cutting or noncutting), and the needle shape (curved or straight) (see Fig. 10.7).

Insertion of Sutures

The medical assistant may be responsible for preparing the suture tray and for assisting the physician during the insertion of the sutures. The physician designates the size and type of suture material and needle required. Because sutures, needles, and suture-needle combinations (swaged needles) are contained in peel-apart packages, they can be added to the sterile field by flipping them onto the sterile field or by placing them there with a sterile gloved hand (Fig. 10.10).

Suture Insertion Setup

The items required for a suture insertion setup are listed next.

Items Placed to the Side of the Sterile Field

- Clean disposable gloves
- Antiseptic solution
- Surgical scrub brush
- Antiseptic swabs
- Sterile gloves
- Local anesthetic
- Antiseptic wipe to cleanse the vial
- Tetanus toxoid with needle and syringe

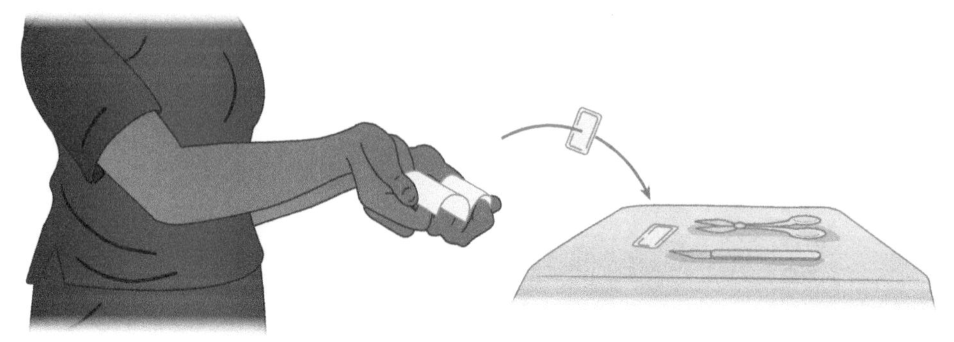

Flipping sutures onto the sterile field.

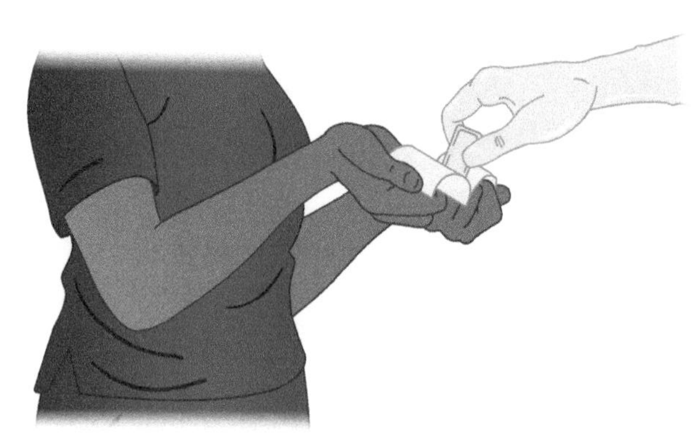

The physician removing the sutures with a sterile gloved hand.

Fig. 10.10 Adding sutures to a sterile field.

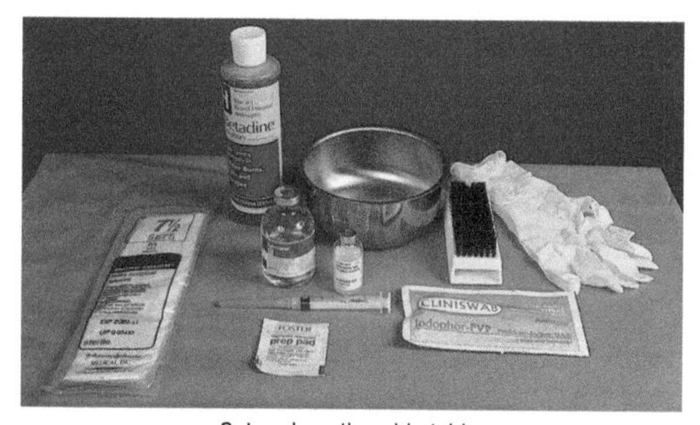

Suture insertion side table.

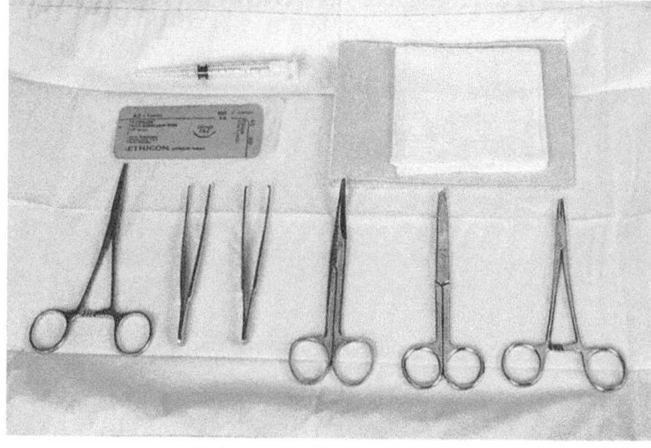

Suture insertion sterile field.

Items Included on the Sterile Field

- Fenestrated drape
- Syringe and needle for drawing up the local anesthetic
- Hemostatic forceps
- Thumb forceps
- Tissue forceps
- Dissecting scissors
- Operating scissors
- Needle holder
- Suture
- Sterile 4 × 4 gauze

Procedure: Suture Insertion

Sutures are inserted as follows:

1. A local anesthetic is used to numb the area.
2. The physician inserts sutures to close a surgical incision or to repair an accidental wound.
3. A sterile dressing may be applied to the operative site.

Postoperative Instructions: Suture Insertion

Postoperative instructions include the following:

1. Keep the dressing clean and dry.

2. Contact the medical office if any signs of infection occur at the incision site, including excessive redness, swelling, discharge, or an increase in pain.
3. Notify the medical office if the sutures become loose or break.

Provide the patient with written instructions on wound care to refer to at home (Box 10.2) and instruct the patient when to return for removal of the sutures.

Suture Removal

When the wound has healed such that it no longer needs the support of nonabsorbable suture material, the sutures must be removed. The length of time the sutures remain in place depends on their location and the amount of healing that must occur. Some areas of the body, such as the head and neck, have a good blood supply; the sutures do not need to remain there as long as they do in other areas because this area heals more rapidly.

Sutures must always be left in place long enough for proper healing to occur. The physician determines the length of time, but in general, skin sutures inserted in the face and neck are removed in 3 to 5 days, and sutures inserted in other areas, such as the skin of the chest, arms, legs, hands, and feet, are removed in 7 to 14 days.

What Would You Do? What Would You *Not* Do?

Case Study 1

Kerry Ventura brings her 6-year-old son Cory to the medical office. Cory got a new bike for his birthday and just learned how to ride it without training wheels. While going around a corner, he lost his balance and fell and cut his left knee. The incision is almost 2 inches long. Cory is going to need sutures to approximate the wound. Mrs. Ventura is very upset and blames herself. She says that she should have been watching him more closely. Mrs. Ventura wants to know why Steri-Strips cannot be used to close the incision. She says that it would be a lot less painful for Cory than having stitches. When asked to sign the consent to treatment form for Cory, Mrs. Ventura says she does not want to sign the form until her husband is back from his weeklong business trip to Japan and has a chance to assess the situation. ■

SURGICAL SKIN STAPLES

Surgical skin staples are often used to close wounds. Stapling is the fastest method of closure of long skin incisions. In addition, trauma to the tissue is reduced because the tissue does not have to be handled much when the staples are inserted. Surgical staples are stainless steel and are inserted

BOX 10.2 Wound Care Instructions

General Wound Care Instructions

Explain the following to the patient regarding wounds:

- The type of wound that the patient has: incision, laceration, puncture, or abrasion.
- If a tetanus toxoid has been administered, explain the purpose of this immunization: to protect against tetanus (lockjaw).

Instruct the patient how to care for the wound, as follows:

- Keep the wound clean and dry, especially for the first 24–48 h.
- Some swelling, redness, and pain are common with all wounds and will go away as the wound heals.
- Apply an ice bag for swelling (if prescribed by the physician).
- Report immediately any signs that the wound is infected. These signs include the following:
  a. Fever
  b. Persistent or increased pain, swelling, drainage, or foul odor
  c. Red streaks radiating away from the wound
  d. Increased redness or warmth
- Avoid any activities that may put strain on the wound. This could cause the wound to re-open.
- Return as instructed by the physician.
- Give the patient written instructions on wound care to refer to at home.

Sutures and Staples

Instruct the patient on how to take care of sutures or staples (in addition to general wound care instructions).

- The purpose of suturing or stapling the wound: to close the skin and protect against further contamination, to facilitate healing, and to leave a smaller scar.
- Do not take a tub bath or swim until the sutures or staples have been removed.
- After showering, gently pad the area dry with a soft towel.
- Do not pick at your sutures or staples.
- Notify the medical office if the sutures become loose or break.
- Return as instructed by the physician for removal of the sutures or staples.

Skin Closure Tape and Tissue Adhesives

Instruct the patient how to take care of skin closure tape and tissue adhesives (in addition to general wound care instructions).

- The purpose of applying skin closure tape or tissue adhesives: to close the skin and protect against further contamination, to facilitate healing, and to leave a smaller scar.
- Do not take a tub bath or swim.
- After showering, gently pad the area dry.
- Do not scratch, pick at or rub the tape or adhesive film.
- Do not apply any topical ointments or creams to the wound.
- Notify the medical office if the wound re-opens.

into the skin using a special skin stapler. Skin staplers are available as reusable or disposable devices. The skin stapler holds a cartridge that contains a prescribed number and size of staples (Fig. 10.11).

The physician inserts the staples by gently approximating the tissues with tissue forceps. The skin stapler is held over the site, and the staple is inserted into the skin. The medical assistant should provide the patient with instructions for caring for the wound (Box 10.2). Skin stapling produces excellent cosmetic results, and the staples are easy to remove with a specially designed staple remover.

The medical assistant is frequently responsible for removing sutures and staples. This procedure should be done only after the physician has given a written or verbal order to the medical assistant. Procedure 10.5 presents the method used to remove sutures and skin staples.

TOPICAL TISSUE ADHESIVES

Topical tissue adhesives (also known as surgical glue) are the newest method of skin closure. In 1998, the Food and Drug Administration (FDA) approved the use of 2-octyl cyanoacrylate which is marketed as Dermabond (Ethicon, Somerville, NJ) and is available in a pre-filled single-use applicator.

Tissue adhesives work by forming a strong transparent flexible bond across the top of the skin that binds the skin edges together. Before applying a tissue adhesive, it is important to make sure the wound is clean and dry. The physician applies the tissue adhesive by approximating the edges of the wound with sterile gloves or forceps. The tissue adhesive is then applied as a liquid to the outer surface of the skin (Fig. 10.12). The liquid quickly dries into a film that holds the edges of the wound together. The film lasts for 5 to 10 days and then naturally falls off on its own. The medical assistant should provide the patient with instructions for caring for the wound (see Box 10.2).

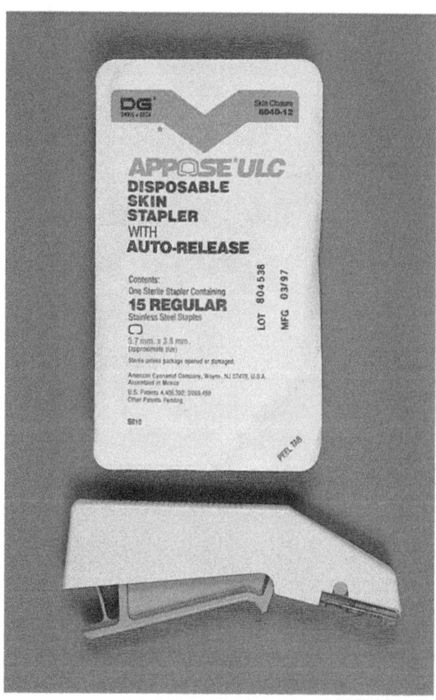

Fig. 10.11 Disposable skin stapler.

Tissue adhesives are best suited to close small superficial lacerations or surgical incisions of the face, torso, and limbs. They cannot be used on wounds of the mucous membranes such as the lips or oral cavity. They also cannot be used on areas that harbor moisture (e.g., palms of the hands, soles of the feet, axillae) and hairy areas of the body (e.g., scalp) and areas that are subjected to too much tension or flexion (e.g., joints). The advantages of tissue adhesives are that they eliminate the need for sutures and a local anesthetic, are easy to apply, form a water-resistant protective covering over the wound, and result in less scarring than sutures.

SKIN CLOSURE TAPE

Skin closure tape may be used for wound repair to approximate the edges of a laceration or incision. Skin closures consist of sterile, hypoallergenic adhesive tape that is commercially available in a variety of widths and lengths and is strong enough to approximate a wound until healing occurs. Brand names for skin closure tape are Steri-Strip (3M Corporation, St Paul, Minn) and Proxi-Strip (Ethicon, Bridgewater, NJ) (Fig. 10.13).

Skin closure tape may be used when not much tension exists on the skin edges. The strips of tape are applied transversely across the line of incision to approximate the skin

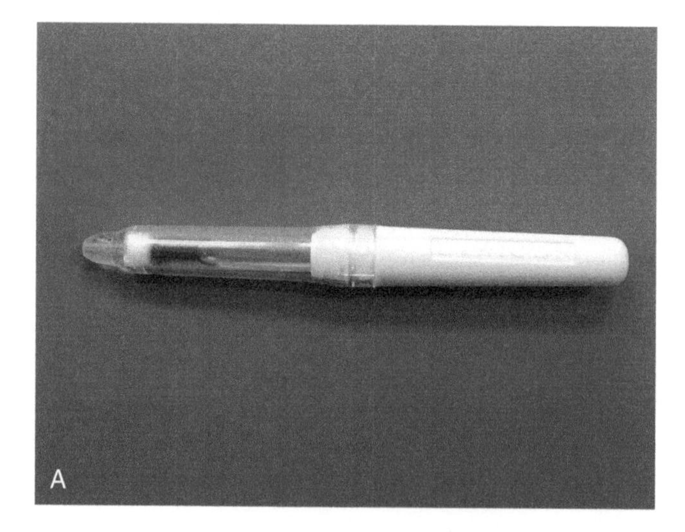

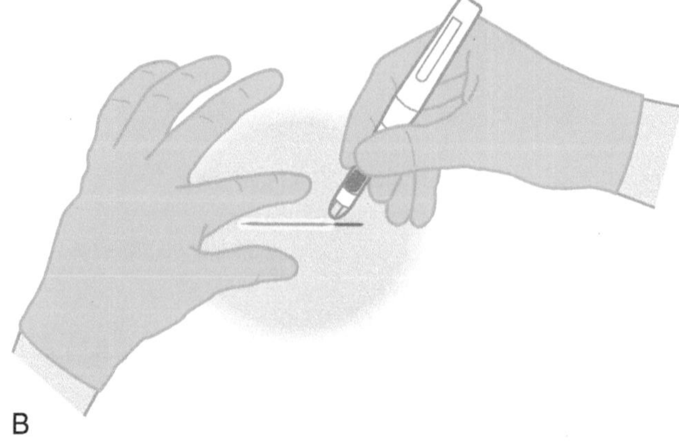

Fig. 10.12 (A and B) Topical tissue adhesive. (From Bonewit-West K, Hunt SA: *Today's medical assistant*, ed 4, St Louis: Elsevier; 2021.)

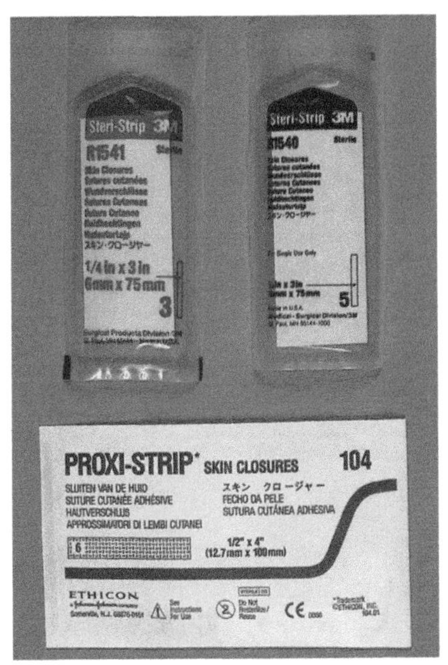

Fig. 10.13 Skin closure tape in different sizes.

edges. The advantages of skin closure tape are that they eliminate the need for sutures and a local anesthetic, are easy to apply and remove, have a lower incidence of wound infection compared with sutures, and result in less scarring than sutures. The disadvantage of this method is that there is less precision in bringing the wound edges together compared with suturing the wound. In addition, skin closure tape cannot be used on certain areas of the body where the tape has difficulty adhering to the skin. This includes areas that harbor moisture (e.g., palms of the hands, soles of the feet, axillae) and hairy areas of the body (e.g., scalp, a man's chest).

The medical assistant frequently is responsible for applying skin closure tape (Procedure 10.6) and for providing the patient with instructions for caring for the wound (see Box 10.2). Approximately 5 to 10 days after application, the skin closures usually loosen and fall off on their own. If they require removal by the medical assistant, the method presented at the end of Procedure 10.6 should be followed.

ASSISTING WITH MINOR OFFICE SURGERY

TRAY SETUP

Assisting with minor office surgery requires a thorough knowledge of the instruments and supplies for each tray setup and the type of assistance required by the physician during the surgery. The medical assistant must be able to work quickly and efficiently and to anticipate the physician's needs.

The instruments and supplies for the surgery must be set on a sterile field. Many offices maintain index cards indicating the appropriate instruments and supplies for each minor office surgery tray setup. The card also may include information regarding the type of skin preparation, position of the patient, physician's glove size, type of suture material, preoperative instructions, and postoperative instructions. In general, the index cards are kept in a file box and are filed alphabetically by the type of surgery. The medical assistant should pull the card before setting up for the minor office surgery and use it as a guide to ensure that all required articles are placed on the sterile field. The medical assistant may set up the sterile tray before or after preparing the patient's skin. The sterile tray setup must not become contaminated. If the medical assistant must turn away from the sterile tray or leave the room after setting up, a sterile towel must be placed over the tray to maintain sterility.

Methods Used to Set up a Sterile Tray

A common method used to set up a sterile tray is to use prepackaged sterile setups wrapped in disposable sterilization paper or muslin that are prepared by the medical office through autoclave sterilization (see Procedure 10.2). These setups are labeled according to use (e.g., suture pack, cyst removal pack) and contain most of the instruments and supplies required for the minor office surgery indicated on the label. The medical assistant opens the wrapped package on a flat surface, such as a **Mayo tray**. A Mayo tray is a broad, flat metal tray placed on a stand that can be used to hold sterile instruments and supplies; the inside of the wrapped package is sterile and serves as the sterile field. Several additional articles not contained in the prepackaged setup (e.g., an antiseptic, sterile 4 × 4 gauze pads, disposable syringes and needles, sutures) may need to be added to the sterile field when the package is opened. Items in peel-apart packages are added by flipping them onto the sterile field or by placing them on the field using a sterile gloved hand.

If an antiseptic solution is poured into a basin on the sterile field, this is performed according to Procedure 10.3.

Another method used to set up a sterile tray is to place all necessary articles on the sterile field by flipping them onto the sterile field from peel-apart packages. With this method, the sterile field is prepared by placing a sterile towel over a tray such as a Mayo tray or another flat surface. The sterile towel must be handled by the corners so as not to contaminate it. It must not be fanned through the air but instead must be laid down gently and slowly to prevent airborne contamination.

Side Table

Some articles required for minor office surgery are not placed on the sterile field but are set on an adjacent table or counter. These articles, such as a surgical scrub brush, are not sterile and must not be placed on the sterile field. The local anesthetic, which is a sterile solution, is in a vial that is not sterile and must *not* be placed on the sterile field. The physician needs to apply gloves to perform the surgery. Although the gloves are sterile, the outside wrapper is not; the package of gloves must not be placed on the sterile field. In addition, it is easier for the physician to apply gloves

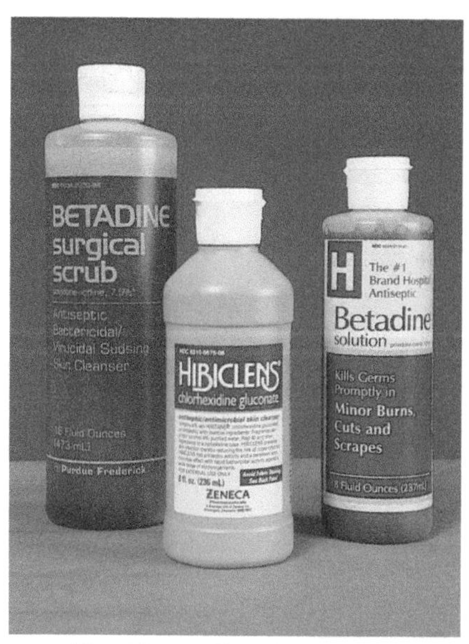

Fig. 10.14 Cleansing solutions.

from a side table or counter. To facilitate application of the gloves, the medical assistant opens the outside wrapper for the physician.

SKIN PREPARATION

The patient's skin must be prepared before the minor office surgery because the skin contains an abundance of microorganisms. If these microorganisms were to enter the body through the operative site, a wound infection could develop. It is impossible to sterilize skin because chemical agents required to kill all living microorganisms are too strong to be placed on the skin surfaces. The operative site and the area surrounding it must be cleaned and prepared in such a way as to remove as many microorganisms as possible to reduce the risk of surgical wound contamination.

Shaving the Site

Hair supports the growth of microorganisms, and the physician may want the medical assistant to shave the skin at and around the operative site. Shave preparation trays are commercially available and include several gauze sponges, a measured amount of antiseptic soap, a container for soapy water, and a disposable safety razor. The skin should be pulled taut as it is shaved, and the medical assistant must be careful to prevent nicks. When all the hair has been removed, the shaved area should be rinsed and dried thoroughly.

Cleansing the Site

The operative site must be cleaned with an antiseptic solution such as povidone-iodine (Betadine Surgical Scrub) or chlorhexidine gluconate (Hibiclens) (Fig. 10.14). The medical assistant should scrub the operative area with a surgical scrub brush using a firm circular motion, moving from the

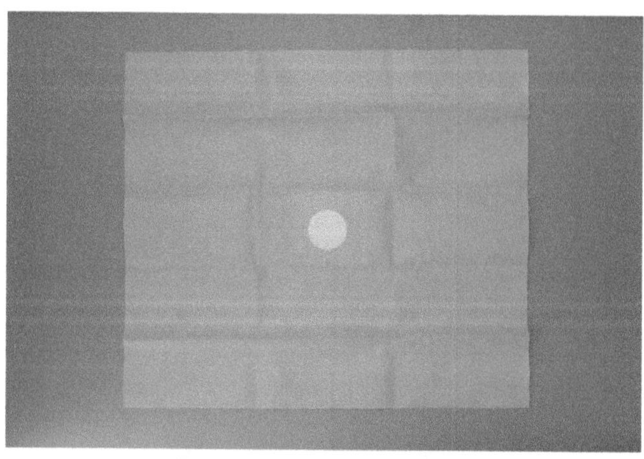

Fig. 10.15 Fenestrated drape.

inside outward. The area is rinsed using gauze pads saturated with water and is blotted dry with sterile gauze.

Antiseptic Application

When the patient's skin has been shaved (if required) and cleansed, an antiseptic is applied to the operative area, followed by the application of a sterile drape. The antiseptic decreases the number of microorganisms on the patient's skin; a common antiseptic is Betadine. A disposable sterile *fenestrated drape* (Fig. 10.15) is the type of drape most commonly used. It has an opening that is placed directly over the operative site. A fenestrated drape covers a wide area of skin around the operative area, leaving only the operative site exposed. This provides a sterile area around the operative site and decreases contamination of the patient's surgical wound.

LOCAL ANESTHETIC

Minor office surgeries often require the use of a local anesthetic; the local anesthetic most frequently used in the medical office is lidocaine hydrochloride (Xylocaine). The physician injects the local anesthetic into the tissue surrounding the operative site, a process termed **infiltration**, to produce a loss of sensation in that area and prevent the patient from feeling pain during the surgery. When first injected into the tissues, lidocaine causes the patient to experience a brief burning or stinging sensation at the injection site. The local anesthetic begins working in 5 to 15 minutes and has a duration of action of 1 to 3 hours, depending on the type of anesthetic.

Some physicians prefer to use a local anesthetic containing *epinephrine.* Epinephrine is a vasoconstrictor that prolongs the local effect of the anesthetic and decreases the rate of systemic absorption of the local anesthetic. It accomplishes this by constricting blood vessels at the operative site. The physician informs the medical assistant of the type, strength, and amount of local anesthetic needed for the minor office surgery. Xylocaine is available in 0.5%, 1%, 1.5%, and 2% solutions. The physician may order 1 mL of

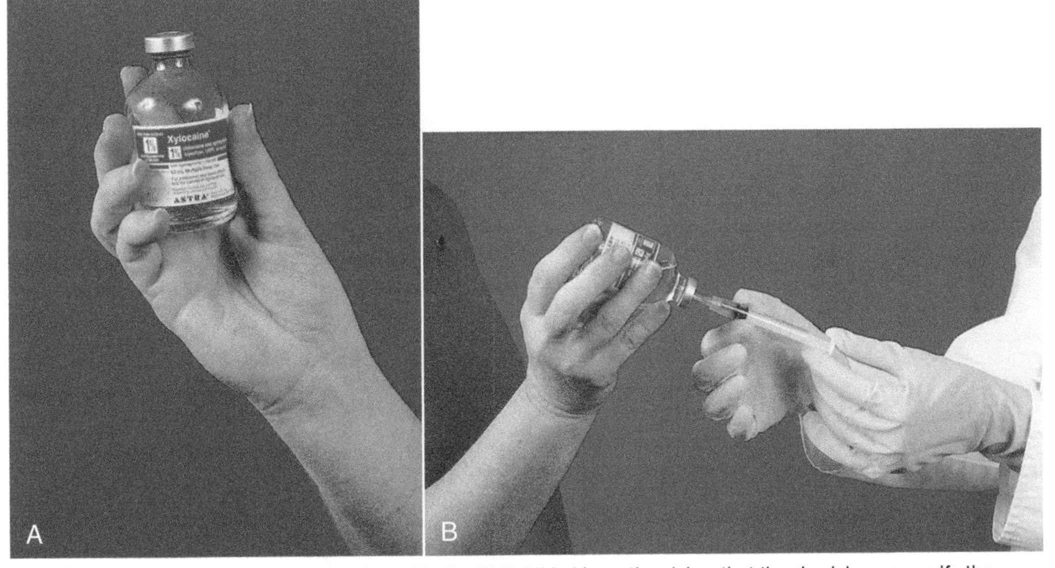

Fig. 10.16 Drawing up the local anesthetic. (A) Heidi holds up the vial so that the physician can verify the name and strength of the local anesthetic. (B) Heidi holds the vial securely, while the physician withdraws the medication.

Xylocaine 2% with epinephrine to suture a laceration of the forearm.

Preparing the Anesthetic

The local anesthetic is drawn up into the syringe from a vial according to the procedure presented in Chapter 11. The vial must first be cleansed using an antiseptic wipe. The correct amount of anesthetic solution is withdrawn into the syringe. This may be performed by the medical assistant or the physician. The medical assistant withdraws the anesthetic into the syringe and hands it to the physician, who has not yet applied sterile gloves. The physician injects the anesthetic into the patient's tissues and then applies sterile gloves to begin the surgery.

The physician may prefer to draw the anesthetic solution into the syringe after he or she has applied sterile gloves. The medical assistant should first show the label of the vial to the physician and should then hold the vial securely while the physician withdraws the medication (Fig. 10.16). The medical assistant must hold the vial because the outside of the vial is medically aseptic and cannot be touched by the physician's sterile gloved hand.

If the medical assistant prepares the anesthetic injection, the needle and syringe are not placed on the sterile field but are assembled off to the side. If the physician withdraws the anesthetic, the needle and syringe are placed on the sterile field.

ASSISTING THE PHYSICIAN

The type of assistance required by the physician during minor office surgery is based on the type of surgery and the physician's preference. Some physicians want the medical assistant to apply sterile gloves and assist directly by handing instruments and supplies from the sterile field. An instrument should be handed to the physician in a firm, confident manner so that the instrument does not slip out of the physician's hand and drop on the floor. The instrument should be placed in the physician's hand in its functional position—that is, the position in which it is to be used (Fig. 10.17). If the instrument is handed correctly, the physician should not have to reposition the instrument to use it.

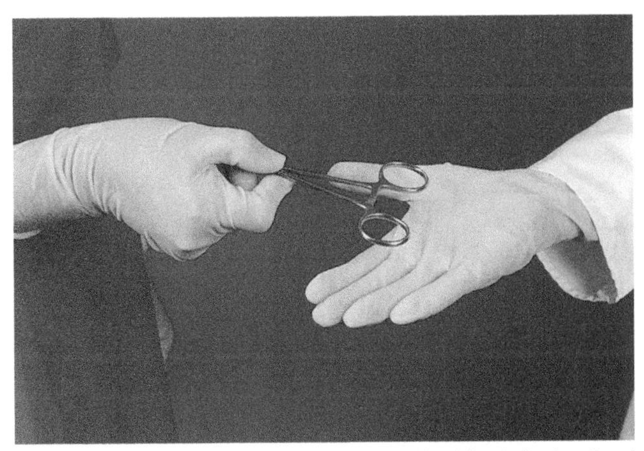

Fig. 10.17 Heidi hands a hemostat to the physician in its functional position.

The medical assistant is responsible for adding any instruments or supplies to the sterile field that the physician requires after the surgery has begun, such as another hemostat, additional 4 × 4 gauze pads, and sutures. This is usually accomplished by using peel-apart packages and either flipping the contents onto the sterile field or holding the package open and allowing the physician to remove the contents with a gloved hand. In assisting with minor office surgery, it is essential to know all steps in the procedure so

DIAGNOSTIC PATHOLOGY ASSOCIATES, INC

HISTOPATHOLOGY/CYTOPATHOLOGY REQUISITION

BILL TO: ☐ ACCOUNT ☐ PATIENT ☐ MEDICARE ☐ MEDICAID ☐ BLUE SHIELD ☐ OTHER | PATIENT NAME (LAST, FIRST, MIDDLE INITIAL) | PATIENT ID | ROOM NO.

SEX | BIRTHDATE / / | DATE COLLECTED | TIME COLLECTED A.M. P.M. | REQUESTING PHYSICIAN | SPECIAL INSTRUCTIONS

RESPONSIBLE PARTY NAME | RESPONSIBLE PARTY ADDRESS | CITY, STATE, ZIP

PHONE | MEDICAID ID NUMBER | MEDICARE HIC NUMBER | INSURANCE COMPANY NAME

INSURANCE COMPANY ADDRESS | GROUP NUMBER | CONTRACT NUMBER | COVERAGE CODE | PATIENT/INSURED RELATIONSHIP ☐ SELF ☐ SPOUSE ☐ DEPEND.

PATIENT AUTHORIZATION: I AUTHORIZE THE RELEASE OF ANY MEDICAL INFORMATION NECESSARY TO PROCESS A CLAIM, I PERMIT A COPY OF THIS AUTHORIZATION TO BE USED IN PLACE OF THE ORIGINAL AND REQUEST PAYMENT OF ANY MEDICAL INSURANCE BENEFITS EITHER TO ME OR TO THE PARTY WHO ACCEPTS ASSIGNMENT. | SIGNED X________ | DATE ________

TISSUE EXAM:
☐ GROSS & MICROSCOPIC
☐ GROSS ONLY
SPECIMEN TYPE:
☐ BIOPSY
☐ SCRAPING
☐ BRUSHING
☐ WASHING
☐ FLUIDS
☐ FINE NEEDLE
☐ OTHER ________

SOURCE OF SPECIMEN:
☐ PHONE REPORT (NEXT WORKING DAY)
COPIES TO:________

CLINICAL DIAGNOSIS:

PATIENT HISTORY:

Fig. 10.18 Biopsy requisition. (Courtesy Diagnostic Pathology Associates, Columbus, OH.)

that the physician's needs can be anticipated and that the surgery proceeds smoothly and efficiently.

The physician may obtain a tissue specimen that is sent to the laboratory for histologic examination. The specimen must be placed in an appropriate-sized container with a preservative. The medical assistant is responsible for labeling the specimen container. An unlabeled specimen is a cause for rejection of the specimen by an outside laboratory. Two *unique identifiers* should be used to label the specimen. A unique identifier is information that clearly identifies a specific patient, such as the patient's name and date of birth. A specimen can be labeled by attaching a computerized bar code label to the specimen. A specimen can also be labeled by hand-writing the information on the label, which should include the patient's name and date of birth, the date and time of collection, the medical assistant's initials, and any other information required by the laboratory, such as the source of the specimen. The information should be printed legibly, and the medical assistant should be certain that the information is accurate to avoid a mix-up of specimens. The medical assistant also must complete a laboratory requisition to accompany the specimen; this is known as a *biopsy requisition* (Fig. 10.18).

When the minor office surgery is completed, the physician may want the medical assistant to place a DSD over the surgical wound to protect it from contamination or injury or to absorb drainage. The medical assistant also is responsible for assisting the patient and cleaning the examining room.

Procedure 10.7 describes the medical assistant's responsibilities while assisting with minor office surgery. Specific instruments and supplies required for the minor office surgery depend on the type of surgery being performed and the physician's preference. Knowing the name and function of the surgical instruments shown in Fig. 10.3 enables the medical assistant to set up for each type of minor surgery performed in the medical office. If the medical office uses prepackaged sterile setups, the medical assistant should have already assembled the instruments and supplies in the package during the sanitization and sterilization process; however, the instruments and supplies should be checked after the pack is opened to ensure that all the sterile articles are included.

What Would You Do? What Would You *Not* Do?

Case Study 2

Abbey Mendy is having a sebaceous cyst removed from her neck. She wants to know why the antiseptic applied to her neck is orange and whether it is going to permanently stain her skin. During the procedure, Abbey reaches her hand up to adjust her hair and accidentally touches the physician's gloved hand. After the procedure, a sterile dressing is applied to her neck, and she is given an appointment to return to have her sutures removed. Abbey becomes alarmed when she is told that the cyst will be sent to the laboratory for a biopsy. She wants to know if the physician is not telling her everything, and is concerned that she might have cancer. Abbey asks if her neighbor can take out her sutures. She says that he has worked as a veterinary assistant for the past 8 years and has lots of experience in removing stitches. ■

HIGHLIGHT on the History of Surgery

Primitive Surgery

Surgery evolved from very primitive beginnings. The first record of a surgical operation dates back to 350,000 BCE. Primitive humans believed that headaches were caused by demons that had gained entrance to the head and were unable to get out. To release the demons, a hole was chiseled through the patient's skull with a sharp flint. Early operating instruments consisted of sharpened flints and crude hammers. Sharpened animal teeth were used for bloodletting and drainage of abscesses. Ancient records show that suturing materials consisted of dried gut, dried tendon, strips of hide, horsehair, and fibers from tree bark. To help form a clot, bleeding wounds were covered with materials such as rabbit fur, shredded tree bark, egg yolk, and cobwebs.

Early 1800s

In the early 1800s, surgical instruments were still almost nonexistent. Kitchen knives and penknives doubled as scalpels, and table forks were used as retractors. Physicians would use household pincushions to hold their suturing needles. The same sponges were used for every patient to wipe away blood and other secretions. Because of these conditions, the most trivial operations were likely to be followed by infection, and death occurred in half of all surgical operations. Joseph Lister, an English surgeon, was one of the first individuals to advocate the use of antiseptics during surgery. Lister insisted on the use of antiseptics on the hands of his surgical team, instruments, wounds, and dressings. Many surgeons ridiculed Lister's ideas, but in 1879, his antiseptic principles were, at long last, formally adopted by the medical profession. Today, Lister is known as the father of modern surgery.

Mid-1800s

Anesthetic agents, such as ether and chloroform, were discovered in the mid-1800s. Before this time, various methods were used to subdue and restrain patients during surgery, such as having the patient consume alcohol before the operation and strapping the patient to the operating table. With the advent of anesthetics, new surgical procedures never before considered possible came into existence. This resulted in new demands for surgical instruments and the necessity for smaller and more delicate instruments.

Late 1800s and Early 1900s

The late 1800s and early 1900s saw dramatic advances in surgical operations and techniques. The most notable include the invention of the steam sterilizer, which permitted sterilization of surgical instruments and supplies; the use of surgical gowns, caps, masks, and gloves during surgery; the monitoring of the condition of patients under anesthesia; the development of stainless steel, which provided a superior material for manufacturing surgical instruments; and the establishment of standards for manufacturing and packaging sutures. Other discoveries important to surgery during this time included the discovery of x-rays by Wilhelm Röntgen; the discovery of penicillin by Alexander Fleming; the discovery by William Halsted that cocaine could be used as a local anesthetic; and the development of endoscopic instruments, such as the laryngoscope, bronchoscope, and sigmoidoscope, for viewing internal structures of the body.

Breakthroughs in surgical technology established through the ages laid the foundation for present-day complex surgical procedures, such as laser surgery, open-heart surgery, microsurgery, robotic surgery, and telesurgery. It is incredible to think that it all started with a sharpened flint! ■

MEDICAL OFFICE SURGICAL PROCEDURES

The most common surgical procedures performed in the medical office are presented on the following pages. A discussion of the procedure and the items required for each tray setup are included. The medical assistant should take into account, however, that the instruments and supplies may vary slightly from those listed here based on the physician's preference.

SEBACEOUS CYST REMOVAL

A **sebaceous cyst** (also known as an *epidermal cyst*) is a thin, closed sac or capsule located just under the surface of the skin. A sebaceous cyst forms when the outlet of a sebaceous (oil) gland becomes obstructed. The cyst contains *sebum,* which is made up of secretions from the sebaceous gland. The built-up secretion of sebum causes swelling, and the lining of the cyst consists of the stretched sebaceous gland. A sebaceous cyst is usually white or yellow in appearance and varies in size from less than ¼ inch (0.6 cm) in diameter to nearly 2 inches (5 cm) in diameter. It is usually a movable, dome-shaped mass with a smooth surface that is filled with a thick, fatty-white, cheesy material that has a foul odor. This type of cyst can occur anywhere on the body except on the palms of the hands and the soles of the feet—these areas do not contain sebaceous glands. Sebaceous cysts tend to occur most frequently on the scalp, face (Fig. 10.19), ears, neck, back, and genital area.

A sebaceous cyst is usually slow-growing, painless, and nontender and may disappear on its own. A sebaceous cyst usually does not require surgical removal unless it becomes infected. An infected cyst is painful, tender, red, and swollen and may have a grayish-white, foul-smelling discharge. Because it is difficult to remove an infected sebaceous cyst, the physician usually drains the cyst and allows it to heal and then performs the cyst excision at a later time. Other reasons for removing a sebaceous cyst include cosmetic concerns and the need to reduce discomfort from a cyst that is located in a body area that is easily irritated, such as the armpit.

Surgical excision of a sebaceous cyst is a simple procedure that involves the complete removal of the sac wall and its contents. Most sebaceous cysts are benign and are not

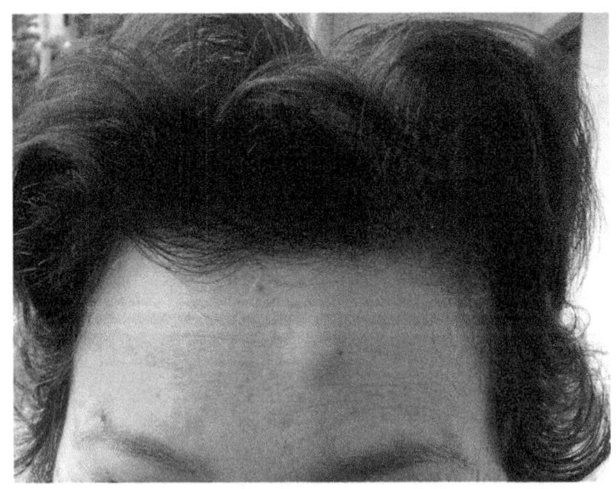

Fig. 10.19 Sebaceous cyst. (From Scully C: *Medical problems in dentistry,* ed 6, Norwalk: Churchill Livingstone; 2010.)

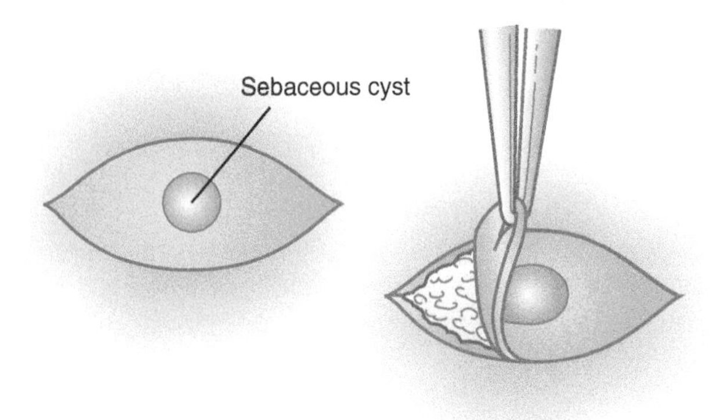

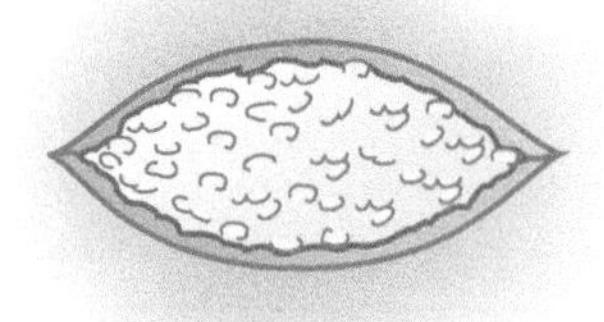

Fig. 10.20 Sebaceous cyst removal. The physician makes an incision, removes the cyst, and sutures the surgical incision. (From Nealon TF, Jr.: *Fundamental skills in surgery,* ed 4, Philadelphia: WB Saunders; 1994.)

usually biopsied unless they have an unusual appearance that may indicate a more serious problem. The side tray setup includes the items needed for a tissue biopsy (specimen container and laboratory request form); however, these items would not be placed on the tray if the physician determines that a biopsy of the sebaceous cyst is not warranted.

Procedure: Sebaceous Cyst Removal

A sebaceous cyst is removed as follows:

1. A local anesthetic is used to numb the area.
2. The physician makes an incision using either a single cut down the center or an oval cut on both sides of the cyst. The physician then removes the cyst and sutures the surgical incision (Fig. 10.20).
3. If the cyst is to be biopsied, it is placed in a specimen container with a preservative and sent to the laboratory for examination by a pathologist.
4. A sterile dressing is applied to the operative site.

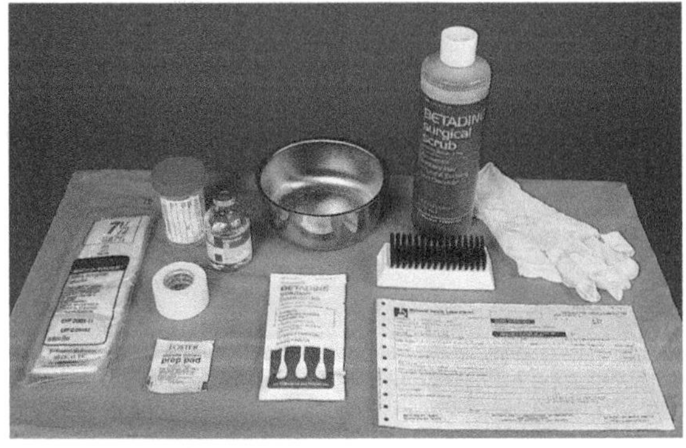

Sebaceous cyst removal side table.

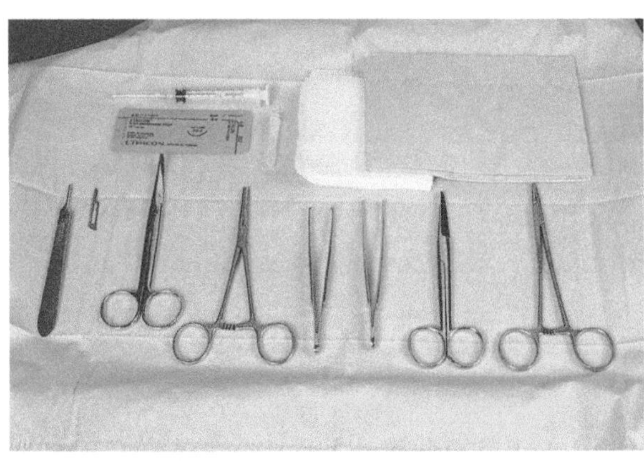

Sebaceous cyst removal sterile field.

Postoperative Instructions: Sebaceous Cyst Removal

Postoperative instructions include the following:

1. Keep the dressing clean and dry.
2. Report any signs that the wound is infected, which include fever, increased pain, swelling, redness, warmth, and discharge.
3. Notify the medical office if the sutures become loose or break.

Provide the patient with written instructions on wound care to refer to at home (see Box 10.2).

SURGICAL INCISION AND DRAINAGE OF LOCALIZED INFECTIONS

An **abscess** is a collection of pus in a cavity surrounded by inflamed tissue (Fig. 10.21A). It is caused by a pathogen that invades the tissues, usually via a break in the skin. An abscess serves as a defense mechanism of the body to keep an infection localized by walling off the microorganisms, preventing them from spreading through the body (see Fig. 10.21B). A **furuncle**, also known as a *boil,* is a localized staphylococcal infection that originates deep within a hair follicle (Fig. 10.22). Furuncles produce pain and itching. The skin initially becomes red and then turns white and necrotic over the top of the furuncle. Erythema and induration usually surround it.

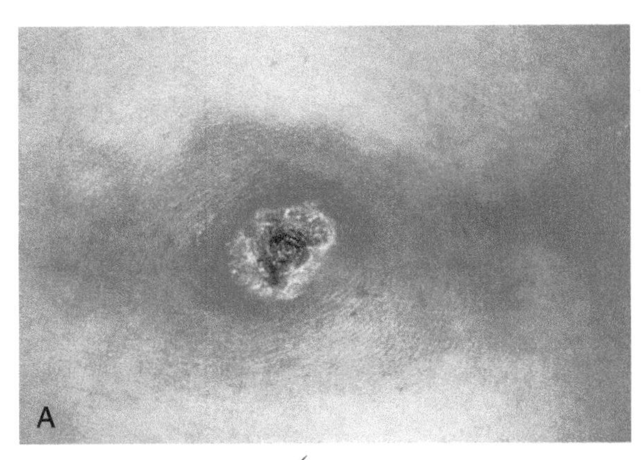

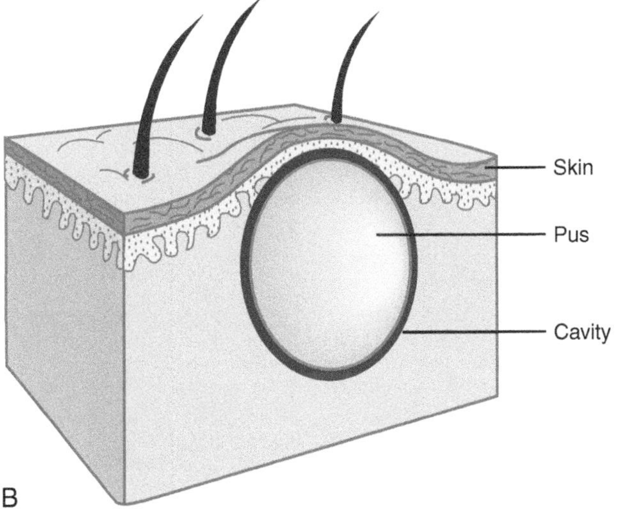

Fig. 10.21 (A) *Staphylococcus* skin abscess. (B) An abscess is a collection of pus in a cavity surrounded by inflamed tissue. (A, From Braverman IM: *Skin signs of systemic disease,* ed 3, Philadelphia: WB Saunders; 1998. B, From Nealon TF, Jr.: *Fundamental skills in surgery,* ed 4, Philadelphia: WB Saunders; 1994.)

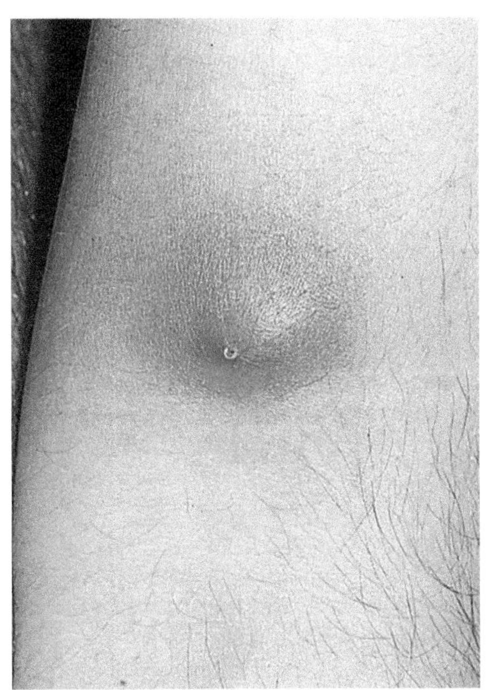

Fig. 10.22 Furuncle (boil) resulting from a *Staphylococcus aureus* infection. (From LaFleur Books M: *Exploring medical language: a student-directed approach,* ed 9, St Louis: Elsevier; 2014.)

Procedure: Incision and Drainage

Localized infections, such as abscesses, furuncles, and infected sebaceous cysts, that do not rupture and drain naturally may need to be incised and drained by the physician as follows:

1. A local anesthetic is typically used for the procedure.
2. A scalpel is used to make the incision. The physician then allows the pus to drain out and uses gauze to absorb pus and blood. Either gauze packing or a rubber Penrose drain is inserted into the wound to keep the edges of the tissues apart; this facilitates drainage of the exudate. The exudate contains pathogenic microorganisms; the medical assistant should be careful to avoid contact with the exudate while assisting with the minor surgery.
3. A sterile dressing of several thicknesses is applied over the operative site to absorb the drainage.

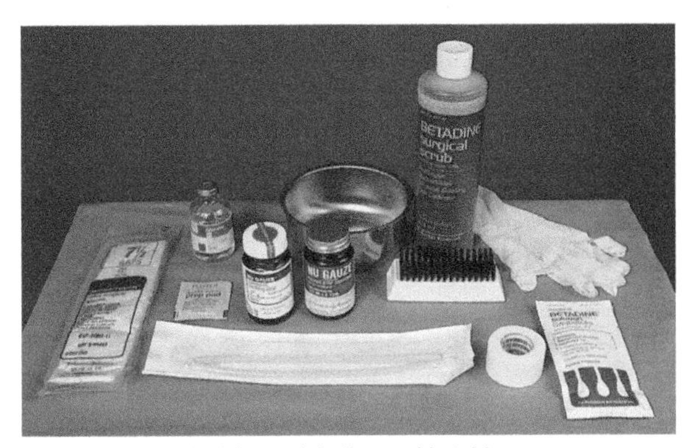

Incision and drainage side table.

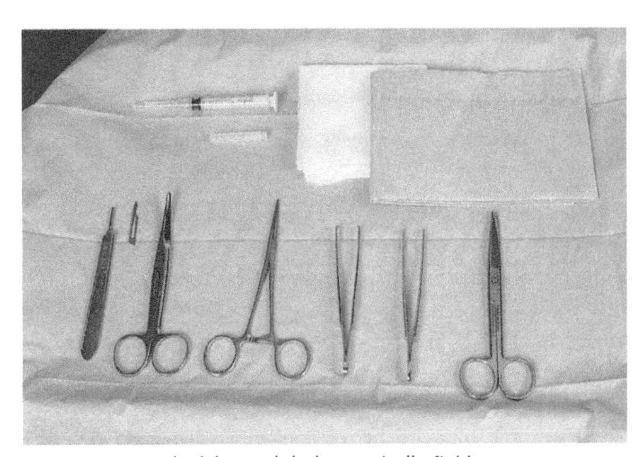

Incision and drainage sterile field.

Postoperative Instructions: Incision and Drainage

Postoperative instructions include the following:

1. Keep the dressing clean and dry.
2. Report any signs that the wound is infected, which include fever, increased pain, swelling, redness, warmth, and discharge.

Provide the patient with written instructions on wound care to refer to at home (see Box 10.2) and instruct the patient when to return for removal of the gauze packing or Penrose drain.

MOLE REMOVAL

A mole (also known as a *nevus*) is a small growth on the human skin. An individual may be born with moles, which are known as *congenital nevi,* but may develop moles over

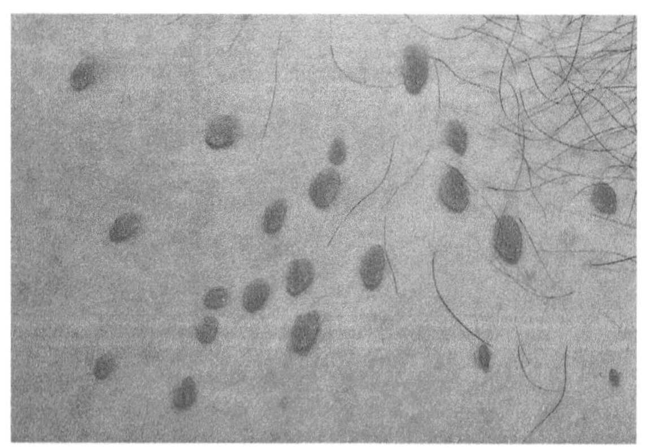

Fig. 10.23 Skin tags. (From White GM, Cox NH: *Diseases of the skin: a color atlas and text,* ed 2, St Louis: Elsevier; 2006.)

time, known as *acquired nevi.* According to the American Academy of Dermatology, the majority of moles appear during the first 20 years of an individual's life. Moles can occur anywhere on the skin, and between 10 and 40 moles on the body is considered normal. Large numbers of moles can be concentrated on the back, chest, and arms. Most moles are benign and exhibit the following characteristics:

- Usually range in color from brown to nearly black but can be a pinkish flesh color to dark blue or even black. Dark-colored moles consist of a cluster of melanocytes. Melanocytes produce the pigment *melanin,* which is responsible for the dark color of moles.
- Shape is usually round or oval and may be smooth or rough.
- Size is usually smaller than a pencil eraser but can range from barely visible to quite a large area.
- May form a raised area on the skin or may be flat.
- May sometimes have hairs growing out of them.

The most common types of moles are skin tags, flat moles, and raised moles. *Skin tags* or *acrochordon* are small, painless, benign growths that project from the skin from a small narrow stalk known as a *peduncle.* They are flesh colored or slightly darker, often appear in groups, and range from 1 to 5 mm in size (Fig. 10.23). Skin tags occur most often during and after middle age in adults who are overweight or have diabetes. Skin tags are most frequently found in body areas where the skin creases, such as the eyelids, neck, armpits, upper chest, and groin. Occasionally a skin tag becomes irritated as a result of shaving or rubbing from clothing or jewelry.

A *flat mole* is any dark spot or irregularity in the skin. A *raised mole,* as the name implies, extends above the skin. It can be a variety of colors and runs deeper than flat moles (Fig. 10.24).

Although most moles are benign, some moles may be precancerous and are known as *dysplastic nevi* (Fig. 10.25). Dysplastic nevi are usually larger than normal moles and have an irregular coloration and shape. The center of dysplastic nevi may be raised and darkened. According to the National Cancer Institute, dysplastic nevi are more likely than ordinary moles to develop into malignant melanoma. Because of this, dysplastic nevi are often biopsied or removed and biopsied to determine whether they are malignant.

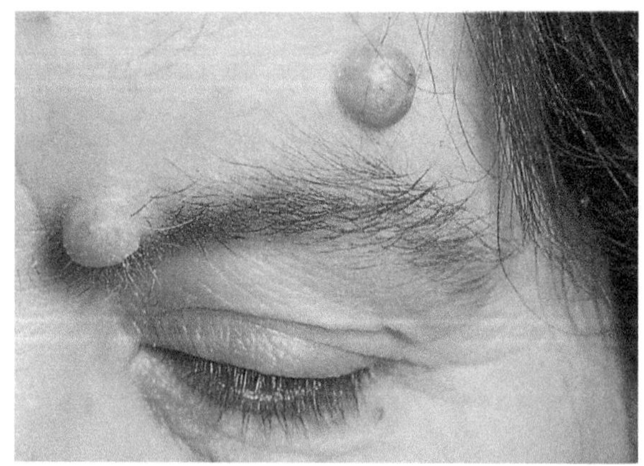

Fig. 10.24 Raised moles. (From Forbes CD: *Color atlas and text of clinical medicine,* ed 3, St Louis: Elsevier; 2003.)

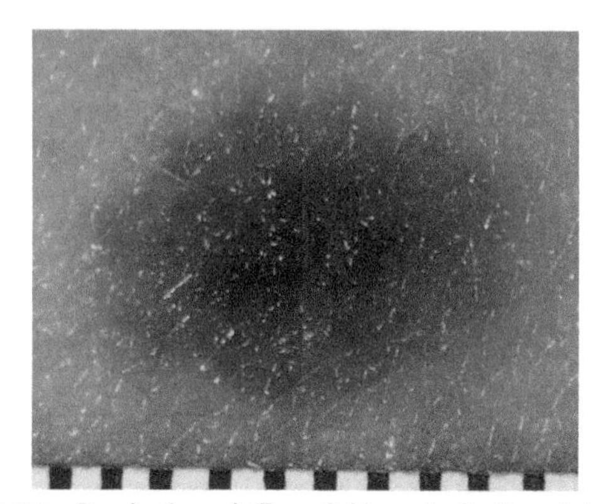

Fig. 10.25 Dysplastic nevi. (From Goldman L: *Cecil medicine,* ed 24, Philadelphia: Elsevier; 2012.)

Melanoma is a very serious type of skin cancer that can sometimes develop within a mole. Melanoma is most apt to be found on the upper backs of men and on the lower legs of women. Studies show that excessive sun exposure, especially severe blistering sunburns early in life, increases the risk of developing certain melanomas. If discovered early, it may be possible to completely remove the melanoma and reduce the spread of skin cancer. Left untreated, melanoma can be fatal.

Any moles exhibiting the following characteristics common to melanoma (Fig. 10.26) should be evaluated by a physician:

- Asymmetric: one-half of the mole is different from the other half.
- Irregular border: the edges of the mole are notched, uneven, or blurred rather than round or distinct.
- Color varies from one area of the mole to another: various shades of tan, brown, and black (and sometimes white, red, or blue) are present.
- Diameter is larger than ¼ inch (6 mm), which is about the diameter of a pencil eraser.
- Other signs: the mole is painful or tender, itches, bleeds, oozes, or has a scaly appearance.

Moles are removed for a variety of reasons, which include cosmetic issues (i.e., to improve an individual's appearance) and reduction of irritation and discomfort from a mole that

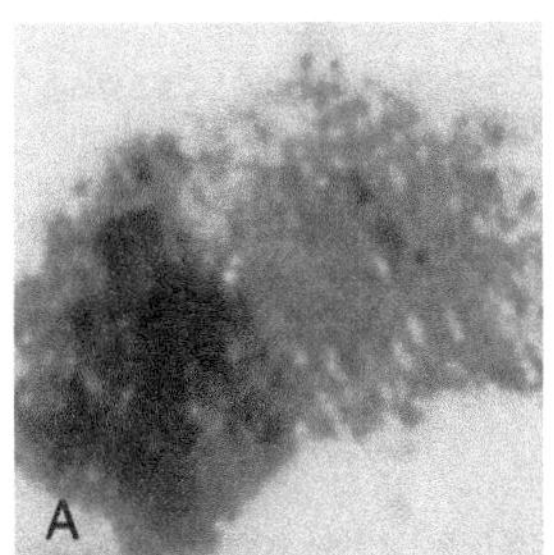

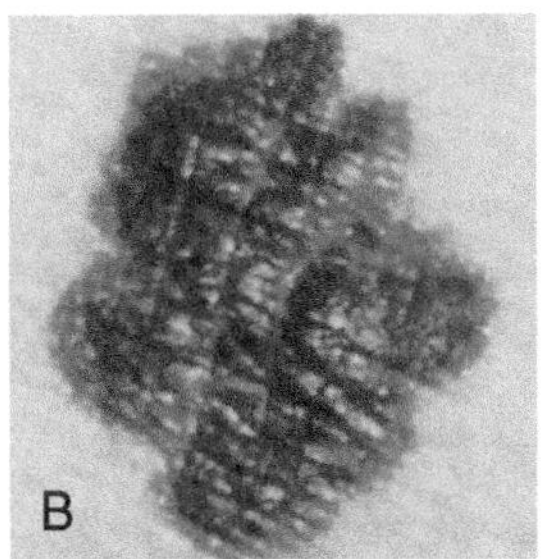

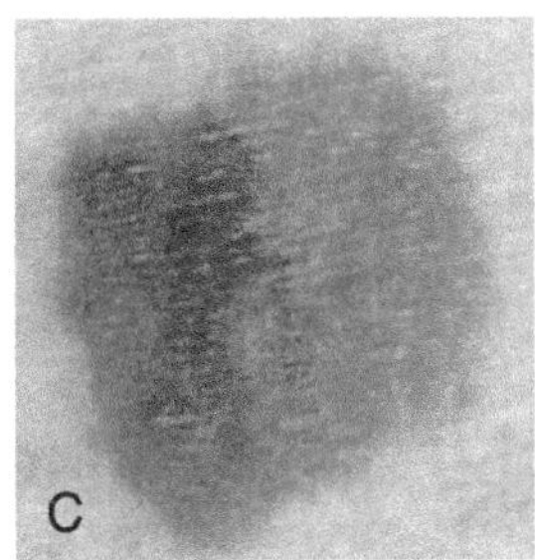

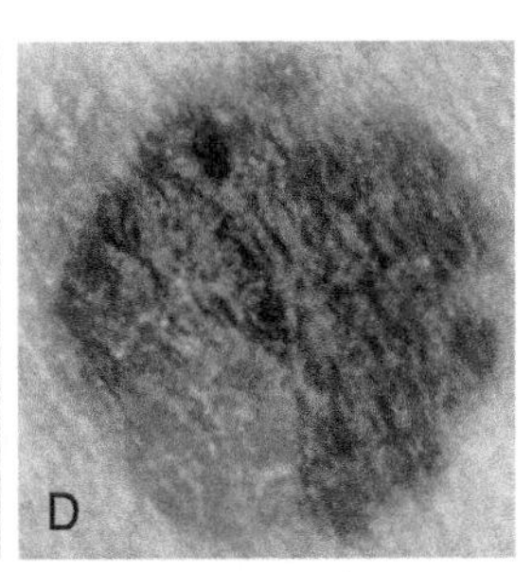

Fig. 10.26 The *ABCDs* of melanoma. (A) Asymmetry (one-half unlike the other half). (B) Border (edges of mole are notched, uneven, or blurred). (C) Color varied from one area to another; shades of tan, brown, and black, and sometimes white, red, or blue. (D) Diameter larger than 1/4 inch or 6 mm (diameter of a pencil eraser). (From Cooper K, Gosnell K: *Adult health nursing,* ed 7, St Louis: Elsevier; 2015.)

is rubbing against clothing or that is in the way when shaving. A more serious reason for removing a mole is that the mole is suspected of being precancerous (dysplastic nevus) or cancerous (melanoma). Several methods may be used for mole removal. The most common methods include shave excision, surgical excision, and laser surgery. The method used depends on the type of mole being removed, including its size, shape, color, and location. In some cases, a biopsy of the mole is performed before the mole is removed to determine whether the mole is benign or malignant.

Procedure: Mole Shave Excision

A shave excision is most commonly used to remove protruding moles. It can also be used to remove skin tags. This procedure is not used to remove dysplastic nevi because it might leave mole cells beneath the surface of the skin, which could cause the mole to grow back again. Sutures are not usually required for a shave excision. After the numbing effect of the anesthetic wears off, the area will be tender and sore. As healing occurs, a scab forms, which usually falls off within 1 to 2 weeks, leaving a red mark. As healing progresses, a flat, white mark usually remains in the place of the mole, which is approximately the same size as the mole. Over time, it fades to a barely visible scar. A mole is removed using the shave excision procedure as follows:

1. The physician numbs the area with a local anesthetic.
2. The physician uses a scalpel to shave off the protruding part of the mole until the area is flush with the level of the surrounding skin.
3. The physician may use an electrocautery instrument to destroy the tissue below the surface of the mole and to control bleeding.
4. A topical antibiotic is applied to the area.
5. A sterile dressing is applied to the operative site.
6. The mole shavings may be placed in a specimen container with a preservative and sent to the laboratory for examination by a pathologist.

Procedure: Surgical Mole Excision

The surgical excision procedure is often used when the physician suspects that a mole is precancerous or cancerous. A scalpel is used to remove the entire mole, as well as a border of surrounding skin and tissue underlying the mole, to remove all the mole cells. A scar commonly forms after this procedure; however, it usually fades over time. A mole is removed using the surgical excision procedure as follows:

1. The physician numbs the area with a local anesthetic.
2. The physician uses a scalpel to cut an oval border surrounding the mole and removes the mole with tissue forceps.
3. The physician may use an electrocautery instrument to control bleeding.
4. The physician inserts sutures to close the surgical incision.
5. A sterile dressing is applied to the operative site.
6. The mole is placed in a specimen container with a preservative and is sent to the laboratory for examination by a pathologist.

Postoperative Instructions: Shave Excision and Surgical Excision

Postoperative instructions for both a shave excision and a surgical excision of a mole include the following:

1. Keep the dressing clean and dry.
2. Report any signs that the wound is infected, which include fever, increased pain, swelling, redness, warmth, and discharge.
3. If sutures have been inserted, notify the medical office if they become loose or break.
4. To reduce scarring, protect the area from the ultraviolet (UV) rays of the sun by staying out of the sun or using a good sunscreen with a sun protection factor (SPF) of 15 or higher.

Provide the patient with written instructions on wound care to refer to at home (see Box 10.2).

LASER MOLE SURGERY

Laser surgery is used to remove small or flat moles that are brown or black in color. This procedure involves the use of a laser beam of light that evaporates the mole tissue. The laser beam also seals off blood vessels, avoiding the need for sutures. Because the laser light cannot penetrate deeply enough, this method usually is not used on raised moles, deep moles, large moles, or dysplastic nevi.

Removing a mole with a laser reduces the amount of tissue destruction in the surrounding tissue, which minimizes scarring. This procedure does not require a local anesthetic. No pain is involved during the procedure; the patient feels only a mild tingling when the laser pulses. A scab forms, which usually falls off within 1 to 2 weeks. Once the scab falls off, the area is usually reddish, and it may take several weeks before normal skin color returns. Repeated treatments (one to three) may be required before the mole is completely removed.

The medical assistant should instruct the patient to keep the area clean and dry. The patient should also protect the area from the UV rays of the sun by staying out of the sun or by using a good sunscreen with an SPF of 15 or higher.

NEEDLE BIOPSY

A **biopsy** is the removal and examination of tissue from the living body. The tissue usually is examined under a microscope. Biopsies are most often performed to determine whether a tumor is malignant or benign; however, a biopsy also may be used as a diagnostic aid for other conditions, such as infections. A **needle biopsy** is a type of biopsy in which tissue from deep within the body is obtained by the insertion of a biopsy needle through the skin. The advantage of a needle biopsy is that a sample of tissue can be obtained that might otherwise require a major surgical operation.

Procedure: Needle Biopsy

1. The procedure is performed with the patient under a local anesthetic, and because an incision is not required, the patient does not have to undergo the discomfort and inconvenience of an operative recovery.
2. The tissue specimen is placed in a container with a preservative and is sent to the laboratory for examination by a pathologist.
3. A small dressing, placed over the needle puncture site, is usually sufficient to protect the operative site and promote healing.
4. After the procedure, the patient should be observed for any evidence of complications related to the procedure.

Postoperative Instructions: Needle Biopsy

1. A bruise typically occurs at the biopsy site and will gradually disappear within several weeks.
2. Keep the dressing clean and dry.
3. Rest and avoid strenuous activity and heavy lifting for 2 days after the procedure.
4. Report any signs that the wound is infected, which include fever, increased pain, swelling, redness, warmth, and discharge.

INGROWN TOENAIL REMOVAL

An ingrown toenail occurs when the edge of the toenail grows deeply into the nail groove and penetrates the surrounding skin, resulting in pain and discomfort (Fig. 10.27A). An ingrown nail can occur in both the nails of the hands and those of the feet; however, it is more apt to occur in the toenails. External pressure, such as from tight shoes, or trauma, improper nail trimming, or infection can cause an ingrown toenail. The protruding nail acts as a foreign body, usually resulting in secondary infection and inflammation. In mild cases, this condition is treated by inserting a small piece of cotton packing under the toenail to raise the nail edge away from the tissue of the nail groove (see Fig. 10.27B). In severe and recurring cases, part of the nail must be surgically removed (see Fig. 10.27C and D). Severe cases cause pain, swelling, redness, and drainage (Fig. 10.28). The toenail removal procedure relieves pain by decreasing nail pressure on the soft tissues.

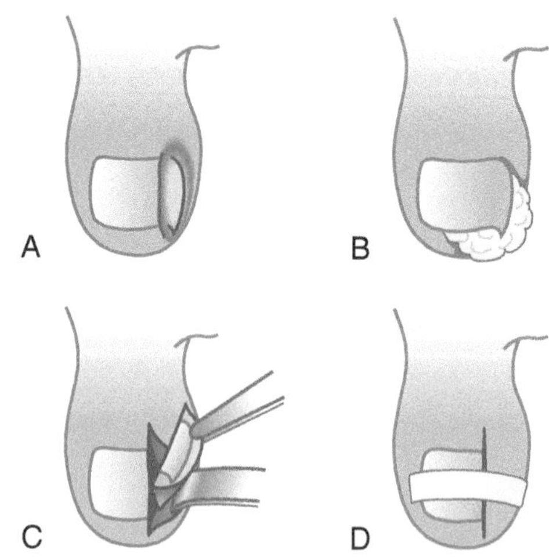

Fig. 10.27 Ingrown toenail. (A) The edge of the toenail grows deeply into the nail groove. (B) In mild cases, treatment consists of inserting a small piece of cotton packing under the toenail. (C) In severe and recurring cases, a wedge of the nail is surgically removed. (D) A strip of surgical tape is applied over the area. (From Nealon TF, Jr.: *Fundamental skills in surgery,* ed 4, Philadelphia: WB Saunders; 1994.)

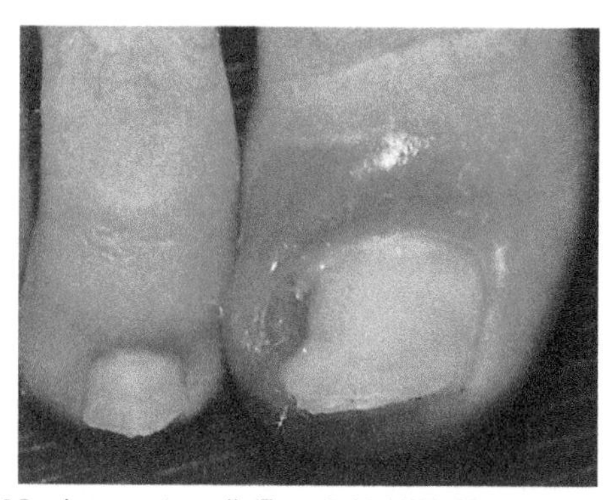
Fig. 10.28 Ingrown toenail. (From Seidel HM: *Mosby's guide to physical examination,* ed 6, St Louis, 2006, Elsevier.)

Procedure: Ingrown Toenail

An ingrown toenail is removed as follows:

1. Before the surgical procedure is performed, the affected foot must be soaked in tepid water containing an antibacterial skin solution for 10 to 15 minutes to soften the nail plate and decrease the possibility of bacterial infection.
2. The patient is placed in a reclining position with the foot adequately supported, and the toe is shaved to remove hair, which would act as a contaminant.
3. An antiseptic is applied to the affected toe, which is then numbed using a local anesthetic.

4. Using surgical toenail scissors, the physician surgically removes a wedge of the nail (see Fig. 10.27C).
5. An antibiotic ointment is applied to the area.
6. A sterile gauze dressing or a strip of surgical tape is applied over the area to protect the operative site and to promote healing (see Fig. 10.27D).

Postoperative Instructions: Ingrown Toenail

Postoperative instructions include the following:

1. Elevate the foot for 24 hours following the procedure.
2. Keep the area clean and dry.
3. Cleanse the toe daily with warm water and gently dry the area.
4. Apply an antibiotic ointment daily until the wound has completely healed.
5. Wear loose-fitting shoes for 2 weeks after the procedure.
6. Avoid strenuous exercise for 2 weeks after the procedure.
7. Contact the medical office if any signs of infection occur, which include increasing pain, redness, swelling, and drainage from the toe.

Provide the patient with written instructions on wound care to refer to at home (see Box 10.2) and instruct the patient on the importance of wearing properly fitting shoes and on the proper procedure for nail trimming. The nail should be cut straight across with the corners of the nail protruding from the end of the toe.

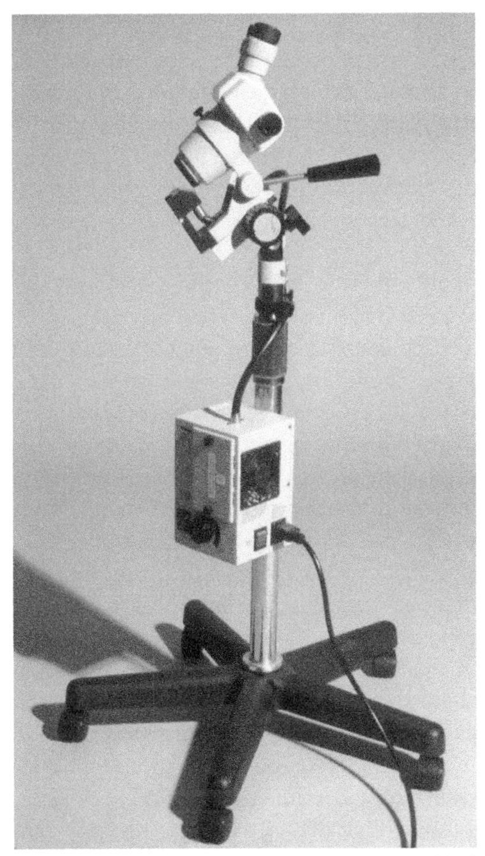

Fig. 10.29 A colposcope. (From Apgar BS, Brotzman GL, Spitzer M: *Colposcopy: principles and practice—an integrated textbook and atlas*, Philadelphia: Elsevier; 2002.)

COLPOSCOPY

Colposcopy is the visual examination of the vagina and cervix by means of a lighted instrument with a binocular magnifying lens, known as a **colposcope** (Fig. 10.29). The purpose of colposcopy is to examine the vagina and cervix to detect areas of abnormal tissue growth that may not be visible with the naked eye (Fig. 10.30). Colposcopy is performed after abnormal Pap test results and to evaluate a vaginal or cervical lesion observed during a pelvic examination. The primary goal of colposcopy is to prevent cervical cancer by detecting precancerous lesions early and treating them.

Blood cells make it more difficult for the physician to observe the cervix; therefore, a colposcopy is usually performed 1 week after the end of the menstrual period. To prepare for the procedure, the patient should be told not to douche; use tampons, vaginal medications, or spermicides; or have intercourse for 24 hours before the examination. The lens of the colposcope is positioned approximately 12 inches (30 cm) from the opening of the vagina. The lens magnifies tissue, facilitating the inspection of cervical cells and the obtaining of a biopsy specimen. For a routine colposcopic examination, a magnification ranging from 6× to 15× is typically used. The colposcope may be placed on an adjustable stand or attached to the side of the examining table and swung out before use.

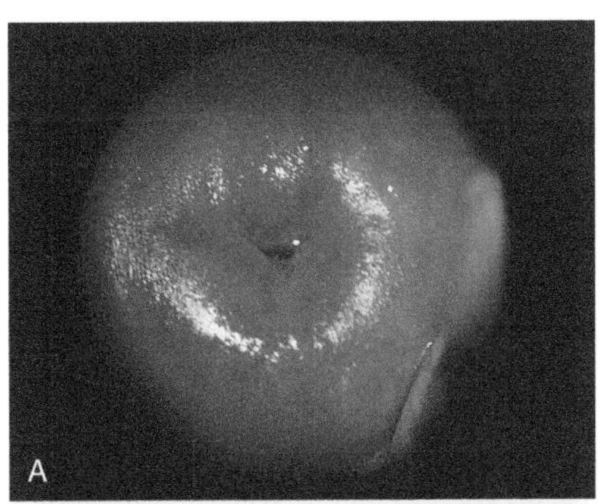

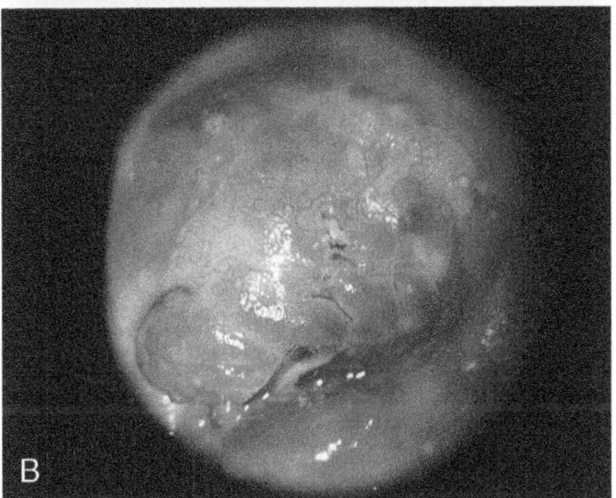

Fig. 10.30 (A) Normal cervix. (B) Abnormal cervix. (From Damjanov I: *Pathology for the health-related professions*, ed 4, St Louis: Elsevier; 2012.)

Procedure: Colposcopy

Colposcopy is performed as follows:

1. The patient is assisted into a lithotomy position and is prepared for a pelvic examination.

2. The physician inserts a vaginal speculum into the vagina.
3. A long, cotton-tipped applicator moistened with saline is used to wipe the cervix to remove the mucous film that normally covers it. The saline also provides better visualization of the cervical epithelium because dry cervical epithelium is not transparent and does not allow satisfactory viewing of the vascular pattern of the cervix.
4. The colposcope is focused on the cervix, and the physician inspects the saline-moistened cervix.
5. The cervix is swabbed with acetic acid using a long, cotton-tipped applicator. The acetic acid dissolves cervical mucus and other secretions. It also causes abnormal tissue to turn white, allowing easier visualization of abnormal areas of the cervix.
6. The cervical epithelium also may be stained with Lugol iodine solution using a long, cotton-tipped applicator. This provides another means to identify unhealthy epithelium. The healthy epithelium of the cervix contains glycogen, which can absorb the iodine, causing the epithelium to stain a dark brown color. Conversely, abnormal epithelium, such as would constitute a malignancy, does not contain glycogen and is unable to absorb the iodine.
7. If an abnormal area is observed, the physician obtains a cervical biopsy specimen using punch biopsy forceps, which is described next.

CERVICAL PUNCH BIOPSY

A cervical biopsy is performed in combination with colposcopy to remove a cervical tissue specimen for examination by a pathologist. The purpose of the biopsy is to detect the presence of cervical dysplasia or cancer of the cervix. *Cervical dysplasia* is an abnormal growth of cells on the surface of the cervix that are precancerous. *Precancerous* means that abnormal cells have the potential to develop into cancer in the future. Cervical dysplasia can range from mild to moderate to severe. A cervical punch biopsy can also be used to diagnose polyps on the cervix and genital warts. Genital warts may indicate infection with human papillomavirus (HPV), which is a risk factor for developing cervical cancer. Performing a cervical punch biopsy helps the physician determine the type of abnormal tissue present on the cervix so that the physician can determine the best form of treatment for the patient's condition.

Cervical biopsies are most frequently performed after abnormal Pap test results. Although an abnormal Pap test result is a cause for concern, the majority of abnormal Pap test results are not caused by cervical cancer, but rather by a vaginal infection. To prevent inaccurate test results, the cervical biopsy is usually performed 1 week after the end of the menstrual period when the cervix is the least vascular. To prepare for the procedure, the patient should be told not to douche; use tampons, vaginal medications, or spermicides; or have intercourse for 24 hours before the procedure to prevent inaccurate test results.

What Would You Do? What Would You *Not* Do?

Case Study 3

Sadira Wisal has been referred to the office by her family physician for a colposcopy. Her last Pap test results came back as abnormal, and a repeat Pap test 3 months later also had abnormal results. While having her vital signs taken, Sadira bursts into tears. She tearfully explains that she is afraid that she has cancer and that no one at her family physician's office told her what to expect from this procedure. Sadira does not understand why she has to have this procedure and does not know what will be done during the procedure. She says that she feels stupid, but she does not even know what a cervix is. Sadira also worries that the procedure will affect her ability to have children. ■

Procedure: Cervical Punch Biopsy

A cervical punch biopsy is performed as follows:

1. The patient is positioned and draped in a lithotomy position. An anesthetic is not needed because the cervix has few pain receptors. The patient may experience no discomfort during the procedure or a certain amount of discomfort ranging from mild to moderate in intensity. Some patients experience mild cramping and pinching when the specimen is being removed from the cervix.
2. The physician inserts a vaginal speculum into the vagina for proper visualization of the cervix.
3. The cervix is wiped with saline and then swabbed with ascetic acid.
4. To assist in obtaining the specimen, the physician may stain the cervix with Lugol iodine solution.
5. The colposcope is focused on the cervix, and the physician inspects the cervix.
6. Using cervical biopsy punch forceps, the physician obtains several tissue specimens (Fig. 10.31A) from the abnormal cervical epithelium (see Fig. 10.31B). The patient may feel a pinching sensation and mild cramps each time a specimen is removed from the cervix.
7. The specimen is placed in a container with a preservative and is sent to the laboratory for examination by a pathologist.
8. If bleeding occurs, the physician controls it with gauze packing, a hemostatic solution (e.g., Monsel solution), or electrocautery.
9. The patient is given a sanitary pad at the office after the procedure to absorb any discharge.

Postoperative Instructions: Cervical Punch Biopsy

Postoperative instructions include the following:

1. A minimum amount of cramping and bleeding may follow the procedure and last up to 1 week. Contact the medical office if the bleeding lasts longer than 2 weeks.
2. A thick, dark-colored vaginal discharge may occur after the procedure (if Monsel solution was used to control bleeding) and may last for several days.

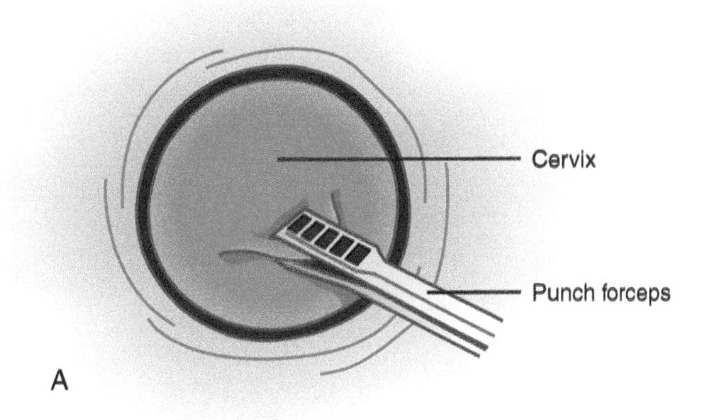

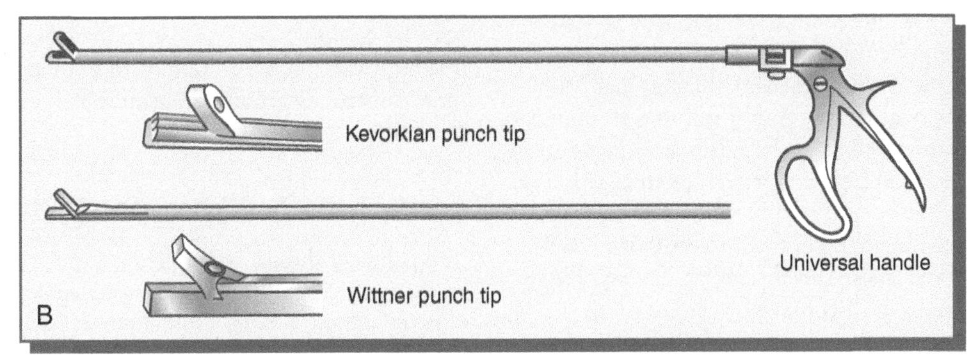

Fig. 10.31 Cervical punch biopsy. (A) Obtaining a tissue specimen from the cervix using cervical biopsy punch forceps. (B) Cervical biopsy punch forceps. (Courtesy Elmed, Addison, IL.)

3. Do not douche, use tampons, or have intercourse for 1 week after the procedure to allow proper healing of the cervix to take place.
4. Contact the medical office if any of the following occurs: bleeding that is heavier than normal menstrual bleeding, a foul-smelling vaginal discharge, fever, or lower abdominal pain.

Provide the patient with written instructions to refer to at home. An appointment is scheduled approximately 1 week after the procedure to make sure that healing is taking place and to discuss the biopsy results.

CRYOSURGERY

Cervical Cryosurgery

Cervical **cryosurgery**, also known as *cryotherapy*, uses freezing temperatures to treat certain gynecologic conditions. Cryosurgery is most often performed as a treatment for cervical dysplasia to destroy abnormal cervical cells that show changes that may lead to cancer. Cryosurgery is done only after a colposcopy confirms the presence of cervical dysplasia. Cryosurgery is also used for the treatment of chronic cervicitis, which is inflammation of the cervix.

Cervical cryosurgery can be performed without an anesthetic, although occasionally a mild analgesic is necessary immediately afterward. The cryosurgery unit consists of a long metal cryoprobe attached to a cooling-agent tank (Fig. 10.32). The principal cooling agents are liquid nitrogen and compressed nitrogen gas. The cryoprobe is inserted into the vagina and placed firmly in contact with the abnormal area. The cooling agent flows through the cryoprobe, freezing the cervical tissue to −20° C. This causes the abnormal cells to die and slough off so that the cervical covering can eventually be replaced with new, healthy epithelial tissue. Regeneration of cervical tissue occurs within approximately 4 to 6 weeks after the procedure. After cryosurgery, the patient will be required to have a Pap test every 3 to 6 months for a period of time determined by the physician.

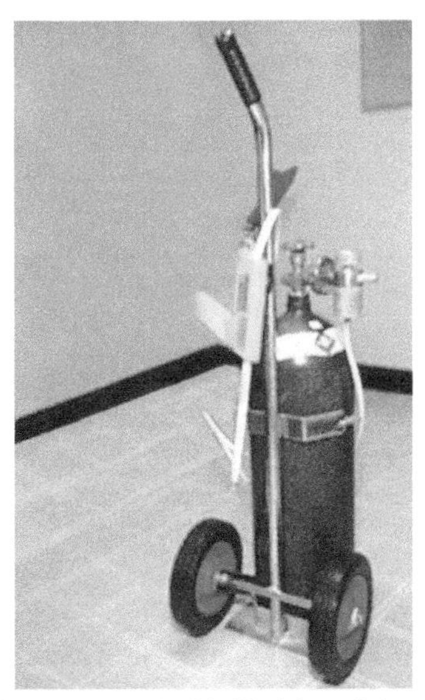

Fig. 10.32 Cryosurgery unit. (Modified from Zakus S: *Clinical skills for medical assistants*, ed 4, Philadelphia: WB Saunders; 2001.)

Procedure: Cervical Cryosurgery

Cryosurgery is performed as follows:

1. The patient is draped and assisted into the lithotomy position.
2. The physician inserts a vaginal speculum for proper visualization of the cervix.
3. The cervix is swabbed with an acid-saline solution to remove mucus and other contaminants.
4. The metal cryoprobe is inserted into the vagina and placed firmly in contact with the affected area, and the cryosurgery unit is turned on.
5. The cooling agent flows through the cryoprobe and causes the metal probe to freeze and destroy superficial abnormal cervical tissue. The physician allows the cryoprobe to come in contact with the cervical area for approximately 3 minutes. During the procedure, the patient may experience some pain resembling menstrual cramping.
6. The cryoprobe is removed for 3 to 5 minutes to permit the cervical tissue to return to its normal temperature. The freezing procedure is then repeated for an additional 3 minutes.
7. When the procedure has been completed, the medical assistant should assist the patient as necessary and observe her for signs of discomfort or vertigo.
8. The patient is given a sanitary pad at the office after the procedure to absorb any discharge.

Postoperative Instructions: Cervical Cryosurgery

Postoperative instructions include the following:

1. Normal activities can be resumed the day after the cryosurgery.
2. On the first postoperative day, a clear, watery vaginal discharge occurs, which lasts for 2 to 4 weeks. The discharge is caused by the shedding of the dead cervical tissue and gradually diminishes as the healing progresses.
3. Use sanitary pads (rather than tampons) to absorb the watery discharge.
4. Do not douche, use tampons, or have intercourse for 2 to 3 weeks after the procedure to allow proper healing of the cervix to take place.
5. Contact the medical office if any of the following occurs: bleeding that is heavier than normal menstrual bleeding, a foul-smelling vaginal discharge, fever, or lower abdominal pain.

Provide the patient with written instructions to refer to at home. The patient must schedule a return visit 6 weeks after the procedure to ensure that proper healing has occurred.

Skin Lesions

In the medical office, cryosurgery also may be used to remove benign skin lesions, such as common warts and skin tags. Only a small amount of cooling agent is required for skin lesions, so the cryosurgery unit is considerably smaller than the one described for cervical cryosurgery. Most physicians use liquid nitrogen contained in a small, pressurized, stainless steel canister with an attached probe. The physician applies the liquid nitrogen to the skin lesion until it turns white, which indicates that freezing of the tissue has occurred. During the procedure, the patient feels a slight burning or stinging sensation as the cooling agent is applied. After cryosurgery, a blister develops and dries to a scab in 1 week to 10 days and eventually sloughs off. The patient should be told to keep the area clean and dry until the scab has sloughed off. In some cases, the treatment may not result in complete destruction of the lesion; two or more treatments may be required to remove the lesion.

BANDAGING

A **bandage** is a strip of woven material used to wrap or cover a part of the body. The function of the bandage may be to apply pressure to control bleeding, to protect a wound from contamination, to hold a dressing in place, or to protect, support, or immobilize an injured part of the body.

GUIDELINES FOR APPLICATION

The bandage should be applied so that it feels comfortable to the patient, and it must be fastened securely with metal clips or adhesive tape. Guidelines for applying a bandage are as follows:

1. Observe the principles of medical asepsis during the application of a bandage.
2. Ensure that the area to which a bandage is applied is clean and dry.
3. Do not apply a bandage directly over an open wound. To prevent contamination of the wound, first apply a sterile dressing and then the bandage. The bandage should extend at least 2 inches (5 cm) beyond the edge of the dressing.
4. To prevent irritation, do not allow the skin surfaces of two body parts (e.g., two fingers) to touch. In addition, the patient's perspiration provides a moist environment that encourages the growth of microorganisms. A piece of gauze should be inserted between the two body parts.
5. Ensure that joints and prominent parts of bones are padded to prevent the bandage from rubbing the skin and causing irritation.
6. Bandage the body part in its normal position with joints slightly flexed to avoid muscle strain.
7. Apply the bandage from the distal to the proximal part of the body to aid the venous return of blood to the heart.
8. As you apply the bandage, ask the patient whether it feels comfortable. The bandage should fit snugly enough that it does not fall off but not so tightly that it impedes circulation.
9. If possible, leave the fingers and toes exposed when bandaging an extremity. This provides the opportunity to check them for signs of impairment in circulation. Signs indicating that the bandage is too tight include coldness, pallor, numbness, cyanosis of the nail beds,

swelling, pain, and tingling sensations. If any of these signs occurs, loosen the bandage immediately.

10. If a bandage roll is dropped during the procedure, obtain a new bandage and begin again.

TYPES OF BANDAGES

Three basic types of bandages are used in the medical office. A *roller bandage* is a long strip of soft material wound on itself to form a roll. It ranges from 1/2 inch to 6 inches (1.3 to 15.2 cm) wide and from 2 to 5 yards (1.83 to 4.57 m) long. The width used depends on the part being bandaged. Roller bandages usually are made of sterilized gauze. Gauze is porous and lightweight, molds easily to a body part, and is relatively inexpensive and easily disposed of. Because it is made of loosely woven cotton, however, it may slip and fray easily. *Kling gauze* is a special type of gauze that stretches; this allows it to cling, and as a result, it molds and conforms better to the body part than does regular gauze.

Elastic bandages are made of woven cotton that contains elastic fibers. One brand name of elastic bandages is the Ace bandage. Although elastic bandages are expensive, they can be washed and used again. The medical assistant must be extremely careful when applying an elastic bandage because it is easy to apply it too tightly and impede circulation. Elastic adhesive bandages also may be used; these have an adhesive backing to provide a secure fit.

BANDAGE TURNS

Five basic bandage turns are used, alone or in combination. The type of turn used depends on which body part is to be bandaged and whether the bandage is used for support or immobilization or for holding a dressing in place.

The *circular turn* is applied to a part of uniform width, such as toes, fingers, or the head. Each turn completely overlaps the previous turn. Two circular turns are used to anchor a bandage at the beginning and end of a spiral, spiral-reverse, figure-eight, or recurrent turn (Fig. 10.33).

The *spiral turn* is applied to a part of uniform circumference, such as the fingers, arms, legs, chest, or abdomen. Each spiral turn is carried upward at a slight angle and should overlap the previous turn by one-half to two-thirds the width of the bandage (Fig. 10.34).

The *spiral-reverse turn* is useful for bandaging a part that varies in width, such as the forearm or lower leg. Reversing each spiral turn allows for a smoother fit and prevents gaping caused by variation in the contour of the limb. The thumb is used to make the reverse halfway through each spiral turn. The bandage is directed downward over the thumb towards the lower edge of the previous turn. Each turn should overlap the previous one by two-thirds the width of the bandage. The reverse turn is used as often as necessary to provide a uniform fit (Fig. 10.35).

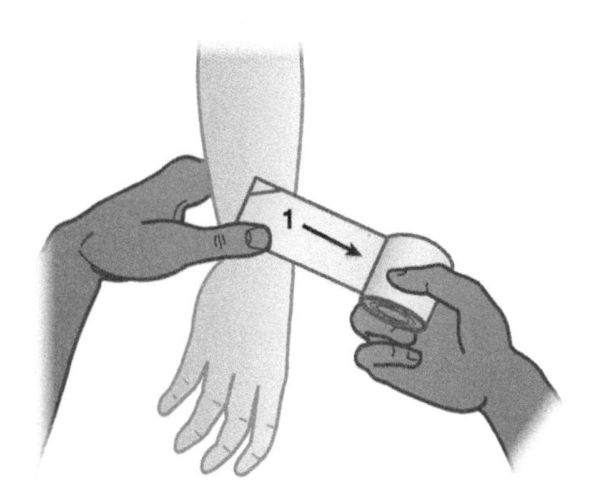

1. Place the end of the roller bandage on a slant.

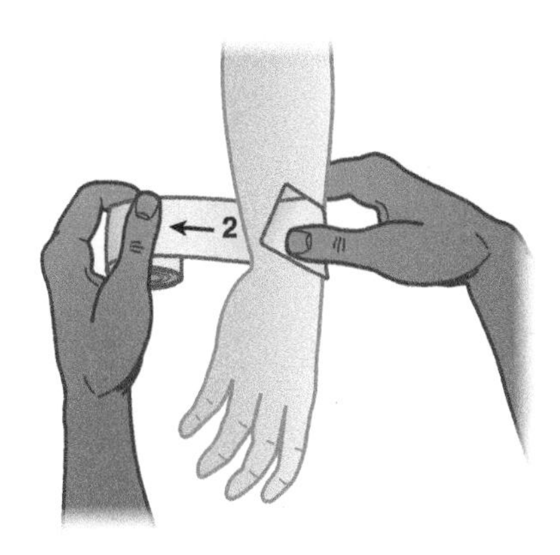

2. Encircle the part while allowing the corner of the bandage to extend.

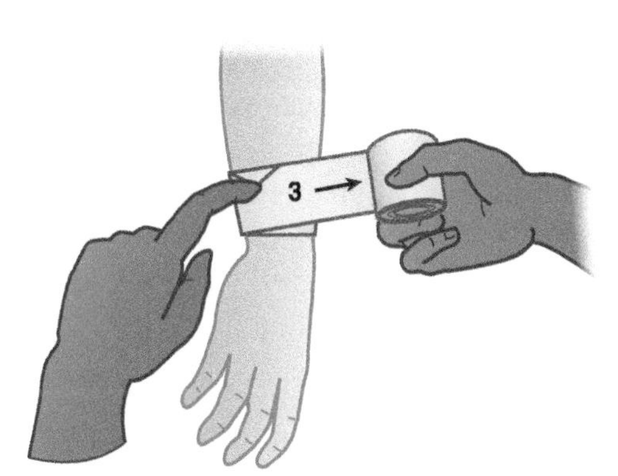

3. Turn down the corner of the bandage.

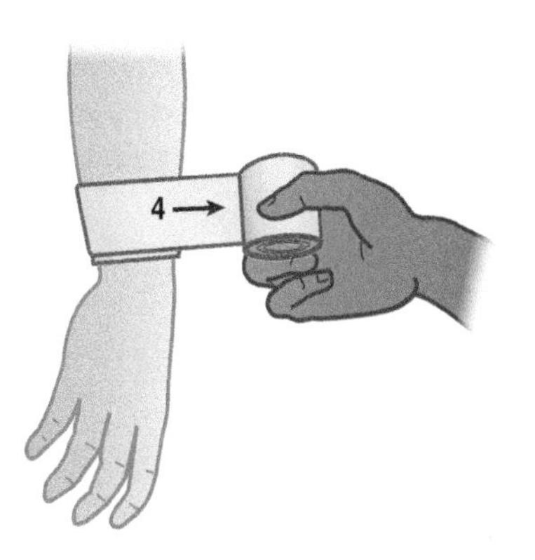

4. Make another circular turn around the part.

Fig. 10.33 Anchoring a bandage.

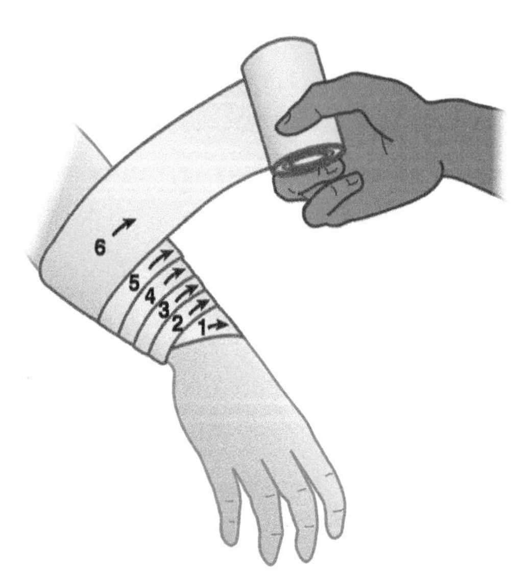

Fig. 10.34 Spiral turn.

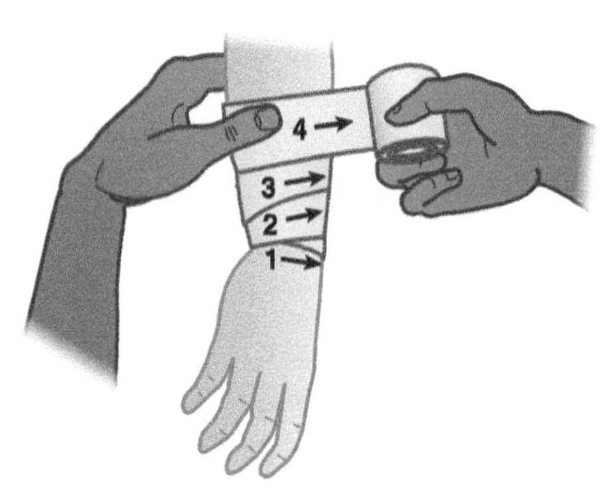

1. Encircle the lower arm while keeping the bandage at a slant.

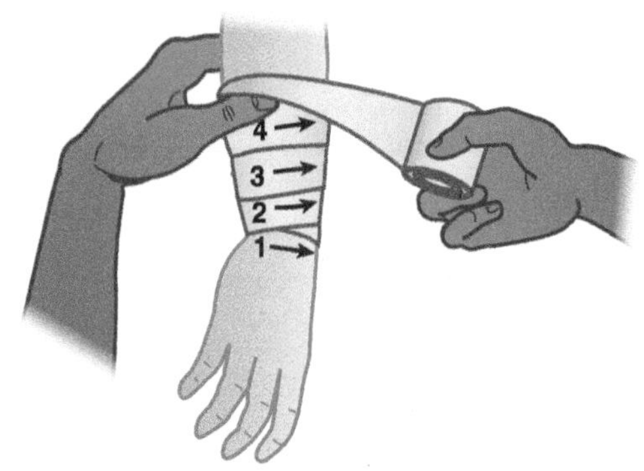

2. Direct the bandage downward over the thumb towards the lower edge of the previous turn.

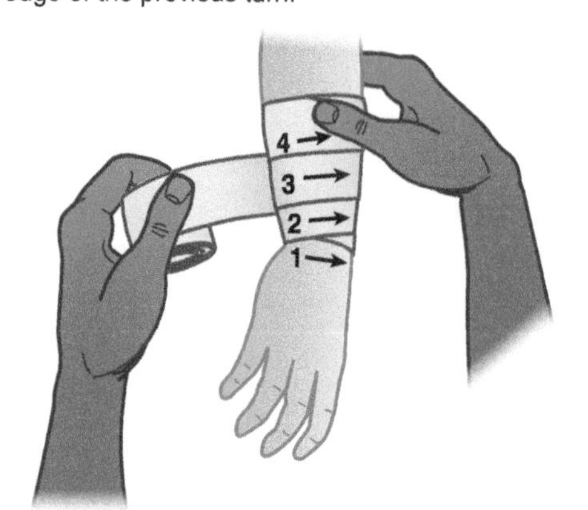

3. Keep the bandage parallel to the lower edge of the previous turn.

Fig. 10.35 Spiral-reverse turn.

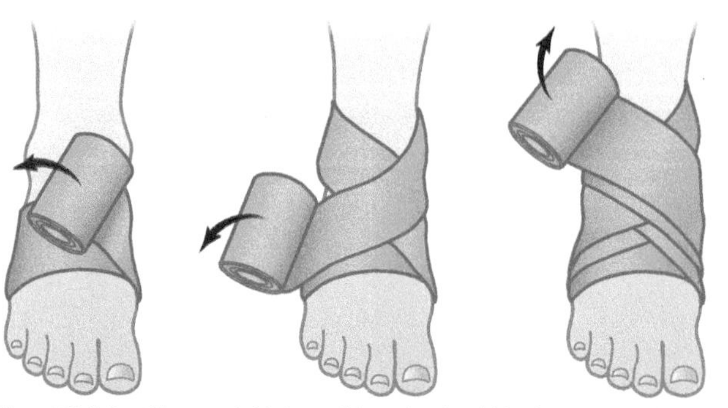

Fig. 10.36 Figure-eight turn. (From Leake MJ: *A manual of simple nursing procedures*, Philadelphia: WB Saunders; 1971.)

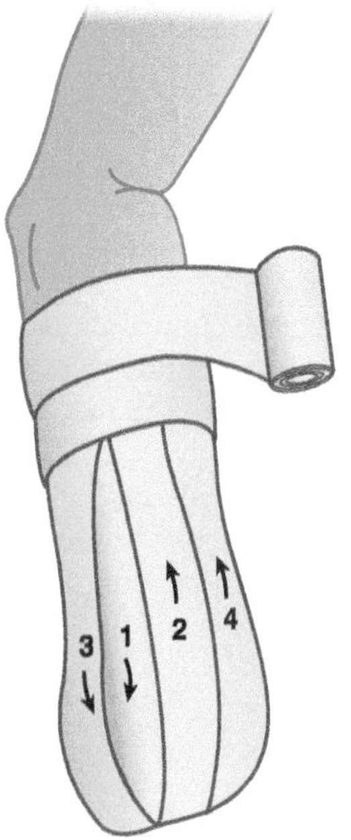

Fig. 10.37 Recurrent turn.

In general, the *figure-eight turn* is used to hold a dressing in place or to support and immobilize an injured joint, such as the ankle, knee, elbow, or wrist. The figure-eight turn consists of slanting turns that alternately ascend and descend around the part and cross over one another in the middle, resembling the figure-eight. Each turn overlaps the previous one by two-thirds the width of the bandage (Fig. 10.36).

The *recurrent turn* is a series of back-and-forth turns used to bandage the tips of fingers or toes, the stump of an amputated extremity, or the head. The bandage is anchored by using two circular turns and is passed back and forth over the tip of the part to be bandaged, first on one side and then on the other side of the first center turn. Each turn should overlap the previous turn by two-thirds the width of the bandage (Fig. 10.37).

What Would You Do? What Would You *Not* Do? RESPONSES

Case Study 1
Page 333

What Did Heidi Do?
- ❑ Tried to calm and reassure Mrs. Ventura. Told her that children at this age are prone to accidents and that she should not blame herself.
- ❑ Told Mrs. Ventura that Cory's wound could not be held together effectively with Steri-Strips. Explained that sutures would help the wound heal better.
- ❑ Told Mrs. Ventura that the doctor could not suture the wound unless she signs the consent form. Explained that Cory's wound should be sutured as soon as possible to prevent infection and to minimize scarring.
- ❑ Asked Mrs. Ventura if she would like to talk with the doctor again before signing the form.

What Did Heidi Not Do?
- ❑ Did not prepare Cory for the suture insertion procedure until Mrs. Ventura signed the consent to treatment form.

Case Study 2
Page 338

What Did Heidi Do?
- ❑ Explained to Abbey that the antiseptic contains iodine, which appears orange when it is applied to the skin. Assured her that the iodine would not stain her skin permanently and that it would wear off in a few days.
- ❑ Calmly and discreetly opened a new pair of sterile gloves so that the physician could reapply sterile gloves. Reminded Abbey not to move during the procedure.
- ❑ Told Abbey that most tissues removed from patients are routinely sent to the laboratory for a biopsy. Reassured her that the doctor has told her everything he knows about her condition.
- ❑ Made it clear to Abbey that her neighbor is not permitted to remove her sutures. Stressed to her that the doctor needs to check her incision before the sutures are removed to ensure that proper healing has occurred.

What Did Heidi Not Do?
- ❑ Did not scold Abbey for contaminating the physician's sterile gloved hand.

Case Study 3
Page 346

What Did Heidi Do?
- ❑ Listened empathetically to Sadira, and tried to calm and reassure her.
- ❑ Spent some time going over the colposcopy procedure and what to expect.
- ❑ Answered as many of Sadira's questions as possible. Reassured her that a lot of people do not know what a cervix is and that she is asking some very good questions.
- ❑ Asked the physician to spend some time talking with Sadira before the procedure to answer questions that Heidi is not qualified to answer.
- ❑ Ensured that Sadira understood all of the information about the procedure before asking her to sign the consent to treatment form.

What Did Heidi Not Do?
- ❑ Did not tell Sadira that her family physician should have explained the procedure to her.
- ❑ Did not tell Sadira that she does not have cancer.

TERMINOLOGY REVIEW

Key Term	Word Parts	Definition
Abrasion		A wound in which the outer layers of the skin are damaged; a scrape.
Ascess		A collection of pus in a cavity surrounded by inflamed tissue.
Absorbable suture		Suture material that is gradually digested and absorbed by the body.
Approximation		The process of bringing two parts, such as tissue, together through the use of sutures or other means.
Bandage		A strip of woven material used to wrap or cover a part of the body.
Biopsy	*bi/o:* life *-opsy:* to view	The surgical removal and examination of tissue from the living body. Biopsies are typically performed to determine whether a tumor is benign or malignant.
Capillary action		The action that causes liquid to rise along a wick, a tube, or a gauze dressing.
Colposcope	*colp/o:* vagina *-scope:* instrument used for visual examination	A lighted instrument with a binocular magnifying lens used to examine the vagina and cervix.

Continued

TERMINOLOGY REVIEW—cont'd

Key Term	Word Parts	Definition
Colposcopy	*colp/o:* vagina *-scopy:* visual examination	The visual examination of the vagina and cervix using a colposcope.
Contaminate		As it relates to sterile technique, to cause a sterile object or surface to become unsterile.
Contusion		An injury to the tissues under the skin that causes blood vessels to rupture, allowing blood to seep into the tissues; a bruise.
Cryosurgery	*cry/o:* cold	The therapeutic use of freezing temperatures to destroy abnormal tissue.
Exudate		A discharge produced by the body's tissues.
Fibroblast	*fibr/o:* fibrous tissue *-blast:* developing cell	An immature cell from which connective tissue can develop.
Forceps		A two-pronged instrument for grasping and squeezing.
Furuncle		A localized staphylococcal infection that originates deep within a hair follicle. Also known as a *boil.*
Hemostasis	*hem/o:* blood *-stasis:* control, stop	The arrest of bleeding by natural or artificial means.
Incision		A clean cut caused by a cutting instrument.
Infection		The condition in which the body, or part of it, is invaded by a pathogen.
Infiltration		The process by which a substance passes into and is deposited within the substance of a cell, tissue, or organ.
Inflammation		A protective response of the body to trauma and the entrance of foreign matter. The purpose of inflammation is to destroy invading microorganisms and to remove damaged tissue debris from the area so that proper healing can occur.
Laceration		A wound in which the tissues are torn apart, leaving ragged and irregular edges.
Ligate		To tie off and close a structure such as a severed blood vessel.
Local anesthetic		A drug that produces a loss of feeling and an inability to perceive pain in only a specific part of the body.
Mayo tray		A broad, flat metal tray placed on a stand and used to hold sterile instruments and supplies when it has been covered with a sterile towel.
Needle biopsy	*bi/o:* life *-opsy:* to view	A type of biopsy in which tissue from deep within the body is obtained by the insertion of a biopsy needle through the skin.
Nonabsorbable suture		Suture material that is not absorbed by the body and either remains permanently in the body tissue and becomes encapsulated by fibrous tissue or is removed.
Postoperative	*post-:* after	After a surgical operation.
Preoperative	*pre-:* before	Before a surgical operation.
Puncture		A wound made by a sharp-pointed object piercing the skin.
Scalpel		A surgical knife used to divide tissues.
Scissors		A cutting instrument.
Sebaceous cyst		A thin, closed sac or capsule that contains fatty secretions from a sebaceous gland.
Serum		The clear, straw-colored part of the blood that remains after the solid elements have been separated out of it.
Sterile		Free of all living microorganisms and bacterial spores.
Surgery		The branch of medicine that deals with operative and manual procedures for correction of deformities and defects, repair of injuries, and diagnosis and treatment of certain diseases.
Surgical asepsis	*a:* without or absence of *-sepsis:* infection	Practices that keep objects and areas sterile or free from microorganisms.
Sutures		Material used to approximate tissues with surgical stitches.
Swaged needle		A needle with suturing material permanently attached to its end.
Wound		A break in the continuity of an external or internal surface caused by physical means.

PROCEDURE 10.1 Applying and Removing Sterile Gloves

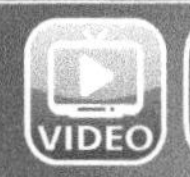

Outcome Apply and remove sterile gloves.

The medical assistant must wear sterile gloves to perform a sterile procedure, such as a dressing change, or to assist the physician during minor office surgery. The medical assistant must learn to put on the gloves using the principles of surgical asepsis so as not to contaminate them.

Gloves must be removed in a manner that protects the medical assistant from contaminating the clean hands with pathogens that might be on the outside of the gloves. This is accomplished by not allowing the bare hands to come in contact with the outside of the gloves.

Equipment/Supplies

- Sterile gloves

Applying Sterile Gloves

1. **Procedural Step.** Remove all rings and put them in a safe place. Wash your hands with antimicrobial soap.
   Principle. Rings may cause the gloves to tear. The warm, moist environment inside gloves provides ideal growing conditions for the multiplication of transient microorganisms on the hands. Washing the hands with an antimicrobial removes these microorganisms and also deposits an antibacterial film on your hands to discourage the growth of bacteria. This prevents the transmission of pathogens.
2. **Procedural Step.** Choose appropriate-sized gloves; they should not be too small or too large. The gloves should fit snugly but not be too tight.
   Principle. If your gloves are too small, they may rip as you apply them or become uncomfortable to wear. If they are too large, you may find it difficult to perform your tasks.
3. **Procedural Step.** Place the glove package on a clean flat surface. Open the glove package without touching the inside of the wrapper. The tops of the gloves are turned down to form a cuff.
   Principle. The hands are not sterile, and the inside of the wrapper is sterile.
4. **Procedural Step.** Pick up the first glove on the inside of the cuff with the fingers of the opposite hand, being sure not to touch the outside of the glove with your ungloved hand.
   Principle. After applying the gloves, the inside of the cuff lies next to your skin and does not remain sterile; therefore, it is permissible to pick up the glove by the cuff. The outside of the glove is sterile, and touching it would contaminate it. If a glove becomes contaminated, you must obtain a new pair of gloves and repeat the procedure.

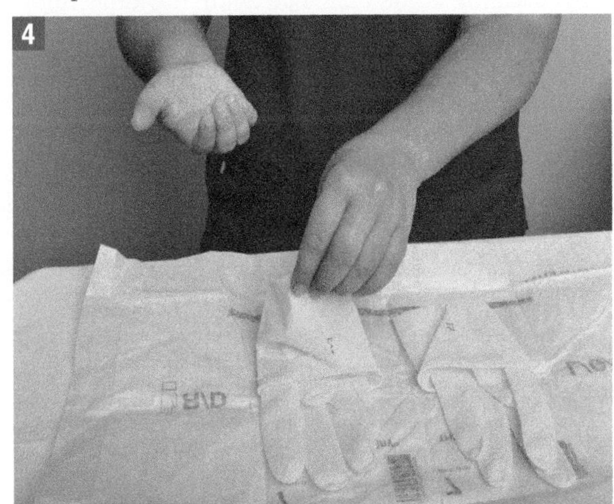

Pick up the first glove on the inside of the cuff.

5. **Procedural Step.** Step back and pull the glove on. Allow the cuff to remain turned back on itself.
   Principle. Stepping back prevents your unsterile hand from passing over the glove still in the glove package, which would contaminate it.
6. **Procedural Step.** Pick up the second glove by slipping your sterile gloved fingers under its cuff.
   Principle. The underside of the cuff is sterile and may be touched by the sterile gloved hand.

Continued

PROCEDURE 10.1 Applying and Removing Sterile Gloves—cont'd

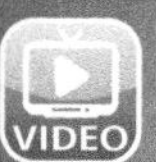

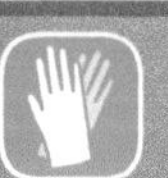

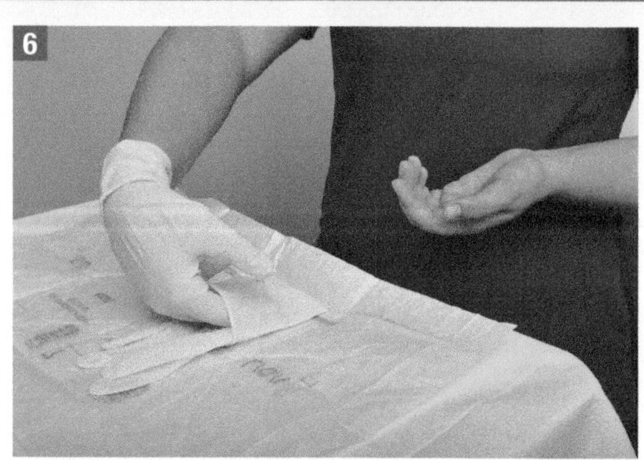

Pick up the second glove.

7. **Procedural Step. Pull the glove onto your hand and turn back the cuff.**
8. **Procedural Step.** Turn back the cuff of the first glove by reaching under the cuff with the other gloved hand. Do not allow your sterile gloved hand to come in contact with the inside of the cuff. Adjust the gloves to a comfortable position. Inspect the gloves for tears.

   Principle. The area under the folded cuff is sterile and may be touched by the sterile gloved hand. The inside of the cuff has previously been touched by your clean hands and is not sterile. If a tear is present, a new pair of gloves must be applied.

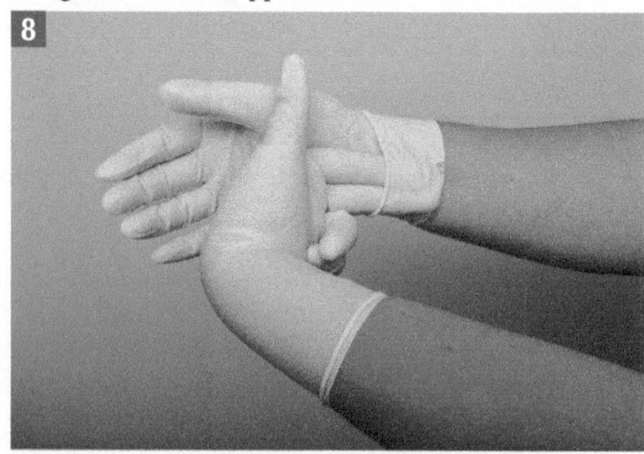

Turn back the cuff of the first glove.

Removing Sterile Gloves

1. **Procedural Step.** With your gloved left hand, grasp the outside of the right glove 1 to 2 inches from the top. (*Note:* It does not matter which glove is removed first—you may start with the left glove if you prefer.)

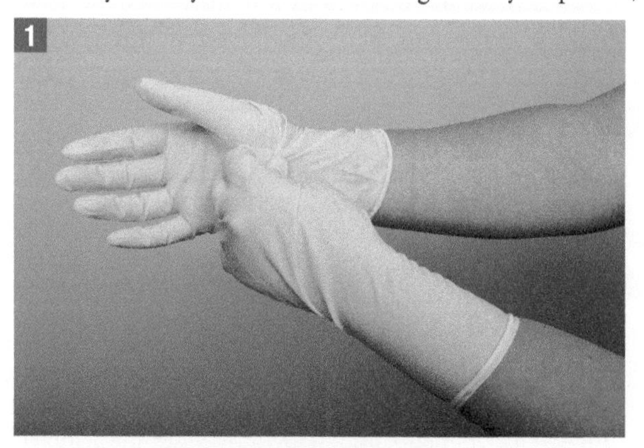

Grasp the outside of the glove.

2. **Procedural Step.** Slowly pull the right glove off the hand. It turns inside out as it is removed from your hand.
3. **Procedural Step.** Pull the right glove free, and scrunch it into a ball with your gloved left hand.

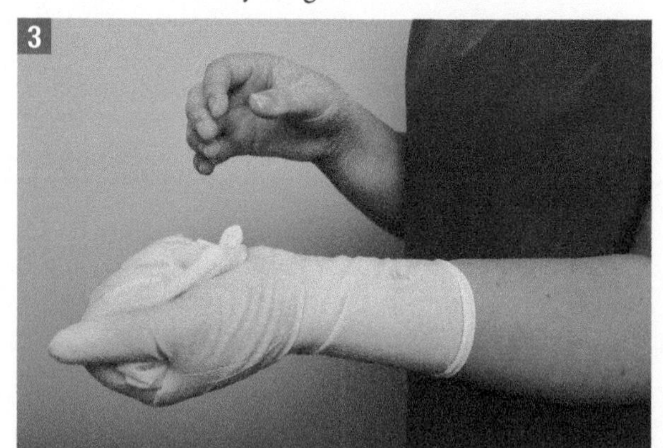

Scrunch the glove into a ball.

4. **Procedural Step.** Place the index and middle fingers of the right hand on the inside of the left glove. Do not allow your clean hand to touch the outside of the glove.

PROCEDURE 10.1 Applying and Removing Sterile Gloves—cont'd

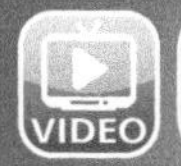

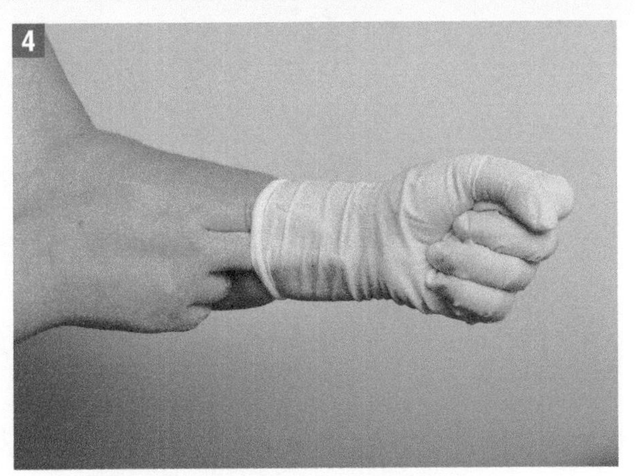

Place the fingers on the inside of the glove.

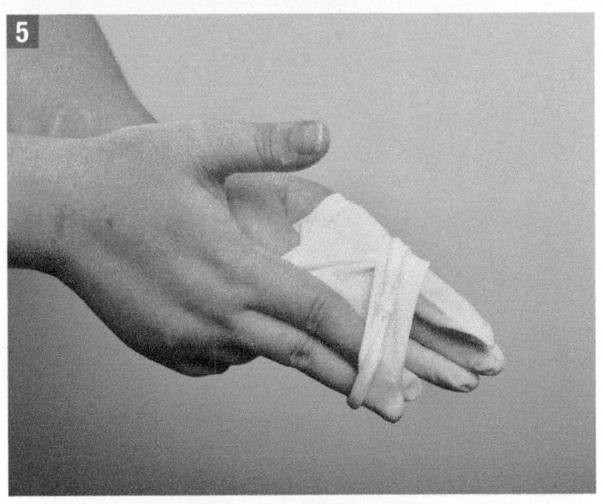

Pull the glove off the hand.

5. **Procedural Step.** Pull the second glove off the left hand. It turns inside out as it is removed from your hand, enclosing the balled-up right glove. Discard both gloves in an appropriate waste container. If your gloves are visibly contaminated with blood or other potentially infectious materials, discard them in a biohazard waste container; otherwise, they can be discarded in a regular waste container.

6. **Procedural Step.** Sanitize your hands thoroughly to remove any microorganisms that may have come in contact with your hands.

PROCEDURE 10.2 Opening a Sterile Package

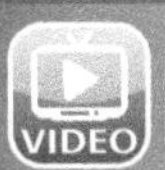

Outcome Open a sterile package. The sterile package may be in the form of a commercially prepared disposable package or a pack that has been assembled and sterilized at the medical office; in both cases, the inside of the sterile wrapper serves as the sterile field.

Equipment/Supplies

- Sterile package

1. **Procedural Step.** Sanitize your hands.
2. **Procedural Step.** Assemble the equipment.
3. **Procedural Step.** Check the pack to make sure it is not wet, torn, or opened. These factors cause contamination of the sterile contents and the pack must not be used. If autoclave tape has been used to close the pack, check to make sure the tape has changed color.

   Principle. Autoclave tape indicates that the pack has been through the sterilization process, but it does not verify that the contents of the pack are sterile.

PROCEDURE 10.2

PROCEDURE 10.2 Opening a Sterile Package—cont'd

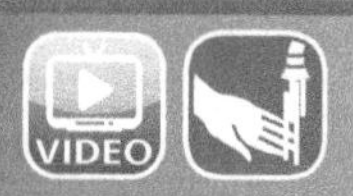

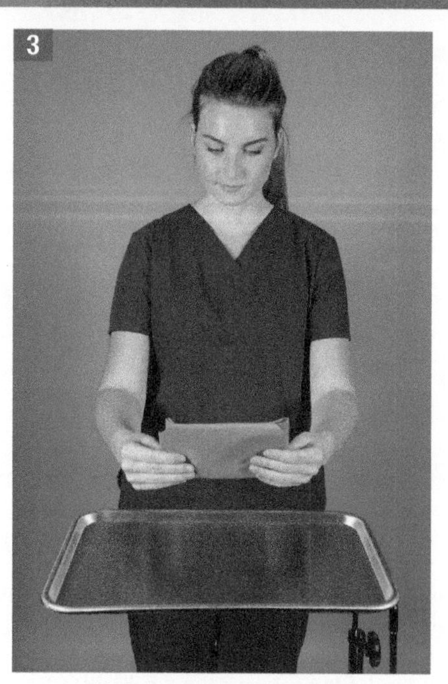

Check the sterilization indicator.

4. **Procedural Step.** Place the wrapped package on the table so that the top flap of the wrapper opens away from you. Always face the sterile field, and do not talk, laugh, cough, or sneeze over the field. These actions contaminate the sterile field.
5. **Procedural Step.** Loosen and remove the fastener on the wrapped package, and discard it in a waste container.
6. **Procedural Step.** Open the first flap away from the body. Handle only the outside of the wrapper.
   Principle. The medical assistant should open the sterile package so as not to reach over the sterile contents. Otherwise, dust or lint from unsterile clothing may fall on the contents of the package and cause contamination.

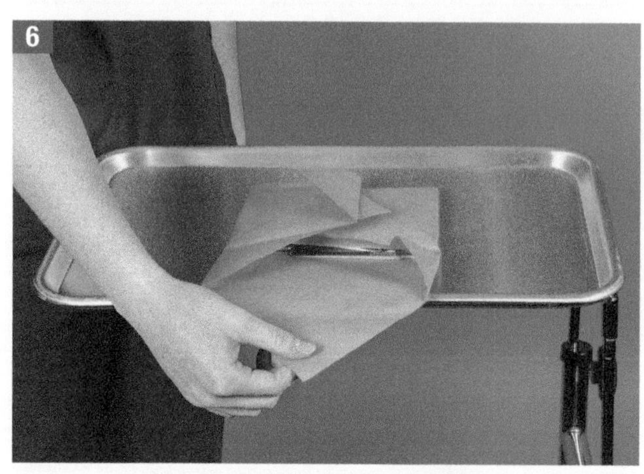

Open the first flap away from the body.

7. **Procedural Step.** Without crossing over the sterile field, open the left and right flaps.

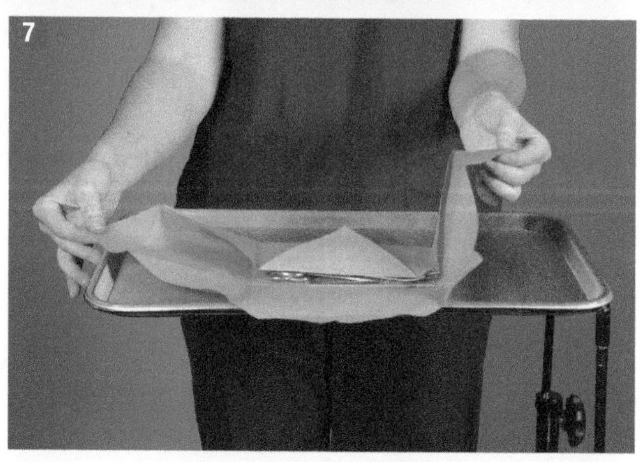

Open the left and right flaps.

8. **Procedural Step.** Open the flap closest to the body by lifting it toward you. Touch only the outside of the wrapper.

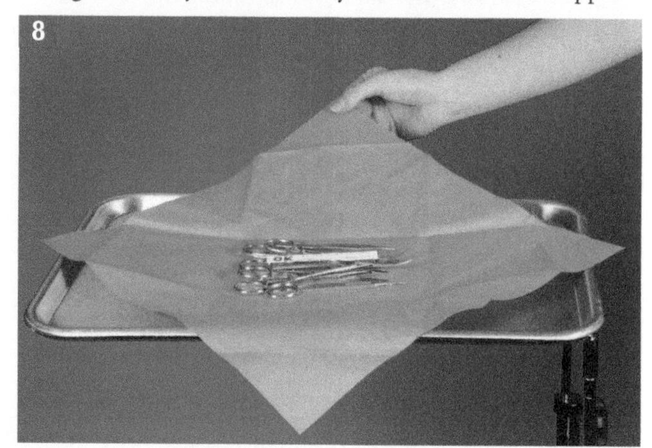

Open the flap closest to the body.

9. **Procedural Step.** Adjust the sterile wrapper by the corners as needed to make sure it lies in proper position on the tray or table.

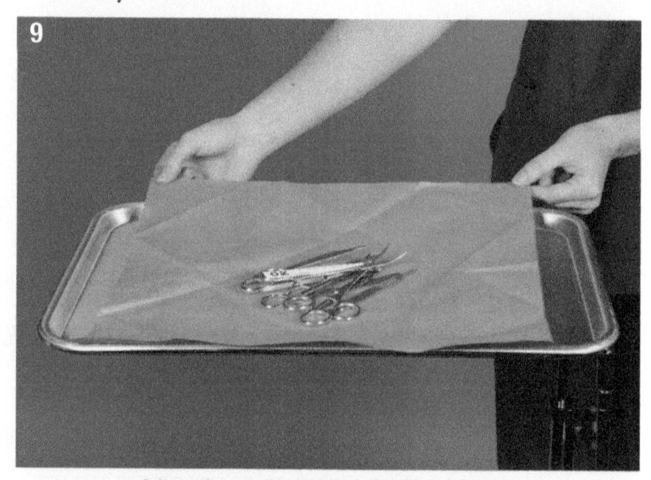

Adjust the sterile wrapper by the corners.

10. **Procedural Step.** Check the sterilization indicator on the inside of the pack to make sure it has changed appropriately. This indicates that the contents of the pack are sterile.

PROCEDURE 10.3 Pouring a Sterile Solution

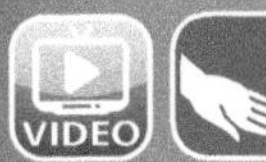
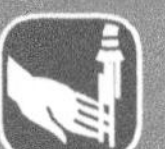

Outcome Pour a sterile solution.

Equipment/Supplies

- Sterile solution
- Sterile container
- Sterile towel

1. **Procedural Step.** Read the label of the solution to ensure that you have the correct solution.
2. **Procedural Step.** Check the expiration date on the solution. Do not use an outdated solution.
   Principle. Outdated solutions may produce undesirable effects and should be discarded.
3. **Procedural Step.** Check the solution label a second time to make sure you have the correct solution.
4. **Procedural Step.** Place the palm of your hand over the label. Remove the cap by touching only the outside, and place the cap on a flat surface with the open end up. Do not place the cap on the sterile field, as the outside of the cap is contaminated.
   Principle. Palming the label prevents the solution from dripping on the label and obscuring it. Handling the cap by the outside prevents contamination of the inside. Placing the cap with the open end up prevents contamination of the inside of the cap by an unsterile surface.
5. **Procedural Step.** Rinse the lip of the bottle (if it has been previously used) by pouring a small amount of solution into a separate container.
   Principle. Rinsing the lip washes away any microorganisms that may be on it.
6. **Procedural Step.** Pour the proper amount of solution into the sterile container at a height of approximately 6 inches. Do not allow the neck of the bottle to come in contact with the sterile container, and be careful not to splash solution onto the sterile field.
   Principle. Pouring from a height of approximately 6 inches reduces splashing and prevents contamination of the sterile container with the outside of the (unsterile) bottle.

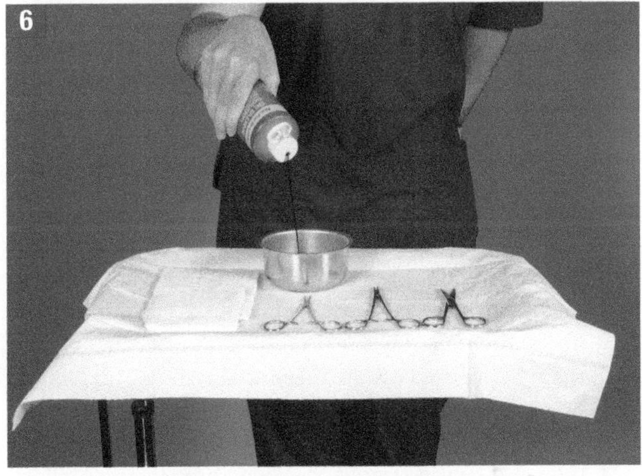

Pour the proper amount of solution.

7. **Procedural Step.** Replace the cap on the container without contaminating it. Check the label a third time to ensure that you have poured the correct solution.

PROCEDURE 10.3

PROCEDURE 10.4 Changing a Sterile Dressing

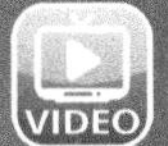

Outcome Change a sterile dressing.

Equipment/Supplies

- Mayo stand
- Biohazard waste container

Side Table

- Clean disposable gloves
- Antiseptic swabs
- Sterile gloves
- Plastic waste bag
- Surgical tape
- Scissors

Sterile Field

- Sterile dressing
- Sterile thumb forceps

Continued

PROCEDURE 10.4 Changing a Sterile Dressing—cont'd

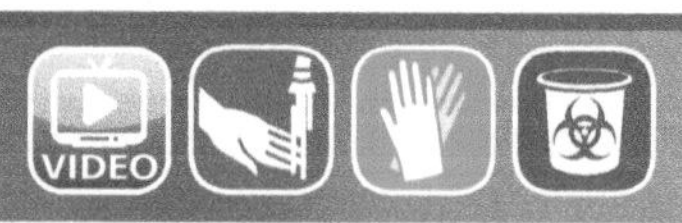

1. **Procedural Step.** Wash your hands with antimicrobial soap.
2. **Procedural Step.** Assemble the equipment. Set up the nonsterile items on a side table or counter. Position the waterproof waste bag in a location convenient for the disposal of contaminated items.

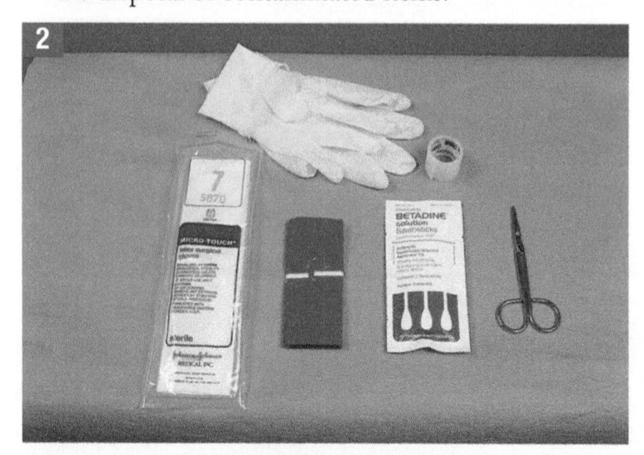

Prepare the side table.

3. **Procedural Step.** Greet the patient and introduce yourself. Identify the patient by full name and date of birth and explain the procedure. Instruct the patient not to move during the procedure. Adjust the light so that it is focused on the dressing.
4. **Procedural Step.** Apply clean gloves. Loosen the tape on the dressing, and pull it toward the wound. Carefully and gently remove the soiled dressing by pulling it upward. Do not touch the inside of the dressing that was next to the open wound. If the dressing is stuck to the wound, it can be loosened by moistening it with a normal saline solution. Place the soiled dressing in the waste bag without allowing the dressing to touch the outside of the bag.
   Principle. Gentle dressing removal avoids unnecessary stress on the wound. Touching the inside of the dressing can transfer an infected discharge to your gloves.

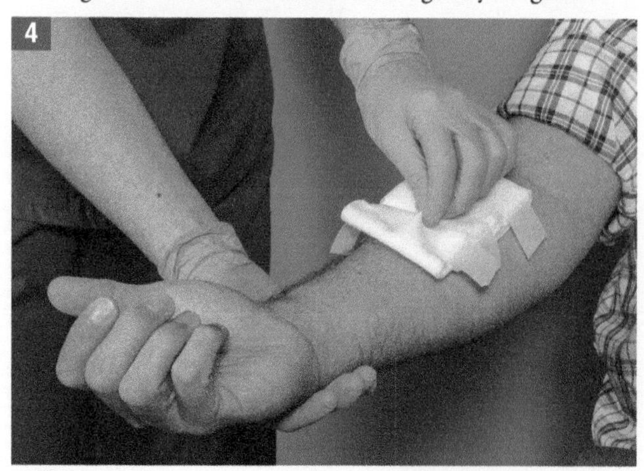

Remove the soiled dressing.

5. **Procedural Step.** Inspect the wound, and observe for the following: amount of healing; presence of inflammation; and presence of drainage, including the amount (scant, moderate, or profuse) and type of drainage.
   Principle. Drainage is classified as serous (containing serum), sanguineous (red and composed of blood), serosanguineous (containing serum and blood), or purulent (containing pus and appearing white with tinges of yellow, pink, or green, depending on the type of infecting microorganism). Purulent drainage is usually thick and has an unpleasant odor.
6. **Procedural Step.** Open the pouch containing the sterile antiseptic swabs, and place it in a convenient location or hold it in your nondominant hand.
7. **Procedural Step.** Using the antiseptic swabs, apply the antiseptic to the wound. Apply the antiseptic from the top to the bottom of the wound, working from the center to the outside of the wound. Use a new swab for each motion. Discard each contaminated swab in the waste bag after use.
   Principle. The purpose of the antiseptic is to decrease the number of microorganisms in the wound.

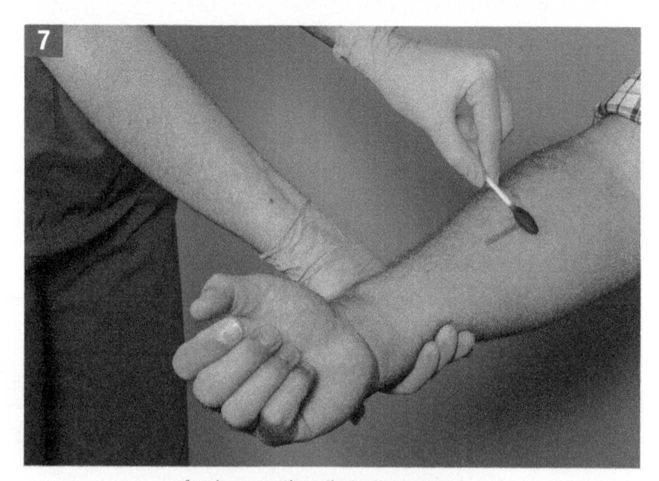

Apply an antiseptic to the wound.

8. **Procedural Step.** Remove the clean disposable gloves, and discard them in the waste bag without contaminating yourself. Sanitize your hands, and prepare the sterile field using surgical asepsis. Items are either placed onto a sterile field or are contained in a prepackaged setup. Instruct the patient not to talk, laugh, sneeze, or cough over the sterile field.
   Principle. Microorganisms are carried in water vapor from the mouth, nose, and lungs and can be transferred onto the sterile field.
9. **Procedural Step.** Open a package of sterile gloves, and apply them.

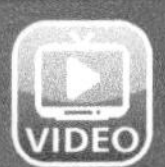

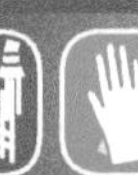

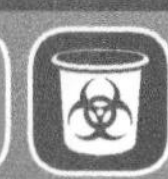

10. Procedural Step. Pick up the sterile dressing with your gloved hand or sterile forceps. Place the sterile dressing over the wound by lightly dropping it in place. Do not move the dressing once you have dropped it into place. Discard the gloves or forceps in the waste bag.
Principle. Dropping the dressing over the wound and not moving it prevent the transfer of microorganisms from the skin to the center of the wound.

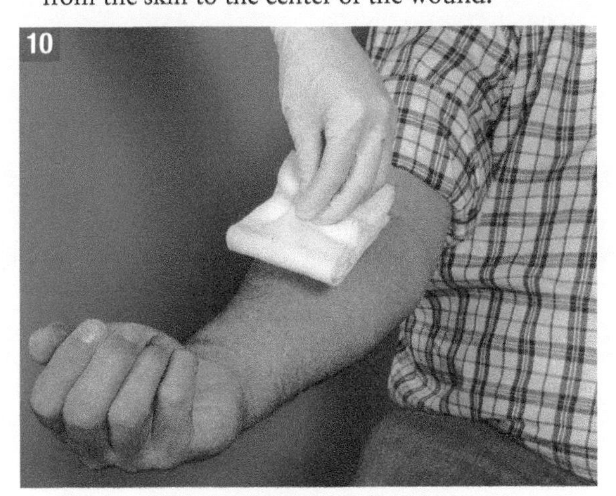

Place the dressing over the wound.

11. Procedural Step. Apply hypoallergenic adhesive tape to hold the dressing in place. The tape must be long enough to adhere to the skin, but not so long that it loosens when the patient moves. The strips of tape should be evenly spaced, with strips at each end of the dressing.

12. Procedural Step. Instruct the patient in wound care as follows:

a. Provide the patient with written wound care instructions (refer to Box 10.2).
b. Explain the wound care instructions and ask the patient whether he or she has any questions. Tell the patient to keep the wound clean and dry and to contact the office if signs of infection occur such as excessive swelling, pain, or discharge.
c. Ask the patient to sign the instruction sheet on the appropriate line.
d. Witness the patient's signature by signing your name in the appropriate space on the form. Include today's date.
e. Before the patient leaves the medical office, make a copy of the instruction sheet. Give a signed copy of the wound care instructions to the patient.
f. File the instruction sheet.

Electronic health record (EHR): Scan the instruction sheet into the patient's electronic record.
Paper-based patient record: File the original instruction sheet in the patient's medical record.
Principle. The filed copy protects the physician legally in the event that the patient fails to follow the instructions and causes further harm or damage to the wound.

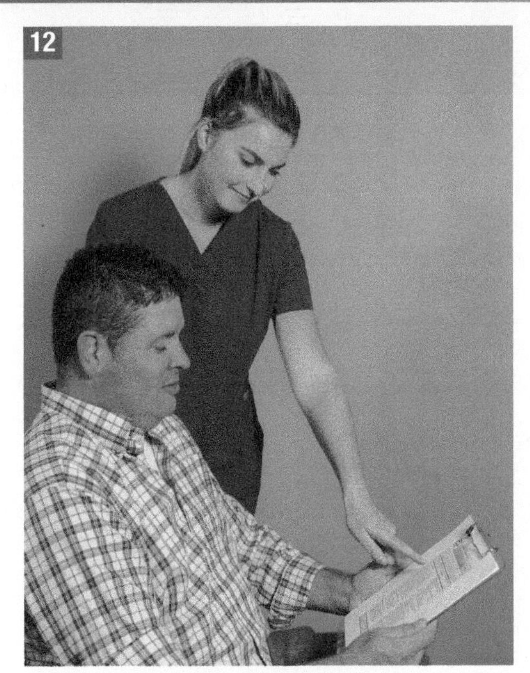

Instruct the patient in wound care.

13. Procedural Step. Return the equipment. Tightly secure the bag containing the soiled dressing and contaminated articles and dispose of it in a biohazard waste container.
Principle. Contaminated items must be disposed of properly to prevent the spread of infection.

14. Procedural Step. Sanitize your hands.

15. Procedural Step. Document the procedure in the patient's medical record.

a. *Electronic health record (EHR):* Document the location of the dressing, condition of the wound, type and amount of drainage, care of the wound, and any problems the patient has experienced with the wound using the appropriate radio buttons, drop-down menus, and free text fields. Also, document the instructions given to the patient on wound care.
b. *Paper-based patient record:* Document the date and time, location of the dressing, condition of the wound, type and amount of drainage, care of the wound, and any problems the patient experienced with the wound. Also, document the instructions given to the patient on wound care (refer to the PPR documentation example).

PPR Documentation Example

Date	
9/20/XX	10:30 a.m. Dressing changed (L) ant forearm.
	Scant amt of serous drainage noted. Sl redness
	around incision line. Sutures intact and suture
	line in good approximation. Incision cleaned c̄
	Betadine and DSD applied. No complaints of pain or
	discomfort. Explained wound care. Written
	instructions provided. Signed copy filed in chart. To
	return in 2 days for suture
	removal. ________ H. Hopstetter, CMA (AAMA)

PROCEDURE 10.5 Removing Sutures and Staples

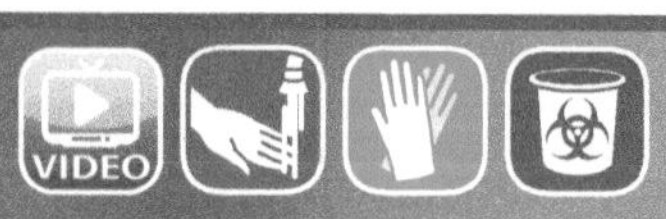

Outcome Remove sutures and staples.

Equipment/Supplies

- Antiseptic swabs
- Clean disposable gloves
- Sterile 4 × 4 gauze
- Surgical tape
- Mayo stand
- Biohazard waste container

For Suture Removal

- Suture removal kit, which includes the following:
  - Suture scissors
  - Thumb forceps
  - Sterile 4 × 4 gauze

For Staple Removal

- Staple removal kit, which includes the following:
- Staple remover
- Sterile 4 × 4 gauze

1. **Procedural Step.** Wash your hands with antimicrobial soap. Assemble the equipment.
   Principle. Washing the hands with antimicrobial soap removes microorganisms from the hands and also deposits an antimicrobial film on your hands to discourage the growth of bacteria.

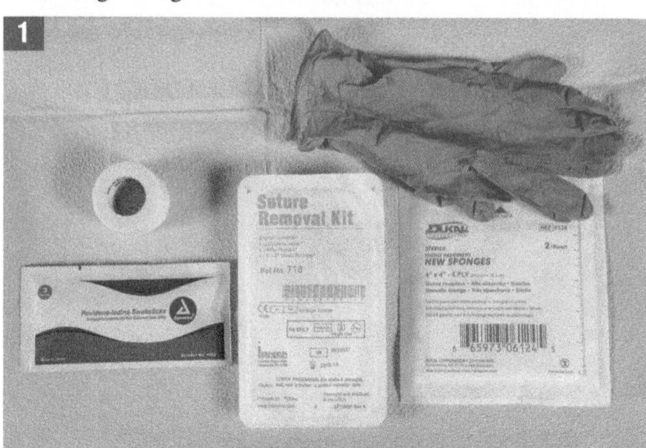

Suture removal setup.

2. **Procedural Step.** Greet the patient and introduce yourself. Identify the patient by full name and date of birth and explain the procedure.
3. **Procedural Step.** Position the patient as required to provide good access to the site. Adjust the light so that it is focused on the wound. Verify that the sutures (or staples) are intact and that the incision line is approximated and not gaping. Check that the incision line is not infected. If the incision line is not approximated, or if redness, swelling, or a discharge is present, do not remove the sutures; notify the physician.
   Principle. The sutures (or staples) should not be removed unless the incision line is approximated and free from infection.
4. **Procedural Step.** Open the suture or staple removal kit, keeping the contents of the kit sterile. Most kits are opened by peeling back a top cover, exposing a plastic tray that holds the necessary instruments and supplies.

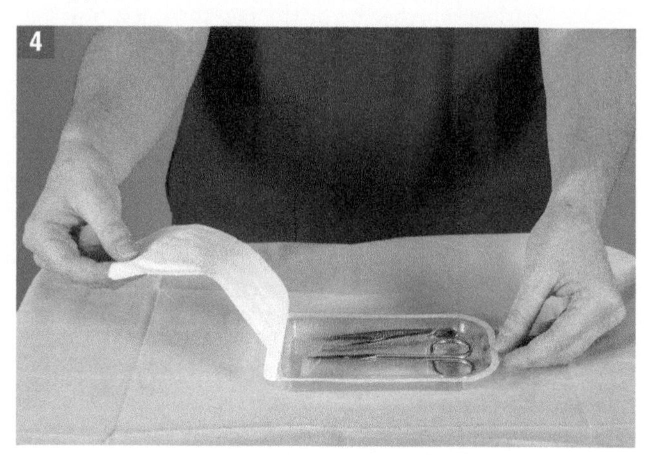

Open the suture removal kit.

PROCEDURE 10.5 Removing Sutures and Staples—cont'd

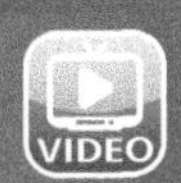

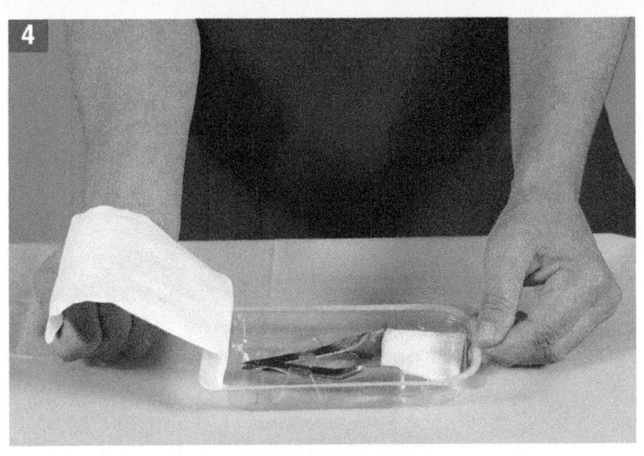

Open the staple removal kit.

5. **Procedural Step.** Apply clean gloves. Cleanse the incision line with an antiseptic swab to destroy microorganisms and to remove any dried exudate encrusted around the sutures or staples. Clean the wound from the top to the bottom, working from the center to the outside of the wound. Use a new swab for each cleansing motion. Allow the skin to dry.
   Principle. Dried exudate must be removed to allow unimpeded removal of the sutures or staples.
6. **Procedural Step.** Remove the sutures or staples. Tell the patient that he or she will feel a pulling or tugging sensation as each suture (or staple) is removed but that it will not be painful. Count the number of sutures or staples removed. Check the patient's medical record to make sure the same number is removed as was inserted by the physician.
7. **To Remove Sutures**
   a. Using the sterile thumb forceps provided in the kit, pick up the knot of the first suture.
   b. Place the curved tip of the suture scissors under the suture. Using the sterile suture scissors, cut the suture below the knot on the side of the suture closest to the skin. Cut the suture as close to the skin as possible.

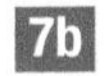

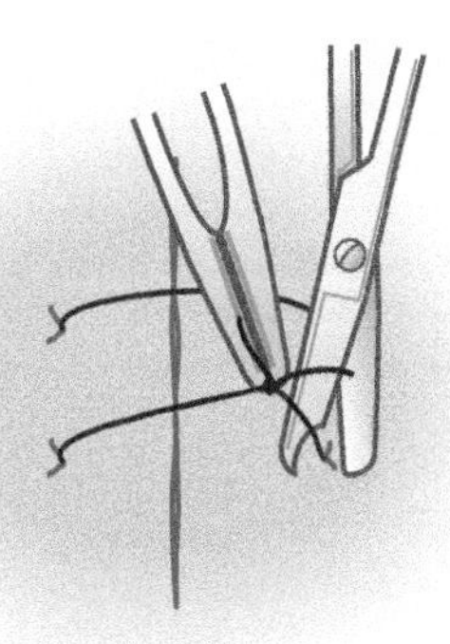

Cut the suture below the knot in the side closest to the skin. (Modified from Nealon TF, Jr.: *Fundamental skills in surgery,* ed 4, Philadelphia: WB Saunders; 1994.)

   c. Using a smooth, continuous motion, gently pull the suture out of the skin. Remove the suture without allowing any portion that was previously outside to be pulled back through the tissue lying beneath the incision line. Place the suture on the 4 × 4 gauze included in the suture kit.

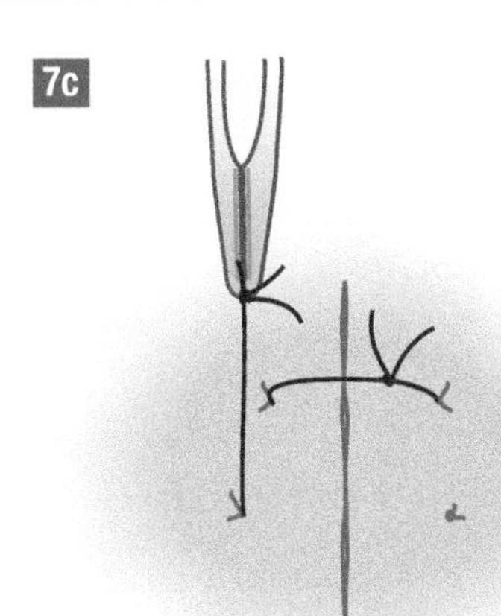

Gently pull the suture out. (Modified from Nealon TF, Jr.: *Fundamental skills in surgery,* ed 4, Philadelphia: WB Saunders; 1994.)

   d. Continue in this manner until all the sutures have been removed.
   Principle. To prevent infection, the suture must be removed without pulling any portion that has been outside the skin back through the tissue lying beneath the incision line.
8. **To Remove Staples**
   a. Gently place the bottom jaws of the staple remover under the staple to be removed.

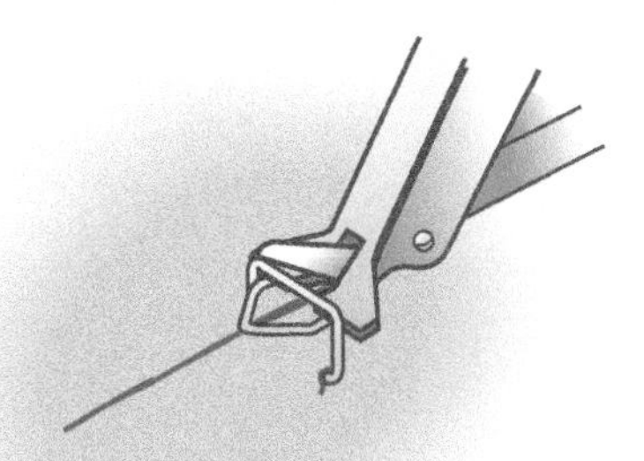

Place the bottom jaws of the staple remover under the staple. (© Ethicon, Inc. 2022. Reproduced with permission.)

Continued

PROCEDURE 10.5 Removing Sutures and Staples—cont'd

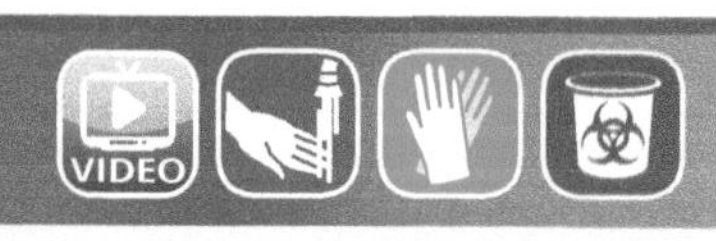

b. Firmly squeeze the staple handles until they are fully closed.

8b

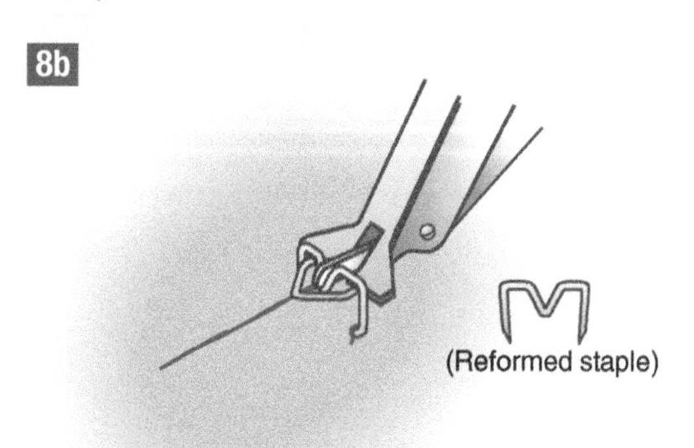

Firmly squeeze the staple handles until they are fully closed. (© Ethicon, Inc. 2022. Reproduced with permission.)

c. Carefully lift the staple remover upward to remove the staple from the incision line. Place the staple on the 4 × 4 gauze included in the staple kit.

d. Continue in this manner until all the staples have been removed.

9. **Procedural Step.** Cleanse the site with an antiseptic swab. Some physicians want the medical assistant to apply skin closure tape after removing the sutures or staples to provide additional support to the wound as it continues to heal.
10. **Procedural Step.** Apply a dry sterile dressing if indicated by the physician.
11. **Procedural Step.** Dispose of the sutures (or staples) and the gauze in a biohazard waste container.
12. **Procedural Step.** Remove the gloves and sanitize your hands.
13. **Procedural Step.** Document the procedure in the patient's medical record.
    a. *Electronic health record (EHR):* Document the status of the sutures (or staples) and incision line, the number of sutures (or staples) removed, the location of the site, the care of the wound (e.g., application of an antiseptic or dressing), and the patient's reaction using the appropriate radio buttons, drop-down menus, and free text fields.
    b. *Paper-based patient record:* Document the date and time, the status of the sutures (or staples) and incision line, the number of sutures (or staples) removed, the location of the site, care of the wound (e.g., application of an antiseptic or dressing), and the patient's reaction. Document any instructions given to the patient (refer to the PPR documentation example).

PPR Documentation Example

Date	
9/20/XX	10:30 a.m. Sutures intact and incision line in
	good approximation. No signs of infection.
	Sutures x6 removed from (R) ant forearm.
	Incision line cleaned c̄ Betadine and DSD applied.
	Instructions provided on dressing care.
	———————— H. Hopstetter, CMA (AAMA)

PROCEDURE 10.6 Applying and Removing Skin Closure Tape

Outcome Apply and remove skin closure tape.

Equipment/Supplies

- Clean disposable gloves
- Sterile gloves
- Antiseptic solution
- Surgical scrub brush
- Antiseptic swabs
- Tincture of benzoin
- Sterile cotton-tipped applicator
- Adhesive skin closure strips
- Sterile 4 × 4 gauze pads
- Surgical tape
- Biohazard waster container

PROCEDURE 10.6 Applying and Removing Skin Closure Tape—cont'd

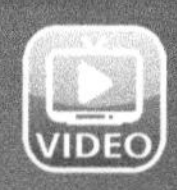

Application of Skin Closure Tape

1. **Procedural Step.** Wash your hands with an antimicrobial soap and assemble the equipment. Check the expiration date on the skin closure tape.

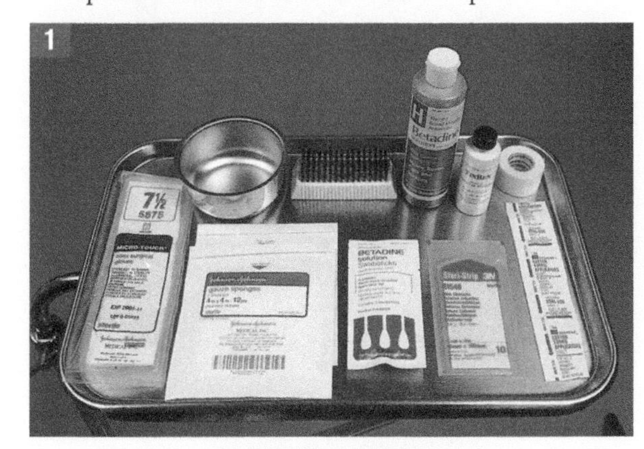

Assemble the equipment.

2. **Procedural Step.** Greet the patient and introduce yourself.
3. **Procedural Step.** Identify the patient by full name and date of birth and explain the procedure.
4. **Procedural Step.** Position the patient as required for application of the strips. Adjust the light so that it is focused on the wound. Apply clean gloves. Inspect the wound for signs of redness, swelling, and drainage. (*Note:* Document this information in the patient's record after completing the procedure.)
5. **Procedural Step.** Gently scrub the wound using an antiseptic solution (e.g., Betadine solution) and a sterile gauze pad or a surgical scrub brush. Clean at least 3 inches around the wound, removing all debris, skin oil, and exudates. Allow the skin to dry or pat dry with gauze pads. (*Note:* Change gloves as needed to maintain cleanliness.)

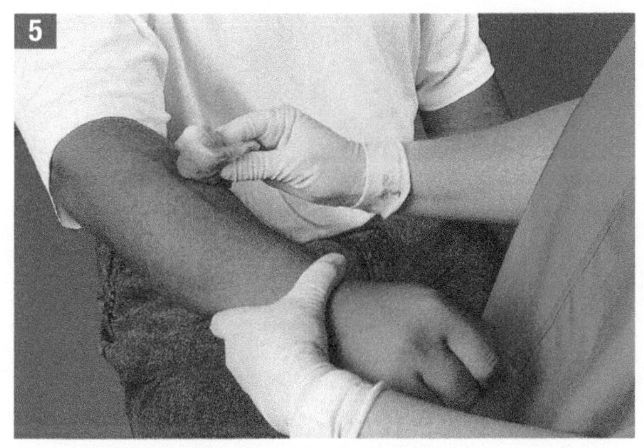

Clean the wound.

6. **Procedural Step.** Apply an antiseptic to the site using antiseptic swabs such as Betadine swabs. Apply the antiseptic from the top to the bottom of the wound, working from the center to the outside of the wound. Use a new swab for each motion. Allow the skin to dry completely.
   Principle. The antiseptic decreases the number of microorganisms in the wound. The skin must be completely dry to ensure adhesion of the skin closures to the skin.

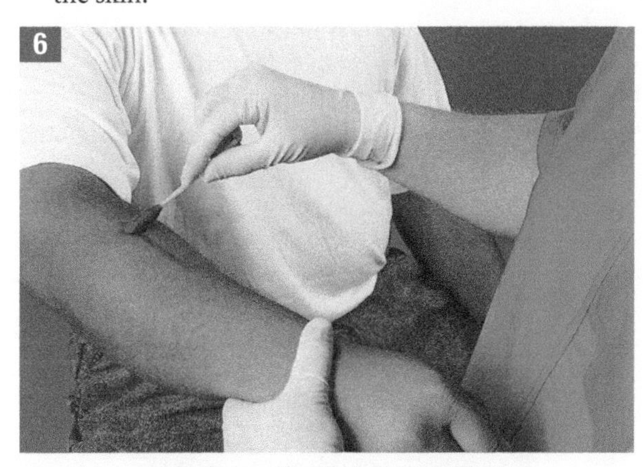

Apply an antiseptic to the wound.

7. **Procedural Step.** If dictated by the medical office policy, apply a thin coat of tincture of benzoin to the skin parallel to each side of the wound with a sterile cotton-tipped applicator. Do not allow the tincture of benzoin to touch the wound. Allow the skin to dry. Remove the gloves, and wash your hands with an antimicrobial soap.
   Principle. Tincture of benzoin facilitates adhesion of the strips to the skin.

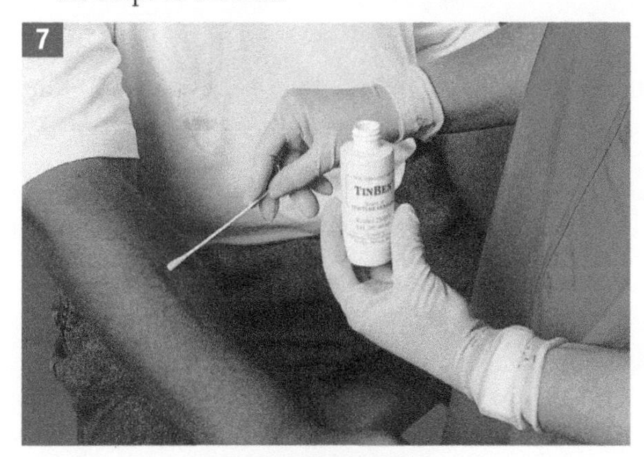

Apply tincture of benzoin.

8. **Procedural Step.** Open the plastic peel-apart package of strips using sterile technique as follows:

Continued

PROCEDURE 10.6 Applying and Removing Skin Closure Tape—cont'd

a. Grasp each flap of the package between the thumbs and bent index fingers. Pull the package apart.
b. Peel back the package until it is completely open.
c. Lay the opened package flat on a clean dry surface. The inside of the package serves as the sterile field.

9. Procedural Step. Apply sterile gloves. Fold the card of strips along its perforated tab, and tear off the tab, which exposes the ends of the tape strips, making them easier to grasp. Peel a strip of tape off the card at a 45-degree angle to the card.

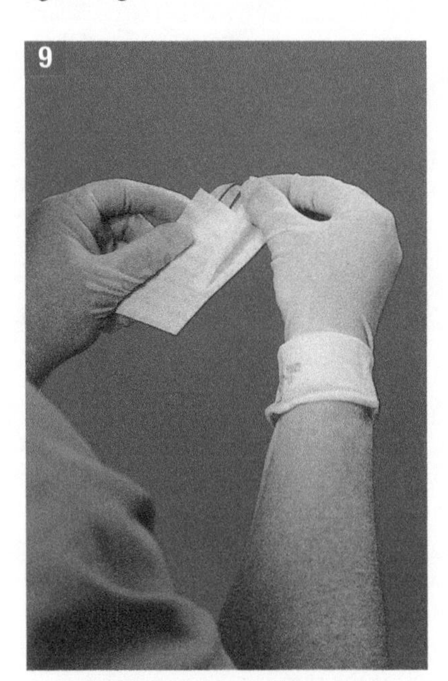
9
Peel a strip of tape off the card.

10. Procedural Step. Check that the skin surface is dry. Position the first strip over the center of the wound as follows:

a. Secure one end of the strip of tape to the skin on one side of the wound by pressing down firmly on the tape.
b. Use your gloved hand to assist in bringing the edges of the wound together as closely as possible.
c. Apply the second half of the strip transversely across the line of the incision making sure the edges of the wound are approximated exactly.
d. Secure the strip on the skin on the other side of the wound by pressing down firmly on the tape.

Principle. Approximating the wound exactly facilitates good healing and minimizes scar formation.

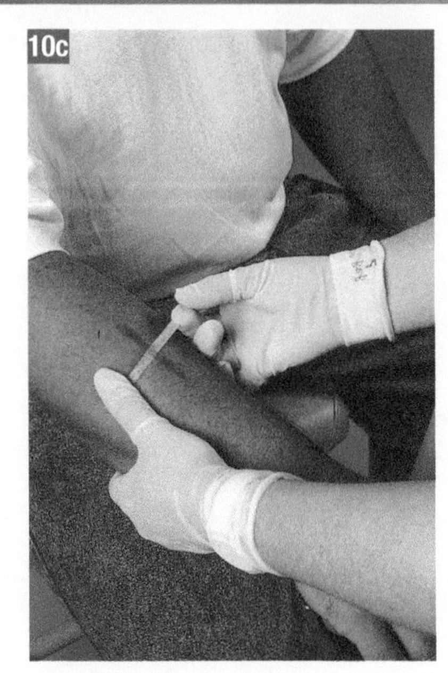
10c
Apply the second half of the strip transversely across the incision.

11. Procedural Step. Apply the second strip perpendicular to the wound on one side of the center strip. The space between the strips should be approximately 1/8 inch. Apply a third strip on the other side of the center strip at a 1/8-inch interval. Continue applying the strips at 1/8-inch intervals until the edges of the wound are approximated. If at any time the skin surfaces become moist with perspiration, blood, or serum, wipe the area dry with a sterile gauze pad before applying the next strip.

Principle. Applying the strips of tape in this manner facilitates good approximation of the wound. Spacing the strips at 1/8-inch intervals allows proper drainage of the wound.

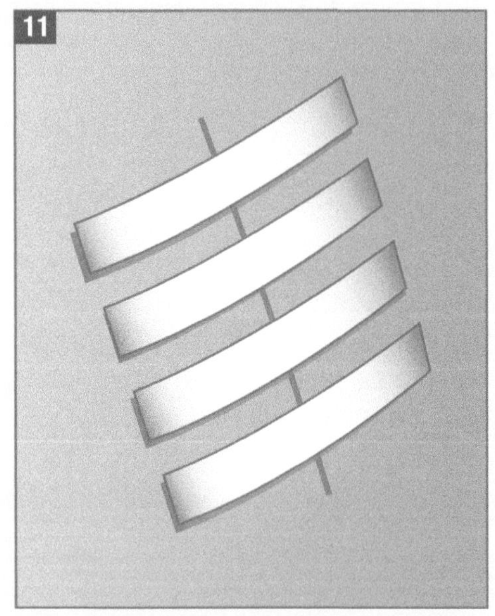
11
Apply the strips until the edges of the wound are approximated.

PROCEDURE 10.6 Applying and Removing Skin Closure Tape—cont'd

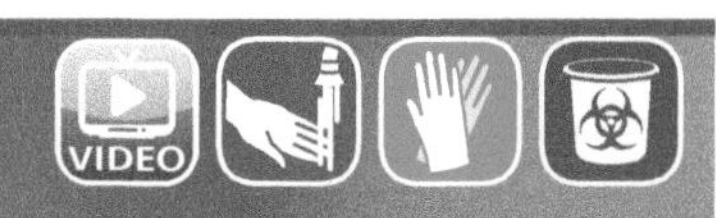

12. Procedural Step. Apply two closures approximately 1/2 inch from the ends of the strips and parallel to the wound (ladder fashion).

Principle. Applying a strip along each edge redistributes the tension and assists in holding the strips firmly in place.

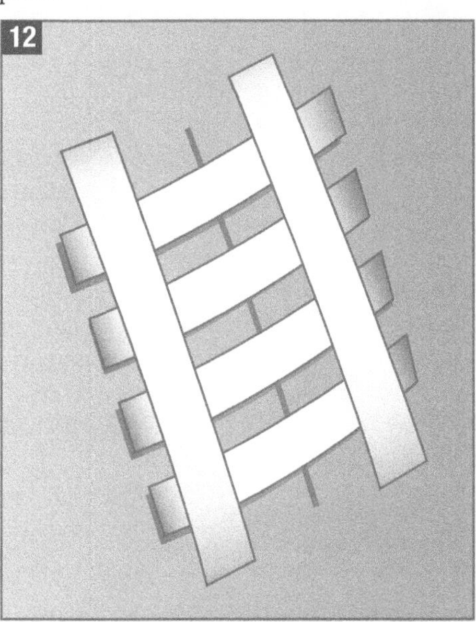

Apply a strip along each edge.

13. Procedural Step. Apply a dry sterile dressing over the strips if indicated by the physician (see Procedure 10.4).

14. Procedural Step. Remove the gloves, and sanitize your hands.

15. Procedural Step. Instruct the patient in wound care as follows:

a. Provide the patient with written wound care instructions (see Box 10.2).
b. Explain the wound care instructions and ask the patient whether he or she has any questions.
c. Ask the patient to sign the instruction sheet on the appropriate line.
d. Witness the patient's signature by signing your name in the appropriate space on the form. Include today's date.
e. Before the patient leaves the medical office, make a copy of the instruction sheet. Give a signed copy of the wound care instructions to the patient.
f. File the instruction sheet.

Electronic health record (EHR): Scan the instruction sheet into the patient's electronic record.

Paper-based patient record: File the original instruction sheet in the patient's medical record.

Principle. An instruction sheet signed by the patient provides legal documentation that wound care instructions were provided to the patient in the event that the patient fails to follow the instructions and causes further harm or damage to the wound.

16. Procedural Step. Document the procedure in the patient's medical record.

a. *Electronic health record (EHR):* Document the appearance of the wound, wound preparation, the number of strips applied, the location of the wound, the care of the wound, and the patient's reaction using the appropriate radio buttons, drop-down menus, and free text fields. Also, document verbal and written instructions given to the patient concerning wound care.
b. *Paper-based patient record:* Document the date and time, the appearance of the wound, the wound preparation, the number of strips applied, the location of the wound, the care of the wound, and the patient's reaction. Document verbal and written instructions given to the patient concerning wound care (refer to the PPR documentation example).

PPR Documentation Example

Date	
9/20/XX	10:30 a.m. Incision approx 5 cm long located on
	post Ⓡ forearm. Redness noted on edge of
	wound. Sl amt of serous drainage noted. Wound
	scrubbed c̄ Betadine sol and Betadine
	antiseptic applied. Applied Steri-Strips x4.
	Incision in good approximation. Applied DSD.
	Explained wound care. Written instructions
	provided. To return in 5 days for removal
	of strips. ———— H. Hopstetter, CMA (AAMA)

Removal of Skin Closure Tape

Skin closure tape usually loosen and fall off on their own approximately 5–10 days after application. If they require removal, the procedure outlined here should be followed by the medical assistant.

1. Procedural Step. Sanitize your hands. Greet the patient and introduce yourself. Identify the patient by full name and date of birth and explain the procedure.

2. Procedural Step. Position the patient as required. Adjust the light so that it is focused on the wound. Check that the skin closures are intact and that the incision line is

Continued

PROCEDURE 10.6 Applying and Removing Skin Closure Tape—cont'd

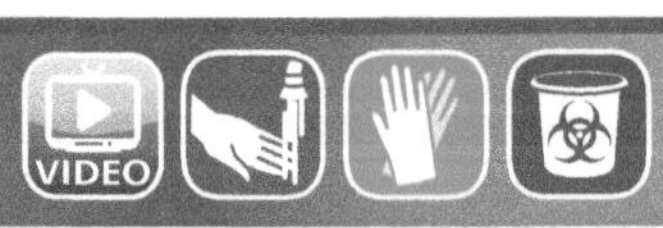

approximated and not gaping. Check that the incision line is not infected. If the incision line is not approximated, or if redness, swelling, or a discharge is present, do not remove the skin closures; notify the physician.

3. **Procedural Step.** Position a 4 × 4 gauze pad in a convenient location. Apply clean gloves.
4. **Procedural Step.** Remove the skin closures as follows:
   a. Gently grasp one end of a strip of tape with the dominant hand.
   b. Stabilize the skin with one finger of the nondominant hand.
   c. Slowly loosen and peel off one-half of the strip of tape from the outside to the wound margin, keeping the peeled-off section of the strip close to the skin surface and pulled back over itself. As you remove the strip from the skin, continue moving the finger as necessary to support the newly exposed skin. Always pull the strip toward the wound. Never pull the strip away from the wound because tension on the wound site could disrupt the healing process.
   d. Remove the other half of the strip of tape from the outside to the wound margin in the manner just described.
   e. When both halves of the strip are completely loosened, gently lift the strip up and away from the wound surface. Place the strip on a 4 × 4 gauze pad.
   f. Continue in this manner until all the skin closures have been removed.
5. **Procedural Step.** Cleanse the site with an antiseptic swab. Apply a dry sterile dressing if indicated by the physician (see Procedure 10.4).
6. **Procedural Step.** Dispose of the strips and gauze in a biohazard waste container. Remove the gloves, and sanitize your hands.
7. **Procedural Step.** Document the procedure in the patient's medical record.
   a. *Electronic health record (EHR):* Document the status of the skin closures, the number of skin closures removed, the location of the site, the care of the wound, and the patient's reaction, using the appropriate radio buttons, drop-down menus, and free text fields. Also, document any instructions given to the patient.
   b. *Paper-based patient record:* Document the date and time, the status of the skin closures, the number of skin closures removed, the location of the site, the care of the wound, and the patient's reaction. Document any instructions given to the patient (refer to the PPR documentation example).

PPR Documentation Example

Date	
9/25/XX	10:30 a.m. Skin closures intact and in good
	approximation. No signs of infection. Strips
	x 4 removed from Ⓡ post forearm. Incision
	line cleaned c̄ Betadine and DSD applied.
	Instructions provided on dressing care.
	____________ H. Hopstetter, CMA (AAMA)

PROCEDURE 10.7 Assisting with Minor Office Surgery

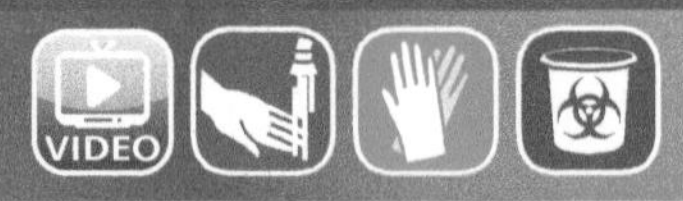

Outcome Set up a surgical tray, and assist with minor office surgery.

Equipment/Supplies

- Mayo stand
- Instruments and supplies for the type of surgery to be performed
- Biohazard waste container

Preparing the Tray

1. **Procedural Step.** Determine the type of minor office surgery to be performed. The physician instructs the medical assistant as to the type of surgery and provides any additional information needed to set up for the surgery, such as the type of local anesthetic and sutures to be used. If the medical office maintains a minor office surgery filing system, pull the file card that indicates the instruments and supplies required for the type of surgery to be performed.
2. **Procedural Step.** Prepare the examining room. Make sure the room is clean and well lighted.

PROCEDURE 10.7

PROCEDURE 10.7 Assisting with Minor Office Surgery—cont'd

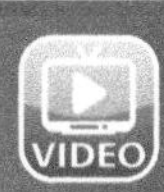

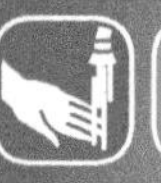
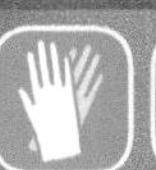

3. **Procedural Step.** Sanitize your hands.
4. **Procedural Step.** Set up nonsterile articles on a side table or counter. If a specimen container is included in the setup, perform one of the following (based on the medical office policy):
   a. Attach a computer-generated bar code label to the specimen container *or*
   b. Clearly label the tubes and containers with the patient's name and date of birth, the date, your initials, and any other information required by the laboratory, such as the source of the specimen.

   Principle. Articles that are not sterile cannot be placed on the sterile field because they would contaminate it. Two unique identifiers should be used when labeling the specimen (e.g., patient's name and date of birth).
5. **Procedural Step.** Wash your hands with an antimicrobial soap and set up the minor office surgery tray on a clean, dry, flat surface, using the principles of surgical asepsis. The sterile tray can be set up as follows:

   Prepackaged Setup

   a. Select the appropriate package from the supply shelf, and place it on a Mayo tray or other flat surface.
   b. Open the sterile pack using the inside of the wrapper as the sterile field. Check the sterilization indicator to make sure the contents of the pack are sterile.

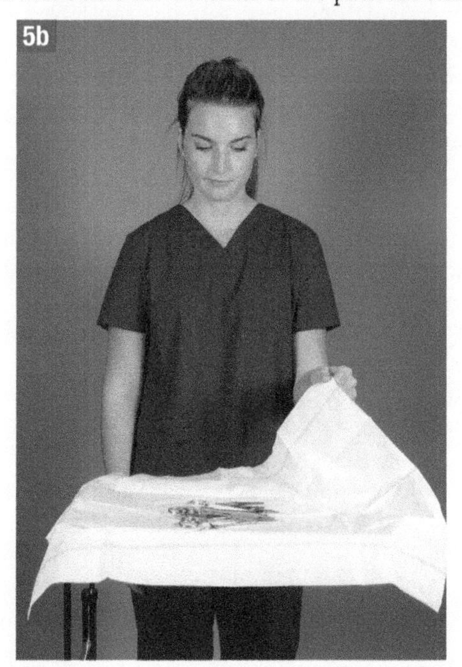

Open the sterile pack using the inside of the wrapper as the sterile field.

   c. Add other articles to the sterile field that are needed for the surgery but not contained in the sterile package, such as 4 × 4 gauze, sutures, and a fenestrated drape. If sutures are required for the setup, make sure to check the expiration date of the sutures.

   Transferring Articles to a Sterile Field

   a. Pick up the folded sterile towel by two corner ends and allow it to unfold; make sure it does not touch an unsterile surface.
   b. Lay the sterile towel down gently and slowly over the Mayo tray, making sure it does not brush against an unsterile surface such as your uniform. Do not allow your arms to pass over the towel as you lay it down because this would result in contamination of the sterile field.

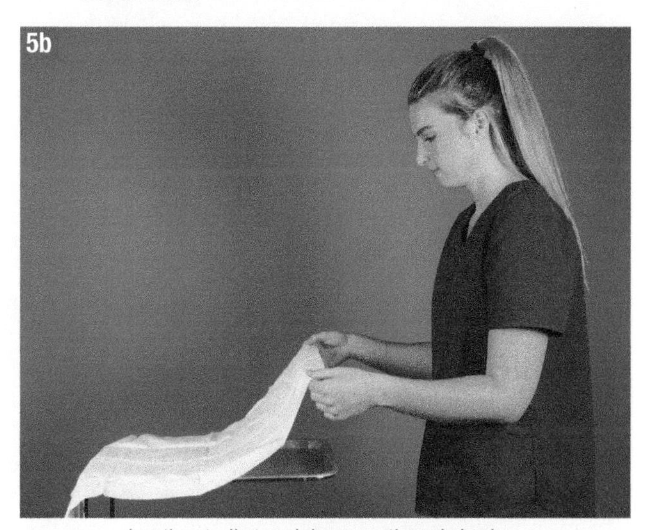

Lay the sterile towel down gently and slowly.

   c. Transfer instruments and supplies to the sterile field from wrapped or peel-apart packages.

   Principle. The principles of surgical asepsis must be followed to prevent contamination of the sterile field.
6. **Procedural Step.** Apply a sterile glove, and arrange the articles neatly on the sterile field. Do not allow one article to lie on top of another. Check that all the instruments and supplies required for the surgery are available on the sterile field.

   Principle. Instruments and supplies can be located quickly and efficiently on a neat and orderly sterile field. Sterile gloves must be used to prevent contamination of the sterile articles.

Continued

PROCEDURE 10.7 Assisting with Minor Office Surgery—cont'd

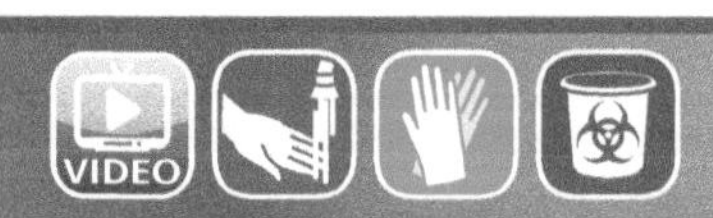

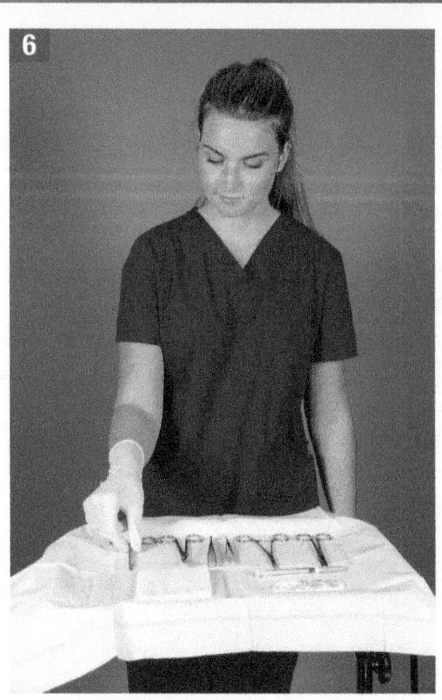

Arrange the articles neatly on the sterile field.

7. **Procedural Step.** Cover the tray setup with a sterile towel by picking up the towel by two corner ends and placing it gently and slowly over the setup. Do not allow your arms to pass over the sterile field as you lay it down.
 Principle. The towel prevents the sterile tray from becoming contaminated. The towel must be picked up by the corner ends to prevent contaminating it and should be moved slowly and not fanned through the air to prevent airborne contamination. Passing the arms over the sterile field results in contamination of the field.

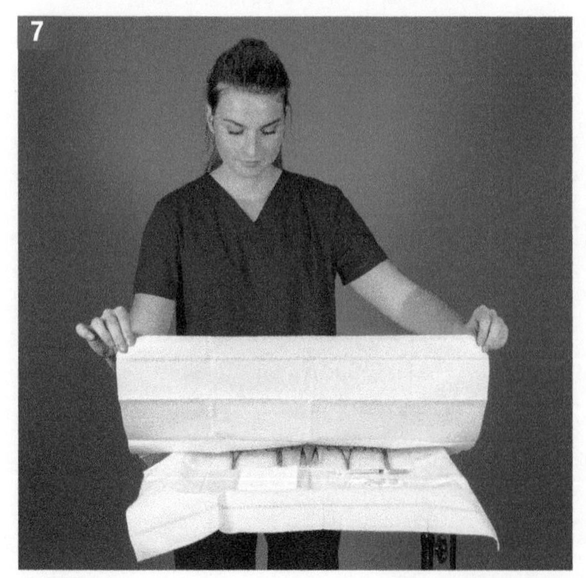

Cover the tray setup with a sterile towel.

Preparing the Patient

8. **Procedural Step.** Greet the patient and introduce yourself. Identify the patient by full name and date of birth. Explain the procedure, and prepare the patient for the minor office surgery as follows:
 a. Try to allay the patient's fear or anxiety.
 b. Ask the patient whether he or she needs to void before the surgery.
 c. Provide instructions to the patient about any clothing that must be removed and putting on an examination gown, if required. Enough clothing must be removed to expose the operative area completely and to avoid getting the antiseptic or blood on the patient's clothing.
 d. Instruct the patient not to move during the procedure and not to talk, laugh, sneeze, or cough over the sterile field.
 Principle. Minor office surgery is often a frightening experience for the patient, and reassurance should be offered to reduce apprehension. The amount of clothing that must be removed depends on the type of minor office surgery being performed. By moving, the patient may accidentally contaminate the sterile field or touch the operative site. Microorganisms are carried in water vapor from the mouth, nose, and lungs and can be transferred onto the sterile field.
9. **Procedural Step.** Position the patient. The position is determined by the type of minor office surgery to be performed. The patient is positioned in such a way as to provide the best possible exposure and accessibility to the operative site. *Note:* If a difficult position must be maintained, such as the knee-chest position, the patient should not be positioned until the physician is ready to begin the minor office surgery.
10. **Procedural Step.** Adjust the light so that it is focused on the operative site.
11. **Procedural Step.** Prepare the patient's skin by performing the following:
 a. Apply clean disposable gloves.
 b. If hair is present, the skin at and around the operative site may need to be shaved. The skin should be pulled taut as it is shaved. The area is rinsed and dried thoroughly.
 c. Cleanse the patient's skin with an antiseptic solution and a surgical scrub brush using a firm, circular motion and moving from the inside outward. Do not return to an area just cleansed. The area is rinsed using gauze pads saturated with water and blotted dry with a sterile gauze pad.

PROCEDURE 10.7 Assisting with Minor Office Surgery—cont'd

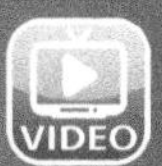

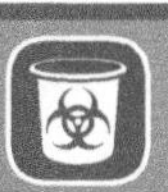

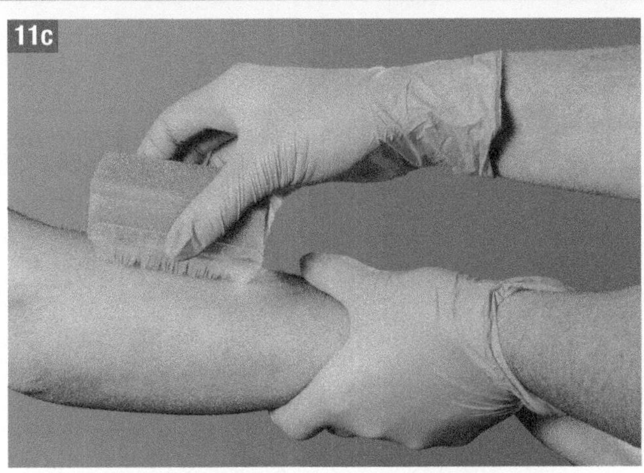

Cleanse the patient's skin with an antiseptic solution.

d. Apply an antiseptic to the site using antiseptic swabs such as Betadine. Allow the skin to dry. Alternatively, the physician may place a fenestrated drape over the operative site and then apply the antiseptic.
e. Remove the gloves, and sanitize your hands.

12. **Procedural Step.** Verify that everything is prepared for the minor office surgery, and inform the physician that the patient is ready.

Assisting the Physician

13. **Procedural Step.** Assist the physician as required during the minor office surgery, following the principles of surgical asepsis. The physician drapes the patient, injects the local anesthetic, and performs the surgery. The responsibilities of the medical assistant may include the following:
a. Uncover the sterile tray setup by picking up the sterile towel covering it. The towel should be picked up by two corner ends and removed slowly and gently without allowing the arms to pass over the sterile field.
b. Open the outer glove wrapper for the physician to facilitate the application of sterile gloves.
c. Withdraw the local anesthetic into a syringe and hand it to the physician, or hold the vial while the physician withdraws the local anesthetic. If lidocaine (Xylocaine) is used, the physician or medical assistant should inform the patient to expect a brief burning or stinging sensation as it is injected into the tissues.
d. Adjust the light as needed by the physician for good visualization of the operative site.
e. Restrain patients such as children.
f. Relax and reassure the patient during the minor office surgery.
g. Hand instruments and supplies to the physician. (Sterile gloves are required.)
h. Keep the sterile field neat and orderly. (Sterile gloves are required.)
i. Hold a basin in which the physician can deposit soiled instruments and supplies, such as hemostats and gauze sponges. (Clean gloves are required.)

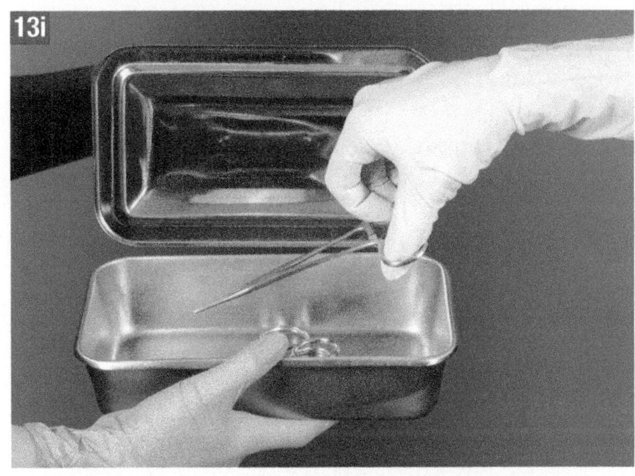

Hold a basin for the physician to deposit soiled instruments.

j. Retract tissue from an area to allow the physician the best access to and visibility of the operative site. (Sterile gloves are required.)
k. Sponge blood from the operative site. (Sterile gloves are required.)
l. Add instruments and supplies to the sterile field as required by the physician.
m. Hold the specimen container to accept a tissue specimen received from the physician. (Clean gloves are required.) Do not touch the inside of the container because it is sterile. After the physician inserts the specimen, replace the container lid and close it tightly.

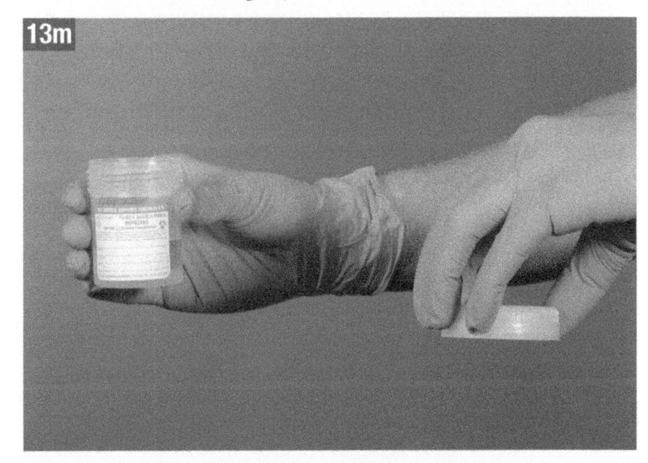

Hold the container to accept a tissue specimen.

Continued

PROCEDURE 10.7 Assisting with Minor Office Surgery—cont'd

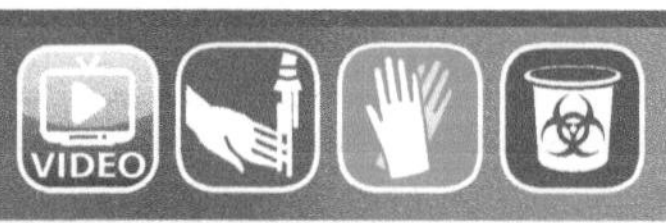

n. After the physician has inserted a suture, cut the ends of the suture material approximately 1/8 inch above the knot of the suture. (Sterile gloves are required.)

14. Procedural Step. Apply a sterile dressing to the surgical wound, if ordered by the physician (see Procedure 10.4).

Principle. The sterile dressing protects the wound from contamination and injury and absorbs drainage.

15. Procedural Step. After the surgery, perform the following:

a. Stay with the patient as a safety precaution and to assist and instruct the patient.

b. Ensure that postoperative instructions regarding any type of medical care to be administered at home are understood. If the patient has a wound or if sutures have been inserted, he or she should be told to keep the area clean and dry and to report any signs of infection, such as excessive redness, swelling, discharge, or increased pain. Provide the patient with written wound care instructions (see Box 10.2). Ask the patient if he or she has any questions. Have the patient sign the instruction sheet. Witness the patient's signature. Before the patient leaves the office, make a copy of the instruction sheet. Give a copy to the patient.

c. File the instruction sheet.

Electronic health record: Scan the instruction sheet into the patient's electronic record.

Paper-based patient record: File the original instruction sheet in the patient's medical record.

d. Relay information regarding the return visit for postoperative care, such as the removal of sutures or a dressing change.

e. Help the patient off the table to prevent falls.

f. Instruct the patient to get dressed, offering assistance if needed.

g. Any instructions or information given must be documented in the patient's medical record.

Principle. The patient (especially an elderly one) may become dizzy after the minor office surgery and may fall when getting off the examining table. The filed copy protects the physician legally, in the event that the patient fails to follow instructions and causes harm or damage to the operative site.

16. Procedural Step. If a specimen was collected, it must be transferred to the laboratory in a tightly closed, properly labeled specimen container. Prepare the specimen for transport. Complete a biopsy request form to accompany the specimen. Place the specimen container in a biohazard specimen bag and seal it. Insert the biopsy request in the outer pocket of the bag and tuck the requisition under the flap. Place the bag in the appropriate location for pickup by the laboratory.

17. Procedural Step. Document specimen transport information in the patient's medical record.

a. *Electronic health record (EHR):* Document the date the specimen was picked up or sent to the laboratory, as well as the name of the laboratory, using the appropriate radio buttons, drop-down menus, and free text fields.

b. *Paper-based patient record:* Document the date the specimen was picked up or sent to the laboratory and the name of the laboratory (refer to the PPR documentation example).

Principle. Documenting information regarding transport of the specimen documents that the specimen was sent to the laboratory.

18. Procedural Step. Clean the examining room. Handle the instruments carefully so as not to damage them. Be especially careful with sharp instruments to prevent cutting yourself. Blood and body secretions should be rinsed off the instruments immediately to prevent them from drying and hardening. The instruments must be sanitized and sterilized when it is convenient to do so; follow the procedures presented in Chapter 3. Discard disposable articles contaminated with blood or other potentially infectious materials in a biohazard waste container.

Principle. Surgical instruments are expensive and must be handled carefully to prolong their life span. Hardened blood and secretions on an instrument are difficult to remove. Disposable articles must be discarded in an appropriate manner to prevent the spread of infection.

PPR Documentation Example

Date	
9/25/XX	2:00 p.m. Applied DSD to Ⓡ post forearm.
	Instructed patient on suture care. Written
	instructions provided. To return in 5 days for
	removal of sutures. Sebaceous cyst
	specimen sent to Medical Center Laboratory
	for biopsy on
	9/25/XX.——— H. Hopstetter, CMA (AAMA)

PROCEDURE 10.7

Administration of Medication and Intravenous Therapy

Check out the Evolve site at http://evolve.elsevier.com/Bonewit/today/ to access additional interactive activities and exercises to help you study and prepare for success.

LEARNING OUTCOMES

Introduction to the Administration of Medication

1. Explain the difference among administering, prescribing, and dispensing medication.
2. State the common routes for administering medication.
3. List and describe the categories of information included in a drug package insert.
4. Describe the Food and Drug Administration's responsibilities with respect to drugs.
5. List and define the four names of drugs.
6. Classify drugs according to preparation.
7. Classify drugs according to the action they have on the body.
8. List the guidelines for writing metric notations.
9. List and describe the five schedules for controlled drugs.
10. List and explain the parts of a prescription.
11. Describe the functions performed by an electronic health record (EHR) prescription program.
12. Explain the purpose of a medication record.
13. List and describe the factors that affect the action of drugs in the body.
14. List and describe the possible adverse effects of medication.
15. List the guidelines for preparing and administering medication.

Oral Administration

16. Explain why the oral route is most frequently used to administer medication.
17. State where the absorption of most oral medications occurs.

Parenteral Administration

18. State the advantages and disadvantages of the parenteral route of administration.
19. Identify the parts of a needle and syringe and explain their functions.
20. State the ranges of gauge and length of needles for each of the following injections: intradermal, subcutaneous, and intramuscular.
21. State the purpose of safety-engineered syringes.
22. Describe the dispensing units available for injectable medications.
23. State which tissue layers of the body are used for intradermal, subcutaneous, and intramuscular injections.
24. List the medications commonly administered through each of the following routes: intradermal, subcutaneous, and intramuscular.
25. Explain the reason for administering medication with the Z-track method.

PROCEDURES

Interpret a drug package insert.
Calculate drug dosage.
Complete a prescription using a paper form and an EHR prescription program.
Complete a medication record form.

Prepare and administer oral medications.

Reconstitute a powdered drug for parenteral administration.
Withdraw medication from a vial.
Withdraw medication from an ampule.
Locate appropriate subcutaneous injection sites.
Administer a subcutaneous injection.
Locate each of the following intramuscular injection sites: deltoid, vastus lateralis, ventrogluteal, and dorsogluteal.
Administer an intramuscular injection.
Administer an injection using the Z-track method.
Administer an intradermal injection.

Tuberculin Testing	
26. Explain the difference between active and latent tuberculosis.	Administer a Mantoux tuberculin skin test, and read the test results.
27. Explain the purpose of tuberculin testing.	Complete a tuberculosis test record card.
28. Identify the categories of individuals who should have a tuberculin test.	
29. Explain the significance of a positive reaction to a tuberculin test.	
30. List the diagnostic procedures that might be performed following a positive tuberculin test.	
31. State the guidelines that should be followed when administering and reading a Mantoux tuberculin skin test.	
32. State the advantages and disadvantages of the tuberculosis blood test.	
Allergy Testing	
33. Define an allergy, and name common allergens.	Perform allergy skin testing.
34. Explain what occurs during an allergic reaction.	
35. List the guidelines for direct skin allergy testing.	
36. State the purpose of each of the following types of allergy tests: patch testing, skin-prick testing, intradermal skin testing, and in vitro blood testing.	
Intravenous Therapy	
37. Explain the advantages of outpatient intravenous (IV) therapy.	
38. Identify the role of the entry-level medical assistant in IV therapy.	
39. State the indications for outpatient IV therapy.	

CHAPTER OUTLINE

KEY TERMS

adverse reaction (AD-vers ree-AK-shun)
allergen (AL-er-jen)
allergy (AL-er-jee)
ampule (AM-pyool)
anaphylactic reaction (an-uh-ful-AK-tik ree-AK-shun)
chemotherapy
controlled drug
conversion (kon-VER-shun)
cubic centimeter (KYOO-bik SEN-tih-mee-ter)
DEA number
dose
drug
gauge (GAYJ)
induration (in-dur-AY-shun)
infusion
inscription (in-SKRIP-shun)
intradermal injection (in-tra-DER-mal in-JEK-shun)
intramuscular (in-tra-MUS-kyoo-lar) injection
intravenous (in-tra-VEE-nus) (IV) therapy
oral (OR-ul) administration
parenteral (par-EN-ter-al)
pharmacology (far-ma-KOL-oh-jee)
prescription
signatura (sig-na-CHUR-ah)
subcutaneous (sub-kyoo-TAY-nee-us) injection
subscription (sub-SKRIP-shun)
superscription (soo-per-SKRIP-shun)
transfusion
vial (VIE-ul)
wheal (WEE-ul)

Introduction to the Administration of Medication

Pharmacology is the study of drugs and includes the preparation, use, and action of drugs in the body. A **drug** is a chemical that is used for the treatment, prevention, or diagnosis of disease. Most drugs are produced synthetically, but they also can be obtained from other sources, such as animals, plants, and minerals.

ADMINISTERING, PRESCRIBING, AND DISPENSING MEDICATION

Medication may be administered, prescribed, or dispensed in the medical office. Medication that is *administered* is actually given to a patient at the office. Medication is *prescribed* when a provider authorizes the dispensing of a drug by a pharmacist. *Dispensed* medication is given to a patient at the office to be taken at home; for example, the provider gives a patient drug samples to take home.

LEGAL ASPECTS

An important responsibility of the medical assistant is the administration of medication. The medical assistant should administer medication only under the direction of the provider. In all states, it is unlawful to administer medication in the medical office without the consent of the provider.

ROUTES OF ADMINISTRATION

Common routes of administration of medication are oral, sublingual, inhalation, buccal, rectal, vaginal, topical, intradermal, subcutaneous (subcut), intramuscular (IM), and intravenous (IV). The route of administration depends on the type of drug being given, the dosage form, the intended action, and the rapidity of response desired. The route by which medication is most commonly administered in the medical office is the parenteral route. **Parenteral** refers to sites outside the gastrointestinal tract; this term is most commonly used to refer to the administration of medication by injection.

DRUG REFERENCES

The medical assistant is obligated to become familiar with the drugs that are most frequently used in his or her office. It is essential to know their indications, adverse reactions, routes of administration, dosage, and storage. With each drug (including drug samples and injectable medications), the manufacturer includes a *package insert* (PI), which contains important information regarding the drug. The information included in a PI is divided into categories which are listed and described in Fig. 11.1. Drug information is also available in drug reference books and on the Internet on certain recognized websites such as the *Prescribers' Digital Reference* (pdr.net).

DRUG PACKAGE INSERT

The categories of information included in a drug package insert are listed and described as follows:

DESCRIPTION: This category consists of a general description of the drug and includes the following information: brand name (with pronunciation), generic name, drug category, dosage form (e.g., tablets, capsules), route of administration, chemical name and structural formula, and the inactive ingredients contained in the drug. This category also indicates if the product requires a prescription (Rx) or if it is available over-the-counter (OTC). The symbol C and a Roman numeral appearing next to the drug indicates that it is a scheduled drug and that a prescription written for this drug requires the physician's DEA number.

CLINICAL PHARMACOLOGY: This category describes how the drug functions in the body to produce its therapeutic effect. Also included is an analysis of the absorption, distribution, metabolism, and excretion of the drug after it enters the body.

INDICATIONS AND USAGE: This category presents a list of the conditions that the drug has been formally approved to treat by the U.S. Food and Drug Administration (FDA).

CONTRAINDICATIONS: This category includes situations in which the drug should not be used because the risk of using the drug in these situations outweighs any possible benefit. Contraindications include administration of the drug to patients known to have a hypersensitivity (allergy) to it and use of the drug in patients who have a substantial risk of being harmed by it because of their particular age, sex, concurrent use of another drug, disease state, or condition (e.g., pregnancy).

WARNINGS: This category describes serious adverse reactions and potential safety hazards that may occasionally occur with the use of the drug and what should be done if they occur.

PRECAUTIONS: This category includes information regarding any special care that needs to be taken by the physician for the safe and effective use of the drug. Information typically presented in this category includes:

- **General Precautions:** Lists any disease states or situations that may require special consideration when the drug is being taken.
- **Information for Patients:** Includes information that should be relayed to the patient to ensure safe and effective use of the drug.
- **Laboratory Tests:** Indicates the laboratory tests that may be helpful in following the patient's response to the drug or in identifying possible adverse reactions to the drug.
- **Drug Interactions:** Lists any known interactions of this drug with other drugs that can affect the proper functioning of the drug.
- **Laboratory Test Interactions:** Includes any laboratory tests that may be affected when taking the medication.
- **Pregnancy:** Indicates the pregnancy category of the drug.

ADVERSE REACTIONS: This category describes the unintended and undesirable effects that may occur with the use of the drug. Some adverse reactions are harmless and therefore often tolerated by the patient in order to obtain the therapeutic effect of the drug. Other adverse reactions may be harmful to the patient and warrant discontinuing the medication.

OVERDOSAGE: This category describes symptoms associated with an overdosage of the drug, as well as the complications that can occur and the treatment to institute for an overdosage.

DOSAGE AND ADMINISTRATION: This category lists the recommended adult dosage, the usual dosage range of the drug, and the route of administration (e.g., by mouth, sublingual, IM). Also included is information about the intervals recommended between doses, the usual duration of treatment, and any modification of dosage needed for special groups such as children, the elderly, and patients with renal or hepatic disease.

HOW SUPPLIED: This category indicates the dosage forms that are available (e.g., 20-mg tablets), the units in which the dosage form is available (e.g., bottles of 100; 5-ml multiple-dose vial), information to help identify the dosage form (shape and color), and the handling and storage conditions for the drug.

Fig. 11.1 Information included in a drug package insert.

FOOD AND DRUG ADMINISTRATION

The US Food and Drug Administration (FDA) is a federal agency in the Department of Health and Human Services. The FDA is responsible for determining whether new food products, drugs, vaccines, medical devices, cosmetics, and other products are safe before they are released for human use.

The FDA determines the safety and effectiveness of prescription and nonprescription (over-the-counter [OTC]) drugs. Pharmaceutical manufacturers are required to submit new drug applications to the FDA for review and approval before products can be released for human use.

The FDA also is responsible for determining whether a medication will be available with or without a prescription. Medications that require a prescription have been determined by the FDA to be safe and effective when used under the guidance of a provider.

Nonprescription medications are drugs that the FDA determines to be safe and effective for use without provider supervision. Nonprescription medications have a low incidence of adverse reactions when the consumer follows the directions and warnings on the label. Examples of nonprescription medications include mild pain relievers; cough, cold, and allergy medications; antacids; topical antibiotics and antifungals; antidiarrheals; and laxatives.

DRUG NOMENCLATURE

Each drug has four names: chemical, generic, official, and brand (also known as *trade*) names.

1. *Chemical name.* The chemical name provides a precise description of the drug's chemical composition; pharmaceutical manufacturers and pharmacists are most concerned with the chemical makeup of a drug.
2. *Generic name.* After a drug has received official approval from the FDA, a generic name is assigned to it by the US Adopted Name (USAN) Council. The responsibility of the USAN Council is to select a simple, short, informative, and unique generic name for each new drug developed by a pharmaceutical manufacturer.
3. *Official name.* The official name is the name under which the drug is listed in official publications, such as the *United States Pharmacopeia* (USP) and the *National Formulary* (NF). Official publications set specific standards to regulate the strength, purity, packaging, safety, labeling, and dosage form of each drug. The generic name is frequently used for the official name.
4. *Brand name.* The brand name is the common or trade name under which a pharmaceutical manufacturer markets a drug. Because a drug may be manufactured by more than one pharmaceutical company, it may have several brand names (but only one generic name). Brand names are usually less complicated and easier to remember than generic names. The generic name of a common analgesic is acetaminophen; brand names for this drug include Tylenol, Tempra, Datril, Exdol, Panadol, and Liquiprin.

The medical assistant should be familiar with the generic and brand names of medications commonly prescribed and administered in the medical office.

What Would You Do? What Would You *Not* Do?

Case Study 1

Carol Okasinski, 56 years old, is a new patient. She was a patient of another physician in the community; however, his receptionist was often rude to her, and she decided not to go there anymore. Mrs. Okasinski is obese and has hypertension, type 2 diabetes, osteoarthritis in her hands and knees, and problems with depression. While filling in the health history form, she says she cannot fill in the names of her medications. She is on a lot of medications prescribed by her previous physician. She says she could not get the childproof pill containers open because of the arthritis in her hands, so she had her husband throw away the childproof containers and transfer each medication into an easy-to-open plastic container. She knows when to take her medications, but she does not know the names of them or why she is taking them. She has brought in a bag with all her medications in their plastic containers. ■

CLASSIFICATION OF DRUGS BASED ON PREPARATION

Drugs are available in two basic forms: liquid and solid. A medication may be available in both these forms (liquid and solid), which permits it to be administered to different types of patients. A liquid preparation of an antibiotic is administered to young children, and the solid preparation (e.g., tablets) of the same medication is administered to older children and adults. The following list includes the common categories of drugs based on preparation.

LIQUID PREPARATIONS

Elixir A drug that is dissolved in a solution of alcohol and water. Elixirs are sweetened and flavored and are taken orally. *Example:* Dimetapp elixir.

Emulsion A mixture of fats or oils in water. *Example:* Durezol ophthalmic emulsion.

Liniment A drug combined with oil, soap, alcohol, or water. Liniments are applied externally, using friction, to produce a feeling of heat or warmth. *Example:* Heet liniment.

Lotion An aqueous preparation that contains suspended ingredients. Lotions are used to treat external skin conditions. They work to soothe, protect, and moisten the skin and to destroy harmful bacteria. *Example:* Caladryl lotion.

Solution A liquid preparation that contains one or more completely dissolved substances. The dissolved substance is known as the *solute,* and the liquid in which it is dissolved is known as the *solvent.* Most drugs administered parenterally (by injection) consist of solutions. *Example:* Depo-Provera injectable solution.

Spirit A drug combined with an alcoholic solution that is volatile (a substance that is volatile evaporates readily). *Example:* Aromatic spirit of ammonia.

Spray A fine stream of medicated vapor, usually used to treat nose and throat conditions. *Example:* Dristan nasal spray.

Suspension A drug that contains solid insoluble drug particles in a liquid; the preparation must be shaken before administration. *Example:* Amoxicillin oral suspension.

Suspension aerosol A pressurized form in which solid aerosol or liquid drug particles are suspended in a gas to be dispensed in a cloud or mist. *Example:* Proventil inhalation aerosol.

Syrup A drug dissolved in a solution of sugar, water, and sometimes a flavoring to disguise an unpleasant taste. *Example:* Robitussin cough syrup.

Tincture A drug dissolved in a solution of alcohol or alcohol and water. *Example:* Tincture of iodine.

SOLID PREPARATIONS

Tablet A powdered drug that has been pressed into a disc. Some tablets are scored—that is, they are marked with an indentation so that they can be broken into halves or quarters for proper dosage. *Example:* Tylenol tablets.

Chewable tablet A powdered drug that has been flavored and pressed into a disc. Chewable tablets are often used for antacids, antiflatulents, and children's medications. *Example:* Pepto-Bismol chewable tablets.

Sublingual tablet A powdered drug that has been pressed into a disc and is designed to dissolve under the tongue, which permits its rapid absorption into the bloodstream. *Example:* Nitroglycerin sublingual tablets (Nitrostat).

Enteric-coated tablet A tablet coated with a substance that prevents it from dissolving until it reaches the intestines. The coating protects the drug from being destroyed by gastric juices and prevents it from irritating the stomach lining. To prevent the active ingredients from being released prematurely in the stomach, enteric-coated tablets must not be crushed or chewed. *Example:* Ecotrin enteric-coated aspirin.

Capsule A drug contained in a gelatin capsule that is water-soluble and functions to prevent the patient from tasting the drug. *Example:* Benadryl capsules.

Sustained-release capsule A capsule that contains granules that dissolve at different rates to provide a gradual and continuous release of medication. This reduces the number of doses that must be administered. (Sustained-release medication also comes in other preparations, such as tablets and caplets.) *Example:* Sudafed 12-hour sustained-release capsules.

Caplet A drug contained in an oblong tablet with a smooth coating to make swallowing easier. *Example:* Advil caplets.

Lozenge A drug contained in a candy-like base. Lozenges are circular and are designed to dissolve on the tongue. *Example:* Chloraseptic throat lozenges.

Cream A drug combined in a base that is usually nongreasy, resulting in a semisolid preparation. Creams are applied externally to the skin. *Example:* Hydrocortisone topical cream.

Ointment A drug with an oil base, resulting in a semisolid preparation. Ointments are applied externally to the skin and are usually greasy. *Example:* Cortisporin topical ointment.

Suppository A drug mixed with a firm base, such as cocoa butter, that is designed to melt at body temperature. A suppository is shaped into a cylinder or a cone for easy insertion into a body cavity, such as the rectum or vagina. *Example:* Preparation H suppositories.

Transdermal patch A patch with an adhesive backing, which contains a drug, that is applied to the skin. The drug enters the circulation after being absorbed through the skin. *Example:* Nitroglycerin patches (Nitro-Dur).

CLASSIFICATION OF DRUGS BASED ON ACTION

Drugs also can be classified according to the action they have on the body. The medical assistant should know in which category a particular drug belongs and its primary uses and major therapeutic effects. Table 11.1 contains classifications based on action and examples of drugs that are commonly administered and prescribed in the medical office.

SYSTEMS OF MEASUREMENT FOR MEDICATION

Two systems of measurement are used in the United States for prescribing, administering, and dispensing medication: the metric system and the household system. The metric system is the most common system used to measure medication because it provides a more exact measurement and is easier to use. The household system is not as accurate as the metric system for the measurement of medication and usually is used only when a patient takes liquid medication at home.

Systems of measurement have units of weight, volume, and length. *Weight* refers to the heaviness of an item, and *volume* refers to the amount of space occupied by a substance. *Length* is a unit of linear measurement of the distance from one point to another. Although length is not used to administer medication, it is used in other aspects of the medical office. The head circumference of infants is measured in centimeters (cm), a metric unit of linear measurement.

To prepare and administer medication properly and to avoid medication errors, the medical assistant must have a thorough knowledge of the specific units of measurement for these two systems and must be able to convert within each system and from one system to another. A basic discussion of the metric and household systems is presented next. A more thorough study of these systems, including conversion of units and dose calculation, is included in Chapter 11 of the Study Guide.

METRIC SYSTEM

The metric system was developed in France in the latter part of the 18th century in an effort to simplify measurement. Most European countries are required by law to use this system for the measurement of weight, volume, and length. Overall, the metric system is used for most scientific and medical measurements. Pharmaceutical companies use the metric system to measure and label medications.

The metric system employs a uniform decimal scale based on units of 10, making it very flexible and logical. The basic metric units of measurement are the gram, liter, and meter. The *gram* is a unit of weight used to measure solids, the *liter* is a unit of volume used to measure liquids, and the *meter* is a linear unit used to measure length or distance. The metric units used most often in the administration of medication in the medical office are the milligram, gram, milliliter, and cubic centimeter. Because a **cubic centimeter** (cc) is the amount of space occupied by 1 milliliter (mL), these two units can be used interchangeably (i.e., 1 mL = 1 cc).

Table 11.1 Classification of Drugs Based on Action

		COMMONLY PRESCRIBED DRUGS	
Drug Category	**Primary Use and Major Therapeutic Effects**	**Generic**	**Brand**
Analgesics (opioid)	*Indications for Use:* Used to manage moderate to severe pain *Desired Effects:* Work by altering perception of and response to painful stimuli *Side Effects:* Sedation, pruritis, dizziness, nausea, vomiting, constipation, physical dependence, tolerance, respiratory depression. **Vicodin** 32.5/5 mg **Darvocet-N** 50/325 mg 100/650 mg	codeine/acetaminophen (APAP)	▸Tylenol w/Codeine (III)
		fentanyl	Duragesic
		hydrocodone/APAP	▸Vicodin (III)
		hydrocodone/aspirin (ASA)	Lortab/ASA (III)
		hydrocodone/ibuprofen	▸Vicoprofen (III)
		meperidine	Demerol (II)
		morphine	MS Contin (II)
		oxycodone	▸OxyContin (II)
		oxycodone/APAP	▸Percocet (II)
		oxycodone/ASA	Percodan (II)
		propoxyphene	Darvon (IV)
		propoxyphene N/APAP	▸Darvocet-N (IV)
		tramadol	▸Ultram
Analgesics (barbiturate)	*Indications for Use:* Used to manage moderate to severe pain of tension headaches *Desired Effects:* Work by relieving pain and relaxing muscle contractions *Side Effects:* Drowsiness, lightheadedness, dizziness, sedation, shortness of breath, nausea, vomiting, abdominal pain, intoxicated feeling	butalbital/APAP/caffeine	▸Fioricet (III)
		butalbital/ASA/caffeine	Fiorinal (III)
Analgesics/ antipyretics	*Indications for Use:* Used to manage mild to moderate pain and to reduce fever *Desired Effects:* Work by relieving pain and reducing fever *Side Effects:* Nausea, dyspepsia, ulceration or bleeding, diarrhea, headache, dizziness.	acetaminophen	Tylenol[a]
		aspirin	Bayer[a] Ecotrin[a]
Analgesics/ antipyretics	**Naprosyn** 250 mg 375 mg 500 mg	**Nonsteroidal Antiinflammatory Drugs (NSAIDs)**	
		diclofenac	Voltaren
		ibuprofen	▸Advil[a] ▸Motrin[a]
		naproxen	Aleve[a] ▸Anaprox ▸Naprosyn
Anesthetics (local)	*Indications for Use:* Used to produce local anesthesia through loss of feeling to a body part *Desired Effects:* Work by preventing initiation and conduction of normal nerve impulses in body part *Side Effects:* Mild bruising, swelling, or itching at the injection site.	lidocaine	Xylocaine
		dibucaine	Nupercainal ointment[a]
Antacids	*Indications for Use:* Used to treat heartburn, hyperacidity, indigestion, and gastroesophageal reflux disease and to promote healing of ulcers *Desired Effects:* Work by neutralizing gastric acid to relieve gastric pain and irritation *Side Effects:* Nausea, constipation, diarrhea, headache, hyperacidity.	aluminum hydroxide/ magnesium hydroxide	Maalox[a] Mylanta[a]
		calcium carbonate	Tums[a]
		sodium bicarbonate/ ASA	Alka-Seltzer[a]
Anthelmintics	*Indications for Use:* Used to treat worm infections (pinworms, roundworms, hookworms)		

Continued

Table 11.1 Classification of Drugs Based on Action—cont'd

		COMMONLY PRESCRIBED DRUGS	
Drug Category	Primary Use and Major Therapeutic Effects	Generic	Brand
	Desired Effects: Work by destroying worms *Side Effects:* Abdominal pain, diarrhea, headache, dizziness	mebendazole	Vermox
Anti-Alzheimer agents	*Indications for Use:* Used to treat mild to moderate dementia associated with Alzheimer disease *Desired Effects:* Work by elevating acetylcholine concentration in the cerebral cortex *Side Effects:* Headache, fatigue, dizziness, nausea, vomiting, diarrhea, loss of appetite, joint pain, insomnia	donepezil memantine rivastigmine	▸Aricept ▸Namenda Exelon
Antianemics	**Iron Supplements**		
	Indications for Use: Used to prevent or cure iron-deficiency anemia *Desired Effects:* Work by increasing amount of iron in body *Side Effects:* Upset stomach, cramps, constipation, diarrhea, nausea, vomiting	ferrous sulfate iron dextran	Feosol[a] Dexferrum INFeD
	Vitamin B_{12}		
	Indications for Use: Used to treat pernicious anemia *Desired Effects:* Work by increasing amount of vitamin B_{12} in body *Side Effects:* Headache, dizziness, weakness, nausea, upset stomach, diarrhea, numbness or tingling, pain, swelling and redness at injection site, joint pain.	cyanocobalamin	Cobex injection Cyanoject injection Nascobal nasal spray
	Folic Acid Supplements		
	Indications for Use: Used to promote normal fetal development *Desired Effects:* Work by stimulating production of red blood cells, white blood cells, and platelets *Side Effects:* Allergic reaction	folic acid	▸Folvite
Antianginals	*Indications for Use:* Used to relieve or prevent angina attacks *Desired Effects:* Work by increasing blood supply to myocardial tissue *Side Effects:* Headache, dizziness, lightheadedness, fainting, fatigue **Imdur** 60 mg **Nitrostat** 0.3 mg 0.4 mg 0.6 mg	**Nitrates**	
		isosorbide dinitrate	Sorbitrate
		isosorbide mononitrate	▸Imdur
		nitroglycerin	Nitro-Bid Nitro-Dur Nitrostat
		Beta-Blockers	
		atenolol	Tenormin
		propranolol	Inderal
		metoprolol	▸Toprol-XL
		Calcium Channel Blockers	
		amlodipine	▸Norvasc
		bepridil	Vascor
		diltiazem	Cardizem Dilacor XR
		nifedipine	Adalat Procardia XL
		verapamil	▸Calan Isoptin Verelan

Table 11.1 Classification of Drugs Based on Action—cont'd

		COMMONLY PRESCRIBED DRUGS	
Drug Category	Primary Use and Major Therapeutic Effects	Generic	Brand
Antianxiety agents	*Indications for Use:* Used to treat anxiety *Desired Effects:* Work at many levels in central nervous system to produce anxiolytic (anxiety-relieving) effect *Side Effects:* Drowsiness, lack of energy, clumsiness, slurred speech, confusion, disorientation, depression, dizziness, impaired thinking, memory loss **Xanax** 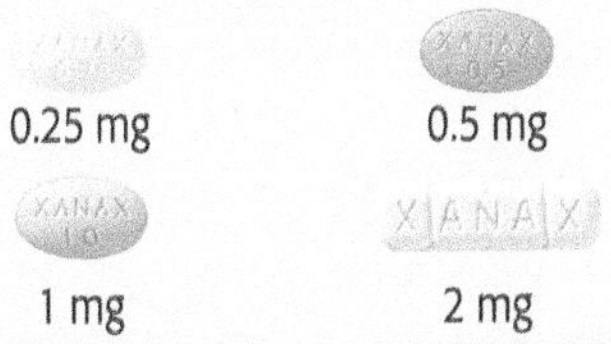 0.25 mg 0.5 mg 1 mg 2 mg	alprazolam buspirone chlordiazepoxide diazepam lorazepam	▸Xanax (IV) BuSpar Librium (IV) ▸Valium (IV) ▸Ativan (IV)
Anticholinergics	*Indications for Use:* Used preoperatively to decrease oral and respiratory secretions *Desired Effects:* Work by blocking effects of acetylcholine in autonomic nervous system *Side Effects:* Dry mouth and eyes, decreased sweating, blurred vision, constipation, flushing of the face, urinary retention	atropine	Atro-Pen
Anticoagulants	*Indications for Use:* Used to prevent and treat venous thrombosis, pulmonary embolism, and myocardial infarction by preventing clot extension and formation *Desired Effects:* Work by delaying or preventing blood coagulation *Side Effects:* Hemorrhaging, hematuria, bruising, bleeding gums, nosebleeds, bloody or black stools, menorrhagia **Coumadin** 1 mg 2 mg	heparin enoxaparin warfarin clopidogrel rivaroxaban apixaban	 ▸Lovenox ▸Coumadin Plavix ▸Xarelto ▸Eliquis
Anticonvulsants	*Indications for Use:* Used to prevent or relieve seizures *Desired Effects:* Work by decreasing incidence and severity of seizures *Side Effects:* Constipation, nausea, vomiting, dizziness, drowsiness **Neurontin** 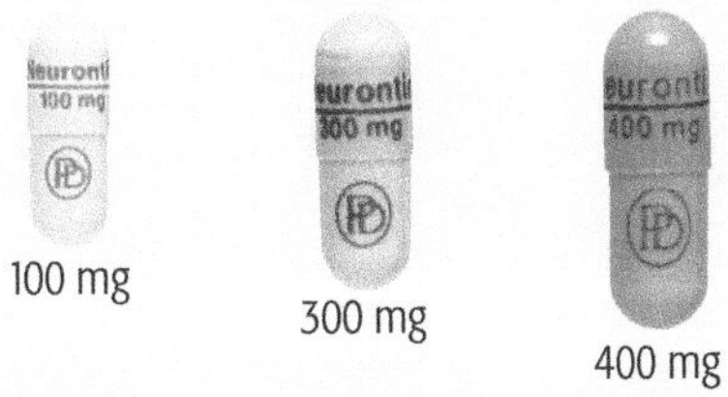 100 mg 300 mg 400 mg	carbamazepine clonazepam divalproex gabapentin lamotrigine phenytoin pregabalin topiramate	Tegretol ▸Klonopin (IV) ▸Depakote ▸Neurontin ▸Lamictal ▸Dilantin ▸Lyrica ▸Topamax

Continued

Table 11.1 Classification of Drugs Based on Action—cont'd

Drug Category	Primary Use and Major Therapeutic Effects	Commonly Prescribed Drugs: Generic	Commonly Prescribed Drugs: Brand
Antidepressants	*Indications for Use:* Used to prevent, cure, or alleviate depression and to treat anxiety disorders (panic attacks) and obsessive-convulsive disorder *Desired Effects:* Work by inhibiting reuptake of neurotransmitters in the central nervous system *Side Effects:* Nausea, increased appetite, weight gain, loss of sexual desire, fatigue, drowsiness **Prozac** 10 mg 20 mg **Wellbutrin-SR** 100 mg 150 mg	**Selective Serotonin Reuptake Inhibitors (SSRIs)**	
		citalopram	▸Celexa
		escitalopram	▸Lexapro
		fluoxetine	▸Prozac
		fluvoxamine	Luvox
		paroxetine	▸Paxil
		sertraline	▸Zoloft
		Serotonin-Norepinephrine Reuptake Inhibitors (SNRIs)	
		desvenlafaxine	Pristiq
		duloxetine	▸Cymbalta
		venlafaxine	▸Effexor XR
		Miscellaneous	
		amitriptyline	▸Elavil
		bupropion	▸Wellbutrin SR
		mirtazapine	▸Remeron
		nefazodone	Serzone
		trazodone	▸Desyrel
Antidiabetics	**Hypoglycemics** *Indications for Use:* Used to manage non–insulin-dependent type 2 diabetes mellitus *Desired Effects:* Work by stimulating release of insulin from pancreas and increasing sensitivity to insulin *Side Effects:* Headache, stomach upset, loss of appetite, nausea, diarrhea, vomiting, hypoglycemia **Amaryl** 2 mg 4 mg **Glucotrol XL** 5 mg 10 mg	glimepiride	▸Amaryl
		glipizide	▸Glucotrol XL
		glyburide	▸Micronase
		metformin	▸Glucophage
		pioglitazone	▸Actos
		rosiglitazone	▸Avandia
		sitagliptin	▸Januvia
		dulaglutide (injectable)	▸Trulicity
Antidiabetics	**Insulins** *Indications for Use:* Used to manage diabetes mellitus *Desired Effects:* Work by reducing blood glucose levels *Side Effects:* Hypoglycemia, headache, weight gain, pain, redness and irritation at the injection site	regular insulin	Humulin R[a] Novolin R[a]
		NPH insulin	Humulin N[a] Novolin N[a]
		NPH/regular insulin	Humulin 70/30[a] Novolin 70/30[a]
		insulin glargine	▸Lantus
		insulin lispro	Humalog
Antidiarrheals	*Indications for Use:* Used to control and relieve diarrhea *Desired Effects:* Work by inhibiting peristalsis, reducing fecal volume, and preventing loss of fluids and electrolytes *Side Effects:* Abdominal pain, constipation, dizziness, dry mouth, drowsiness **Lomotil** 2.5/0.025 mg	bismuth subsalicylate	Pepto-Bismol[a]
		diphenoxylate/atropine	Lomotil (V)
		kaolin/pectin	Kaopectate[a]
		loperamide	Imodium[a]

Table 11.1 Classification of Drugs Based on Action—cont'd

		COMMONLY PRESCRIBED DRUGS	
Drug Category	**Primary Use and Major Therapeutic Effects**	**Generic**	**Brand**
Antidysrhythmics	*Indications for Use:* Used to control or prevent cardiac dysrhythmias *Desired Effects:* Work by decreasing myocardial excitability and slowing conduction velocity *Side Effects:* Dry mouth and throat, dizziness, diarrhea, loss of appetite, lightheadedness, blurred vision **Inderal** 10 mg 20 mg 40 mg 60 mg 80 mg	metoprolol procainamide propranolol	▸Lopressor ▸Toprol-XL Pronestyl Inderal
Antiemetics	*Indications for Use:* Used to prevent or relieve nausea and vomiting *Desired Effects:* Work by depressing chemoreceptor trigger zone in central nervous system to inhibit nausea and vomiting *Side Effects:* Dry mouth, drowsiness, dysuria, dizziness, blurred vision	dronabinol ondansetron prochlorperazine promethazine meclizine	Marinol (III) Zofran Compazine ▸Phenergan Bonine[a]
Antiflatulents	*Indications for Use:* Used to relieve discomfort of excess gas and bloating in gastrointestinal tract *Desired Effects:* Work by causing coalescence of gas bubbles in intestinal tract *Side Effects:* Nausea, constipation, hypersensitivity reaction	simethicone	Gas-X[a] Mylanta Gas[a]
Antifungals	*Indications for Use:* Used to treat fungal infections *Desired Effects:* Work by killing or inhibiting growth of susceptible fungi *Side Effects:* Mild stomach pain, headache, dizziness, unusual or unpleasant taste in the mouth **Diflucan** 50 mg 100 mg 200 mg	amphotericin B clotrimazole fluconazole itraconazole ketoconazole miconazole nystatin terbinafine	Fungizone Gyne-Lotrimin[a] ▸Diflucan Sporanox Nizoral Monistat[a] Mycostatin[a] ▸Lamisil
Antigout agents	*Indications for Use:* Used to prevent attacks of gout *Desired Effects:* Work by inhibiting production of uric acid *Side Effects:* Skin rash, diarrhea, nausea, itching, drowsiness **Zyloprim** 100 mg 300 mg	allopurinol colchicine	▸Zyloprim Colchicine tablets
Antihistamines	*Indications for Use:* Used to relieve symptoms associated with allergies (increased sneezing; rhinorrhea; itchy eyes, nose, and throat) *Desired Effects:* Work by blocking effects of histamine at histamine receptor sites *Side Effects:* Dry mouth, drowsiness, dizziness, nausea, vomiting, blurred vision, urinary retention **Allegra** 60 mg 180 mg	brompheniramine cetirizine chlorpheniramine desloratadine diphenhydramine fexofenadine/ pseudoephedrine levocetirizine loratadine promethazine	Dimetane[a] ▸Zyrtec[a] Chlor-Trimetron[a] Teldrin[a] ▸Clarinex Benadryl[a] ▸Allegra Xyzal ▸Claritin[a] ▸Phenergan

Continued

Table 11.1 Classification of Drugs Based on Action—cont'd

Drug Category	Primary Use and Major Therapeutic Effects	COMMONLY PRESCRIBED DRUGS Generic	 Brand
Antihypertensives	*Indications for Use:* Used to manage hypertension *Desired Effects:* Work by causing systemic vasodilation to reduce blood pressure *Side Effects:* Constipation, dehydration, dizziness, lightheadedness, drowsiness	**Angiotensin-Converting Enzyme (ACE) Inhibitors**	
		benazepril	Lotensin
		captopril	Capoten
		enalapril	▸Vasotec
		lisinopril	▸Prinivil
		quinapril	▸Accupril
		ramipril	▸Altace
		Peripherally Acting Adrenergic Blockers	
		clonidine	▸Catapres
		doxazosin	Cardura
		prazosin	Minipress
		Angiotensin II Receptor Antagonists	
		Candesartan	Atacand
		irbesartan	▸Avapro
		losartan	▸Cozaar
		olmesartan	▸Benicar
		telmisartan	Micardis
		valsartan	▸Diovan
		Beta-Blockers	
		atenolol	▸Tenormin
		carvedilol	▸Coreg
		metoprolol	▸Lopressor ▸Toprol-XL
		nebivolol	▸Bystolic
		propranolol	▸Inderal
		sotalol	Betapace
		Calcium Channel Blockers	
		amlodipine	▸Norvasc
		diltiazem	▸Cardizem
		felodipine	Plendil
		Vasodilator	
		hydralazine	Apresoline
		Miscellaneous	
		amlodipine/atorvastatin	Caduet
		amlodipine/benazepril	▸Lotrel
		bisoprolol/ hydrochlorothiazide	Ziac
		irbesartan/ hydrochlorothiazide	▸Avalide
		lisinopril/ hydrochlorothiazide	▸Zestoretic
		losartan/ hydrochlorothiazide	▸Hyzaar
		olmesartan/ hydrochlorothiazide	▸Benicar HCT
		triamterene/ hydrochlorothiazide	▸Maxzide
		valsartan/ hydrochlorothiazide	Diovan HCT

Accupril
5 mg
10 mg
20 mg
40 mg

Cozaar
25 mg
50 mg

Topro XL
50 mg
100 mg
200 mg

Cardizem
30 mg
60 mg
90 mg
120 mg

Table 11.1 Classification of Drugs Based on Action—cont'd

Drug Category	Primary Use and Major Therapeutic Effects	COMMONLY PRESCRIBED DRUGS Generic	Brand
Anti-Impotence agents	*Indications for Use:* Used to treat erectile dysfunction *Desired Effects:* Work by promoting increased blood flow to penis *Side Effects:* Headache, flushing, indigestion, stuffy or runny nose, temporary vision changes **Viagra** 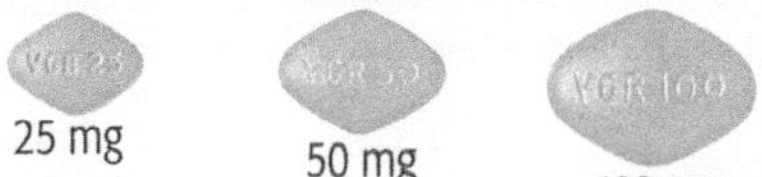 25 mg, 50 mg, 100 mg	sildenafil	▸Viagra
		tadalafil	▸Cialis
		vardenafil	Levitra
Anti-Infectives	*Indications for Use:* Used to treat infections *Desired Effects:* Work by killing or inhibiting growth of bacteria *Side Effects:* Vomiting, diarrhea, allergic reaction, abdominal cramps, vaginal itching or discharge, white patches on the tongue **Amoxil** 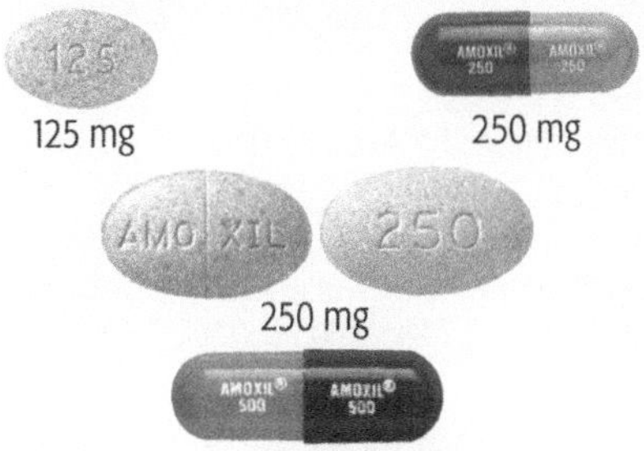 125 mg, 250 mg, 250 mg, 500 mg **Zithromax** 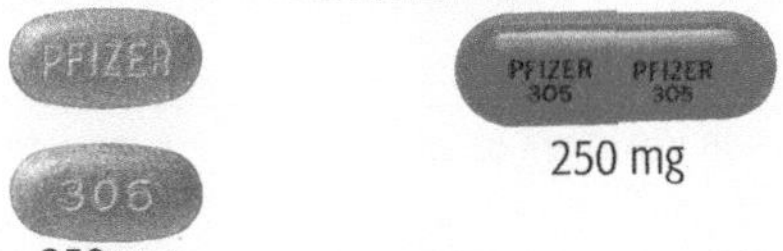 250 mg, 250 mg **Keflex** 250 mg, 500 mg **Cipro** 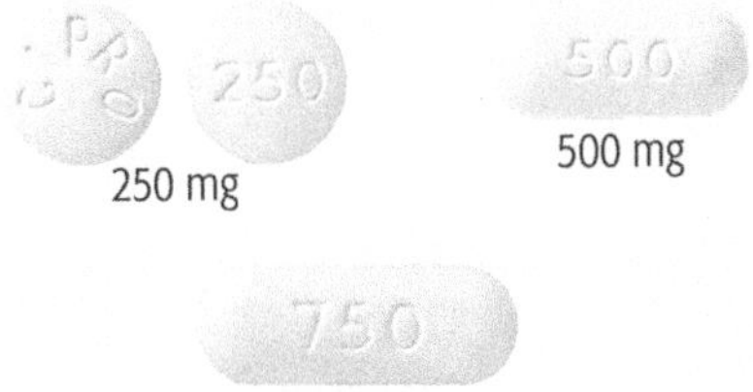 250 mg, 500 mg, 750 mg **Macrobid** 100 mg	**Penicillins**	
		amoxicillin	▸Amoxil ▸Trimox
		amoxicillin/clavulanate	▸Augmentin
		ampicillin	Omnipen
		benzathine penicillin	Bicillin
		penicillin VK	▸Pen-VK
		procaine penicillin	Wycillin
		Macrolides	
		azithromycin	▸Zithromax (Z-Pak)
		clarithromycin	Biaxin
		erythromycin	Ery-Tab
		Cephalosporins	
		cefaclor	Ceclor
		cefdinir	▸Omnicef
		cefprozil	▸Cefzil
		ceftriaxone	Rocephin
		cefuroxime	Ceftin
		cephalexin	▸Keflex
		Fluoroquinolones	
		ciprofloxacin	▸Cipro
		levofloxacin	▸Levaquin
		moxifloxacin	Avelox
		ofloxacin	Floxin
		Tetracyclines	
		doxycycline	Doryx ▸Vibramycin
		minocycline	Arestin
		tetracycline	Achromycin Sumycin
		Aminoglycosides	
		gentamicin	Garamycin
		kanamycin	Kantrex
		neomycin	Neobiotic
		tobramycin	Nebcin
		Sulfonamides	
		sulfamethoxazole	Gantanol
		trimethoprim/sulfamethoxazole	▸Bactrim
		Miscellaneous	
		clindamycin	Cleocin
		chloramphenicol	Chloromycetin
		nitrofurantoin	▸Macrobid Macrodantin
		vancomycin	Vancocin

Continued

Table 11.1 Classification of Drugs Based on Action—cont'd

		COMMONLY PRESCRIBED DRUGS	
Drug Category	Primary Use and Major Therapeutic Effects	Generic	Brand
Anti-Inflammatories	*Indications for Use:* Used to relieve signs and symptoms of osteoarthritis and rheumatoid arthritis in adults *Desired Effects:* Work by decreasing pain and inflammation *Side Effects:* Vomiting, nausea, constipation, reduced appetite, headache, dizziness, rash, drowsiness **Celebrex** 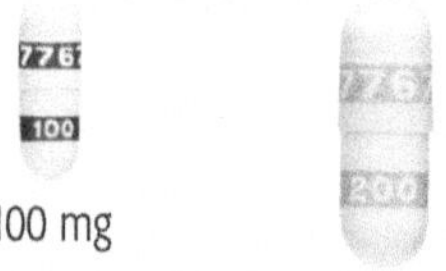 100 mg 200 mg	aspirin celecoxib etodolac ibuprofen indomethacin meloxicam nabumetone naproxen piroxicam valdecoxib	Bayer[a] Ecotrin[a] ▸Celebrex Lodine Advil[a] Motrin[a] Indocin ▸Mobic ▸Relafen Aleve[a] Anaprox Naprosyn Feldene Bextra
Antimanics	*Indications for Use:* Used to treat bipolar affective disorders *Desired Effects:* Work by altering cation transport in nerves and muscles *Side Effects:* Restlessness, mild tremor of hands, mild thirst, loss of appetite, stomach pain, flatulence, indigestion, weight gain or loss **Eskalith** 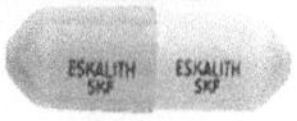 300 mg **Eskalith CR** 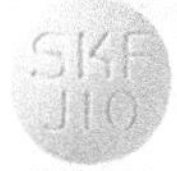 450 mg	lithium	Eskalith Eskalith CR
Antimigraine agents	*Indications for Use:* Used in acute treatment of migraine attacks *Desired Effects:* Work by causing vasoconstriction in large intracranial arteries *Side Effects:* Dizziness, flushing, nausea, vomiting, sore throat, tingling sensation, abdominal pain	sumatriptan topiramate	▸Imitrex ▸Topamax
Antineoplastics	*Indications for Use:* Used to treat tumors *Desired Effects:* Work by preventing development, growth, or proliferation of malignant cells *Side Effects:* Nausea, vomiting, loss of appetite, diarrhea, hair loss, bone marrow depression	cyclophosphamide methotrexate	Cytoxan Mexate Folex
Anti-Parkinson agents	*Indications for Use:* Used to treat symptoms of Parkinson disease *Desired Effects:* Work by restoring balance between acetylcholine and dopamine in central nervous system *Side Effects:* Nausea, vomiting, sleepiness, dizziness, headache, low blood pressure **Sinemet** 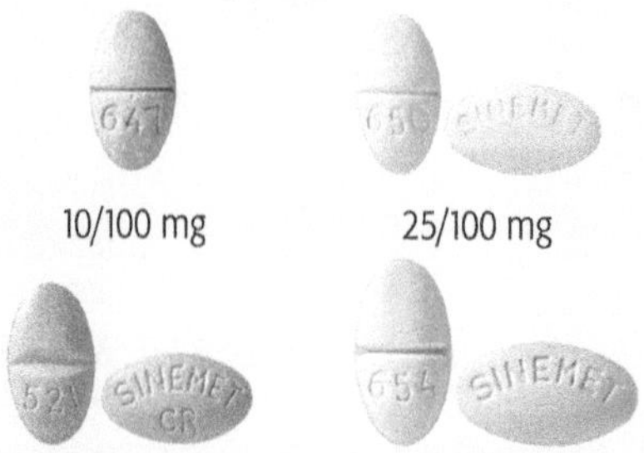 10/100 mg 25/100 mg 50/200 mg 25/250 mg	carbidopa/levodopa ropinirole	Sinemet Requip

Table 11.1 Classification of Drugs Based on Action—cont'd

Drug Category	Primary Use and Major Therapeutic Effects	COMMONLY PRESCRIBED DRUGS: Generic	COMMONLY PRESCRIBED DRUGS: Brand
Antiprotozoals	*Indications for Use:* Used to treat protozoal infections *Desired Effects:* Work by destroying protozoa *Side Effects:* Diarrhea, nausea, vomiting, stomach pain **Flagyl** 250 mg, 500 mg, 375 mg	metronidazole	Flagyl
Antipsychotics	*Indications for Use:* Used to treat psychotic disorders *Desired Effects:* Work by blocking dopamine and serotonin receptors in central nervous system *Side Effects:* Drowsiness, rapid heartbeat, dizziness, weight gain **Risperdal** 1 mg, 2 mg, 3 mg, 4 mg	haloperidol	Haldol
		aripiprazole	▸Abilify
		olanzapine	▸Zyprexa
		risperidone	▸Risperdal
		quetiapine	▸Seroquel
Antiretrovirals	*Indications for Use:* Used to manage human immunodeficiency virus (HIV) infections and to reduce maternal-fetal transmission of HIV *Desired Effects:* Work by inhibiting replication of retroviruses *Side Effects:* Nausea, diarrhea, loss of appetite, headache, fatigue, peripheral neuropathy, lipodystrophy **Retovir** 100 mg	efavirenz	Sustiva
		emtricitabine	Emtriva
		lamivudine	Epivir
		ritonavir	Norvir
		tenofovir	Viread
		zidovudine	Retrovir
Antispasmodics	*Indications for Use:* Used to control hypermotility in irritable bowel syndrome, spastic colitis, spastic bladder, and pylorospasm *Desired Effects:* Work by preventing or relieving spasms of gastrointestinal or genitourinary tract *Side Effects:* Flatulence, bloating, dizziness, heartburn, dry mouth, constipation,	dicyclomine	Bentyl
		hyoscyamine	Levsin
Antituberculars	*Indications for Use:* Used to treat tuberculosis *Desired Effects:* Work by killing or inhibiting growth of mycobacteria *Side Effects:* Diarrhea, stomach pain, nausea, vomiting, loss of appetite, unusual tiredness or weakness	isoniazid	INH
		rifampin	Rifadin
Antitussives	*Indications for Use:* Used in prevention or relief of coughs caused by minor viral upper respiratory infections or inhaled irritants *Desired Effects:* Work by suppressing cough reflex by direct effect on cough center in central nervous system *Side Effects:* Irritability, dizziness, drowsiness, nausea, vomiting	benzonatate	Tessalon
		chlorpheniramine/ hydrocodone	Tussionex (III)
		dextromethorphan	Robitussin DM[a]
		guaifenesin/codeine	Robitussin A-C (V)
Antiulcer agents	*Indications for Use:* Used to manage ulcers, gastroesophageal reflux disease, heartburn, indigestion, and gastric hyperacidity *Desired Effects:* Work by decreasing the amount of acid produced by the stomach. *Side Effects:* Headache, mild diarrhea, nausea, stomach pain, flatulence, constipation, dry mouth **Prevacid** 15 mg, 30 mg	**Proton Pump Inhibitors**	
		esomeprazole	▸Nexium
		lansoprazole	▸Prevacid
		omeprazole	▸Prilosec[a]
		pantoprazole	▸Protonix
		rabeprazole	▸AcipHex
		H_2-Receptor Antagonists	
		cimetidine	Tagamet[a]
		famotidine	▸Pepcid AC[a]
		ranitidine	▸Zantac[a]

Continued

Table 11.1 Classification of Drugs Based on Action—cont'd

Drug Category	Primary Use and Major Therapeutic Effects	COMMONLY PRESCRIBED DRUGS	
		Generic	Brand
Antivirals	*Indications for Use:* Used to manage viral infections *Desired Effects:* Work by inhibiting viral replication *Side Effects:* Nausea, vomiting, dizziness, diarrhea, headache, insomnia **Valtrex** 500 mg 1 g	acyclovir famciclovir valacyclovir oseltamivir	▸Zovirax Famvir ▸Valtrex Tamiflu
Bone resorption inhibitors	*Indications for Use:* Used to treat and prevent osteoporosis *Desired Effects:* Work by inhibiting reabsorption of bone *Side Effects:* Nausea, vomiting, stomach pain, diarrhea, headache, dizziness, pain in the extremities, loss of voice **Fosamax** 5 mg 10 mg 40 mg	alendronate ibandronate raloxifene risedronate	▸Fosamax Boniva ▸Evista ▸Actonel
Bronchodilators	*Indications for Use:* Used to manage reversible airway obstruction caused by asthma or chronic obstructive pulmonary disease *Desired Effects:* Work by relaxing smooth muscle of respiratory tract resulting in bronchodilation *Side Effects:* Dry mouth, constipation, diarrhea, headache, heart palpitations, dizziness, trembling, nervousness, muscle aches or cramps **Singulair** 4 mg 5 mg 10 mg	albuterol budesonide/formoterol fluticasone formoterol ipratropium/albuterol levalbuterol montelukast salmeterol theophylline tiotropium	▸Proventil ▸ProAir HFA ▸Symbicort ▸Advair Diskus ▸Breo Ellipta Foradil ▸Combivent Xopenex ▸Singulair Serevent Bronkodyl ▸Spiriva
Cardiac glycosides	*Indications for Use:* Used to treat congestive heart failure and cardiac arrhythmias *Desired Effects:* Work by increasing strength and force of myocardial contractions and slowing heart rate *Side Effects:* Cardiac arrhythmias, nausea, vomiting, diarrhea, loss of appetite, dizziness, weakness, headache, blurred vision, depression **Lanoxicaps** 0.1 mg	digitoxin digoxin	Crystodigin ▸Digitek Lanoxicaps ▸Lanoxin

Table 11.1 Classification of Drugs Based on Action—cont'd

		COMMONLY PRESCRIBED DRUGS	
Drug Category	**Primary Use and Major Therapeutic Effects**	**Generic**	**Brand**
Central nervous system stimulants	*Indications for Use:* Used to treat narcolepsy and manage attention-deficit/hyperactivity disorder *Desired Effects:* Work by increasing level of catecholamines in central nervous system *Side Effects:* Loss of appetite, increased anxiety level, weight loss, dizziness, headache, irritability, facial tics, restlessness, panic attacks, insomnia, tachycardia **Adderall (II)** 5 mg 10 mg 20 mg 30 mg	atomoxetine	▸Strattera
		dextroamphetamine	Dexedrine (II)
		dextroamphetamine saccharate and sulfate	▸Adderall (II)
		lisdexamfetamine	Vyvanse (II)
		methylphenidate	▸Ritalin (II) ▸Concerta
Contraceptives (hormonal)	*Indications for Use:* Used to prevent pregnancy and to regulate menstrual cycle *Desired Effects:* Work by inhibiting ovulation *Side Effects:* Headache, dizziness, lightheadedness, stomach upset, bloating, nausea, weight gain, metrorrhagia, breast tenderness, mood changes **Ortho-Novum** 7/7/7 1/35	**Oral Contraceptives**	
		ethinyl estradiol/ drospirenone	▸Yasmin Yaz
		ethinyl estradiol/ levonorgestrel	Alesse Levlen
		ethinyl estradiol/ norethindrone	Kariva ▸Ortho-Novum ▸Loestrin Fe
		ethinyl estradiol/ norgestimate	▸Ortho Tri-Cyclen Tri-Sprintec
		Injectable Contraceptives	
		medroxyprogesterone	▸Depo-Provera
		Transdermal Contraceptives	
		ethinyl estradiol/ norelgestromin	▸Ortho Evra
		Vaginal Ring Contraceptives	
		ethinyl estradiol/ etonogestrel	NuvaRing
Corticosteroids	**Systemic Corticosteroids** *Indications for Use:* Used to treat inflammation, allergies, asthma, and autoimmune disorders and as replacement therapy in adrenal insufficiency *Desired Effects:* Work by suppressing inflammation and modifying normal immune response *Side Effects:* Increased appetite, weight gain, sudden mood swings, easy bruising, muscle weakness, blurred vision, increased growth of body hair, swollen face	cortisone	Cortone
		fluticasone	▸Flovent
		hydrocortisone	Cortef
		methylprednisolone	Medrol Depo-Medrol
		prednisone	▸Deltasone
		triamcinolone	Aristocort
	Nasal Corticosteroids *Indications for Use:* Used to treat chronic nasal inflammatory conditions (e.g., allergic rhinitis) *Desired Effects:* Work by suppressing inflammation and reducing hypersecretions of respiratory tract *Side Effects:* Nosebleed, sinus pain, sore throat, burning, dryness or irritation inside the nose	fluticasone	▸Flonase
		mometasone	▸Nasonex
		triamcinolone	▸Nasacort
Decongestants	*Indications for Use:* Used to decrease nasal congestion *Desired Effects:* Work by producing vasoconstriction in respiratory tract mucosa *Side Effects:* Irritation of the lining of the nose, headache, nausea, dry mouth, nervousness, insomnia, dizziness	oxymetazoline	Afrin[a] Dristan[a]
		phenylephrine	Neo-Synephrine[a]
		pseudoephedrine	Sudafed[a]

Continued

Table 11.1 Classification of Drugs Based on Action—cont'd

		COMMONLY PRESCRIBED DRUGS	
Drug Category	**Primary Use and Major Therapeutic Effects**	**Generic**	**Brand**
Diuretics	*Indications for Use:* Used to manage hypertension, edema in congestive heart failure, and renal disease *Desired Effects:* Work by removing excess fluid from the body by increasing urine output *Side Effects:* Dry mouth, increased thirst, weakness, lethargy, drowsiness, muscle pain or cramps, confusion, oliguria, headache, dizziness **Lasix** 20 mg 40 mg 80 mg	**Loop Diuretics**	
		bumetanide	Bumex
		furosemide	‣Lasix
		Thiazide Diuretics	
		Chlorthalidone	Hygroton
		hydrochlorothiazide	‣Microzide
		Potassium-Sparing Diuretics	
		spironolactone	Aldactone
		triamterene	Dyrenium
Electrolyte replacements	*Indications for Use:* Used to treat or prevent electrolyte depletion *Desired Effects:* Work by replacing electrolytes in body *Side Effects:* Nausea, vomiting, diarrhea, flatulence, high blood pressure, arrhythmias **Klor-Con** 600 mg 750 mg	**Potassium Supplements**	
		potassium chloride	‣K-Dur ‣Klor-Con
Emetics	*Indications for Use:* Used to treat poisoning *Desired Effects:* Work by inducing vomiting *Side Effects:* Diarrhea, lethargy, stomach cramps, prolonged vomiting	syrup of ipecac	
Expectorants	*Indications for Use:* Used to manage coughs by expelling mucus *Desired Effects:* Work by decreasing viscosity of bronchial secretions to promote clearance of mucus from respiratory tract *Side Effects:* Nausea, vomiting, stomach upset, dizziness, headache, drowsiness, diarrhea, constipation	guaifenesin	Robitussin[a] Mucinex[a] Naldecon[a]
Hormone replacements	*Indications for Use:* Used to treat moderate to severe vasomotor symptoms of menopause *Desired Effects:* Work by restoring hormonal balance *Side Effects:* Headache, nausea, vaginal discharge, fluid retention, weight gain, breast tenderness **Premarin** 0.3 mg 0.625 mg 0.9 mg 1.25 mg 2.5 mg	conjugated estrogens	‣Premarin
		conjugated estrogen/progesterone	‣Prempro
		estradiol	‣Estrace
		estradiol/norethindrone	Activella

Table 11.1 Classification of Drugs Based on Action—cont'd

		COMMONLY PRESCRIBED DRUGS	
Drug Category	**Primary Use and Major Therapeutic Effects**	**Generic**	**Brand**
Immunizations	*Indications for Use:* Used to prevent (vaccine-preventable) diseases *Desired Effects:* Work by stimulating body to produce antibodies *Side Effects:* Pain, redness, tenderness and swelling at the injection site, fatigue, headache, nausea, dizziness, fever	diphtheria, tetanus toxoids, and acellular pertussis vaccine	Acel-Imune Certiva Daptacel Infanrix Tripedia
		Haemophilus b conjugate vaccine	ActHIB HibTITER
		hepatitis A vaccine	Havrix Vaqta
		hepatitis B vaccine	Engerix-B Recombivax HB
		human papillomavirus vaccine	Gardasil
		inactivated polio vaccine	IPOL
		influenza virus vaccine types A and B	Afluria Flushield Fluzone FluMist
		measles, mumps, and rubella vaccine	M-M-R II
		meningococcal conjugate vaccine	Menactra
		pneumococcal conjugate vaccine	Prevnar Pneumovax II
		rotavirus	Rotarix RotaShield
		rubella vaccine	Meruvax II
		varicella vaccine	Varivax
Immunosuppressants	*Indications for Use:* Used to treat severe rheumatoid arthritis and to prevent and treat rejection of transplanted organs *Desired Effects:* Work by inhibiting body's normal immune response *Side Effects:* Abdominal discomfort, swollen and painful gums, acne, increased hair growth, headache, diarrhea, nausea, flushing, cramps	cyclosporine	Sandimmune Neoral
		methotrexate	Rheumatrex
Laxatives	*Indications for Use:* Used to relieve constipation *Desired Effects:* Work by promoting defecation of normal, soft stool *Side Effects:* Bloating, cramping, flatulence, diarrhea, nausea, dehydration	bisacodyl	Dulcolax[a]
		docusate	Colace[a]
		phenolphthalein	Phenolax[a]
		psyllium	Metamucil[a]
Lipid-lowering agents	*Indications for Use:* Used to lower cholesterol to reduce risk of myocardial infarction and stroke *Desired Effects:* Work by inhibiting enzyme needed to synthesize cholesterol in body *Side Effects:* Headache, diarrhea, constipation, muscle aches and weakness, nausea, vomiting, stomach upset, bloating, cramping **Lipitor** 10 mg 20 mg 40 mg	atorvastatin	▸Lipitor
		ezetimibe	▸Zetia
		ezetimibe/simvastatin	▸Vytorin
		fenofibrate	▸Tricor
		fluvastatin	Lescol
		gemfibrozil	Lopid
		lovastatin	▸Mevacor
		pravastatin	▸Pravachol
		rosuvastatin	▸Crestor
		simvastatin	▸Zocor

Continued

Table 11.1 Classification of Drugs Based on Action—cont'd

		COMMONLY PRESCRIBED DRUGS	
Drug Category	**Primary Use and Major Therapeutic Effects**	**Generic**	**Brand**
Muscle relaxants (skeletal)	*Indications for Use:* Used to treat acute painful musculoskeletal conditions *Desired Effects:* Work by relaxing skeletal muscles *Side Effects:* Headache, drowsiness, dizziness, dry mouth, nausea, blurred vision, stomach upset **Flexeril** 10 mg	baclofen carisoprodol cyclobenzaprine metaxalone methocarbamol tizanidine	▸Lioresal ▸Soma ▸Flexeril Skelaxin Robaxin ▸Zanaflex
Ophthalmic anti-infectives	*Indications for Use:* Used to treat eye infections *Desired Effects:* Work by destroying bacteria *Side Effects:* Temporary blurred vision, tearing, eye redness, eye discomfort, allergic reaction	dexamethasone/ tobramycin moxifloxacin polymyxin/bacitracin polymyxin/neomycin polymyxin/trimethoprim tobramycin	Tobradex Vigamox Polysporin Neosporin Polytrim Tobrex
Otic preparations	*Indications for Use:* Used to treat ear conditions		
	Analgesics *Desired Effects:* Work by relieving ear pain *Side Effects:* Allergic reaction	benzocaine	Auralgan
	Anti-infectives *Desired Effects:* Work by treating otitis externa *Side Effects:* Temporary stinging or burning in the ear, allergic reaction	neomycin/polymyxin/ hydrocortisone ofloxacin	Cortisporin Otic Floxin Otic
	Cerumenolytics *Desired Effects:* Work by softening cerumen *Side Effects:* Temporary decrease in hearing and feeling of fullness in the ear	carbamide peroxide	Debrox[a]
Platelet inhibitors	*Indications for Use:* Used to reduce incidence of myocardial infarction and stroke *Desired Effects:* Work by interfering with ability of platelets to adhere to each other *Side Effects:* Itching, eczema, rash, head or joint pain, bruising, diarrhea, stomach upset	clopidogrel salicylates	▸Plavix Aspirin[a]
Sedatives and hypnotics	*Indications for Use:* Used for short-term treatment of insomnia *Desired Effects:* Work by promoting sleep by central nervous system depression *Side Effects:* Burning or tingling in the extremities, change in appetite, constipation, diarrhea, dizziness, daytime drowsiness, loss of coordination, headache, mental slowing, stomach pain, unusual dreams **Ambien** 5 mg 10 mg	eszopiclone flurazepam hydroxyzine phenobarbital temazepam zolpidem	▸Lunesta (IV) Dalmane (IV) Atarax Vistaril Luminal (IV) ▸Restoril (IV) ▸Ambien (IV)
Smoking deterrents	*Indications for Use:* Used to manage nicotine withdrawal to cease cigarette smoking *Desired Effects:* Work by providing nicotine during controlled withdrawal from cigarette smoking *Side Effects:* Dry mouth, nausea, stomach pain, headache, dizziness, vision changes, sore throat, muscle pain	bupropion nicotine varenicline	Zyban Nicorette Gum[a] Nicotrol Inhaler NicoDerm Patch[a] Commit Lozenges[a] Chantix
Thrombolytic agents	*Indications for Use:* Used for acute management of coronary thrombosis (myocardial infarction) *Desired Effects:* Work by dissolving existing clots *Side Effects:* Bleeding, arrhythmias, dizziness, headache, shortness of breath, allergic reaction	alteplase anistreplase reteplase streptokinase	Activase Eminase Retavase Streptase

Table 11.1 Classification of Drugs Based on Action—cont'd

Drug Category	Primary Use and Major Therapeutic Effects	COMMONLY PRESCRIBED DRUGS Generic	Brand
Thyroid preparations	**Thyroid Hormones** *Indications for Use:* Used as replacement or substitute therapy for diminished or absent thyroid functioning of many causes *Desired Effects:* Work by increasing basal metabolic rate *Side Effects:* Hair loss, fast or irregular heart rate, hot flashes, irritability, sweating, mood changes, insomnia, vomiting, diarrhea, appetite changes, weight changes **Levoxyl** 0.05 mg	levothyroxine	▸Levoxyl ▸Synthroid ▸Levothroid
	Antithyroid Agents *Indications for Use:* Used to treat hyperthyroidism *Desired Effects:* Work by inhibiting thyroid hormone synthesis, reducing basal metabolic rate *Side Effects:* Headache, drowsiness, dizziness, nausea, vomiting, stomach upset, itching, muscle, joint or nerve pain, hair loss	methimazole	Tapazole
Urinary tract antispasmodics	*Indications for Use:* Used to treat overactive bladder function *Desired Effects:* Work by inhibiting bladder contractions *Side Effects:* Dry mouth, dry eyes, blurred vision, dizziness, drowsiness, constipation, diarrhea, stomach pain or upset, joint pain, headache	oxybutynin tolterodine	Ditropan ▸Detrol
Vasopressors	*Indications for Use:* Used to treat severe allergic reactions and cardiac arrest *Desired Effects:* Work by increasing blood pressure and cardiac output and by dilating bronchi *Side Effects:* Sweating, nausea, vomiting, pale skin, feeling short of breath, dizziness, weakness or tremors, headache, feeling nervous or anxious	epinephrine	Adrenalin EpiPen
Weight control agents	*Indications for Use:* Used to manage obesity **Appetite Suppressants** *Desired Effects:* Work by suppressing appetite center in central nervous system *Side Effects:* Nausea, vomiting, diarrhea, upset stomach, headache, blurred vision, nervousness, insomnia, dizziness, fatigue, dry mouth **Meridia** 5 mg 10 mg 15 mg	diethylpropion phentermine sibutramine orlistat	Tenuate (IV) Fastin (IV) Meridia (IV) Xenical
	Lipase Inhibitors *Desired Effects:* Work by inhibiting action of lipase to decrease absorption of dietary fats *Side Effects:* Oily or fatty stools, orange or brown-colored oil in stool, flatulence with an oily discharge, loose stools, increased number of bowel movements, stomach pain, nausea, vomiting		Alli[a]

▸Top 200 most prescribed drugs.
[a]Available OTC (over the counter).
(II), Schedule II drug; *(III)*, schedule III drug; *(IV)*, schedule IV drug.

BOX 11.1 Metric Notation Guidelines

Follow these guidelines when using the metric notation of measurement and dosage.

1. The units of metric measurement are written using the following abbreviations.

Weight
- microgram: mcg
- milligram: mg
- gram: g
- kilogram: kg

Volume
- milliliter: mL
- liter: L

2. Do not use a period with the abbreviations for metric units because the period might be mistaken for another letter or symbol.
   Correct: mg
   mL
   Incorrect: mg.
   mL.
3. Place the numeral that expresses the quantity of the dose in front of the abbreviation. To make it easier to read, leave a (single) space between the quantity and the abbreviation.
   Correct: 5 mL
   Incorrect: mL 5
   5mL
4. Write a fraction of a dose as a decimal and not a fraction.
   Correct: 0.5 g
   Incorrect: 1/2 g
5. If the dose is a fraction of a unit, place a zero before the decimal point as a means of focusing on the fractional dose. This reduces the possibility of misreading the dose as a whole number.
   Correct: 0.5 g (reduces the possibility of not seeing the decimal point and reading the dose as 5 grams)
   Incorrect: .5 g
6. Do not place a decimal point and a zero after a whole number. The decimal point may be overlooked, resulting in a 10-fold overdose error.
   Correct: 1 mL (reduces the possibility of not seeing the decimal point and reading the dose as 10 mL)
   Incorrect: 1.0 mL

Metric System: Conversion of Equivalent Values

Weight
- 1000 micrograms = 1 milligram
- 1000 milligrams = 1 gram
- 1000 grams = 1 kilogram

Volume
- 1000 milliliters = 1 liter
- 1000 liters = 1 kiloliter
- 1 milliliter = 1 cubic centimeter

Prefixes added to the words *gram, liter,* and *meter* designate smaller or larger units of measurement in the metric system. The same prefixes are used with all three units. For example, *milli-* is used as follows: *milli*gram, *milli*liter, and *milli*meter. A prefix changes the value of the basic unit of measurement by the same amount. The prefix *milli-* describes a unit that is 1/1000 of the basic unit: 1 gram is equal to 1000 milligrams, 1 liter is equal to 1000 milliliters, and 1 meter is equal to 1000 millimeters. Box 11.1 lists the metric units of measurement and equivalent values in different units. Specific guidelines are used in the medical notation of metric units and doses, which also are presented in the box. To read prescriptions and medication orders, to document medication administration, and, most important, to avoid medication errors, the medical assistant must be familiar with and be able to follow these guidelines.

HOUSEHOLD SYSTEM

The household system is more complicated and less accurate for administering liquid medication than the metric system. Nevertheless, most individuals are familiar with this system because of its frequent use in the United States. This system of measurement may be the only one the patient can understand and safely use to take liquid medication at home. Most patients are more comfortable measuring medication in teaspoons than in milliliters. In addition, the patient is more likely to have household measuring devices on hand than to have metric measuring devices. If a precise measurement is needed, however, the metric system must be used, and the medical assistant should instruct the patient in the use of the metric measuring device.

Volume is the only household unit of measurement used to administer medication. The basic unit of liquid volume in the household system is the *drop (gtt),* which is approximately equal to 0.6 mL in the metric system. These two units cannot be considered exact equivalents because the size of the drop varies based on temperature, the viscosity of the liquid, and the size of the dropper. The remaining units, in order of increasing volume, are *teaspoon, tablespoon, ounce (fluid ounce), cup,* and *glass.* Table 11.2 lists the units of liquid volume measurement in the household system and equivalent values in different units.

CONVERTING UNITS OF MEASUREMENT

Changing from one unit of measurement to another is known as **conversion.** Conversion is required when medication

Table 11.2 Household System: Conversion of Common Values

Abbreviations	
Drop	gtt
Teaspoon	tsp
Tablespoon	T
Ounce	oz
Cup	c
Volume	
60 gtt =	1 tsp
3 tsp =	1 T
6 tsp =	1 oz
2 T =	1 oz
6 oz =	1 teacup
8 oz =	1 glass

is ordered in a unit of measurement that differs from the medication's label. The dose quantity must be mathematically translated or converted to the unit of measurement of the medication on hand. If the provider orders 5 g of an oral solid medication, and the medication label expresses the drug strength in milligrams, the medical assistant would need to convert the grams into milligrams to know how much medication to administer. Converting units of measurement can be classified into the following categories: (1) conversion of units within a measurement system, and (2) conversion of units from one measurement system to another.

Converting units within a measurement system allows a quantity to be expressed in two different but equal units of measurement within *one* system. An example of converting units of weight within the metric system is as follows: 1 g is equal to 1000 mg. Converting from one measurement system to another allows a quantity written in one measurement system to be expressed in an equivalent unit of measurement in *another* system. An example of a conversion from the metric system to the household system is as follows: 5 mL (metric system) is equivalent to 1 teaspoon (household system).

Conversion requires the use of a conversion table to indicate the equivalent values of various units of measurement. Conversion tables of equivalent values are included in this chapter:

- Metric conversion—Box 11-1: Metric Notation Guidelines
- Household conversion—Table 11.2: Household System

Tables used to convert from one system to another consist of approximate rather than exact equivalents, and a 10% error usually occurs in making these conversions. Conversion tables used to convert from the household system to the metric system are presented in Table 11.3.

The medical assistant must be careful to avoid errors in interpolation when using conversion tables. The numbers on conversion tables are small and close together; it is easy to misread the chart from one column to the other. To reduce this possibility, a straightedge, such as a ruler, should be used when reading a conversion table.

Table 11.3 Equivalences in Household and Metric Units (Volume)

Household	Metric
1 gtt	= 0.06 mL
15 gtts	= 1 mL (1 cc)
1 tsp	= 5 (4) mL[a]
1 T	= 15 mL
2 T	= 30 mL
1 oz	= 30 mL
1 teacup	= 180 mL
1 glass	= 240 mL

[a]The American standard teaspoon is accepted as 5 mL; however, 4 mL can be used as the equivalent to provide a more accurate conversion.

CONTROLLED DRUGS

As a result of federal and state legislation, restrictions are placed on drugs that have potential for abuse. These drugs are known as **controlled drugs**. They are classified into five categories, called *schedules,* which are based on their abuse potential. Table 11.4 lists, describes, and provides examples of the schedules for controlled drugs.

To administer, prescribe, or dispense controlled drugs, a provider must register every 3 years with the Drug Enforcement Administration (DEA). The provider is assigned a registration number known as the **DEA number**. Every time a prescription for a controlled drug is authorized, the provider must include his or her DEA number on the prescription.

PRESCRIPTION

A **prescription** is an order from a licensed provider (e.g., physician, physician's assistant, nurse practitioner) authorizing the dispensing of a drug by a pharmacist. Prescriptions can be authorized in different forms, including handwritten and computer-generated printed prescriptions, or they can be sent electronically, telephoned, or faxed, to a pharmacy. Over the past decade, there has been a substantial increase in the electronic prescribing of medication, known as *e-prescribing,* which is discussed in more detail later in this section.

Abbreviations and symbols are usually used to write a prescription. They also are used to document medication information in the patient's medical record. Common abbreviations used in the medical office for writing prescriptions are included in Table 11.5.

The medical assistant should ensure that all prescription pads are kept in a safe place and out of reach of individuals who may want to obtain drugs illegally. The stock supply of prescription pads should be locked in a drawer.

Table 11.4 Classification of Controlled Drugs

		EXAMPLES	
Classification	**Description and Prescription Regulations**	**Generic**	**Brand**
Schedule I	High potential for abuse Currently no accepted medical use in treatment in the United States There is a lack of accepted safety for use of the drug under medical supervision Use may lead to severe physical or psychological dependence May be used for research with appropriate limitations Not available for prescribing	GHB heroin LSD MDMA ("ecstasy") mescaline methaqualone (Quaalude) psilocybin	
Schedule II	High potential for abuse Currently accepted medical use in treatment in the United States or a currently accepted medical use with severe restrictions Abuse may lead to severe psychological or physical dependence Prescription must be in writing in indelible ink or typed Emergency telephone order permitted only for immediate amount needed to treat patient; written prescription must be provided to pharmacist within 7 days No refills allowed Prescription expires 7 days from issue date Manufacturer's label marked C-II	**ANALGESICS**	
		cocaine	
		codeine	
		fentanyl	Duragesic
		hydrocodone combined with nonopioid analgesic	Vicodin, Lortab, Lorcet, Tussionex, Vicoprofen
		hydromorphone	Dilaudid
		meperidine	Demerol
		methadone	Dolophine
		morphine	MS Contin
		oxycodone	OxyContin
		oxycodone/acetaminophen (APAP)	Percocet
		oxycodone/aspirin (ASA)	Percodan
		CENTRAL NERVOUS SYSTEM STIMULANTS	
		dextroamphetamine	Adderall
		lisdexamfetamine	Vyvanse
		methylphenidate	Ritalin, Concerta
		methamphetamine	Desoxyn
		SEDATIVES/HYPNOTICS	
		amobarbital	Amytal
		glutethimide	Doriden
		pentobarbital	Nembutal
		secobarbital	Seconal
Schedule III	Less potential for abuse than drugs in Schedules I and II Currently accepted medical use in treatment in the United States Abuse may lead to moderate or low physical dependence or high psychological dependence Telephone and fax orders permitted If authorized by provider, prescription can be refilled five times within 6 months from issue date Prescription expires 6 months from issue date Manufacturer's label marked C-III	**ANABOLIC STEROIDS**	
		oxandrolone	Anavar
		oxymetholone	Anapolon
		ANALGESICS	
		buprenorphine	Suboxone Buprenex
		butalbital compound	Fioricet, Fiorinal
		codeine combined with nonopioid analgesic	Tylenol w/Codeine, Empirin w/ Codeine
		CENTRAL NERVOUS SYSTEM STIMULANT	
		benzphetamine	Didrex
		MALE HORMONE	
		testosterone	Depotest, Delatestryl
		SEDATIVE/HYPNOTIC	
		butabarbital	Butisol

Table 11.4 Classification of Controlled Drugs—cont'd

Classification	Description and Prescription Regulations	EXAMPLES: Generic	EXAMPLES: Brand
Schedule IV	Lower potential for abuse than drugs in Schedule III Currently accepted medical use in treatment in the United States Abuse may lead to limited physical or psychological dependence Telephone and fax orders permitted If authorized by provider, prescription can be refilled five times within 6 months of issue date Prescription expires 6 months from issue date Manufacturer's label marked C-IV	**ANALGESICS**	
		butorphanol	Stadol
		pentazocine	Talwin
		propoxyphene	Darvon, Darvocet-N
		ANTIANXIETY AGENTS	
		alprazolam	Xanax
		chlordiazepoxide	Librium
		diazepam	Valium
		halazepam	Paxipam
		lorazepam	Ativan
		meprobamate	Equanil
		oxazepam	Serax
		ANTICONVULSANT	
		clonazepam	Klonopin
		CENTRAL NERVOUS SYSTEM STIMULANTS	
		modafinil	Provigil
		pemoline	Cylert
		SEDATIVES/HYPNOTICS	
		chloral hydrate	Noctec
		eszopiclone	Lunesta
		ethchlorvynol	Placidyl
		flurazepam	Dalmane
		midazolam	Versed
		phenobarbital	Luminal
		temazepam	Restoril
		triazolam	Halcion
		zaleplon	Sonata
		zolpidem	Ambien
		WEIGHT CONTROL AGENTS	
		diethylpropion	Tenuate
		phentermine	Fastin
		sibutramine	Meridia
Schedule V	Low potential for abuse Accepted medical use in United States Abuse may lead to limited physical or psychological dependence Telephone and fax orders permitted Prescribing policies determined by state and local regulations. In most states: • Number of refills determined by provider • Prescription expires 1 year from issue date • Some are available without prescription to patients older than 18 years of age (with proper identification) • Manufacturer's label marked C-V	Cough suppressants with small amounts of codeine	Robitussin A-C, Cheracol syrup
		Antidiarrheals containing paregoric	Parepectolin, Kapectolin PG
		diphenoxylate/atropine	Lomotil

GHB, Gamma hydroxybutyrate; *LSD*, lysergic acid diethylamide; *MDMA*, 3,4-methylenedioxymethamphetamine.

Table 11.5 Common Abbreviations and Symbols Used in Medication Documentation

Abbreviation or Symbol	Meaning	Abbreviation or Symbol	Meaning
a̅a̅	of each	OTC	over the counter
ac	before meals	oz	ounce
ad lib	as desired		after
aq	water	pc	after meals
admin	administer, administration	Pt or pt	patient
AM or a.m.	morning	per	by
APAP	acetaminophen	PM or p.m.	evening
ASA	aspirin	po or PO	by mouth
bid	twice a day	prn	as needed
c̅	with	qAM	every morning
cap(s)	capsule(s)	qh	every hour
DAW	dispense as written	q(2, 3, 4)h	every (2, 3, 4) hours
dil	dilute	qid	four times a day
g	gram	qs	of sufficient quantity
gtt(s)	drop(s)	Rx	prescription
h or hr	hour	s̅	without
ID	intradermal	subcut	subcutaneous
IM	intramuscular	SL	sublingual
IV	intravenous	sol	solution
kg	kilogram	STAT	immediately
L	liter	T	tablespoon
liq	liquid	tab(s)	tablet(s)
mcg	microgram	tid	three times a day
med(s)	medication(s)	tsp	teaspoon
mg	milligram	#	number
min	minute	×	times
mL	milliliter	∅	no, none
NPO	nothing by mouth		

Putting It All Into Practice

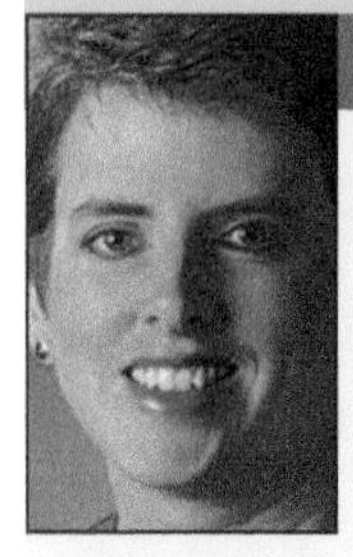

My name is Theresa, and I work for four physicians in a family practice medical office. I have worked there ever since I graduated from college with an associate's degree in medical assisting. One experience that I will never forget taught our entire office staff a valuable lesson. It involved a woman who came to our office because she had lacerated her wrist while using a butcher knife. After the wound was sutured, I gave her a tetanus injection because she was past due for one. Shortly thereafter, she became very nauseated and dizzy, and I made her lie down on the examining table. She asked me to get her a cold drink of water, and I left the room to do so. Apparently, while I was gone, she must have tried to sit up or turn over because she rolled off the table and struck the back of her head on the floor. She sustained a laceration to her scalp, which also had to be sutured. Owing to her persistent symptoms of severe nausea, vomiting, and headache, it was decided that she should be admitted to the hospital for neurologic observation and x-ray studies.

The vital lesson that this experience taught everyone in our office was that you must never leave a patient alone, not even for a minute to get something, if there is the slightest indication that he or she is not feeling perfectly fine. Another staff member should be called to obtain whatever is needed. From that point on, this has been our office policy and procedure. ■

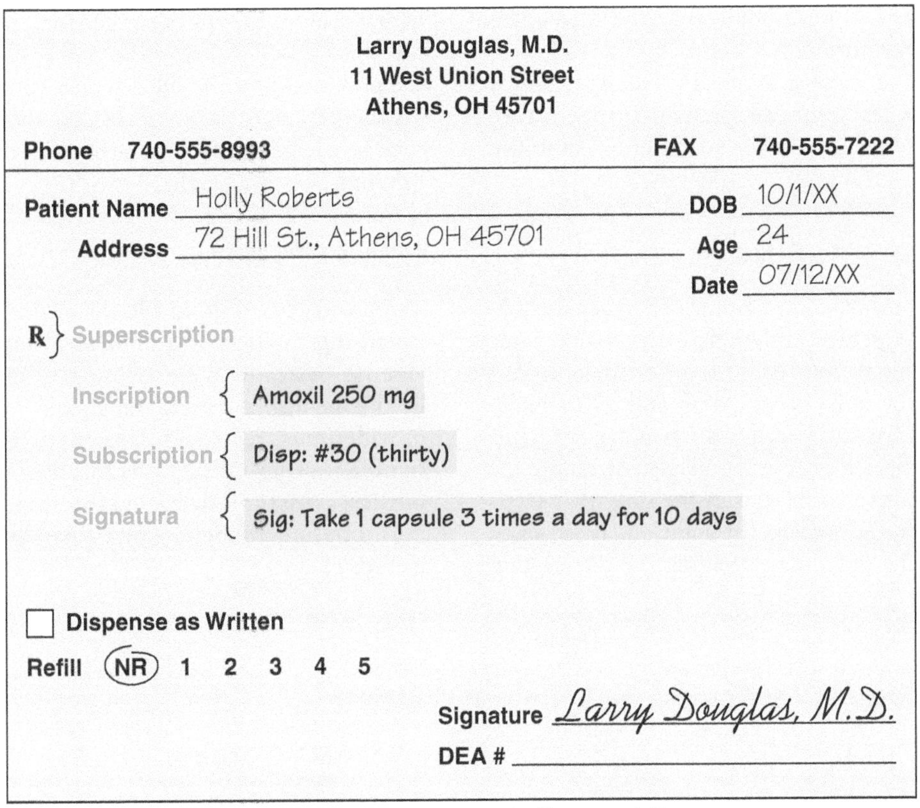

Larry Douglas, M.D.
11 West Union Street
Athens, OH 45701

Phone 740-555-8993 FAX 740-555-7222

Patient Name Holly Roberts DOB 10/1/XX
Address 72 Hill St., Athens, OH 45701 Age 24
Date 07/12/XX

℞ } Superscription

Inscription { Amoxil 250 mg

Subscription { Disp: #30 (thirty)

Signatura { Sig: Take 1 capsule 3 times a day for 10 days

☐ Dispense as Written

Refill (NR) 1 2 3 4 5

Signature Larry Douglas, M.D.

DEA # ____________

Fig. 11.2 Example of a handwritten prescription.

PARTS OF A PRESCRIPTION

A prescription consists of directions to the pharmacist for filling the prescription and instructions to the patient for taking the medication (Fig. 11.2). A prescription must include the following specific information:

- *Prescription date.* A pharmacist cannot fill a prescription unless the date the prescription was issued is indicated on the prescription. The reason for this is that a prescription expires after a certain length of time. In most states, a prescription for a drug (with the exception of controlled drugs) expires 1 year from the date of issue. A prescription for a schedule III, IV, and V drug expires in 6 months from the issue date. After this time, the prescription (or any refills left on the prescription) cannot be filled.
- *Provider's name, address, telephone number, and fax number.* This information is preprinted on prescription forms that are handwritten and automatically printed on forms that are computer generated. This information identifies the provider issuing the prescription and provides the necessary information should the pharmacist have a question and need to contact the medical office.
- *Patient's name and address.* This information is important for insurance billing and for properly dispensing the medication.
- *Patient's date of birth and age.* It is important to include the patient's age on the prescription so that the pharmacist can double-check the provider's order to ensure the proper dose is being dispensed based on the patient's age. The most common errors in dosage occur among children and the elderly, who may not require the standard dose of a drug because patients in these age groups metabolize drugs differently. Knowing the patient's age also allows the pharmacist to double-check that the drug is age appropriate for the patient. For example, ciprofloxacin (e.g., Cipro) should not be taken by children and adolescents because this antibiotic can damage cartilage in individuals younger than 18 years.
- *Superscription.* The **superscription** consists of the abbreviation *Rx.* This symbol comes from the Latin word *recipe* and means "take."
- *Inscription.* The **inscription** identifies the name of the drug and the dose (e.g., Amoxil 250 mg). Most drugs are available in various strengths; therefore, it is important that the correct dosage strength be prescribed. For example, Amoxil comes in the following strengths: 125, 250, and 500 mg.
- *Subscription.* The **subscription** designates the quantity of the drug to be dispensed. To prevent a prescription from being altered illegally, it is recommended that numbers and letters be used to indicate the quantity to be dispensed (e.g., #30 [thirty]).
- *Signatura.* The **signatura** (abbreviated *Sig.*) comes from the Latin term *signa,* which means "write" or "label." The signatura indicates the information to be included on the medication label. It consists of directions to the patient for taking the medication. The name of the medication also is included on the label so that the patient can identify the medication.
- *Refill.* This part of the prescription indicates the number of times the prescription may be refilled.

- *Provider's signature.* A prescription cannot be filled unless it is signed by the provider.
- *DEA number.* The number assigned to the provider by the DEA must appear on the prescription for a controlled drug. See Table 11.4 for examples of controlled drugs.

GENERIC PRESCRIBING

Generic prescribing means that the provider writes the prescription using the generic rather than the brand name of the drug. Because many pharmaceutical manufacturers may produce the same generic drug and sell it under different brand names, price competition often results. If the provider prescribes a drug using its generic name, the pharmacist is permitted to fill it with the drug that offers the best savings to the patient. In addition, most states allow the pharmacist the option of filling the prescription with a chemically equivalent generic drug, even if the drug has been prescribed by brand name. If the provider wants the prescription to be filled with a specific brand of drug, instructions must be indicated on the prescription form, such as "Dispense as Written (DAW)," or words of a similar meaning (see Fig. 11.2).

COMPLETING A PRESCRIPTION FORM

The provider is responsible for having accurate and pertinent information on the prescription form. If the provider so delegates, a prescription form can be completed by the medical assistant and signed by the provider. The provider must review the prescription thoroughly before signing it to ensure all of the information is correct. If the medical assistant is delegated this responsibility, he or she must carefully follow the important guidelines presented in Box 11.2.

BOX 11.2 Guidelines for Completing a Prescription Form

Using a Paper Form

- Work in a quiet, well-lit area that is free of distractions.
- Use an indelible black ink pen to write on the form.
- Print all information on the form.
- Ensure that all information is spelled correctly.
- Review the metric notation guidelines presented in Box 11-1: *Metric Notation Guidelines.* (Most prescriptions are written in metric units.)
- Always ask the provider if you have questions about the prescription.
- Complete all of the required information on the form; it includes the following:
  1. Patient's name, address, date of birth, and age
     - Clearly print all of this information on the form. Never leave the address, date of birth, and age categories blank.
  2. Date
     - Indicate today's date on the prescription form.
  3. Name of the medication
     - The provider may prescribe the medication using either the generic or the brand name.
     - Make sure to spell the name of the drug correctly. If you are unsure, use a drug reference to find the correct spelling of a drug.
  4. Medication dosage
     - Never leave a decimal point "naked." If the dosage is a fraction of a unit, a zero must be placed before the decimal point as a means of focusing on the fractional dose. This reduces the possibility of misreading the dose as a whole number. *Example:* 0.5 mL (not .5 mL).
     - Never place a decimal point and a zero after a whole number because the decimal point may be overlooked, resulting in a 10-fold overdose error. *Example:* 5 mg (not 5.0 mg).
  5. Quantity to dispense
     - Use numbers and letters to indicate the quantity to be dispensed. *Example:* Disp: #30 (thirty).
     - Ensure that the quantity is correct. The number of prescribed pills should match the duration of treatment. *Example:* If the patient has been prescribed 3 tablets a day for 7 days, the quantity should be written as follows: Disp: #21 (twenty-one).
  6. Directions for taking the medication
     - Clearly indicate the directions for taking the medication. Many authorities recommend writing the directions without abbreviations. *Example:* Sig: Take 1 capsule orally 3 times a day for 10 days.
  7. Refills
     - Never leave this category blank.
     - If there are no refills, indicate this clearly on the form. The method for doing this is based on the setup of the preprinted form.
       Example: Refill: (NR) 1 2 3 4 5
       (on this form, the information is circled)
       Example: Refill: 0
       (on this form, the information is written in)
  8. Dispense as written
     - If the provider does not allow a substitution (e.g., generic equivalent) for this medication, check this category.
  9. DEA number
     - If the prescription is for a controlled drug, clearly indicate the provider's DEA number on the form.
  10. Group practice
     - If there is more than one provider in the practice, circle (or check) the name of the provider prescribing the medication. This avoids confusion if the pharmacist cannot read the provider's signature.

BOX 11.2 Guidelines for Completing a Prescription Form—cont'd

Example:
James Ortman, MD, (Mark Rothstein, MD), Richard Bontrager, MD

- Give the prescription to the provider to review and sign.
- Document the prescription order in the patient's medication record if directed by the provider. Give the prescription to the patient. Provide the patient with guidelines for taking the medication (see the Patient Coaching box on prescription medications).
- Ask the patient whether he or she has any questions about the medication.

Using an EHR Prescription Program

1. Access the patient's electronic health record.
2. Access the prescription screen and verify the auto-filled information (i.e., date, patient name, date of birth, address, and age).
3. Select the correct medication from the drop-down menu.
4. The program will display a list of available dosage strengths (e.g., 250 mg, 500 mg) and dosage forms for that medication (e.g., tablets, oral suspension). Select the dosage strength and dosage form ordered by the provider using drop-down lists or check-boxes.
5. Select the dosage frequency and the route of administration using drop-down lists, check-boxes, or fill-in boxes.
6. Enter the correct information in the Refills field. This field should not be left blank; there should be either a number indicated or "no refills."
7. If the provider has indicated that there should be no substitution for this medication, the "Dispense as Written" radio button should be selected.
8. Forward the prescription to the provider for review and his or her electronic signature.
9. Save the prescription in the patient's record.
10. Send the prescription electronically to the pharmacy or print a copy, have the physician sign it, and give it to the patient.

PATIENT COACHING Prescription Medications

To avoid adverse reactions, teach patients the proper guidelines for taking prescription medication. These guidelines are as follows:

- Know the names of all your prescription and nonprescription medications. Know the generic and brand names of each of your medications. Nonprescription drugs are known as over-the-counter (OTC) drugs; they are drugs that can be purchased without a prescription. Vitamin supplements and herbal products are considered OTC drugs.
- *Know why you are taking each medication.* It is important to know the desired therapeutic outcome, dose, frequency and time of administration, and common side effects of each medication, and guidelines ("dos and don'ts") to follow when taking the medication. Never take your medication in the dark or without your reading glasses (if needed for close vision).
- *Take your medication exactly as prescribed, at the right times, and in the right amounts.* The medication may not work properly if it is not taken as directed. If the dose is too small, the drug may not produce its intended therapeutic effect; exceeding the recommended dose could result in a toxic effect. Make sure you know what to do if you are late in taking a dose or miss a dose of your medication. It is also important to know if any other medication or food interferes with your medication and should be avoided.
- *Inform the provider if new symptoms or adverse effects develop when you are taking the medication.* The provider may need to change your dose or prescribe a different medication. There are usually alternative medications that the provider can prescribe to treat your condition.
- *Take the medication for the prescribed duration of time, even after you begin to feel better.* If you do not complete the entire course of drug therapy, your condition may recur. Not taking all of a prescribed antibiotic may cause an infection to return, and it may be worse than the first infection.
- *Tell the provider if you decide not to take your medication.* Otherwise, the provider may think your medication is not working. Not taking a medication prescribed by the provider could be serious because this may allow your condition to worsen.
- *Do not take additional medications, including OTC medications, without checking with the provider.* All drugs, including OTC medications, are designed to have an effect on the body. Vitamin supplements and herbal products are considered OTC drugs. Some combinations of drugs cause serious reactions. In some cases, one drug cancels the effects of another and prevents it from working.
- *Never take a medication that was prescribed for someone else.* Providers prescribe medication based on an individual's age, weight, sex, and condition. Taking a medication prescribed for someone else can have serious results.
- *Keep all medications in their original containers to avoid taking the wrong medication by mistake.* Store your medications in their original containers from the pharmacy. Basic information about your medication is on the original container. Medications that are not clearly marked may be taken inadvertently by the wrong person.
- *Store your medications in a safe place, away from the reach of children.* If you have young children, make sure your medication is dispensed in containers with child-resistant safety closures. After taking your medication, make sure that the cap of the container is closed tightly. Accidental drug poisoning in children is a common and preventable problem. Also, do not take your medication in front of young children because they may want to mimic your behavior.

Continued

PATIENT COACHING Prescription Medications—cont'd

- *Store medications in a cool, dry place or as stated on the label.* Do not store capsules or tablets in the bathroom or kitchen because heat or moisture may cause the medication to break down.
- *Properly discard unused portions of prescription medications and outdated OTC medications.* Unused or expired medication should be disposed of as soon as possible to reduce the chance that individuals may accidentally take or misuse the medication. Because unwanted medications may pose a risk to human health and the environment, they should be disposed of properly. If a drug take-back program (described below) is not available, unused or expired medication should not be flushed down the toilet or drain unless the drug label or accompanying product package insert specifically instructs you to do so.

Disposal of Unwanted Medication

Medication can be safely disposed in the following ways:

1. **Drug Take-Back Programs**
   a. *Collection Events:* Federal, state, or local law enforcement may periodically host a community drug take-back day where residents drop off unwanted medication at a designated location during a specific time period.
   b. *On-Site Collection Receptacle:* Drug collection receptacles permanently located in specific locations such as pharmacies, health departments, and law enforcement locations allow individuals to safely dispose of unwanted medication.
   c. *Mail-Back Program:* Some pharmacies may offer mail-back envelopes to assist consumers in safely disposing of unwanted medication. The consumer places the medication in a specially-designed envelope which is shipped directly to a destruction facility.
2. **Household Disposal:** If a take-back program is not available in the community, the following steps should be followed to dispose of unwanted medication:
   a. Remove the medication from its original container.
   b. Mix the medication with an undesirable substance, such as kitty litter or coffee grounds.
   c. Place the mixture in a disposable container such as a sealable plastic bag or an empty plastic container with a lid and discard it in the household trash.
   d. Remove personal information (including the prescription number) from an empty prescription medication container before discarding the container in the trash to protect the privacy of your personal health information. This can be accomplished by covering the information with a permanent marker or scratching it off. ■

Electronic Prescribing

Electronic health record (EHR) software includes a prescription program for the electronic prescribing (*e-prescribing*) of medication. E-prescribing greatly reduces the amount of time needed to prescribe and refill medication. The program can transmit the prescription electronically to the patient's pharmacy. The prescription program can also generate and print out a prescription, which is then signed by the provider and given to the patient (Fig. 11.3). Both of these features eliminate the need for the pharmacist to decipher the provider's handwriting.

To use an EHR prescription program, the provider first selects the medication. The program then displays a list of available dosage strengths (e.g., 150 mg, 300 mg) and dosage forms (e.g., tablets, capsules, oral suspension) for that medication. The provider indicates the dosage strength and dosage form desired and enters the information into the computer. Next, the provider selects additional information related to the prescription, including dosage frequency and number of refills using fill-in boxes, drop-down lists, and check-boxes. The program automatically checks the prescription against any drug allergies the patient may have. It also checks for potential interactions with other medications being taken by the patient. The EHR prescription program usually has the capability to compare the prescription against the *formulary* or list of drugs covered by the patient's insurance plan. If the prescription is not in the patient's formulary, the provider is advised of alternative drugs that are covered by the patient's insurance plan.

Once the provider has entered the prescription into the computer, the medication is recorded in the patient's medication record. The prescription is then sent electronically to the pharmacy or printed out, signed by the provider, and given to the patient. The EHR prescription program also has the capability to quickly refill a prescription and print a list of medications being taken by the patient. The patient can use this list to keep track of the medication he or she is taking (Fig. 11.4).

MEDICATION RECORD

A medication record (Fig. 11.5) includes detailed information about each medication so that the provider can tell at a glance what medications and how much the patient is taking. Both prescription medications and OTC medications, including vitamin supplements and herbal products, must be documented in the medication record.

The medication record is part of the patient's medical record. The medical assistant is often responsible for documenting medication information in the medication record. Care must be taken to ensure the information is correct and clearly stated.

In a paper-based patient record (PPR), the medical office may use a preprinted form to document the medication that a patient is taking. With an EHR, the medical assistant enters this information into a digital form on the screen of the monitor using free text entry, drop-down lists, and check-boxes.

A medication record typically includes the following information:

- Patient's name and date of birth

PRESCRIPTION: (Give to the pharmacist)	PRESCRIPTION: (Give to the pharmacist)
Huntington Clinic 701 Concord Ave Lexington, KY 48710 614-871-0033	Huntington Clinic 701 Concord Ave Lexington, KY 48710 614-871-0033
Doctor: John Blauser, MD	Doctor: John Blauser, MD
For: Danielle Travis Age: 28 DOB: 08/08/XX	For: Danielle Travis Age: 28 DOB: 08/08/XX
Date: 10/27/20XX	Date: 10/27/20XX
Address: 101 Coventry Lane Lexington, KY 48710	Address: 101 Coventry Lane Lexington, KY 48710
Rx: Amoxil (Generic - amoxicillin) (Dose/unit - 250 mg) (Form - Caps) (Disp - #30) (Frequency - One three times daily for 10 days) (Route - By mouth) (Refills-0).	Rx: Tylenol-3 (Generic - Acetaminophen/Codeine) (Dose/unit - 1 to 2) (Form - Tabs) (Disp - #15) (fifteen) (Frequency - Every 4 hours as needed for moderate to severe pain) (Route - By mouth) (Refills-0).
Dr: *John Blauser, MD*	Dr: *John Blauser, MD*

Fig. 11.3 Example of a computer-generated prescription.

Huntington Clinic
701 Concord Ave
Lexington, KY 48710
614-871-0033

Patient: Clare Andrews
352 Pinewood Dr.
Lexington, KY 48710

Age/DOB: 12/25/XX
EMRN: 7016780

Medication List

Medication	Refills	Start
Abilify 15 mg tablet TAKE 1 TABLET DAILY	0	24Sep20XX
Acetaminophen-Codeine #3 300-30 mg tablet TAKE 1 TABLET EVERY 6 TO 8 HOURS AS NEEDED FOR PAIN	0	23Sep20XX
Clonazepam 1 mg tablet TAKE 1 TABLET EVERY 8 HOURS PRN	0	24Sep20XX
Etodolac CR 500 mg tablet extended release 24 hour 1-2 TABLETS PO ONCE DAILY WITH FOOD	0	21Sep20XX
Fish Oil 1000 mg capsule TAKE 1 CAPSULE DAILY	11	7Apr20XX
Flovent HFA 44 mcg/act aerosol INHALE 2 PUFFS TWICE DAILY	3	6Jan20XX
Fluticasone Propionate 50 mcg/act suspension USE 2 SPRAYS IN EACH NOSTRIL ONCE DAILY	3	9Sep20XX
Lamictal 200 mg tablet TAKE 2 TABLETS DAILY	0	24Sep20XX
Omeprazole 20 mg capsule delayed release TAKE 1 TABLET DAILY	11	24Sep20XX
Pamine 2.5 mg tablet TAKE 1 TABLET 3 TIMES DAILY	0	6Jan20XX
Proventil HFA 108 (90 base) mcg/act aerosol solution INHALE 1-2 PUFFS EVERY 4-6 HOURS AS NEEDED AND AS DIRECTED	3	21Jul20XX
Tramadol HCl 50 mg tablet TAKE 1 TABLET EVERY 6 HOURS	0	29Apr20XX
Voltaren 1% gel APPLY 2 GRAMS TOPICALLY 4 TIMES DAILY	6	24Sep20XX
WelChol 625 mg tablet TAKE 3 TABLETS TWICE DAILY WITH MEALS	11	29Apr20XX

Fig. 11.4 Example of a computer-generated patient medication list.

MEDICATION RECORD

Patient John Walsh

Birthdate 6/10/XX

ALLERGY Ø

DATE	MEDICATION AND DOSAGE	FREQUENCY	RX	OTC	REFILLS	STOP
2/18/XX	Cipro 250 mg	ī q 12 h po x 10 days	X			2/28/XX
6/10/XX	Prevacid 15 mg	ī daily po	X			7/10/XX
6/10/XX	Lipitor 10 mg	ī daily po	X		1/6/XX	
6/10/XX	Prozac 20 mg	ī daily po	X		1/6/XX	
12/3/XX	Tobrex Ophthalmic Solution	ī drop q3h Ⓡ eye	X			12/10/XX
2/5/XX	Echinacea	ī daily po		X		
3/15/XX	Nitrostat 0.4 mg	ī prn pain SL Rep q 5 min prn pain, not to exceed 3 tabs	X			
3/15/XX	Inderal 40 mg	ī bid po	X			
3/15/XX	St. Joseph's ASA Enteric Coated 81 mg	ī daily po		X		

Fig. 11.5 Example of a medication record.

- Any drug allergies
- Date the medication was prescribed (for prescription medications) or date the patient started taking the medication (for OTC medications)
- Name and dose of the medication
- Frequency of administration of the medication
- Route of administration
- Prescription or OTC medication category
- Refills (prescription medication only)
- Date the patient stopped taking the medication

FACTORS AFFECTING DRUG ACTION

THERAPEUTIC EFFECT

Each drug has an intended therapeutic effect—the reason the patient takes the medication. Certain factors affect the therapeutic action of drugs in the body, causing patients to respond differently to the same drug. Because of this, the drug therapy may need to be adjusted to meet these variations, which include the following.

What Would You Do? What Would You *Not* Do?

Case Study 2

Linda Cardwell calls the medical office. Her daughter Rachel, 9 years old, was seen in the office 10 days ago. Rachel was diagnosed with strep throat, and the provider ordered Amoxil 250 mg tid × 7 days. Mrs. Cardwell says that after 3 days of taking the medication, Rachel was much better, so she stopped giving her the Amoxil because it was causing her to have diarrhea. Mrs. Cardwell says that her 12-year-old son started feeling achy all over and she gave him the Amoxil for 2 days, and it seemed to help. She also says that her husband started complaining of sinus problems, so she also gave him the Amoxil for 2 days. Mrs. Cardwell says that now Rachel's throat is hurting again, and she has a fever. She wants to know whether Rachel has developed another case of strep throat. Mrs. Cardwell says she does not know what to do because she does not have any Amoxil left to give Rachel. ■

Age

Children and the elderly tend to respond more strongly to drugs than young and middle-aged adults. The provider may calculate smaller doses for very young and geriatric patients.

Route of Administration

Medications administered by different routes are absorbed at different rates. Drugs administered orally are absorbed slowly because they must be digested first. Parenterally administered drugs are absorbed more quickly than orally administered drugs because they are injected directly into the body.

Size

A patient's body size has an effect on drug action. A thin individual may require a smaller quantity of a drug, and an obese individual may require more.

Time of Administration

A drug administered by the oral route is absorbed more rapidly when the stomach is empty than when it contains food. A drug may not produce the desired effect or may be absorbed too slowly if it is taken when food is present. Some drugs irritate the stomach's lining, however, and must be taken with food. The drug PI or a drug reference should always be consulted to determine when a drug should be taken.

Tolerance

A patient taking a certain drug over a period of time may develop a tolerance to it. This means that the same dose of a drug no longer produces the desired effect after prolonged administration. The provider should be notified to determine whether a change of drug or dosage is needed.

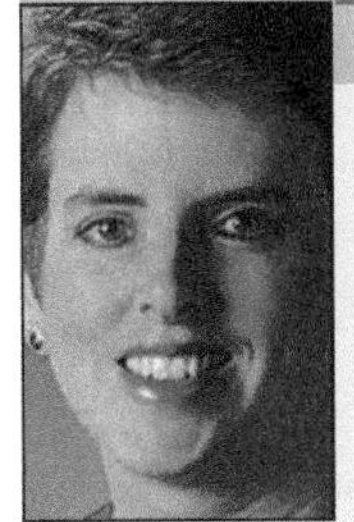

Memories *from* Practicum

Theresa: I can clearly remember the first time I gave an injection at my practicum site. I was worried that I would forget how to give an injection and look bad in front of my practicum supervisor and the patient. What made things worse is that the patient was a woman with very thin arms. I was giving her a flu shot, and I was so scared that the needle would hit her bone even though I was only using a 1-inch needle. When I walked into the room, my supervisor told the woman that I was a student and asked her if it was alright if I gave her the flu injection. The woman laughed and said, "Well, I guess so." That made me feel even more nervous. The patient then asked if it was my first shot. I told her "yes" and she said, "Just don't hurt me." When it came time to give the injection, everything that I had ever learned about injections came back to me. I gave the injection, and the woman told me I did a good job and that she didn't even feel it. That made me feel so good! My supervisor said, "If you can give a shot to her, you can give a shot to anyone." Every injection after that was a "piece of cake." I've learned just to take a deep breath before each difficult situation encountered in the office, and everything will work out. ■

UNDESIRABLE EFFECTS OF DRUGS

A drug may cause undesirable effects, which may occur immediately or may be delayed hours or even days after administration of the medication.

Adverse Reactions

Most drugs produce unintended and undesirable effects known as **adverse reactions**. Adverse reactions are secondary effects that occur along with the therapeutic effect of the drug. Some adverse reactions, referred to as *side effects,* are harmless and are often tolerated by the patient to obtain the therapeutic effect of the drug. Most patients are willing to tolerate the dry mouth and drowsiness that may accompany an antihistamine to obtain its therapeutic effect. Other adverse reactions, such as a decrease in blood pressure or an allergic reaction, can be harmful to the patient and warrant discontinuing the medication.

Drug Interactions

When certain medications are used at the same time, drug interactions may produce undesirable effects. The medical assistant should inquire about other medications the patient is taking and document this information in the patient's medical record for review by the provider.

Allergic Drug Reaction

The patient may exhibit an allergic reaction to a drug. The reaction is usually mild and takes the form of a rash, rhinitis, or pruritus. Occasionally, a patient has a severe allergic reaction that occurs suddenly and immediately. This is known as an **anaphylactic reaction**.

An anaphylactic reaction is the least common but the most serious type of allergic reaction. Symptoms begin with sneezing, urticaria (hives), itching, erythema, angioedema, and disorientation. Erythema is reddening of the skin caused by dilation of superficial blood vessels in the skin. Angioedema is a localized urticaria of the deeper tissues of the body. If not treated, the symptoms of anaphylaxis quickly increase in severity and progress to dyspnea, cyanosis, and shock. Blood pressure decreases, and the pulse becomes weak and thready. Convulsions, loss of consciousness, and death may occur if treatment is not initiated promptly.

To prevent an anaphylactic reaction to a drug or to reduce its danger, the medical assistant should stay with the patient after administration of the medication. The medical assistant should be especially alert for signs of an anaphylactic reaction after administering allergy skin tests or a penicillin or allergy injection. If a reaction occurs, the provider should be notified immediately so that he or she can begin treatment immediately. In general, treatment consists of one or more injections of epinephrine, depending on the severity of the reaction. Epinephrine goes to work immediately to reverse the life-threatening symptoms of anaphylaxis. When the patient's condition has been stabilized, he or she is usually given an injection of an antihistamine. The antihistamine takes longer to begin working but helps alleviate urticaria, itching, angioedema, and erythema. The medical assistant must ensure that an ample supply of epinephrine is on hand at all times. Many offices maintain emergency crash carts for this purpose.

Idiosyncratic Reaction

An idiosyncratic reaction is an abnormal or peculiar response to a drug that is unexplained and unpredictable. Elderly patients are most prone to idiosyncratic reactions to drugs and should be monitored closely when they are taking a new medication.

GUIDELINES FOR PREPARATION AND ADMINISTRATION OF MEDICATION

To prevent medication errors, the medical assistant should follow these guidelines when preparing and administering any drug:

1. Work in a quiet, well-lit atmosphere that is free of distractions.
2. Always ask if you have a question about the medication order.
3. Know the drug to be given.
4. Select the proper drug. Check the label of the medication three times—as it is taken from its storage location, before preparing the medication, and after preparing the medication. Do not use a drug if the label is missing or is difficult to read.
5. Do not use a drug if the color has changed, if a precipitate has formed, or if it has an unusual odor.
6. Check the expiration date before preparing the drug for administration.
7. Prepare the proper dose of the drug. The term **dose** refers to the quantity of a drug to be administered at one time. Each medication has a dose range, or range of quantities of the drug that can produce therapeutic effects. It is important to administer the exact dose of the drug. A dose that is too small would not produce a therapeutic effect, and a dose that is too large could be harmful or even fatal to the patient.
8. Correctly identify the patient so that the drug is administered to the intended patient. When medication is administered, the patient should be identified by his or her full name and date of birth.
9. Before administering the medication, check the patient's records or question the patient to ensure that he or she is not allergic to the medication.
10. If you are giving an injection, determine the appropriate route and site at which to administer the injection; the route and site are dictated by the type of injection being given. An allergy injection is given by the subcutaneous route, and an antibiotic injection is given by the IM route. The site must be free from abrasions, lesions, bruises, and edema.
11. Use the proper technique to administer the medication.
12. Stay with the patient after administering the medication.
13. Document information properly in the patient's medical record immediately after administering the drug. If using a PPR, include the date and time, the name of the medication, the manufacturer and lot number (if required), the dose given, the route of administration, the site of administration, and any unusual observations or patient reactions. Sign the recording with your name and credentials. If you administer a medication that contains a fraction of a unit, place a 0 before the decimal point (e.g., 0.5 mg, not .5 mg) so that the dose is not misread as 5 mg. A decimal point and a zero should never be placed after a whole number. The decimal point may be overlooked and misread, resulting in a 10-fold overdose error (e.g., 20 mg, not 20.0 mg). If using an EHR, document the name of medication, the manufacturer and lot number (if required), the dose given, the route of administration, and any unusual observations or patient reactions using the appropriate radio buttons, drop-down menus, and free text fields.
14. Always follow the seven "rights" of preparing and administering medication in the medical office:
    Right patient
    Right medication
    Right dose
    Right route
    Right time
    Right technique
    Right documentation

ORAL ADMINISTRATION

The oral route is the most convenient and most used method of administering medication. **Oral administration** means that the drug is given by mouth in either a solid form (e.g., tablet, capsule) or a liquid form (e.g., suspension, syrup). Absorption of most oral medications occurs in the small intestine, although some may be absorbed in the mouth and stomach.

Many patients find it easier to swallow a tablet or a capsule with a glass of water. Water should not be offered after the patient has received a cough syrup, however, because the water would dilute the medication's beneficial effects. Unless the patient has a malabsorption problem or is unable to swallow, the oral route is considered the safest and most desirable route for administering medication. Procedure 11.1 outlines the procedure for the administration of oral medications.

PARENTERAL ADMINISTRATION

The parenteral route of drug administration has several advantages. Medications given subcutaneously, intramuscularly, and intravenously are absorbed more rapidly and completely than medications given orally. In some cases, the parenteral route is the only way a drug can be given (e.g., insulin, most immunizations). If the patient is unconscious or has a gastric disturbance, such as nausea or vomiting, the parenteral route may be used to administer medication. Medical assistants are usually responsible for administering subcutaneous, IM, and intradermal injections in the medical office. IV medications are sometimes administered in the medical office and are discussed in greater detail later in the section on IV therapy.

The parenteral route also has disadvantages, such as pain and the possibility of infection as a result of breaking the skin. The medical assistant can minimize pain by inserting and withdrawing the needle quickly and smoothly and by withdrawing the needle at the same angle as for insertion. If injections are given repeatedly (e.g., allergy injections), the sites should be rotated to prevent the overuse of one site, which may cause irritation and tissue damage. Rotating sites also allows for better absorption of the drug.

When documenting the administration of a medication in the patient's medical record, the medical assistant must include the site of injection (e.g., right upper arm, left ventrogluteal). This assists in proper site rotation for patients who receive repeated injections. In addition, the information provides a reference point should a problem arise with the injection site.

Medical asepsis must be used when parenteral medications are administered. In addition, the needle and the inside of the syringe must remain sterile. These practices reduce the danger of microorganisms entering the patient's body during the administration of medication. The medical assistant must follow the OSHA standard when administering medication as a means of protecting himself or herself from bloodborne pathogens (see Chapter 2). Procedure 11.2 describes how to prepare an injection.

PARTS OF A NEEDLE AND SYRINGE

Needle

The needle consists of several parts (Fig. 11.6). The *hub* of the needle fits onto the top of the syringe. The *shaft* is inserted into the body tissue. The opening in the shaft of the needle, known as the *lumen,* is continuous with the needle hub. Medication flows from the syringe and through the lumen of the needle. The *point* of the needle is located at the end of the needle shaft. The point is sharp so that it can penetrate body tissues easily. The top of the needle is slanted and is called the *bevel.* The bevel is designed to make a narrow, slit like opening in the skin. This narrow opening closes quickly when the needle is removed to prevent leakage of medication, and it heals quickly.

The length of the needle ranges between 3/8 and 3 inches; the length used is based on the type of injection being administered. For example, the needle used to administer an IM injection must be longer than the one used for a subcutaneous injection so that the needle can penetrates deeply enough to reach muscle tissue. The length of the needle required also depends on the size of

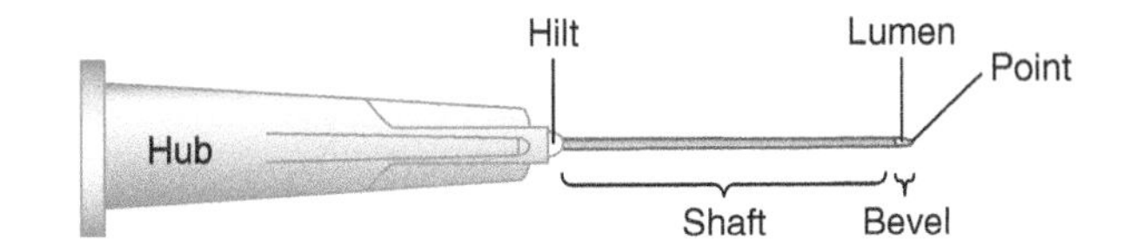

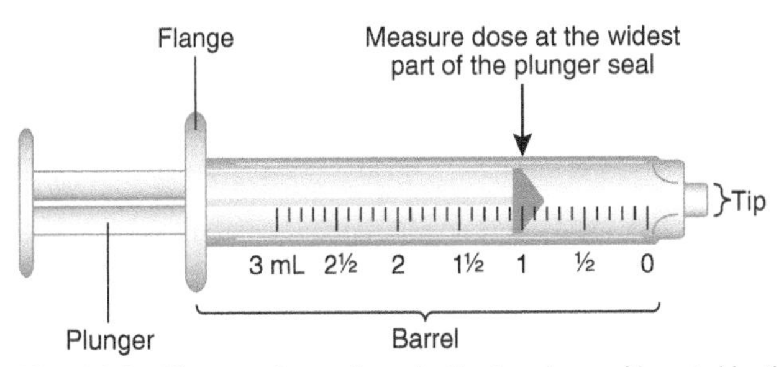

Fig. 11.6 Diagram of a needle and a 3-mL syringe, with parts identified. (From Bonewit-West K, Hunt SA: *Today's medical assistant,* ed 4, St. Louis: Elsevier; 2021.)

the patient. Administering an IM injection to an obese adult requires a longer needle to reach the muscle tissue than would be required for a normal-size adult. Administering an IM injection to a thin patient requires a shorter needle to avoid inserting a needle too deeply and possibly penetrating the bone. Refer to Fig. 11.7 for examples of various needle lengths.

Each needle has a certain **gauge;** needle gauges for administering medication range between 18 G and 27 G. The gauge of a needle refers to the diameter of the lumen of the needle: As the size of the gauge increases, the diameter of the lumen decreases (see Fig. 11.7). A needle with a gauge of 23 has a smaller lumen diameter than a needle with a gauge of 21. The gauge of the needle selected depends on the viscosity (thickness) of the medication being administered. Aqueous medications are thin and can be administered with a smaller lumen (higher gauge) needle. Thick or oily medications must be given with a large lumen (lower gauge) needle because they are too thick to pass through a smaller one. A needle with a larger lumen makes a larger needle track in the tissues. To reduce pain and tissue damage, a needle lumen with the smallest diameter appropriate for the solution and route of administration is always chosen.

Syringe

The syringe is used for inserting fluids into the body. It is made of plastic and must be disposed of after one use. The syringe with an attached needle is packaged in a cellophane wrapper or a rigid plastic container. Information regarding the syringe's capacity and the needle's length and gauge is printed on the wrapper of the syringe and needle (Fig. 11.8). Syringes and needles also are available in separate packages. In this case, the medical assistant must attach a needle to the syringe before withdrawing medication into the syringe.

The parts of a syringe are the tip, barrel, flange, and plunger (see Fig. 11.6). The *tip* is the end of the syringe to which the needle hub attaches. The *barrel* of the syringe

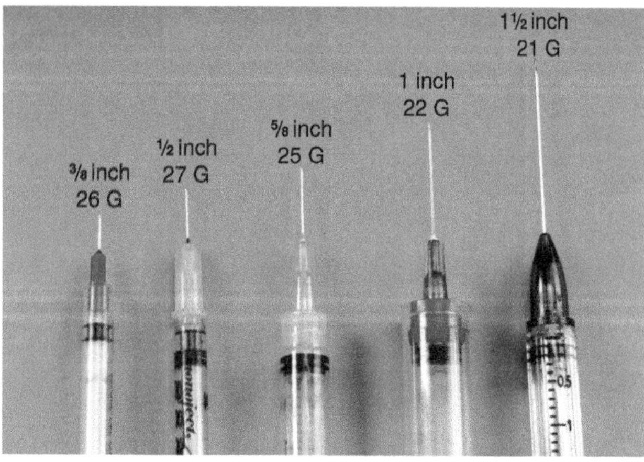

Fig. 11.7 Needle lengths and gauges.

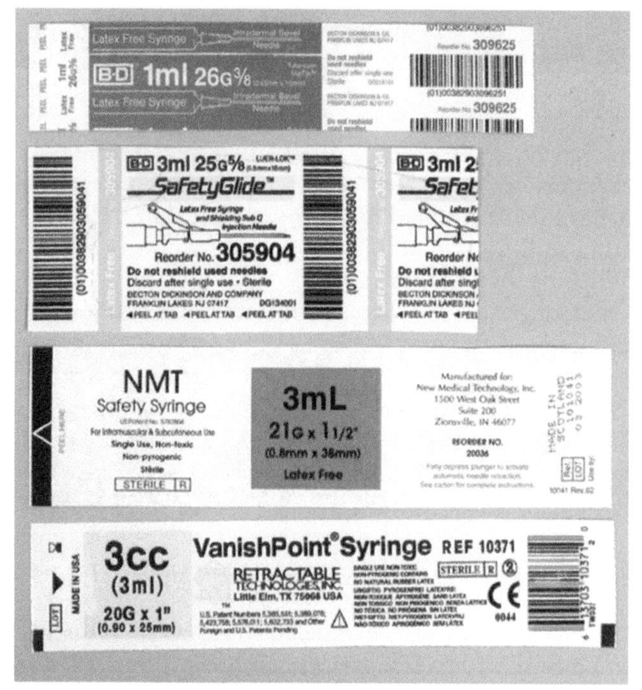

Fig. 11.8 Examples of syringe and needle packages labeled according to contents.

holds the medication and contains calibrated markings to measure the proper amount of medication. Syringes are usually calibrated in milliliters (mL), which is the unit of measurement used most often to administer parenteral medication. The medical assistant should become familiar with reading the graduated scales on syringes. At the end of the barrel is a rim known as the *flange,* which helps in injecting the medication. The flange also prevents the syringe from rolling when it is placed on a flat surface. The *plunger* is a movable cylinder with a seal tip that slides back and forth in the barrel. It is used to draw medication into the syringe when an injection is prepared and to push medication out of the syringe when an injection is administered. The medication should be measured at the widest part of the plunger seal closest to the needle (see Fig. 11.6).

Various types of syringes are available to administer injections. The choice is based on the type of injection being administered (e.g., tuberculin skin test [TST], insulin injection, antibiotic injection) and the amount of medication being administered. The types of syringes used most often in the medical office include hypodermic, insulin, and tuberculin (Fig. 11.9).

Hypodermic syringes are available in 2-, 2.5-, 3-, and 5-mL sizes and are calibrated in milliliters (or cubic centimeters). They are commonly used to administer IM injections.

The *insulin syringe* is designed especially for the administration of an insulin injection, and the barrel is calibrated in units. The most common type is the U-100 syringe, which is calibrated into 100 units in increments of 2.

Tuberculin syringes are employed to administer a small dose of medication, such as when administering a TST. The tuberculin syringe has a capacity of 1 mL, and the calibrations are divided into tenths (0.10) and hundredths (0.01) of a milliliter.

Syringes also are available with capacities of 10, 20, 30, 50, and 60 mL; however, they are not used for administering medication, but rather for medical treatments, such as irrigating wounds and draining fluid from cysts.

SAFETY-ENGINEERED SYRINGES

OSHA stipulates requirements to reduce needlestick and other sharps injuries among health care workers. As discussed in Chapter 2, employers are required to evaluate and implement commercially available safer medical devices that reduce occupational exposure to the lowest extent feasible.

Safer medical devices include safety-engineered syringes. *Safety-engineered syringes* incorporate a built-in safety feature to reduce the risk of a needlestick injury. The three types of safety-engineered syringes most commonly used include protective shield, sliding-sleeve, and retractable needle syringes. Fig. 11.10 illustrates three types of safety-engineered syringes and the procedures for activating them.

PREPARATION OF PARENTERAL MEDICATION

Medication used for injections is available in various types of dispensing units—vials, ampules, and prefilled syringes and cartridges.

Vials

A **vial** is a closed glass or plastic container with a rubber stopper; a soft metal or plastic cap protects the rubber stopper and must be removed the first time the medication is used. An injectable medication may be available in a single-dose vial, a multiple-dose vial, or both (Fig. 11.11). A vial is labeled with specific information as illustrated in Fig. 11.12.

Before the medication can be withdrawn, some vials require mixing (e.g., reconstituting a powdered drug, mixing a vial that separates on standing). Vials that require mixing should be rolled between the hands rather than shaken because shaking would cause the medication to foam, creating

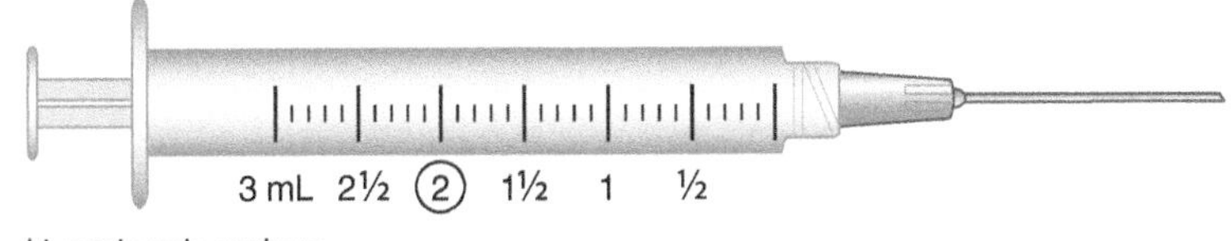

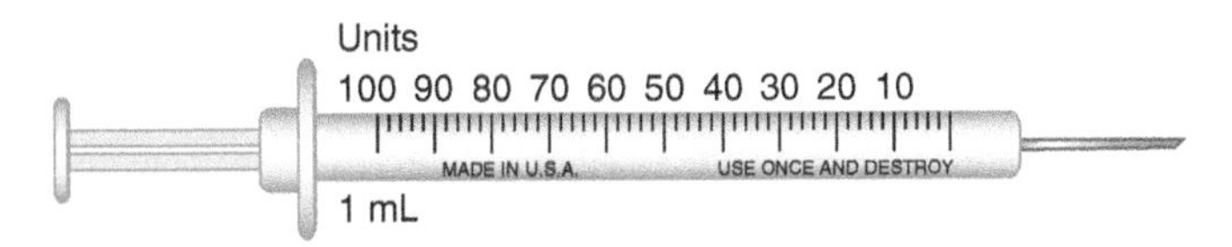

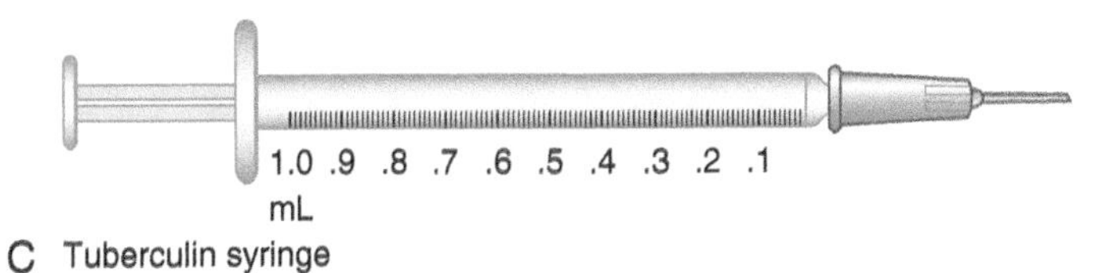

Fig. 11.9 Various syringes used to administer injections. (A) Hypodermic. (B) Insulin (U-100). (C) Tuberculin.

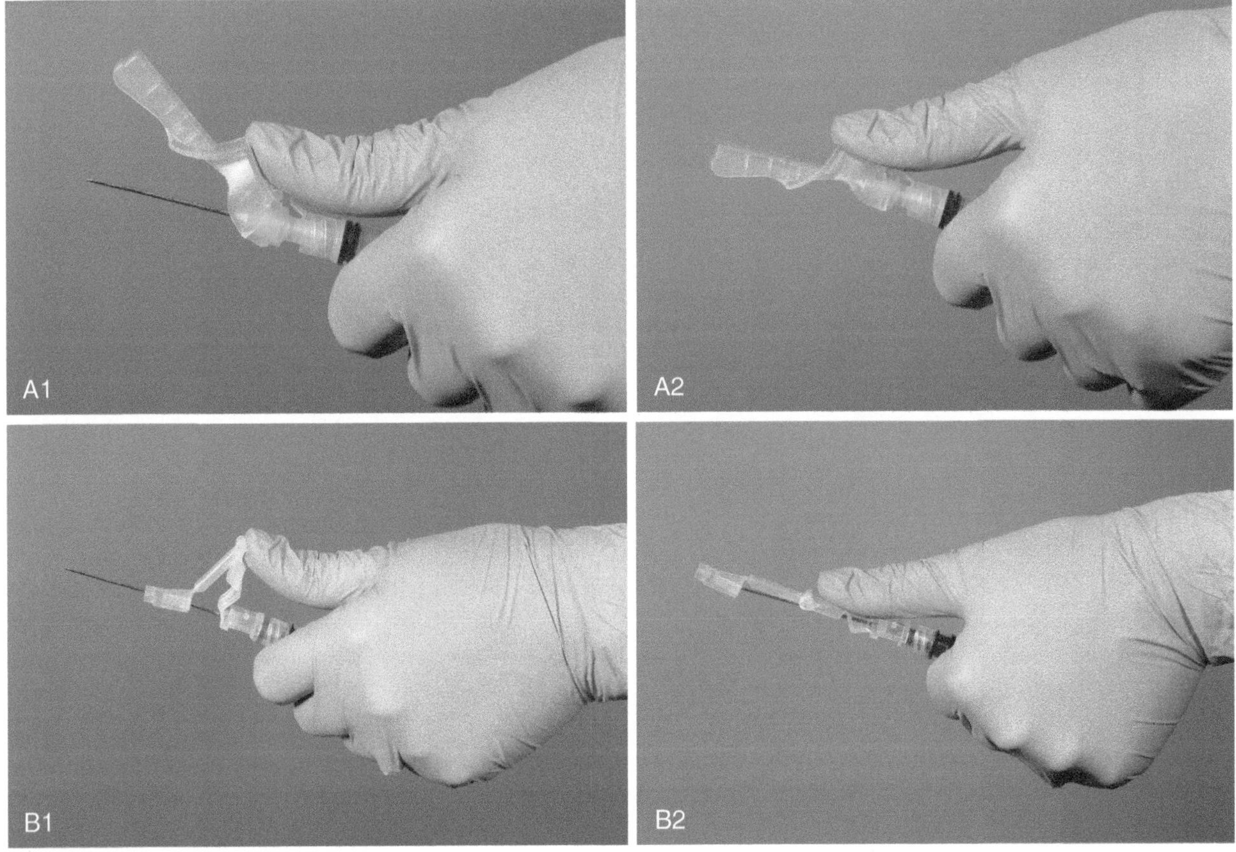

Fig. 11.10 Activation of safety-engineered syringes.

(A) Pivoting-shield syringe (Becton-Dickinson Eclipse Syringe).

1. After administering the injection, hold the syringe and needle away from yourself and others. Center your thumb (or forefinger) on the textured finger pad of the shield.
2. Push the shield forward until you hear a click and then visually confirm that the shield has fully encased the needle. Discard the syringe in a biohazard sharps container.

(B) Hinged-shield syringe (BD Safety Glide Syringe).

1. After administering the injection, hold the syringe and needle away from yourself and others. Push the lever arm forward.
2. Continue pushing until the lever arm is fully extended and the needle tip is completely covered. Visually confirm that the needle tip is covered. Discard the syringe in a biohazard sharps container.

Continued

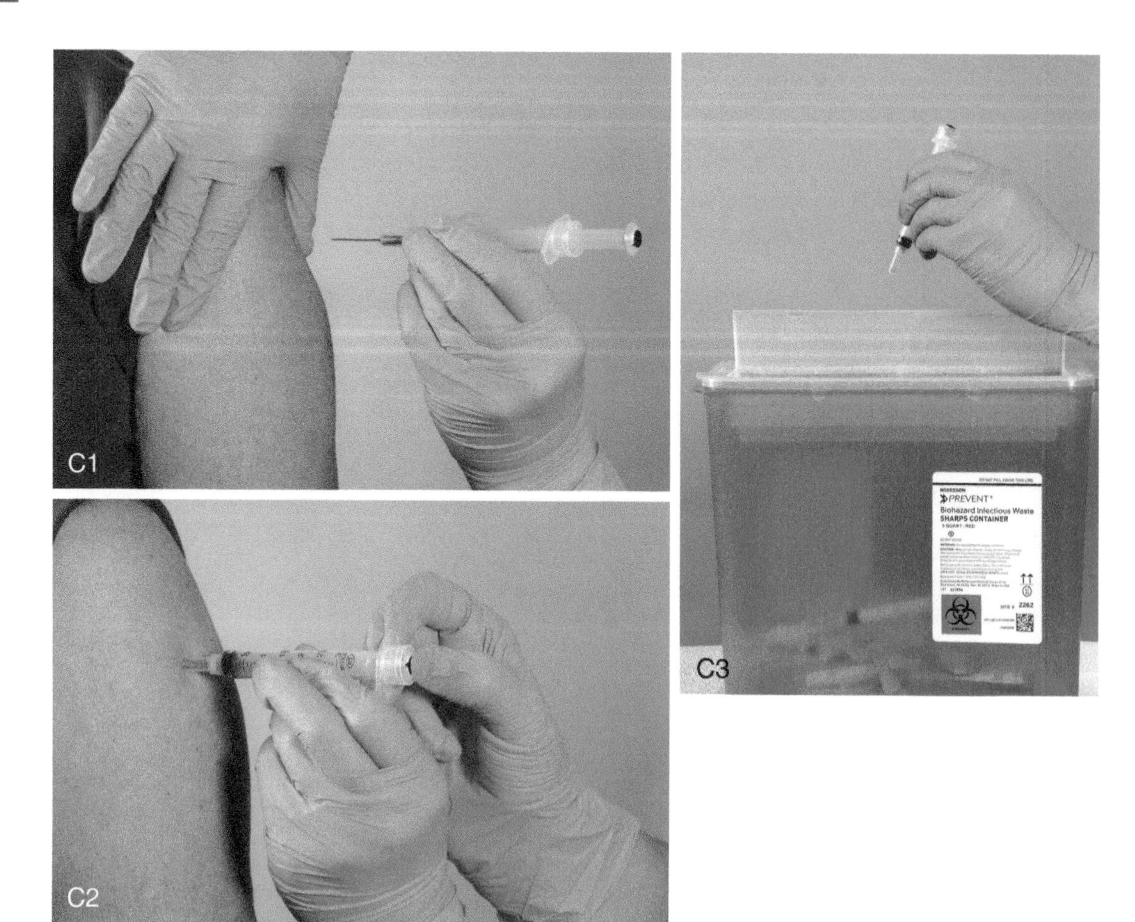

Fig. 11.10, cont'd

(C) Retractable syringe (Vanish Point Syringe).

1 Administer the injection by following the proper technique.
2 After administering the medication, continue depressing the plunger with the thumb. Use firm pressure past the point of initial resistance. This action delivers the full dose of medication to the patient and activates the needle retraction device, causing the needle to retract automatically from the patient's skin and into the barrel of the syringe.
3 Discard the syringe in a biohazard sharps container.

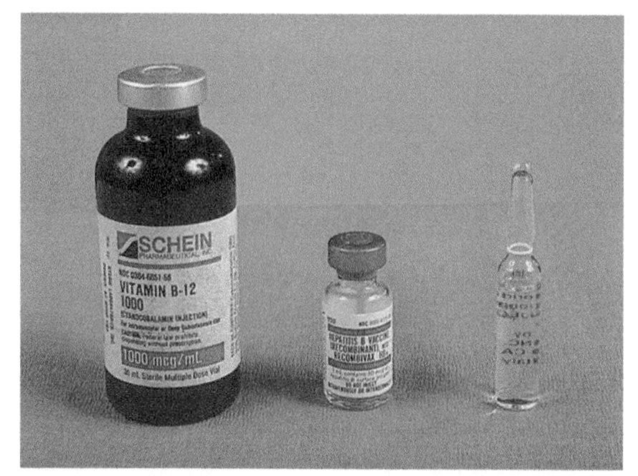

Fig. 11.11 The multiple-dose vial *(left)* and the single-dose vial *(middle)* consist of a closed glass container with a rubber stopper. The ampule *(right)* consists of a small, sealed glass container that holds a single dose of medication.

air bubbles that may enter the syringe when the medication is withdrawn.

To remove medication from a vial, an amount of air exactly equal to the amount of liquid to be removed is injected into the vial. The air should be inserted above the fluid level to avoid creating bubbles in the medication. If air is not injected first, a partial vacuum is created, and it is difficult to remove the medication. During the withdrawal of medication, the needle opening should be inserted below the fluid level to prevent the entrance of air bubbles. Air bubbles can be removed by tapping the barrel of the syringe with the fingertips. If the bubbles are allowed to remain, they take up space that the medication should occupy, which would prevent the patient from receiving the full dose of medication.

Ampules

An **ampule** is a small, sealed glass container that holds a single dose of medication (see Fig. 11.11). An ampule has a constriction in the stem, known as the *neck,* which helps in opening it. Before opening, the medical assistant must ensure that there is no medication in the stem by tapping it lightly. A colored ring around the neck indicates where the ampule is prescored for easy opening. The ampule is opened by holding it firmly with gauze and breaking off the stem with a strong steady pressure.

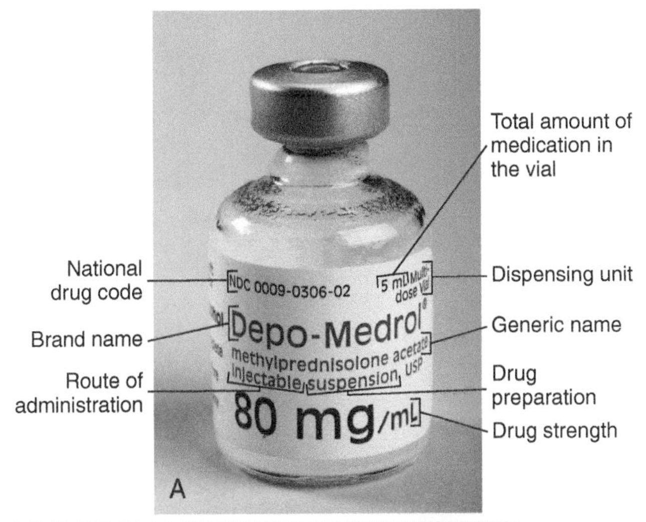

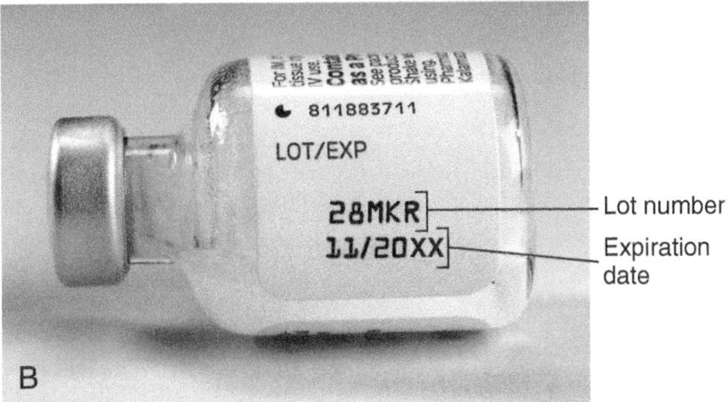

Fig. 11.12 (A and B) Information included on the label of a medication vial.

A hazard with medication in ampules is the possibility of small glass particles getting into the ampule as the stem is broken off. When the medication is withdrawn into the syringe, the glass particles also might be withdrawn. To prevent this problem, a needle with a filter should be used that filters out small glass particles (Fig. 11.13).

The needle opening is inserted into the base of the ampule below the fluid level to withdraw medication. To prevent contamination, the needle should not be permitted to touch the outside of the ampule. Air should never be injected into the ampule because it could force out some of the medication.

Prefilled Syringes

Some drugs come in *prefilled disposable syringes.* Using this type of dispensing unit does not require drawing up the medication. The name of the drug, the dose, and the expiration date are printed on the syringe (Fig. 11.14).

STORAGE

The medical assistant should always read the drug PI to determine the proper method for storing each parenteral medication because improper storage may alter the effectiveness of the medication.

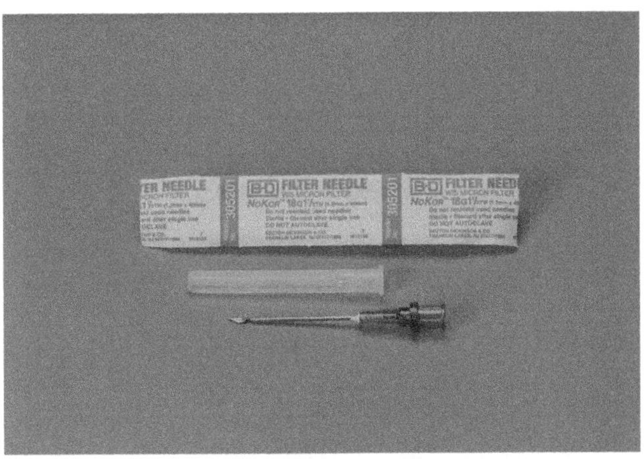

Fig. 11.13 Filter needle used to withdraw medication from an ampule.

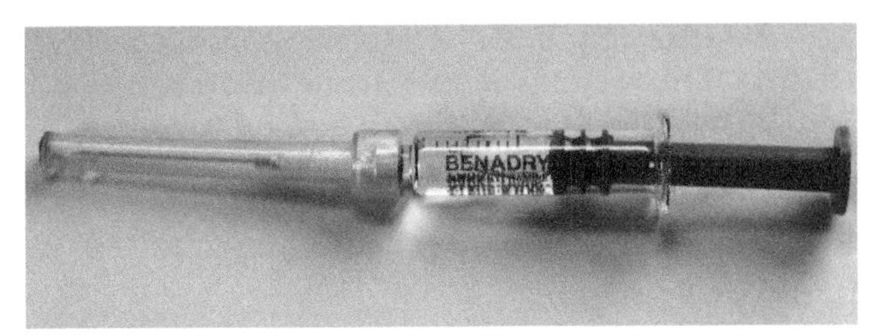

Fig. 11.14 A prefilled disposable syringe of medication.

RECONSTITUTION OF POWDERED DRUGS

Some parenteral medications are stable for only a short time in liquid form; these medications are prepared and stored in powdered form and require the addition of a liquid before administration. The process of adding a liquid to a powdered drug is known as *reconstitution.* The liquid used to reconstitute a powdered drug is known as the *diluent* and usually consists of sterile water or normal saline. The powdered drug is contained in a single-dose or multiple-dose vial and is accompanied by specific instructions for reconstitution. An example of a parenteral medication that requires reconstitution is the measles, mumps, and rubella (MMR) immunization (Fig. 11.15). The procedure for reconstituting powdered drugs is outlined in Procedure 11.3.

SUBCUTANEOUS INJECTIONS

A **subcutaneous injection** is made into the subcutaneous tissue, which consists of adipose (fat) tissue and is located just under the skin (Fig. 11.16). Subcutaneous tissue is located all over the body; however, certain sites are more commonly used because they are located where bones and blood vessels are not near the surface of the skin. These sites include the upper lateral part of the arms, the anterior thigh, the upper back, and the abdomen (Fig. 11.17). Absorption of medication from a subcutaneous injection occurs mainly through capillaries, resulting in a slower absorption rate than with IM injections. To ensure proper absorption, tissue that is grossly adipose, hardened, inflamed, or edematous should not be used as an injection site.

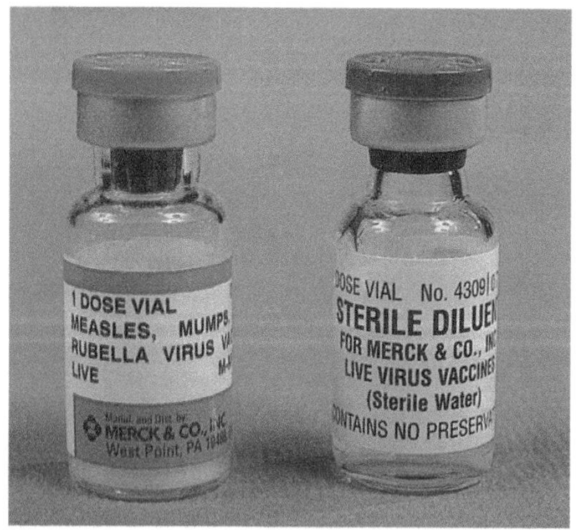

Fig. 11.15 The measles, mumps, and rubella (MMR) vaccine is a parenteral medication that requires reconstitution before administration. The vial on the left contains the medication in powdered form, and the vial on the right contains the sterile diluent.

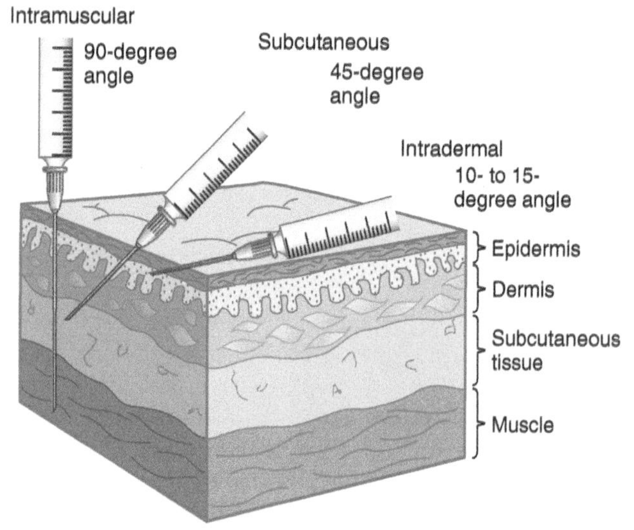

Fig. 11.16 Angle of insertion for intradermal, subcutaneous, and intramuscular injections.

The needle length varies from 1/2 to 5/8 inch, and the gauge ranges from 23 G to 25 G. Elderly and dehydrated patients tend to have less subcutaneous tissue, and obese patients have more. The length of the needle should be adjusted accordingly to ensure the medication is administered into the subcutaneous tissue and not into muscle tissue.

Subcutaneous tissue is sensitive to irritating solutions and large volumes of medications; therefore, drugs given subcutaneously must be isotonic, nonirritating, nonviscous, and water soluble. The amount of medication injected through the subcutaneous route should not exceed 1 mL. More than this amount results in pressure on sensory nerve endings, causing discomfort and pain.

Medications commonly administered through the subcutaneous route include epinephrine, insulin, and allergy injections. Patients who receive allergy injections must wait in the medical office for 15 to 20 minutes after the injection to be observed for an allergic reaction. Procedure 11.4 outlines the administration of a subcutaneous injection.

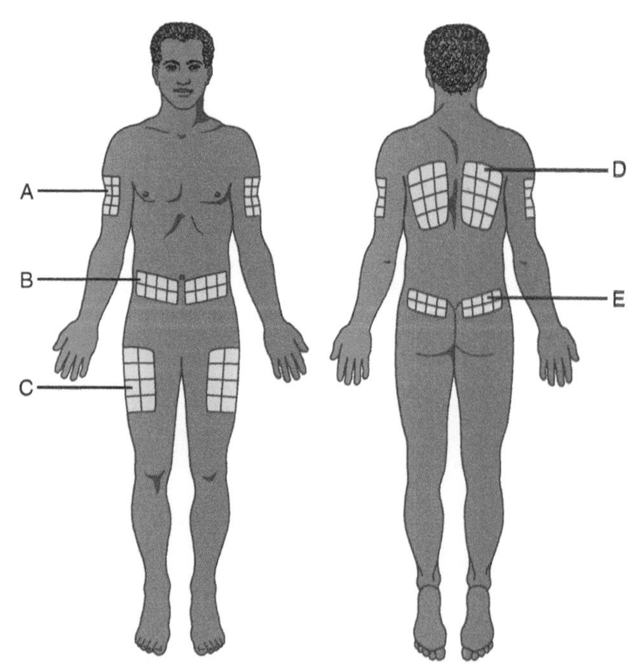

Fig. 11.17 Common sites for subcutaneous injections. *A*, Upper outer arm. *B*, Lower abdomen. *C*, Upper outer thigh. *D*, Upper back. *E*, Flank region.

INTRAMUSCULAR INJECTIONS

Intramuscular injections are made into the muscular layer of the body, which lies below the skin and subcutaneous layers (see Fig. 11.16). The amount of medication that can be injected into muscle tissue is more than the amount that can be injected into subcutaneous tissue. An amount of up to 3 mL can be injected into the ventrogluteal or vastus lateralis muscles of an adult, although older and very thin adults are able to tolerate only 2 mL or less in these sites.

Absorption is more rapid by this route than by the subcutaneous route because there are more blood vessels in muscle tissue. Medication that is irritating to subcutaneous tissue is often given intramuscularly because there are fewer nerve endings in deep muscle tissue. Most parenteral medications administered in the medical office are given through the IM route; examples include antibiotics, injectable contraceptives, vitamin B_{12}, corticosteroids, and many immunizations.

The needle for an adult must be long enough to reach muscle tissue and varies in length from 1 to 3 inches. A 11/2-inch needle is typically used for an average-sized adult, whereas a 1-inch needle is often used for a thin adult or a child, and a needle length of 2 to 3 inches may be needed for an obese adult. The gauge of the needle used ranges from 18 G to 23 G, depending on the viscosity of the medication. Procedure 11.5 outlines the technique for the administration of an IM injection.

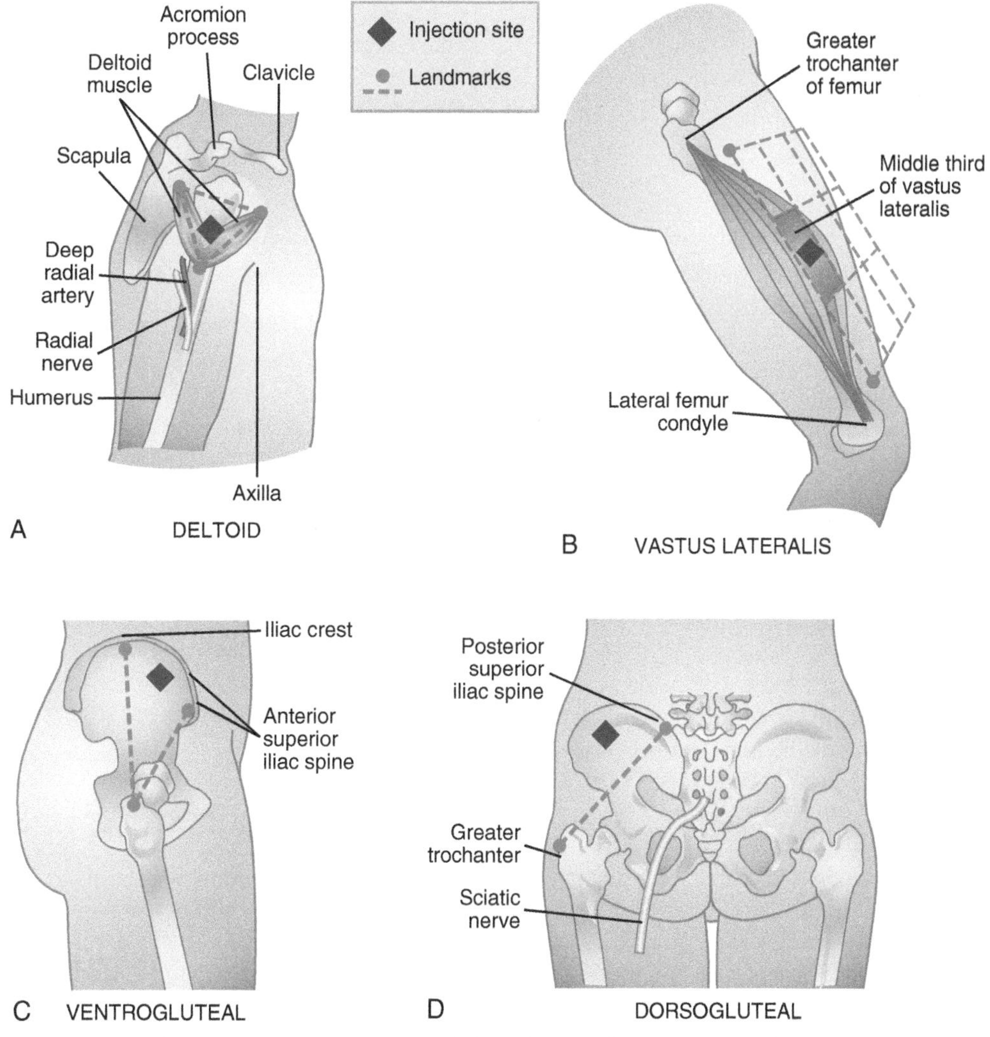

Fig. 11.18 Sites of intramuscular injections. (A) Deltoid muscle. (B) Vastus lateralis. (C) Ventrogluteal muscle. (D) Dorsogluteal muscle. (Modified from Leahy JM, Kizilay PE: *Foundations of nursing practice: a nursing process approach.* Philadelphia: WB Saunders; 1988.)

Intramuscular Injection Sites

The sites chosen for IM injections are away from large nerves and blood vessels. The medical assistant should practice locating these sites to become familiar with them. The area should always be fully exposed to permit clear visualization of the injection site.

Deltoid Site

The deltoid site can be used to administer an injection to an adult and children that are 3 years of age and older. This site is easily accessible and can be used when the patient is sitting or lying down. In most individuals the deltoid site is small and large amounts of medication (no more than 1 mL) and repeated injections should not be given in this area. This is the most common site used to administer vaccines (e.g., influenza vaccine).

When using the deltoid site, the medical assistant should make sure the entire arm is exposed by having the patient's sleeve completely pulled up or by removing the sleeve from the arm if it cannot be pulled up. A tight sleeve constricts the arm and causes unnecessary bleeding from the puncture site. In an adult, the deltoid site is located by palpating the lower edge of the acromion process and going two finger widths down from the acromion process. This forms the base of an inverted triangle with the midpoint of the triangle on the lateral side of the arm in line with the axilla. The injection is administered into the center of the triangle (Fig. 11.18A).

Vastus Lateralis Site

The vastus lateralis site is used because it is not near major nerves and blood vessels and is a relatively thick muscle. This site can be used for both children and adults and is particularly desirable for infants and children younger than 3 years of age. The area is bounded by the midanterior thigh on the front of the leg and the midlateral thigh on the side. In an adult, the proximal boundary is a handbreadth below the greater trochanter, and the distal boundary is a handbreadth above the knee. It is easier to give an injection in the vastus lateralis if the patient is lying down, but a sitting position also can be used.

The vastus lateralis site is located by dividing the front thigh into thirds both vertically and horizontally to make 9 squares. The injection is administered to the outer middle square (see Fig. 11.18B).

Ventrogluteal Site

The ventrogluteal site can be used to administer an injection to both children and adults. It is considered an ideal IM injection site because the subcutaneous layer over this site is relatively thin and the muscle layer is thick allowing it to absorb a large amount of medication. It is also located away from major nerves and blood vessels.

To locate the ventrogluteal site, the patient is placed on his or her side with the injection site facing upward. If the injection is being made into the patient's right side, the palm of the left hand is placed over the greater trochanter with the fingers pointing toward the patient's head and the thumb pointing toward the front of the leg. The index finger is then placed on the anterior superior iliac spine. The middle finger is spread posteriorly as far as possible away from the index finger toward the iliac crest to form a "V." (The hand position is reversed if the injection is being made into the patient's left side.) The injection is administered into the center of the "V" at the level of the knuckles between the index and middle fingers (see Fig. 11.18C).

Dorsogluteal Site

The dorsogluteal site has been used for many years by health care workers to administer IM injections because it is a large muscle and can absorb a large amount of medication. Many researchers, however, no longer recommend the dorsogluteal site because of its close proximity to the sciatic nerve and the superior gluteal artery. Despite these recommendations, health care workers continue to use this site in adults.

To locate this site, the patient lies on the abdomen with the toes pointed inward, which aids in relaxation of the gluteal muscles. The medication is injected into the upper outer quadrant of the gluteal area. This site is located by palpating the greater trochanter and the posterior superior iliac spine. An imaginary line is then drawn between these two points, and the injection is administered above and outside of this area (see Fig. 11.18D). The dorsogluteal site can also be located by dividing the buttocks into quadrants. The site is located in the upper outer quadrant approximately 2 to 3 inches below the iliac crest. The medical assistant must be *extremely* careful to maintain the proper boundary lines to avoid injection into the sciatic nerve or superior gluteal artery. Damage to the sciatic nerve can result in pain, numbness, and temporary or permanent leg paralysis.

Z-Track Method

Medications that are irritating to subcutaneous and skin tissue or that discolor the skin must be given intramuscularly using the Z-track method; one medication that is administered by this method is iron dextran (Imferon). The ventrogluteal and vastus lateralis sites can be used as areas to administer a Z-track injection.

The Z-track method is similar to the IM injection procedure except that the skin and subcutaneous tissue at the injection site are pulled to the side before the needle is inserted. This causes a zigzag path through the tissues when the needle is removed and the skin is released. The zigzag path prevents the medication from reaching the subcutaneous layer or skin surface by sealing off the needle track (Fig. 11.19). The procedure for administering medication using the Z-track method is outlined in Procedure 11.6.

What Would You Do? What Would You *Not* Do?

Case Study 3

Danielle Roush, 16 years old, has come to the office with her mother. Danielle is complaining of a painful sore throat, fever, and severe aching in both of her ears. The physician diagnoses her with strep throat and otitis media and prescribes a parenteral antibiotic to be given deep IM in the ventrogluteal site. Danielle says that she's a basketball player and on the varsity team at her high school. She says that she is always too embarrassed to change or take a shower in front of the other girls because she's so skinny. Danielle would like to have the injection in her arm because it would be too embarrassing to have it in her hip. ■

INTRADERMAL INJECTIONS

An **intradermal injection** is given into the dermal layer of the skin, at an angle almost parallel to the skin (see Fig. 11.16). Absorption is slow; only a small amount of medication may be injected (0.01 to 0.2 mL). The sites most often used for an intradermal injection are areas where the skin is thin, such as the anterior forearm and the middle of the back. The upper arm also is used to administer an intradermal injection.

The needle used is short, usually 3/8 to 5/8 inch long, and the lumen has a small diameter, usually 25 G to 27 G. A tuberculin syringe is often used for administering the injection. The capacity of the syringe is small (1 mL), and the calibrations are divided into tenths and hundredths of a milliliter. The fine calibrations allow a very small amount of medication to be administered, which is required with an intradermal injection. Procedure 11.7 outlines the technique for the administration of an intradermal injection.

The most frequent use of intradermal injections is to administer a skin test, such as an allergy test or a TST. The medication for the appropriate test is placed into the skin layers, and a small, raised area known as a **wheal** is produced at the injection site, owing to distention of the skin (Fig. 11.20). At a time dictated by the type of test being administered, the results are read and interpreted. Most allergy tests can be read and interpreted at the medical office a short time (usually 15 to 20 minutes) after administration of the test, whereas tuberculin testing requires 48 hours before the results can be read.

The skin testing medication interacts with the body tissues; if no reaction occurs, the wheal disappears within a

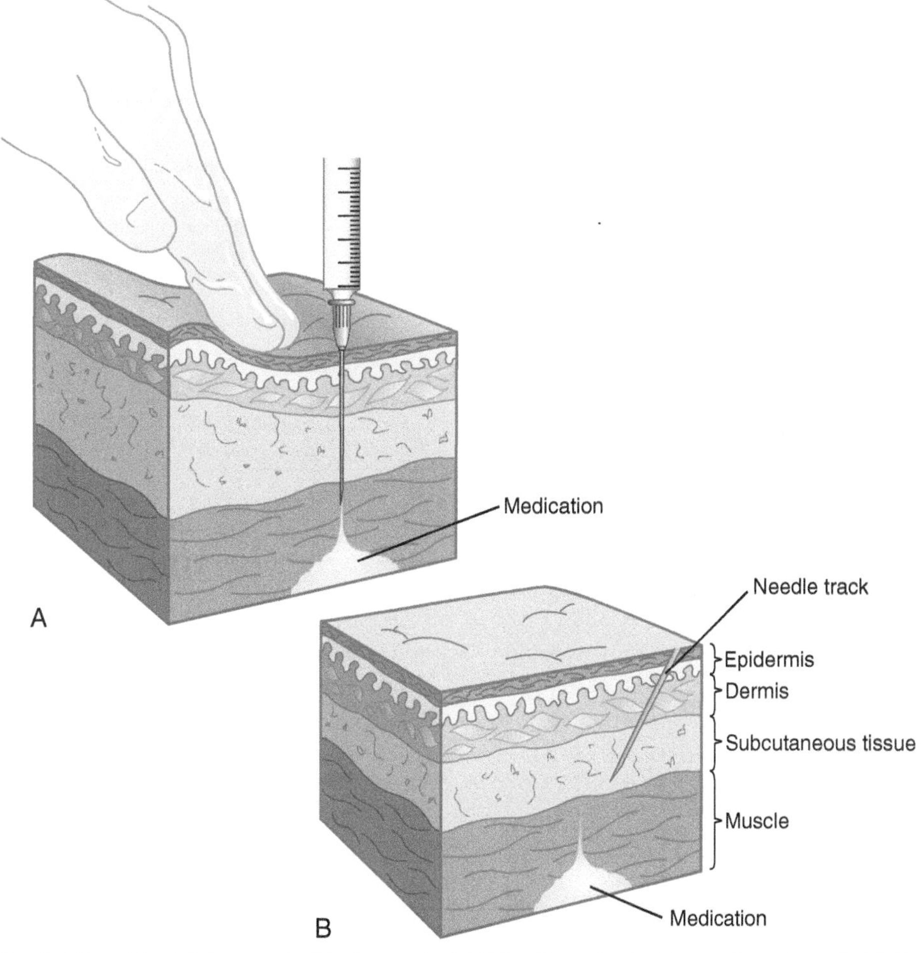

Fig. 11.19 Z-track intramuscular injection method. (A) The skin and subcutaneous tissue are pulled to the side before the needle is inserted. (B) This causes a zigzag path through the tissue when the skin is released, which seals off the needle track.

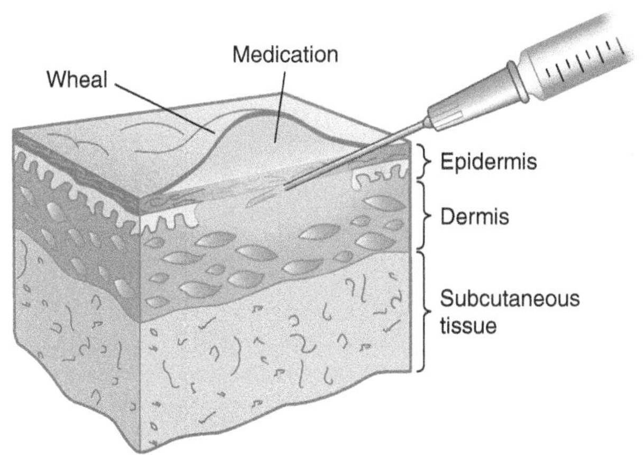

Fig. 11.20 Intradermal injections are used to administer skin tests. Enough medication must be deposited in the skin layers to form a wheal.

short time, and the only visible sign left is the puncture site. If a reaction to the skin test occurs, induration results, indicating a positive reaction. Erythema also may be present at the test site; however, for most skin tests the extent of induration is the only criterion used to assess a positive reaction.

TUBERCULIN TESTING

TUBERCULOSIS

Tuberculosis (TB) is an infectious bacterial disease that can occur in almost any part of the body but usually attacks the lungs. Tuberculosis affecting the lungs is known as *pulmonary tuberculosis,* whereas tuberculosis occurring in other parts of the body is known as *extrapulmonary tuberculosis* and is most apt to occur in the brain, spine, kidneys, bones, and joints. The name of the bacterium that causes tuberculosis is *Mycobacterium tuberculosis,* which is a rod-shaped bacterium. Shortly (within weeks) after infection, a small percentage of individuals infected with TB bacteria develop active pulmonary tuberculosis.

Active Tuberculosis

Active tuberculosis develops when TB bacteria are able to overcome the body's defense system which occurs in 10% of infected individuals. Active tuberculosis is most apt to occur in young children and individuals with a weakened immune system. The TB bacteria then begin to multiply and attack the body, resulting in the destruction of tissue. Symptoms of

Table 11.6 Differences Between Active and Latent Tuberculosis

Characteristics	Active TB	Latent TB
Symptoms	Patient usually feels sick and has symptoms of TB such as cough, fever, and weight loss.	Patient feels fine and has no symptoms.
TB bacterial status	Active TB bacteria are present in the body.	TB bacteria are present in the body that are alive but inactive.
TB test results	Patient usually has a positive TST or QFT-G blood test result.	Patient usually has a positive TST or QFT-G blood test result.
Diagnostic tests	Patient may have an abnormal chest radiograph and a positive sputum test result.	Patient has a normal chest radiograph and a negative sputum test result.
Ability to infect others	Patient is infectious and may spread the disease to others.	Patient is not infectious and cannot spread TB to others.
Treatment	Patient needs treatment for active TB.	Provider may consider treatment for latent TB to prevent active TB disease.

QFT-G, QuantiFERON-TB Gold; *TB,* tuberculosis; *TST,* tuberculin skin testing.

active pulmonary tuberculosis include a chronic cough lasting 3 weeks or longer that produces a mucopurulent sputum, occasional hemoptysis (coughing up blood), and chest pain. Systemic symptoms include fatigue, loss of appetite, weakness, unexplained weight loss, chills, low-grade fever, and sweating at night. If active tuberculosis is left untreated, it can result in serious complications such as permanent lung damage and even death.

Latent Tuberculosis

Most people (90%) infected with the TB bacterium do not develop the active disease because their body defenses protect them. Body defenses may be able to destroy the TB bacteria immediately after they enter the body and completely clear them from the body. If this is not possible, the TB bacteria are engulfed by white blood cells known as macrophages. The body then builds a fibrous wall of tissue around these macrophages (infected with TB bacteria) to encapsulate them. Some of the TB bacteria may remain alive inside the capsule in a dormant or inactive state. During this time, the individual experiences no symptoms and cannot spread the disease to others. Individuals are said to have a latent tuberculosis infection (LTBI), and the only sign indicating that they have been infected with tuberculosis is a positive reaction to a TB test.

Individuals with latent tuberculosis may go on to develop active tuberculosis. This occurs in approximately 10% of individuals with LTBI. About half of these individuals develop active tuberculosis within 2 years after the initial infection, and the other half develop tuberculosis many years, even decades, after having become infected. The TB bacteria break out of the capsule and cause the symptoms of active tuberculosis (described previously). The development of LTBI into active tuberculosis is most apt to occur when the body's immune system is weakened, such as during a serious illness, or in patients who have an immune disorder such as human immunodeficiency virus (HIV) infection. The difference between active tuberculosis and latent tuberculosis is outlined in Table 11.6.

PURPOSE OF TUBERCULIN TESTING

The purpose of tuberculin testing is to identify individuals who are infected with *M. tuberculosis.* Early identification of individuals with active infectious tuberculosis leads to early treatment and prevents the spread of tuberculosis.

A tuberculin test is recommended for individuals who are at higher risk for tuberculosis exposure or infection, or at higher risk for progressing from latent tuberculosis to active tuberculosis. Examples include individuals who have close day-to-day contact with someone with active tuberculosis, individuals who have immigrated from a country with a high incidence of TB, and individuals who work or reside in facilities or institutions with people who are at high risk for TB (e.g., hospitals and other health care facilities, correctional facilities, and nursing homes). Tuberculin testing may also be required as a prerequisite for employment, college entrance, entrance into the military service, and so on. A positive reaction to a tuberculin test occurs 2 to 10 weeks after an individual is infected with tuberculosis. Because of this, a patient recently infected with TB bacteria may show a false-negative test result and should be retested 10 weeks later.

There are two main types of tuberculin tests. They include the TST and the tuberculin blood test that are described in more detail in this section.

MANTOUX TUBERCULIN SKIN TEST

The Mantoux test is most commonly used for tuberculin skin testing and is named after Charles Mantoux, the French physician who developed the test. The Mantoux TST is administered through an intradermal injection using a tuberculin syringe with a capacity of 1.0 mL and a short (3/8 to 1/2 inch) needle with a gauge of 26 to 27. The substance used for the test is tuberculin, which consists of a purified protein derivative (PPD) extracted from a culture of *M. tuberculosis* (the causative agent of tuberculosis), to test for sensitivity to the TB organism. The tuberculin PPD solution contains no live tuberculosis organisms and is completely harmless, making it safe to administer to people of all ages.

The standard injected dose is 0.1 mL of tuberculin PPD solution containing 5 TU (tuberculin units). Brand names for Mantoux tests include Tubersol and Aplisol. Once opened, a vial of tuberculin PPD solution expires after 30 days and must be discarded. This is because oxidation and degradation of tuberculin reduce its potency, which can lead to inaccurate test results. The medical assistant should write the expiration date on the vial on opening. Before withdrawing tuberculin from the vial, the medical assistant should check both the manufacturer's expiration date and the 30-day expiration date marked by the medical assistant on the vial.

It is important to properly store the tuberculin PPD solution because it can be adversely affected by exposure to light and heat. The vial should be stored in the dark as much as possible; exposure to bright light should be avoided because this can diminish the potency of the PPD solution. A vial that has been exposed to light for an extended period of time should be discarded. The vial must be stored in the refrigerator at a temperature between 35° F to 46° F (2° C to 8° C). The vial should be returned to its refrigerated storage area as soon as possible after the proper dose has been drawn up into a syringe.

It is important that the medical assistant draw up the proper amount of tuberculin PPD solution. Injecting too much of the solution might elicit a reaction not caused by a tuberculous infection and injecting too little of the solution results in insufficient solution being injected into the skin to elicit a reaction. This will invalidate the test because if no reaction occurs, it cannot be accepted as a negative reaction.

The medical assistant must make sure to inject the tuberculin solution into the superficial skin layers to form a tense, pale, raised area known as a **wheal.** If the injection is made into the subcutaneous layer, a wheal will not form and the test will yield a false-negative result, whereas a too-shallow injection may cause leakage of the tuberculin solution onto the skin. In either case, the medical assistant must repeat the TST at a site at least 2 inches (5 cm) away.

The medical assistant should not apply pressure to the site after injecting the tuberculin PPD solution because the solution is not intended to be absorbed into the tissues. In addition, applying pressure may cause leakage of the solution through the needle puncture site. The wheal will disappear on its own within a few minutes and should not be covered with an adhesive bandage.

TUBERCULIN SKIN TEST REACTIONS

When PPD solution is introduced into the skin of an individual with an active or latent case of tuberculosis, it causes localized thickening of the skin, resulting in induration. **Induration,** which indicates a positive reaction, is an abnormally raised hardened area with clearly defined margins caused by an accumulation of small, sensitized lymphocytes (a type of white blood cell) that occurs in the area in which the tuberculin was injected into the skin (Fig. 11.21). TST reactions are based on the amount of induration present and are interpreted according to the manufacturer's instructions that accompany the test.

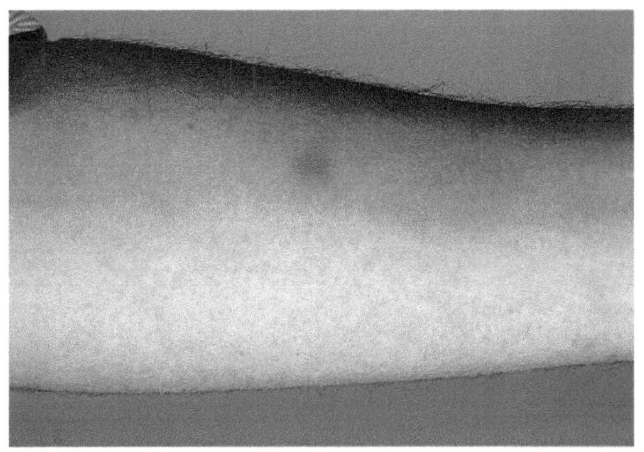

Fig. 11.21 Positive tuberculin skin test result. (From Nairn R: *Immunology for medical students,* ed 2, Philadelphia: Elsevier; 2007.)

A positive reaction to a TST indicates the presence of a tuberculous infection; however, it does not differentiate between active and latent forms of the infection. Therefore, a positive reaction warrants additional diagnostic procedures before the provider can make a final diagnosis. Other procedures used to detect an active tuberculous infection include chest x-ray and microbiologic examination and culture of the patient's sputum for TB bacteria.

Guidelines for Administering a Mantoux Tuberculin Skin Test

1. Use the anterior forearm, approximately 4 inches (10 cm) below the bend in the elbow, as the site of administration of the test. Avoid the following areas because they make the test harder to perform and interfere with good visualization and palpation of test reactions:
   - Hairy areas of the skin
   - Areas with visible veins
   - Scar tissue
   - Red or swollen areas
   - Bruised areas
   - Areas with lesions, dermatitis, or other skin irritations
   - Muscle ridges
2. Cleanse the skin thoroughly with an antiseptic wipe and allow it to dry completely before administering the test.
3. Be sure to inject the PPD tuberculin solution slowly into the superficial layers of the skin. If the injection is performed correctly, a wheal should appear that is approximately 6 to 10 mm (3/8 inch) in diameter. If blood appears at the puncture site once the TST has been administered, this is not significant and will not interfere with the test. The blood can be removed by gently blotting the area with a gauze pad, making sure not to apply pressure.
4. Once the TST has been administered, the results must be read within 48 to 72 hours.

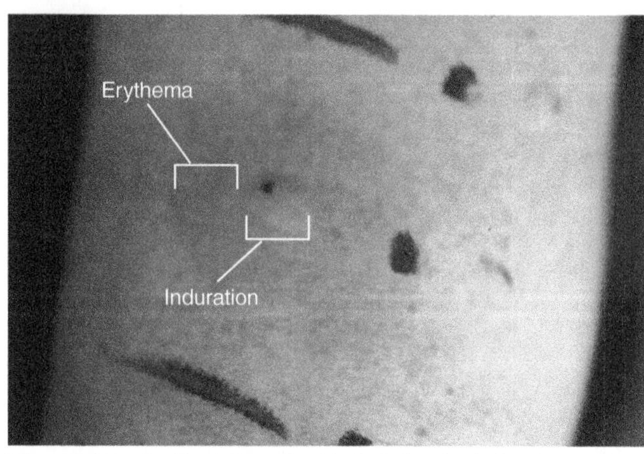

Fig. 11.22 Positive tuberculin skin test showing induration and erythema. Induration is the only criterion used to determine a positive reaction. (From Abbas AK, Lichtman AH, Pillai, S: *Basic immunology functions and disorders of the immune system,* ed 4, Philadelphia: Elsevier; 2014.)

Guidelines for Reading Mantoux Tuberculin Skin Test Results

1. The TST results must be read in good lighting within 48 to 72 hours.
2. Use both inspection and palpation to read the TST results. Induration may not always be visible and therefore must be assessed through palpation.
3. If induration is present, rub your fingertip lightly from the area of normal skin (without induration) to the indurated area to assess its size. The diameter of induration must be assessed and measured transversely to the long axis of the forearm (left to right, not up and down). Measure the widest diameter of induration in millimeters using a flexible millimeter ruler. (*Note:* If you have difficulty locating the edges of the induration, the following technique will help. Take a ballpoint pen and place the tip of it on normal skin adjacent to the induration at a 45-degree angle. Then push the pen toward the indurated area. The pen will make an ink line on the normal skin and then will stop at the edge of the induration. Repeat this technique on the opposite side of the induration.
4. The extent of induration present is the only criterion used to determine a positive TST reaction (Fig. 11.22). If erythema is present without induration, the results are interpreted as negative.
5. Document all reactions in millimeters to the nearest millimeter. If no induration is present, the TST results should be documented as 0 mm. Results should never be documented as positive or negative.
6. The interpretation of the TST test results depends on the following:
   a. Measurement (in mm) of the induration
   b. The individual's risk of being infected with tuberculosis (e.g., close contact with an individual with active TB increases the risk of being infected)
   c. The individual's risk of progression to disease if infected (e.g., HIV-infected individuals are more apt to progress from LTBI to active TB)
7. Mantoux TST results are interpreted according to the guidelines presented in Box 11.3. The procedure for administering and reading a Mantoux TST is presented in Procedure 11.7.

TWO-STEP TUBERCULIN SKIN TEST

The two-step TST is recommended by the Centers for Disease Control and Prevention (CDC) for the initial baseline testing of adults who are required to undergo periodic tuberculin skin testing. For example, most health care workers are required to have an initial TST when hired and then a yearly TST thereafter. On employment, the initial TST should consist of a baseline two-step test.

To understand the purpose of a two-step TST, it is first necessary to understand what can sometimes occur in individuals who were infected with tuberculosis many years ago. Over a period of years, the ability of the immune system of an individual with a previous TB infection to react to the tuberculin solution may gradually diminish. When a TST is administered to such an individual, the body does not react at all or only weakly reacts, resulting in a false-negative test result. For example, a 42-year-old individual who was infected with tuberculosis during childhood may have a negative test result to an initial TST.

Administering a TST to an individual with a previous TB infection causes stimulation or "boosting" of the patient's immune system that takes place over several days after administration of the test. Basically, the first test "jogs the memory" of the immune system to recognize and react to the tuberculin. If another TST is administered after the first TST, there is often a strong reaction to the tuberculin, resulting in a positive test result. This boosted reaction is caused by an old TB infection and should not be interpreted as a newly acquired infection. Misinterpretation could result in an unnecessary investigation to identify the source of the infection and unnecessary treatment of individuals. Although the booster effect can occur in an individual in any age group, it is most apt to occur in older individuals who were infected with tuberculosis at a younger age.

To perform a two-step TST, the medical assistant administers the Mantoux TST and instructs the patient to return to have the test result read within 48 to 72 hours as outlined in Procedure 11.7. If the TST result is positive, the individual is considered infected with TB bacteria, and further skin testing is not warranted. If the TST result is negative, a second test is performed 1 to 3 weeks after the first test. If the second TST result is negative, the patient is classified as noninfected, and a positive reaction later to a subsequent TST is likely to represent a new infection. If the second TST result is positive, this is most likely caused by a boosted reaction indicating the patient was previously infected with *M. tuberculosis.* Refer to Fig. 11.23 for a diagram to assist in interpreting two-step TST results.

When periodic TB testing is required, the two-step TST needs to be completed only *once*. The initial test (consisting of two tests) indicates the true baseline reading of the

BOX 11.3 Interpretation of the Tuberculin Mantoux Skin Test[a]

Interpretation of the Mantoux skin test results is based on the individual's risk of being infected with tuberculosis (TB) and the risk of progression to disease if infected. Individuals with impaired immunity are more likely to have a weaker response to a tuberculin skin test. Because of this, there are three cutoff points for identifying a positive reaction to a Mantoux test.

Positive Reaction

An induration of 5 mm or more is classified as positive in individuals with the following high-risk factors for developing TB:

1. Individuals infected with HIV
2. Individuals who have had recent close contact with individuals who have active TB
3. Individuals who have fibrotic changes on a chest radiograph consistent with previously healed TB
4. Individuals who have had organ transplants
5. Individuals on immunosuppressive drug therapy (e.g., prolonged high-dose corticosteroid therapy, TNF-α–antagonist drug therapy [Remicade, Enbrel, Humira])

Negative Reaction

An induration of 4 mm or less

Positive Reaction

An induration of 10 mm or more is classified as positive in individuals who do not meet the aforementioned criteria but who have other risk factors for TB, including the following:

1. Individuals who inject illegal drugs
2. Individuals with the following conditions that weaken the immune system: diabetes mellitus; chronic renal failure; body weight that is 10% or more below ideal body weight; silicosis; gastrectomy; jejunoileal bypass; certain hematologic disorders such as leukemias and lymphomas; carcinoma of the head, neck, or lungs
3. Residents and employees of the following high-risk congregate settings: hospitals and other health care facilities, correctional facilities, nursing homes, homeless shelters, drug rehabilitation centers, residential facilities for patients with AIDS
4. Recent immigrants from countries with a high incidence of TB (countries in Asia, Africa, the Caribbean, Latin America, and Eastern Europe and Russia)
5. Children younger than 4 years
6. Infants, children, and adolescents exposed to adults at high risk for developing TB
7. Mycobacteriology laboratory personnel

Negative Reaction

An induration of 9 mm or less

Positive Reaction

An induration of 15 mm or more is classified as positive in individuals at low risk for developing TB, including individuals with no known risk factors for TB

Negative Reaction

An induration of 14 mm or less

[a]The cutoff point may sometimes vary from state to state from those presented in this box.

AIDS, Acquired immunodeficiency syndrome; *HIV,* human immunodeficiency virus; *TNF,* tumor necrosis factor.

individual's tuberculosis status. Any subsequent TST performed on a periodic basis (after a two-step test) needs to consist of only one skin test.

TUBERCULIN BLOOD TEST

Interferon gamma release assays (IGRAs) are blood tests used to identify individuals who are infected with *M. tuberculosis* (the causative agent of tuberculosis). Currently, there are two IGRAs approved for use by the FDA; these include the QuantiFERON-TB Gold In-Tube test (QFT-GIT) manufactured by Cellestis, Inc. and the T-SPOT TB test (T-SPOT) manufactured by Oxford Immunotec, Ltd. As with the TST, IGRAs cannot differentiate between active and latent forms of the infection. Therefore, a positive result warrants additional diagnostic procedures, such as a chest radiograph and microbiologic examination and culture of the patient's sputum before the provider can make a diagnosis.

If the blood specimen for the IGRA test is drawn in the medical office, it is important for the medical assistant to carefully follow the test manufacturer's instructions for the collection of the specimen to ensure accurate test results. Following collection, the blood specimen for an IGRA must be stored at room temperature and transported to the laboratory within a specified time period for processing. The blood specimen for a QFT-GIT test must be transported within 14 hours following collection while the blood specimen for a T-SPOT must be transported within 8 hours following collection.

When an individual is infected with *M. tuberculosis,* certain lymphocytes in their blood become sensitized and release a substance known as interferon γ (IFN-γ). IGRA tests are able to detect the presence of INF-γ in a patient infected with *M. tuberculosis.* The patient is likely to be infected with *Mycobacterium* if he or she registers an IFN-γ level above the positive cutoff value. On the other hand, if the patient is not infected with *M. tuberculosis,* his or her blood will not contain sensitized lymphocytes and there will not be a release of IFN-γ. In this case, the test result is documented as negative, indicating that the patient is unlikely to be infected with *M. tuberculosis.*

IGRA test results are interpreted as follows:

Positive: Individuals who test positive are likely to be infected with *M. tuberculosis* and should be evaluated further for latent TB or active TB.

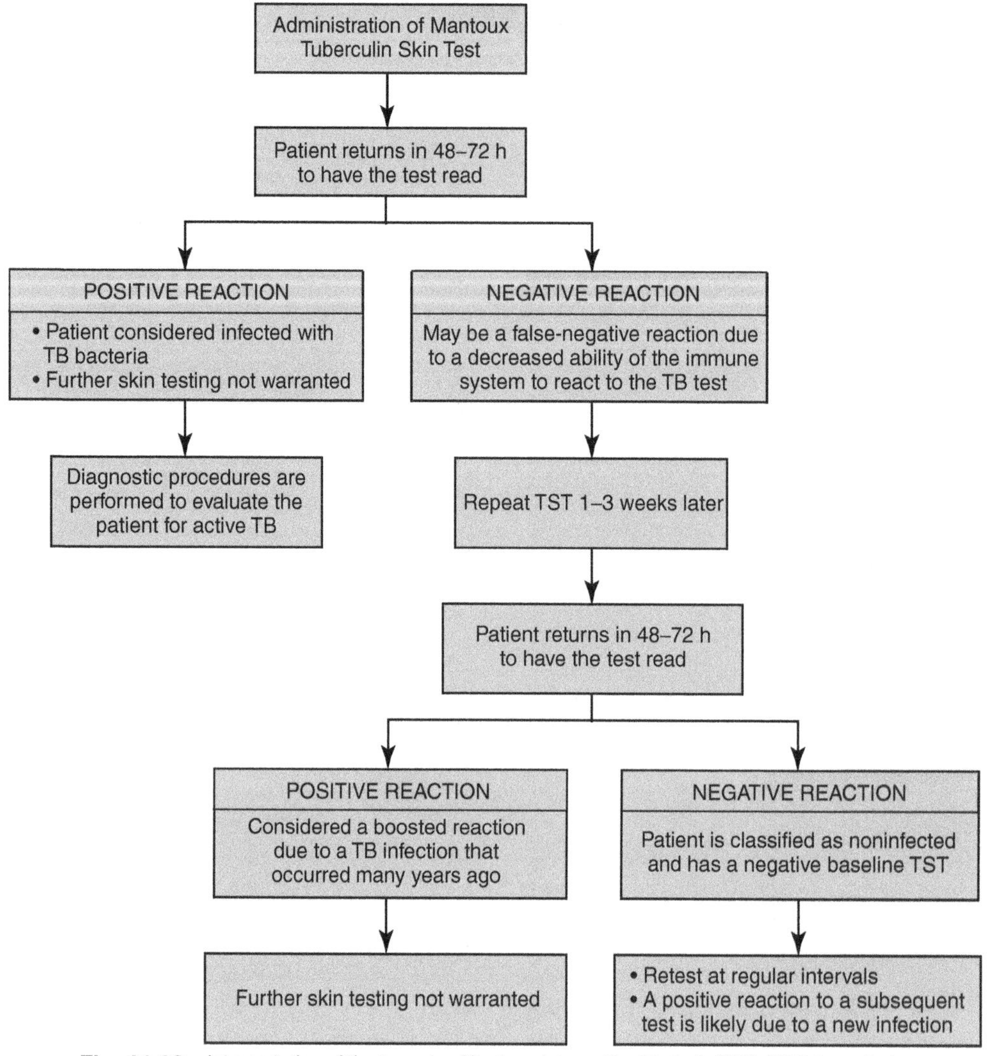

Fig. 11.23 Interpretation of the two-step Mantoux tuberculin skin test *(TST)*. *TB,* Tuberculosis.

Negative: Healthy adults who test negative are unlikely to have an *M. tuberculosis* infection and usually do not require further evaluation.

Indeterminate/borderline: An indeterminate/borderline result indicates that the *M. tuberculosis* infection status cannot be determined because of factors that invalidate the test results. These factors include the following: improper technique used in the collection, handling, and storage of the blood specimen; a delay in transporting the specimen to the laboratory; and the inability of the patient's blood to respond to the test because of a severely weakened immune system, such as in a patient undergoing chemotherapy. If a test result is indeterminate/borderline, the IGRA test should be repeated using a fresh blood specimen.

IGRA tests offer several advantages over the Mantoux TST, which include the following:

1. The patient needs to visit the office only one time to have his or her blood drawn. This alleviates the problem that sometimes occurs with patients undergoing a TST, in which a patient does not return for the second visit to have the results read.
2. The results are available within 24 hours compared with the 48 to 72 hours required for a TST.
3. IGRA tests provide an objective evaluation, whereas the TST is a subjective evaluation. If the TST test is not measured correctly, inaccurate test results may occur.
4. IGRA tests are not affected by the booster effect, which can occur with TST, thus eliminating the need for two-step tuberculin skin testing.
5. IGRA tests provide a positive or negative test result, and risk factors do not have to be taken into consideration when positive reactions are interpreted, as is required with the TST.
6. An individual who has been vaccinated for tuberculosis with the bacillus Calmette-Guérin (BCG) vaccine does not show a false-negative result with IGRA tests, as can occur with a TST.

IGRA tests have some disadvantages that are outlined as follows:

1. The patient's blood specimen must be delivered within a specified time period following collection. This is because the lymphocytes in the blood specimen begin to die after this time period has elapsed.

2. Errors in the collection, handling, or storage of the specimen can affect the accuracy of IGRA tests
3. The cost of IGRA tests are significantly higher than that of a TST.

ALLERGY TESTING

ALLERGY

An **allergy** is an abnormal hypersensitivity of the immune system of the body to substances that are ordinarily harmless; these substances are known as **allergens.** Allergens enter the body by being inhaled, by being swallowed, by being injected, or by coming into contact with the skin. Almost any substance in the environment can be an allergen. Some common allergens are plant pollens, mold, house dust, animal dander, latex, dyes, soaps, detergents, cosmetics, certain foods and medications, and venom from insect stings.

The exact cause of allergies is not fully understood. In many cases, the tendency to develop allergies seems to be inherited because children of allergic parents tend to exhibit more allergic symptoms than children of nonallergic parents. Although allergies can develop at any age, children are more apt to develop allergies than are older individuals.

ALLERGIC REACTION

The immune system of an individual with allergies interprets certain allergens (e.g., pollen, mold, house dust) as invaders. The first time the allergen enters the body of an allergic individual, it stimulates the body to produce antibodies to that allergen. These antibodies are usually of a type known as *immunoglobulin E (IgE) antibodies.* After the initial sensitization, allergic antibodies combine with the allergen in the body, resulting in an allergen-antibody reaction. When such a reaction occurs, histamine is released in significant amounts, causing allergic symptoms (e.g., sneezing, watery eyes, runny nose). Allergen-antibody reactions may involve any system of the body; however, they most frequently affect the respiratory and integumentary systems. Allergic symptoms can range from mild to very severe, as is the case with the potentially fatal anaphylactic reaction.

Depending on the allergen and the body system affected, allergies appear in different forms in an individual and commonly include hay fever (allergy to mold and pollen), allergic rhinitis (runny and inflamed nose), asthma, urticaria, contact dermatitis, eczema, and food allergies. Symptoms exhibited by an allergic individual depend on an individual's form of allergy. Table 11.7 lists the common clinical forms of allergies and symptoms of allergies.

Table 11.7 Clinical Forms of Allergies

Hay fever (seasonal allergic rhinitis)	Caused by allergy to mold or the pollen of trees, grasses, or weeds. The term ***hay fever*** is misleading because hay fever is not caused by hay, and it does not result in fever. English physicians first used the term ***hay fever*** in the early 1800s when treating patients with allergies to grass pollens. Symptoms of hay fever and the common cold are almost identical: episodes of sneezing, itching, and watery eyes; runny and stuffy nose; and burning sensation of the palate and throat. Hay fever is seasonal, occurring when there is pollen in the air. Depending on geographic location, hay fever may occur in spring, summer, or fall, and last until first frost.
Perennial allergic rhinitis	Inflammation of mucous membranes of the nose caused by allergies. Symptoms include nasal congestion, sneezing, and runny nose. With perennial rhinitis, the nasal mucosa is inflamed year-round. This type of allergic rhinitis is commonly caused by allergens that are always present in the environment, such as house dust and animal dander.
Allergic asthma	Condition characterized by coughing, chest tightness, shortness of breath, and wheezing. During an asthma attack, the bronchiole tubes constrict and become clogged with mucus, which accounts for many of the symptoms of allergic asthma. Asthma can occur at any age but is more common in children and young adults and, if not treated, can lead to serious complications such as permanent lung damage. It is frequently, but not always, associated with a family history of allergy. Any common allergen, such as house dust, pollens, mold, or animal dander, may trigger an allergic asthma attack.
Urticaria	Urticaria, or hives, is an outbreak on the skin of welts of varying sizes that are redder or paler than surrounding skin and are accompanied by intense itching. When swellings are large and invade deeper tissues, the condition is known as ***angioedema.*** Hives may develop on the face or lips or even internally. Allergies to food or drugs (especially penicillin and aspirin) and insect bites often cause hives, but they also may result from underlying disease or occur after exercise. In many cases the exact causes of urticaria cannot be determined. 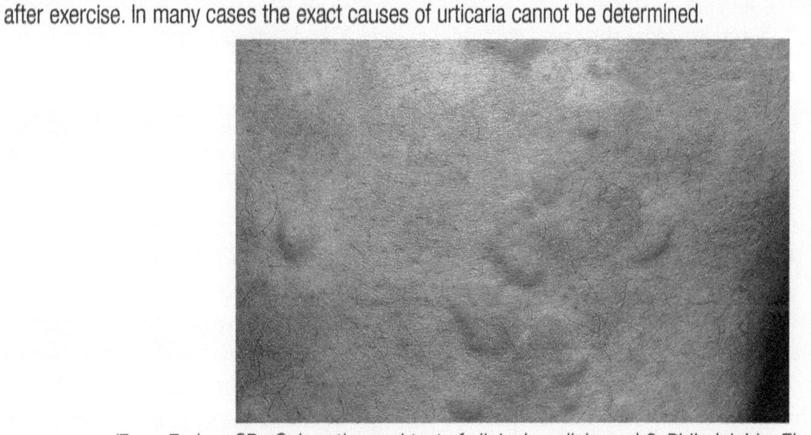 (From Forbes CD: *Color atlas and text of clinical medicine*, ed 3, Philadelphia: Elsevier; 2002.)

Continued

Table 11.7 Clinical Forms of Allergies—cont'd

Contact dermatitis	Rash caused by direct contact of the skin with an allergen, such as cosmetics, perfumes, deodorants, latex, plastics, certain plants, and clothing treated with certain preservatives or dyes. Symptoms include swelling, blistering, oozing, and scaling. Rash usually occurs only on the areas of the body that have been in contact with the allergen. The most common causes of contact dermatitis are poison ivy, poison oak, and sumac. 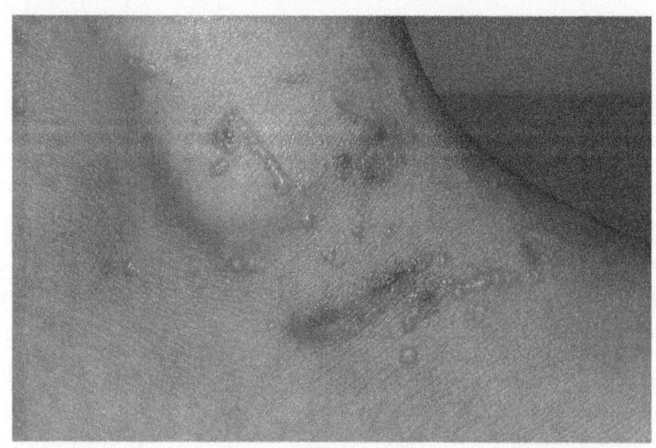 (From Forbes CD: *Color atlas and text of clinical medicine*, ed 3, Philadelphia: Elsevier; 2002.)
Eczema	Noncontagious rash accompanied by redness, itching, vesicles, oozing, crusting, and scaling. Eczema is a common allergic reaction in children, but it also may occur in adults, usually in a more severe form. A rash commonly appears on the face, neck, and folds of the elbows and knees. Eczema frequently is associated with allergies, and substances to which a person is allergic may aggravate it. Foods may be important factors, particularly milk, fish, or eggs. Allergens that are inhaled, such as dust and pollen, rarely cause eczema. 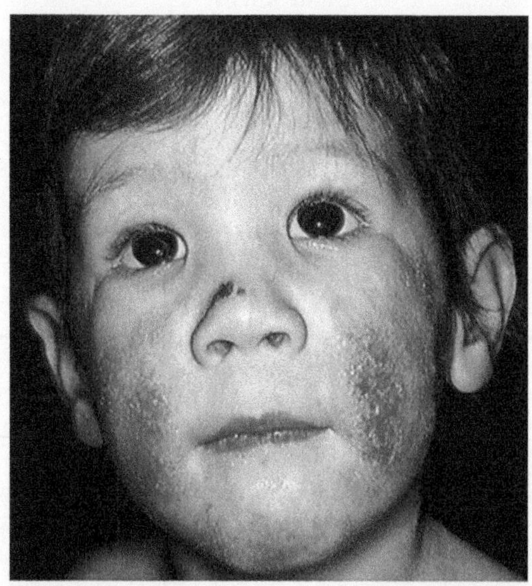 (From Leifer G: *Introduction to maternity and pediatric nursing*, ed 5, St Louis: Elsevier; 2009.)
Food allergy	An immune system reaction that occurs soon after eating a food to which an individual is allergic. The most common symptoms that occur when a patient has a food allergy are urticaria (hives), asthma symptoms (such as wheezing and shortness of breath), gastrointestinal symptoms (such as nausea, vomiting, diarrhea, abdominal pain), and swelling of the lips, face, tongue, or throat. The most common foods that cause allergies are milk, soy, eggs, peanuts, tree nuts (e.g., walnuts), fish, shellfish, and wheat. The primary treatment for a food allergy involves avoidance of the food. If the individual has a severe allergy to a food, such as peanuts, consuming the food can cause an anaphylactic reaction, which can be life threatening. Treatment involves the immediate injection of epinephrine.

DIAGNOSIS AND TREATMENT

The best way to prevent allergic symptoms is to identify and avoid the offending allergen or allergens. The first and most important step in this process is the completion of a careful and detailed medical history by the provider. Of particular importance to the diagnosis of an allergy are the patient's home and work environments, diet, and living habits. The provider also performs a thorough physical examination to detect conditions resulting from allergies, such as nasal polyps, wheezing, skin rashes, and urticaria.

When the medical history and physical examination have been completed, the provider may order diagnostic tests. Allergy testing is performed to confirm information obtained through the medical history and physical examination. The allergy tests ordered most often are direct skin testing and in vitro blood testing, which are described in greater detail in the following section. The general treatment of allergies includes avoiding the allergen(s) (if possible); alleviating the symptoms through drug therapy such as antihistamines, decongestants, bronchodilators, and inhaled steroids; and decreasing the sensitivity of the body to the allergen by the administration of allergy injections, or desensitization injections (known as *immunotherapy*).

TYPES OF ALLERGY TESTS

The purpose of allergy testing is to determine the specific substances or allergens that are causing the patient's allergic symptoms. The two main categories of allergy tests are direct skin tests and the in vitro blood test. The medical assistant is often responsible for performing direct skin testing in the medical office. The in vitro blood test is performed on a blood specimen by an outside laboratory. The medical assistant may be responsible for performing a venipuncture to obtain the blood specimen.

Direct Skin Testing

Direct skin testing involves applying extracts of common allergens to the skin and observing the body's reaction to them. The extract is applied either topically to the skin (patch testing) or into the superficial skin layers (skin-prick testing and intradermal testing). The advantage of direct skin testing is that test results are obtained immediately. This in vivo administration of allergens has the potential, however, to cause adverse reactions, the least common but most serious being an anaphylactic reaction. The medical assistant should have a thorough knowledge of the signs of an anaphylactic reaction and should alert the provider immediately if the patient begins to exhibit them.

Regardless of the specific type of direct skin test used (patch, skin-prick, or intradermal), some general guidelines should be followed:

1. Instruct the patient to discontinue the use of antihistamines for 3 days before the skin testing. Antihistamines block the response of histamine, which may suppress skin testing reactions and lead to false-negative test results. Certain medications decrease the immune response of the body to skin testing, which could cause a false-negative test result. These medications include tricyclic antidepressants, corticosteroids, theophylline, beta-blockers, angiotensin-converting enzyme (ACE) inhibitors, and nifedipine. If the patient is taking any of these medications, the provider must determine if it is possible to take the patient off of the medication. If it is not feasible, the provider may order in vitro allergy blood testing, which is not affected by medication.
2. Verify that the area of application is free from hair, scar tissue, and dermatitis to permit good visualization and palpation of test reactions. Recommended sites include the anterior forearm, the upper arm, and the middle of the back. The back is usually used for patch and skin-prick testing, and the upper arm and forearm are typically used for intradermal skin testing.
3. Cleanse the area of application thoroughly with an antiseptic wipe, and allow it to dry completely.
4. Wear gloves when the allergy testing involves puncture of the skin, which includes skin-prick testing and intradermal skin testing. Gloves protect the medical assistant from exposure to bloodborne pathogens, as required by the OSHA standard.
5. Space the allergen extracts at least 1 inch apart to provide enough surface area for a sizable reaction. If not enough surface area is available, large adjacent reactions may run together, making it difficult to read test results.
6. Label the test sites so that the application site of each allergen extract can be identified later when reading results.
7. Closely observe the patient after the procedure for a systemic reaction to the skin testing. The patient should remain at the office for at least 30 minutes after the procedure for observation.
8. Make the patient aware that the skin testing may cause a mild allergic reaction, such as a runny nose, sneezing, and mild wheezing 8 to 24 hours after skin-prick and intradermal skin testing. Instruct the patient to contact the provider immediately if a more severe reaction than this occurs, such as difficulty in breathing, dizziness, or swelling of the face, lips, or mouth.

Quality Control

Positive and negative controls should be performed with each skin testing procedure to ensure reliable and valid test results. Controls are performed at the same time and in the same way that the allergy skin testing is performed.

Negative Control

To perform a negative skin test control, a substance that should not cause a reaction in a normal person is inserted into the patient's superficial skin layers. The negative control usually consists of normal saline. Some patients have a condition known as *dermographism,* which causes them to have a reaction just from the irritating effect of a needle pricking their skin. Running a negative control ensures that positive skin test reactions are truly positive and are not the result of another factor, such as dermographism.

Positive Control

For a positive control, a substance that should cause a reaction in a nonallergenic patient is inserted into the patient's superficial skin layers. The substance used for the positive control is histamine. The positive control should produce a reaction that consists of at least 3 mm of induration surrounded by erythema. Patients who are taking an antihistamine or who have a depressed immune system because of a disease or immunosuppressive medication may have a false-negative reaction to a skin test. Running a positive control ensures that negative skin test reactions are truly negative and are not just the result of another factor, as in a patient who has taken an antihistamine.

HIGHLIGHT on Allergens

House Dust

There are many components in house dust to which an individual may be allergic; the most significant of these is the house dust mite. Dust mites thrive in warm humid conditions and feed on scales shed from human skin; they are often found in mattresses, carpets, stuffed animals, and upholstered furniture. An individual who is allergic to house dust reacts to the waste products of these dust mites.

There is no shortage of food for the dust mite because one person sheds up to 1 g of scales per day, which is enough to feed thousands of mites for months. *Dermatophagoides pteronyssinus* and *Dermatophagoides farinae* are the most common house dust mites and are present in varying numbers in virtually every home. Mites occur in greatest numbers in bedding, particularly in mattresses; there may be 5000 mites in each gram of dust from a mattress. Sufferers often notice that symptoms become much worse when the bedding is disturbed and allergenic material becomes airborne. Practices that eliminate dust also reduce the number of dust mites in a household.

Insect Stings

It is estimated that 1 of every 125 Americans is allergic to the venom from insect stings. Approximately 40 people in the United States die each year from a severe allergic reaction to insect venom. The incidence of deaths is low because most people know they need to obtain medical attention immediately if an allergic reaction begins.

Almost all insects whose venom can cause allergic reactions belong to the order Hymenoptera, which includes honeybees and bumblebees, wasps, yellow jackets, and hornets. When a honeybee stings, its stinger remains embedded in the victim's skin, causing the bee to die as it tries to tear itself away. Wasps, yellow jackets, and hornets are more aggressive than bees and can sting repeatedly. Hornets are the most aggressive of the group and may sting even when not provoked. Yellow jackets are close behind in aggressiveness, but wasps usually sting only if someone interferes with them near their nest.

If an insect sting does not cause an allergic reaction within 30 minutes, chances are excellent that no problem will occur. A normal reaction to an insect sting includes localized pain, redness, swelling, and itching lasting 1 to 2 days. Any generalized reaction not arising directly from the area of the sting is almost certain to be an anaphylactic reaction, which begins with such symptoms as sneezing, urticaria, itching, angioedema, erythema, and disorientation and progresses to difficulty in breathing, dizziness, faintness, and loss of consciousness. Medical care should be sought immediately because most fatalities occur within 2 hours after the sting. Because time is a factor, individuals who are known to have a severe allergy to insect stings are provided with an anaphylactic emergency treatment kit that contains epinephrine in a prefilled syringe and oral antihistamines. They can carry the kit with them so that treatment for a severe allergic reaction can be started as soon as possible.

Penicillin

Penicillin is a common cause of allergic drug reactions. Approximately 2% to 5% of individuals are allergic to penicillin. The reaction may be mild and completely overlooked or confused with the symptoms of the disease being treated with penicillin, or it can be more serious and take the form of severe dermatitis or an anaphylactic reaction. Death as a result of a severe anaphylactic reaction is rare, occurring in only 0.01% of patients being treated with penicillin.

Penicillin was discovered in 1929 by Sir Alexander Fleming, but it was not used as a therapeutic drug until 1940. By 1944, it was evident that some of the side effects of penicillin were allergic reactions; the first documented death as a result of an anaphylactic reaction to penicillin occurred in 1945.

Oral administration of penicillin is safer than a penicillin injection because it has a lower frequency of severe allergic reactions. There have been only six reported deaths from oral administration of penicillin.

Approximately 95% of serious reactions occur within 1 hour after a penicillin injection. The best preventive measure is to keep the patient under direct observation for at least 30 minutes after administration of the injection. ■

Types of Direct Skin Tests

Patch Testing

Patch testing is primarily used to identify allergens that cause contact dermatitis. Patch testing involves the topical application of each allergen to the skin, using a "patch." A patch consists of a small piece of gauze or filter paper impregnated with the allergen, which is applied to the skin and taped in place with hypoallergenic tape (Fig. 11.24). Allergens commonly applied include plants, topical drugs, latex, resins, metals, cosmetics, dyes, and chemicals. The patient should be instructed to leave the patches in place, keep them dry, and return to the medical office in 48 hours to have the results read. When the patient returns to the office, the patches are carefully

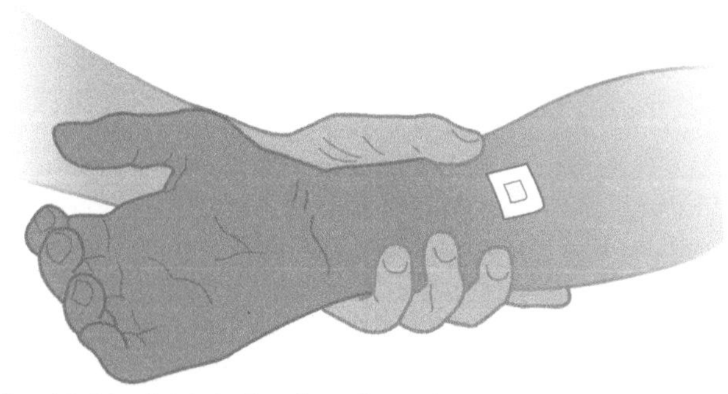

Fig. 11.24 Patch testing. A patch consists of a small piece of gauze or filter paper impregnated with the allergen, which is applied to the skin and taped in place.

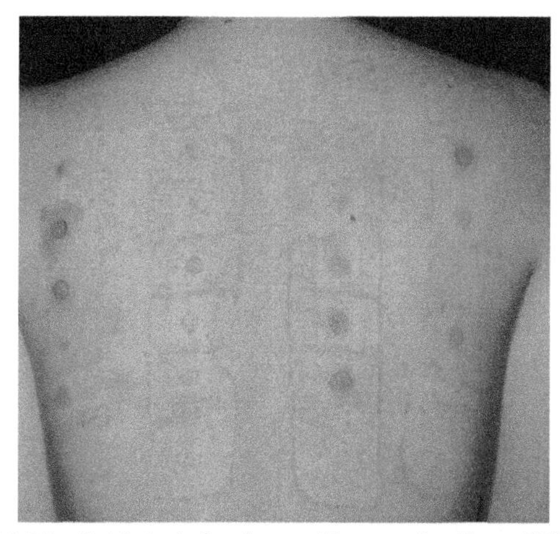

Fig. 11.25 Patch test showing positive results. (From Shiland BJ: *Mastering healthcare terminology,* ed 4, St Louis: Elsevier; 2013.)

removed, and the results are read 20 minutes later. The delayed reading time allows lessening of redness that may occur from the tape removal.

Test results are documented as positive or negative. Positive reactions cause a small area of contact dermatitis characterized by itching, erythema, induration, and vesiculation (Fig. 11.25). In strongly positive responses, the reaction may extend beyond the margins of the patch. Positive results are graded further on a quantitative 1+ to 3+ scoring system according to the type of reaction (Table 11.8).

Table 11.8 Guidelines for Documenting Direct Skin Test Results

Patch Test	
—	No reaction
+1	Presence of erythema and edema, possibly papules
+2	Presence of erythema, edema, and vesicles, possibly papules
+3	Erythema, vesicles, and severe edema
Skin-Prick Testing and Intradermal Testing	
—	No reaction
±1	Induration 1 mm or less
+1	Induration greater than 1 mm and up to 5 mm in diameter
+2	Induration greater than 5 mm and up to 10 mm in diameter
+3	Induration greater than 10 mm and up to 15 mm in diameter
+4	Induration greater than 15 mm in diameter

Skin-Prick Testing

Skin-prick testing usually is performed to diagnose allergies to common allergens, particularly those that are inhaled, such as house dust, pollens, and molds. It is also used to test for food allergies; the most common foods that cause allergies are milk, soy, eggs, peanuts, tree nuts (e.g., walnuts), fish, shellfish, and wheat.

Skin-prick testing involves the application of numerous allergen extracts to the skin, followed by the pricking of each with a sterile needle or another sharp instrument (Fig. 11.26). The number of allergen extracts applied during one office visit usually ranges between 20 and 30. Pricking the skin deposits the allergens in the outer layers of the skin to allow each to react with the body tissues.

The following guidelines should be followed for skin-prick testing: The extracts should be placed on the skin in rows in a specific pattern. This, along with labeling the test sites with a felt-tipped pen, tracks the location of each extract. Only a single drop of extract should be placed on the skin; more than this amount may cause the extracts to diffuse and run together. A sterile needle should be passed through the drop, and the point should lightly lift the top layer of skin without causing bleeding. It is important to wipe the needle dry with a sterile swab between pricks to prevent one extract from mixing with the next, leading to inaccurate test results.

The maximum reaction is usually seen in 15 to 20 minutes. During this time, the test sites should be left uncovered,

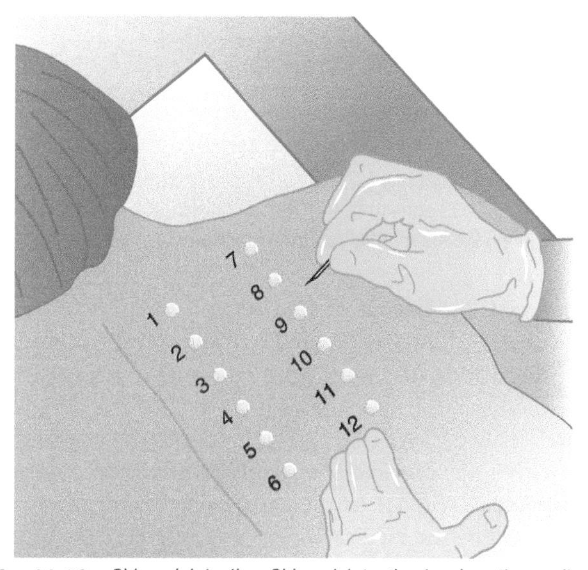

Fig. 11.26 Skin-prick testing. Skin-prick testing involves the application of numerous allergen extracts to the skin, followed by the pricking of each with a sterile needle.

and the patient should be instructed not to touch them. These areas should not be wiped because this removes the allergen extract, resulting in false-negative results. The results are read (after 15 to 20 minutes) using a millimeter ruler.

An area of induration surrounded by redness and itching characterizes a positive reaction. Positive results are documented by measuring the size of the induration in millimeters and converting it to a numeric scale based on the extent of the induration (see Table 11.8). Any redness should be ignored. See Fig. 11.27 for an illustration of skin test results. If a negative or only a mild reaction occurs and the provider still suspects the presence of an allergy, the provider may order intradermal skin testing.

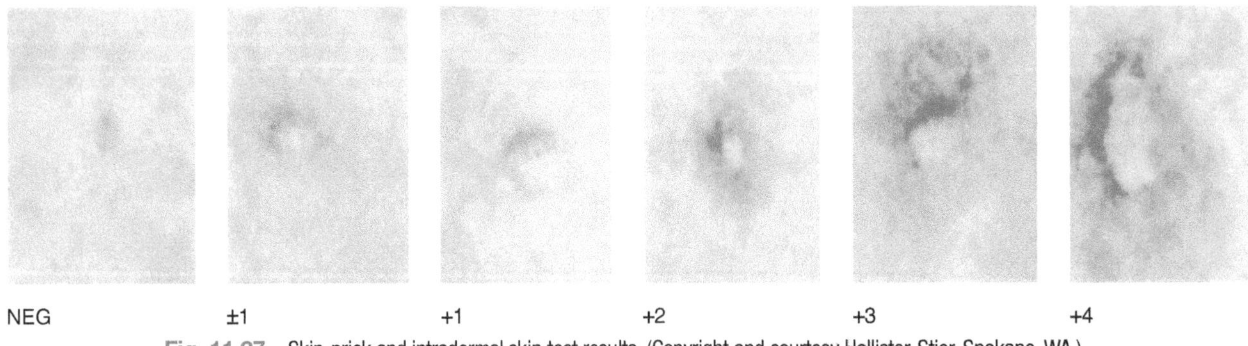

Fig. 11.27 Skin-prick and intradermal skin test results. (Copyright and courtesy Hollister-Stier, Spokane, WA.)

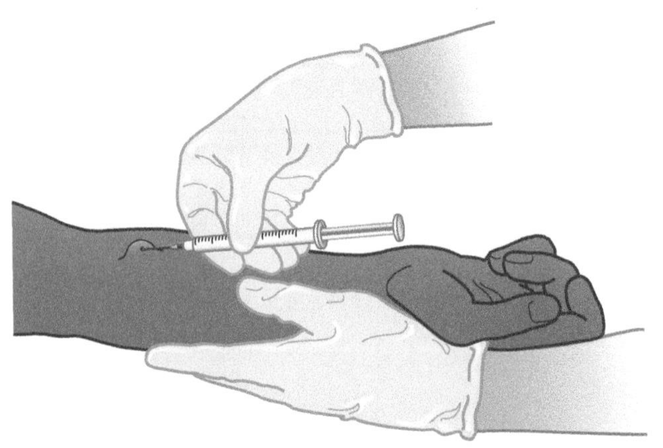
Fig. 11.28 Intradermal skin testing. Intradermal testing involves the injection of a small amount of allergen extract into the superficial skin layers through the intradermal route of administration.

Intradermal Skin Testing

Intradermal skin testing is similar to skin-prick testing but is more sensitive. The number of skin tests performed during one office visit ranges from 5 to 30. Because there is a greater chance of adverse allergic reactions to intradermal skin testing, the provider often starts with skin-prick testing in individuals who are suspected of being highly allergic as determined by the medical history and results of the physical examination.

Intradermal skin testing involves the injection of a small amount (0.02 to 0.05 mL) of allergen extract into the superficial skin layers through the intradermal route of administration (Fig. 11.28). A tuberculin syringe is used to administer the test, and the allergen extract is injected until a wheal forms (see Procedure 11.7). After 15 to 20 minutes, the test sites are observed for reactions. Positive reactions are characterized by an area of induration surrounded by redness and itching. As with skin-prick testing, positive results are documented by measuring the size of the induration in millimeters and converting it to a numeric scale based on the amount of induration present (see Fig. 11.27; see Table 11.8).

In Vitro Allergy Blood Testing

An in vitro allergy blood test measures the amount of IgE antibodies in the blood that respond to common allergens. Examples of in vitro blood tests include enzyme-linked immunosorbent assay (ELISA), the radioallergosorbent test (RAST), and ImmunoCAP. For an in vitro allergy blood test, a sample of the patient's blood is sent to an outside laboratory, where it is exposed to allergens suspected of causing an allergic reaction in that patient. A detection device is used to measure the level of IgE antibodies that respond to each allergen being tested, and the results are reported as a numeric value. An elevated level of IgE antibodies responding to an allergen indicates the patient is allergic to that allergen.

Advantages of the in vitro blood test over direct skin testing are as follows: The results are not affected by medication (e.g., antihistamines); there is no danger of adverse allergic reactions because the test is performed in vitro, meaning outside the body; and in vitro blood testing can be performed on patients who have skin eruptions and are unable to undergo direct skin testing because of the lack of an intact skin surface area. In vitro blood testing is expensive, however, and does not provide immediate test results, which are available with direct skin testing. Blood testing is often used to test for allergies when it is not possible to perform skin testing. These situations include the following:

1. The provider does not want the patient to be taken off of a medication that interferes with skin test results.
2. The provider suspects that skin testing could result in an anaphylactic reaction in that patient.
3. The patient has a severe skin condition such as widespread dermatitis.
4. The skin testing may be difficult to perform, as in a child younger than 4 years.

INTRAVENOUS THERAPY

Intravenous (IV) therapy is the administration of a liquid agent directly into a patient's vein, where it is distributed throughout the body by way of the circulatory system (Fig. 11.29). The veins most commonly used for IV therapy are the peripheral veins of the arm and hand. The liquid agent may consist of basic fluids, medication, nutrients, blood, or blood products. When fluids, medications, or nutrients are administered by the IV route, the technique is called an **infusion.** When whole blood or blood products are administered by the IV route, the procedure is called a **transfusion.**

Most IV therapy occurs in a hospital setting on both an inpatient and an outpatient basis. IV therapy also is administered in outpatient ambulatory settings, such as medical

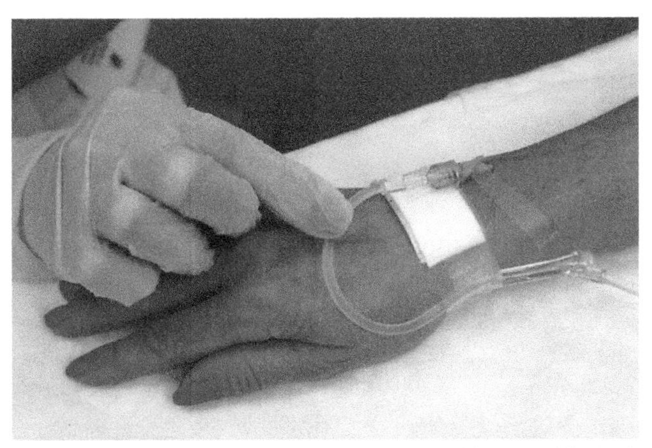

Fig. 11.29 Intravenous therapy. (From Potter PA, Perry AG: *Basic nursing: essentials for practice,* ed 7, St Louis: Elsevier; 2011.)

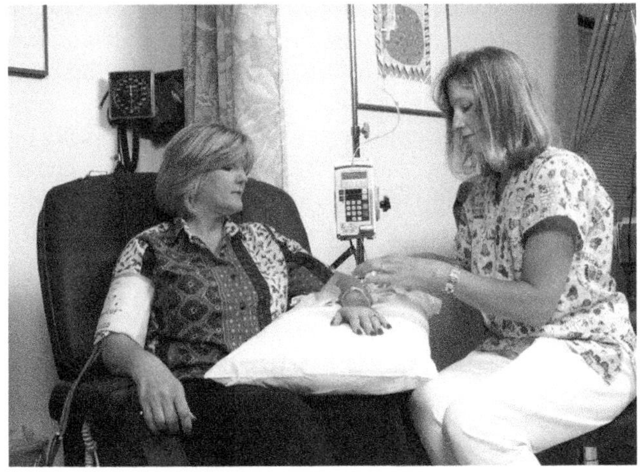

Fig. 11.30 Patient receiving intravenous therapy in an outpatient setting. (Photo by Margaret Hartshorn. Courtesy Arizona Arthritis Center [www.arthritis.arizona.edu].)

offices and clinics, urgent care centers, ambulatory infusion clinics, and the patient's home (Fig. 11.30).

ADVANTAGES OF OUTPATIENT INTRAVENOUS THERAPY

Administration of IV therapy in an outpatient setting is growing in acceptance by patients and the medical community. IV therapy may be administered in an outpatient setting for a variety of reasons. which include the following:

- Administration of IV medication
- Replacement of fluids and electrolytes
- Administration of nutritional supplements
- Administration of blood products
- Emergency administration of IV medication and fluids

Outpatient IV therapy is more convenient for the patient and reduces medical costs through earlier discharge from the hospital or avoidance of hospitalization altogether.

Earlier Hospital Discharge

When a hospitalized patient is receiving IV therapy and requires continued therapy, it is not always necessary or cost-effective to keep the patient in the hospital. If the patient is medically stable, he or she may no longer need the careful observation and daily nursing care provided by a hospital. By receiving IV therapy in an outpatient setting, the patient can be discharged earlier. Most patients, particularly children, are more comfortable in their home environment, which often contributes to faster healing. An example of this is a hospitalized patient with an infection who still needs IV antibiotic therapy but no longer needs to be hospitalized and who receives the therapy at an infusion clinic.

Avoidance of Hospitalization

Outpatient IV therapy provides an alternative to patients with an acute or chronic illness that requires IV therapy. Patients who do not require hospitalization for their condition are able to obtain their IV therapy in an outpatient setting. This allows patients the option of being able to continue their daily routine without major interruptions and provides them with greater independence and control over their condition. An example of this is a patient with rheumatoid arthritis who needs IV infliximab (Remicade) therapy and receives that therapy at the rheumatology medical office.

MEDICAL OFFICE–BASED INTRAVENOUS THERAPY

Some medical offices provide outpatient IV therapy. Outpatient IV therapy may be provided in an oncology office for the administration of IV chemotherapy. **Chemotherapy** refers to the treatment of cancer using antineoplastic medications. With the advent of newer rheumatology medications that must be given intravenously, some rheumatology offices have started to provide this service. There are distinct advantages to medical office–based IV therapy. It allows the provider to provide closer monitoring of a patient's response to the IV therapy and any adverse reactions exhibited by the patient. These benefits have prompted more providers to consider office-based IV therapy.

Based on the potential future growth of IV therapy in the medical office and the current growth of other IV outpatient settings, such as infusion clinics and the patient's home, there is a need for medical assistants to acquire some basic knowledge in IV therapy. The medical assistant is often responsible for scheduling IV therapy and providing the patient with IV therapy instructions and information, such as the length of time required for the therapy. In addition, patients may have questions that the medical assistant may need to answer (or refer to the proper individual for answering) regarding their outpatient IV therapy. The entry-level medical assistant should be familiar with the basic theory of outpatient IV therapy, which is presented here.

Advanced IV theory and initiating, maintaining, and discontinuing IV therapy are not entry-level medical assisting competencies and are not addressed in this text. Certain requirements must be met before the medical assistant can perform IV therapy in the medical office. The medical assistant first should check the laws of his or her state to determine whether it is legally permissible for the medical assistant to perform this procedure. The medical assistant must acquire the proper training (theory and skills) by completing a recognized IV therapy training program, including supervised clinical practice. Although the IV procedure can appear simple when performed by an expert, it is a difficult skill that requires considerable practice to perfect.

INDICATIONS FOR OUTPATIENT INTRAVENOUS THERAPY

Outpatient IV therapy has been shown to be a safe and effective alternative to inpatient IV therapy for the treatment of certain conditions. Before prescribing outpatient IV therapy, the provider assesses the need for the therapy by determining whether the following criteria are met: The patient's condition warrants the use of IV therapy, no alternative routes are feasible or appropriate to deliver the therapy, and the patient does not need to be hospitalized to receive the IV therapy. After determining the need for outpatient IV therapy, the provider prescribes the appropriate medication or fluid and treatment plan, orders laboratory tests to monitor the patient's progress, and assesses the patient after the IV therapy.

Scheduling the Intravenous Therapy

If the patient receives the IV therapy at an outpatient site other than the medical office (e.g., an infusion clinic), the medical assistant may be responsible for scheduling the necessary services and providing the patient with IV therapy instructions, such as the length of time required for the therapy, any dietary restrictions, whether to wear loose-fitting comfortable clothing, and whether someone needs to transport the patient to and from the appointment.

Medical Office Guidelines

Medical offices that provide IV therapy on-site usually set up a special room to deliver the therapy, which often includes a lounge chair to provide for patient comfort during the therapy. With office-based IV therapy, the entry-level medical assistant is responsible for scheduling the IV therapy and providing the patient with the IV therapy instructions listed previously. The medical office employs an IV practitioner, such as a nurse or a specially trained medical assistant, to initiate, maintain, and discontinue the IV therapy. This practitioner must be completely familiar with all aspects of the IV therapy, including indications and uses, actions, dose and rate of infusion, incompatibilities, contraindications and precautions, antidote, and adverse effects. During the IV therapy, the practitioner must carefully monitor the patient's response to the therapy and be alert for adverse or allergic reactions. After the therapy is completed, the IV practitioner provides the patient with follow-up instructions, such as information on normal side effects that may occur when the patient returns home and any adverse reactions that need to be reported to the medical office.

What Would You Do? What Would You *Not* Do? RESPONSES

Case Study 1
Page 375

What Did Theresa Do?

- ❑ Asked Mrs. Okasinski what pharmacy she uses. Called the pharmacy and ask them to send an electronic copy of Mrs. Okasinski's medications to the medical office. Used the information to identify Mrs. Okasinski's medications.
- ❑ Documented the medications in her medical record for the physician to review.
- ❑ Explained to Mrs. Okasinski that when she has her prescriptions filled, she should request non-childproof containers so that she will be able to use the original containers, which have the name and prescription information on them. This will make it easier to tell her medications apart.
- ❑ After the physician was finished with Mrs. Okasinski, printed out a list of all the medications she would be taking based on the physician's orders. Reviewed each medication with Mrs. Okasinski, and told her to keep the list a reference.

What Did Theresa Not Do?

- ❑ Did not criticize Mrs. Okasinski for taking her medications out of their original containers.

Case Study 2
Page 402

What Did Theresa Do?

- ❑ Explained to Mrs. Cardwell that for the infection to be completely eliminated from Rachel's body, she needed to be given all of the medication.
- ❑ Stressed to Mrs. Cardwell that medication prescribed to one person should never be given to someone else because it might cause him or her to have a bad reaction.
- ❑ Explained to Mrs. Cardwell that if side effects of medication ever occur, it is important to call the medical office for information on what to do.
- ❑ Told Mrs. Cardwell that Rachel needs to be seen by the doctor again, and scheduled an appointment for her. Asked if any other family members needed an appointment with the doctor.

What Did Theresa Not Do?

- ❑ Did not scold Mrs. Cardwell for giving Rachel's antibiotic to the other family members.

Case Study 3
Page 412

What Would You Do? What Would You *Not* Do? RESPONSES—cont'd

What Did Theresa Do?

- ❑ Explained to Danielle that if the injection were given in her arm, it would not be absorbed very well and she might not get better.
- ❑ Explained to Danielle that injections are given to patients every day in the hip at the office and that Danielle does not need to be embarrassed.
- ❑ Told Danielle that she would be draped extra well and that it would only take a minute to give the injection.

What Did Theresa Not Do?

- ❑ Did not disregard Danielle's concerns.
- ❑ Did not give the injection in the deltoid.

TERMINOLOGY REVIEW

Key Term	Word Parts	Definition
Adverse reaction		An unintended and undesirable effect produced by a drug.
Allergen		A substance that is capable of causing an allergic reaction.
Allergy		An abnormal hypersensitivity of the body to substances that are ordinarily harmless.
Ampule		A small, sealed glass container that holds a single dose of medication.
Anaphylactic reaction		A serious allergic reaction that requires immediate treatment.
Chemotherapy	*chem/o-:* chemical *-therapy:* treatment	The use of chemicals to treat disease. The term *chemotherapy* is most often used to refer to the treatment of cancer using antineoplastic medications.
Controlled drug		A drug that has restrictions placed on it by the federal government because of its potential for abuse.
Conversion		Changing from one system of measurement to another.
Cubic centimeter		The amount of space occupied by 1 milliliter (1 mL = 1 cc).
DEA number		A registration number assigned to providers by the Drug Enforcement Administration for prescribing or dispensing controlled drugs.
Dose		The quantity of a drug to be administered at one time.
Drug		A chemical used for the treatment, prevention, or diagnosis of disease.
Enteral nutrition	*enter/o:* intestines *-al:* pertaining to	The delivery of nutrients through a tube inserted into the gastrointestinal tract.
Gauge		The diameter of the lumen of a needle used to administer medication.
Hemophilia	*hem/o:* blood *-philia:* love	An inherited bleeding disorder caused by a deficiency of a clotting factor needed for proper coagulation of the blood.
Immune globulin		A blood product consisting of pooled human plasma containing antibodies.
Induration		An abnormally raised, hardened area of the skin with clearly defined margins.
Infusion		The administration of fluids, medications, or nutrients into a vein.
Inhalation administration		The administration of medication by way of air or other vapor being drawn into the lungs.
Inscription		The part of a prescription that indicates the name of the drug and the drug dosage.
Intradermal injection	*intra-:* within *derm/o:* skin *-al:* pertaining to	Introduction of medication into the dermal layer of the skin.
Intramuscular injection	*intra-:* within *muscul/o:* muscle *-ar:* pertaining to	Introduction of medication into the muscular layer of the body.
Intravenous (IV) therapy	*intra-:* within *ven/o:* vein *-ous:* pertaining to	The administration of a liquid agent directly into a patient's vein, where it is distributed throughout the body by way of the circulatory system.
Oral administration		Administration of medication by mouth.
Parenteral		Administration of medication by injection.
Pharmacology	*pharmac/o:* drugs *-ology:* study of	The study of drugs.

Continued

TERMINOLOGY REVIEW—cont'd

Key Term	Word Parts	Definition
Prescription		An order from a licensed provider authorizing the dispensing of a drug by a pharmacist.
Signatura		The part of a prescription that indicates the information to print on the medication label.
Subcutaneous injection	*sub-:* under, below *cutane/o:* skin *-ous:* pertaining to	Introduction of medication beneath the skin, into the subcutaneous or fatty layer of the body.
Sublingual administration	*sub-:* under, below *lingu/o:* tongue *-al:* pertaining to	Administration of medication by placing it under the tongue, where it dissolves and is absorbed through the mucous membrane.
Subscription	*sub-:* under, below	The part of the prescription that gives directions to the pharmacist and usually designates the number of doses to be dispensed.
Superscription	*super-:* over, above	The part of a prescription consisting of the abbreviation (from the Latin word *recipe,* meaning "take").
Topical administration		Application of a drug to a particular spot, usually for a local action.
Transfusion	*trans-:* through, across	The administration of whole blood or blood products by the intravenous route.
Vial		A closed glass container with a rubber stopper that holds medication.
Wheal		A tense, pale, raised area of the skin.

PROCEDURE 11.1 Administering Oral Medication

Outcome Administer oral solid and liquid medications.

Equipment/Supplies

- Medication ordered by the provider
- Medication order
- Medicine cup
- Medication tray

1. **Procedural Step.** Sanitize your hands.
2. **Procedural Step.** Assemble the equipment.
3. **Procedural Step.** Work in a quiet, well-lit atmosphere.
   Principle. Good lighting aids the medical assistant in reading the medication label.
4. **Procedural Step.** Select the correct medication from the shelf. Compare the medication with the provider's instructions and medication order. Check the drug label three times—while removing the medication from storage, while preparing the medication, and after preparing the medication. Check the expiration date.
   Principle. If the medication is outdated, consult the provider because it may produce undesirable effects for which the medical assistant could be held responsible. To prevent a drug error, the medication should be carefully compared with the provider's instructions.

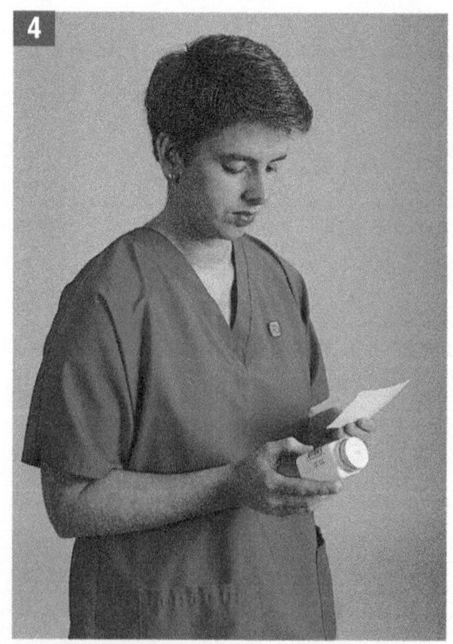

Compare the medication with the provider's instructions.

PROCEDURE 11.1 Administering Oral Medication—cont'd

5. **Procedural Step.** Calculate the correct dose to be given, if necessary.
6. **Procedural Step.** Remove the bottle cap, touching the outside of the lid only.
   Principle. Touching the inside of the lid contaminates it.
7. **Procedural Step.** Check the drug label again, and pour the medication.
   Solid medications: Pour the correct number of capsules or tablets into the bottle cap. Transfer the medication to a medicine cup, being careful not to touch the inside of the cup.
   Principle. Pouring the medication into the lid prevents contamination of the medication and lid.
   Liquid medications: Place the lid of the bottle on a flat surface with the open end facing up. Palm the surface of the label.
   With the opposite hand, place the thumbnail at the proper calibration on the medicine cup, and hold the cup at eye level. Pour the medication, and read the dose at the lowest level of the meniscus. (The meniscus is the curved surface of the liquid in a container. When a liquid is poured into a medicine cup, capillary action causes the liquid in contact with the cup to be drawn upward, resulting in a curved surface in the middle.)
   Principle. Placing the bottle cap with the open end up prevents contamination of the inside of the cap. Palming the medication label prevents the medication from dripping on the label and obscuring it.

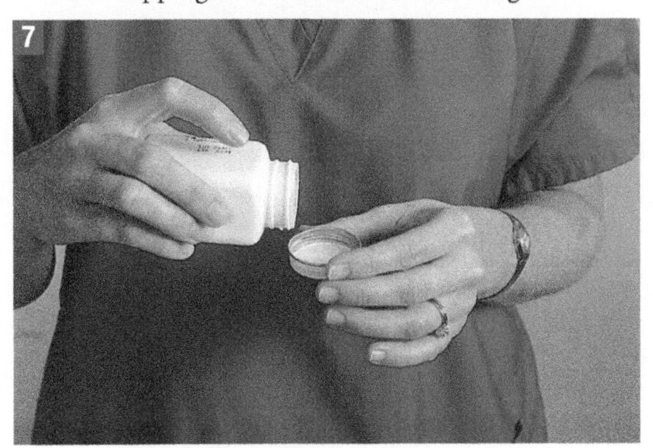

Pour the correct number of capsules or tablets into the bottle cap.

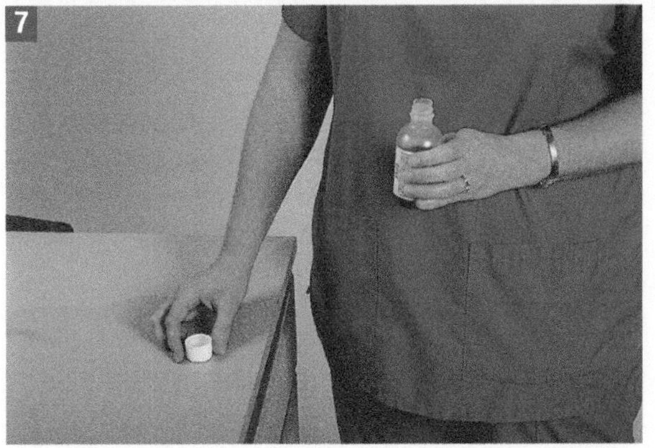

Place the lid of the bottle on a flat surface with the open end facing up.

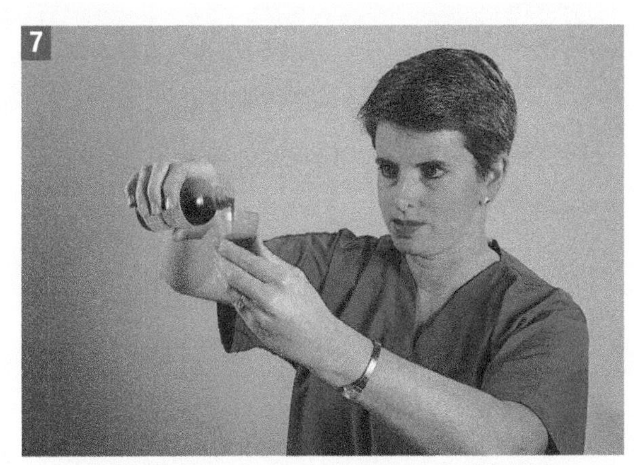

Hold the cup at eye level, and pour the medication.

8. **Procedural Step.** Replace the bottle cap, and check the drug label a third time to ensure it is the correct medication. Return the medication to its storage location.
9. **Procedural Step.** Greet the patient and introduce yourself. Identify the patient by full name and date of birth and explain the procedure. Explain the purpose of administering the medication.
   Principle. It is crucial that no error be made in patient identity.
10. **Procedural Step.** Hand the medicine cup containing the medication to the patient, along with a glass of water. (If the medication is a cough syrup, do not offer water.)
    Principle. Water helps the patient swallow the medication.
11. **Procedural Step.** Remain with the patient until the medication is swallowed. If the patient experiences any unusual reaction, notify the provider.
12. **Procedural Step.** Sanitize your hands.

Continued

PROCEDURE 11.1 Administering Oral Medication—cont'd

13. **Procedural Step.** Document the procedure in the patient's medical record.
    a. *Electronic health record (EHR):* Document the name of the medication, the dose given, the route of administration, and any significant observations or patient reactions, using the appropriate radio buttons, drop-down menus, and free text fields.
    b. *Paper-based patient record:* Document the date and time, the name of the medication, the dose given, the route of administration, and any significant observations or patient reactions. The Latin abbreviation *po,* which means "by mouth," can be used to indicate the route of administration (refer to the PPR documentation example).

PPR Documentation Example

Date	
2/12/XX	9:30 a.m. Acetaminophen, 650 mg, po.
	——————— T. Cline, CMA (AAMA)

PROCEDURE 11.2 Preparing an Injection

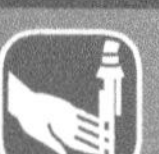

Outcome Prepare an injection from an ampule and a vial.

Equipment/Supplies

- Medication ordered by the provider
- Medication order
- Appropriate needle and syringe
- Antiseptic wipe
- Medication tray

1. **Procedural Step.** Sanitize your hands.
2. **Procedural Step.** Assemble the equipment.
3. **Procedural Step.** Work in a quiet and well-lit atmosphere.
   Principle. Good lighting aids the medical assistant in reading the medication label.
4. **Procedural Step.** Select the proper medication. Compare the medication with the provider's instructions. Check the drug label three times—while removing the medication from storage, before withdrawing the medication into the syringe, and after preparing the medication. Check the expiration date.
   Principle. The medication should be carefully identified to prevent administration of the wrong medication. Outdated medication should not be used because it could produce undesirable effects.

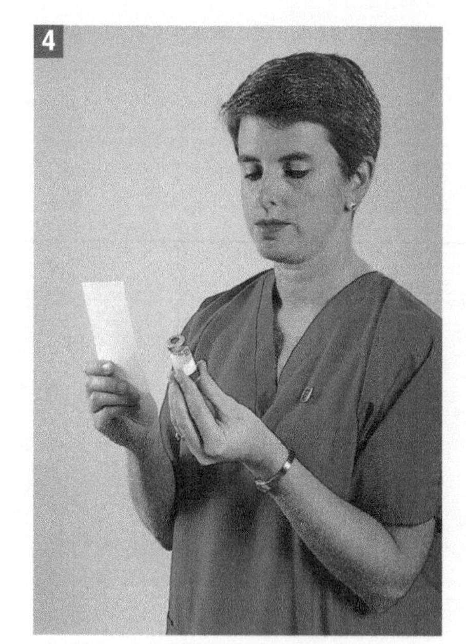

Compare the medication with the provider's instructions.

PROCEDURE 11.2 Preparing an Injection—cont'd

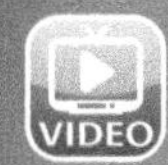

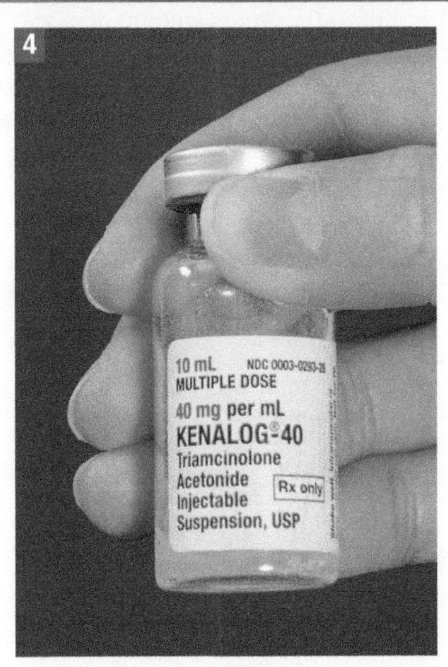

Check the drug label three times.

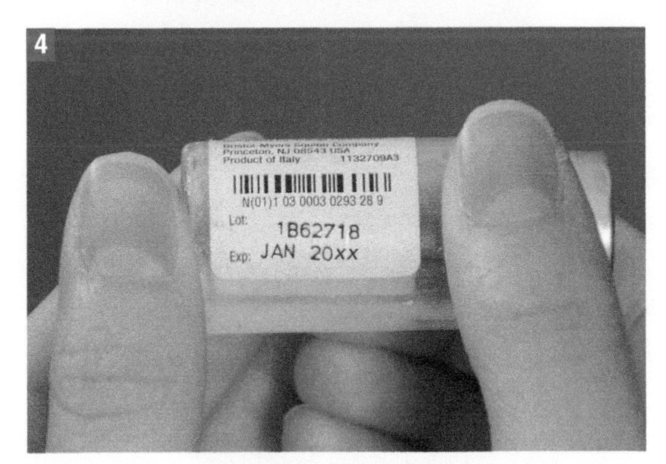

Check the expiration date.

5. Procedural Step. Calculate the correct dose to be given, if necessary. If you have any questions regarding the administration of the medication, check the package insert accompanying the drug.

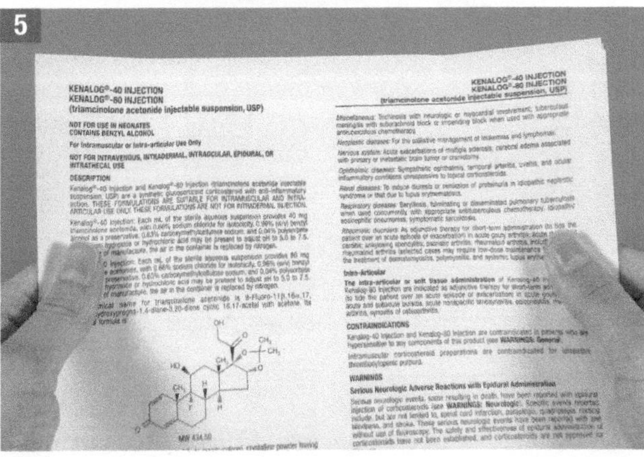
KENALOG®-40 INJECTION
KENALOG®-80 INJECTION
(triamcinolone acetonide injectable suspension, USP)
NOT FOR USE IN NEONATES
CONTAINS BENZYL ALCOHOL
For Intramuscular or Intra-articular Use Only
NOT FOR INTRAVENOUS, INTRADERMAL, INTRAOCULAR, EPIDURAL, OR INTRATHECAL USE
DESCRIPTION
Intra-Articular
CONTRAINDICATIONS
WARNINGS

Check the package insert.

6. Procedural Step. Open the syringe and the needle package. If necessary, assemble the needle and syringe.
Principle. Disposable needles and syringes may come already assembled together in a package or in separate packages that require assembly of the needle and syringe.

7. Procedural Step. Check to ensure that the needle is attached firmly to the syringe by loosening the guard on the needle, grasping the needle at the hub, and tightening it. Break the seal on the syringe by moving the plunger back and forth several times.

8. Procedural Step. Check the drug label again to ensure it is the correct medication. If required, mix the medication by rolling the vial between your hands to obtain a uniform suspension of the medication.

9. Procedural Step. Withdraw the medication following these steps.

Withdrawing Medication from a Vial

a. Procedural Step. Remove the soft metal or plastic cap protecting the rubber stopper of an unused vial to expose the rubber stopper. Open the antiseptic; wipe and cleanse the rubber stopper and allow it to dry.
Principle. Cleansing the top of the vial removes dust and bacteria. The alcohol must be allowed to dry to prevent it from adhering to the needle and mixing with the medication.

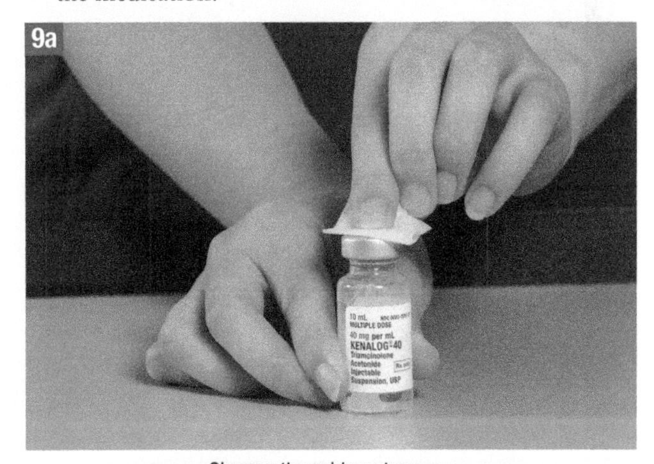

Cleanse the rubber stopper.

b. Procedural Step. Place the vial in an upright position on a flat surface. Remove the needle guard. Pull back on the plunger to draw an amount of air into the syringe equal to the amount of medication to be withdrawn from the vial.
Principle. Air must be injected into the vial first to prevent the formation of a partial vacuum in the vial, which would make it difficult to remove medication.

Continued

Procedure 11.2

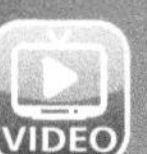

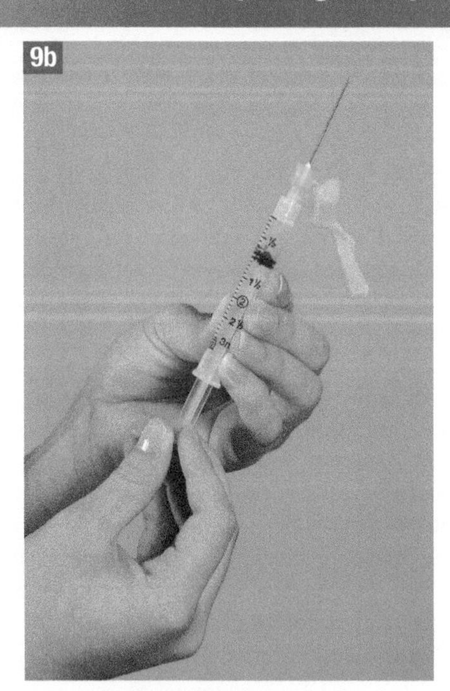

Draw the air into the syringe.

c. Procedural Step. With the vial on a flat surface, use moderate pressure on the barrel of the syringe to insert the needle through the center of the rubber stopper at a 90-degree angle. Continue to apply pressure until the needle reaches the empty space between the stopper and fluid level. Be careful not to bend the needle. Push down on the plunger to inject the air into the vial, keeping the needle opening above the fluid level. (*Note:* If you are using a retractable safety syringe, do not push too hard on the plunger to avoid activating the retracting mechanism prematurely.)

Principle. The center of the rubber stopper is thinner and easier to penetrate. The air must be inserted above the fluid level to avoid creating air bubbles in the medication.

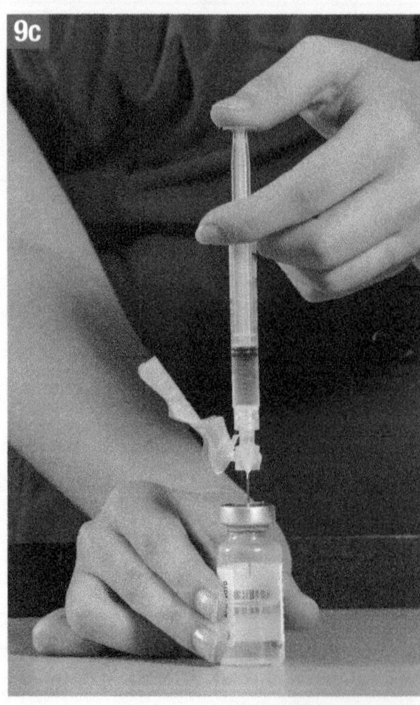

Inject air into the vial.

d. Procedural Step. Invert the vial while holding onto the syringe and plunger. Hold the syringe at eye level, and withdraw the proper amount of medication. The medication should be measured at the widest part of the plunger seal closest to the needle. Make sure to keep the needle opening below the fluid level.

Principle. The needle opening must be below the fluid level to prevent the entrance of air bubbles into the syringe.

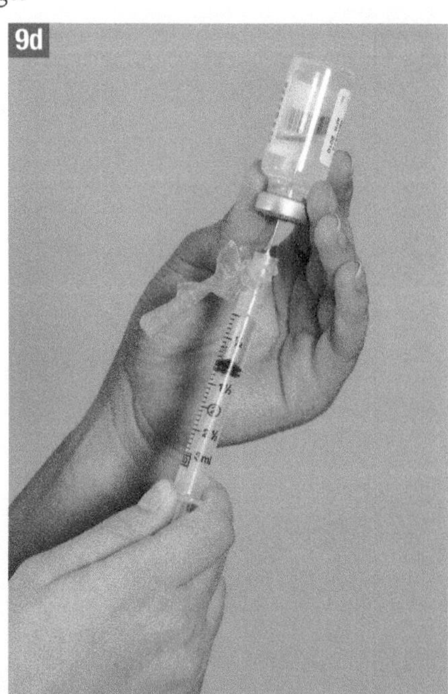

Withdraw the proper amount of medication.

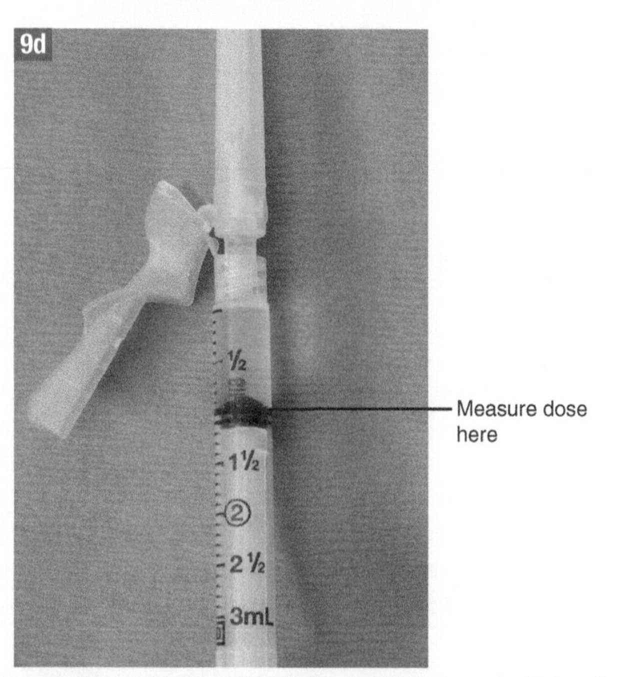

Measure the medication at the widest part of the plunger seal closest to the needle.

e. Procedural Step. Remove any air bubbles in the syringe by holding the syringe in a vertical position

PROCEDURE 11.2 Preparing an Injection—cont'd

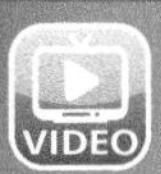

and tapping the barrel carefully with the fingertips until they disappear.

Principle. Tapping the barrel too forcefully could cause the needle to bend. Air bubbles take up space the medication should occupy, preventing the patient from getting the proper dose of medication.

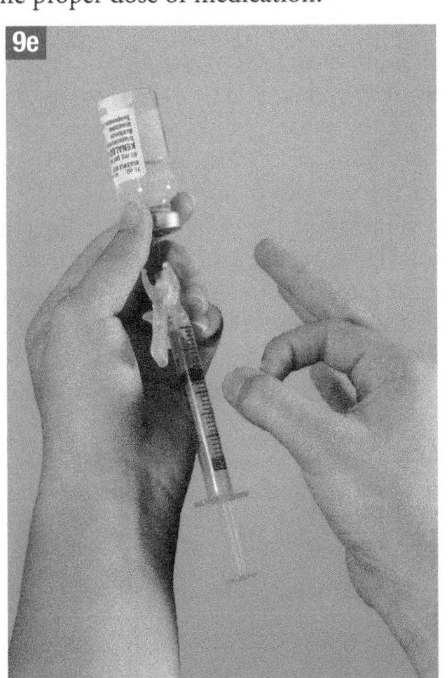

Tap the barrel with the fingertips to remove air bubbles.

f. **Procedural Step.** Remove any air remaining at the top of the syringe by slowly pushing the plunger forward and allowing the air to flow back into the vial.

g. **Procedural Step.** Holding the syringe at eye level, check again to make sure you have drawn up the proper amount of medication. Carefully remove the needle from the rubber stopper, and replace the needle guard. (*Note:* After drawing up the medication, some facilities require that the needle used to draw up the medication be removed from the syringe and replaced with a new sterile needle. This is because the point of the needle may not be as sharp after it has been inserted into rubber stopper of the medication vial. The medical assistant should follow the policy set forth by his or her medical office.)

Principle. The needle must remain sterile. The needle guard prevents the needle from becoming contaminated.

h. **Procedural Step.** Check the drug label for the third time, and return the medication to its proper storage location.

Withdrawing Medication from an Ampule

a. **Procedural Step.** Remove the needle (and needle guard) from the syringe, and attach a filter needle (and needle guard).

b. **Procedural Step.** Open the antiseptic wipe, and cleanse the neck of the ampule.

Principle. Cleansing the neck of the ampule removes dust and bacteria.

c. **Procedural Step.** Tap the stem of the ampule lightly to remove any medication in the neck of the ampule.

d. **Procedural Step.** Check the medication label a second time and place a piece of gauze around the neck of the ampule. Hold the base of the ampule between the first two fingers and the thumb of one hand. Hold the neck of the vial between the first two fingers and the thumb of the other hand. Apply a strong steady pressure with the thumbs, and break off the stem by snapping it quickly and firmly away from the body. Discard the stem and gauze in a biohazard sharps container.

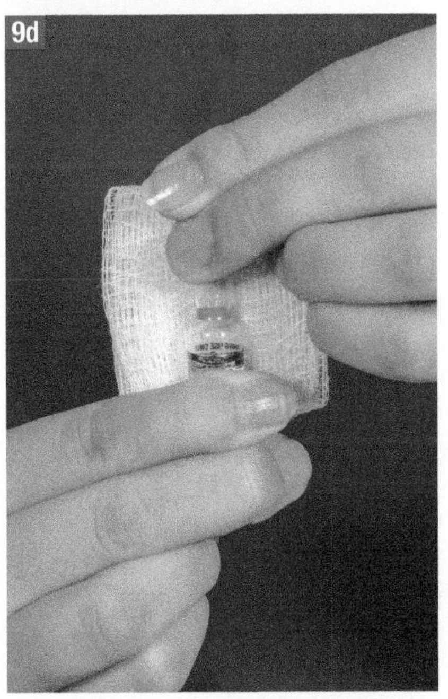

Snap the stem away from the body.

e. **Procedural Step.** Place the ampule on a flat surface. Remove the needle guard. Insert the filter needle opening below the fluid level.

Principle. The filter needle prevents glass particles from being withdrawn into the syringe.

f. **Procedural Step.** Withdraw the proper amount of medication by pulling back on the plunger. The medication should be measured at the widest part of the plunger seal closest to the needle. Make sure to keep the needle opening below the fluid level to prevent the entrance of air bubbles into the syringe. Tilt the ampule as needed to keep the needle opening immersed in the fluid.

Note: There is another method that can be used to remove medication from an ampule. Choose the method that is easiest for you. To perform this method, invert the

Continued

PROCEDURE 11.2 Preparing an Injection—cont'd

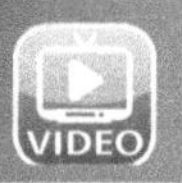

ampule, making sure to keep the needle opening below the fluid level. Withdraw the proper amount of medication by pulling back on the plunger. Move the needle downward as necessary to keep the needle opening immersed in the fluid.

Principle. Air bubbles take up space the medication should occupy, resulting in an inaccurate measurement of medication.

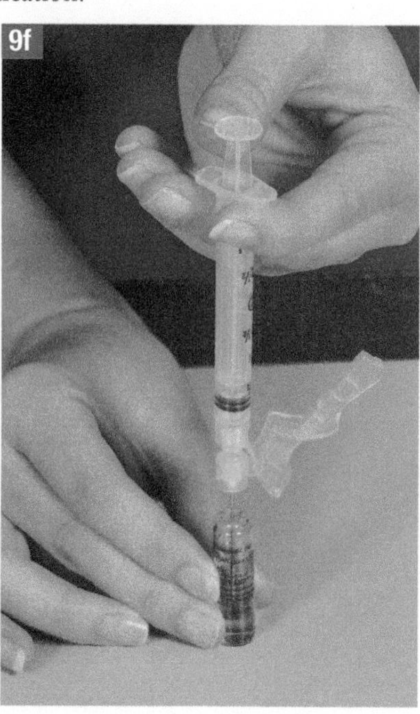

Withdraw the medication.

g. **Procedural Step.** Remove the needle from the ampule, and replace the needle guard. Check the drug label for the third time, and dispose of the glass ampule in a biohazard sharps container.

h. **Procedural Step.** Remove the filter needle (and guard) from the syringe, and discard it in a biohazard sharps container. Reapply the needle (and guard) for administering the medication.

i. **Procedural Step.** If air bubbles are in the syringe, remove the needle guard, hold the syringe in a vertical position, and tap the barrel with the fingertips until the bubbles disappear. Remove the air at the top of the syringe by slowly pushing the plunger forward. If the syringe contains excess fluid, hold the syringe vertically over a sink with the needle tip up and slanted toward the sink. Slowly eject the excess fluid into the sink. Holding the syringe at eye level, check again to make sure you have drawn up the proper amount of medication. Replace the needle guard.

PROCEDURE 11.3 Reconstituting Powdered Drugs

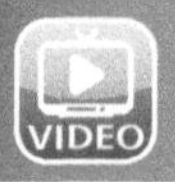

Outcome Reconstitute a powdered drug for parenteral administration.

Equipment/Supplies

- Medication ordered by the provider
- Medication order
- Appropriate needle and syringe
- Antiseptic wipe
- Medication tray

1. **Procedural Step.** Follow steps 1 through 8 of Procedure 11.2.
2. **Procedural Step.** From the vial of the powdered drug, withdraw an amount of air equal to the amount of liquid to be injected into the vial.

   Principle. Removing air from the powdered drug vial allows room for injection of the diluent.
3. **Procedural Step.** Inject the air removed from the powdered drug vial into the vial of diluent.

   Principle. Air must be injected into the vial to prevent formation of a partial vacuum in the vial, which would make it difficult to remove the diluent.
4. **Procedural Step.** Invert the diluent vial, and withdraw the proper amount of liquid into the syringe. Remove air bubbles from the syringe. Holding the syringe at eye level, check again to make sure you have drawn up the proper amount of diluent. Carefully remove the needle from the vial.

PROCEDURE 11.3 Reconstituting Powdered Drugs—cont'd

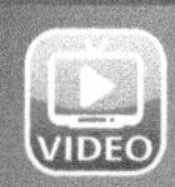

5. Procedural Step. Insert the needle into the powdered drug vial, and inject the diluent into the vial. Remove the needle from the vial, and replace the needle guard.

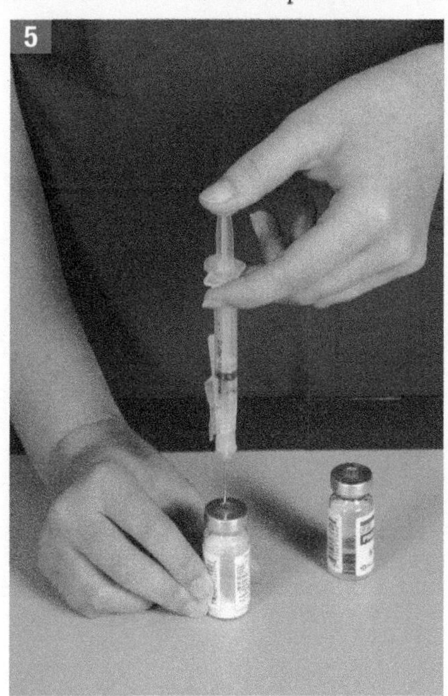

Inject the diluent into the vial.

6. Procedural Step. Roll the vial between the hands to mix the powdered drug and liquid (unless indicated otherwise by the drug package insert).

Principle. Shaking the vial may cause air bubbles to form.

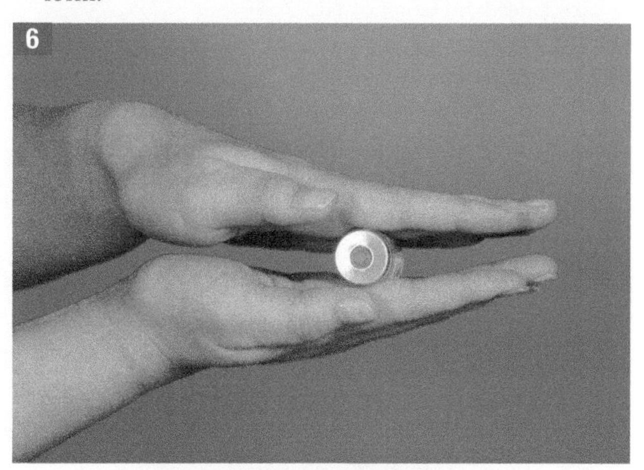

Roll the vial between the hands.

7. **Procedural Step.** Label multiple-dose vials with the date of preparation and your initials.
8. **Procedural Step.** Prepare the medication and administer the injection.
9. **Procedural Step.** Store multiple-dose vials as indicated by the manufacturer's instructions. Because reconstituted drugs are stable for a short time, carefully check the date of preparation on the multiple-dose vial before administering the medication again.

PROCEDURE 11.4 Administering a Subcutaneous Injection

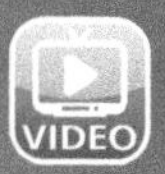

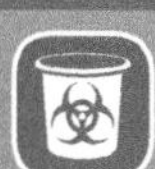

Outcome Administer a subcutaneous injection.

Equipment/Supplies

- Medication ordered by the provider
- Medication order
- Appropriate needle and syringe
- Antiseptic wipe
- Sterile 2 × 2 gauze pad
- Disposable gloves
- Biohazard sharps container

1. **Procedural Step.** Sanitize your hands, and prepare the injection (see Procedure 11.2).
2. **Procedural Step.** Greet the patient and introduce yourself. Identify the patient by full name and date of birth. Explain the procedure and the purpose of the injection.

   Principle. It is crucial that no error be made in patient identity. An apprehensive patient may need reassurance.
3. **Procedural Step.** Select an appropriate injection site. The upper arm, thigh, back, and abdomen are recommended sites for a subcutaneous injection. See Fig. 11.17.

   Principle. The entire area should be exposed to ensure a safe and comfortable injection.
4. **Procedural Step.** Prepare the injection site. Cleanse the area with an antiseptic wipe. Using a circular motion, start with the injection site and move outward. Do not touch the site after cleansing it.

   Principle. Using a circular motion carries contaminants away from the injection site. Touching the site

Continued

PROCEDURE 11.4 Administering a Subcutaneous Injection—cont'd

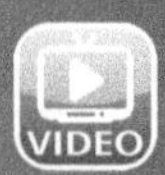

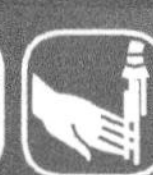

after cleansing contaminates it, and the cleansing process needs to be repeated.

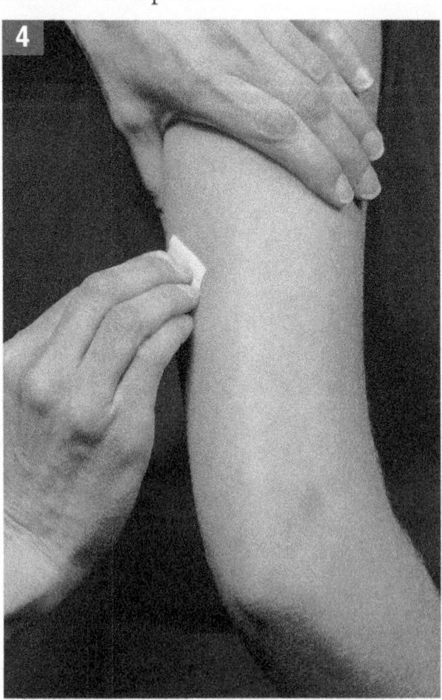

Cleanse the area with an antiseptic wipe.

5. **Procedural Step.** Allow the area to dry completely.
   Principle. If the area is not permitted to dry, the antiseptic may enter the tissues when the skin is pierced, resulting in irritation and patient discomfort.
6. **Procedural Step.** Apply gloves, and remove the needle guard. Position your nondominant hand on the area surrounding the injection site. The skin may be held taut, or the area surrounding the injection site may be grasped and held in a cushion fashion.
   Principle. Gloves provide a barrier against bloodborne pathogens. In normal adults the needle enters the subcutaneous tissue when the skin is held taut. Grasping the area around the injection site is recommended for a thin or dehydrated patient. This ensures that the subcutaneous tissue, and not muscle tissue, is entered.

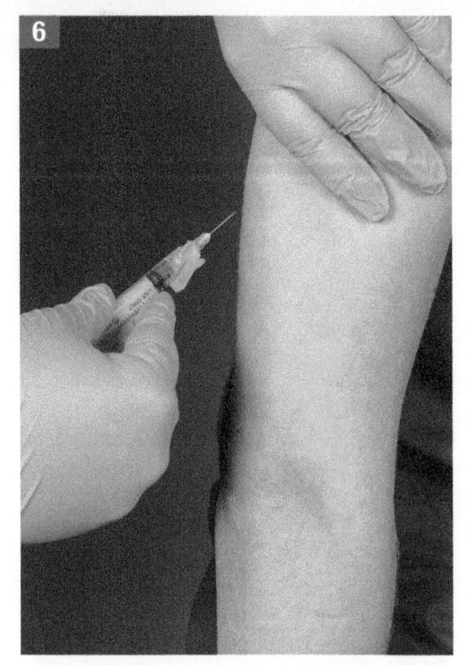

Grasp the area surrounding the injection site.

7. **Procedural Step.** Hold the barrel of the syringe between your thumb and index finger. Insert the needle quickly and smoothly at a 45-degree or 90-degree angle, depending on the length of the needle. With a 1/2-inch needle, a 90-degree angle should be used; with a 5/8-inch needle, a 45-degree angle should be used. Insert the needle to the hub.
   Principle. Inserting the needle quickly and smoothly minimizes tissue trauma and pain. Needle length determines the angle of insertion to ensure placement of the medication in subcutaneous tissue.

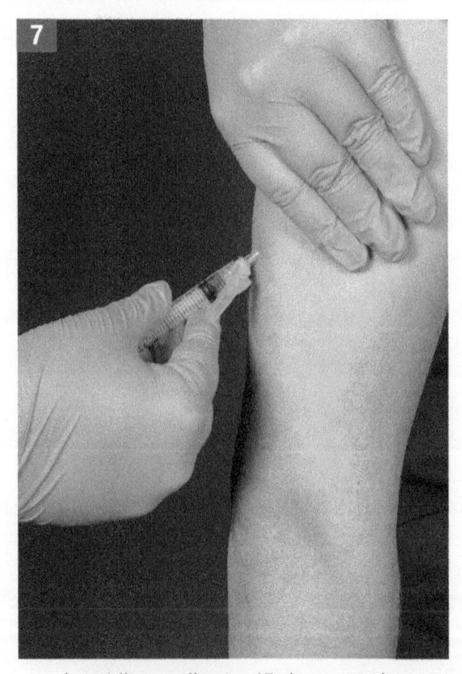

Insert the needle at a 45-degree angle.

Procedure 11.4

PROCEDURE 11.4 Administering a Subcutaneous Injection—cont'd

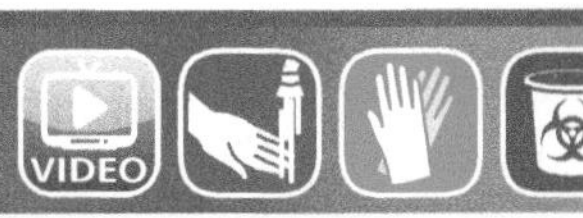

8. **Procedural Step.** Remove your hand from the skin.
   Principle. Medication injected into compressed tissue causes pressure against nerve fibers and is uncomfortable for the patient.
9. **Procedural Step.** Inject the medication slowly and steadily by depressing the plunger while holding the syringe steady. If you are using a retractable safety syringe, activate it at this time by following the steps outlined in Fig. 11.10C, and continue to Step 12.

(*Note:* Unless otherwise required by the package insert accompanying the medication to be administered or by your medical office policy, aspiration of the syringe for blood is not necessary because there are no large blood vessels located in subcutaneous tissue).

Principle. Rapid injection creates pressure and destroys tissue, both of which are uncomfortable for the patient. Moving the syringe after the needle has entered the tissue causes patient discomfort.

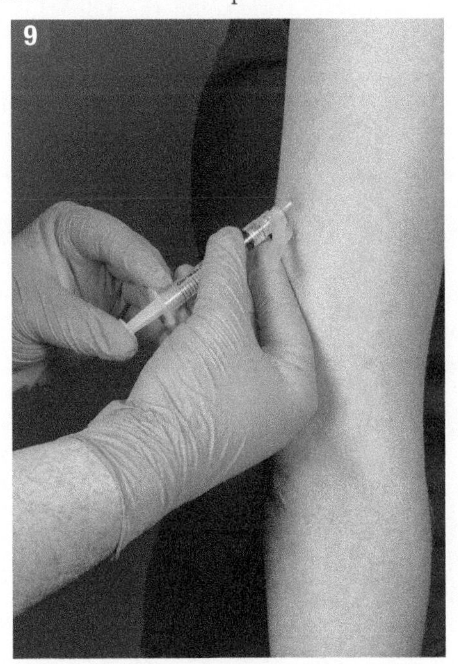

Inject the medication slowly and steadily.

10. **Procedural Step.** Place a gauze pad gently over the injection site and quickly remove the needle, keeping it at the same angle as for insertion.
    Principle. Withdrawing the needle quickly and at the same angle as for insertion reduces patient discomfort. The gauze pad placed over the injection site helps prevent tissue movement as the needle is withdrawn, reducing patient discomfort.
11. **Procedural Step.** Apply gentle pressure to the injection site with a gauze pad. If you are using a safety syringe with a shield or sliding-sleeve, activate the safety feature at this time by following the steps outlined in Fig. 11.10.
    Principle. Gentle pressure helps distribute the medication so that it is completely absorbed. Avoid vigorous massaging because this could damage underlying tissue.
12. **Procedural Step.** Properly dispose of the needle and syringe in a biohazard sharps container.
    Principle. Proper disposal is required by the OSHA standard to prevent accidental needlestick injuries.
13. **Procedural Step.** Remove gloves, and sanitize your hands.
14. **Procedural Step.** Document the procedure in the patient's medical record.
    a. *Electronic health record (EHR):* Document the name of the medication, the manufacturer and lot number (if required), the dose given, the route of administration, the injection site used, and any significant observations or patient reactions, using the appropriate radio buttons, drop-down menus, and free text fields.
    b. *Paper-based patient record:* Document the date and time, the name of the medication, the manufacturer and lot number (if required), the dose given, the route of administration, the injection site used, and any significant observations or patient reactions (refer to the PPR documentation example).

    Principle. The lot number indicates the batch in which the medication was made. Should a problem arise with that batch, the drug can be recalled, and the individuals who received it can be identified.
15. **Procedural Step.** Stay with the patient to ensure that he or she is not experiencing any unusual reactions. (*Note:* If an allergy injection has been given, the patient should remain at the medical office for 15–20 min to ensure that an allergic reaction does not occur.) Check the patient's arm after the waiting period, and observe for induration and redness. If the patient experiences such a reaction, notify the provider immediately. Document the inspection of the injection site in the patient's medical record.

PPR Documentation Example

Date	
2/17/XX	3:30 p.m. Ragweed allergy inj, 0.20 mL, subcut, Ⓡ
	upper arm. Arm checked 15 min. after admin. No
	reaction noted. ______T. Cline, CMA (AAMA)

PROCEDURE 11.5 Administering an Intramuscular Injection

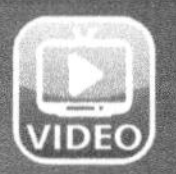

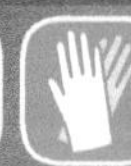

Outcome Administer an intramuscular injection.

Equipment/Supplies

- Medication ordered by the provider
- Medication order
- Appropriate needle and syringe
- Antiseptic wipe
- Sterile 2 × 2 gauze pad
- Disposable gloves
- Biohazard sharps container

1. **Procedural Step.** Sanitize your hands, and prepare the injection (see Procedure 11.2).
2. **Procedural Step.** Greet the patient and introduce yourself. Identify the patient by his or her full name and date of birth. Explain the procedure and purpose of the injection.
   Principle. Make sure that you administer the medication to the right patient. Explain the purpose of the injection. Assistance may be needed for restraining infants and children.
3. **Procedural Step.** Select an appropriate intramuscular (IM) injection site. See Fig. 11.18 for the recommended intramuscular injection sites. Remove the patient's clothing as necessary to ensure the entire area is exposed.
   Principle. The medical assistant should develop skill and accuracy in locating the proper sites.
4. **Procedural Step.** Prepare the injection site. Cleanse the area with an antiseptic wipe. Using a circular motion, start with the injection site and move outward. Do not touch the site after cleansing it.
   Principle. Using a circular motion carries contaminants away from the injection site. Touching the site after cleansing contaminates it, and the cleansing process needs to be repeated.

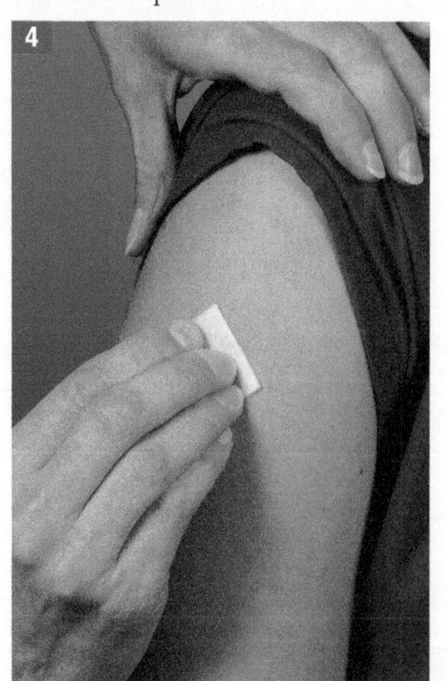
4

Cleanse the site with an antiseptic wipe.

5. **Procedural Step.** Allow the area to dry completely.
   Principle. If the area is not permitted to dry, the antiseptic may enter the tissues when the skin is pierced, resulting in irritation and patient discomfort.
6. **Procedural Step.** Apply gloves, and remove the needle guard. Using the thumb and first two fingers of the nondominant hand, stretch the skin taut over the injection site.
   Principle. Gloves provide a barrier against bloodborne pathogens. Stretching the skin taut permits easier insertion of the needle and helps ensure that the needle enters muscle tissue.
7. **Procedural Step.** Hold the barrel of the syringe like a dart, and insert the needle quickly and smoothly at a 90-degree angle to the patient's skin with a firm motion. Insert the needle to the hub.
   Principle. The needle is inserted at a 90-degree angle and to the hub to ensure that it reaches muscle tissue. Inserting the needle quickly and smoothly minimizes tissue trauma and pain.

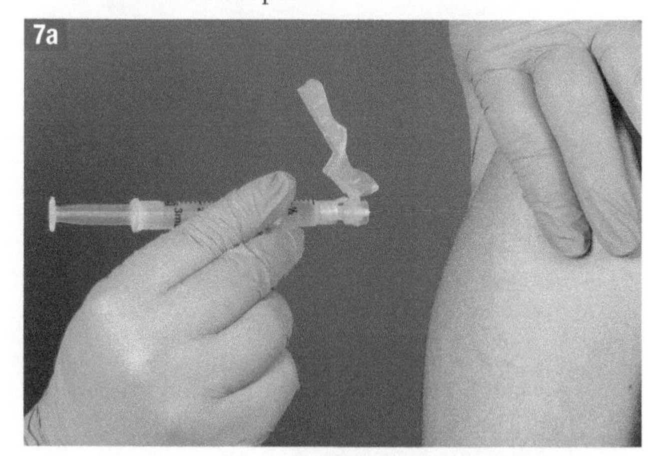
7a

Insert the needle at a 90-degree angle (deltoid site).

PROCEDURE 11.5 Administering an Intramuscular Injection—cont'd

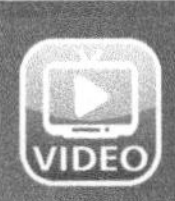

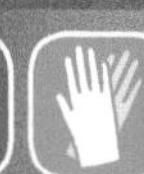

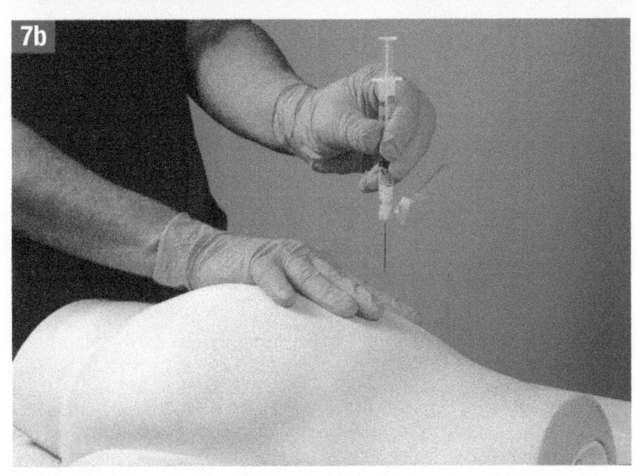

7b Insert the needle at a 90-degree angle (ventrogluteal site).

8. Procedural Step. Hold the syringe steady, and pull back gently on the plunger for 5–10 s to determine whether the needle is in a blood vessel. If blood appears, withdraw the needle, prepare a new injection, and begin again. (Note: Some IM injections (e.g., vaccines) do not require aspiration. The medical assistant should review the drug package insert and follow the aspiration recommendations stated by the manufacturer).

Principle. Moving the syringe after the needle has penetrated the tissue causes patient discomfort. If the needle is in a small blood vessel, it takes 5–10 s for the blood to appear in the syringe. If drugs intended for intramuscular administration are injected into a blood vessel, the result is faster absorption of the medication. This may produce undesirable results.

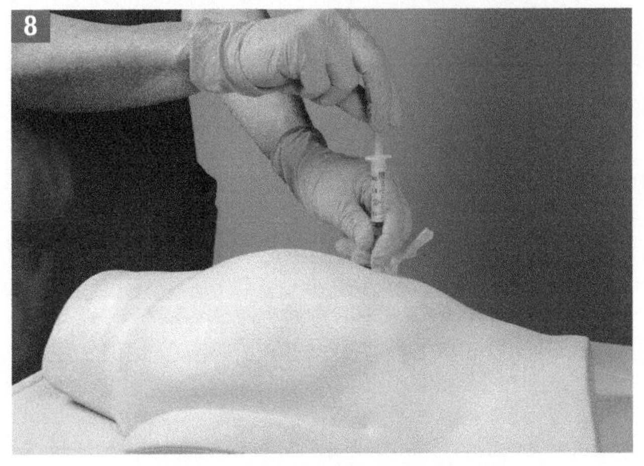

8 Aspirate to determine if the needle is in a blood vessel.

9. Procedural Step. Inject the medication slowly and steadily by depressing the plunger. If you are using a retractable safety syringe, activate it at this time while following the steps outlined in Fig. 11.10, *C*, and continue to Step 11.

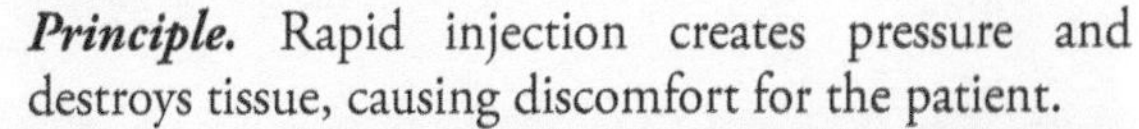

Principle. Rapid injection creates pressure and destroys tissue, causing discomfort for the patient.

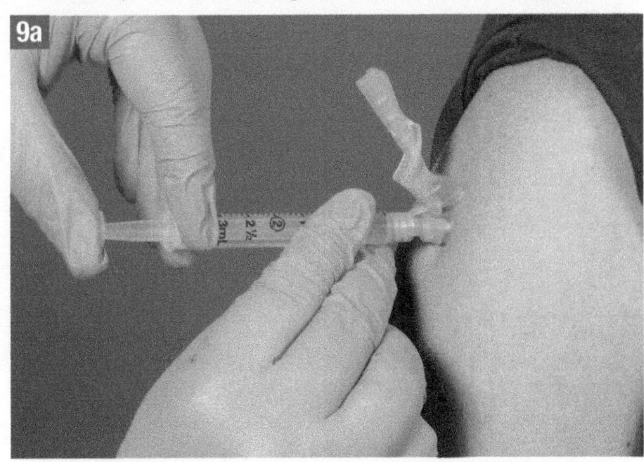

9a Inject the medication slowly and steadily (deltoid site).

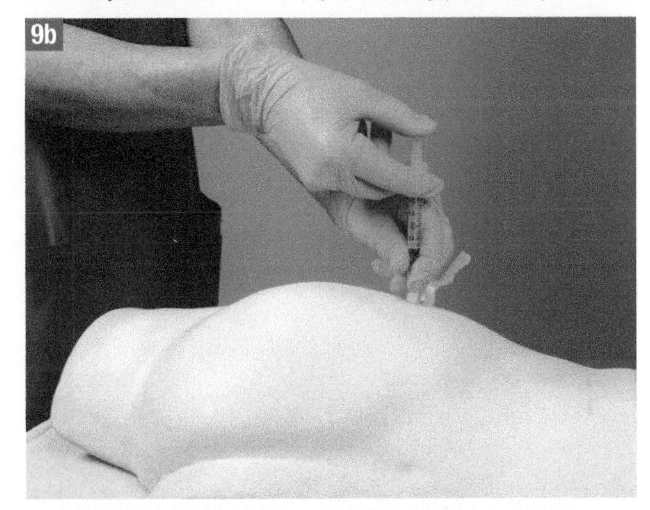

9b Inject the medication slowly and steadily (ventrogluteal site).

10. Procedural Step. Place a gauze pad gently over the injection site and remove the needle quickly, keeping it at the same angle as for insertion.

Principle. Withdrawing the needle quickly and at the same angle as for insertion reduces patient discomfort. Placing a gauze pad over the injection site helps prevent tissue movement as the needle is withdrawn, also reducing patient discomfort. Using a gauze pad prevents a stinging sensation from the alcohol.

11. Procedural Step. Apply gentle pressure to the injection site with a gauze pad. If you are using a safety syringe with a shield or sliding-sleeve, activate the safety feature at this time by following the steps outlined in Fig. 11.10.

Principle. Gentle pressure helps distribute the medication so that it is absorbed by the muscle tissue. Avoid vigorous massaging because this could damage underlying tissues.

Continued

PROCEDURE 11.5 Administering an Intramuscular Injection—cont'd

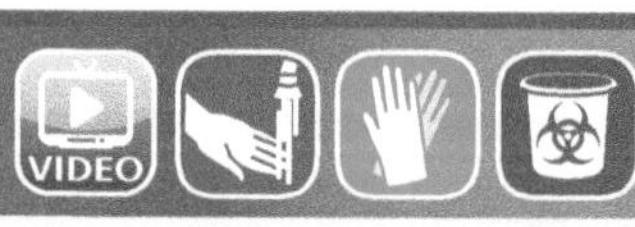

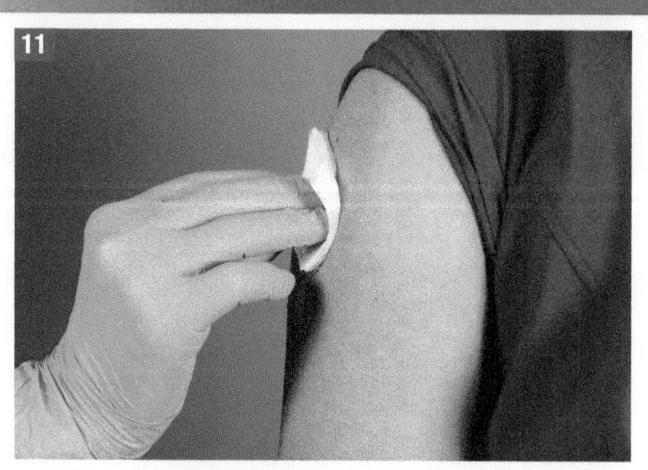

Apply gentle pressure to the injection site.

12. **Procedural Step.** Properly dispose of the needle and syringe in a biohazard sharps container.
    Principle. Proper disposal is required by the OSHA standard to prevent accidental needlestick injuries.
13. **Procedural Step.** Remove the gloves, and sanitize your hands.
14. **Procedural Step.** Document the procedure in the patient's medical record.
    a. *Electronic health record (EHR):* Document the name of the medication, the manufacturer and lot number, the dose given, the route of administration, the injection site used, and any significant observations or patient reactions, using the appropriate radio buttons, drop-down menus, and free text fields.
    b. *Paper-based patient record:* Document the date and time, the name of the medication, the manufacturer and lot number, the dose given, the route of administration, the injection site used, and any significant observations or patient reactions (refer to the PPR documentation example).

    Principle. The lot number indicates the batch in which the medication was made. Should a problem arise with that batch, the drug can be recalled, and individuals who received it can be identified.
15. **Procedural Step.** Stay with the patient to ensure he or she is not experiencing any unusual reactions. If the patient experiences an unusual reaction, notify the provider immediately.

PPR Documentation Example

Date	
2/20/XX	9:30 a.m. Rocephin (Hoffmann-LaRoche, Lot #: U6261).
	Admin 1 gram, IM, Ⓡ deltoid. Tolerated
	injection well.——————T. Cline, CMA (AAMA)

PROCEDURE 11.6 Z-Track Intramuscular Injection Technique

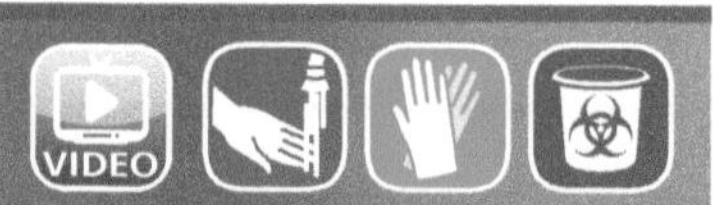

Outcome Administer an intramuscular injection using the Z-track method.

Equipment/Supplies

- Medication ordered by the provider
- Medication order
- Appropriate needle and syringe
- Antiseptic wipe
- Disposable gloves
- Biohazard sharps container

1. **Procedural Step.** Follow steps 1 through 5 of Procedure 11.5.
2. **Procedural Step.** Apply gloves, and remove the needle guard. With the nondominant hand, pull the skin away laterally from the injection site approximately 1–1 1/2 inches.
3. **Procedural Step.** Insert the needle quickly and smoothly at a 90-degree angle.
4. **Procedural Step.** If required, spirate for 5–10 s to determine whether the needle is in a blood vessel. If blood appears, withdraw the needle and discard the needle and syringe. Prepare another injection and begin again.
5. **Procedural Step.** Inject the medication slowly and steadily.
6. **Procedural Step.** After injecting the medication, wait 10 seconds before withdrawing the needle to allow initial absorption of the medication.
7. **Procedural Step.** Withdraw the needle quickly, keeping it at the same angle as for insertion.

PROCEDURE 11.6 Z-Track Intramuscular Injection Technique—cont'd

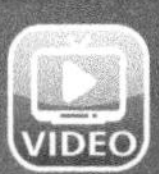
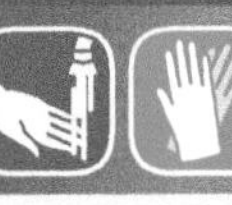

8. **Procedural Step.** Release the traction on the skin to seal off the needle track; doing so prevents the medication from reaching the subcutaneous tissue and skin surface.
9. **Procedural Step.** Do not apply pressure to the site because this could cause the medication to seep out.
10. **Procedural Step.** If you are using a safety syringe with a shield, activate the safety feature at this time by following the steps outlined in Fig. 11.10.
11. **Procedural Step.** Properly dispose of the needle and syringe in a biohazard sharps container.
12. **Procedural Step.** Remove your gloves, and sanitize your hands.
13. **Procedural Step.** Document the procedure in the patient's medical record.
    a. *Electronic health record (EHR):* Document the name of the medication, the manufacturer and lot number, the dose given, the route of administration, the injection site used, and any significant observations or patient reactions using the appropriate radio buttons, drop-down menus, and free text fields.
    b. *Paper-based patient record:* Document the date and time, the name of the medication, the manufacturer and lot number, the dose given, the route of administration, the injection site used, and any significant observations or patient reactions (refer to the PPR documentation example).
14. **Procedural Step.** Stay with the patient to ensure he or she is not experiencing any unusual reactions. If the patient experiences an unusual reaction, notify the provider immediately.

PPR Documentation Example

Date	
2/20/XX	10:30 a.m. Iron dextran (Watson Pharmaceuticals,
	Lot #: 1445). Admin 100 mg, IM, Z-track into Ⓡ
	ventrogluteal. No complaints of discomfort.———
	———————————— T. Cline, CMA (AAMA)

PROCEDURE 11.7 Administering an Intradermal Injection

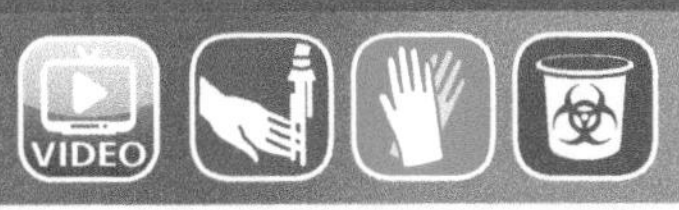

Outcome Administer an intradermal injection and read the test results.

Equipment/Supplies

- Skin test solution ordered by the provider
- Medication order
- Appropriate needle and syringe
- Antiseptic wipe
- Sterile 2 × 2 gauze pad
- Disposable gloves
- Millimeter ruler
- Tuberculosis (TB) skin test record card
- Biohazard sharps container

1. **Procedural Step.** Sanitize your hands and prepare the injection (see Procedure 11.2).
2. **Procedural Step.** Greet the patient and introduce yourself. Identify the patient by full name and date of birth. Explain the procedure and purpose of the injection.
   Principle. It is crucial that no error be made in patient identity. Explain the purpose of the injection to reassure an apprehensive patient.
3. **Procedural Step.** Select an appropriate injection site. The anterior forearm and the middle of the back are recommended sites for an intradermal injection. If using the anterior forearm, position the arm on a firm surface with the palm facing upward.
   Principle. The entire area should be exposed to ensure a safe and comfortable injection.
4. **Procedural Step.** Prepare the injection site. Cleanse the area with an antiseptic wipe. Using a circular motion, start with the injection site and move outward. Do not touch the site after cleansing it.
   Principle. Using a circular motion will carry material away from the injection site. Touching the site after cleansing will contaminate it, and the cleansing process will need to be repeated.
5. **Procedural Step.** Allow the area to dry completely.
   Principle. If the area is not permitted to dry, the antiseptic may enter the tissue when the skin is pierced, resulting in irritation and patient discomfort. In

Continued

PROCEDURE **11.7** **Administering an Intradermal Injection—cont'd**

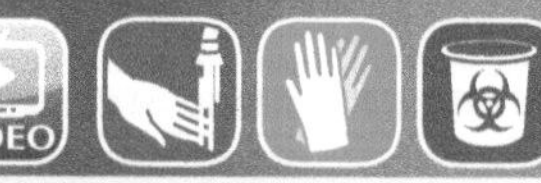
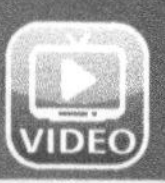

addition, the antiseptic may cause a reaction that could be mistaken for a positive test response.

6. **Procedural Step.** Apply gloves, and remove the needle guard. With the nondominant hand, stretch the skin taut at the proposed site of administration. Insert the needle at a 10- to 15-degree angle (almost parallel to the skin), with the bevel upward. The needle should be inserted about 1/8 inch until the bevel of the needle just penetrates the skin. Slight resistance may be felt as the needle is inserted. No aspiration is needed.
   Principle. Gloves provide a barrier against bloodborne pathogens. Stretching the patient's skin taut will permit easier insertion of the needle. The needle should be inserted at an angle almost parallel to the skin, to ensure penetration within the dermal layer of the skin. The needle must be inserted with the bevel facing up to allow proper wheal formation. If the needle is inserted with the bevel facing down, the skin test solution will be absorbed into the underlying subcutaneous tissue, and a wheal will not form.

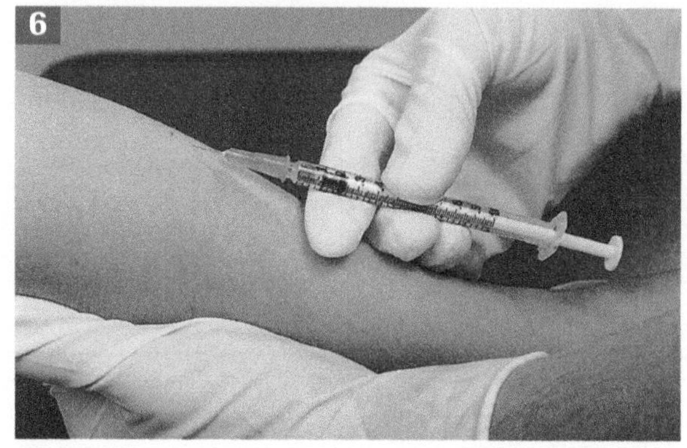

Insert the needle at a 10- to 15-degree angle with the bevel upward.

7. **Procedural Step.** Release the stretched skin. Hold the syringe steady, and inject the skin test solution slowly and steadily by depressing the plunger until a firm, tense, pale wheal forms (approximately 6–10 mm in diameter). Expect to feel a certain amount of resistance as you inject the solution; this helps in indicating that the needle is properly located in the superficial skin layers rather than in the deeper subcutaneous tissue. If a wheal does not form, the test must be repeated at another site that is at least 2 inches (5 cm) from the first site. If you are using a retractable safety syringe, activate it at this time by following the steps outlined in Fig. 11.10C, and continue to Step 9.
   Principle. Moving the syringe once the needle has entered the skin causes patient discomfort. Test results are considered reliable only if a wheal forms.

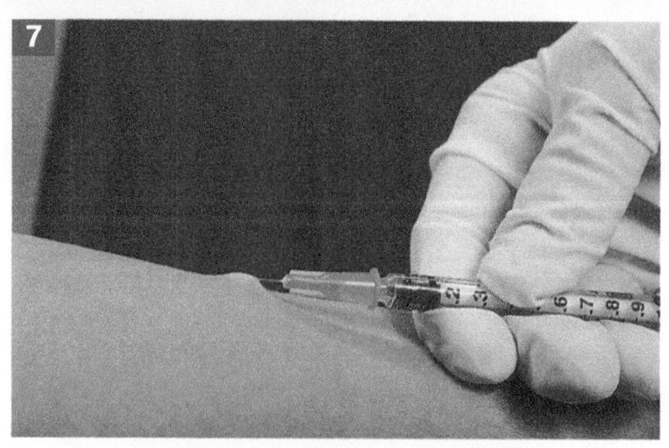

Inject the medication to form a wheal.

8. **Procedural Step.** Place a gauze pad gently over the injection site and remove the needle quickly and at the same angle as for insertion.
   Principle. Withdrawing the needle quickly and at the angle of insertion reduces patient discomfort. The gauze pad placed over the injection site helps prevent tissue movement as the needle is withdrawn, also reducing patient discomfort.
9. **Procedural Step.** Do not apply pressure to the injection site. If blood appears at the injection site, blot the site lightly with a gauze pad. If you are using a safety syringe with a shield or sliding-sleeve, activate the safety feature at this time by following the steps outlined in Fig. 11.10.
   Principle. Applying pressure may cause leakage of the testing solution through the needle puncture site, resulting in inaccurate test results.
10. **Procedural Step.** Properly dispose of the needle and syringe in a biohazard sharps container.
   Principle. Proper disposal of the needle and syringe is required by the OSHA standard to prevent accidental needlestick injuries.
11. **Procedural Step.** Remove gloves and sanitize your hands.
12. **Procedural Step.** Stay with the patient to make sure that he or she is not experiencing any unusual reactions. The medical assistant should be especially careful and alert for any sign of a patient reaction when administering allergy skin tests. If the patient experiences an unusual reaction, notify the provider immediately.
13. **Procedural Step.** Perform one of the following, based on the type of skin test being administered.

Allergy Skin Tests

a. Read the test results within 20–30 min, using inspection and palpation at the site of the injection to assess the presence of and to determine the amount of

PROCEDURE 11.7 Administering an Intradermal Injection—cont'd

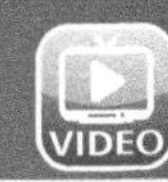

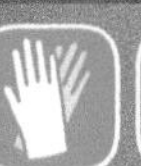
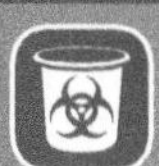

induration. Interpret the skin test results according to the information outlined in Table 11.8.

b. Document the procedure in the patient's medical record.
   (1) *Electronic health record:* Document the injection site, the names of the skin tests, the skin test results, and any significant observations or patient reactions using the appropriate radio buttons, drop-down menus, and free text fields.
   (2) *Paper-based patient record:* Document the date and time, the injection site used, the names of the skin tests, the skin test results, and any significant observations or patient reactions (refer to the PPR documentation example).

PPR Documentation Example

Date	
2/15/XX	Allergy skin tests, ID, Ⓡ ant forearm.
	Results: House dust +2
	Cat dander +4
	Dog dander – No reaction
	Ragweed +4
	Mixed fungi +3
	——————T. Cline, CMA (AAMA)

Mantoux Tuberculin Skin Test

1. Inform the patient of the date and time to return to the medical office to have the results read. Results must be read within 48–72 h after the test has been administered. Stress the importance of returning to the office to have the results read, even if the test site does not exhibit a reaction. Failure to return warrants having to repeat the test.
2. Document the procedure in the patient's medical record.
   a. *Electronic health record:* Document the name of the tuberculin purified protein derivative (PPD) solution, the dose given, the manufacturer and lot number, the route of administration, the injection site used, and any significant observations or patient reactions, using the appropriate radio buttons, drop-down menus, and free text fields.
   b. *Paper-based patient record:* Document the date and time, the name of the tuberculin PPD solution, the dose given, the manufacturer and lot number, the route of administration, the injection site used, and any significant observations or patient reactions (refer to the PPR documentation example).

   Principle: The lot number indicates the batch in which the tuberculin solution was made. Should a problem arise with that batch, the tuberculin solution can be recalled and the individuals who received it can be identified.
3. Instruct the patient in the care of the test site as follows:
   - Continue your normal daily personal hygiene activities.
   - Do not cover the test site with an adhesive bandage.
   - Avoid the use of ointments, lotions, and sunscreens.
   - Mild itching, swelling, or irritation may normally occur at the test site.
   - Do not touch, scratch, press on, or rub the test site. This could alter the test results. If the test site itches, apply a cold compress to the area.
   - Pat the arm dry after washing it. Do not rub it dry.

PPR Documentation Example

Date	
2/15/XX	10:00 a.m. Tubersol Mantoux test 5 TU,
	0.10 mL, ID. (Connaught Laboratories,
	Lot #: C0832AA). Admin Ⓡ ant forearm.
	Pt to return on 2/17/XX to have results
	read. ——————T. Cline, CMA (AAMA)

Reading Mantoux Tuberculin Skin Test Results

Equipment/Supplies

- Millimeter ruler
- Disposable gloves
- Tuberculin test record card

1. **Procedural Step.** Greet the patient and introduce yourself. Identify the patient by full name and date of birth and explain the procedure.
2. **Procedural Step.** Work in a quiet well-lit atmosphere. Check the patient's medical record to determine which arm was used to administer the test.
3. **Procedural Step.** Sanitize your hands and apply gloves.
4. **Procedural Step.** Position the patient's arm on a firm surface with the arm flexed at the elbow.
5. **Procedural Step.** Locate the application site. The result should be read transversely to the long axis of the forearm, meaning "across" the forearm.
6. **Procedural Step.** Gently rub your fingertip over the test site and lightly palpate for the presence of induration. If induration is present, the area should be lightly rubbed from the area of normal skin (without induration) to the indurated area to assess the size of the area of induration. If the margins of induration

Continued

PROCEDURE 11.7 Administering an Intradermal Injection—cont'd

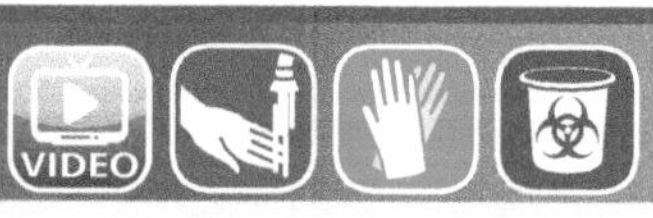

are irregular, assess the widest diameter of induration across the forearm.
Principle. Induration is the only criterion used in determining a positive reaction. If erythema is present without induration, the results are interpreted as negative.

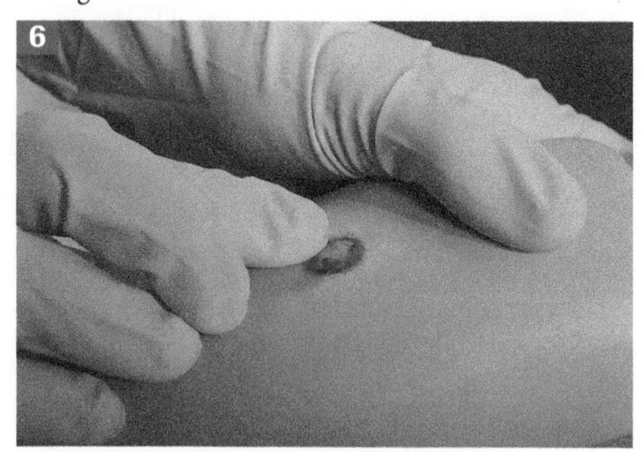

Lightly palpate for induration.

7. Procedural Step. Measure the diameter of the induration with a flexible millimeter ruler (supplied by the manufacturer).

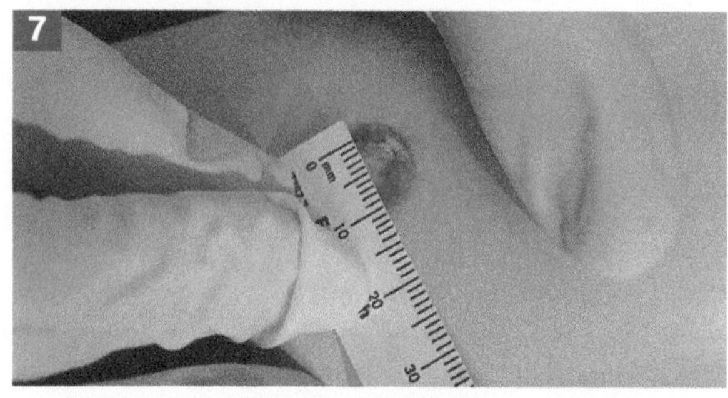

Measure the induration.

8. Procedural Step. Remove gloves and sanitize your hands.

9. Procedural Step. Document the results in the patient's medical record.

a. *Electronic health record (EHR):* Document the name of the test (Mantoux TST) and the test results (documented in millimeters) using the appropriate radio buttons, drop-down menus, and free text fields. If no induration is present, 0 mm should be documented. The results of the Mantoux TST are interpreted according to the guidelines outlined in Box 11.3.

b. *Paper-based patient record:* Document the date and time, the name of the test, and the test results (documented in millimeters). If no induration is present, 0 mm should be documented (refer to the PPR documentation example). The results of the Mantoux TST are interpreted according to the guidelines outlined in Box 11.3.

10. Procedural Step. Complete a tuberculin test record card and give it to the patient.
Principle. The record card provides the patient with a permanent record of the test results.

10

TUBERCULOSIS TEST RECORD

Name	Date Admin: 2/15/XX
Carrie Fee	Date Read: 2/17/XX
MANTOUX TEST	**RESULT**
Tubersol, 5 TU	9 mm

Logan Family Practice
401 St. George St.
St. Augustine, FL 32084
(904) 555-3933

Performed by T. Cline, CMA (AAMA)

PPR Documentation Example

Date	
2/17/XX	3:00 p.m. Tubersol Mantoux test: 9 mm.
	Pt provided c̄ TB record card. Scheduled
	for TB retesting on 2/28/XX. ————
	————T. Cline, CMA (AAMA)

Cardiopulmonary Procedures

Check out the Evolve site at http://evolve.elsevier.com/Bonewit to access additional interactive activities and exercises to help you study and prepare for success.

LEARNING OUTCOMES

Electrocardiography

1. Trace the path of the blood through the heart, starting with the right atrium.
2. Describe the heart's conduction system.
3. State the purpose of electrocardiography.
4. Identify each of the following components of the ECG cycle:
   - P wave
   - QRS complex
   - T wave
   - P-R segment
   - ST segment
   - P-R interval
   - Q-T interval
   - Baseline following the T wave
5. State the purpose of the standardization mark.
6. State the functions of the electrodes, amplifier, and output device.
7. List the 12 leads that are included in an ECG.
8. Describe the function served by each of the following:
   - Three-channel recording capability
   - Interpretive electrocardiography
   - Electronic medical record connectivity
   - Teletransmission
9. Identify each of the following types of artifact, and state its causes:
   - Muscle
   - Wandering baseline
   - 60-cycle interference
   - Interrupted baseline

Holter Monitor Electrocardiography

10. List the reasons for applying a Holter monitor.
11. State the guidelines for wearing a Holter monitor.
12. Explain the use of the patient diary in Holter monitor electrocardiography.

Cardiac Dysrhythmias

13. Identify each of the following cardiac dysrhythmias, and explain its causes:
    - Premature atrial contraction
    - Paroxysmal atrial tachycardia
    - Atrial flutter
    - Atrial fibrillation
    - Premature ventricular contraction
    - Ventricular tachycardia
    - Ventricular fibrillation

PROCEDURES

Record a 12-lead, three-channel ECG.

Instruct a patient in the guidelines for wearing a Holter monitor.

Apply a Holter monitor.

Identify cardiac dysrhythmias on a 12-lead ECG.

Pulmonary Function Testing

14. Identify the different pulmonary function tests.
15. List indications for performing spirometry testing.
16. Describe each of the following: FVC, FEV_1, and FEV_1/FVC ratio.
17. Explain the difference between predicted values and measured values.
18. Describe patient preparation for spirometry.
19. Explain how to calibrate a spirometer.
20. Explain the purpose of post-bronchodilator spirometry.

Perform a spirometry test.

Peak Flow Measurement

21. Identify the symptoms of an asthma attack.
22. List examples of asthma triggers.
23. Explain the difference between long-term control and quick-relief asthma medications.
24. Describe the purpose of a peak flow meter.
25. State the purpose of a peak flow chart.
26. Identify the information included in an asthma action plan.

Measure a patient's peak flow expiratory rate.

Home Oxygen Therapy

27. Explain why the body needs oxygen.
28. Describe what occurs when the body cannot maintain an adequate blood oxygen level.
29. Identify the conditions that may require home oxygen therapy.
30. List and describe the information that is included on a prescription for home oxygen therapy.
31. List and describe the three common types of oxygen delivery systems along with the advantages and disadvantages of each.
32. List and describe the two types of devices used to administer home oxygen therapy.
33. State the usage and safety guidelines that should be followed by a patient on home oxygen therapy.

CHAPTER OUTLINE

INTRODUCTION TO ELECTROCARDIOGRAPHY

Structure of the Heart

Conduction System of the Heart

Cardiac Cycle

- Waves
- Baseline, Segments, and Intervals

Electrocardiograph Paper

Standardization of the Electrocardiograph

Electrocardiograph Leads

- Electrodes
- Bipolar Leads
- Augmented Leads
- Chest Leads

Patient Preparation

Maintenance of the Electrocardiograph

Electrocardiographic Capabilities

- Three-Channel Recording Capability
- Interpretive Electrocardiograph
- Electronic Health Record Connectivity
- Teletransmission

Artifacts

- Muscle Artifact
- Wandering Baseline Artifact
- 60-Cycle Interference Artifact
- Interrupted Baseline Artifact

Holter Monitor Electrocardiography

- Purpose
- Digital Holter Monitor
- Patient Preparation
- Electrode Placement
- Patient Diary
- Event Marker
- Evaluating Results
- Maintenance of the Holter Monitor

Cardiac Dysrhythmias

- Premature Atrial Contraction
- Paroxysmal Supraventricular Tachycardia
- Atrial Flutter
- Atrial Fibrillation
- Premature Ventricular Contraction
- Ventricular Tachycardia
- Ventricular Fibrillation

Pulmonary Function Tests

- Spirometry
- Post-Bronchodilator Spirometry

Peak Flow Measurement

KEY TERMS

amplitude (AM-pli-tood)
artifact (AR-tih-fakt)
atherosclerosis (ath-roe-skler-OH-sus)
baseline
cardiac cycle
dysrhythmia (dis-RITH-mee-ah)
ECG cycle
electrocardiogram (ee-LEK-troe-KAR-dee-oh-gram) (ECG)
electrocardiograph (ee-LEK-troe-KAR-dee-oh-graf)
electrode (ee-LEK-trode)
electrolyte (ee-LEK-troe-lite)
flow rate
hypoxemia
hypoxia
interval (IN-ter-val)
ischemia (is-KEEM-ee-ah)
normal sinus rhythm
oxygen therapy
peak flow rate
segment
spirometer (spih-ROM-ih-ter)
spirometry (spih-ROM-ih-tree)
wheezing

Introduction to Electrocardiography

The **electrocardiograph** is an instrument used to record the electrical activity of the heart. The **electrocardiogram** (ECG) is the graphic representation of this activity. The ECG exhibits the amount of electrical activity produced by the heart and the time required for the impulse to travel through the heart.

Cardiovascular disorders can cause abnormal changes to occur on the ECG. Because of this, electrocardiography is used for the following purposes:

- To evaluate the following symptoms: chest pain, shortness of breath, dizziness, or heart palpitations
- To detect an abnormality in the heart's rate or rhythm (**dysrhythmia**)
- To detect the presence of impaired blood flow to the heart muscle known as myocardial ischemia. The term **ischemia** refers to a deficiency of blood in a body part usually caused by a blocked artery.
- To help diagnose damage to the heart caused by a myocardial infarction
- To determine the presence of hypertrophy (enlargement) of the heart
- To detect inflammation of the heart muscle (myocarditis) or the lining of the heart (pericarditis)
- To assess the effect on the heart of digitalis and other cardiac drugs
- To determine the presence of electrolyte disturbances
- To assess the progress of rheumatic fever
- To detect congenital heart defects
- Performed before surgery to assess cardiac risk during surgery
- As part of a complete physical examination

A 12-lead resting ECG cannot detect all cardiovascular disorders, nor can it always detect impending heart disease such as a myocardial infarction. An ECG is taken with the patient in a resting state and records only about 10 seconds of the heart's electrical activity. If a patient has a dysrhythmia that occurs intermittently, the abnormal heartbeat may not occur during this brief time period. A patient who experiences angina pectoris does not typically have symptoms while in a resting state (see the box Patient Coaching: Angina Pectoris, presented later), and an ECG run on such a patient may appear normal. Because of this, an ECG must be used in combination with the patient's symptoms, health history, physical examination, and other diagnostic and laboratory tests to obtain a complete assessment of cardiac functioning.

The medical assistant is frequently responsible for recording ECGs in the medical office. The medical assistant must acquire knowledge, and skill must be acquired in the following aspects of electrocardiography: preparation of the patient, operation of the electrocardiograph, identification and elimination of artifacts, and care and maintenance of the electrocardiograph.

STRUCTURE OF THE HEART

The human heart consists of four chambers. The right and left atria are the small upper chambers of the heart, and the right and left ventricles are the large lower chambers (Fig. 12.1). Blood enters the right atrium from two large veins—the superior vena cava and the inferior vena cava—which bring it back from its circulation through the body. The blood entering the right atrium is

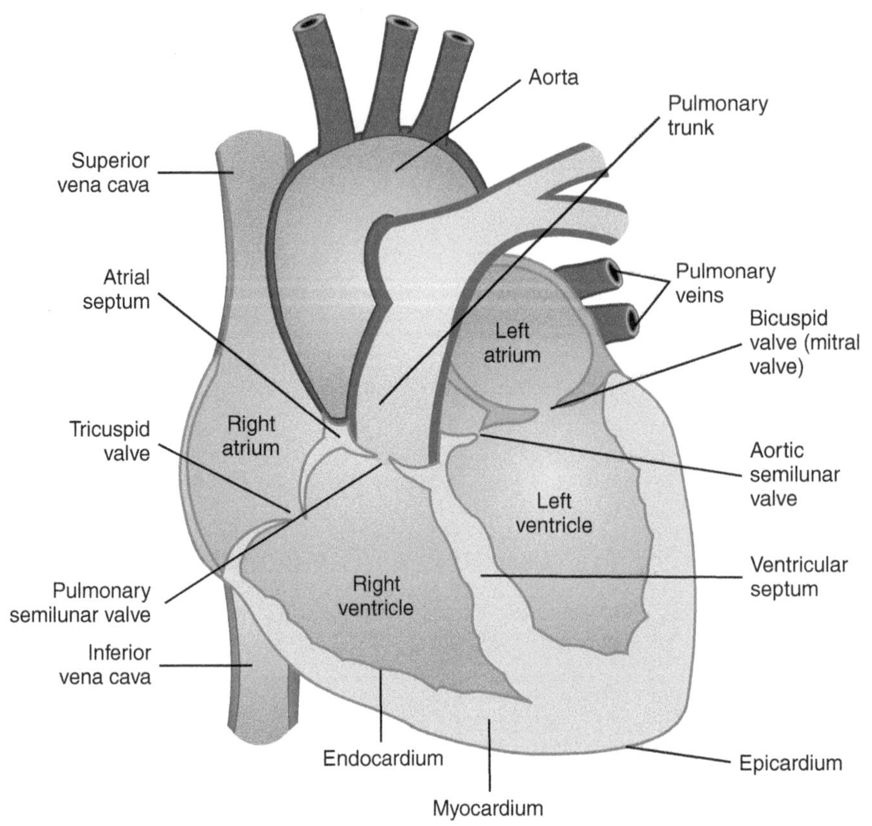

Fig. 12.1 Diagram of the heart.

deoxygenated, meaning it contains very little oxygen and is high in carbon dioxide.

From the right atrium, the blood enters the right ventricle. It is pumped from here to the lungs by way of the pulmonary artery. The blood picks up oxygen in the lungs in exchange for carbon dioxide and returns to the left atrium of the heart through the pulmonary veins. From the left atrium, the blood enters the left ventricle. This is the most muscular and powerful chamber of the heart and pumps blood to the entire body. Blood exits from the left ventricle through the aorta, which distributes it to all parts of the body to nourish the tissues with oxygen and nutrients. The coronary arteries consist of two small arteries that branch off the aorta and innervate the heart (Fig. 12.2). These arteries have numerous branches, which supply the heart itself with oxygen and nutrients.

CONDUCTION SYSTEM OF THE HEART

The *sinoatrial (SA) node* is located in the upper portion of the right atrium, just below the opening of the superior vena cava. It consists of a knot of modified myocardial cells that have the ability to send out an electrical impulse without an external nerve stimulus. In this way, the SA node initiates and regulates the heartbeat and is often referred to as the "pacemaker" of the heart. In a normal individual, the SA node generates electrical impulses at a rate of 60 to 100 times per minute.

Each electrical impulse discharged by the SA node is distributed to the right and left atria and causes them to contract. This contraction forces blood through the open cuspid valves and into the ventricles. The impulse is picked up by the *atrioventricular (AV) node,* another knot of modified myocardial cells located at the base of the right atrium. The AV node delays the impulse momentarily to allow for complete contraction of the atria and filling of the ventricles with blood from the atria. The AV node then transmits the electrical impulse to the *bundle of His.* The bundle of His divides into right and left branches known as the *bundle branches,* which relay the impulse to the *Purkinje fibers.* The Purkinje fibers distribute the impulse evenly to the right and left ventricles, causing them to contract; this forces blood out of the right ventricle and into the pulmonary trunk and out of the left ventricle into the aorta. Ejection of blood into the aorta causes the blood pressure and pulse to be produced. The entire heart then relaxes momentarily. The SA node initiates a new impulse, and the cycle repeats (Fig. 12.3).

CARDIAC CYCLE

The **cardiac cycle** represents one complete heartbeat. It consists of the contraction of the atria, the contraction of the ventricles, and the relaxation of the entire heart (as described previously). The electrocardiograph records the electrical

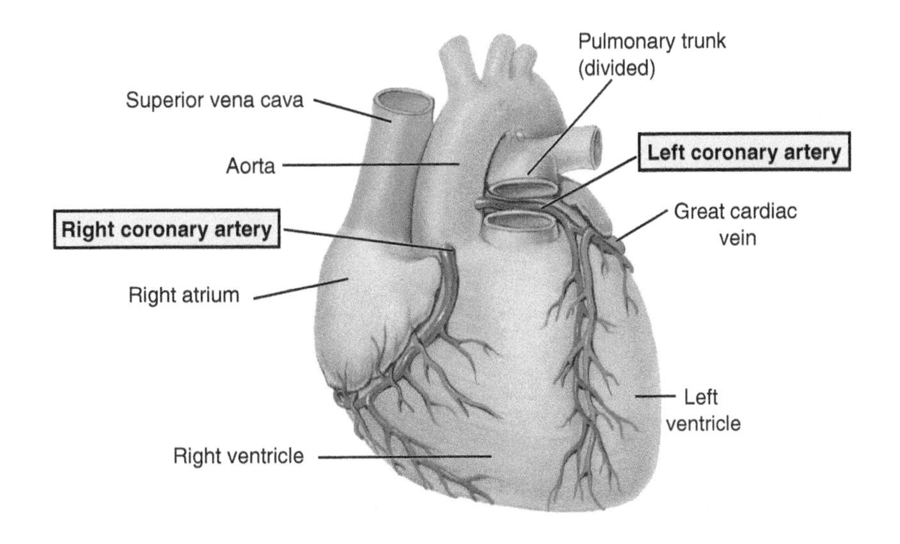

Fig. 12.2 Coronary arteries. (From Applegate EJ: *The anatomy and physiology of the learning system,* ed 4, St Louis: Elsevier; 2011.)

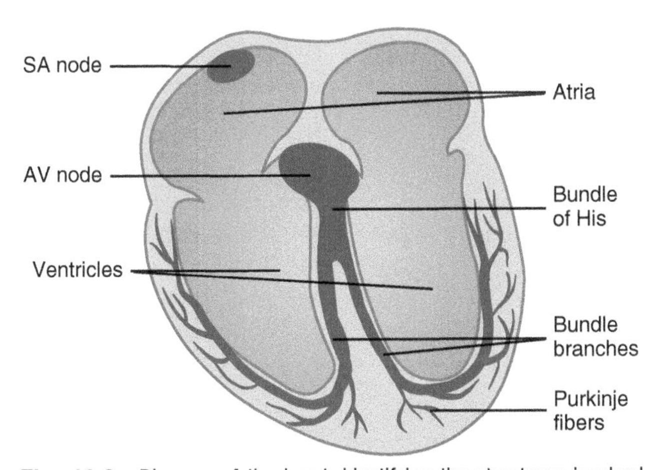

Fig. 12.3 Diagram of the heart, identifying the structures involved with the conduction of an electrical impulse through the heart. *AV,* Atrioventricular; *SA,* sinoatrial.

activity that causes these events in the cardiac cycle. The **ECG cycle** is the graphic representation of the cardiac cycle (Fig. 12.4).

WAVES

The normal ECG cycle consists of a P wave; the Q, R, and S waves (known as the *QRS complex*); and a T wave. The ECG cycle is recorded from left to right, beginning with the P wave.

P wave The P wave represents the electrical activity associated with the contraction of the atria, or *atrial depolarization.*

QRS complex The QRS complex represents the electrical activity associated with the contraction of the ventricles, or *ventricular depolarization,* and consists of the Q wave, the R wave, and the S wave. The ventricles are larger than the atria and therefore require a stronger electrical stimulus to depolarize the ventricles. That is why the R wave is taller than the P wave on the ECG graph cycle.

T wave The T wave represents the electrical recovery of the ventricles, or *ventricular repolarization.* The muscle cells are

Putting It All Into Practice

My name is Anitra, and I work in the medical laboratory of an internal medicine office. I also run electrocardiograms, apply and remove Holter monitors, perform pulmonary function tests, and assist with cardiac stress testing.

One of my most rewarding experiences was when a young woman came into the office with severe chest pain. I immediately helped her back to an examining room. I ran an electrocardiogram, as ordered by the physician. After the physician read the electrocardiogram, he indicated the results did not look good and that the patient would have to be transported to the hospital. I went into the patient's room to comfort her. She asked me if she was going to have to go to the hospital. I replied, "Possibly." She immediately said, "I don't want to go!" Then I began to explain to her how important it was to have more tests to make sure she would be all right. She finally agreed to go. After being taken to the hospital by an ambulance, she was later transferred to another hospital for the insertion of a stent. A few weeks passed, and she came into the office. She hugged me and thanked me for possibly saving her life. It felt so good that I could help make a difference in a patient's life. ■

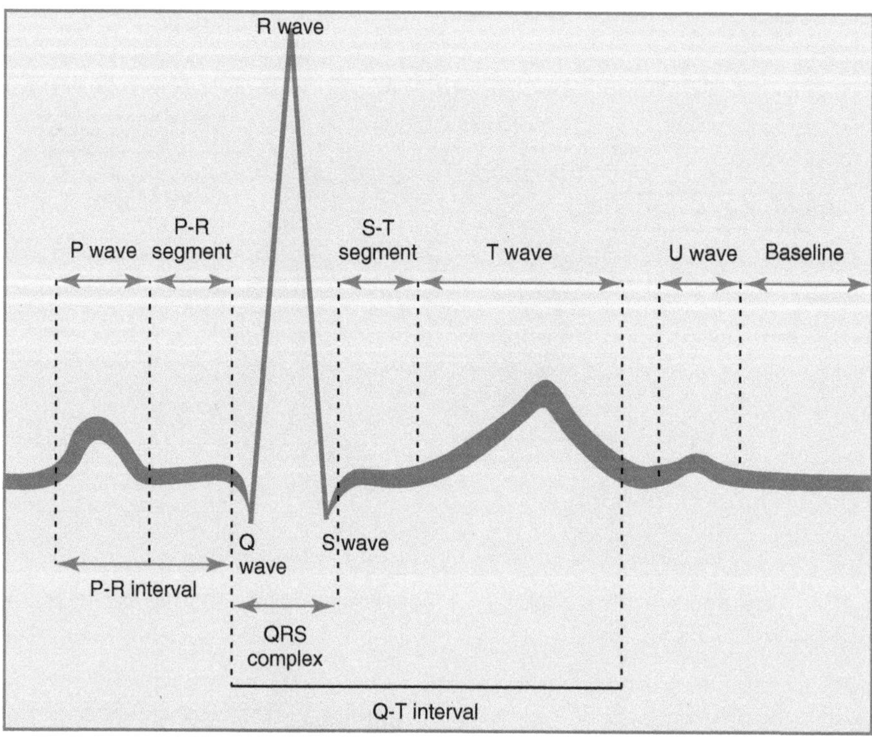

Fig. 12.4 ECG cycle.

recovering in preparation for another impulse. (*Note:* Electrical recovery, known as *atrial repolarization,* follows the P wave. This repolarization occurs at the same time as ventricular depolarization [QRS complex]. Because of this, atrial repolarization is masked or hidden by the QRS complex and does not appear as a separate wave on the ECG cycle.)

U wave Occasionally a U wave follows a T wave. It is a small round wave that is associated with repolarization of the Purkinje fibers in the papillary muscle of the heart.

BASELINE, SEGMENTS, AND INTERVALS

The flat, horizontal line that separates the various waves is known as the **baseline.** Following the U wave, the heart is at rest or *polarized.* Because no electrical activity is occurring in the heart during this time, the electrocardiograph does not have anything to record, which is why the baseline is flat.

The waves deflect either upward (positive deflection) or downward (negative deflection) from the baseline. The ECG cycle between the P wave and the T wave is divided into segments and intervals for the purpose of interpretation and analysis of the ECG by the provider. A **segment** is the portion of the ECG between two waves, and an **interval** is the length of one or more waves and a segment.

Segments

PR segment The PR segment represents the time interval from the end of the atrial depolarization to the beginning of the ventricular depolarization. It is the time needed for the impulse to be delayed at the AV node and then travel through the bundle of His and Purkinje fibers to the ventricles.

ST segment The ST segment represents the time interval from the end of the ventricular depolarization to the beginning of repolarization of the ventricles.

Intervals

PR interval The PR interval represents the time interval from the beginning of the atrial depolarization to the beginning of the ventricular depolarization.

QT interval The QT interval is the time interval from the beginning of the ventricular depolarization to the end of repolarization of the ventricles.

Baseline The baseline after the T wave (or U wave, if present) represents the period when the entire heart returns to its resting, or polarized, state.

ELECTROCARDIOGRAPH PAPER

Electrocardiograph paper is divided into two sets of squares for the accurate and convenient manual measurement of the waves, intervals, and segments (Fig. 12.5). Each small square is 1 mm high and 1 mm wide. Each large square (made up of 25 small squares) is 5 mm high and 5 mm wide. By manually measuring the various waves, intervals, and segments of the ECG graph cycle with ECG calipers or an ECG ruler, the provider is able to determine whether the electrical activity of the heart falls within normal limits.

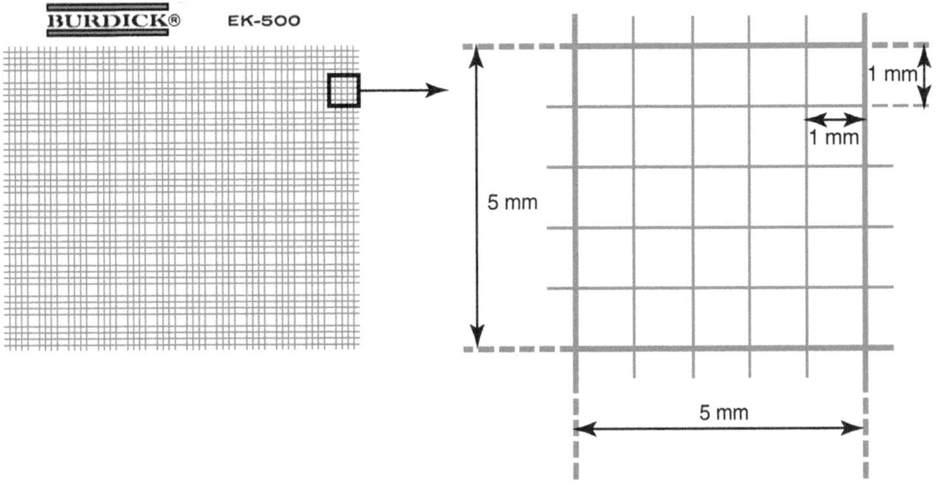

Fig. 12.5 Diagram of ECG paper with a section enlarged to indicate the sizes of the large and small squares.

Heart disease can trigger abnormal changes in the ECG cycle, causing the results to fall outside of normal limits. For example, myocardial ischemia (often caused by coronary artery disease [CAD]) can cause a depressed ST segment and an inverted T wave. A myocardial infarction can cause a larger-than-normal Q wave and an elevated ST segment.

Electrocardiograph paper contains a thermosensitive coating. A black or red graph is printed on top of this coating. The electrocardiograph uses a thermal print head to produce the ECG tracing. The print head has the ability to generate heat in a prescribed pattern. When the thermosensitive paper comes in contact with the heated print head, the coating turns black in the areas where it is heated, producing the ECG tracing. In addition to being heat sensitive, ECG paper is pressure sensitive and should be handled carefully to avoid making impressions that would interfere with proper reading of the ECG.

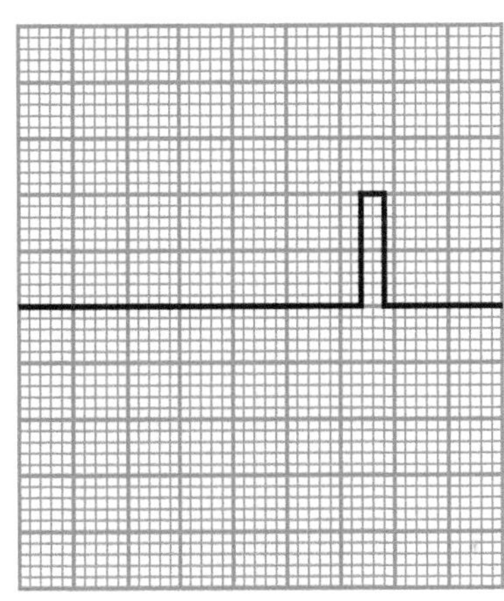

Fig. 12.6 Standardization mark.

STANDARDIZATION OF THE ELECTROCARDIOGRAPH

The electrocardiograph must be standardized, or calibrated, when an ECG is recorded. This is a quality control measure that ensures an accurate and reliable recording. It also means that an ECG run on one electrocardiograph compares in accuracy with a recording run on another machine. An ECG run on a properly calibrated electrocardiograph results in an accurate and reliable representation of the electrical activity of the patient's heart.

By international agreement, 1 mV of electricity should cause the stylus to move 10 mm high in **amplitude** (10 small squares). During the recording, the machine allows 1 mV to enter the electrocardiograph, which should result in an upward deflection of 10 mm. The marking that occurs on the ECG paper is known as a *standardization mark* (Fig. 12.6). The width of the mark made by the machine is approximately 2 mm (two small squares). The electrocardiograph automatically records standardization marks on the ECG; a standardization mark is recorded at the beginning and end of each of the ECG strips (see Fig. 12.11, presented later). If the standardization mark is more or less than 10 mm in amplitude, the electrocardiograph must be adjusted; otherwise, the ECG recording may not be accurate. The manufacturer's operating manual must be consulted for proper adjustment information.

ELECTROCARDIOGRAPH LEADS

The standard ECG consists of 12 leads. A *lead* is a tracing of the electrical activity of the heart between two electrodes.

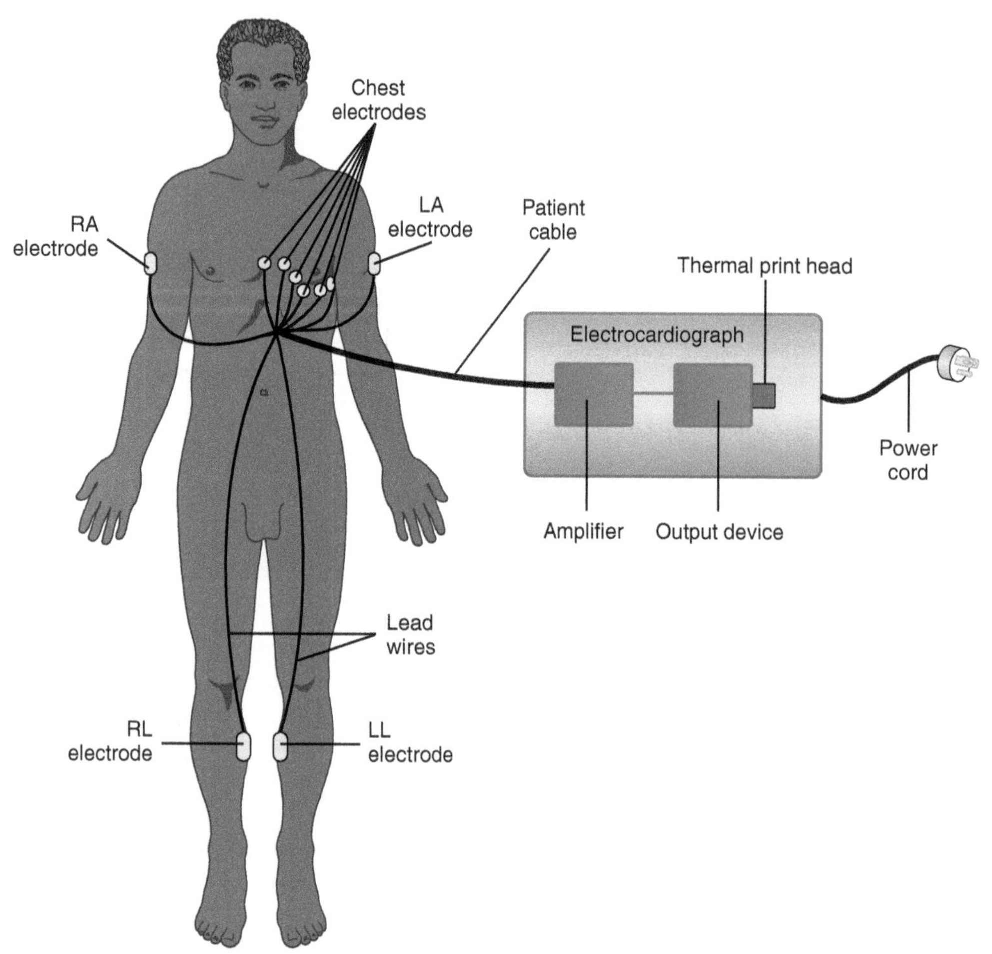

Fig. 12.7 Diagram of the basic components of the electrocardiograph. The limb electrodes are attached to the fleshy parts of the limbs, and the lead wires are arranged to follow body contour. The patient cable is not dangling, and the power cord points away from the electrocardiograph.

Each lead provides an electrical "photograph" of the heart's activity from a different angle. Together, the 12 leads, or "photographs," facilitate a thorough interpretation of the heart's activity.

Ten lead wires are attached to the patient and are used to take the 12 electrical "photographs" of the heart. There are four limb lead wires: the right arm lead wire (RA), the left arm lead wire (LA), the right leg lead wire (RL), and the left leg lead wire (LL). The right leg lead wire is known as the *ground.* It is not used for the actual recording but serves as an electrical reference point. There are six chest lead wires; each is abbreviated with a "V" and includes V_1, V_2, V_3, V_4, V_5, and V_6.

ELECTRODES

The electrical impulses given off by the heart are picked up by **electrodes** and conducted into the machine through lead wires. Electrodes are composed of a substance that is a good conductor of electricity. The electrical impulses given off by the heart are very small (0.0001 to 0.003 V). To produce a readable ECG, they must be made larger, or amplified, by a device known as an *amplifier,* located within the electrocardiograph. The amplified voltages are then relayed to an *output device.* The output device graphically records the images on ECG paper using a thermal print head or electronically sends the recording to a computer where it is displayed on the screen of the computer (Fig. 12.7).

Disposable electrodes are used to record a resting 12-lead ECG. The electrode contains a thin layer of a metallic substance; this metallic substance is a good conductor of electricity. The electrode is square in shape and has a tab extending from one end (Fig. 12.8A). The tab allows for the firm attachment of an alligator clip (see Fig. 12.8B). The back of the electrode contains an electrolyte gel combined with an adhesive (see Fig. 12.8C). An **electrolyte** is a substance that facilitates the transmission of the heart's electrical impulse. Skin is a poor conductor of electricity; therefore, an electrolyte must be used when recording an ECG. The adhesive allows for firm adherence of the electrode to the patient's skin. There is no adhesive on the tab of the electrode, to allow for attachment of the alligator clip. The electrode is applied to the skin and held in place with its adhesive backing; it is thrown away after use.

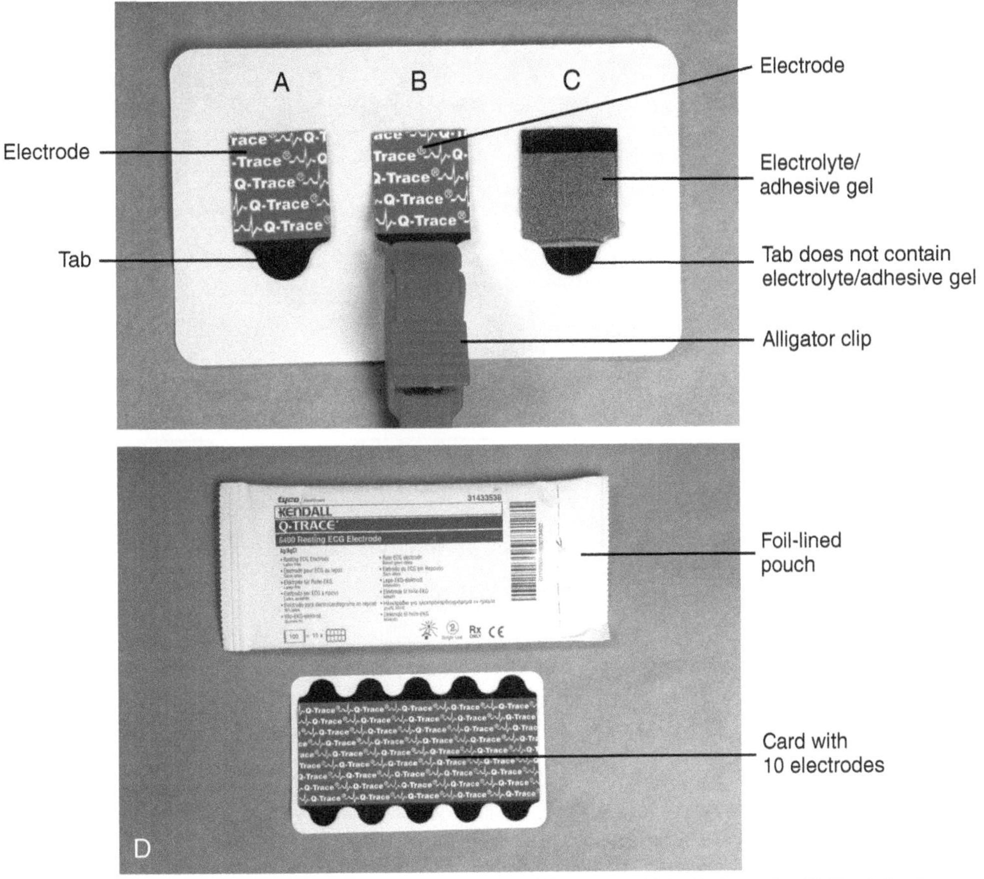

Fig. 12.8 Resting 12-lead ECG electrodes. (A) Disposable resting 12-lead electrode. (B) The tab allows for attachment of the alligator clip. (C) The back of the electrode contains an electrolyte gel combined with an adhesive. (D) Disposable 12-lead electrodes are packaged in a foil-lined pouch and come on a card that contains 10 electrodes.

Disposable 12-lead electrodes come on a card containing 10 electrodes (see Fig. 12.8D). A foil-lined pouch is used to hold 10 cards of electrodes (or 100 electrodes per pouch). The foil-lined pouch preserves moisture to prevent the electrolyte from drying out. Each electrode pouch (and the box containing the pouches) is stamped with an expiration date. The medical assistant must always check the expiration date of the electrodes before applying them. The electrolyte gel on outdated electrodes may be dried out; a dried-out electrolyte is unable to transmit a good ECG signal.

Electrodes are sensitive to environmental conditions and must be stored properly to prevent electrolyte drying. They should be stored in a cool area (less than 75°F or 24°C) away from sources of heat. When an electrode pouch is opened, the medical assistant should seal the pouch by folding over the end of it and then place the pouch (containing the remaining electrode cards) in a zipper-lock plastic bag to preserve moisture.

BIPOLAR LEADS

The first three leads of the 12-lead ECG are the bipolar leads; they are leads I, II, and III. The bipolar leads use two of the limb electrodes to record the heart's electrical activity. Lead I records the electric current traveling between the right arm and the left arm electrodes, lead II records the electric current traveling between the right arm and the left leg electrodes, and lead III records the electric current traveling between the left arm and the left leg electrodes (Fig. 12.9).

Lead II shows the heart's rhythm more clearly than the other leads. Because of this, the provider often requests a *rhythm strip,* which is a longer recording (approximately 12 inches) of lead II (see Fig. 12.11, presented later).

AUGMENTED LEADS

The next three leads are the augmented leads: aVR (augmented voltage—right arm), aVL (augmented voltage—left arm), and aVF (augmented voltage—left leg or foot). Lead aVR records the electric current traveling between the right arm electrode and a central point between the left arm and left leg electrodes. Lead aVL records the electric current traveling between the left arm electrode and a central point between the right arm and left leg electrodes. Lead aVF records the electric current traveling between the left leg electrode and a central point between the right and left arm electrodes. Leads I, II, III, aVR, aVL, and aVF provide an electrical "photograph" of the heart's activity from side to side and from the top to the bottom of the heart (see Fig. 12.9).

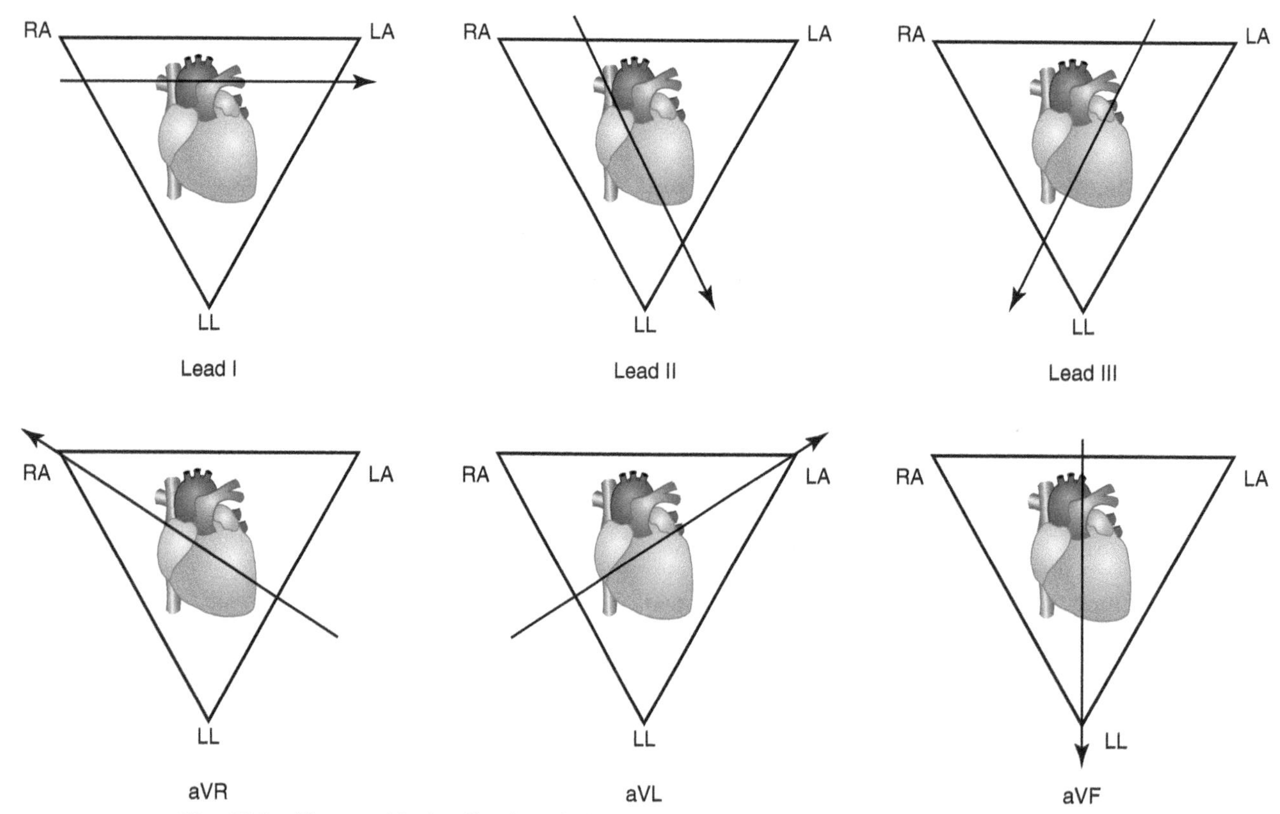

Fig. 12.9 Diagram of the heart's voltage for leads I, II, III, aVR (augmented voltage—right arm), aVL (augmented voltage—left arm), and aVF (augmented voltage—left leg or foot). *LA,* Left arm electrode; *LL,* left leg electrode; *RA,* right arm electrode; *RL,* right leg electrode.

CHEST LEADS

The last six leads are the chest, or precordial, leads (V_1, V_2, V_3, V_4, V_5, and V_6). These leads record the heart's voltage from front to back. The electric current traveling through the heart is recorded from a central point "inside" the heart to a point on the chest wall where the electrode is placed. These points correspond to the chest electrode placement sites. Fig. 12.10 shows the proper location of the electrodes

What Would You Do? What Would You *Not* Do?

Case Study 1

Camilla Rossi is 22 years old and works at a Waffle House during the day and goes to business school at night. She comes to the office because she has been experiencing some heart problems. Over the past month, she has had three episodes of tachycardia, palpitations, difficulty in breathing, and profuse sweating. She is really scared that she has heart disease because her grandfather just died from a heart attack. The physician orders an ECG, but Camilla is reluctant to have the procedure. She is embarrassed about having to disrobe from the waist up, and she is worried that all the wires coming out of the machine will shock her. She says that she does not have health insurance, and she does not know how she would pay for the test. She wants to know whether there is a less expensive way to find out what is wrong with her. ■

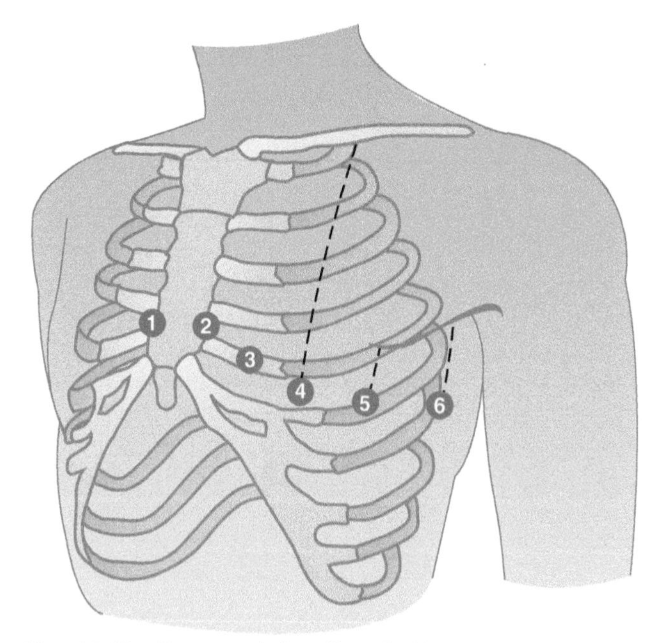

Fig. 12.10 Recommended positions for ECG chest electrodes. V_1, Fourth intercostal space at right margin of sternum; V_2, fourth intercostal space at left margin of sternum; V_3, midway between positions 2 and 4; V_4, fifth intercostal space at junction of left midclavicular line; V_5, at horizontal level of position 4 at left anterior axillary line; V_6, at horizontal level of position 4 at left midaxillary line.

HIGHLIGHT on Cardiac Stress Testing

Description

A cardiac stress test (also known as an *exercise tolerance test* or *exercise electrocardiogram* [ECG]) is a diagnostic procedure used to evaluate the cardiovascular health of individuals with known heart disease and individuals at high risk for developing heart disease, particularly coronary artery disease (CAD). Cardiac stress testing is usually performed in a hospital under the direction of a cardiologist and a cardiac technician so that emergency equipment and trained personnel are available to deal with any unusual situations that might arise. (*Note:* A *nuclear cardiac stress test* is a type of stress test that employs the use of a radioactive material injected through an intravenous line and is described in Chapter 14.)

Purpose

The purpose of cardiac stress testing is as follows:

1. To evaluate symptoms of ischemic heart disease that cannot be assessed by a resting ECG. Ischemic heart disease occurs as a result of an inadequate blood supply to the myocardium, which is most commonly caused by atherosclerosis. **Atherosclerosis** is a condition in which fibrous plaques of fatty deposits and cholesterol build up on the inner walls of arteries. This causes narrowing and partial blockage of the lumen of these arteries, along with hardening of the arterial wall. Atherosclerosis in the coronary arteries is called *coronary artery disease.* During rest, the myocardium supplied by the partially blocked artery may receive an adequate blood supply. If the individual exercises, however, the artery may not be able to supply enough blood to the myocardium, resulting in myocardial ischemia. Myocardial ischemia can cause chest discomfort and certain abnormal changes on the ECG.
2. To assist in evaluating symptoms indicating the presence of cardiac dysrhythmias.
3. To assess the effectiveness of cardiac drug therapy.
4. To follow the course of rehabilitation after a myocardial infarction or a cardiac surgical procedure, such as a coronary bypass operation or a coronary stent placement.
5. To determine an individual's fitness level for a strenuous exercise program, such as jogging.

Patient Preparation

Patient preparation for a cardiac stress test includes the following:

1. Refrain from smoking for 4 hours before the test.
2. Avoid strenuous physical activities for 8–12 hours before the test.
3. Do not consume alcohol or food and beverages containing caffeine for 12 hours before the test. These substances may interfere with obtaining accurate results.
4. Do not eat or drink anything except water for 4 hours before the test. This reduces the likelihood of nausea that may accompany strenuous activity after a meal.
5. Certain cardiac medications may need to be discontinued 1–2 days before the test; the provider makes this determination.
6. Wear loose, comfortable clothing and sports shoes suitable for exercising.

How the Test Works

- Cardiac stress testing involves the continuous electrocardiographic monitoring of an individual during physical exercise. During exercise, the body's need for oxygen places added demands or "stress" on the heart, making it work harder. A cardiac stress test evaluates the response of the heart to maximum or near-maximum exertion.
- A resting 12-lead ECG is usually performed before a cardiac stress test, and the results of the resting ECG are compared with the results of the cardiac stress test.
- The stress test is accomplished by having the patient use a treadmill while connected to an electrocardiograph machine through lead wires and electrodes (see illustration).
- The intensity of the physical exertion starts with a slow warm-up walk on the treadmill. The speed and incline of the treadmill are gradually increased every 3 minutes until the patient's target heart rate is reached. During this time the ECG is continuously displayed on a computer screen. The patient's blood pressure, heart rate, and physical symptoms are also monitored during the test.
- If the signs and symptoms of myocardial ischemia appear, the test is stopped. These symptoms include severe dyspnea, chest discomfort or pain, pallor, weakness, and dizziness. The test is also stopped if the ECG shows abnormal changes, if a serious, irregular heartbeat occurs, or if there is an abnormal change in blood pressure.
- Once the exercising is complete, the patient's blood pressure, heart rate, and ECG are monitored until they return to normal.

Interpretation of Results

The patient's response to the cardiac stress test is used to determine normal or abnormal results. A normal response is a gradual increase in the patient's blood pressure as physical exertion increases, whereas an abnormal response is a sudden increase or decrease in the patient's blood pressure. The ECG of a normal individual undergoing exercise exhibits a shortened PR interval and a compressed QRS complex. An abnormal tracing indicative of myocardial ischemia results in a depressed ST segment and an inverted T wave. An abnormal cardiac stress test result usually warrants further testing, such as coronary angiography, to assess the extent and severity of the heart disease.

Continued

HIGHLIGHT on Cardiac Stress Testing—cont'd

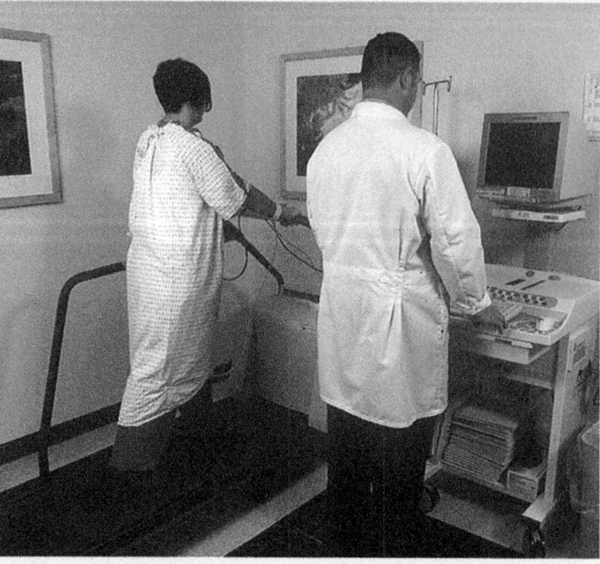

Cardiac treadmill stress test. (From deWit SC: *Medical-surgical nursing: concepts and practice,* St. Louis: Elsevier; 2008.)

for the six chest leads. To ensure an accurate and reliable recording, the medical assistant must be able to locate these electrode placement sites accurately (by palpating the patient's chest). For example, if V_1 and V_2 are placed in the third intercostal space (instead of the fourth intercostal space), changes can occur to the P and T waves, which can falsely indicate heart disease. When first learning to locate the electrode sites for each chest lead, it helps to mark their locations on the patient's chest with a felt-tipped pen.

PATIENT PREPARATION

Minimal preparation is required for an ECG. The medical assistant should instruct the patient in the following guidelines, which facilitate placement of the electrodes and ensure good adhesion of the electrodes to the patient's skin.

1. Do not apply body lotion, oil, or powder on the day of the test. This may make it more difficult to apply the electrodes.
2. Wear comfortable clothing and a shirt or blouse that can be removed easily.
3. Avoid wearing tights since the electrodes need to be placed on the lower legs.

MAINTENANCE OF THE ELECTROCARDIOGRAPH

Electrocardiographs require periodic maintenance. The casing of the electrocardiograph should be cleaned frequently with a soft cloth, slightly dampened with a mild detergent, to remove dust and dirt. Commercial solvents and abrasives should not be used because they can damage the finish of the casing.

The patient cables, lead wires, and power cord should be cleaned periodically with a cloth moistened with a disinfectant cleaner. The cables should never be immersed in the cleaning solution because this could damage them. Inspect the cables frequently for cracks or fraying, and replace them if needed. Check the metal tip of each lead wire for adhesive/electrolyte gel residue, which can interfere with the transmission of a good ECG signal from the electrode. Remove any residue with an alcohol wipe using pressure and friction.

The reusable alligator clips should be cleaned thoroughly with an alcohol wipe after patient use. Check the alligator clips periodically to make sure they fit snugly on the metal tip of each lead wire.

ELECTROCARDIOGRAPHIC CAPABILITIES

Electrocardiographs have a variety of capabilities that permit specific recording and transmittal options.

THREE-CHANNEL RECORDING CAPABILITY

Most medical offices use a three-channel electrocardiograph. An electrocardiograph with a three-channel recording capability can record the electrical activity of the heart through three leads simultaneously. This is in contrast to a single-channel electrocardiograph, which records only one lead at a time. The advantage of a three-channel electrocardiograph

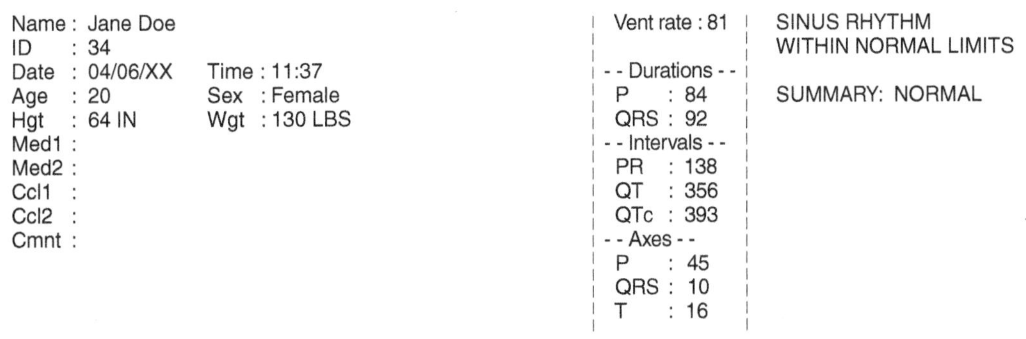

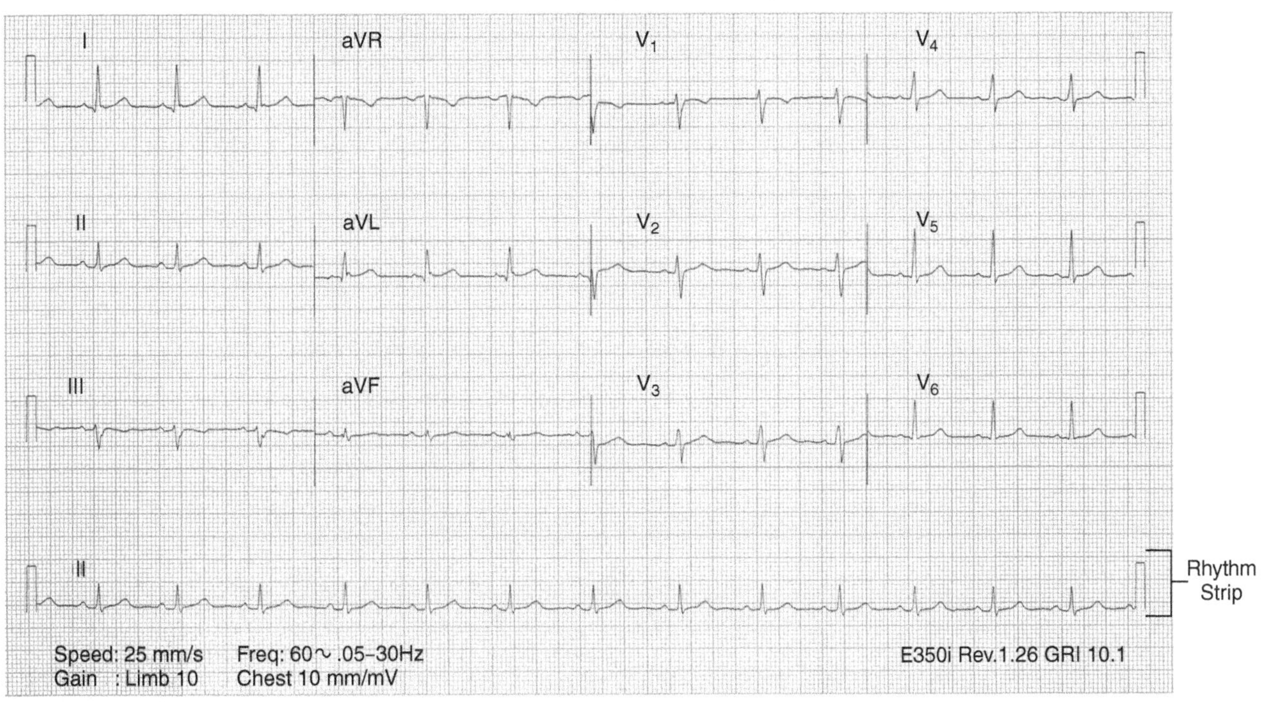

Fig. 12.11 A three-channel ECG with a rhythm strip.

is that an ECG can be produced in less time than would be required if each lead were recorded separately.

The leads that are recorded simultaneously are leads I, II, and III; followed by aVR, aVL, and aVF; followed by V_1, V_2, and V_3; followed by V_4, V_5, and V_6. Each lead is automatically labeled by the electrocardiograph with its appropriate abbreviation. Fig. 12.11 is an example of a three-channel ECG recording that also includes a rhythm strip. Procedure 12.1 describes how to run a 12-lead three-channel ECG.

INTERPRETIVE ELECTROCARDIOGRAPH

An electrocardiograph with interpretive capabilities has a software program that analyzes the recording as it is being run. Interpretive electrocardiographs provide immediate information on the heart's activity, leading to earlier diagnosis and treatment. Patient data are used in the interpretation of the ECG and must be entered into the electrocardiograph using a keyboard before running the recording. The data generally required are the patient's age, sex, height, weight, and medications, which are presented at the top of the recording. The computer analysis of the ECG is also printed at the top of the recording, along with the reason for each interpretation (Figs. 12.11 and 12.12). The results are reviewed and interpreted further by the provider before a diagnosis is made and treatment is initiated.

ELECTRONIC HEALTH RECORD CONNECTIVITY

Electronic health record (EHR) connectivity allows the electrocardiograph to be linked with a computer system. The electrical activity of the heart is converted into a digital format which is sent electronically to a computer where it is displayed on the screen of the computer. If needed, a copy of the ECG report can be printed out on a regular sheet of paper. The ECG report is reviewed and interpreted by the provider and then stored electronically in the patient's EHR.

TELETRANSMISSION

An ECG that has been recorded in a digital format can be transmitted electronically to an ECG data interpretation site. The recording is interpreted by a cardiologist (often along with a computer analysis) at the interpretation site,

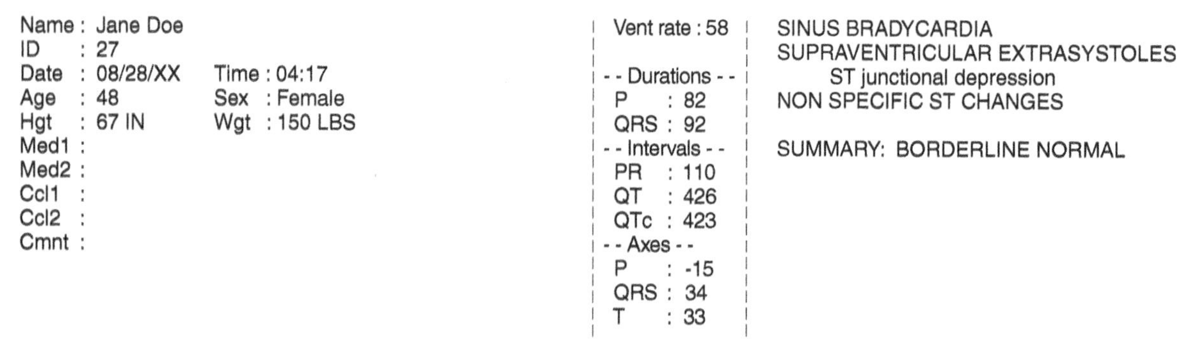

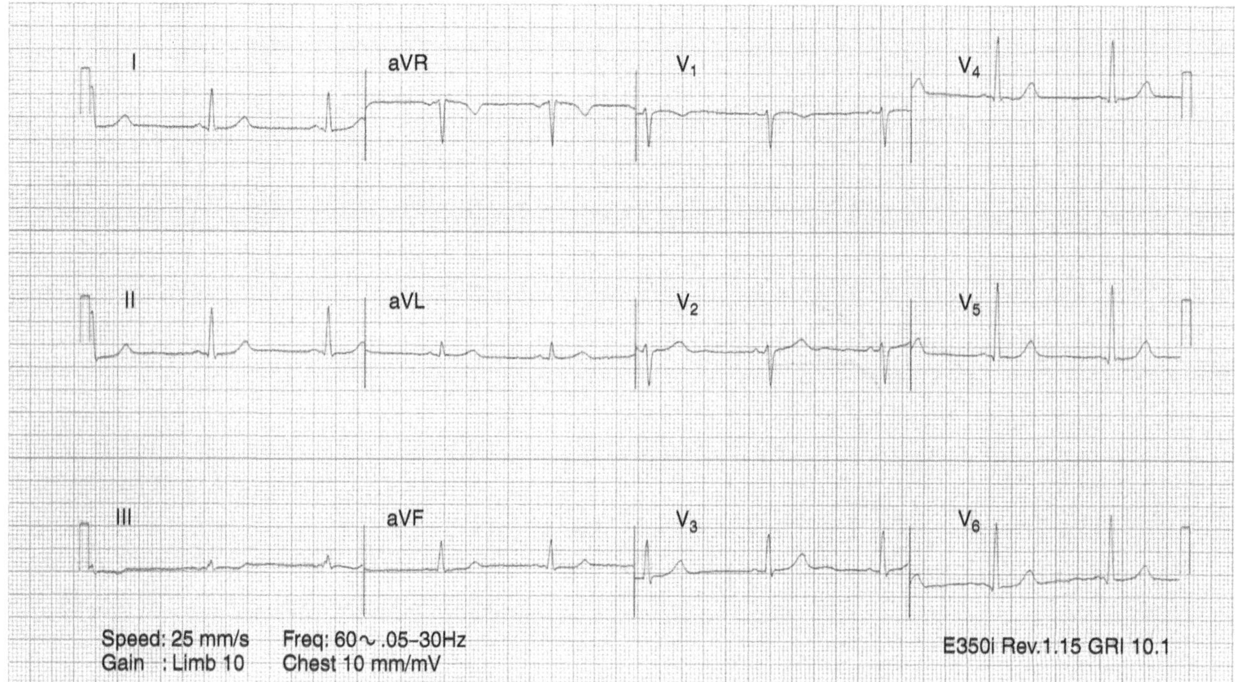

Fig. 12.12 An ECG recording that has been analyzed by an interpretive electrocardiograph. The computer analysis is printed at the top of the recording, along with the reason for each interpretation.

and the ECG recording and its interpretation is electronically transmitted to the sending office the same day.

ARTIFACTS

The medical assistant is responsible for producing a clear and concise ECG recording that can be read and interpreted by both a computer and the provider. Structures sometimes appear in the recording that are not natural and interfere with the normal appearance of the ECG cycles. They are known as **artifacts** and represent additional electrical activity that is picked up by the electrocardiograph. The presence of artifacts affects the quality of the recording, making it difficult to manually measure the ECG cycles. Artifacts can also sometimes cause a false-positive result on an ECG that is analyzed by a computer. The medical assistant should be able to identify artifacts and eliminate them. There are several types of artifacts; the most common are muscle, wandering baseline, and 60-cycle interference.

If the medical assistant is unable to correct an artifact, it is possible that the machine is broken. If an electrocardiograph service technician needs to be contacted, the medical assistant should have the following information available to aid the technician in locating the problem:

1. What already has been done to locate and correct the problem
2. Leads in which the artifact occurs
3. A sample of the artifact recorded by the machine

MUSCLE ARTIFACT

A muscle artifact (Fig. 12.13A) can be identified by its fuzzy, irregular baseline. There are two types of muscle artifacts: those caused by involuntary muscle movement (somatic tremor) and those caused by voluntary muscle movement. The cause of muscle artifacts and the action to take to eliminate them is presented as follows:

1. *An apprehensive patient.* To reduce the patient's apprehension and relax muscles, explain the procedure and

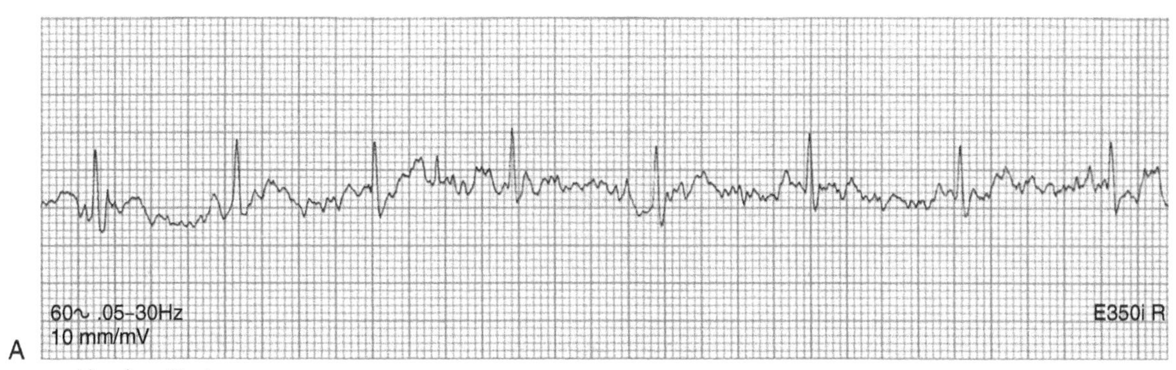

Muscle artifact

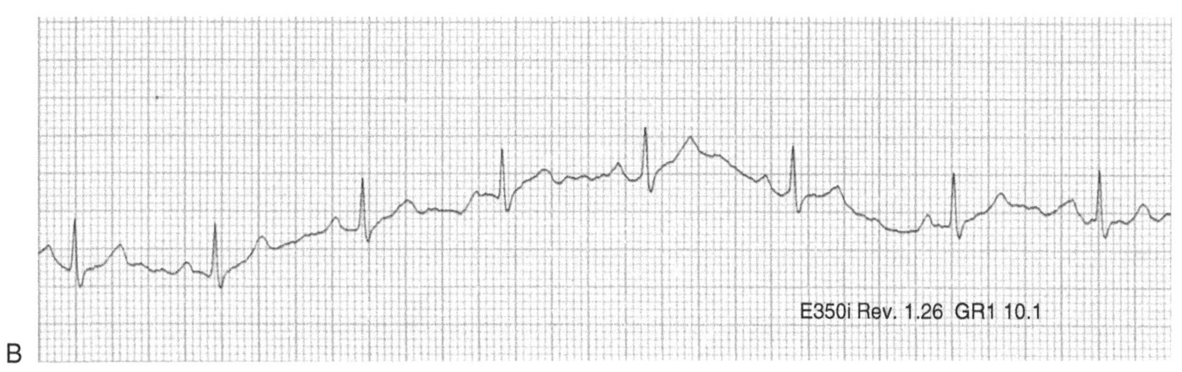

Wandering baseline artifact

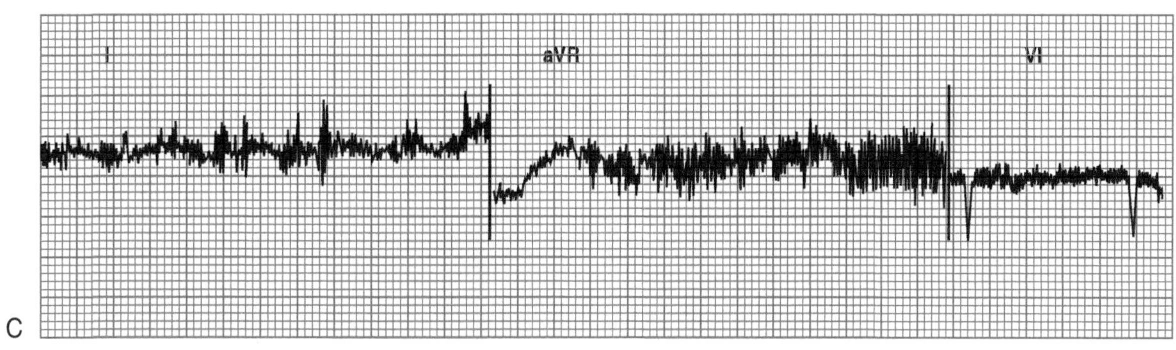

60-Cycle interference artifact

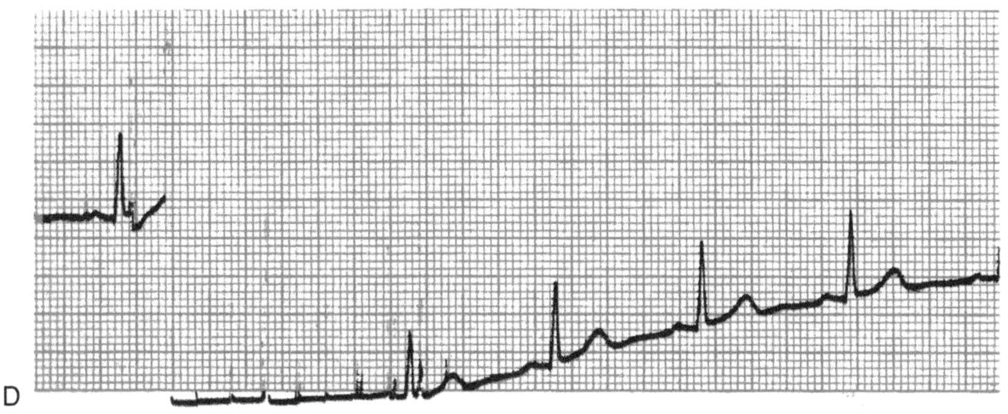

Interrupted baseline artifact

Fig. 12.13 (A–D) Examples of ECG artifacts. (D, From Long BW: *Radiography essentials for limited practice*, ed 3, St Louis: Elsevier; 2010.)

reassure the patient that having an ECG recorded is a painless procedure.

2. *Patient discomfort.* Ensure that the table is wide enough to support the patient's arms and legs adequately. The patient can be made more comfortable by placing a pillow under his or her head. Check that the room temperature is comfortable for the patient. A temperature that is warm enough for the medical assistant may be too cold for the patient who has removed clothing. This could result in shivering, which also would produce a muscle artifact on the ECG.
3. *Patient movement.* The patient must be instructed to lie still and not talk during the recording.
4. *A physical condition.* Several nervous system disorders, such as Parkinson disease, prevent relaxation, and the patient trembles continually. For these individuals, it is difficult to obtain an ECG that is free of artifacts. The artifacts can be reduced, however, by asking the patient to place his or her hands under the buttocks with the palms facing downward.

WANDERING BASELINE ARTIFACT

A wandering baseline artifact appears as a slow wavy baseline on the ECG (see Fig. 12.13B). The cause of wandering baseline artifacts and the action to take to eliminate them is presented below:

1. *Loose electrodes.* The medical assistant should ensure that the electrodes are attached firmly to the patient's skin. A loose electrode results in poor transmission of the electrical impulse from the patient's skin to the electrode. If an electrode pulls loose, it can be reattached with hypoallergenic tape or replaced with a new electrode. The alligator clips should be attached firmly to the tabs of the electrodes. To prevent pulling of the lead wires on the electrodes, the patient cable should be well supported on the table or the patient's abdomen and should not be allowed to dangle. Pulling on the electrodes can cause the electrodes to pull away from the patient's skin.
2. *Dried-out electrolyte.* If the electrolyte gel on an electrode is dried out, the medical assistant must replace it with a new electrode. Always check the expiration date stamped on the electrode pouch (or box) to make sure the electrodes are within their expiration date.
3. *Body creams, oils, or lotions on the skin in the area where the electrode is applied.* Creams, oils, or lotions prevent good adhesion of the electrodes to the patient's skin. The medical assistant should remove these substances by rubbing with alcohol, using friction.
4. *Excessive movement of the chest wall during respiration.* The medical assistant should encourage the patient to relax and breathe more calmly, using the diaphragm rather than expanding the chest.

60-CYCLE INTERFERENCE ARTIFACT

A 60-cycle interference artifact (also known as an *AC artifact*) is caused by electrical interference. Electric current can "leak" or spread out from the power used by electrical appliances in the room in which the ECG is being run. This current may be picked up by the patient and carried into the electrocardiograph, where it would show up on the ECG recording as a 60-cycle interference artifact. This type of artifact appears as small, straight, spiked lines that are consistent (see Fig. 12.13C), causing the baseline to be thick and unreadable. The cause of 60-cycle interference artifacts and the action to take to eliminate them is presented below:

1. *Lead wires not following body contour.* Dangling lead wires can pick up electric current. Arrange the wires to follow body contour and to lie flat.
2. *Other electrical equipment in the room.* Lamps, autoclaves, electrically powered examining tables, or other electrical equipment that is plugged in may be leaking electric current. Unplug all nearby electrical equipment. (*Note:* Jewelry and watches do not interfere with the recording; therefore it is not necessary for the patient to remove these items unless they interfere with proper placement of the electrodes.)
3. *Wiring in the walls, ceilings, or floors.* Try moving the patient table away from the walls.
4. *Improper grounding of the electrocardiograph.* The machine is automatically grounded when it is plugged in. Check the three-pronged plug of the ECG machine to make sure the prongs are not loose or damaged. Ensure that the plug is securely in the wall outlet. The right leg electrode is not used for recording the leads, but it picks up electric current that has "leaked" onto the patient and carries it into the electrocardiograph. The electric current is carried away by the machine's grounding system.

INTERRUPTED BASELINE ARTIFACT

Occasionally, an interrupted baseline artifact (see Fig. 12.13D) occurs that may be caused by the metal tip of a lead wire becoming detached or by a frayed or broken patient cable. If the latter is the case, a new patient cable should be ordered from the manufacturer.

HOLTER MONITOR ELECTROCARDIOGRAPHY

A Holter monitor is also known as an *ambulatory electrocardiographic monitor* (AEM). A Holter monitor is a portable ambulatory monitoring system for the continuous recording of the electrical activity of the heart for 24 hours or longer (Fig. 12.14). The monitor is named for Dr. Norman Holter, an American biophysicist who invented this cardiac monitoring device. The original Holter monitor consisted of a large pack of equipment worn on the patient's back.

The purpose of a Holter monitor is to detect cardiac abnormalities that occur while the patient is engaged in his or her normal daily routine. Because of this, the Holter system is designed so that the patient is able to maintain his or

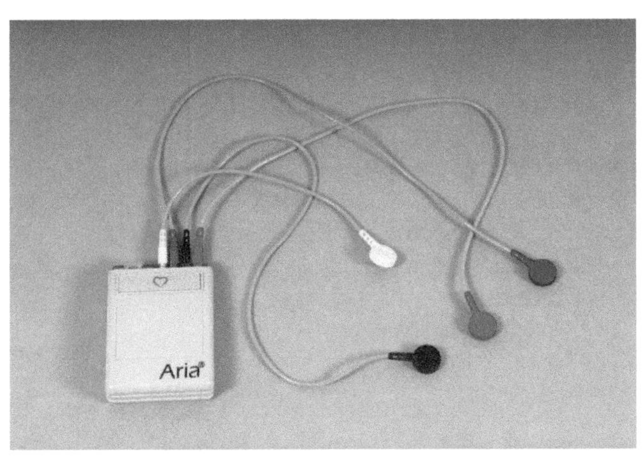

Fig. 12.14 Digital Holter monitor.

her usual daily activities with minimal inconvenience while being monitored.

A Holter monitor is similar to a resting 12-lead ECG in that the electrical impulses given off by the heart are picked up by electrodes and transmitted through lead wires to a recording device. It is different from a resting 12-lead ECG in that only about 10 seconds of the heart's activity are recorded with a 12-lead ECG, whereas a Holter monitor records the heartbeat continuously for an extended period of time. This allows the Holter monitor to pick up cardiac abnormalities that do not occur during the brief recording period of a resting 12-lead ECG.

PURPOSE

Holter monitor electrocardiography is an important noninvasive procedure used to diagnose cardiac rate, rhythm, and conduction abnormalities. Specifically, it is most frequently used for the following purposes:

- To assess the rate and rhythm of the heart during daily activities.
- To evaluate patients with unexplained chest pain, dizziness, or syncope (fainting).
- To discover intermittent cardiac dysrhythmias not picked up on a routine resting 12-lead ECG. A resting ECG records only 40 to 50 heartbeats, whereas a Holter monitor records approximately 100,000 heartbeats in a 24-hour period.
- To detect myocardial ischemia.
- To assess the effectiveness of antidysrhythmic medications (e.g., digitalis, antianginal medications).
- To assess the effectiveness of a pacemaker.

DIGITAL HOLTER MONITOR

A digital Holter monitor is lightweight and battery powered that uses a memory card to document the heart's activity (see Fig. 12.14). The monitor can be clipped onto a belt around the patient's waist. It can also be held in a protective pouch, which is hung around the patient's neck with a strap known as a *lanyard*. Digital monitors can continuously record the electrical activity of the heart for 24 hours, 48 hours, or 72 hours. Most providers order a 24-hour recording, but they may occasionally order a 48- or 72-hour recording when the heart's activity needs to be recorded for a longer period of time. Throughout the monitoring period, the system continuously records the electrical activity of the heart and stores it on the memory card. The monitor may have a small liquid crystal diode (LCD) screen that displays the date and time along with the remaining recording time. The Holter monitor automatically stops recording after the monitoring period has been completed.

Some providers have Holter monitors in their medical offices. The medical assistant is responsible for preparing the patient, applying and removing the monitor, and instructing the patient in patient preparation requirements and the guidelines that must be followed during the monitoring period (see Box 12.1). Procedure 12.2 describes how to apply a Holter monitor.

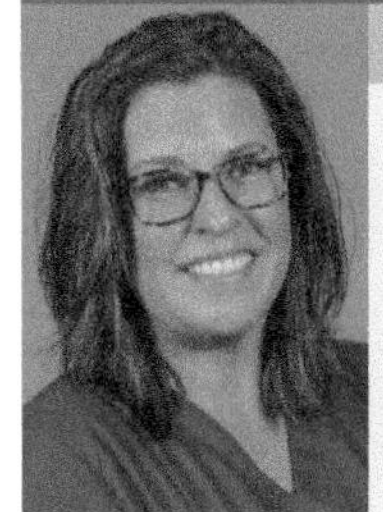

Memories *from* Practicum

Anitra: During my practicum, I was at an office where electrocardiograms were one of the many procedures performed. For my first electrocardiogram, the patient was a man who had a lot of hair on his chest, and I would need to shave the electrode placement sites on his chest. I was very nervous, but the procedure went well. When the electrocardiogram was run, he told me that I did a wonderful job and that it did not hurt at all to have his chest shaved. I realized then that it was not so bad after all. That patient made me feel so good about what I do and helped me feel confident in the procedures I had ahead of me. ■

PATIENT PREPARATION

The medical assistant should instruct the patient in the preparation required for the test, which includes the following:

1. Take a shower or bath before coming to the medical office to have the Holter monitor applied. You will not be able to shower or bathe again until the monitor is removed.
2. Do not apply body lotion, oil, or powder to your chest before or during the test. This may make it more difficult to apply the electrodes.
3. Take your usual medications unless the provider specifies otherwise.
4. Wear loose, comfortable clothing with a shirt or blouse that buttons down the front for easier application of the electrodes and to prevent the electrodes from rubbing against clothing and becoming loose.

ELECTRODE PLACEMENT

The purpose of the electrodes is to pick up the electrical impulses given off by the heart. The impulses are then transmitted through the lead wires and patient cable to the monitor. A special type of electrode is used with the Holter

BOX 12.1 Holter Monitor Patient Guidelines

Most routine activities can be performed while wearing a Holter monitor, except those that can damage the monitor or cause artifacts on the recording. Artifacts affect the quality of the recording and can lead to false-positive results on ECG recordings analyzed by a computer. The following guidelines must be relayed to the patient to ensure an accurate and reliable electrocardiographic recording:

1. Participate in your normal everyday activities during the monitoring period. The purpose of Holter monitoring is to determine how your heart functions during your usual daily activities. Avoid engaging in activities, however, that cause excessive sweating (such as vigorous physical exercise), which might cause the electrodes to become loose or fall off.
2. Do not shower, bathe, or swim while wearing the monitor because water can damage the monitor and loosen the electrodes. A sponge bath can be taken if needed.
3. Check periodically to make sure the monitor indicator light is still on and that all the electrodes and lead wires are still attached to the chest.
4. Do not touch or move the electrodes or lead wires during the monitoring period to prevent artifacts from appearing in the recording.
5. If a lead wire detaches from an electrode, snap it back onto the electrode as soon as possible, and record this information in the patient diary.
6. If an electrode comes loose, press down around the edges of the electrode and apply tape to the electrode to restore the contact. Document this information in the patient diary. Contact the medical office if an electrode comes off and cannot be replaced.
7. Do not handle the monitor or take it out of its pouch.
8. Do not use an electric blanket, hair dryer, electric shaver, heating pad, microwave oven, or electric toothbrush while wearing the monitor. Other items and areas to avoid during the testing period include magnets, metal detectors, and areas with high-voltage electrical wires. These items or areas can cause electrical interference artifacts, which may affect the quality of the recording.
9. Document your activities and emotional states in the patient diary. With each entry, note the time that the activity or emotional state occurred. The following activities should be documented:
   - Physical exercise associated with daily activities (e.g., walking, housework, gardening, employment-related activities)
   - Walking up or down stairs
   - Periods of inactivity (e.g., sitting in a chair, lying on a couch)
   - Driving
   - Smoking
   - Urination
   - Bowel movements
   - Meals (including alcohol and caffeinated beverages)
   - Sexual intercourse
   - Medications consumed
   - Sleep periods (including naps)

   The following are examples of emotional states that should be documented:
   - Anger
   - Excitement
   - Anxiety
   - Fear
   - Laughter
10. Document the physical symptoms experienced during each activity. If you do not experience anything abnormal during an activity, leave that symptom space blank. The following are examples of physical symptoms that should be documented:
    - Shortness of breath
    - Chest pain
    - Neck, arm, or face pain
    - Heart palpitations
    - Nausea
    - Dizziness
    - Faintness

monitor. It usually consists of foam and is round or rectangular in shape with an electrode plate and a snap for attaching a lead wire. The electrode has an adhesive backing and a central sponge pad that contains an electrolyte gel (Fig. 12.15). This type of electrode is disposable and must be discarded after use.

Most Holter monitors are three-channel recording systems. This means that the monitor can record three leads at one time. Depending on the brand and model of monitor, a three-channel monitor uses between four and seven electrodes that are placed at various locations on the patient's chest. Information on the number of electrodes and their locations is diagrammed in an electrode placement chart included in the operating manual that accompanies the Holter monitor. To reduce artifacts during the recording period, these electrodes are typically placed over bone, such as on the sternum or ribs. The medical assistant should make sure the electrodes are properly placed to ensure an accurate recording. When first learning to place these electrodes, it may help to mark their locations on the patient's chest with a felt-tipped pen.

The monitor's effectiveness should be checked after hooking up the patient to ensure that a clear signal is being relayed from the electrodes to the monitor. This check is performed by accessing the *Lead Status* screen on the LCD display screen located on the monitor. The quality of the ECG signal for each lead is displayed on the screen. The ECG signal should be clear and strong. If the signal is "noisy," this may indicate that an electrode does not have a good connection with the patient's skin. The medical assistant should apply gentle pressure to each electrode to improve contact

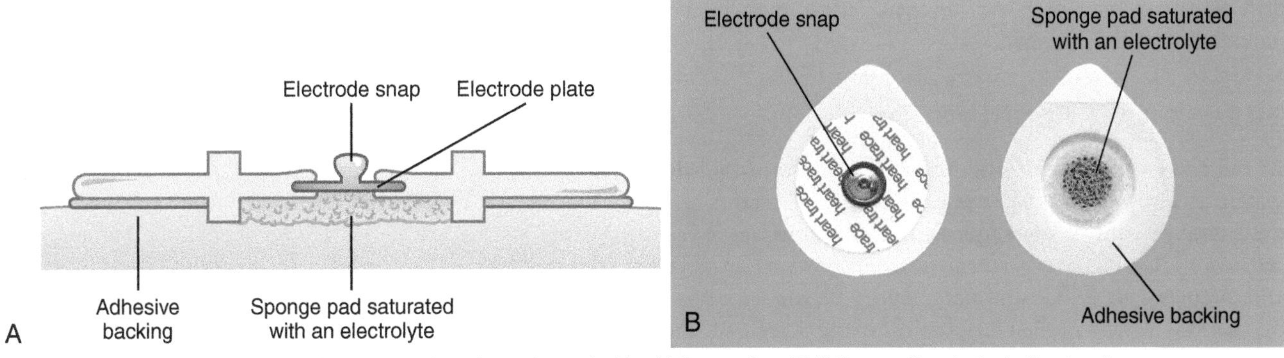

Fig. 12.15 (A) Diagram of an electrode used with a Holter monitor. (B) Holter monitor electrode (front and back).

PATIENT DIARY		
TIME	ACTIVITY	SYMPTOM
AM PM	*Start recording*	
8:30 AM	*Ate breakfast* *Smoked cigarette*	
9:15 AM	*Driving freeway*	*Chest pounding*
10:35 AM	*Argued with boss*	*Chest pain*
10:45 AM	*Took medication*	
12:30 PM	*Ate lunch*	
1:15 PM	*Walked up two flights of stairs*	*Stomach burning* *Pain in left arm*

Page 1

PATIENT DIARY		
TIME	ACTIVITY	SYMPTOM

Page 2

Fig. 12.16 Holter monitor patient diary.

with the patient's skin. If a problem still exists, the monitor may be malfunctioning and in need of repair.

PATIENT DIARY

An important aspect of the Holter monitor procedure is the completion of a diary by the patient (Fig. 12.16). All activities and emotional states must be documented during the monitoring period, along with the time of their occurrence. In addition, any physical symptoms experienced by the patient during the activity must be indicated next to each activity. A dysrhythmia or ECG change recorded by the Holter monitor can then be compared with the information in the patient's diary. This allows the provider to correlate patient activities, emotional states, and symptoms with cardiac activity to determine if a certain activity triggers an ECG abnormality.

EVENT MARKER

Some Holter monitor models have an *event marker* button, which is used along with the patient diary for patient evaluation. When the event marker button is pressed, a beep may sound as an audible feedback. The patient should be told to depress the button momentarily when experiencing a symptom and then document the time and nature of the symptom in the Holter diary. Depressing the button places an electronic signal on the recording. This signal highlights the specific portion of the recording where the symptom occurred. When a computer analyzes the patient data, the time of the event along with an *ECG event strip* will be included in the ECG report.

EVALUATING RESULTS

At the end of the monitoring period, the Holter monitor system is removed from the patient. The information on the memory card is then uploaded to a computer. Specialized ECG software performs calculations on the data and prepares an ECG summary report of the monitoring period, which is then displayed on the screen of the computer.

The computer-generated ECG report summarizes information about the patient's heart rate and rhythm and any abnormalities that occurred during the monitoring period. The report also includes selected samples of the patient's cardiac activity, including patient event strips and any abnormal cardiac activity exhibited by the patient, such as dysrhythmias. The results of the ECG summary report are reviewed and interpreted further by the provider. The provider also reviews the patient's diary to determine if there is a correlation between any of the patient's activities, emotional states, or symptoms and ECG abnormalities. The ECG summary report can be printed out and stored in a paper-based patient record (PPR) or stored electronically in the patient's EHR.

MAINTENANCE OF THE HOLTER MONITOR

At the end of each recording period, the battery should be removed from the monitor and discarded. Leaving a battery in the monitor could corrode the battery, which could damage the monitor. The casing of the monitor should be cleaned frequently, using a soft cloth moistened with a mild disinfectant to remove dust and dirt. Commercial solvents and abrasives should not be used because they can damage the finish of the casing. The patient cable and lead wires should be cleaned periodically with a cloth moistened with a mild disinfectant. The cable and lead wires should never be immersed in the cleaning solution because this could damage them. The snap of each lead wire should be cleaned with alcohol and a small brush to eliminate any trace of gel remaining after the use of disposable electrodes. The monitor should be stored in a dry, dust-free area.

CARDIAC DYSRHYTHMIAS

The normal ECG graph cycle consists of a P wave, a QRS complex, and a T wave, which repeat in a regular pattern (see Fig. 12.4). The term **normal sinus rhythm** refers to an ECG that is within normal limits. This means that the waves, intervals, segments, and cardiac rate fall within the normal range. The normal heart rate ranges from 60 to 100 beats per minute. A rate slower than 60 beats per minute is *sinus bradycardia,* and a rate faster than 100 beats per minute is *sinus tachycardia.*

Cardiac **dysrhythmia** is the term used to describe abnormal electrical activity in the heart causing an irregular heartbeat. Cardiac dysrhythmias can be classified into one of the following categories: (1) extra beats, (2) an abnormal rhythm, or (3) an abnormal heart rate. Most cardiac dysrhythmias are harmless; however, some can be serious or even life threatening. The medical assistant should be able to recognize basic cardiac dysrhythmias on an electrocardiographic recording for the purpose of alerting the provider of their presence. The dysrhythmias the medical assistant should be able to identify are presented next, along with brief descriptions and significant clinical aspects.

PREMATURE ATRIAL CONTRACTION

Description

A premature atrial contraction (PAC) is characterized by a beat that comes before the next normal beat is due. The most distinguishing feature is that the P wave of the premature beat has a different shape from the P wave of the normal beat. The PAC has a normal QRS complex and a normal T wave, similar to the other ECG graph cycles.

Clinical Significance

PACs are common in healthy individuals and are often associated with the intake of stimulants, such as caffeine and tobacco. They also can be associated with more serious atrial dysrhythmias and structural heart disease.

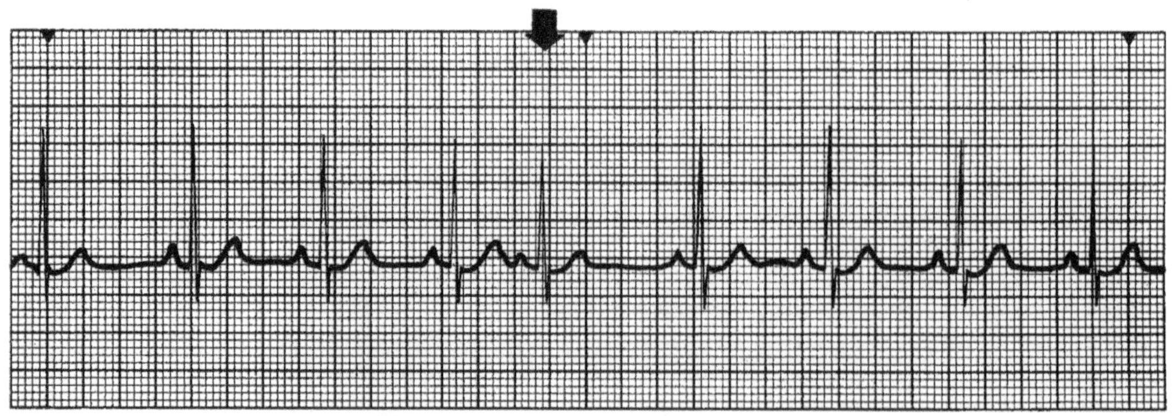

Premature atrial contraction. (From Huang SH, Kessler CA, McCulloch CD, Dasher LA: *Coronary care nursing,* Philadelphia, PA: WB Saunders; 1989.)

PAROXYSMAL SUPRAVENTRICULAR TACHYCARDIA

Description

Paroxysmal supraventricular tachycardia (PSVT) is an abrupt episode of tachycardia with a constant heart rate that usually falls between 150 and 250 beats per minute. PSVT is characterized by a rhythm that has a sudden onset and termination. The sudden increase in rate occurs in short bursts and lasts only a few seconds, after which the rate returns to what it was before the PSVT occurred. Because of the increase in heart rate, the ECG graph cycles are very close together. With PSVT, the patient experiences a sudden pounding or fluttering of the chest associated with weakness, breathlessness, and acute apprehension. Occasionally, the patient experiences syncope.

Clinical Significance

PSVT is one of the most common rhythm disorders, often occurring in healthy patients with no underlying heart disease and young adults with normal hearts. It also can occur in individuals with organic heart disease.

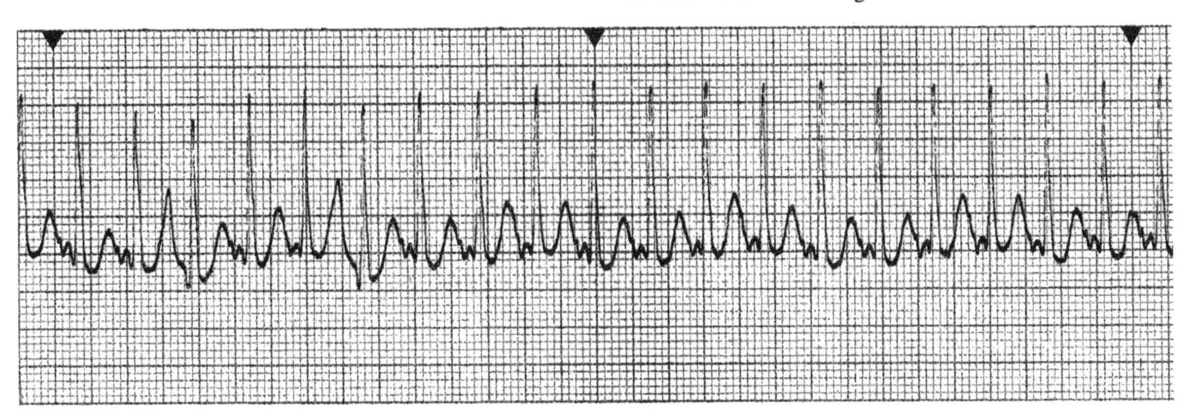

Premature supraventricular tachycardia. (From Huang SH, Kessler CA, McCulloch CD, Dasher LA: *Coronary care nursing,* Philadelphia, PA: WB Saunders; 1989.)

PATIENT COACHING Angina Pectoris

Answer questions the patient has about angina pectoris.

What is angina pectoris?

Angina pectoris is a symptom, or a set of symptoms, rather than a disease. Its name is a Latin term that means "pain in the chest." Angina pectoris occurs when the muscle tissue of the heart does not receive enough oxygenated blood, resulting in discomfort or pain under the sternum.

What causes angina pectoris?

For most patients, the cause of angina is atherosclerosis. *Atherosclerosis* is a condition in which fibrous plaques of fatty deposits and cholesterol build up on the inner walls of the arteries. This causes narrowing and partial blockage of the lumen of these arteries, along with hardening of the arterial wall. Atherosclerosis in the coronary arteries is called coronary artery disease (CAD). CAD results in a reduction in oxygenated blood flow to the heart muscle. Despite the narrowing, enough oxygen may still reach the heart muscle for normal needs. More oxygen is needed, however, when situations occur that increase the workload of the heart, such as physical activity, emotional stress, a heavy meal, and exposure to cold weather. If the coronary arteries cannot deliver enough oxygen to the heart muscle during these times of increased need, angina pectoris results.

What happens during an angina episode?

Individuals experience angina in different ways, including the following: severe indigestion, tightness or burning, heaviness, ache, and squeezing or crushing pressure in the center of the chest. Other symptoms that may occur with an angina episode include shortness of breath, sweating, nausea, weakness, fatigue, heart palpitations, and dizziness. The chest discomfort that occurs with an angina episode varies greatly. It can feel only mildly uncomfortable, or it may be intense and accompanied by a feeling of suffocation and doom. Pain is usually felt beneath the sternum and may radiate to the neck, throat, jaw, left shoulder, arm, or back. In most cases, the pain lasts no longer than a few minutes and is relieved by resting. Severe and prolonged anginal pain generally suggests a myocardial infarction (heart attack) caused by complete blockage of the coronary arteries and requires immediate medical attention.

What tests might the provider order?

For patients who exhibit angina pectoris, the provider may order one or more of the following: an electrocardiogram, cardiac stress test, echocardiogram, nuclear stress test, chest x-ray, blood tests, coronary angiography, cardiac CT scan, or a cardiac MRI. These tests assist in detecting coronary artery narrowing and blockage. To determine the exact location and extent of blockage, a more specific test, known as *coronary angiography,* may be performed.

What type of treatment might the provider prescribe?

The goal of treating angina is to reduce the workload of the heart and increase the oxygen supply to the heart. This is accomplished by resting when an angina attack occurs. In addition, the provider often

Continued

prescribes medications, the most common one being nitroglycerin. Nitroglycerin is usually taken sublingually. It works by reducing the workload of the heart and increasing the oxygen supply to the heart by dilating the coronary arteries. Nitroglycerin also can be administered through patches worn on the skin or an ointment rubbed into the skin.

To help prevent more serious heart disease from developing, the provider generally recommends lifestyle changes, such as a diet low in cholesterol and saturated fat, weight reduction, controlling high blood pressure, smoking cessation, exercise, and stress reduction. For patients with severe blockage of the coronary arteries, balloon angioplasty with coronary stent placement or coronary artery bypass surgery may be recommended.

Provide the patient with educational materials on angina pectoris and coronary artery disease. ■

ATRIAL FLUTTER

Description

Atrial flutter (AFL) is a rapid, regular fluttering of the atrium in which the heart rate falls between 250 and 350 beats per minute. More than one P wave precedes each QRS complex, and the P waves appear as saw-toothed spikes between the QRS complexes. The number of waves can range from just one extra P wave to eight falling in rapid succession, but all have the same size and shape. The QRS complexes of an AFL configuration are normal; however, the T wave is usually lost in the P waves.

Clinical Significance

AFL rarely occurs in healthy individuals. It is found in patients with underlying heart disease. AFL is not specific to any particular heart disease; it can occur in patients with mitral valve disease, CAD, acute myocardial infarction, chronic lung disease, hypertensive heart disease, and pulmonary emboli, and in patients who have undergone cardiac surgery.

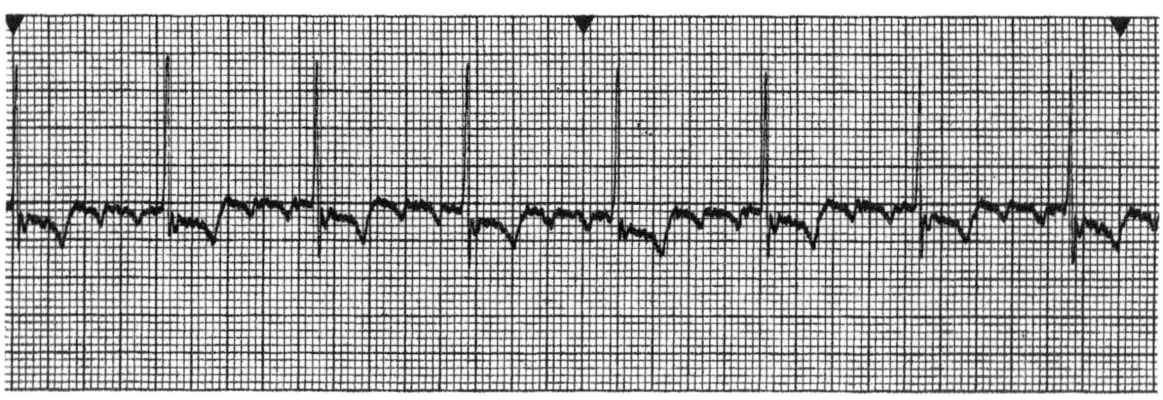

Atrial flutter. (From Johnson R, Swartz MH: *A simplified approach to electrocardiography,* Philadelphia, PA: WB Saunders; 1986.)

ATRIAL FIBRILLATION

Description

Atrial fibrillation (A-fib) is characterized by an ECG in which the P waves have no definite pattern or shape. The P waves appear as irregular wavy undulations between the QRS complexes. The QRS complexes in A-fib are normal but do not have a definite pattern. It is difficult to measure accurately the atrial rate because the P waves are not discernible; however, the atria are contracting between 400 and 600 times per minute. The ventricular rate may be rapid (150 to 180 beats per minute) or relatively normal. A-fib can cause blood to pool in the atrium of the heart; the pooled blood may cause formation of a blood clot, which can travel to the brain, resulting in a stroke.

Clinical Significance

A-fib is a common dysrhythmia that can occur in healthy individuals and in patients with a variety of cardiac diseases. In healthy individuals, it can be initiated by emotional stress, excessive alcohol consumption, and vomiting. In individuals younger than 50 years old, the common causes of A-fib are congenital heart disease and rheumatic heart disease with mitral valve involvement. In individuals older than 50, A-fib

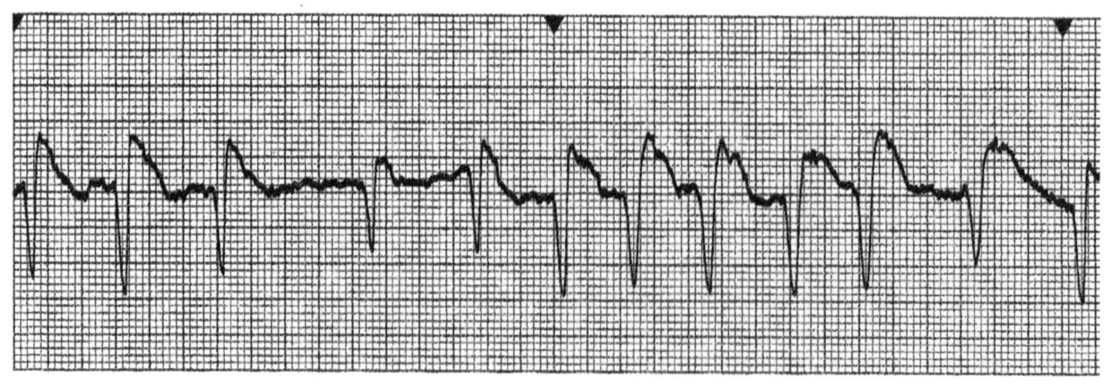

Atrial fibrillation. (From Huang SH, Kessler CA, McCulloch CD, Dasher LA: *Coronary care nursing,* Philadelphia, PA: WB Saunders; 1989.)

is caused by diseases capable of producing either ischemia or hypertrophy of the atria, such as CAD, mitral valve disease, and hypertensive heart disease.

PREMATURE VENTRICULAR CONTRACTION

Description

Premature ventricular contractions (PVCs) are among the most common rhythm disturbances seen on an ECG. The PVC is characterized by a beat that comes early in the cycle, is not preceded by a P wave, has a wide and distorted QRS complex, and has a T wave opposite in direction to the R wave of the QRS complex. Because of the unusual configuration of the QRS complex, the PVC easily stands out from the normal ECG graph cycles. The baseline distance after the PVC is usually longer than the normal distance between the other cycles. In other words, the PVC is followed by a pause before the next normal beat.

Clinical Significance

PVCs are seen in normal individuals in all age groups and are caused by anxiety, smoking, caffeine, alcohol, and certain medications (e.g., epinephrine, isoproterenol, aminophylline). PVCs can occur with virtually any type of heart disease but are seen most often in patients with hypertensive heart disease, ischemic heart disease, lung disease with hypoxia, and digitalis toxicity. PVCs also are common in individuals with mitral valve prolapse.

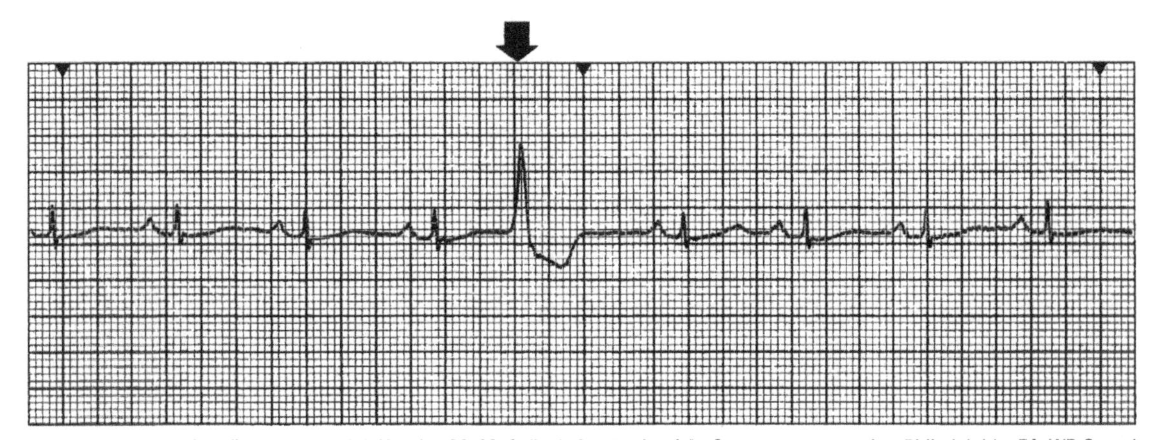

Premature ventricular contraction. (From Huang SH, Kessler CA, McCulloch CD, Dasher LA: *Coronary care nursing,* Philadelphia, PA: WB Saunders; 1989.)

VENTRICULAR TACHYCARDIA

Description

Ventricular tachycardia (V-tach) consists of a series of three or more consecutive PVCs that occur at a rate of 150 to 300 per minute. The tachycardia may occur paroxysmally and last only a short time, or it may persist for a long time. The QRS complexes are bizarre and widened, and no P waves are present. Sustained V-tach is a life-threatening dysrhythmia because the rapid ventricular rate prevents adequate filling time for the heart, leading to reduced cardiac output that often degenerates into ventricular fibrillation (V-fib) and cardiac arrest.

Clinical Significance

V-tach is usually seen in patients with acute or chronic heart disease. Runs of V-tach indicate CAD. V-tach also occurs as a complication of a myocardial infarction.

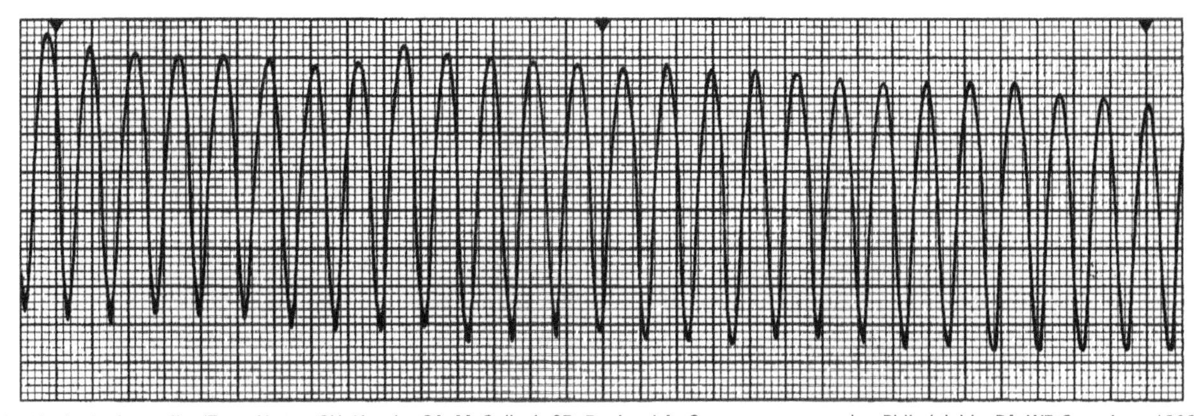

Ventricular tachycardia. (From Huang SH, Kessler CA, McCulloch CD, Dasher LA: *Coronary care nursing,* Philadelphia, PA: WB Saunders; 1989.)

VENTRICULAR FIBRILLATION

Description

V-fib is the most serious dysrhythmia. With this type of dysrhythmia, the ventricles do not beat in a coordinated manner, but instead they quiver or fibrillate. Because of this, virtually no blood is ejected into the systemic circulation. On an ECG, V-fib is characterized by irregular, chaotic undulations of the baseline. There are no recognizable P waves, QRS complexes, or T waves in the irregular line of jagged spikes. Because the ventricles are quivering irregularly, there is no effective ventricular pumping action, resulting in no circulation. V-fib is a serious dysrhythmia that must be treated immediately because it can lead to sudden death.

Clinical Significance

The most common cause of V-fib is an acute myocardial infarction. It also can occur in patients with organic heart disease and cardiac dysrhythmias. It may be preceded by a dysrhythmia such as PVCs or V-tach, or it may occur spontaneously.

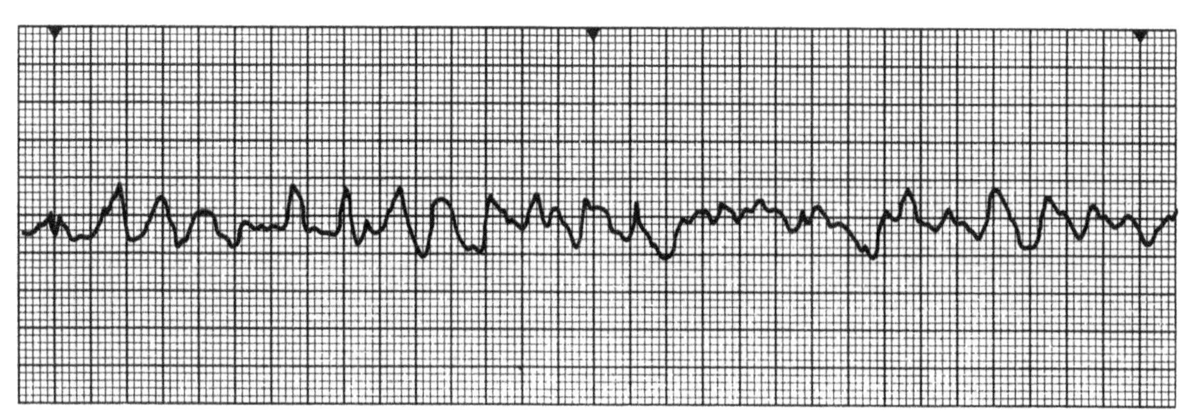

Ventricular fibrillation. (From Huang SH, Kessler CA, McCulloch CD, Dasher LA: *Coronary care nursing,* Philadelphia, PA: WB Saunders; 1989.)

PULMONARY FUNCTION TESTS

The purpose of a pulmonary function test (PFT) is to assess lung functioning, assisting in the detection and evaluation of pulmonary disease. PFTs include spirometry, lung volumes, diffusion capacity, arterial blood gas (ABG) studies, pulse oximetry, and cardiopulmonary exercise tests. The most frequently performed PFT is spirometry, which is described in detail in the next section. Procedure 12.3 presents the procedure for performing a spirometry test.

SPIROMETRY

Spirometry is a simple, noninvasive screening test that is often performed in the medical office. A computerized electronic instrument known as a **spirometer** is used to conduct the test. A spirometer measures how much air is pushed out of the lungs and how fast it is pushed out. The spirometry report is printed out as a table and graph. Spirometry is considered a screening test, and abnormal test results require that the patient undergo additional PFTs and possibly a computed tomography scan before a diagnosis can be made. Indications for performing spirometry include the following:

1. Patients who exhibit symptoms of lung dysfunction such as dyspnea
2. Individuals at high risk for lung disease because of smoking or exposure to environmental pollutants such as coal dust, asbestos, and exhaust fumes
3. Patients with lung disease, such as asthma, chronic bronchitis, and emphysema
4. Patients who are to undergo surgery (to assess probable lung performance during an operation)
5. Patients who need to be evaluated for lung disability or impairment for a compensation program (e.g., coal miners)

Spirometry Test Results

The results obtained from spirometry testing provide numerous measurements that help the provider assess lung functioning. The most important parameters are described next.

Forced Vital Capacity

Forced vital capacity (FVC) is the maximum volume of air (measured in liters) that can be expired when the patient exhales as forcefully and rapidly as possible and for as long as possible. FVC is obtained by having the patient perform a breathing maneuver. The patient is instructed to take a deep breath until the lungs are completely full. Following this, the patient is told to blow all the air out of the lungs and into the mouthpiece as hard and as fast as possible until no more air can be expelled. To be considered an adequate test, the patient must forcibly blow out all the air from the lungs and continue smooth, continuous exhaling for at least 6 seconds. To be considered a valid test, a minimum of three acceptable efforts must be obtained.

Some patients have difficulty performing the FVC breathing maneuver because they have a physical impairment or poor motivation, or they do not understand the instructions. The medical assistant should be patient and work with these individuals to help them perform the maneuver. If patients are unable to perform the maneuver after eight attempts, however, testing should be discontinued. At this point, fatigue may affect the accuracy of the results, and additional efforts are not recommended.

What Would You Do? What Would You *Not* Do?

Case Study 2

Joel Matthews, 48 years old, is at the office for a checkup. Joel had a mild heart attack two years ago. Since then, he has made significant changes to his lifestyle. He's become a vegetarian and practices yoga every morning before going to work. After he gets home, he jogs 10 miles. He also lifts weights every other day and takes herbal vitamin supplements. Since his heart attack, he has lost 40 pounds and says that he has never felt better. The only thing he cannot seem to do is give up smoking. He started smoking when he was 17 years old and has cut back from two packs to one pack a day. He keeps trying to stop but says that he has been smoking so long that it might not be possible. Besides, with all the other healthy stuff he is doing, he thinks it probably cancels out the bad effect of the cigarettes. Joel is very concerned that if he does stop smoking, he will gain back all of the weight that it took him so long to lose. ■

Forced Expiratory Volume after 1 Second

Forced expiratory volume after 1 second (FEV_1) is the volume of air (in liters) that is forcefully exhaled during the first second of the FVC breathing maneuver. The spirometer automatically determines this parameter from the FVC maneuver.

FEV_1/FVC Ratio

In patients with healthy lungs, 70% to 75% of the air exhaled (FVC) is exhaled in the first second (FEV_1) of the breathing maneuver. This comparison is known as the *FEV_1/FVC ratio,* and it is expressed as a percentage. A patient with healthy lungs may have a FEV_1/FVC ratio of 85%. This means that 85% of the exhaled air was exhaled during the first second of the breathing maneuver.

In patients with chronic obstructive pulmonary disease (COPD), the FEV_1/FVC ratio is less than 70% to 75%. These patients are unable to move most of their exhaled air out of the lungs during the first second because of an obstruction to the airflow, such as inflammation or damaged lung tissue. Based on the FEV_1/FVC ratio, the obstruction is characterized as mild (61% to 69%), moderate (45% to 60%), or severe (less than 45%). Fig. 12.17 shows a graph of spirometry parameters in a patient with healthy lungs and in a patient with obstructive pulmonary disease.

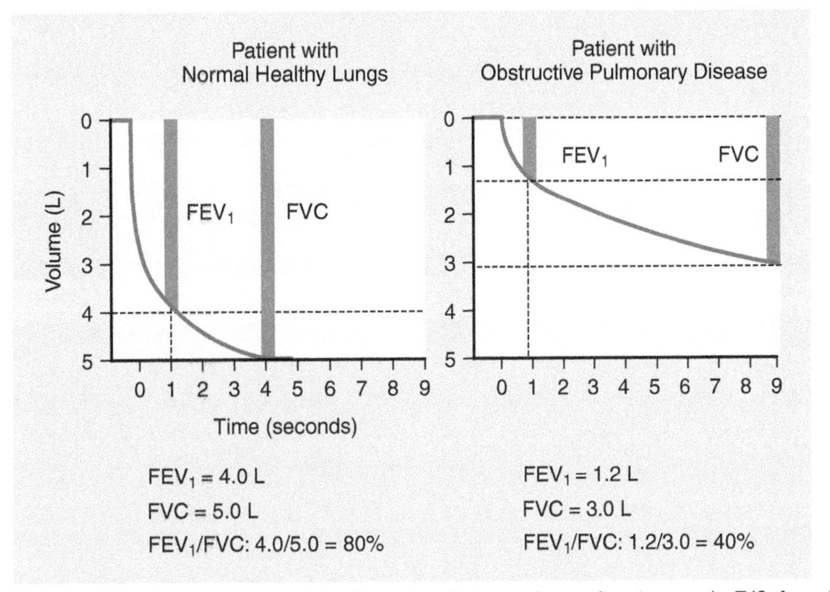

Fig. 12.17 Spirometry parameters. *FEV_1*, Forced expiratory volume after 1 second; *FVC,* forced vital capacity.

Evaluation of Results

To evaluate the spirometry test results fully, certain demographic factors must be taken into consideration, including the patient's age, sex, weight, and height. These demographic factors are used to calculate the *predicted values,* which is what the results should be for a patient with healthy lungs. When the test is run, the provider compares the patient's *measured values* with the predicted values. For example, the FVC predicted value is 6 L, and the FVC measured value is 4 L. This means that the patient should have been able to exhale 6 L of air (based on age, sex, weight, and height), but he or she was able to exhale only 4 L of air.

The computerized spirometer automatically calculates predicted values using demographic information entered into the machine by the medical assistant. The predicted values and the measured values are printed on the spirometry report. Fig. 12.18 shows an example of these results. Comparing the

Parameter	Predicted Values	Measured Values
FVC	6.00 L	4.00 L
FEV_1	5.00 L	2.00 L
FEV_1/FVC	83%	50%

Fig. 12.18 Predicted values compared with measured values. This individual exhibits a moderate airflow obstruction. *FEV_1*, Forced expiratory volume after 1 second; *FVC,* forced vital capacity.

measured values with the predicted values assists the provider in detecting the presence of pulmonary disease.

Patient Preparation

Patient preparation is essential to obtain accurate test results. To prepare for the test, the patient should be instructed to do the following:

1. Do not eat a heavy meal for 8 hours before the test. (The patient must exert the diaphragm muscles, and a full stomach may interfere with this action.)
2. Stop smoking at least 8 hours before the test.
3. Do not take bronchodilators for 4 hours before the test.
4. Do not engage in strenuous activity for 4 hours before the test.
5. Wear loose, nonrestrictive clothing to keep the chest area as free as possible, which makes it easier to perform the breathing maneuver.

Calibration of the Spirometer

To ensure accurate and valid test results, the spirometer should be calibrated each day that the machine is used. Calibration is performed by injecting a known quantity of air into the spirometer. A large 3-L spirometry syringe is used to inject 3 L of air into the machine. The output should read 3 L, and the reading should not vary by more than 3%. If the machine is not properly calibrated, the medical assistant should consult the operating manual and adjust the machine as required.

POST-BRONCHODILATOR SPIROMETRY

If the results of the spirometry test indicate a possible obstruction, the provider usually orders a post-bronchodilator spirometry test. This test is performed by having the patient inhale a bronchodilator and running a spirometry test approximately 10 to 15 minutes later. The purpose of this test is to inform the provider as to how treatment would work in patients whose airways are obstructed. If the FVC or FEV_1 parameter increases by at least 15%, the result is reported as positive for bronchodilator responsiveness. This means that the obstruction may be reversible or partially reversible through the use of medication.

What Would You Do? What Would You *Not* Do?

Case Study 3

Walter Conrad, 62 years old, comes to the office because he gets short of breath when he goes up and down stairs. He has worked in the coal mines his whole life and has just retired. The physician orders a pulmonary function test. Walter tries to breathe like he is supposed to during the spirometry test, but he cannot do it, and he is getting dizzy from trying so hard. He also is having problems with the nose clips. He says they pinch his nose, and he feels like he is being smothered. After four attempts, he puts down the spirometer in frustration and wants to know if he can come back some other time. He says that he is thinking his symptoms are not that bad after all, and maybe he will just wait and see what happens and will come back if they get worse. ■

HIGHLIGHT on Smoking and Chronic Obstructive Pulmonary Disease

Chronic Obstructive Pulmonary Disease Defined

COPD is a chronic airway obstruction that results from emphysema or chronic bronchitis or a combination of these conditions. COPD is a chronic, debilitating, irreversible, and sometimes fatal disease.

More than 16 million Americans have been diagnosed with COPD; however, it is estimated that an additional 8 million Americans have the disease and remain undiagnosed. Smoking tobacco is the primary cause of COPD. In the United States, approximately 85% to 90% of deaths from COPD are caused by smoking. According to the American Lung Association, COPD is the fourth leading cause of death in the United States, behind heart disease, cancer, and stroke. COPD claims the lives of more than 140,000 Americans each year.

Emphysema

Emphysema is most often seen in older individuals with a long history of smoking. Emphysema due to smoking is caused by irreversible damage to the alveoli in the lungs from toxins present in cigarette smoke (see illustration). As alveoli continue to be damaged, the lungs are able to transfer less and less oxygen to the bloodstream. In addition, air becomes trapped in the damaged alveoli, making it difficult to remove during exhalation. Because of this, the primary symptom of emphysema is shortness of breath. Other symptoms include chronic cough, tiredness, and limited exercise tolerance. More than 3 million people in the United States currently have been diagnosed with emphysema. The reason is not yet understood, but only 15% to 20% of long-term smokers develop emphysema.

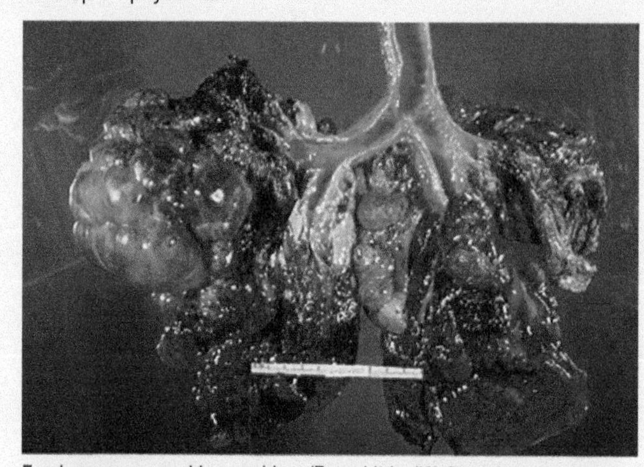

Emphysema caused by smoking. (From Little JW: Dental management of the medically compromised patient, ed 7, St Louis: Elsevier; 2008. Courtesy McLay RN, etal. Tulane gross pathology tutorial. Last modified July 15, 1997, Tulane University School of Medicine, New Orleans, LA.)

HIGHLIGHT on Smoking and Chronic Obstructive Pulmonary Disease—cont'd

Chronic Bronchitis

Chronic bronchitis is an inflammation of the lining of the bronchiole tubes that causes swelling and excess production of mucus. Swelling and excess mucus narrow the bronchiole tubes and restrict airflow into and out of the lungs. Symptoms include chronic cough, shortness of breath, and coughing up of mucus. To be classified as chronic bronchitis, the symptoms must last 3 or more months out of the year for at least 2 years. As the disease progresses, the lips and skin may exhibit cyanosis resulting from lack of oxygen in the blood. Chronic bronchitis is most often caused by long-term irritation of the bronchial tubes as a result of cigarette smoking; other causes include air pollution and exposure to dust or toxic gases in the workplace (e.g., coal mines). Chronic bronchitis often precedes or accompanies emphysema. It is estimated that 10 million Americans have chronic bronchitis. This condition affects individuals of all ages but has a higher incidence in individuals older than 45 years. Women are more than twice as likely to be diagnosed with chronic bronchitis as men.

Symptoms of Chronic Obstructive Pulmonary Disease

Damage to the lungs caused by COPD occurs gradually over many years. In fact, more than 90% of patients who have COPD are over the age of 45 at the time of their diagnosis. Because there are no early symptoms, many people do not know they have COPD. By the time an individual experiences symptoms, it is usually a sign that irreversible lung damage has already occurred. The first symptoms of COPD include mild shortness of breath on exertion and occasional coughing. The disease slowly becomes more pronounced with severe episodes of dyspnea and coughing after even modest activity. As the disease progresses, the heart also can be affected and shortness of breath is present all the time, even while the patient is sitting quietly. At this point the individual's quality of life is greatly diminished. When the lungs and the heart are no longer able to deliver oxygen to the body's tissues, death occurs.

Treatment for Chronic Obstructive Pulmonary Disease

The best treatment for COPD caused by smoking is for the patient to stop smoking. Continued smoking makes the COPD worse; quitting smoking slows the disease process. There are programs, support groups, nicotine replacement aids (e.g., nicotine patch, gum, lozenges, inhalers, nasal sprays), and prescription medications (e.g., Chantix, Zyban) to help individuals quit smoking. Other forms of treatment depend on the patient's condition and degree of lung impairment and may include the following:

1. Bronchodilators to relax and widen the bronchial tubes to increase airflow. They may be inhaled as aerosol sprays or taken orally.
2. Expectorants to thin the mucus so that it is easier to expel.
3. Antibiotics to treat infections that could interfere further with breathing and lung function.
4. Corticosteroids to reduce inflammation in the airways.
5. Breathing exercises to strengthen the muscles used to breathe.
6. Maintenance of overall good health habits, which include proper nutrition, adequate sleep, and regular exercise.
7. Oxygen therapy for patients with low blood oxygen to help with shortness of breath, allowing them to be more active.
8. Special measures including avoiding extremes of temperature (heat and cold), getting an annual influenza immunization, avoiding individuals with respiratory infection, and reducing exposure to air pollution.
9. Lung transplantation surgery is being performed on some patients who are in the later stages of COPD. ■

PEAK FLOW MEASUREMENT

ASTHMA

Asthma is a chronic inflammatory lung disease that affects the airways of the lungs. Asthma is characterized by recurrent episodes of coughing, chest tightness, shortness of breath, and wheezing known as an *asthma attack* or *flare-up*. **Wheezing** is a continuous, high-pitched, whistling, musical sound heard particularly during exhalation and sometimes during inhalation.

Asthma can develop at any age but is more common in children and young adults. In the United States, there are approximately 20 million individuals with asthma; of these, 6 million are children. Each year, more than 4000 deaths result from asthma.

The exact cause of asthma is not known. It is thought to be caused by a combination of factors, including genetics, certain childhood respiratory infections, and contact with allergens or exposure to certain viral infections in infancy or early childhood.

Asthma Triggers

In a normal individual, the airways to the lungs are fully open, allowing air to move easily into and out of the lungs. In a patient with asthma, the airways are always inflamed and hypersensitive to certain stimuli that do not affect the airways of normal individuals. These stimuli are known as *asthma triggers* because they can "trigger" an asthma attack. Asthma triggers vary from one patient to another and may also vary from one season to the next. Examples of common allergens that may trigger an asthma attack include dust mites, pollens, molds, animal dander, and cockroaches. Asthma attacks can also be triggered by environmental irritants, activities, or events, including air pollutants, tobacco smoke, chemical fumes (e.g., perfume, paint, and gasoline), vigorous physical exercise, upper respiratory viral infections, exposure to cold, and emotional stress. It is sometimes

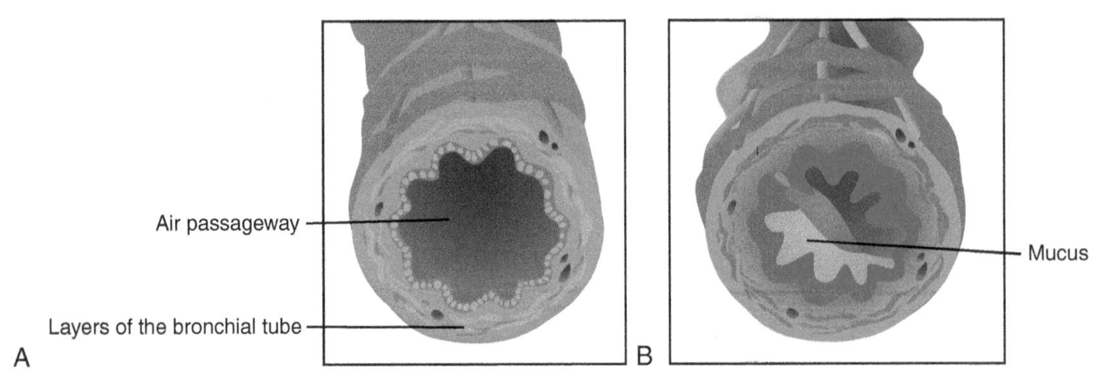

Fig. 12.19 (A) Normal bronchial tube. (B) Bronchial tube during an asthma attack.

difficult to determine what specific triggers cause a patient's asthma attacks.

Asthma Attack

When the inflamed airways of a patient with asthma are stimulated by a trigger, the inflamed airways become even more inflamed causing a series of reactions occur. The bronchial tubes begin to constrict and swell, causing the patient to experience the symptoms of an asthma flare-up. Sometimes the symptoms are mild and go away, either on their own or with treatment with medication. At other times, the symptoms become worse, leading to a severe asthma attack. During a severe attack the bronchial tubes continue to constrict and swell and become clogged with mucus (Fig. 12.19). This results in less air moving into and out of the lungs, which leads to a decrease in the amount of oxygen available to the body. The narrowed bronchial tubes and decreased oxygen supply cause the patient to experience coughing, chest tightness, shortness of breath, and wheezing, making it hard to breathe. A severe asthma attack that does not improve with medication therapy can become a life-threatening emergency.

Depending on the patient, asthma attacks vary in frequency and severity and may come on suddenly or gradually. An asthma attack may last for only 10 to 15 minutes or it may last for hours or even days.

Diagnosis and Treatment

The provider diagnoses asthma through a careful and detailed medical history. Of particular importance to the diagnosis of asthma are the patient's symptoms, family history of asthma, home and work environment, and living habits. The provider also performs a thorough physical examination to detect symptoms resulting from asthma, such as wheezing. When the medical history and physical examination have been completed, the provider usually orders laboratory and diagnostic tests, which may include PFTs (e.g., spirometry), allergy testing, and ABG studies.

Although asthma is a chronic disease with no cure, most patients with asthma are able to lead a normal life through proper management and treatment. It is important to treat symptoms when they first begin to occur to prevent them from getting worse and causing a severe asthma attack, which may require emergency treatment. The general treatment of asthma includes identifying and avoiding asthma triggers (if possible) and preventing and alleviating asthma symptoms through medication therapy. Two general categories of medication are prescribed for asthma: long-term–control medication and quick-relief medication.

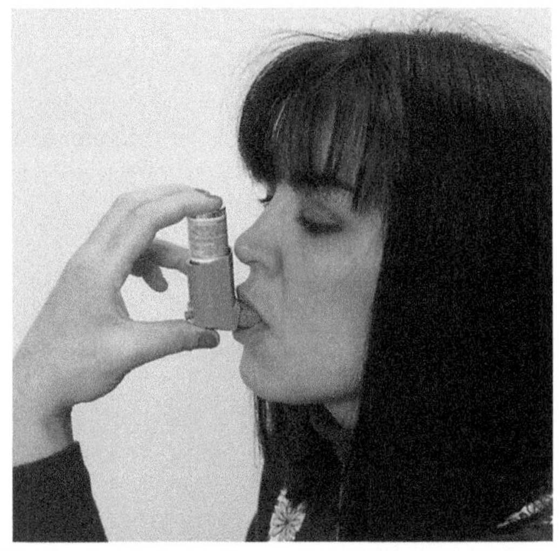

Fig. 12.20 An inhaler is often used to deliver asthma medication to the bronchial tubes of the lungs. (From Potter PA: *Basic nursing: essentials for practice*, ed 7, St Louis: Elsevier; 2011.)

- **Long-term–control medication** helps relieve bronchial inflammation and prevents symptoms from occurring. Control medication helps the patient have fewer and milder asthma attacks and is typically taken every day. Corticosteroids are an example of a control medication; brand names include Flovent, Pulmicort, Asmanex, Qvar, and AeroBid. Other examples of long-term control medication include Singulair, Accolate, Serevent, Zyflo, and Advair.
- **Quick-relief medication** (also called *rescue medication*) opens the airways quickly by dilating the bronchial tubes. It is taken when the patient is experiencing symptoms to prevent or control an asthma attack. Fast-acting bronchodilators are an example of quick-relief medication; brand names include Proventil, Ventolin, and Xopenex.

Many asthma medications are delivered through an *inhaler* (Fig. 12.20), which allows the medication to go directly to the lungs. Quick-relief medications can be used in a breathing machine known as a *nebulizer* to treat an asthma

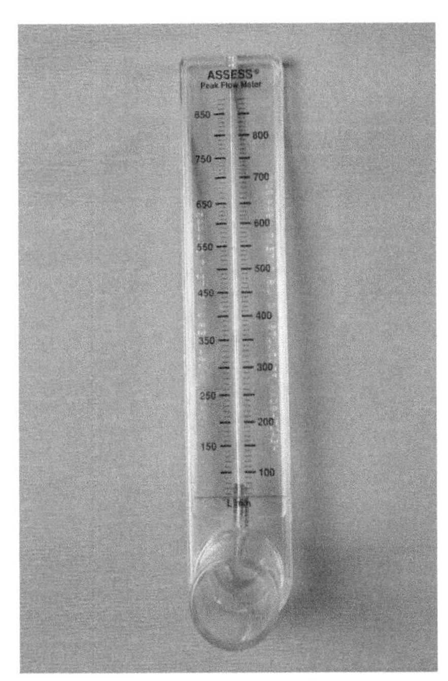

Fig. 12.21 Manual peak flow meter.

attack at home. Other asthma medications are administered orally; however, they take longer to work because they first have to travel through the digestive and circulatory systems before reaching the lungs.

PEAK FLOW METER

A peak flow meter is a portable, handheld device used to measure a breathing maneuver performed by the patient. It is recommended that a peak flow meter be used on a regular schedule by patients with moderate to severe asthma to determine how well their asthma is being controlled. The measurements obtained from a peak flow meter are not as accurate as those obtained by spirometry; however, a peak flow meter can be used easily by a patient at home. The provider determines each patient's schedule of use based on the severity and frequency of asthma symptoms. Most providers recommend that the patient use a peak flow meter at least once a day, preferably in the morning before taking asthma medication. A peak flow measurement should also be obtained when the patient is having symptoms. If the patient has a more severe form of asthma, the provider may want the patient to use a peak flow meter twice a day—in the morning and in the evening.

Peak flow meters can be purchased over the counter and are available in two types: manual and digital. *A manual peak flow meter* consists of a plastic tube with a sliding indicator that manually moves along a scale of numbers when the patient performs the breathing maneuver (Fig. 12.21). They are available in two ranges: a low range and a full range. The *low-range meter* has a range from 0 to 300 and is used by young children and some older patients. The *full-range meter* has a range from 0 to 800 and is used by older children, teenagers, and adults (Fig. 12.22). An adult has much larger bronchial tubes than a child and needs the

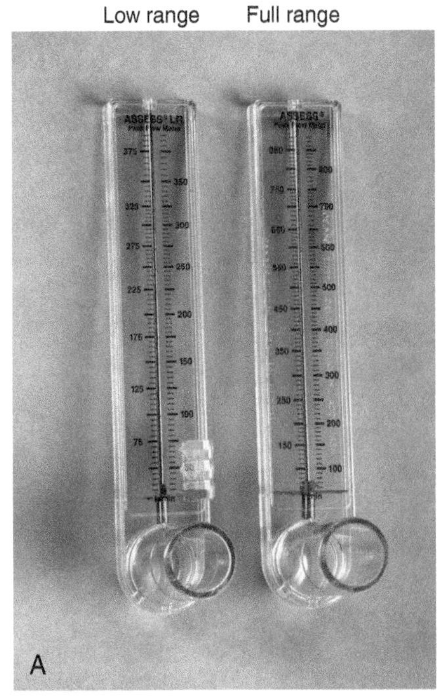

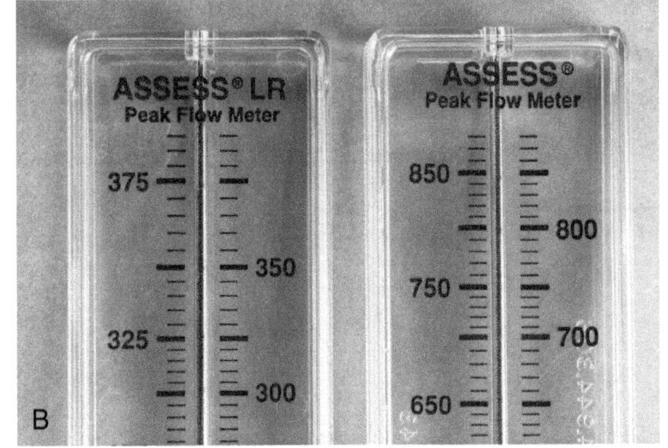

Fig. 12.22 Comparison of a low-range (A, B: *left*) and full-range (A, B: *right*) peak flow meter.

wider range. A *digital peak flow meter* automatically measures the breathing maneuver and displays the measurement digitally on a screen (Fig. 12.23).

Several different brands of peak flow meters are available, and peak flow measurements may vary among brands. Because of this, a patient who purchases more than 1 m should always use the same brand to attain consistency among measurements.

PEAK FLOW MEASUREMENT

The peak flow measurement obtained from the breathing maneuver is known as the **peak expiratory flow rate** (PEFR). The PEFR is the maximum volume of air measured in liters per minute (L/min) that can be exhaled when the patient blows into a peak flow meter as forcefully and as rapidly as possible. To obtain the most accurate PEFR, the patient should perform three acceptable breathing

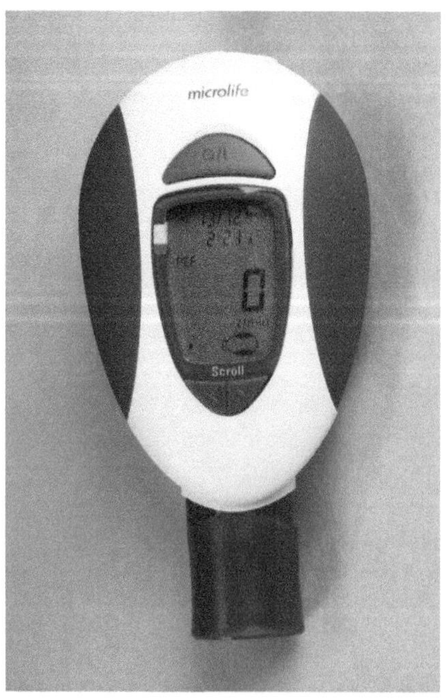

Fig. 12.23 Digital peak flow meter.

maneuvers and then record the highest of the three measurements. The three measurements should be about the same to show that an acceptable breathing maneuver was performed each time. Peak flow measurements provide patients with important information such as the severity of an asthma attack and when to take medication.

Peak flow measurements may show changes before the patient feels them. A patient's PEFR may drop hours or even days before any asthma symptoms occur. For example, the patient may feel fine, but when a peak flow measurement is taken, the reading is slightly decreased. By taking medication before symptoms occur, it may be possible to stop the attack quickly to avoid a severe asthma attack.

Peak Flow Chart

Peak flow measurements may be recorded on a peak flow chart (Fig. 12.24), which allows the patient and the provider to track changes in the patient's lung function over a period of time. A peak flow chart consists of graph paper with a range of peak flow numbers (usually from 50 to 800 L/min) listed in a vertical column on the left side of the

PEAK FLOW CHART

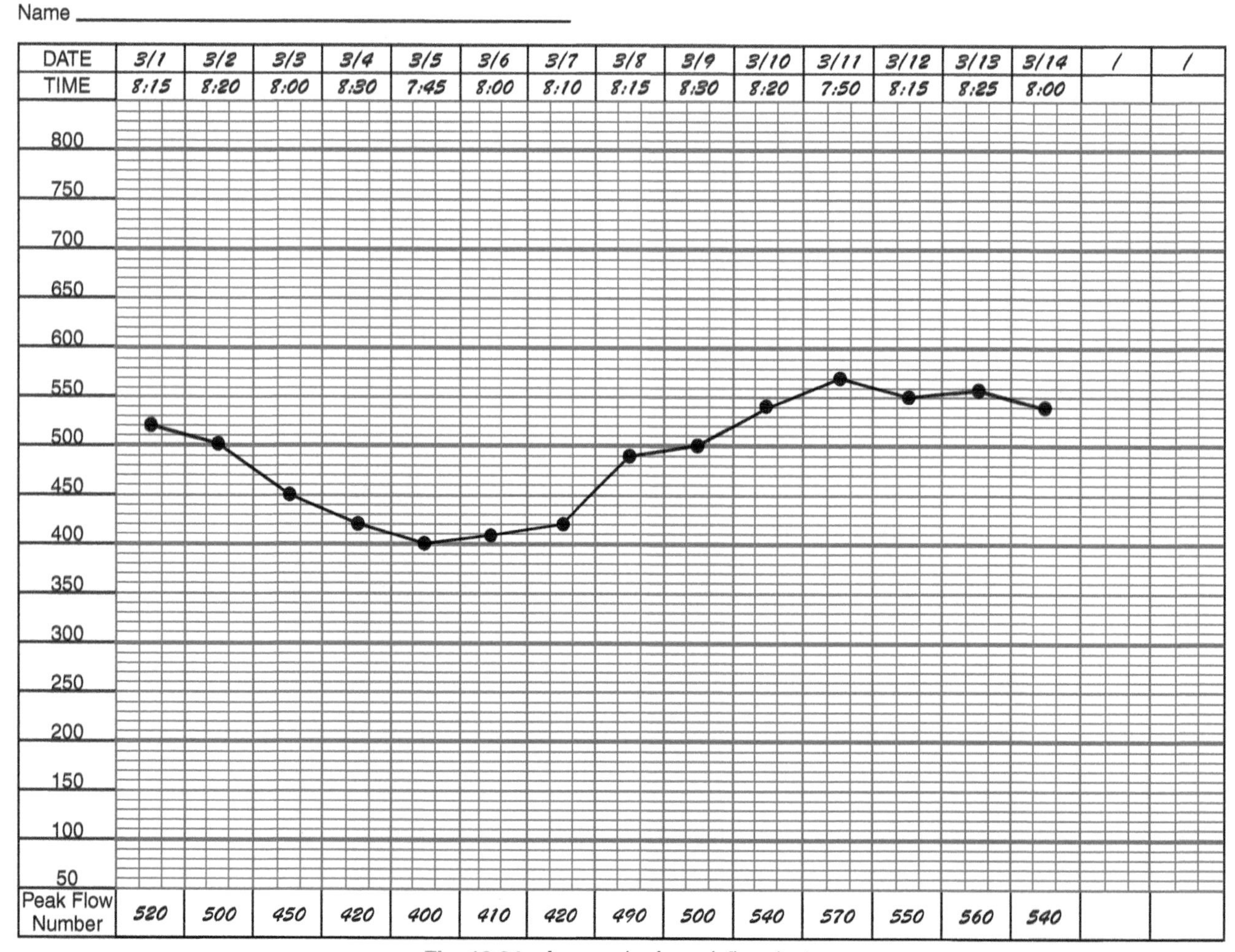

Fig. 12.24 An example of a peak flow chart.

graph paper. The patient indicates the date and time at the top of the chart. After obtaining a peak flow measurement, the patient places a dot across from the peak flow number in the appropriate column. A sample peak flow chart usually accompanies a peak flow meter and can be photocopied for ongoing use or download from the Internet.

Peak flow charts allow providers and patients to monitor changes in the patient's airflow over time to determine how well the patient's asthma is being controlled. They also help the provider determine if a patient's daily medications need to be adjusted or changed. If the patient is doing well as indicated by high peak flow measurements, the provider may be able to lower the dosage of the patient's medication or discontinue certain medications altogether.

The medical assistant is often responsible for instructing a newly diagnosed asthma patient in the procedure for using a peak flow meter and recording results on a peak flow chart. In addition, the medical assistant may be responsible for obtaining the PEFR of a patient with asthma at the medical office. The procedure for measuring PEFR is outlined in Procedure 12.4.

ASTHMA ACTION PLAN

An *asthma action plan* (AAP) is a written individualized management plan developed jointly by the provider and the patient. The goal of an AAP is to provide the patient with guidelines to follow for the control and treatment of his or her asthma which usually leads to fewer asthma attacks.

An AAP typically includes the following information:

- A list of possible asthma triggers that should be avoided
- Instructions for taking asthma medications
- Guidelines for determining the severity of an asthma attack based on symptoms and peak flow measurements
- Recommendations on what to do during an asthma attack
- Instructions on when to call a doctor and/or obtain emergency care
- Emergency telephone numbers

Zones

An AAP is divided into three asthma zones that can be compared to the colors on a traffic light (green, yellow, and red). The threshold level for each zone is based on the patient's symptoms and percentage determinations of the patient's personal best peak flow measurement. The *personal best measurement* is the highest peak flow measurement a patient can achieve over a two-to-three-week period when under good asthma control. The patient must obtain a peak flow measurement (i.e., the highest of three acceptable measurements) twice a day; in the morning upon awakening and in the late afternoon or early evening. The highest measurement (personal best) during this time period is then used to determine the threshold level for each of the patient's three asthma zones. As an example, the threshold level for the green zone is 80% to 100% of the patient's personal best measurement. Therefore, if a patient's personal best is 500 L/min, the threshold level for his or her green zone would be between 400 L/min *(80% of 500 L/min)* and 500 L/min *(100% of 500 L/min)*. An overview of the three asthma zones is outlined in Box 12.2 and an example of an individualized AAP developed by the American Lung Association is presented in Fig. 12.25.

BOX 12.2 Asthma Zones

Green Zone: Doing Well

- Peak flow measurement is 80%–100% of the patient's personal best measurement
- No asthma symptoms are present
- The patient is doing well and under reasonably good control
- Patient should take their daily control medication as usual

Yellow Zone: Caution

- Peak flow measurement is 50%–79% of the patient's personal best measurement
- Asthma symptoms may not be present
- If symptoms are present, they are mild to moderate resulting in some breathing problems
- Patient should take their quick-relief medication in addition to daily control medication

Red Zone: Get Help Now

- Peak flow measurement is less than 50% of the patient's personal best measurement
- Asthma symptoms are severe resulting in extreme breathing difficulties
- Asthma medication is not working
- Signals a medical emergency
- Call 911

HOME OXYGEN THERAPY

Oxygen is a colorless, odorless, and tasteless gas that is vital to the human body. Oxygen is transported by the blood to various tissues of the body. When it reaches the tissues, oxygen is taken into the cells, where it combines with glucose to produce energy. Energy is necessary to the body for carrying out all metabolic processes that sustain life such as breathing and beating of the heart.

When the lungs cannot deliver enough oxygen to the body, there is a reduction in the amount of oxygen in the blood, resulting in hypoxemia. **Hypoxemia** is defined as a decrease in the oxygen saturation of the blood. Hypoxemia, in turn, leads to **hypoxia,** which is a reduction in the oxygen supply to the tissues of the body. Failure to maintain an adequate blood oxygen level can result in progressive deterioration of the patient, beginning with the death of cells and, if prolonged, continuing to organ failure and eventually body system failure and death.

Provider: ______ Clinic: ______

American Lung Association.

My Asthma **Action Plan**

Name: ______ DOB: ___/___/___

Severity classification: ☐ Intermittent ☐ Mild persistent ☐ Moderate persistent ☐ Severe persistent

Asthma triggers (list): ______

Peak flow meter personal best: ______

Green zone: Doing well

Symptoms: Breathing is good – No cough or wheeze – Can work and play – Sleeps well at night
Peak flow meter ______ (more than 80% of personal best)

Flu vaccine–Date received: ______ Next flu vaccine due: ______ COVID19 vaccine–Date received: ______

Control medicine(s)	Medicine	How much to take	When and how often to take it
	______	______	______
	______	______	______

Physical activity ☐ Use albuterol/levalbuterol ___ puffs, 15 minutes before activity
☐ With all activity ☐ When you feel you need it

Yellow zone: Caution

Symptoms: Some problems breathing – Cough, wheeze, or tight chest – Problems working or playing – Wake at night
Peak flow meter ______ to ______ (between 50% and 79% of personal best)

Quick-relief medicine(s) ☐ Albuterol/levalbuterol ___ puffs, every 20 minutes for up to 4 hours as needed
Control medicine(s) ☐ Continue green zone medicines
☐ Add ______ ☐ Change to ______

You should feel better within 20–60 minutes of the quick–relief treatment. If you are getting worse or are in the yellow zone for more than 24 hours, THEN follow the instructions in the RED ZONE and call the doctor right away!

Red zone: Get help now!

Symptoms: Lots of problems breathing – Cannot work or play – Getting worse instead of better – Medicine is not helping
Peak flow meter ______ (less than 50% of personal best)

Take quick-relief medicine NOW! ☐ Albuterol/levalbuterol ___ puffs, ______ (how frequently)

Call 911 immediately if the following danger signs are present:
- Trouble walking/talking due to shortness of breath
- Lips or fingernails are blue
- Still in the red zone after 15 minutes

Emergency contact Name ______ Phone (___) ___-____

Date: ___/___/___ 1-800-LUNGUSA | Lung.org

ALA Asthma AP V2 6 10 2021

Fig. 12.25 Asthma Action Plan. (From the American Lung Association, 2020.)

There are certain conditions, such as severe COPD, that reduce the amount of oxygen in the body, resulting in hypoxemia. In these cases, the provider may write a prescription for home oxygen therapy. **Oxygen therapy** is the administration of supplemental oxygen at concentrations greater than room air to treat or prevent hypoxemia. Oxygen therapy increases the oxygen supply to the lungs, which in turn raises blood oxygen to normal levels and increases the availability of oxygen to the tissues. Oxygen therapy helps to alleviate the effects of low oxygen levels such as shortness of breath and fatigue and helps the patient have a better quality of life and live longer.

Home oxygen therapy is most commonly prescribed for patients with severe COPD caused by smoking. Other common causes of hypoxemia that may require home oxygen therapy include asthma, occupational lung disease, lung cancer, cystic fibrosis, and congestive heart failure.

OXYGEN PRESCRIPTION

The provider determines a patient's need for oxygen therapy through clinical observation of the patient and by measuring the oxygen level of the patient's blood. Clinical signs of hypoxemia include cyanosis, dyspnea, tachypnea, tachycardia, and anxiety. The oxygen level of the blood is typically measured by ABG analysis and through pulse oximetry. A normal individual should have an ABG analysis of 75 to 100 mmHg and a pulse oximetry reading above 94%. An ABG analysis less than or equal to 55 mmHg and a pulse oximetry reading of 88% or less warrants the use of supplemental oxygen. The goal of oxygen therapy is to maintain a blood oxygen level of 65 mmHg (as measured through ABG analysis) and 90% to 93% (as measured through pulse oximetry).

Once the need for supplemental oxygen has been determined, the provider must write a prescription for oxygen therapy that is filled by a home medical supply company. The prescription must include the amount and duration of supplemental oxygen needed by the patient, which are based on the severity of the patient's condition. In addition, the prescription includes the recommended oxygen delivery system and the administration device, which are described in the next section.

The amount of supplemental oxygen prescribed for a patient is known as the **flow rate**, which is measured in L/min. For example, if a patient has been prescribed 2 L/min, each minute, 2 L of oxygen will flow from the patient's oxygen delivery system into tubing, and then into the patient's upper airway. As previously described, the flow rate prescribed by the provider is targeted at raising the patient's ABG analysis to 65 mmHg and the pulse oximetry measurement to 90% to 93%. Most people with COPD start out with a flow rate of 1 to 2L/min. As their COPD worsens over time, the flow rate might increase to 3 to 6 L/min.

The duration of oxygen therapy refers to the number of hours per day oxygen therapy is administered and, depending on the patient's lung function, can vary from a few hours a day up to 15 or more hours per day. Some patients need oxygen only when sleeping or exercising, whereas other patients with more severe hypoxemia may require continuous oxygen therapy. *Continuous oxygen therapy* refers to the use of oxygen for more than 15 hours a day.

Once oxygen therapy is initiated, periodic assessment of the patient's blood oxygen level is required. This assessment is necessary to make sure that the patient still requires oxygen therapy, and that the amount and duration of oxygen are adequate to meet the patient's oxygen needs.

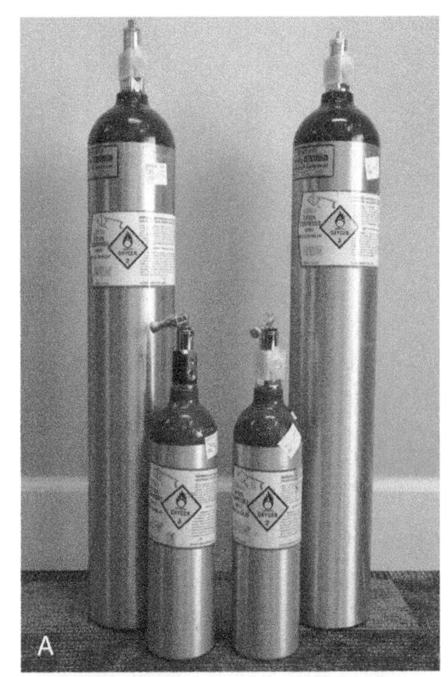

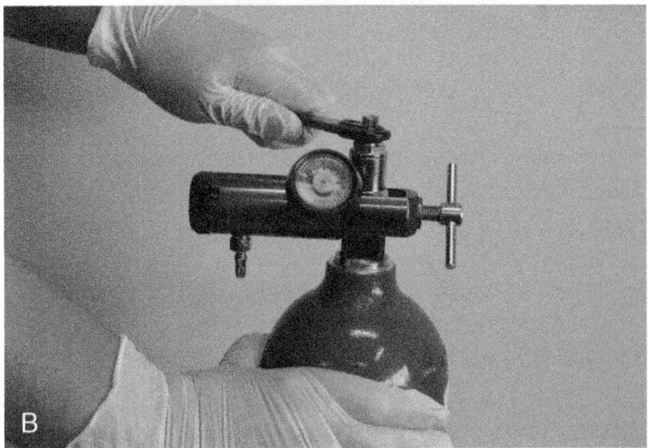

Fig. 12.26 (A) Compressed oxygen cylinders. (B) Oxygen cylinder with regulator and flow meter attached. (Courtesy of Family Oxygen and Medical Equipment, Athens, OH.)

OXYGEN DELIVERY SYSTEMS

There are three common delivery systems for providing supplemental oxygen to a patient: compressed oxygen gas, liquid oxygen, and an oxygen concentrator. The type of delivery system prescribed by the provider is based on the patient's condition, the patient's personal preference, the ease of equipment use, and cost. Each of these delivery systems can be used alone or in combination with another system to meet the oxygen needs of the patient. These systems are described in greater detail in the next section.

Compressed Oxygen Gas

Compressed oxygen gas is oxygen gas compressed under high pressure and then stored in a container referred to as a *cylinder* or *tank*. Compressed oxygen cylinders vary in size from very large stationary cylinders to small portable cylinders that can be carried around (Fig. 12.26A). The patient uses a large cylinder of compressed oxygen at home. When

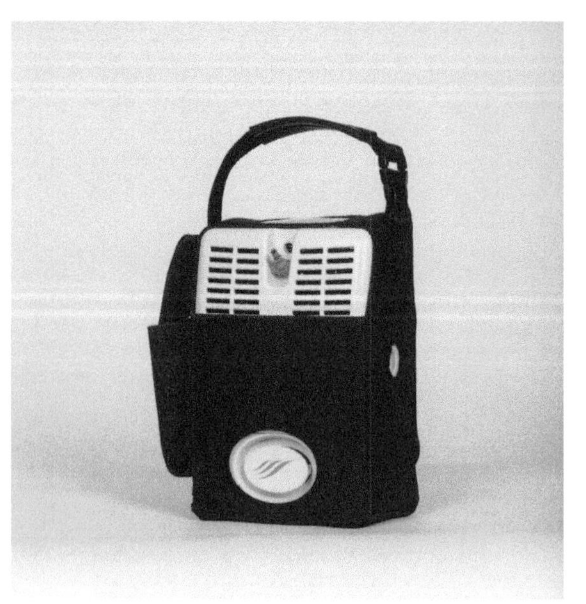

Fig. 12.27 Liquid oxygen portable tank. (From Perry AG: *Clinical nursing skills and techniques*, ed 8, St Louis: Elsevier; 2014.)

the patient goes outside of the home, he or she uses a small cylinder that has been placed in a carrying device such as a shoulder bag.

The cylinder is equipped with a regulator and a flow meter that control the flow rate of the oxygen (see Fig. 12.26B). The flow of oxygen out of the cylinder is constant. To conserve oxygen and avoid waste, an oxygen-conserving device may be attached to the system. An oxygen-conserving device releases the oxygen gas only when the patient inhales and cuts off the release of oxygen when the patient exhales. Advantages and disadvantages of compressed oxygen gas include the following:

Advantage

- Compressed oxygen gas is less expensive than liquid oxygen.

Disadvantages

- The oxygen cylinders must be refilled frequently.
- A compressed oxygen gas cylinder cannot be taken on a commercial airliner.

Liquid Oxygen

When oxygen gas is subjected to an extremely cold temperature, it changes from a gas to a very cold liquid. The liquid oxygen is stored in an insulated tank with a lining similar to a Thermos. Oxygen in a liquid form takes up much less space than compressed oxygen gas—for example, 1 L of liquid oxygen is equal to 860 L of compressed oxygen gas. Because of this, a container of liquid oxygen lasts four times longer than compressed oxygen gas of the same weight.

A liquid oxygen system consists of a large stationary tank that serves as the primary reservoir of oxygen. A small portable tank weighing between 5 and 13 pounds is filled from the large primary tank for use outside the home (Fig. 12.27). The portable tank can be hung over the shoulder or pulled on a roller cart. When liquid oxygen is released from its tank, it changes into a gas and the patient breathes it in, similar to breathing in compressed oxygen gas. Advantages and disadvantages of liquid oxygen include the following.

Advantage

- Because it takes up less space and is easier to transport than compressed oxygen gas, liquid oxygen is often preferred by individuals who want to maintain an active life.

Disadvantages

- Liquid oxygen is more expensive than compressed oxygen gas.
- The contents of a liquid oxygen tank evaporate, making it necessary to have the tank refilled often.
- A liquid oxygen portable tank cannot be taken on a commercial airliner.

Oxygen Concentrator

An oxygen concentrator is an electrically powered device that weighs about 35 pounds and is about the size of a large suitcase (Fig. 12.28A). It works by separating oxygen out of the air, concentrating it, and then storing it for use by the patient. The oxygen concentrator is equipped with a built-in flow meter, which allows the prescribed flow rate to be set.

Small, portable, battery-powered oxygen concentrator systems weighing about 10 pounds have been developed (see Fig. 12.28B). They can provide a patient with oxygen for about 8 hours when used at a flow rate of 2 L/min. For many patients, portable oxygen concentrators have replaced liquid oxygen or compressed gas cylinders for mobility. Advantages and disadvantages of oxygen concentrators include the following:

Advantages

- Oxygen concentrators do not need to be resupplied with oxygen from a home medical supply company.
- Oxygen concentrators are less expensive and safer than oxygen cylinders.
- Portable oxygen concentrators that are battery powered offer the patient even greater freedom and mobility than other oxygen delivery systems.
- Some portable oxygen concentrators have been approved by the Federal Aviation Administration (FAA) for use on commercial airlines.

Disadvantage

- Because oxygen concentrators use electricity, if the power goes out, the patient must have a compressed oxygen gas cylinder for use as a backup.

OXYGEN ADMINISTRATION DEVICES

A device must be used to administer the oxygen to the upper airway of the patient from the delivery system. The device used depends on the expected duration of therapy and the personal preference and needs of the patient. The most commonly used

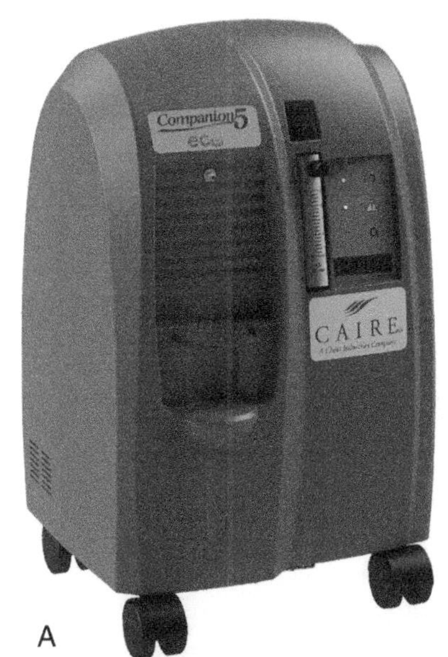

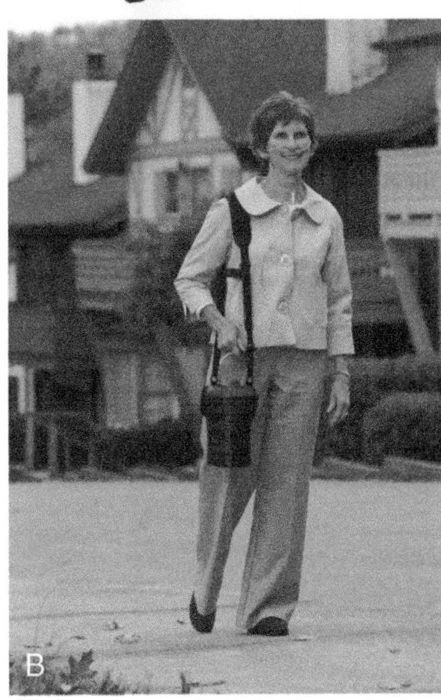

Fig. 12.28 (A) The CAIRE Companion 5 is a 5 LPM compact stationary oxygen concentrator designed specifically for quality, performance, and reliability. (B) Portable oxygen concentrator. (A, Courtesy of CAIRE, a Chart Industries company. B, Courtesy AirSep Corporation.)

devices to administer home oxygen therapy are a nasal cannula and a face mask, which are described in greater detail here.

Nasal Cannula

A nasal cannula is the most frequently used device for administering home oxygen therapy. A nasal cannula consists of soft plastic tubing with a two-pronged device that is inserted into the patient's nose (Fig. 12.29A). The tubing of the prongs loops over the patient's ears and is secured under the chin (see Fig. 12.29B). The tubing connects to the delivery system (i.e., compressed oxygen cylinder, liquid oxygen, or oxygen concentrator). The primary advantage of a nasal cannula is that it does not interfere with the patient's ability to talk, eat, or drink.

The concentration of oxygen inhaled by the patient depends on the flow rate prescribed by the provider. A nasal cannula can deliver oxygen at a flow rate between 0.25 and 6 L/min. If the flow rate is greater than 4 L/min, it can dry out the patient's nasal passages. To prevent this from occurring, a humidifier should be used to provide moisture for a flow rate above 4 L/min.

The cannula should be washed once or twice a week using liquid soap and water, rinsed thoroughly, and allowed to air-dry. The cannula should be replaced with a new cannula every 2 to 4 weeks.

Face Mask

A face mask consists of plastic and fits over the patient's nose and mouth. A face mask strap is then tightened around the patient's head to ensure a secure fit (Fig. 12.30). Oxygen tubing is used to connect the face mask to the oxygen delivery system. A face mask is not used as frequently as a nasal cannula to administer oxygen because it is bulky and must be removed for eating or drinking and to communicate effectively.

A face mask is often used for patients who need a high flow of oxygen. It can deliver oxygen to the patient at a flow rate between 5 and 15 L/min. Wearing a nasal cannula for an extended period of time can irritate the nose. Because of this, the patient might prefer to wear a nasal cannula during the day and a face mask at night to reduce the irritation that may occur from a nasal cannula. The patient who has nasal congestion from a cold will also prefer a face mask.

The face mask should be washed once or twice a week using liquid soap and water, then rinsed thoroughly and dried. The face mask should be replaced with a new one every 2 to 4 weeks, or sooner if it becomes cracked or discolored.

OXYGEN GUIDELINES

The home medical supply company that provides the patient with the oxygen equipment gives the patient specific instructions on safe use, care, and maintenance of the equipment. Listed below are general usage and safety guidelines that the patient should follow.

Usage

1. Contact the provider if any of the symptoms of a low blood oxygen level occur, which include frequent headaches, anxiety, cyanosis of the lips or fingernails, drowsiness, confusion, restlessness, and slow, shallow, difficult, or irregular breathing.
2. Keep the oxygen delivery system clean and free from dust.
3. Do not change the oxygen flow rate unless directed to do so by the provider.
4. Do not use alcohol or take any other sedating drugs, as these substances will slow the breathing rate.
5. Order more oxygen from a home medical company in a timely manner.

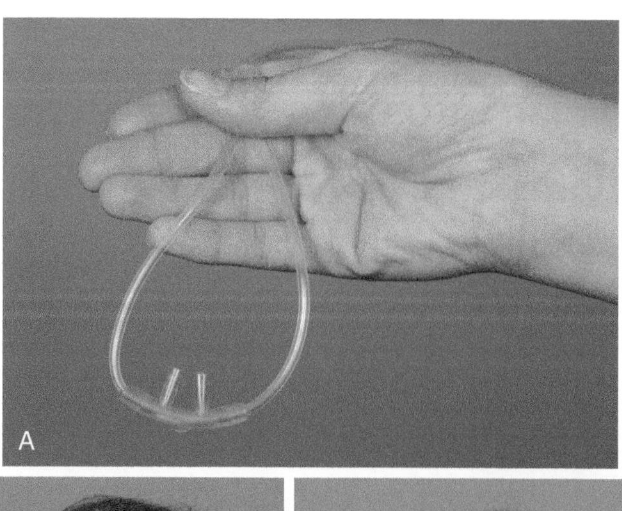

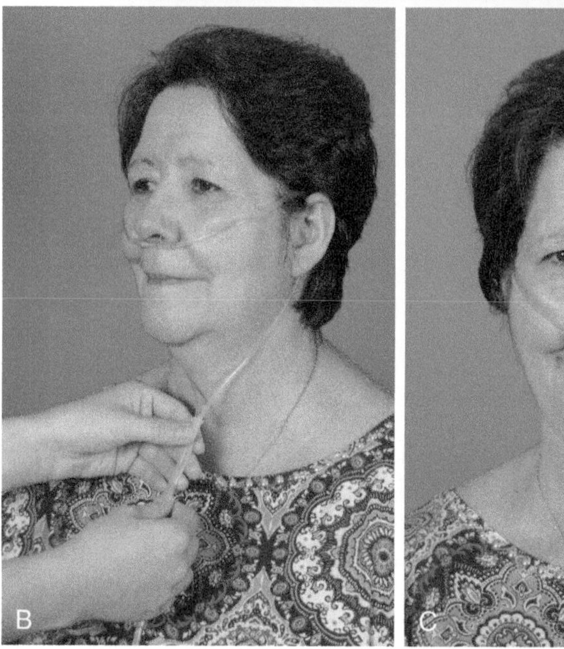

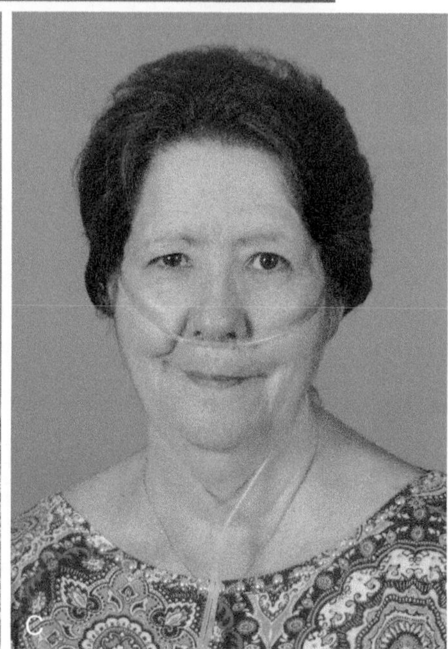

Fig. 12.29 (A) Nasal cannula showing prongs. (B and C) The tubing of the prongs loops over the patient's ears and is secured under the chin.

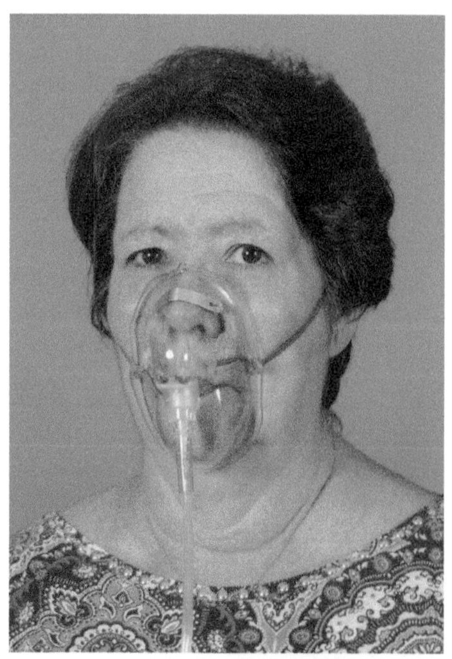

Fig. 12.30 Face mask.

6. To prevent the cheeks or skin behind the ears from becoming irritated from the tubing, tuck some gauze under the tubing. If you have persistent redness under your nose, contact the provider.
7. Oxygen therapy dries out the inside of the patient's nose and mouth. Use water-based lubricants (e.g., K-Y Jelly) on the lips or nostrils to relieve the drying effect. Do not use oil-based products such as petroleum jelly.
8. Do not use more than 40 to 50 feet of tubing with the oxygen delivery system to avoid bending or twisting of tubing to ensure unobstructed oxygen flow.
9. People are not allowed to bring compressed oxygen cylinders or liquid oxygen tanks on board an airplane. Many airlines will provide oxygen if notified 48 to 72 hours in advance.

Safety

Oxygen is a safe gas as long as it is used properly. Oxygen itself is not flammable, nor will it explode; however, it greatly increases the combustion rate of a fire. If something catches fire, oxygen will make the flame hotter and cause it to burn faster and more vigorously. The result is that a fire involving oxygen can appear explosive-like.

1. Store oxygen in a clean, dry, well-ventilated room. If kept in a closed area such as a closet, the small amount of oxygen gas that is continually vented from these units can accumulate in a confined space and become a fire hazard.
2. Compressed oxygen cylinders and liquid oxygen tanks must remain upright at all times. Secure oxygen cylinders and tanks to a fixed object, or place in a stand.
3. Never smoke while using oxygen. Do not allow smoking in the room where the oxygen is kept. Post "No Smoking: Oxygen in Use" signs where oxygen is kept.
4. Keep the oxygen supply at least 6 to 8 feet away from open flames such as gas stoves, lighted fireplaces, and candles.
5. Keep the oxygen supply at least 6 to 8 feet away from intense heat such as radiators, furnaces, and space heaters.
6. Keep the oxygen supply away from flammable products such as cleaning fluid, paint thinner, and aerosol sprays.
7. Do not lubricate oxygen equipment with oil or grease, as these substances are flammable.
8. Be sure to have functioning smoke detectors in the home.
9. Buy a fire extinguisher, and be familiar with how to use it.

Check out the Evolve site to access interactive activities, procedure videos, and other helpful study resources.

What Would You Do? What Would You *Not* Do? RESPONSES

Case Study 1

Page 454

What Did Anitra Do?

- ❑ Tried to reduce Camilla's fears by talking with her calmly and quietly.
- ❑ Explained to Camilla that an ECG is the best screening test available to check for heart problems.
- ❑ Reassured Camilla that she would be draped during the procedure and that she would be exposed as little as possible.
- ❑ Told Camilla that the wires may look a little scary, but there is no chance of being shocked by them. Explained that she will not feel anything when the test is being run.
- ❑ Told Camilla that she could talk with the billing clerk about setting up a payment plan for the test. Provided her with information about community resources that might help her pay for the test.

What Did Anitra Not Do?

- ❑ Did not tell Camilla that she was too young to have heart problems.
- ❑ Did not tell Camilla that she needed to be more mature about being tested.

Case Study 2

Page 469

What Did Anitra Do?

- ❑ Commended Joel on his weight loss and lifestyle changes.
- ❑ Shared a positive story with Joel about a patient who stopped smoking and did not gain weight.
- ❑ Asked Joel whether he would like any of the latest information on smoking cessation.

What Did Anitra Not Do?

- ❑ Did not agree that Joel's lifestyle changes would counteract the bad effects of smoking.
- ❑ Did not lecture Joel on the dangers of smoking, because if he has been smoking since age 17 and has been trying to quit, he already knows what they are.

Case Study 3

Page 470

What Did Anitra Do?

- ❑ Removed the nose clips and empathized with Mr. Conrad that the test is hard to do and that the nose clips do fit snugly.
- ❑ Explained to Mr. Conrad that it is normal to feel dizzy and that it is only temporary.
- ❑ Allowed Mr. Conrad to rest for a while. Tried to relax and calm him by talking with him about his family and interests.
- ❑ Talked to Mr. Conrad about the importance of performing the test. Told him that detecting a problem early would help him get the treatment he needs as soon as possible so that his condition will not get worse.
- ❑ Asked Mr. Conrad to try the test one more time.

What Did Anitra Not Do?

- ❑ Did not criticize Mr. Conrad for not being able to perform the test.
- ❑ Did not force Mr. Conrad to stay if he did not want to, but scheduled another pulmonary function test for him before he left the office. ■

TERMINOLOGY REVIEW

Key Term	Word Parts	Definition
Amplitude		Refers to amount, extent, size, abundance, or fullness.
Artifact		Additional electrical activity picked up by the electrocardiograph that interferes with the normal appearance of the ECG cycles.
Atherosclerosis	*ather/o:* yellowish, fatty plaque *-sclerosis:* hardening of	Buildup of fibrous plaques of fatty deposits and cholesterol on the inner walls of an artery that causes narrowing, obstruction, and hardening of the artery.
Baseline		The flat horizontal line that separates the various waves of the ECG cycle.
Cardiac cycle	*cardi/o:* heart	One complete heartbeat.
Dysrhythmia	*dys-:* difficult, painful, abnormal *rhythm*: rhythm *-ia:* condition of diseased or abnormal state	An irregular heart rate or rhythm; also termed *arrhythmia.*
ECG cycle		The graphic representation of a heartbeat.
Electrocardiogram (ECG)	*electr/o:* electrical, electrical activity *cardi/o:* heart *-gram:* record of	The graphic representation of the electrical activity of the heart.
Electrocardiograph	*electr/o:* electrical, electrical activity *cardi/o:* heart *-graph:* instrument used to record	The instrument used to record the electrical activity of the heart.
Electrode	*electr/o:* electrical, electrical activity	A conductor of electricity, which is used to promote contact between the body and the electrocardiograph.
Electrolyte	*electr/o:* electrical, electrical activity	A chemical substance that promotes conduction of an electric current.
Flow rate		The number of liters of oxygen per minute that come out of an oxygen delivery system.
Hypoxemia	*hypo-:* below, deficient *ox/i:* oxygen *-emia:* blood condition	A decrease in the oxygen saturation of the blood.
Hypoxia	*hypo-:* below, deficient *ox/i:* oxygen *-ia:* condition of diseased or abnormal state	A reduction in the oxygen supply to the tissues of the body.
Interval		The length of one or more waves and a segment.
Ischemia	*isch/o:* deficiency, blockage *-emia:* blood condition	Deficiency of blood in a body part.
Normal sinus rhythm		Refers to an ECG that is within normal limits.
Oxygen therapy		The administration of supplemental oxygen at concentrations greater than room air to treat or prevent hypoxemia.
Peak flow rate		The maximum volume of air that can be exhaled when the patient blows into a peak flow meter as forcefully and as rapidly as possible.
Segment		The portion of the ECG between two waves.
Spirometer	*spir/o:* breathe, breathing *-meter:* instrument used to measure	An instrument for measuring air taken into and expelled from the lungs.
Spirometry	*spir/o:* breathe, breathing *-metry:* measurement	Measurement of an individual's breathing capacity by means of a spirometer.
Wheezing		A continuous, high-pitched whistling musical sound heard particularly during exhalation and sometimes during inhalation.

PROCEDURE 12.1 Recording a 12-Lead Electrocardiogram

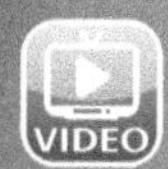

Outcome Record a 12-lead electrocardiogram (ECG).

Equipment/Supplies

- Three-channel electrocardiograph
- Disposable electrodes
- ECG paper

1. **Procedural Step.** Work in a quiet, relaxing atmosphere away from sources of electrical interference.
2. **Procedural Step.** Sanitize your hands, and assemble the equipment. Check the expiration date of the electrodes. Greet the patient and introduce yourself. Identify the patient by full name and date of birth.
   Principle. The electrolyte gel on outdated electrodes may be dried out, which can cause artifacts on the ECG.
3. **Procedural Step.** Help the patient relax by explaining the procedure. Tell the patient that having an ECG recording is painless. Explain that he or she must lie still, breathe normally, and not talk while the ECG is being recorded so that an accurate ECG can be obtained.
   Principle. Explaining the procedure helps reassure apprehensive patients. The patient should be mentally and physically relaxed for an accurate ECG recording; an apprehensive or moving patient produces muscle artifacts. Heavy breathing or sighing can cause a wandering baseline artifact.
4. **Procedural Step.** Prepare the patient. Ask him or her to remove clothing from the waist up. The lower legs also must be uncovered. Provide a female patient with a gown, and instruct her to put it on with the opening in front. Assist the patient into a supine position on the table. The table should support the arms and legs adequately so that they do not dangle. Properly drape the patient to prevent exposure and to provide warmth. A pillow can be used to support the patient's head.
   Principle. The chest, upper arms, and lower legs must be uncovered to allow proper placement of the electrodes. The patient should be kept warm, and the arms and legs should not be allowed to dangle; otherwise, muscle artifacts could result.
5. **Procedural Step.** Position the electrocardiograph so that the power cord points away from the patient and does not pass under the table. It is usually easier for the medical assistant to work on the left side of the patient.
   Principle. Proper positioning of the electrocardiograph reduces 60-cycle interference artifacts.
6. **Procedural Step.** Prepare the patient's skin for application of the disposable electrodes. If the patient has sweaty or oily skin or has used lotion, rub the area to which the electrode will be applied with alcohol, and allow it to dry. If the patient's chest is hairy, dry shave it at each electrode site before applying the electrode.
   Principle. The patient's skin must be dry and free of oil and body hair so that the adhesive backing of the electrodes sticks to the patient's skin and stays on during the procedure.
7. **Procedural Step.** Remove a card containing 10 electrodes from its foil-lined pouch and reseal the pouch. Apply the limb electrodes. Firmly apply the adhesive backing of the electrodes to the fleshy part of each of the four limbs (upper arms and lower legs). The electrode tabs should point toward the center of the body. The tabs of the arm electrodes should point downward, and the tabs of the leg electrodes should point upward. The adhesive backing of the electrode allows it to adhere firmly to the patient's skin.
   Principle. The pouch should be resealed to preserve moisture and prevent the electrolyte on the remaining electrodes from drying out. The electrodes must be firmly attached to permit good transmission of the electrical impulse from the patient's skin to the electrode. Loose electrodes can cause artifacts to occur on the recording, making it difficult to analyze the recording. The tabs of the electrodes should be positioned toward the center of the body to provide a more stable connection when the lead wire is attached to the electrode and to prevent the lead wires from pulling onto the electrodes and causing artifacts.

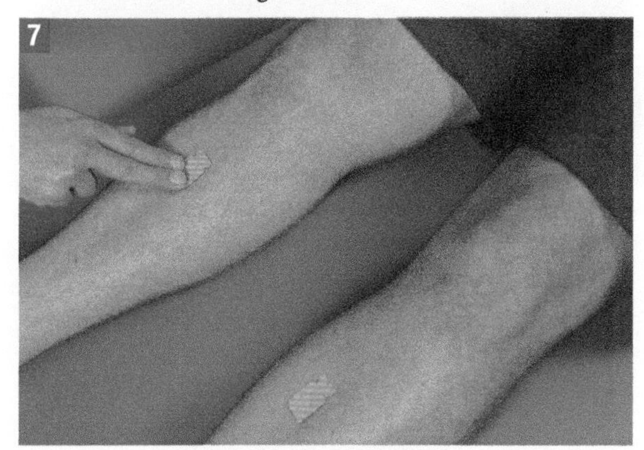

Apply the leg electrodes.

Continued

PROCEDURE 12.1 Recording a 12-Lead Electrocardiogram—cont'd

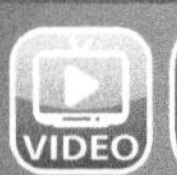

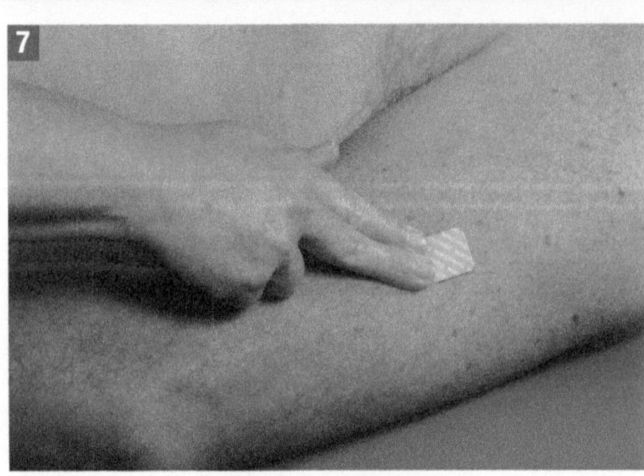

Apply the arm electrodes.

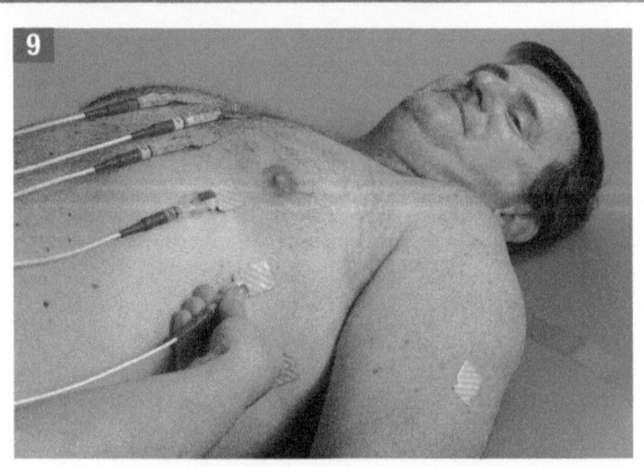

Connect the lead wires to the electrodes.

8. Procedural Step. Apply the chest electrodes. Properly locate each electrode placement site using palpation, and apply the electrode with the tab pointing downward. Continue until all six of the chest electrodes have been applied.

Principle. Positioning the tabs of the electrodes downward prevents the lead wires from pulling and causing artifacts.

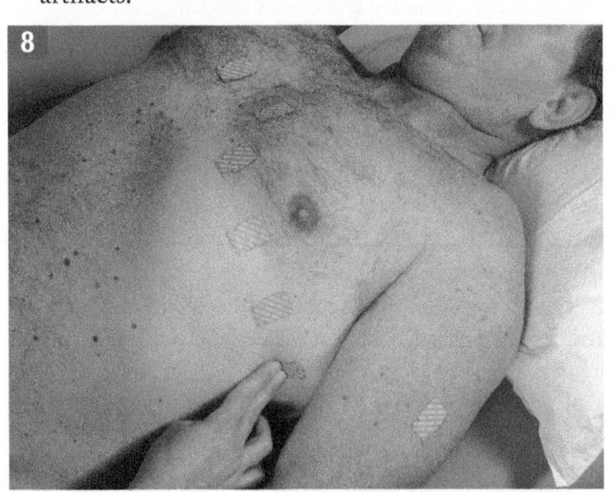

Apply the chest electrodes.

9. Procedural Step. Connect the lead wires to the electrodes. This is accomplished by inserting an alligator clip onto the metal tip of each lead wire. Next, firmly attach an alligator clip to the tab of each electrode. The ends of the lead wires are usually color coded (e.g., red for the arms and green for the legs) and identified with abbreviations to help the medical assistant connect the proper lead to each electrode. Arrange the lead wires to follow body contour.

Principle. The lead wires must be attached correctly to ensure an accurate and reliable ECG. Arranging the lead wires to follow body contour reduces the possibility of 60-cycle interference artifacts.

10. Procedural Step. Plug the patient cable into the machine. The cable should be supported on the table or on the patient's abdomen to prevent pulling of the lead wires on the electrodes.

Principle. Pulling of the lead wires on the electrodes can cause the electrodes to pull away from the skin, resulting in artifacts.

11. Procedural Step. Turn on the electrocardiograph. Enter patient data using the soft-touch keypad. Always use your fingertips to enter the data. Pencils and other sharp objects can damage the keyboard. As the data are entered, they are displayed on the liquid crystal diode (LCD) screen. Patient data to be entered typically include the patient's name, a patient identification number, age, sex, height, weight, and medications.

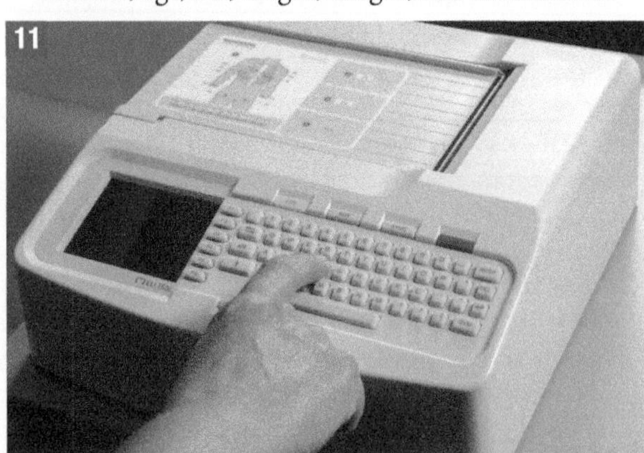

Enter patient data.

12. Procedural Step. Remind the patient to lie still, breathe normally, and not talk. Press the AUTO (automatic) button, and run the recording. The machine automatically inserts a standardization mark at the beginning of each ECG strip, followed by the recording of the 12-lead ECG in a three-channel format. Another standardization mark is inserted at the end of each ECG strip.

PROCEDURE 12.1 Recording a 12-Lead Electrocardiogram—cont'd

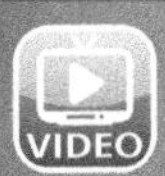

(*Note:* With most three-channel electrocardiographs, the machine checks for a clear ECG signal after the AUTO button is pressed. If the signal is "noisy," this may indicate that an electrode does not have a good connection with the patient's skin. The machine usually indicates which electrode is causing the problem (e.g., "V_6 noisy"). Apply firm pressure to the electrode causing the problem. If this does not correct the problem, replace the electrode with a new one and/or place a piece of nonallergenic tape over the electrode.)

13. Procedural Step. After the ECG has been recorded:

a. Check the printout to ensure that the standardization mark is 10 mm high. If it is more or less than 10 mm, adjust the standardization mark according to the manufacturer's instructions, and run another ECG.

b. Check the direction of the R wave in lead I. If your patient's limb leads are attached correctly, the R wave on lead I should have a positive deflection. If it has a negative deflection, the limb leads are not attached correctly. Reattach the limb leads properly and run another recording.

c. Observe the recording for artifacts. If an artifact is present, determine the cause of the artifact, correct the problem, and run another ECG.

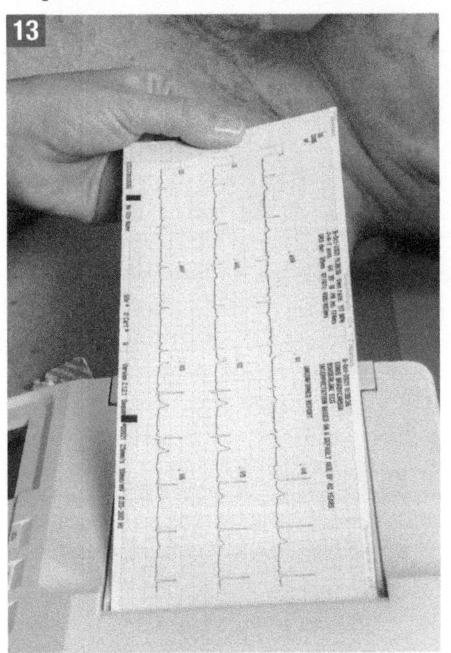

Check the standardization mark.

14. Procedural Step. Inform the patient that you are finished and he or she can now talk or move. Turn the machine off. Disconnect the lead wires. Remove and discard the electrodes.

15. Procedural Step. Assist the patient in stepping down from the table.

16. Procedural Step. Sanitize your hands.

17. Procedural Step. Document the procedure in the patient's medical record.

a. *Electronic health record (EHR):* Document the procedure performed (12-lead ECG) using the appropriate radio buttons, drop-down menus, and free text fields.

b. *Paper-based patient record:* Document the date and time and the name of the procedure (12-lead ECG). Refer to the PPR documentation example.

18. Procedural Step. Return all equipment to its proper storage place.

PPR Documentation Example

Date	
6/12/XX	10:30 a.m. Completed a 12-lead ECG.
	Recording to physician for review. ———
	——————— A. Martin, CMA (AAMA)

PROCEDURE 12.1

PROCEDURE 12.2 Applying a Holter Monitor

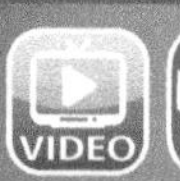
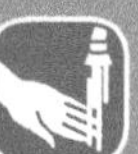

Outcome Apply a Holter monitor.

Equipment/Supplies

- Holter monitor (with an internal memory card)
- Battery
- Disposable pouch and lanyard or a belt clip
- Disposable electrodes
- Razor
- Antiseptic wipes
- Gauze pads
- Abrasive pad
- Nonallergenic tape
- Patient diary

1. **Procedural Step.** Assemble the equipment.

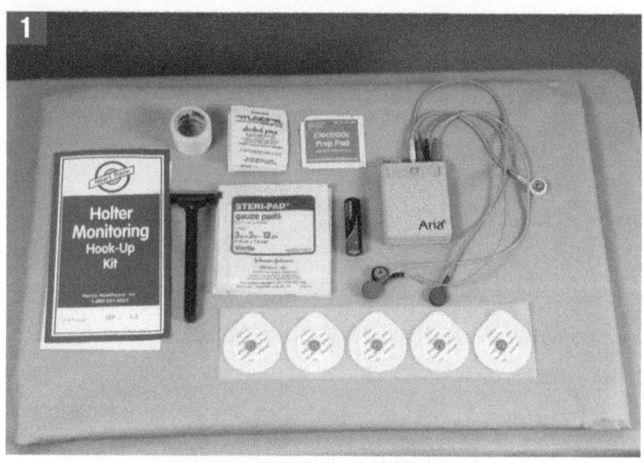

Assemble the equipment.

2. **Procedural Step.** Prepare the equipment. Install a new high-quality alkaline battery according to the markings on the battery holder to ensure correct battery polarity. Check the expiration date on the electrodes.
   Principle. A new battery must be installed each time the monitor is used to ensure sufficient power throughout the monitoring period. The electrolyte on outdated electrodes may be dried out, which can cause artifacts on the ECG.

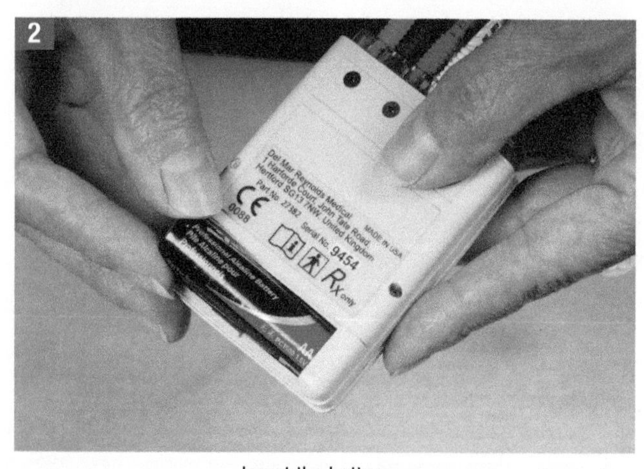

Insert the battery.

3. **Procedural Step.** Connect the Holter monitor to the computer using a docking station or a computer cable connected to a USB port. Enter patient demographic data into the computer. Patient data to be entered generally include the patient's name and date of birth and a patient identification number. Download this information to the Holter monitor.
   Principle. The data are used to identify the recording. They are also used in computer-assisted interpretation of the ECG.
4. **Procedural Step.** Sanitize your hands. Greet the patient and introduce yourself.
5. **Procedural Step.** Identify the patient by full name and date of birth, and explain the procedure. Tell the patient that the Holter monitor will record the heartbeat without interfering with his or her daily activities. Tell the patient that, because of its small size, the monitor will be fairly inconspicuous. Instruct the patient in the guidelines for wearing a Holter monitor (see Box 12.1). Emphasize to the patient that it is important to maintain daily activities during the monitoring period.
   Principle. The patient must follow the guidelines carefully to ensure an accurate recording.
6. **Procedural Step.** Prepare the patient by asking him or her to remove clothing from the waist up.
   Principle. Clothing must be removed for placement of the chest electrodes.
7. **Procedural Step.** Place the patient in a sitting position.
8. **Procedural Step.** Locate the chest electrode sites by following the electrode placement diagram included in the operating manual. Prepare an area of skin slightly larger than an electrode at each placement site as follows:
   a. If the patient's chest is hairy, dry shave it at each electrode site.

PROCEDURE 12.2 Applying a Holter Monitor—cont'd

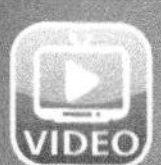

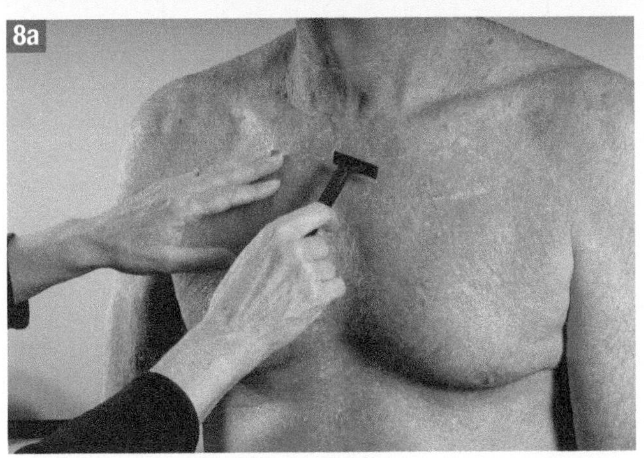

Shave the chest.

b. Rub the skin with an alcohol wipe to remove any dirt, perspiration, or body oils that might be on the skin. Allow the area to dry completely.

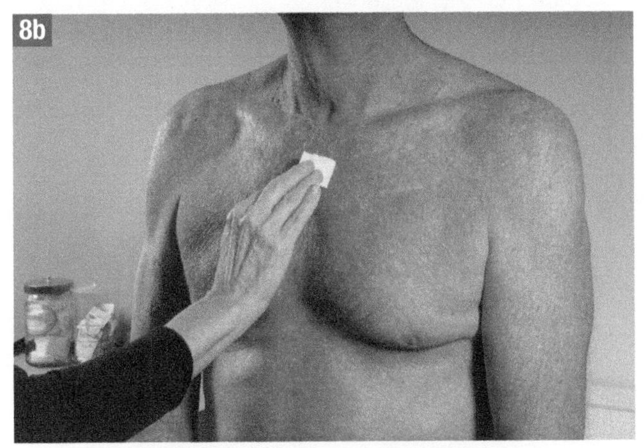

Rub the skin with an alcohol wipe.

c. Slightly abrade the skin with a gauze pad or an abrasive pad until the skin is reddened. This is accomplished by rubbing the skin lightly with six or seven small circular motions. On a patient with normal skin, use about the same pressure used to file the fingernails with a fingernail file. Use less pressure on geriatric patients and patients with sensitive skin or poor skin condition.

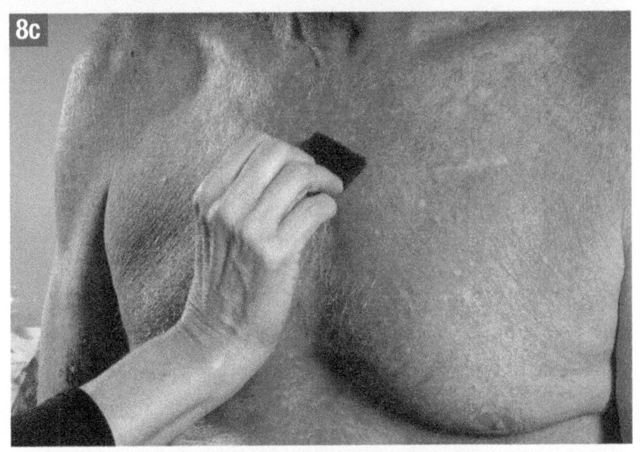

Slightly abrade the skin with a skin abrader.

Principle. Shaving the chest improves the adherence of the electrodes and makes them easier to remove. The placement sites should be rubbed with a skin abrasive to remove dry, dead skin, which improves adherence of the electrodes and increases conductivity of the electrical signal from the skin surface to the electrode.

9. **Procedural Step.** Attach a color-coded lead wire to the snap of each electrode.

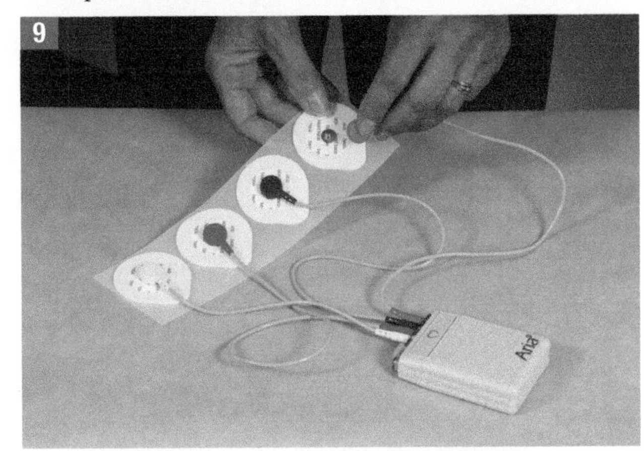

Snap the color-coded lead wires onto the electrodes.

10. **Procedural Step.** Apply the chest electrodes as follows: Determine the first electrode to be applied by looking at the color-coded chest electrode placement chart. Grasp the first electrode by the colored lead wire snap cover, and remove the electrode from its protective backing. Avoid touching the adhesive to prevent

Continued

PROCEDURE 12.2 Applying a Holter Monitor—cont'd

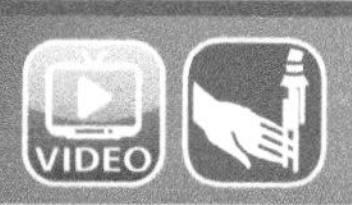

loss of its stickiness. Check that the electrolyte gel is moist. If it is dry, obtain a new electrode.

Principle. The ends of the lead wires are color coded for proper placement of each lead. The electrolyte gel should be moist to ensure good conduction of electrical impulses.

11. Procedural Step. Apply the electrode (with attached lead wire) to the first chest electrode site. Ensure a firm seal by running your finger around the outer edge of the electrode with a firm pressure until it is firmly attached to the skin. Do not press down in the middle of the electrode.

Principle. The electrodes must be firmly attached to permit good transmission of the electrical impulse from the patient's skin to the electrode. Loose electrodes can cause artifacts on the recording, making it difficult to analyze the recording. Pressing down on the middle of the electrode may cause some of the electrolyte gel to be forced out from under the electrode, interfering with good conduction of the electrical signal from the patient's heart.

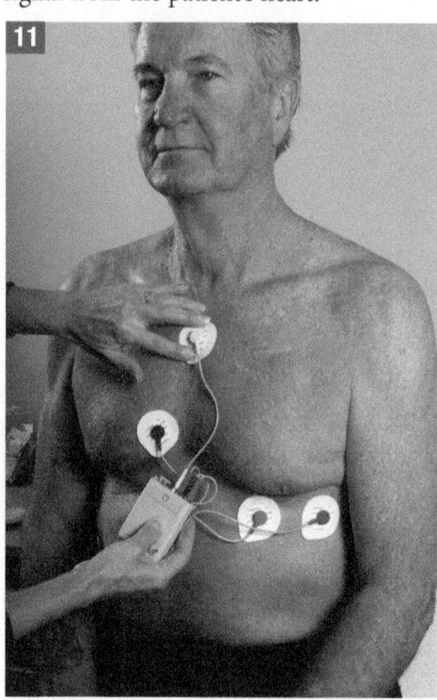

Ensure a firm seal of each electrode.

12. Procedural Step. Repeat steps 10 and 11 until all the chest electrodes have been applied.

Principle. The electrodes pick up and conduct the electrical impulses given off by the heart. The impulses are transmitted through the lead wires and the patient cable to the monitor.

13. Procedural Step. Plug the patient cable into the monitor, and turn on the monitor. Check the ECG signal quality by accessing the *Lead Status* screen on the LCD display screen located on the monitor. The quality of the ECG signal for each lead is displayed on the screen. The ECG signal should be clear and strong. If the signal is "noisy," this may indicate that an electrode does not have a good connection with the patient's skin. Apply gentle pressure to each electrode to improve contact with the patient's skin.

Principle. A clear signal ensures an accurate and reliable ECG recording.

14. Procedural Step. Place a strip of nonallergenic tape over each electrode and cover of the lead wire.

Principle. Applying tape prevents the lead wire from detaching from the electrode.

15. Procedural Step. Check to make sure the date and time displayed on the screen of the monitor are accurate, and start the monitor.

16. Procedural Step. Place the disposable lanyard and pouch around the patient's neck, and insert the monitor into the pouch.

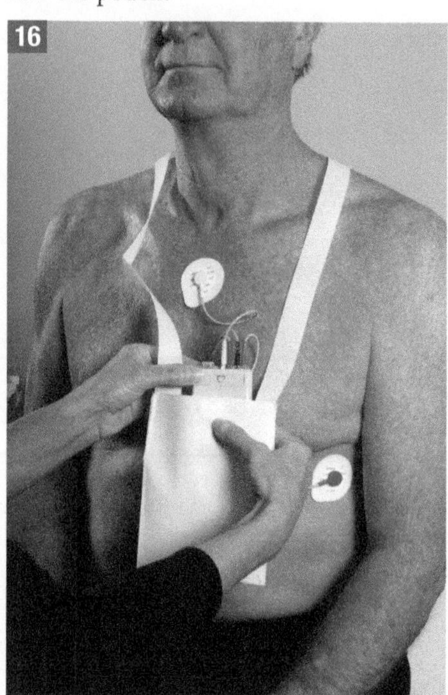

Insert the monitor into a disposable pouch.

17. Procedural Step. Tell the patient to redress while being careful not to pull on the lead wires.

18. Procedural Step. Complete the patient information section of the patient diary, and document the starting time in the patient diary. Give the diary to the patient, and provide him or her with instructions on completing it.

Principle. The beginning time must be documented for later correlation of the patient diary with cardiac activity. The patient diary is used to correlate patient symptoms with cardiac activity.

PROCEDURE 12.2 Applying a Holter Monitor—cont'd

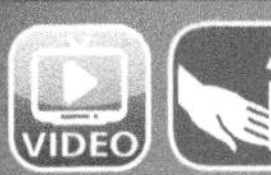

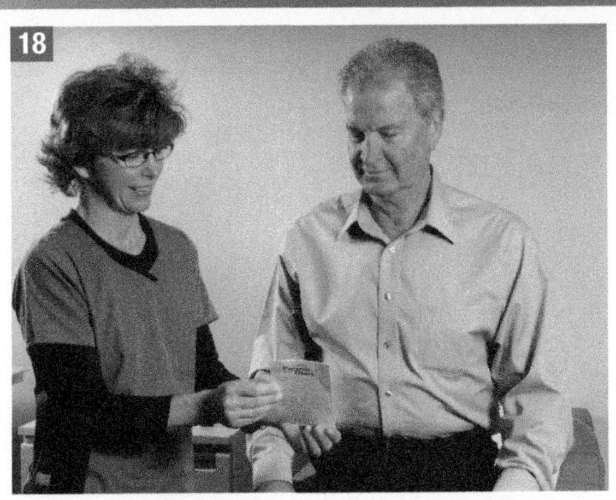

Provide the patient with instructions on completion of the diary.

19. **Procedural Step.** Instruct the patient when to return for removal of the monitor. Remind the patient not to forget to bring the diary.
20. **Procedural Step.** Sanitize your hands.
21. **Procedural Step.** Document the procedure in the patient's medical record.
    a. *Electronic health record (EHR):* Document the procedure performed (application of a Holter monitor) and the beginning time using the appropriate radio buttons, drop-down menus, and free text fields. Also document instructions given to the patient.
    b. *Paper-based patient record:* Document the date and time, the name of the procedure (application of a Holter monitor), and the beginning time. Also document instructions given to the patient (refer to the PPR documentation example).

PPR Documentation Example

Date	
6/15/XX	2:00 p.m. Applied Holter monitor.
	Starting time: 2:15 p.m. Instructed pt on
	recording data in diary. To return on
	6/16/XX at 2:30 p.m. for removal of
	monitor ——— D. Arnold, CMA (AAMA)

PROCEDURE 12.3

PROCEDURE 12.3 Spirometry Testing

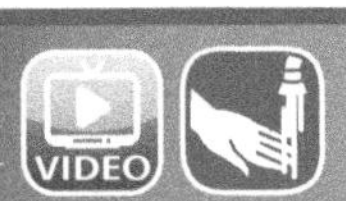

Outcome Perform a spirometry test.

Equipment/Supplies

- Spirometer
- Disposable tubing
- Disposable mouthpiece
- Disposable nose clips
- Waste container

1. **Procedural Step.** Sanitize your hands. Assemble and prepare the equipment. Calibrate the spirometer according to the manufacturer's instructions. Apply a disposable mouthpiece to the mouthpiece holder, which is attached to the spirometer by a cable.
   Principle. Calibration of the spirometer ensures accurate and valid test results.
2. **Procedural Step.** Greet the patient and introduce yourself. Identify the patient and explain the procedure. Tell the patient that he or she will be wearing nose clips and performing a breathing maneuver several times to see how well his or her lungs are functioning. Ask the patient whether he or she prepared properly for the procedure.
3. **Procedural Step.** Prepare the patient. Have the patient remove any heavy or constricting clothing, such as a jacket or a sweater. Also, ask the patient to loosen tight clothing, such as a necktie or a tight collar. If the patient is chewing gum, ask him or her to discard it in a waste container.
   Principle. Heavy outer clothing, tight clothing, or gum may make it difficult for the patient to perform the breathing maneuvers.
4. **Procedural Step.** Measure the patient's weight and height precisely.
   Principle. Precise weight and height measurements are required for the accurate calculation of predicted values.
5. **Procedural Step.** Have the patient sit near the machine. The patient should be seated to prevent dizziness or possible fainting during the procedure. Enter the following data into the computer database of the spirometer: patient's age, sex, weight, and height, and any other information required, such as the patient's

Continued

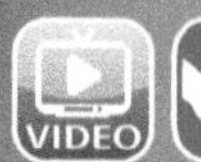

identification number and whether the patient smokes.

Principle. Demographic data need to be entered for the computer to calculate the predicted values.

6. **Procedural Step.** Instruct the patient in the breathing maneuver. The following procedure should be described and demonstrated to the patient:
   a. Relax and take the deepest breath possible until your lungs are completely filled with air.
   b. Place the mouthpiece in your mouth, and seal your lips tightly around it.
   c. Blow out as hard as you can and for as long as possible until your lungs are completely empty. Do not block the opening of the mouthpiece with your tongue.
   d. Remove the mouthpiece.

   Principle. The lips must be tightly sealed around the mouthpiece so that all of the air leaving the mouth enters the mouthpiece.
7. **Procedural Step.** Tell the patient you will repeat the instructions during the test. Encourage the patient to remain calm during the procedure. Gently apply nose clips to the patient's nose. Hand the mouthpiece to the patient, and tell him or her to hold it close to the mouth.

   Principle. Fear or anxiety can make the results less reliable. Nose clips prevent air from escaping from the nostrils and ensure that all breathing is done through the mouth.
8. **Procedural Step.** Begin the test. When the patient is ready, press the start button on the spirometer. Actively coach the patient as follows:
   a. "Now relax and take in a big breath—in—in—in—more—keep inhaling."
   b. "Put the mouthpiece in your mouth and blow hard. Keep going—keep going—keep going—more—more—more—you're almost there—a little more. That's good. You can stop now."
   c. "Take out the mouthpiece and rest for a while. You did a great job."

   Principle. Coaching the patient helps to obtain accurate test results.

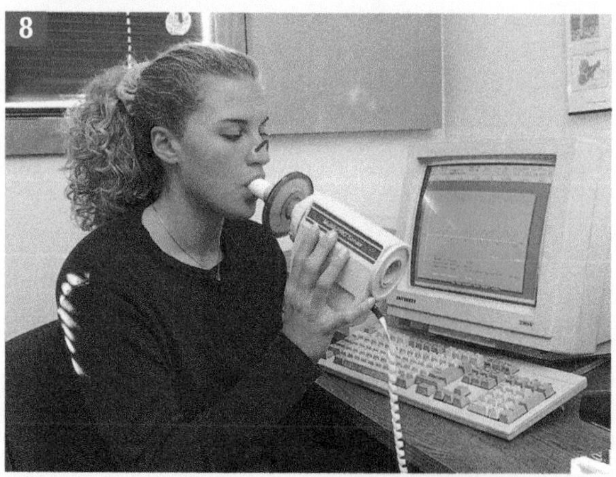

Instruct the patient to blow into the mouthpiece.

9. **Procedural Step.** If the patient does not perform the breathing maneuver correctly, inform him or her of what modifications are needed for the next effort. Continue until three acceptable efforts have been obtained.

   Principle. Three acceptable efforts must be obtained to ensure valid test results.
10. **Procedural Step.** Gently remove the nose clips from the patient's nose. Remove the mouthpiece from the mouthpiece holder. Dispose of the mouthpiece and nose clips in a regular waste container.
11. **Procedural Step.** Allow the patient to remain seated for a few minutes.

    Principle. The patient may feel light-headed after the procedure.
12. **Procedural Step.** Sanitize your hands. Print the report, and label it with the patient's name, the date, and your initials.
13. **Procedural Step.** Document the procedure in the patient's medical record.
    a. *Electronic health record (EHR):* Document the name of the procedure performed and the patient's reaction using the appropriate radio buttons, drop-down menus, and free text fields.
    b. *Paper-based patient record:* Document the date, the time, the name of the procedure, and the patient's reaction (refer to the PPR documentation example).
14. **Procedural Step.** Clean the spirometer according to the manufacturer's instructions.

PPR Documentation Example

Date	
6/20/XX	9:00 a.m. Spirometry test run. Obtained
	3 acceptable efforts. Pt stated she was
	tired following the test. Report to
	physician for review. ————
	———— A. Martin, CMA (AAMA)

PROCEDURE 12.4 Measuring Peak Flow Expiratory Rate

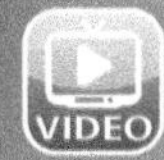

Outcome Measure a patient's peak flow expiratory rate.

Equipment/Supplies

- Peak flow meter
- Disposable mouthpiece
- Waste container

1. **Procedural Step.** Sanitize the hands. Assemble and prepare the equipment. Move the sliding indicator on the peak flow meter to the bottom of the numbered scale. Apply a disposable mouthpiece to the mouthpiece holder.
   Principle. Not placing the marker at the bottom of the numbered scale leads to inaccurate test results. The disposable mouthpiece prevents the spread of microorganisms from one patient to another.

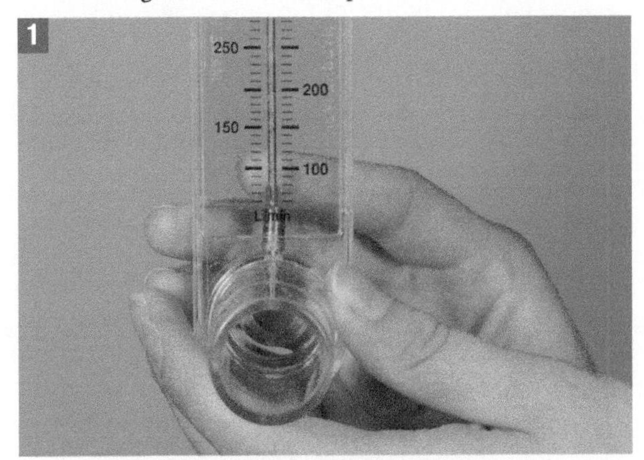

Move indicator to bottom of scale.

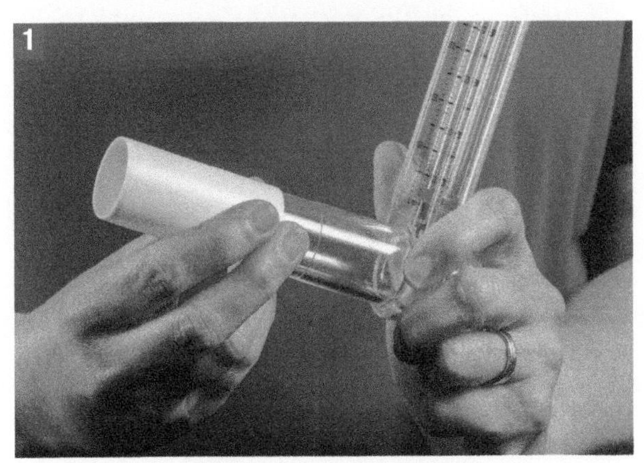

Apply a disposable mouthpiece.

2. **Procedural Step.** Greet the patient and introduce yourself. Identify the patient and explain the procedure. Tell the patient that he or she will be performing a breathing maneuver several times to see how well his or her lungs are functioning.
3. **Procedural Step.** Prepare the patient. Have the patient remove any heavy or constricting clothing, such as a jacket or a sweater. Also, ask the patient to loosen tight clothing, such as a necktie or a tight collar. If the patient is chewing gum, ask him or her to discard it in a waste container.
   Principle. Heavy outer clothing, tight clothing, or gum may make it difficult for the patient to perform the breathing maneuver.
4. **Procedural Step.** Instruct the patient in the breathing maneuver. The following procedure should be described and demonstrated to the patient:
   a. Relax and take the deepest breath possible until your lungs are completely filled with air.

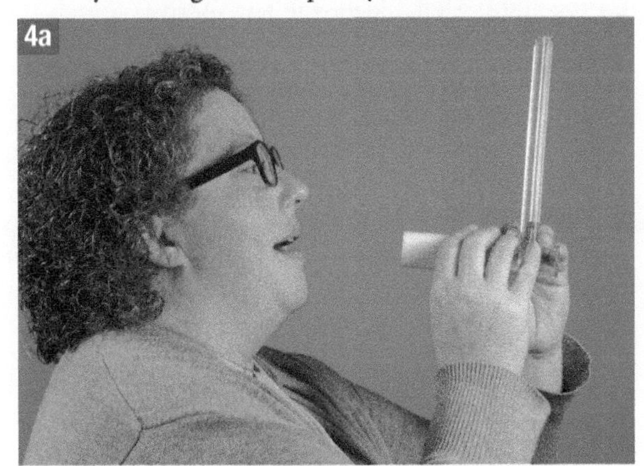

The patient takes a deep breath.

   b. Place the mouthpiece in your mouth, and seal your lips tightly around it.
   c. Blow out as hard and fast as you can until your lungs are completely empty. Try to move the marker as high as you can on the numbered scale. Do not block the opening of the mouthpiece with your tongue.

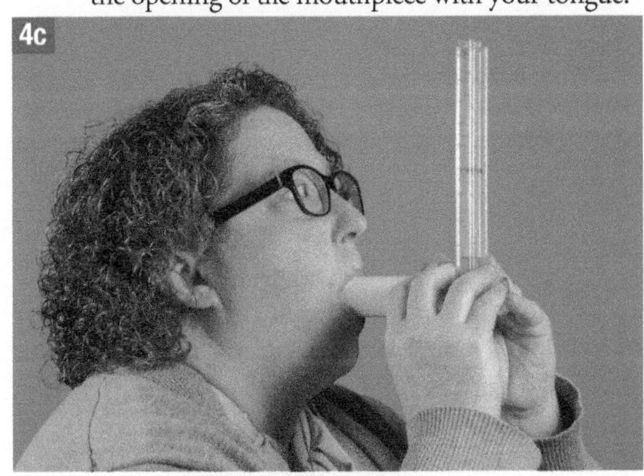

The patient blows out hard and fast.

Continued

PROCEDURE 12.4

PROCEDURE 12.4 Measuring Peak Flow Expiratory Rate—cont'd

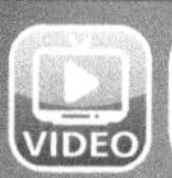

d. Remove the mouthpiece from your mouth.

Principle. The lips must be tightly sealed around the mouthpiece so that all of the air leaving the mouth enters the mouthpiece. The force of the air coming out of the patient's lungs causes the marker to move upward on the scale. The reading depends on how hard the patient blows out the air in his or her lungs.

5. **Procedural Step.** Tell the patient you will repeat the instructions during the test. Encourage the patient to remain calm during the procedure.

   Principle. Fear or anxiety can make the results less reliable.

6. **Procedural Step.** Place a new disposable mouthpiece on the peak flow meter, and slide the marker to the bottom of the numbered scale. Hand the peak flow meter to the patient.

7. **Procedural Step.** Instruct the patient to stand up straight and look straight ahead.

8. **Procedural Step.** Begin the test. Actively coach the patient as follows:
   a. "Now relax and take in a big breath—in—in—in—"
   b. "Put the mouthpiece in your mouth and blow hard."
   c. "Take out the mouthpiece and rest for a while. You did a great job."

9. **Procedural Step.** Note the number at which the indicator stopped on the scale of the peak flow meter. Jot down the number on a piece of paper.

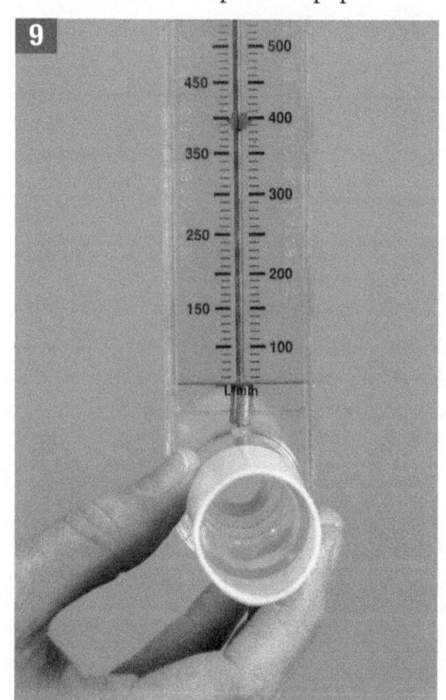

Note where the indicator stopped on the scale.

10. **Procedural Step.** If the patient coughs or does not perform the breathing maneuver correctly, do not write down the number. Inform the patient of what modifications are needed for the next effort.

11. **Procedural Step.** Continue until three acceptable breathing maneuvers have been obtained. Make sure to slide the marker to the bottom of the scale before each measurement.

    Principle. Three acceptable efforts must be obtained to ensure valid test results. If the patient performs the breathing maneuver correctly, the measurements from the three tests should be about the same.

12. **Procedural Step.** Take the peak flow meter from the patient, and remove the mouthpiece from the mouthpiece holder. Dispose of the mouthpiece in a regular waste container.

13. **Procedural Step.** Sanitize your hands. Note the highest of the three peak flow measurements. (Do not calculate an average.)

14. **Procedural Step.** Document the procedure in the patient's medical record.
    a. *Electronic health record (EHR):* Document the name of the procedure and the highest of the three acceptable peak flow measurements using the appropriate radio buttons, drop-down menus, and free text fields.
    b. *Paper-based patient record:* Document the date, the time, the name of the procedure, and the highest of the three acceptable peak flow measurements (refer to the PPR documentation example).

15. **Procedural Step.** Clean the peak flow meter by washing it in warm soapy water, rinsing it thoroughly, and allowing it to dry completely.

PPR Documentation Example

Date	
6/21/XX	10:30 a.m. PFR: 400 L/min. Pt stated she
	was tired following the test. ————
	———— A. Martin, CMA (AAMA)

Colorectal and Male Reproductive Tests and Procedures

Check out the Evolve site at http://evolve.elsevier.com/Bonewit to access additional interactive activities and exercises to help you study and prepare for success.

LEARNING OUTCOMES	PROCEDURES
Colorectal Tests and Procedures	
Stool-Based Colorectal Screening Tests	
1. List the symptoms of colorectal cancer.	
2. Identify the recommended colorectal cancer screening guidelines.	
3. Identify three types of stool-based colorectal screening tests.	
4. Explain the recommended follow-up for a positive stool-based colorectal screening test.	
5. State the purpose of a guaiac fecal occult blood test (gFOBT).	
6. Identify the patient preparation required for a gFOBT.	Instruct a patient in the preparation requirements and the collection procedure for a gFOBT.
7. Describe the quality control measures that should be used with a gFOBT.	Develop and interpret the results of a gFOBT.
8. State the purpose of a fecal immunochemical test (FIT).	
9. Identify the two types of tests included in the FIT-DNA (fecal immunochemical and DNA) test.	
10. Describe the meaning of a positive FIT-DNA test.	
Sigmoidoscopy	
11. Explain the purpose of sigmoidoscopy.	Instruct a patient in the preparation required for a sigmoidoscopy.
12. Explain the importance of proper bowel preparation prior to a sigmoidoscopy.	Assist the provider with a sigmoidoscopy.
13. Explain the purpose of a digital rectal examination (DRE) prior to a sigmoidoscopy.	
Colonoscopy	
14. Explain the purpose of a colonoscopy.	Instruct a patient in the preparation required for a colonoscopy.
15. List the conditions that can be detected and assessed during a colonoscopy.	
16. Describe the procedure for a colonoscopy.	
Male Reproductive Tests and Procedures	
Prostate Cancer Screening Tests and Procedures	
17. List the symptoms of prostate cancer.	
18. Explain how the DRE is used to screen for prostate cancer screening.	Assist the provider with a DRE.
19. Explain the purpose of the prostate-specific antigen (PSA) test.	Instruct a patient in the preparation for a PSA test.
Testicular Cancer Screening Procedure	
20. State the risk factors for testicular cancer.	Teach a patient how to perform a testicular self-examination.
21. Identify the testicular self-examination schedule.	

CHAPTER OUTLINE

KEY TERMS

biopsy (BIE-op-see)
colonoscope (KOL-un-oh-skope)
colonoscopy (KOL-un-OS-koe-pee)
endoscope (EN-doe-skope)
insufflate (IN-suf-flate)
occult (ah-KULT) blood
peroxidase (per-OKS-ih-dase)
polyp
screening
sigmoidoscope (sig-MOYD-oh-skope)
sigmoidoscopy (sig-moyd-OS-koe-pee)

Introduction to Colorectal Tests and Procedures

Colorectal tests and procedures are often performed for the early detection of colorectal cancer and precancerous polyps. Other, less serious conditions, including hemorrhoids, anal fissures, diverticulitis, peptic ulcers, ulcerative colitis, gastroesophageal reflux disease (GERD), and Crohn disease, can also be detected through these tests and procedures. The most commonly used tests and procedures include stool-based colorectal screening tests, sigmoidoscopy, and colonoscopy.

The medical assistant is often responsible for coaching the patient on any advance preparation required for these tests and procedures. The medical assistant should make sure the patient thoroughly understands the instructions. If the patient does not prepare properly, inaccurate results may occur.

STRUCTURE OF THE LARGE INTESTINE

To completely understand colorectal tests and procedures, the medical assistant should be familiar with the structure of the large intestine. The large intestine is divided into three parts, which include the *cecum, colon,* and *rectum* (Fig. 13.1). The *cecum* is the first part of the large intestine. It consists of a blind pouch to which the appendix is attached. The cecum leads into the ascending colon and joins with the *ileum,* which is the last part of the small intestine.

The colon makes up most of the large intestine. It averages 60 inches in length and is divided into four sections, which include the *ascending colon,* the *transverse colon,* the *descending colon,* and the *sigmoid colon.* The sigmoid colon makes up the lower third of the colon. It is identified by its S-shaped curve and connects the descending colon with the rectum. The *rectum* is located between the colon and the anus. The anus contains sphincter muscles and opens to the outside as a means of expelling waste from the body.

The primary functions of the large intestine include absorption of water and preparation of fecal material for elimination. Mucus is secreted from glands embedded in the intestinal wall (mucosa) of the large intestine. The mucus binds the fecal material together and protects the wall of the large intestine from the irritating effects of substances moving through it.

COLORECTAL CANCER

Colorectal cancer (CRC) is used to describe both cancer of the colon (Fig. 13.2) and cancer of the rectum. Although colorectal cancer may occur in young adults, the majority of cases (90%) occur in individuals older than 50 years of age. Colorectal cancer is the third most common type of cancer in the United States and the second leading cause of cancer-related deaths for both men and women. According to the American Cancer Society (ACS), every year more than 140,000 people are diagnosed with colorectal cancer and approximately 50,000 of these individuals die from this disease.

Colorectal cancer usually starts from small precancerous polyps in the colon or rectum. A colorectal **polyp** is an

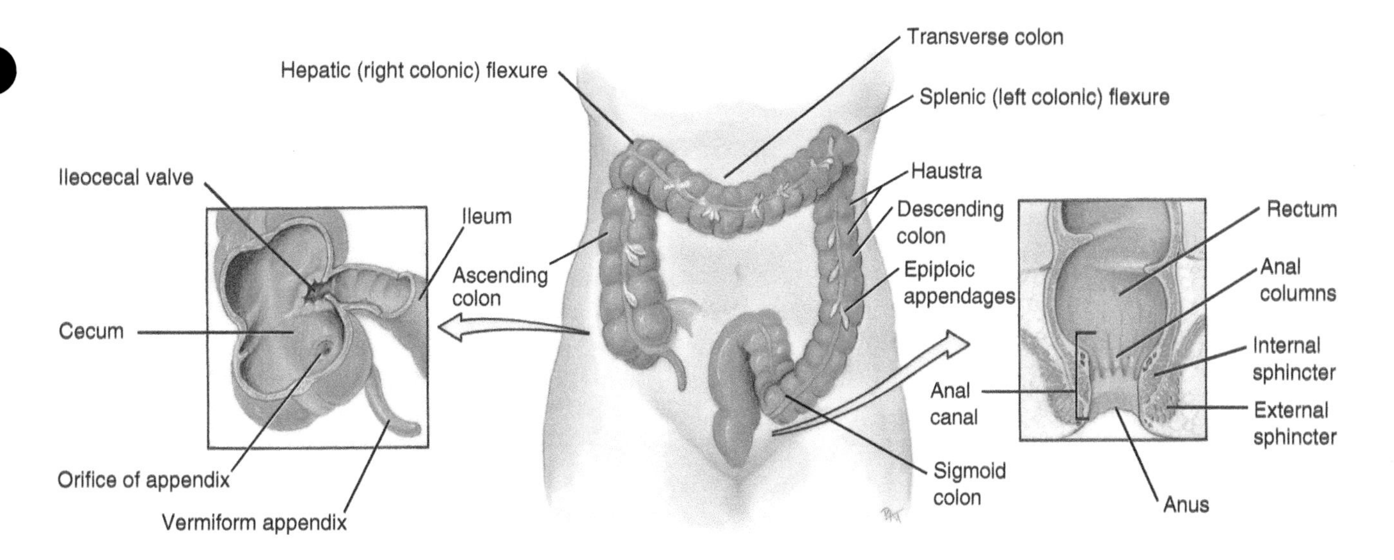

Fig. 13.1 Large intestine. (From Applegate E: *The anatomy and physiology learning system*, ed 4, St Louis: Elsevier; 2011.)

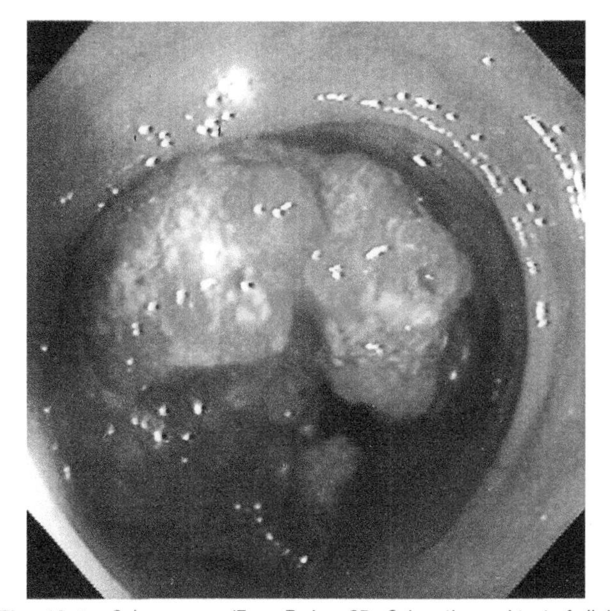

Fig. 13.2 Colon cancer. (From Forbes CD: *Color atlas and text of clinical medicine*, ed 3, Philadelphia: Mosby; 2003.)

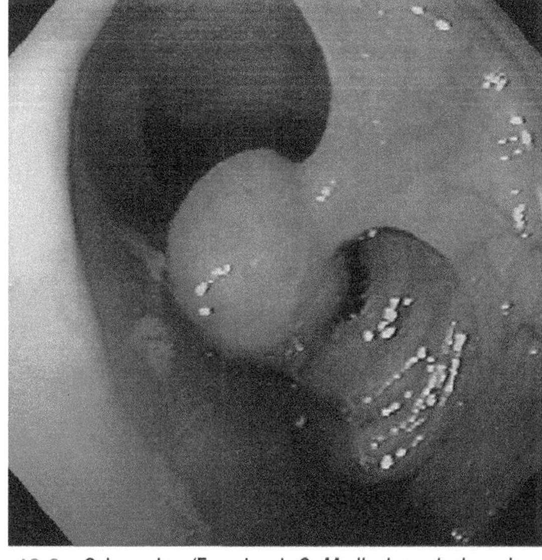

Fig. 13.3 Colon polyp. (From Lewis S: *Medical-surgical nursing*, ed 9, St Louis: Elsevier; 2014.)

abnormal growth that protrudes from the mucous membrane of the large intestine (Fig. 13.3). Most cases of colorectal cancer arise from a type of polyp known as an *adenomatous polyp* that gradually increases in size and becomes malignant and spreads to other parts of the body over a long period of time (typically 10 to 15 years). Adenomatous polyps usually cause no symptoms, and there is no way to prevent them. However, detecting polyps early through colorectal cancer screening allows them to be removed before they can develop into cancer and spread to other parts of the body. Once a polyp is removed, it is examined by a pathologist to determine if it is benign or malignant which then dictates whether further treatment is necessary.

SYMPTOMS

No symptoms or very few symptoms occur during the early stages of colorectal cancer. If colorectal cancer is detected and treated while the patient is still asymptomatic, the patient has a 90% chance of 5-year survival. By comparison, the 5-year survival rate for patients in whom colorectal cancer is diagnosed after symptoms appear is only 40% and the 5-year survival rate when the cancer has spread to distant organs (metastasized) such as the liver or lungs is only 11%.

Symptoms that occur when colorectal cancer is more developed include the following:
- Bleeding from the rectum
- Blood in or on the stool
- A change in the shape of the stool (e.g., stools that are narrower than usual)
- A change in bowel habits (e.g., diarrhea, constipation)
- General abdominal discomfort (e.g., aches, pains, cramps that do not go away)
- Unexplained weight loss
- Constant fatigue

RISK FACTORS FOR COLORECTAL CANCER

The exact cause of colorectal cancer is not known, but certain factors increase the risk of developing this disease. A *risk factor* is anything that increases an individual's chance of developing a disease such as cancer. Although colorectal cancer risk factors often influence the development of cancer, most do not directly cause it. For example, some people with several colorectal risk factors never develop cancer, whereas others with no known risk factors do. Some colorectal risk factors can be changed (e.g., smoking, diet, and physical activity), whereas others cannot be changed (e.g., age and family history). The risk factors for colorectal cancer are outlined in Box 13.1.

BOX 13.1 Colorectal Cancer Risk Factors

The following factors may increase the risk of developing colorectal cancer:
- ***Age.*** The risk of colorectal cancer increases significantly after 50 years of age and reaches a peak from ages 60–75 years.
- ***Gender.*** Men have a slightly higher risk of developing colorectal cancer than women.
- ***Personal history of adenomatous polyps.*** Individuals with adenomatous polyps have an increased risk of developing colorectal cancer. Approximately 10% of adenomatous polyps become cancerous if not removed. Adenomatous polyps that become cancerous are known as *adenocarcinomas.*
- ***Personal or family history of colorectal cancer.*** Individuals who have been diagnosed previously with colorectal cancer are at higher risk for developing it in other parts of the colon and rectum, even if it was completely removed. Individuals with colorectal cancer in a first-degree relative (e.g., parent, sibling) are also at increased risk for developing the disease.
- ***Personal history of inflammatory bowel disease:*** Individuals with inflammatory bowel disease of long duration such as ulcerative colitis and Crohn disease are at increased risk for colorectal cancer.
- ***Personal or family history of an inherited genetic syndrome.*** Approximately 5%–10% of individuals who develop colorectal cancer have an inherited genetic colorectal cancer syndrome. These syndromes occur when a genetic mutation associated with colon or rectal cancer is passed down through a family's genes. The most common of these syndromes include familial adenomatous polyposis (FAP) and hereditary nonpolyposis colon cancer (Lynch syndrome).
- ***Racial and ethnic background.*** African Americans have the highest incidence of colorectal cancer and mortality rates of all racial groups in the United States. The reasons for this are not fully understood.
- ***Other factors*** that have been associated with a higher incidence of colorectal cancer include:
  - Type 2 diabetes
  - Smoking
  - Moderate to heavy alcohol consumption
  - Physical inactivity and obesity
  - Diet high in fat, red meat (e.g., beef, pork, lamb), and processed meats (e.g., hot dogs, bacon, cold cuts)
  - Low intake of fresh fruits and vegetables

COLORECTAL CANCER SCREENING GUIDELINES

Screening refers to the process of testing to detect disease in an individual who is not yet experiencing symptoms. For certain types of cancer (e.g., colorectal cancer and breast cancer), screening allows the cancer to be discovered early, when it is more treatable, which increases the patient's survival rate.

For the early prevention and detection of colorectal cancer, the ACS recommends that all adults ages 45 to 75 years who are at average risk be screened for colorectal cancer. Prior to this, the ACS stipulated 50 as the age to begin screening. However, in recent years, there has been an increase in colorectal cancer among younger adults, resulting in the recommendation to begin screening at 45 years of age. Individuals are considered to be at *average risk* for colorectal cancer if they do not have any of the following: personal or family history of colorectal cancer, adenomatous polyps, or an inherited genetic syndrome; inflammatory bowel disease of long duration; or personal history of getting radiation to the abdomen or pelvic area to treat a prior cancer. Individuals with these conditions have an increased risk for developing colorectal cancer and should be screened at an earlier age and with greater frequency following the recommendations of their providers.

There are many colorectal cancer screening options available; therefore individuals should talk with their health care providers to determine which option is best for them. Colorectal cancer screening guidelines and options are outlined in Box 13.2.

BOX 13.2 American Cancer Society Colorectal Cancer Screening Guidelines

Individuals between the ages of 45 and 75 at average risk for colorectal cancer:

Stool-Based Tests

- Guaiac fecal occult blood test: every year[a]
- Fecal immunochemical test: every year[a]
- Fecal immunochemical–DNA test: every 3 years[a]

Visualization Examination Procedures

- Colonoscopy: every 10 years
- Computed tomography colonography (virtual colonoscopy): every 5 years[a]
- Sigmoidoscopy: every 5 years[a]

Individuals between the ages of 76 and 85:

The decision to be screened should be based on an individual's preferences, life expectancy, overall health, and prior screening history.

Individuals older than the age of 85:

No longer need to be screened

[a] Colonoscopy should be performed if the results are positive.

Data from Wolf A, Fontham E, Church T, et al: Colorectal cancer screening for average-risk adults: 2018 guideline update from the American Cancer Society. *CA Cancer J Clin* 68(4):250–281, 2018.

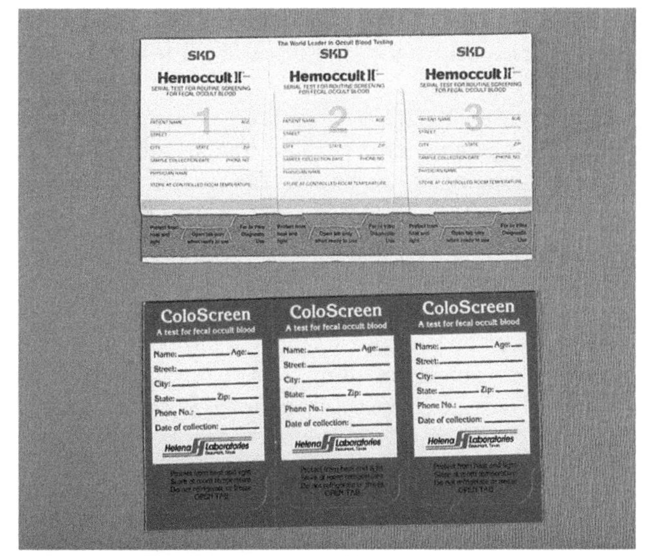

Fig. 13.4 Examples of fecal occult blood testing kits. Hemoccult *(top)* and ColoScreen *(bottom)*.

STOOL-BASED COLORECTAL SCREENING TESTS

Stool-based tests are used to screen for the possible presence of colorectal cancer and polyps. They require that a patient collect a stool specimen at home and return it to the medical office or an outside laboratory for testing. The medical assistant is often responsible for providing the patient with instructions on any patient preparation required, collection of the stool specimen, and the proper care and storage of the specimen. Some patients initially may be reluctant to comply with the patient preparation and specimen collection requirements. The medical assistant can help by explaining the purpose of the test to patients to help them understand the benefits to be derived from the test.

Most stool-based colorectal screening tests work by detecting the presence of blood in the stool. During the early asymptomatic stages, almost all cancers and large polyps of the colon and rectum bleed a small amount on an intermittent basis. This is because the blood vessels in cancer or polyps are often fragile and easily damaged by the passage of stool. The damaged vessels usually bleed into the colon or rectum, but only rarely is there enough bleeding for it to be seen by the unaided eye. This hidden, or nonvisible, blood is termed **occult blood**, and its presence can be detected with a stool-based test.

The patient should be instructed *not* to collect a stool specimen when any of the following conditions are present: diarrhea, blood in the urine or stool, bleeding cuts or wounds on the hands, rectal bleeding, and menstruation. These conditions may cause blood to appear in the stool resulting in a false-positive test result.

A positive test result for a stool-based colorectal screening test does not mean the patient has colorectal cancer. It indicates only the presence of blood in the stool; the source and cause of the bleeding must still be determined. This means that further diagnostic procedures must be performed before the provider can make a diagnosis. These procedures may include colonoscopy, computed tomography (CT) colonography (virtual colonoscopy), and sigmoidoscopy. A negative result does not guarantee the absence of cancer, and the patient should continue to follow the colorectal cancer screening guidelines outlined in Box 13.2.

TYPES OF TESTS

There are three types of stool-based colorectal screening tests commonly used to screen for colorectal cancer which include the following:

- Guaiac fecal occult blood test (gFOBT)
- Fecal immunochemical test (FIT)
- Fecal immunochemical–DNA test (FIT-DNA test)

Guaiac Fecal Occult Blood Test

The gFOBT is a CLIA-waived test that uses guaiac to screen for occult blood in the stool. Guaiac is a chemical that changes to a blue color if blood is present. Brand names for the gFOBT (Fig. 13.4) include Hemoccult *(Beckman Coulter, Inc., Brea CA)* and ColoScreen *(Helena Laboratories, Beaumont, CA)*. The gFOBT is designed to detect the presence of occult blood in three stool specimens collected on 3 different days. The purpose of using three specimens is to allow detection of blood from colorectal lesions that exhibit intermittent bleeding. The gFOBT is an inexpensive test that is easy to perform; however, care must be taken to prevent false-positive and false-negative test results.

Patient Instructions

Patient instructions for a gFOBT play an important role in ensuring accurate test results. The patient must follow a special diet, beginning 3 days before the test, and must continue the diet until all three specimens have been collected. The patient is placed on a high-fiber diet that is free of red meat. Red meat contains animal blood, which could lead to a false-positive test result. A high-fiber diet is used because it encourages bleeding from colorectal lesions that may bleed only occasionally. In addition, fiber adds bulk to the stool, which promotes bowel elimination and ensures adequate specimen collection.

Certain medications irritate the gastrointestinal (GI) tract, which can result in a small amount of bleeding that could cause a false-positive result on a gFOBT. Medications that should be avoided before testing include ibuprofen, naproxen, and more than one adult aspirin per day. In addition, vitamin C (>250 mg/day) from supplements and citrus fruits and juices can cause a false-negative test result. An iron supplement will not affect the test results. Table 13.1 lists patient instructions for fecal occult blood testing using the gFOBT.

Quality Control

Quality control methods must be used with a gFOBT to ensure reliable and valid results. It is important to properly store the testing kit containing the gFOBT cardboard collection slides and developing solution. Adverse storage conditions can result in deterioration of the developing solution and the active reagents impregnated on the filter paper of the slides, leading to inaccurate test results. The testing kit must be stored at a room temperature that is between 59°F and 86°F (15°C and 30°C). The contents of the kit must be protected from heat, sunlight, and strong fluorescent light. In addition, the testing kit should not be stored in close proximity to volatile chemicals such as ammonia, bleach, bromine, iodine, and disinfectant cleaners. If stored properly, the slides and developing solution will remain effective until the expiration date that is stamped on the side of the testing kit, each slide itself, and the container of developing solution.

A quality control procedure must be performed *after* the patient's test has been developed, read, and interpreted.

Putting It All Into Practice

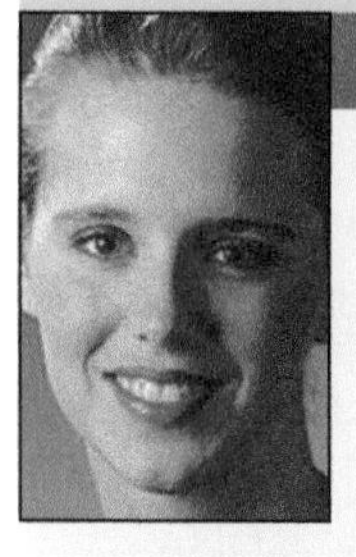

My name is Megan, and I work in a large clinic that includes the specialties of family practice, gastroenterology, immunology, and dermatology. I am the clinical supervisor and oversee all of the clinical medical assistants and our "in-house" laboratory. I work closely with all physicians to meet the growing needs of the clinic.

Working with a gastroenterologist has been interesting and educational. When preparing patients for a sigmoidoscopy, you must help them feel relaxed. This is an embarrassing situation for patients, so you need them to feel as comfortable as possible and maintain their privacy and modesty. During the procedure, I talk to patients about the weather, their pets, and other interests to make them feel more relaxed and comfortable. This can help take their minds off of the procedure.

One day I was assisting with a sigmoidoscopy, and a few minutes into the procedure the look on the physician's face told me something was wrong. When the examination was finished, the physician and I left the room and went back to his office. He informed me that what he saw on his examination was rectal cancer in an advanced stage, and at this stage, not much could be done for the patient. The worst thing a physician has to do is give unpleasant news to a patient and see the look on the patient's face. Going into the room of a patient who has just received life-threatening information is something you do not forget. All you can do is be sympathetic, understanding, and a good listener. You have to be strong and not show your emotions even though your heart is breaking for the patient and their family. Always let patients know you are there for them.

Being with a patient who receives bad news about his or her health can make you think about your own life and how it affects not only you but also your family and friends. I often think of how I would feel about receiving such news. I try to put myself in the patient's place and to be sincere and understanding and willing to lend an ear. ■

What Would You Do? What Would You *Not* Do?

Case Study 1

Beatrice Bernard is 52 years old and has come to the office for a physical examination. The physician wants Mrs. Bernard to collect a stool specimen for a Hemoccult test. After being told the purpose of the test, how to prepare for it, and how to collect the stool specimen, Mrs. Bernard expresses some concerns. She does not like the idea of collecting a stool specimen because it does not seem sanitary to her. She also thinks it will hard for her to follow the diet and medication modifications. She says she has red meat for dinner at least 4 times a week, and she does not understand why she has to eliminate it for 3 days. She says she takes a "baby" aspirin every day for "heart health" and would prefer not to stop taking it. Mrs. Bernard says that she has always taken very good care of herself, and she has never had any problems with her colon. She also says there is no history of colorectal cancer in her family. Mrs. Bernard is too embarrassed to talk about this topic with the physician. She says she may just throw the test away when she gets home. ■

This ensures that the test results are accurate and valid. The Hemoccult test includes an on-slide performance monitor that consists of a positive and negative monitor area. Failure of the expected control results to occur indicates an error, and the test results are not considered valid; possible causes include the use of an outdated test or developing solution; an error in technique; and subjection of the test to heat, sunlight, strong fluorescent light, or volatile chemicals. Procedure 13.1 outlines the procedure for coaching a patient in the collection of a specimen for a Hemoccult test. Procedure 13.2 describes the development and interpretation of a Hemoccult test.

Fecal Immunochemical Test

The fecal immunochemical test (FIT) is a CLIA-waived fecal occult blood test that uses antibodies to detect human hemoglobin, which is a component of red blood cells. Examples of brand names for this test (Fig. 13.5) are QuickVue iFOB *(Quidel Inc., San Diego, CA)* and Hemoccult ICT *(Beckman-Coulter, Inc.)*. The stool specimen for a FIT is collected by the patient at home and then returned to the medical office for processing and interpretation. The method used to collect and process the stool specimen and interpret the test results varies based on the brand of test used. Because of this, it is important for the medical assistant to become completely familiar with the FIT test brand used in his or her office by reading the product instructions that accompanies the testing kit. The medical assistant is responsible for providing the patient with instructions for collection of the specimen and the proper care and storage of the specimen until it is returned to the medical office.

Although the FIT is more expensive than the gFOBT, it is more sensitive to the presence of lower GI bleeding than is the gFOBT test. It is also not affected by drugs or food and therefore does not require any medication or dietary modifications. In addition, FIT has fewer false-positive test results than the gFOBT. When a FIT test is positive, the patient must undergo further testing such as a colonoscopy.

Fecal Immunochemical–DNA Test

A FIT-DNA test is the newest type of stool-based colorectal screening test. It is approved by the US Food and Drug Administration (FDA) for use in the United States only under the brand name of *Cologuard (Exact Sciences Laboratories, Madison WI)*. The Cologuard test is much more expensive than other stool-based colorectal screening tests; however, most insurance companies will cover the cost of it. Cologuard is a combination of two tests: a FIT and a DNA test. As previously discussed, the FIT detects the presence of human hemoglobin in the stool. The DNA test detects altered DNA in the stool shed from cells that may be associated with colorectal cancer or precancerous polyps. Studies show that Cologuard detects 92% of colorectal cancers and 42% of precancerous polyps.

The Cologuard test must be prescribed by a health care provider. A Cologuard collection kit is shipped directly to the patient from a Cologuard laboratory. The kit includes step-by-step instructions for the proper collection and processing of the stool specimen. No special patient preparation (e.g., dietary or medication modifications) is required for the test; however, certain guidelines must be followed which are outlined in Fig. 13.6.

Cologuard Procedure

The general procedure for the collection and processing of the stool specimen by the patient is summarized as follows:

1. Collect an entire bowel movement in the large container (included in the kit).
2. Remove the grooved probe from the collection tube (included in the kit).
3. Obtain a small stool sample from the bowel movement in the large container by scraping the surface of the stool with the probe making sure to cover the grooves at the end of the probe (Fig. 13.7A).
4. Place the probe in the collection tube, and seal it tightly with the screw cap (see Fig. 13.7B).
5. Immediately pour the preservative over the stool specimen in the large container, and seal it tightly with the screw-on lid (see Fig. 13.7C).
6. Label the collection container and tube.
7. Place the large container and the tube in the shipping box, and mail it back to the Cologuard laboratory within 24 hours.

The laboratory tests the specimen and sends the test results to the patient's provider. A positive test result indicates the presence of altered DNA and/or human hemoglobin in the stool sample; however, it does not confirm the presence of colorectal cancer or precancerous polyps. It is therefore recommended that patients with positive test results undergo a colonoscopy. A negative result does not guarantee the absence of cancer or precancerous polyps, and the patient should continue following the colorectal cancer screening guidelines outlined in Box 13.2.

DIAGNOSTIC COLORECTAL PROCEDURES

FLEXIBLE SIGMOIDOSCOPY

Sigmoidoscopy is the visual examination of the mucosa of the rectum and sigmoid colon (lower third of the colon) using a flexible fiberoptic **sigmoidoscope** (Fig. 13.8). The sigmoidoscope consists of a control head and a long flexible insertion tube attached to a light source (Fig. 13.9). The insertion tube is ½ inch (1.3 cm) in diameter and 24 inches (60 cm) long. The sigmoidoscope has a tiny video camera attached to the distal end of the flexible insertion tube. The camera magnifies and transmits images of the sigmoid colon to a video screen for viewing by the provider.

Before a patient undergoes a sigmoidoscopy, the provider explains the nature of the procedure and any risks to the

Table 13.1 Patient Instructions for the Guaiac Fecal Occult Blood Test

For 3 days before and during the collection period:	
Meats	• Eat no red or rare meat (beef and lamb) or liver. • Small amounts of well-cooked pork, poultry, and fish are permitted.
Fruits and Vegetables	• Eat moderate amounts of raw and cooked fruits and vegetables. • Do not consume melons, horseradish, turnips, broccoli, cauliflower, and radishes. *(These foods contain* ***peroxidase,*** *which can cause a false-positive test result).*
High-Fiber Foods	• Eat moderate amounts of whole-wheat bread, bran cereal, and popcorn. Foods high in fiber provide roughage to promote bowel elimination and encourage bleeding from "silent" lesions that bleed only occasionally.
Vitamins	• Do not take vitamin C in excess of 250 mg from supplements or citrus fruits and juices. • An iron supplement will not affect the test results.
Medications	**For 7 days before and during the collection period:** Avoid nonsteroidal antiinflammatory drugs (NSAIDs) and more than one adult aspirin a day. • Examples of NSAIDs include ibuprofen (Advil, Motrin) and naproxen (Aleve). • Acetaminophen (Tylenol) can be taken as needed.
Special Guidelines	• Do not consume any of the food items listed previously if you know, from past experience, that they cause you severe gastrointestinal discomfort or serious diarrhea. • The provider may stipulate additional medication restrictions. • Do not initiate the test during a menstrual period or in the first 3 days after a menstrual period. • Do not conduct the test when blood is visible in the stool or urine, such as from bleeding from hemorrhoids or a urinary tract infection. These conditions result in false-positive test results. • Store the slides with the flaps in a closed position at room temperature, and protect them from heat, sunlight, and fluorescent light. • Store the slides away from volatile chemicals such as ammonia, bleach, and other household cleaners.

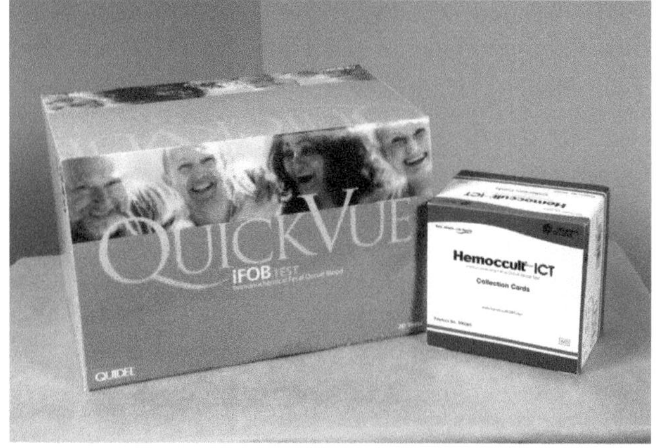

Fig. 13.5 FIT tests: QuickVue iFOB *(left)* and Hemoccult ICT *(right).*

patient and offers to answer questions. The medical assistant is responsible for obtaining the patient's signature on a written consent form, which grants the provider permission to perform the procedure.

Purpose

Sigmoidoscopy may be performed following a positive stool-based colorectal screening test to determine the source and cause of the bleeding. It is also performed to evaluate patient symptoms related to the colon such as lower abdominal pain, diarrhea, or constipation. Conditions that can be detected and assessed during a sigmoidoscopy include lesions (benign or malignant tumors), polyps, hemorrhoids, fissures, infection, and inflammation. It is especially valuable

Cologuard Patient Guidelines

The following guidelines should be followed when using a Cologuard kit:

1. Check the expiration date on the collection kit to make sure it has not expired. If the kit has expired, request a new collection kit.
2. Store the collection kit at room temperature which is between 59°F and 86°F (15°C and 30°C) and keep it away from direct sunlight.
3. Do not collect a stool specimen when any of the following are present:
   - Diarrhea
   - Blood in the urine or stool
   - Bleeding cuts or wounds on the hands
   - Rectal bleeding
   - Menstrual period
4. Avoid getting urine or toilet paper into the collection container.
5. Do not let the liquid preservative touch your skin or eyes. If this occurs, flush the area with water.
6. To ensure the integrity of the stool specimen, it must be received by the laboratory within 72 h (3 days) of collection. This means that the specimen must be mailed back within 24 h following collection to ensure enough delivery time.

Fig. 13.6 Cologuard patient guidelines.

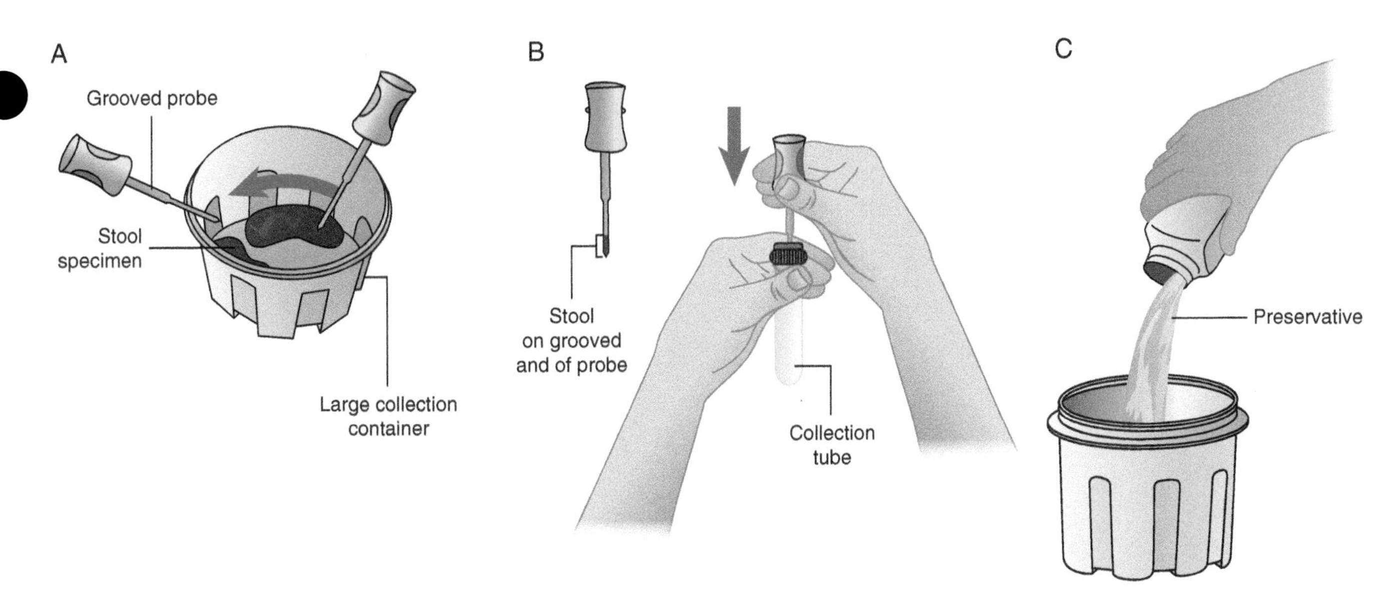

Fig. 13.7 Collection of specimens for the Cologuard test. (A) Scrape the surface of the stool with the grooved probe. (B) Place the probe in the collection tube. (C) Immediately pour the preservative over the stool specimen.

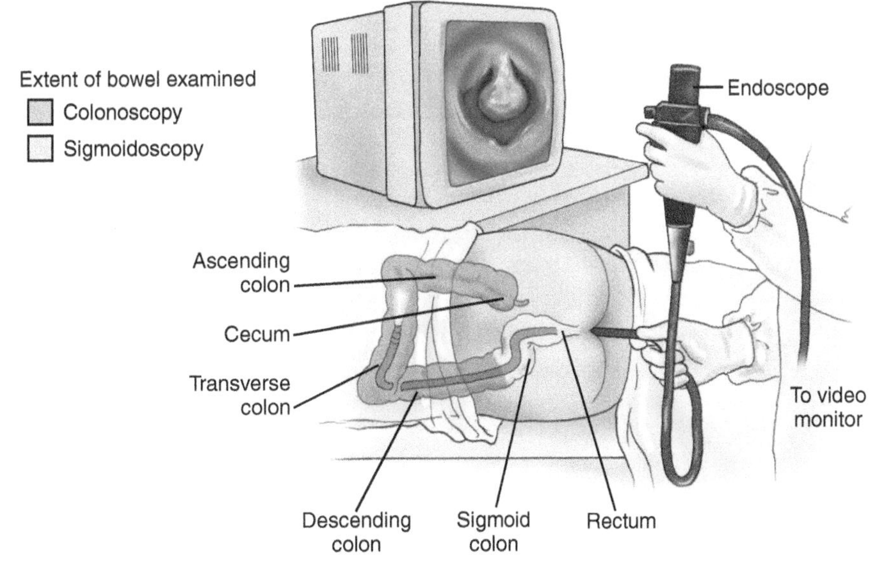

Fig. 13.8 Sigmoidoscopy and colonoscopy. (From Lafleur Brooks M: *Exploring medical language: a student-directed approach,* ed 9, St Louis: Elsevier; 2014.)

as a diagnostic procedure for detecting inflammatory bowel disease such as ulcerative colitis and Crohn disease.

A sigmoidoscopy has certain limitations. Because a sigmoidoscopy reaches only the lower third of the colon, the provider may not be able to determine the cause of the patient's symptoms or fecal occult bleeding. In this situation, the provider may order a colonoscopy to be performed at a later date. If the sigmoidoscopy detects the presence of a precancerous polyp or colorectal cancer, a colonoscopy must be performed to detect additional polyps or cancer that may be present in the rest of the colon.

Patient Preparation for Flexible Sigmoidoscopy

The patient is required to prepare the colon before the sigmoidoscopy. The lower third of the colon must be flushed out completely, so that it is empty and free of fecal material; this is known as a *partial bowel prep* because only a portion of the colon needs to be prepared. Bowel preparation is one of the most important parts of the sigmoidoscopy. Fecal material can interfere with good visualization of the wall of the sigmoid colon, making it difficult for the provider to detect abnormalities.

The medical assistant is responsible for providing the patient with instructions on preparing the colon. The medical assistant should encourage the patient to follow the instructions exactly. If the patient does not prepare properly, the sigmoidoscopy is usually canceled and must be rescheduled, which requires the patient to go through the bowel preparation procedure again. The patient preparation instructions may vary slightly from one facility to another.

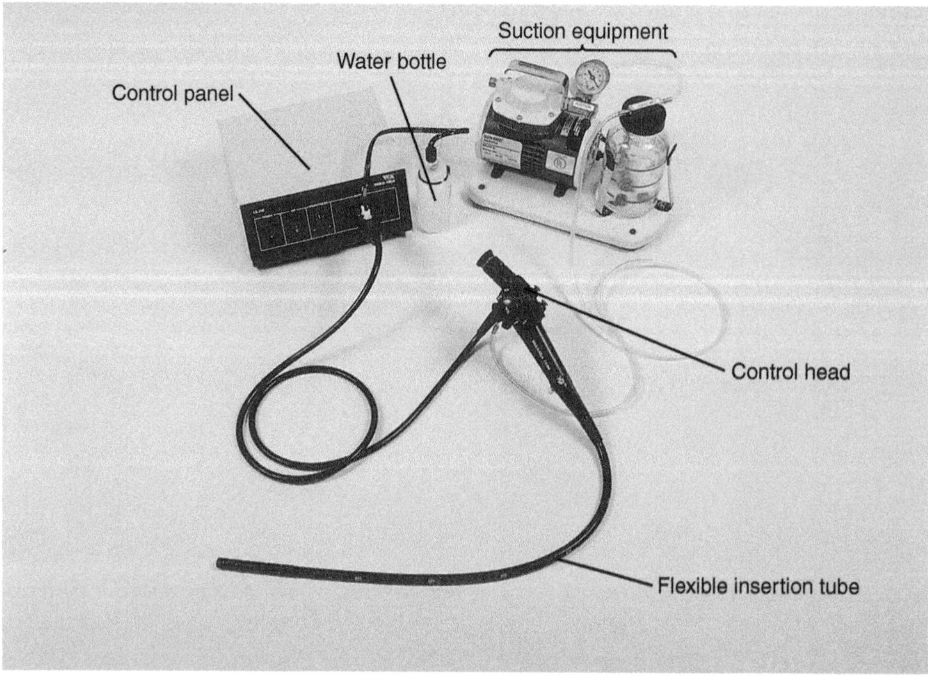

Fig. 13.9 Flexible fiberoptic sigmoidoscope.

Table 13.2 Patient Preparation for Sigmoidoscopy

Beginning 7 days before the procedure	• Discontinue taking iron, aspirin, and aspirin products. • Iron can alter the color of the wall of the colon • Aspirin may cause bleeding if a polyp is removed from the colon.
Beginning 5 days before the procedure	• Discontinue taking nonsteroidal anti-inflammatory drugs such as ibuprofen and naproxen to minimize the risk of bleeding if a polyp is removed.
The day before the procedure	• Do not consume any solid food. • Drink only clear liquids (water, apple juice, sport drinks [e.g., Gatorade], soft drinks, clear broth). • Do not drink alcohol. • Consume only gelatin (Jell-O) or Popsicles (except purple or red, which could be mistaken for blood in the colon). • Coffee or tea is permitted with no milk or cream.
The evening before the procedure	• Drink a laxative solution (e.g., magnesium citrate) as directed by your provider. • Continue drinking plenty of clear liquids.
The day of the procedure	• Continue drinking clear liquids until 4 h before the procedure. • Two hours before the examination: Use an over-the-counter enema kit to cleanse out the lower colon following the package instructions. • One hour before the procedure: Perform another enema.

General patient preparation recommendations for a sigmoidoscopy are outlined in Table 13.2.

DIGITAL RECTAL EXAMINATION

A digital rectal examination (DRE) of the anal canal and rectum is performed before a sigmoidoscopy. Using a well-lubricated, gloved index finger, the provider palpates the rectum for the presence of tenderness, hemorrhoids, polyps, and tumors. Any palpable abnormality is viewed directly when the endoscope is inserted. An **endoscope** is an instrument (e.g., sigmoidoscope and colonoscope) that consists of a tube and an optical system used for direct visual inspection of organs or cavities. The digital examination also helps relax the sphincter muscles of the anus and prepares the patient for the insertion of the endoscope.

Procedure

When the sigmoidoscopy is performed, the patient is placed on his or her left side in the modified left lateral recumbent position. The distal end of the sigmoidoscope is lubricated and inserted into the anus and rectum and then slowly advanced into the colon until it reaches the sigmoid colon. A small amount of air is usually blown, or **insufflated**, into the colon

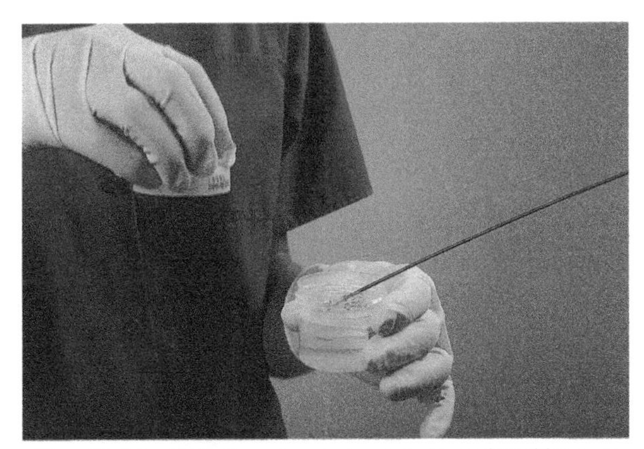

Fig. 13.10 Collection of a specimen during a sigmoidoscopy.

through tubing attached to the air control valve located on the head of the sigmoidoscope. The function of the air is to distend (expand) the lumen of the colon for better visualization. In addition, suction equipment can be used to remove secretions, such as mucus, blood, and liquid feces, which interfere with proper visualization of the intestinal mucosa. The provider then slowly withdraws the sigmoidoscope while carefully observing the mucosa of the sigmoid colon for abnormalities.

If an abnormal lesion is discovered during the examination, the provider will perform a biopsy using a long thin instrument passed through the lumen of the endoscope to obtain a specimen (Fig. 13.10). A **biopsy** is the surgical removal and examination of tissue from the body to determine whether a lesion is benign or malignant. If a polyp is discovered, the provider may remove it (polypectomy) and/or perform a biopsy. Removal of a precancerous polyp prevents it from developing into colon cancer.

The medical assistant must prepare the patient for the procedure and assist the provider during the sigmoidoscopy. These responsibilities include the following:

1. Determine whether the patient has prepared properly for the sigmoidoscopy.
2. Ask the patient to void before the procedure.
3. Position and drape the patient in modified left lateral recumbent position.
4. Reassure the patient, and help the patient to relax.
5. Lubricate the provider's gloved index finger for the digital rectal examination (DRE).
6. Lubricate the distal end of the sigmoidoscope before the provider inserts it (Fig. 13.11).
7. Assist with suction equipment.
8. Hold the specimen container to accept a specimen (if required).
9. Assist the patient after the examination.
10. Prepare the specimen for transport to the laboratory.
11. Clean the examining room.
12. Sanitize and disinfect the sigmoidoscope.

COLONOSCOPY

A **colonoscopy** is the visual examination of the mucosa of the rectum and the entire length of the colon (sigmoid colon, descending colon, transverse colon, and ascending colon) using a flexible fiberoptic **colonoscope**. The colonoscope has a tiny video camera attached to the distal end of the flexible insertion tube. The camera magnifies and transmits images of the colon to a video screen for viewing by the provider (see Fig. 13.8).

Before a patient undergoes a colonoscopy, the provider explains the nature of the procedure and any risks to the patient and offers to answer questions. The medical assistant may be responsible for obtaining the patient's signature on a written consent form, which grants the provider permission to perform the procedure.

Purpose

Colonoscopy is often performed following a positive stool-based colorectal screening test to determine the source and cause of the bleeding. It is also performed to evaluate patient symptoms related to the colon, such as lower abdominal pain, rectal bleeding, chronic constipation, and chronic diarrhea. Colonoscopy is considered the "gold standard" for assessing abnormalities of the colon. Conditions that can be detected and assessed during a colonoscopy include the following:

What Would You Do? What Would You *Not* Do?

Case Study 2

Mr. Frederick Mitchell is 57 years old and is the president of a bank. Two weeks ago, he collected a specimen for a Hemoccult test at home, and two of the three slides were positive. His physician ordered a sigmoidoscopy as a follow-up to help determine whether a problem could be identified. Mr. Mitchell has come to the office for his sigmoidoscopy. Mr. Mitchell says that he was called out of town unexpectedly on business and was not able to prepare for the test, but he says it is fine for the physician to go ahead and perform the procedure anyway. ■

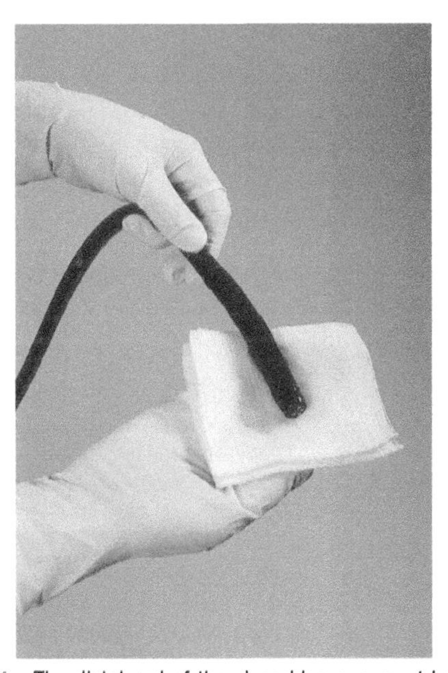

Fig. 13.11 The distal end of the sigmoidoscope must be lubricated before insertion.

- Lesions of the colon or rectum (e.g., benign or malignant growths)
- Colorectal polyps
- Hemorrhoids
- Fissures
- Infection and inflammation

Colonoscopy is particularly valuable for the detection of symptomatic and asymptomatic colorectal cancer. Early detection of colorectal cancer leads to early diagnosis and treatment, which increases the chance of survival for patients with this disease.

Patient Preparation for Colonoscopy

A colonoscopy is usually performed in a hospital on an outpatient basis or in a large medical clinic. The rectum and the entire colon must be flushed out completely so that it is empty and free of fecal material; this is known as a *full bowel prep*. This is one of the most important parts of the colonoscopy. Fecal material can interfere with good visualization of the wall of the colon, making it difficult for the provider to detect abnormalities.

The medical assistant may be responsible for providing the patient with instructions on preparing the colon which includes a strong laxative and a liquid diet. The patient should be encouraged to follow the instructions exactly. If the patient does not prepare properly, the colonoscopy is usually canceled and must be rescheduled, which requires the patient to go through the bowel preparation procedure again. The patient preparation instructions may vary from one facility to another. General patient preparation recommendations for a colonoscopy are outlined in Table 13.3, along with patient instructions following the procedure.

Procedure

A sedative is administered intravenously before the colonoscopy. The sedative causes the patient to become relaxed, sleepy, and less aware of what is taking place. Some patients do not remember the procedure at all afterward.

The procedure itself is similar to a sigmoidoscopy. The patient is placed on his or her left side in modified left lateral recumbent position. The provider performs a DRE before inserting the colonoscope. The colonoscope is advanced all

Table 13.3 Patient Preparation for Colonoscopy

Beginning 7 days before the procedure	• Discontinue taking iron, aspirin, and aspirin products.
Beginning 5 days before the procedure	• Discontinue taking nonsteroidal antiinflammatory drugs such as ibuprofen and naproxen to minimize the risk of bleeding if a polyp is removed.
Beginning 3 days before the procedure	• Eat only low-fiber foods which can be cleared easily from the colon. • High-fiber foods that should be avoided include: seeds, nuts, popcorn, raw vegetables, and fruits with skin, dried beans, and whole grains. These foods are not easily removed from the colon and may interfere with proper visualization of the colon.
Beginning 1 day before the procedure	• Do not consume any solid food. • Drink only clear liquids (water, apple juice, sport drinks [e.g., Gatorade], soft drinks, clear broth). • Do not drink alcohol. • Consume only gelatin (Jell-O) or Popsicles (except purple or red, which could be mistaken for blood in the colon). • Coffee or tea is permitted with no milk or cream.
Begin bowel preparation 1 day before the procedure	• Drink a laxative solution as directed by your provider; examples include GoLytely, NuLytely, MoviPrep, Visicol, and Suprep. • It is best to drink the solution quickly rather than slowly sipping it. • You may experience nausea and a bloated feeling. This is temporary and will disappear once you start having bowel movements. • Liquid stools will usually start within a few hours after you begin drinking the solution. You will have the urge to have a bowel movement approximately 10–15 times. • If you have prepared properly, your stool will be a clear or yellow liquid. • Continue drinking plenty of clear liquids.
The day of the procedure	• You may be asked to drink another laxative solution the morning of the procedure. • Continue drinking clear liquids until 4 h before the procedure.
Following the procedure	• Arrange to have someone drive you home following the procedure. You will be sedated during the procedure and cannot drive yourself. • It takes about an hour to recover from the sedative. • You may experience some bloating, abdominal cramping, and flatulence for several hours following the procedure. • If you had a polyp removed or a biopsy taken, it is normal to experience traces of blood in the stool for 1–2 days. • Contact your provider if you experience significant rectal bleeding, abdominal pain, fever, faintness, dizziness, shortness of breath, or heart palpitations.

the way through the entire colon (approximately 4 to 5 feet) until it reaches the cecum. The provider then slowly withdraws the colonoscope while carefully observing the mucosa of the colon for abnormalities.

If an abnormal lesion is discovered during the examination, the provider will perform a biopsy using a long thin instrument passed through the lumen of the endoscope to obtain a specimen. If a polyp is discovered, the provider may remove it and/or perform a biopsy. Removal of a precancerous polyp prevents it from developing into colon cancer in the future.

Male Reproductive Tests and Procedures

Important tests and procedures related to male reproductive health include prostate cancer screening tests and testicular self-examination (TSE), which assist in the early detection of prostate and testicular cancers.

PROSTATE CANCER

The prostate is a small gland that surrounds the urethra and is located just below the bladder and in front of the rectum (Fig. 13.12). It is approximately the size and shape of a large walnut, and its function is to secrete fluid that transports sperm.

According to the ACS, prostate cancer is the most common type of cancer in American males and is the second most common cause of cancer deaths in men, with lung cancer being the most common. Every year, an estimated 200,000 men are diagnosed with prostate cancer, and more than 33,000 men die from this disease. The incidence of prostate cancer increases with age; approximately 60% of cases are diagnosed in men older than the age of 65. Prostate cancer is found more often in African American men and men with a family history of prostate cancer.

In the early stages, prostate cancer often causes no symptoms. Symptoms that occur when the cancer is more developed include the following:

- Frequent urination, especially at night
- Difficulty in starting or holding back urination
- Weak or interrupted urinary flow
- Painful or burning urination
- Difficulty in having an erection
- Blood in the urine or semen
- Pain or stiffness in the lower back, hips, pelvis, or thighs

PROSTATE CANCER SCREENING

The purpose of prostate cancer screening is to detect prostate cancer at an early stage when it is more treatable. The primary screening tests for prostate cancer are the DRE and the prostate-specific antigen (PSA) test.

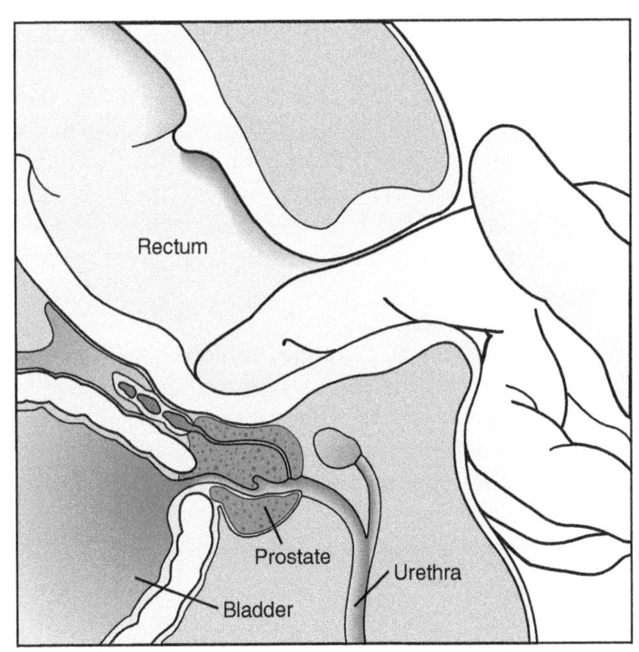

Fig. 13.12 Digital rectal examination.

DIGITAL RECTAL EXAMINATION

The DRE is a quick and simple procedure that causes only momentary discomfort. During the examination, the provider inserts a lubricated gloved finger into the patient's rectum. Because the prostate gland is located in front of the rectum, the provider is able to palpate the surface of the prostate through the rectal wall (see Fig. 13.12). The provider palpates the prostate to determine whether it is enlarged or has an abnormal consistency. Normally, the prostate gland should feel soft, whereas malignant tissue is firm and hard. However, the sensitivity of the DRE is limited because the provider can palpate only the posterior and lateral aspects of the prostate gland.

PROSTATE-SPECIFIC ANTIGEN TEST

The PSA test is a screening test primarily used to screen for the presence of prostate cancer in healthy men without symptoms. PSA is a protein produced by cells in the prostate gland (both normal cells and cancer cells) and is mostly found in semen, but a small amount is also found in blood.

The PSA test measures the amount of PSA in the blood, in units called nanograms per milliliter (ng/mL). When there is a problem with the prostate gland, such as prostate cancer, more PSA is released into the blood. The possibility of having prostate cancer increases as the PSA level goes up; however, there is no set cut-off value that indicates whether or not a man might have prostate cancer. Most men without prostate cancer have a PSA level less than 4 ng/mL. A PSA level of 4 to 10 ng/mL is considered borderline high, and the chance of having prostate cancer is 25%. Men with a PSA level greater than 10 ng/mL have a 50% chance of having prostate cancer. The higher the PSA level, the more likely that cancer is present. Other conditions that can cause an elevated PSA level include benign prostatic hyperplasia (BPH) and prostatitis.

The PSA level may normally increase after vigorous exercise (e.g., jogging and biking); therefore the patient should be instructed to engage only in normal activity for 2 days before having blood drawn for a PSA test. The patient also should be instructed not to have sexual intercourse for 2 days before the test because ejaculation can cause a significant increase in the PSA level.

If the DRE is abnormal and/or the PSA test is elevated, further testing may be performed to determine if prostate cancer is present. To make this assessment, one or more of the following tests may be performed: transrectal ultrasound (TRUS), biopsy of the prostate gland, magnetic resonance imaging (MRI), bone scan, and CT scan.

What Would you do? What Would you *Not* do?

Case Study 3

Peter Bota, a 62-year-old retired male, came to the medical office 1 week ago for a physical examination. The physician performed a digital rectal examination but did not palpate anything abnormal. At that visit, Mr. Bota's blood was drawn for a prostate-specific antigen test, and the results came back as borderline high (8 ng/mL). Mr. Bota was informed of the test results, has returned to the office, and is waiting to talk with the provider about the results and possible follow-up testing. Mr. Bota is extremely worried that he has cancer and wants to know the symptoms of prostate cancer. He also wants to know whether he did anything to cause prostate cancer. He says he does not smoke, drinks very little, and walks his dog twice a day for exercise.■

PROSTATE CANCER SCREENING GUIDELINES

The DRE and PSA screening tests for prostate cancer have certain limitations. Abnormal results from these tests do not necessarily indicate that cancer is present. Furthermore, normal results from these tests do not mean that cancer is *not* present. An abnormal DRE and/or an elevated PSA test may lead to further testing and the detection of cancer in an individual, which can pose a dilemma. Most types of prostate cancer grow very slowly and do not result in death. In fact, many men with this disease live long and healthy lives without ever knowing they have prostate cancer. Fast-growing prostate cancer is less common but is more serious and often life-threatening. The follow-up tests used to diagnose the presence of prostate cancer can be invasive, stressful, and expensive and lead to a diagnosis of a type of cancer that would never have caused a man any harm. Treatment of a man with prostate cancer can have major side effects such as erectile dysfunction, urinary incontinence, and problems with bowel function.

The ACS believes that available evidence does not currently support routine testing for prostate cancer. The ACS recommends that health care providers discuss the potential benefit and harm of prostate cancer screening and treatment with men older than 50 years of age. Following this discussion, the PSA test and the DRE should be offered annually to men 50 years and older who are at average risk for prostate cancer and have at least a 10-year life expectancy. Those men who indicate a preference for testing should be tested. The ACS recommendation provides men with knowledge of the advantages and disadvantages of early detection and treatment of prostate cancer, which then allows them to share in the decision of whether or not to be tested.

TESTICULAR SELF-EXAMINATION

The purpose of TSE is early detection of testicular cancer. Although testicular cancer can develop at any age, it is most common in males 15 to 34 years old. If detected early, it has a very high cure rate. Most cases of testicular cancer are detected by men themselves, either by accident or when performing a TSE. Certain risk factors increase a man's chance of getting testicular cancer, including the following:

- History of cryptorchidism (undescended testicles)
- Family history of testicular cancer
- Cancer of the other testicle
- White race (testicular cancer is five times more common in white men than in African American men).

Memories *From* Practicum

Megan: While on practicum in an office specializing in internal medicine, I had an experience that made me feel that all my schooling and hard work were worthwhile. A patient who had a colostomy had an embarrassing "accident." I took her into a room and cleaned her up, rinsed her colostomy bag, and helped her put it back on. She apologized profusely and asked me if I minded or felt repulsed. I replied that I was learning and getting experience in helping people. She told me that at the nursing home where she lived, she overheard some of the aides saying that it was disgusting and that it made them sick. She said she could not help it and that she felt very ashamed. I reassured her that it was nothing to be ashamed about. She then told me that she wished I could be the one to take care of her all the time. When I reached out to shake her hand and say goodbye, she pulled me down and whispered in my ear that she loved me. I was very moved and knew at that moment that I had chosen the right profession.■

TSE should be performed monthly, starting at 15 years of age. A good idea is for the patient to choose an easy-to-remember date each month, such as the first day of the month. The best time to perform the examination is after taking a warm bath or shower. Heat allows the scrotal skin to relax and become soft, making it easier to palpate the underlying testicular tissues.

TESTICULAR SELF-EXAMINATION

1
Take a warm bath or shower.

2
Stand in front of a mirror. Look for any swelling of the skin of the scrotum.

3
Place the index and middle fingers of both hands on the underside of one testicle and the thumbs on top of the testicle.

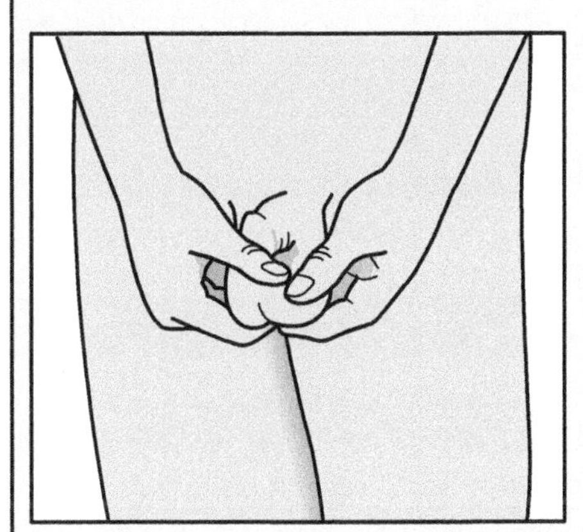

4
Apply a small amount of pressure and gently roll the testicle between the thumb and fingers of both hands, feeling for lumps, swelling, or any change in the size, shape, or consistency of the testicle. A normal testicle should feel smooth, egg-shaped and rather firm. It is also normal for one testicle to be larger or hang lower than the other testicle.

5
Find the epididymis so that you do not confuse it with a lump. The epididymis is a soft tubular cord, located behind the testicle, that functions in storing and carrying sperm.
(Note: Tenderness in the area of the epididymis is considered normal.)

6
Repeat the examination outlined above on the other testicle.

7
Report any of the following abnormalities to the physician: any unusual lump, a feeling of heaviness in the scrotum, a dull ache in the lower abdomen or groin, enlargement of one of the testicles, tenderness or pain in a testicle, or any change in the way the testicle feels.

Fig. 13.13 Testicular self-examination.

The most common sign of testicular cancer is a small, hard, painless lump (approximately the size of a pea) located on the front or side of the testicle. Any abnormality of the testicles should be reported to the provider immediately. It does not mean that the patient has cancer; however, the provider must make that determination. Fig. 13.13 outlines the procedure for a TSE.

Check out the Evolve site to access interactive activities, procedure videos, and other helpful study resources.

What Would You Do? What Would You *Not* Do? RESPONSES

Case Study 1
Page 498

What Did Megan Do?
- ❑ Relayed to Mrs. Bernard that this is not the most fun test to perform but that if colorectal cancer is detected early, the cure rate is very high.
- ❑ Explained to Mrs. Bernard that colorectal cancer increases after age 50 and that an individual can develop colorectal cancer without a family history of it.
- ❑ Told Mrs. Bernard that during the early stages of colorectal cancer no symptoms occur, so it is possible to feel fine but still have a problem.
- ❑ Explained to Mrs. Bernard in greater detail the reason for not eating red meat or taking aspirin during the testing period.
- ❑ Told Mrs. Bernard that disposable gloves could be given to her wear when she collects the specimens.
- ❑ Explained to Mrs. Bernard that the physician talks with patients every day about these types of things, and it is important to talk with him about all aspects of her health so that she receives the best care possible.
- ❑ Told Mrs. Bernard that the office would call her in 3 days to see whether she has any questions or is having any problems with the test.

What Did Megan Not Do?
- ❑ Did not tell Mrs. Bernard that she is getting older and needs to be more concerned about performing health screening tests.

Case Study 2
Page 503

What Did Megan Do?
- ❑ Told Mr. Mitchell that the physician cannot perform a sigmoidoscopy unless the colon has been properly prepared.
- ❑ Explained that the colon needs to be cleaned out, so the physician can see the wall of the colon to check for abnormalities.

Continued

What Would You Do? What Would You *Not* Do? RESPONSES—cont'd

- ❑ Went over the preparation instructions with Mr. Mitchell again, and gave him another instruction sheet to take home.
- ❑ Rescheduled his appointment, and told him that he would be called the day before the examination to be reminded of his appointment and to see whether he has any questions regarding the preparation.

What Did Megan Not Do?

- ❑ Told Mr. Mitchell that an entire office hour had been scheduled for his examination and that other patients could have been seen during this time.

Case Study 3
Page 506

What Did Megan Do?

- ❑ Listened patiently and tried to reassure and calm Mr. Bota. Told him that physicians do not yet know what causes prostate cancer.
- ❑ Explained that the prostate-specific antigen test is a screening test and that he should not jump to conclusions about the results.
- ❑ Told Mr. Bota that the physician would talk with him about his test results in a short while.
- ❑ Commended Mr. Bota on his healthy lifestyle habits, and encouraged him to continue with them.
- ❑ Gave Mr. Bota some brochures on male reproductive health to read while he waited to be seen by the physician.

What Did Megan Not Do?

- Did not tell Mr. Bota that there was nothing to worry about. ■

TERMINOLOGY REVIEW

Medical Term	Word Parts	Definition
Biopsy	*bi/o-:* life *-opsy:* to view	The surgical removal and examination of tissue from the living body. Biopsies generally are performed to determine whether a tumor is benign or malignant.
Colonoscope	*colon/o-:* colon *-scope:* instrument used for visual examination	An endoscope that is specially designed for passage through the anus to permit visualization of the rectum and the entire length of the colon.
Colonoscopy	*colon/o-:* colon *-scopy:* visual examination	The visualization of the rectum and the entire colon using a colonoscope.
Endoscope	*endo-:* within *-scope:* instrument used for visual examination	An instrument that consists of a tube and an optical system used for direct visual inspection of organs or cavities.
Insufflate		To blow a powder, vapor, or gas (e.g., air) into a body cavity.
Occult blood		Blood in such a small amount that it is not detectable by the unaided eye.
Peroxidase	*-oxia:* oxygen *-ase:* enzyme	(As it pertains to the guaiac-based fecal occult blood test [gFOBT]) A substance that is able to transfer oxygen from hydrogen peroxide to oxidize guaiac, causing the guaiac to turn blue.
Polyp (colorectal)		An abnormal noncancerous growth that protrudes from the mucous membrane of the large intestine
Screening		The process of testing to detect disease in an individual who is not yet experiencing symptoms.
Sigmoidoscope	*sigmoid/o-:* sigmoid (colon) *-scope:* instrument used for visual examination	An endoscope that is specially designed for passage through the anus to permit visualization of the rectum and sigmoid colon.
Sigmoidoscopy	*sigmoid/o-:* sigmoid (colon) *-scopy:* visual examination	The visual examination of the rectum and sigmoid colon using a sigmoidoscope.

PROCEDURE 13.1 Patient Coaching: Collection of a Specimen for a Hemoccult Test

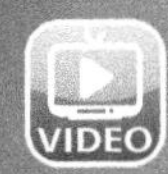

Outcome Coach a patient in specimen collection for a Hemoccult test.

Equipment/Supplies

- Hemoccult kit

1. Procedural Step. Obtain a Hemoccult kit and check the expiration date.

Principle. An outdated kit can lead to inaccurate test results.

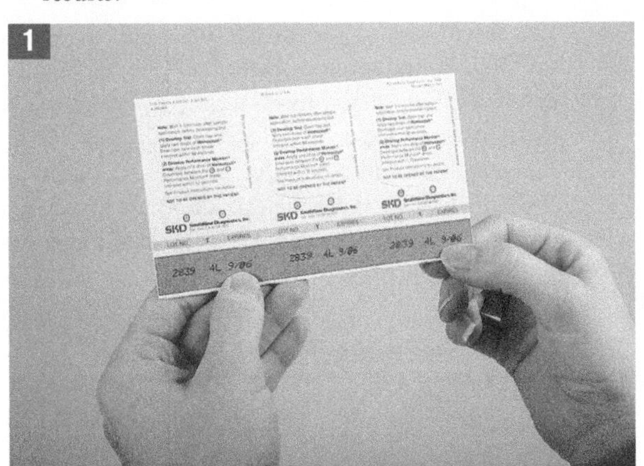

Check the expiration date.

2. Procedural Step. Greet the patient and introduce yourself. Identify the patient and explain the purpose of the Hemoccult test. Tell the patient that the stool specimens should not be collected during a menstrual period, when hemorrhoids are bleeding, or when a urinary tract infection is present.

Principle. Bleeding from other (identifiable) sources causes a false-positive test result.

3. Procedural Step. Provide patient instructions for the test following the guidelines in Box 13.1. Instruct the patient to begin the diet modifications 3 days before collecting the first stool specimen and to continue them throughout the collection period. Encourage the patient to adhere to the diet modifications.

Principle. The diet modifications may discourage patient compliance. The medical assistant should reinforce the importance of adhering to the diet requirements. Improper patient preparation can lead to inaccurate test results.

4. Procedural Step. Provide the patient with the Hemoccult kit. The kit consists of three identical cardboard slides attached to one another; each slide contains two squares, labeled "A" and "B." Three wooden applicator sticks and written instructions also are included in the testing kit.

Principle. Three slides are provided so that three stool specimens can be collected. The two squares in each slide (A and B) contain filter paper impregnated with guaiac, a chemical necessary for detection of blood in the stool.

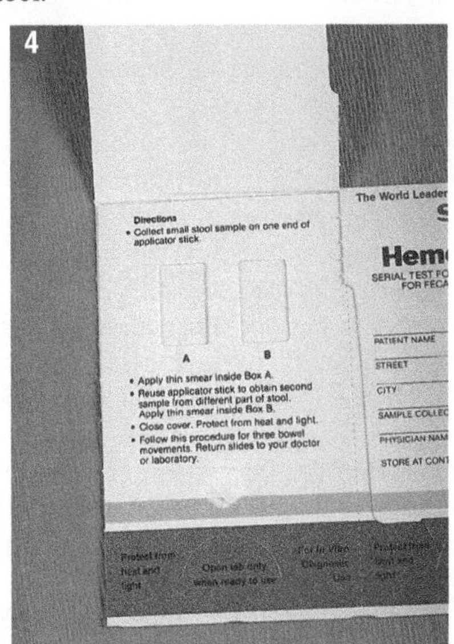

Each slide contains two squares labeled "A" and "B."

5. Procedural Step. Instruct the patient on completion of the information required on the front flap of each collection slide. This includes the patient's name, address, phone number, and age and the date of the specimen collection. A pen should be used to write this information.

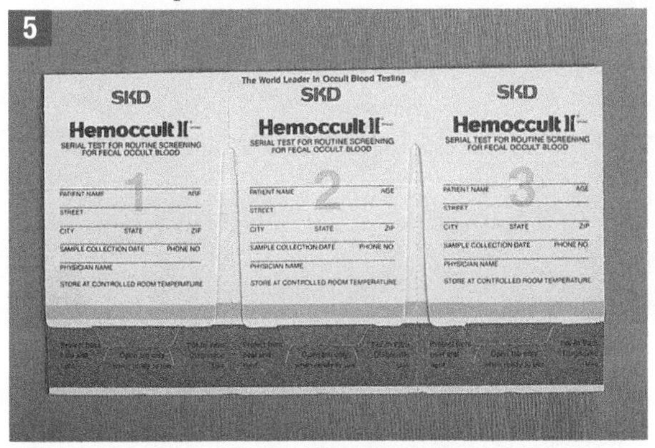

Instruct the patient on how to complete the information section on the slides.

6. Procedural Step. Provide instructions on proper care and storage of the cardboard slides. Make it clear that the slides must be stored (with the flaps in a closed position) at room temperature and protected from heat, sunlight, strong fluorescent light, and volatile chemicals.

Continued

PROCEDURE 13.1 Patient Coaching: Collection of a Specimen for a Hemoccult Test—cont'd

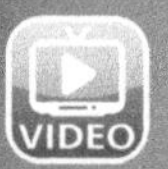

Principle. Adverse storage conditions can result in deterioration of the active reagents impregnated on the filter paper of the slides, leading to inaccurate test results.

7. **Procedural Step.** Instruct the patient on the initiation of the test by telling him or her to begin the diet modifications and then to collect a stool specimen from the first bowel movement after the 3-day preparatory period.

8. **Procedural Step.** Instruct the patient on proper collection of the stool specimen:
   a. Right before a bowel movement, fill in the collection date on the front flap of the first cardboard slide.
   b. Use a clean, dry container to collect the stool specimen. The specimen must be collected before it comes in contact with toilet bowl water. Allow the stool to fall into the collection container.
   c. Use one of the wooden applicators to obtain a specimen from one part of the stool sample.
   d. Open the front flap of the first cardboard slide (located on the left in the series of three).
   e. Spread a very thin smear of the specimen over the filter paper in the square labeled "A."
   f. Using the same wooden applicator, obtain another specimen from a different area of the stool.
   g. Spread a thin smear of the specimen over the filter paper in the square labeled "B."

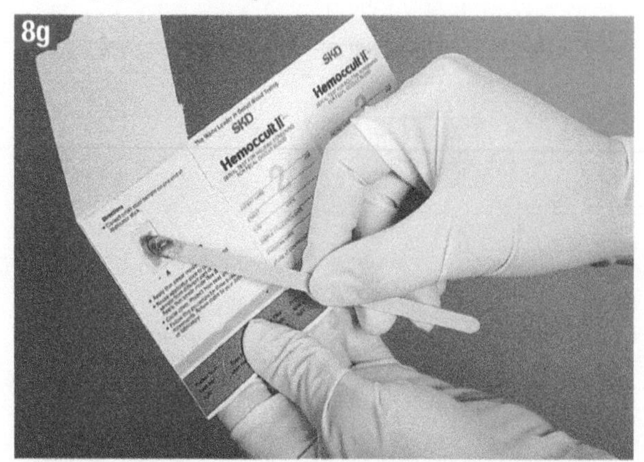

Spread a thin smear of the specimen over the filter paper.

   h. Close the front flap of the cardboard slide.
   i. Discard the wooden applicator in a waste container. Do not flush it down the toilet.
   j. Place the slides in a regular paper envelope to air-dry overnight.

Principle. Two squares are included in each slide to allow specimen collection from different parts of the stool because occult blood is not always uniformly distributed throughout the stool. Thick specimens prevent adequate light penetration through the filter paper, making it difficult to interpret the test results.

9. **Procedural Step.** Instruct the patient to continue the collection period on 3 different days until all three specimens have been obtained as follows.
   a. Repeat Procedural Step 8 after the second bowel movement the next day. If you do not have a bowel movement on the next day, then collect the specimen on the following day. The specimens should be collected on 3 different days. Use the cardboard slide located in the middle of the series of three.
   b. Repeat Procedural Step 8 after the third bowel movement, using the cardboard slide located to the right in the series of three.
   c. Allow the completed slides to air-dry overnight in the paper envelope.

10. **Procedural Step.** Instruct the patient to place the cardboard slides in the envelope lined with foil, seal carefully, and return them as soon as possible to the medical office. Emphasize to the patient that only the foil-lined envelope can be used to mail the slides; a standard envelope cannot be used. Inform the patient that the slides must be returned to the medical office as soon as possible but no later than 10 days after the first specimen is collected.

Principle. Standard paper envelopes are not approved by US postal regulations for mailing fecal occult blood testing slides. Slides should not be developed after 10 days because the test results may not be accurate.

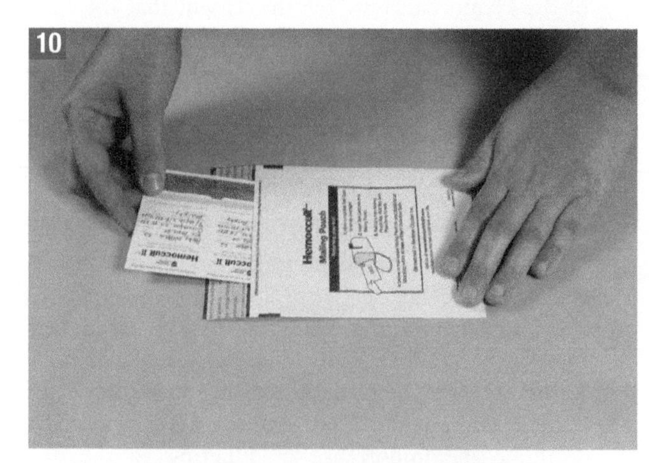

Place the cardboard slides in the envelope.

11. **Procedural Step.** Give the patient an opportunity to ask questions; ensure that the patient understands the instructions for patient preparation and collection of the stool specimen and for storage of the slides.

Principle. Improper patient preparation and poor collection technique can lead to inaccurate test results.

12. **Procedural Step.** Document in the patient's medical record.
   a. *Electronic health record (EHR):* Document that the Hemoccult kit and instructions were given to the

PROCEDURE 13.1 Patient Coaching: Collection of a Specimen for a Hemoccult Test—cont'd

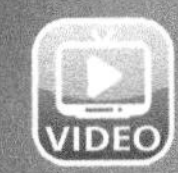

patient using the appropriate radio buttons, drop-down menus, and free text fields.

b. *Paper-based patient record (PPR):* Document the date and verification that the Hemoccult kit and instructions were given to the patient (refer to the PPR documentation example).

PPR Documentation Example

Date	
9/08/XX	9:00 a.m. Pt provided with a Hemoccult
	test and instructions for the procedure.
	——————— M. Baer, CMA (AAMA)

PROCEDURE 13.2 Developing a Guaiac Fecal Occult Blood Test

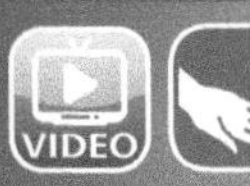

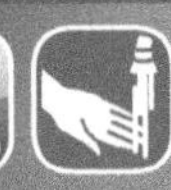

Outcome Develop a Hemoccult test.

Equipment/Supplies

- Disposable gloves
- Prepared cardboard slides
- Hemoccult developing solution
- Waste container

1. **Procedural Step.** Assemble the equipment. Check the expiration date on the developing solution bottle. The developing solution contains hydrogen peroxide and must be stored away from heat and light. It must be tightly capped when not in use.
   Principle. Outdated solution should not be used because it can lead to inaccurate test results. The solution should be stored properly because it is flammable and evaporates easily.
2. **Procedural Step.** Sanitize your hands and apply gloves. Open the back flap of the cardboard slides. Apply 2 drops of the developing solution to the filter paper underlying the back of each smear.
   Principle. The developing solution is absorbed through the filter paper and into the stool specimen. This solution could irritate the skin and eyes; if contact occurs, immediately rinse the area with water.

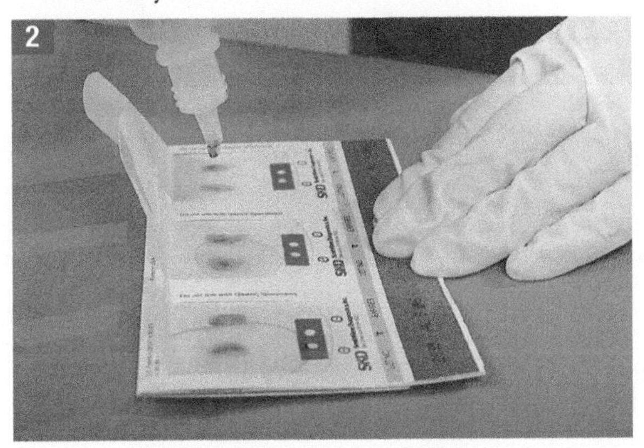

Apply 2 drops of developing solution.

3. **Procedural Step.** Read and interpret the results within 60 s. Fecal blood loss greater than 5 mL/day results in a positive reaction, which is indicated by any trace of blue on or at the edge of the fecal smear. If no detectable color change occurs, the result is considered negative.
   Principle. In the presence of hydrogen peroxide, the heme compound in hemoglobin oxidizes the guaiac, causing it to turn blue within 60 s after the developer is added. The reading time is important because the color reaction may fade after 2–4 min.
4. **Procedural Step.** Perform the quality control procedure as follows:
   a. Apply 1 drop of developing solution between the positive and negative control performance indicators on each of the three slides.

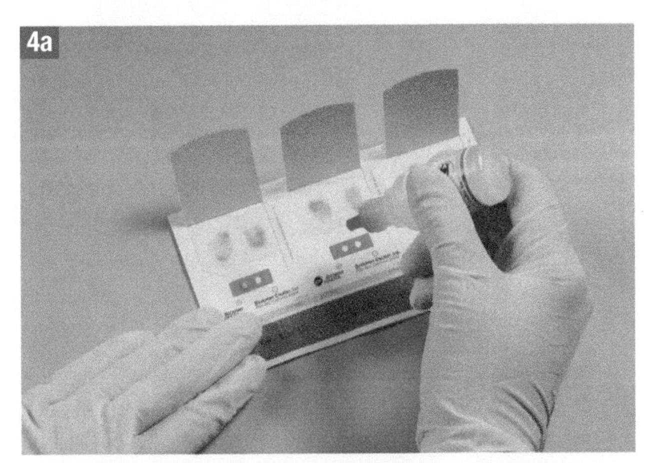

Apply 1 drop of developing solution to the control area.

Continued

PROCEDURE 13.2 Developing a Guaiac Fecal Occult Blood Test—cont'd

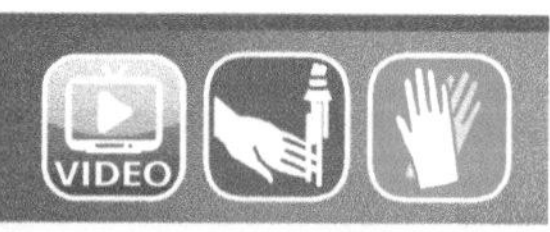

b. Read the results within 10 s.

c. The positive area should turn blue and the negative area should show no color change. Failure of the expected control results to occur indicates an error and that the test results are invalid.

Principle. The quality control procedure must be performed after developing, reading, and interpreting the slides. Quality control procedures ensure the accuracy and reliability of the test results.

4c

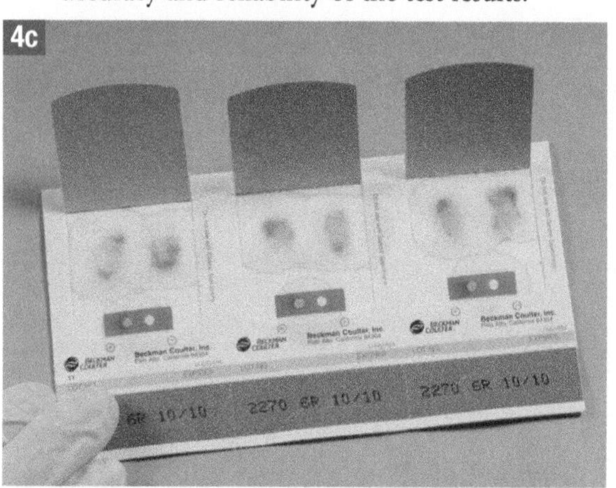

The positive area should turn blue, and the negative area should show no color change.

4

INTERPRETING THE HEMOCCULT® TEST

Negative Smears

Sample report: negative
No detectable blue on or at the edge of the smears indicates the test is negative for occult blood. (See **LIMITATIONS OF PROCEDURE**.)

Negative and Positive Smears

Positive Smears

Sample report: positive
Any trace of blue on or at the edge of one or more of the smears indicates the test is positive for occult blood.

SKD **SmithKline Diagnostics, Inc.**
A SMITHKLINE BECKMAN COMPANY
San Jose, CA 95134-1622

5. **Procedural Step.** Properly dispose of the Hemoccult slides in a regular waste container.

   Principle. Fecal material is not considered regulated medical waste and can be discarded in a regular waste container.

6. **Procedural Step.** Remove gloves and sanitize your hands.

7. **Procedural Step.** Document the results in the patient's medical record.

   a. *Electronic health record (EHR):* Document the brand name of the test (Hemoccult) and the test results for each slide (documented as positive or negative).

   b. *Paper-based patient record (PPR):* Document the date and time, the brand name of the test (Hemoccult), and the test results for each slide (documented as positive or negative). Refer to the PPR documentation example.

PPR Documentation Example

Date	
9/08/XX	9:00 a.m. Pt provided with a Hemoccult
	test and instructions for the procedure.
	——————— M. Baer, CMA (AAMA)
9/14/XX	10:30 a.m. Hemoccult test:
	Slide 1: Negative
	Slide 2: Negative
	Slide 3: Negative
	——————— M. Baer, CMA (AAMA)

PROCEDURE 13.2

Radiology and Diagnostic Imaging

Check out the Evolve site at http://evolve.elsevier.com/Bonewit/today/ to access additional interactive activities and exercises to help you study and prepare for success.

LEARNING OUTCOMES

Radiology

1. State the function of radiographs in medicine.
2. Explain the importance of proper patient preparation for a radiographic examination.
3. Explain the difference between film-based radiography and digital radiography.
4. State the advantages of digital radiography.
5. Explain the function of a contrast medium.
6. Describe the purpose of a fluoroscope.
7. Explain the purpose of each of the following types of radiographic examinations:
   - Mammography
   - Bone density scan
   - Upper gastrointestinal radiography
   - Lower gastrointestinal radiography
   - Intravenous pyelography

Diagnostic Imaging

8. Explain the purpose of each of the following diagnostic imaging procedures:
   - Ultrasonography
   - Computed tomography
   - Magnetic resonance imaging
   - Nuclear medicine imaging
9. Explain how nuclear medicine is used to produce an image of a body part.
10. State the purpose of a bone scan.
11. State the purpose of a nuclear cardiac stress test.
12. Describe a PET scan.

PROCEDURES

Instruct a patient in the proper preparation necessary for each of the following types of radiographic examinations:
- Mammography
- Bone density scan
- Upper gastrointestinal examination
- Lower gastrointestinal examination
- Intravenous pyelography

Instruct a patient in the guidelines for the following diagnostic imaging procedures:
- Ultrasonography
- Computed tomography
- Magnetic resonance imaging
- Nuclear medicine imaging

CHAPTER OUTLINE

INTRODUCTION TO RADIOLOGY
Film-Based Radiography
Digital Radiography
Contrast Media
Fluoroscopy
Positioning the Patient
Radiographic Examinations
  Mammography
  Bone Density Scan
  Gastrointestinal Series
  Intravenous Pyelography
  Other Types of Radiographs
INTRODUCTION TO DIAGNOSTIC IMAGING
Ultrasonography
  Patient Guidelines
Computed Tomography

KEY TERMS

contrast medium
echocardiogram (EK-oh-KAR-dee-oh-gram)
enema (EN-em-ah)
fluoroscope (FLOOR-oh-skope)
fluoroscopy (floor-OS-koe-pee)
radiograph (RAY-dee-oh-graf)
radiography (ray-dee-OG-rah-fee)
radiologist (ray-dee-AH-lah-jist)
radiology (ray-dee-AH-lah-jee)
radiolucent (ray-dee-oh-LOO-sent)
radiopaque (ray-dee-oh-PAYK)
sonogram (SON-oh-gram)
ultrasonography (ul-trah-son-AH-grah-fee)

Introduction to Radiology

Radiology is the branch of medicine that uses radiation and other imaging techniques to diagnose and treat disease; examples include x-rays, ultrasound, computed tomography (CT), magnetic resonance imaging (MRI), and nuclear medicine imaging. A **radiologist** is a provider who specializes in the diagnosis and treatment of disease using radiation and other imaging techniques.

Wilhelm Konrad Röntgen, a German physicist, discovered x-rays on November 8, 1895, while working with a cathode ray tube. He noticed that these rays could pass through solid materials, such as paper, wood, and human skin. Because he did not know what they were, he named them *x-rays*. The rays have since been renamed *roentgen rays* after their discoverer; however, they are better known as "x-rays."

X-rays are high-energy electromagnetic waves that are invisible and have a short wavelength that enables them to penetrate solid materials in varying degrees. **Radiography** is the taking of permanent images of internal body organs and structures by passing x-rays through the body to act on a radiosensitive receptor device such as a digital detector or radiographic film. A **radiograph** is a term used for the permanent image produced by x-rays acting on a radiosensitive receptor device.

X-rays are used to visualize internal organs and structures which assist in detecting the presence of disease. They are especially useful for detecting abnormal conditions associated with the skeletal system, such as fractures. X-rays also are used in the treatment of disease conditions, such as for the radiation therapy of malignant neoplasms.

An orthopedic medical office may have its own radiographic equipment, but more often radiographs are taken in a hospital or large medical clinic on an outpatient basis. Some radiographs, such as a chest x-ray, require no advance preparation, whereas others, such as a lower gastrointestinal (GI) study, require a great deal of special preparation. Medical assistants are usually responsible for patient instruction in the type of preparation necessary for a particular radiographic examination and for ensuring that the patient understands the importance of the preparation. If the patient does not prepare properly, the radiograph may be of poor quality, and the procedure may need to be rescheduled. This section introduces the study of radiographs, with a focus on the patient preparation necessary for common radiographs.

FILM-BASED RADIOGRAPHY

X-rays can be taken using the conventional film-based method or digitally using a computer and digital detectors. With film-based radiography, radiographic film is loaded into a device known as an *x-ray cassette*. The cassette is placed behind the part being examined, and a shadow or image of the internal body structure photographed is produced on the film. After the x-ray has been taken, the film must be processed in order to develop the image on the film. A radiologic technician takes the cassette into a darkroom and develops the image using an x-ray processor. The image on the film is then reviewed by a radiologist on a high-intensity lightbox.

DIGITAL RADIOGRAPHY

Advances in digital imaging technology have made inroads into the field of radiology. The result is the transformation of film-based radiography into a system of computer-displayed and stored digital images. To assist in understanding digital radiography, this transformation can be compared with the replacement of film cameras with digital cameras.

With digital radiography, permanent images of internal body organs and structures are obtained by passing x-rays through the body to act on a digital detector. A *digital detector* converts x-rays into electronic signals which are sent to a computer to produce a digital image. The radiologist then reviews the digital image on a high-resolution computer

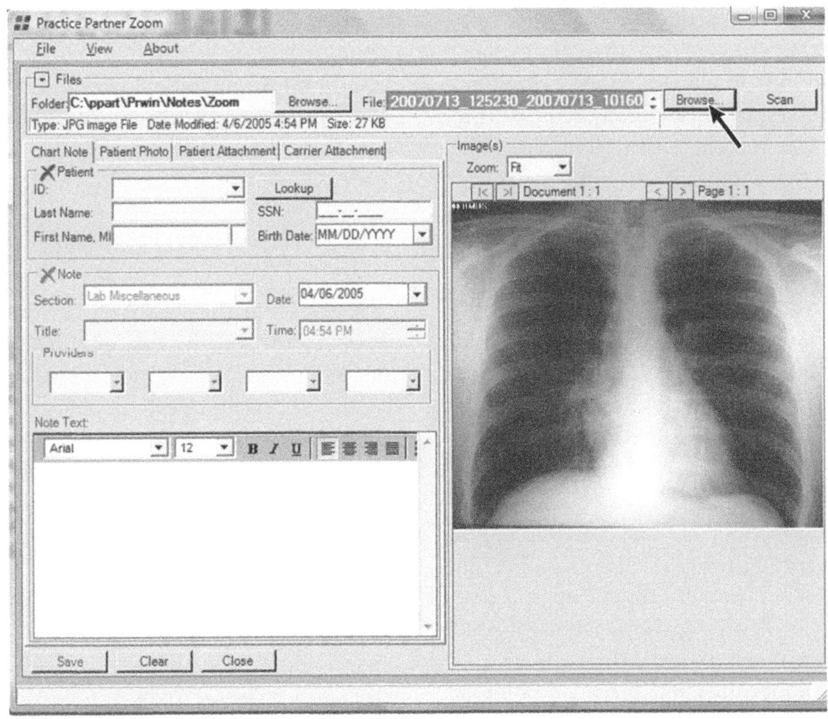

Fig. 14.1 Digital image of a chest x-ray. (Screenshot used by permission of MCKESSON Corporation. All rights reserved. © MCKESSON Corporation, 2011. From Buck CJ: *Electronic health record booster kit for the medical office*, St Louis: Elsevier; 2009.)

monitor. Digital radiography allows images to be taken and viewed immediately and also allows them to be sent electronically to a network of computers.

Important benefits of digital radiography include a shorter radiation exposure time, higher-quality images, the ability to manipulate the images (e.g., enhance and enlarge the image), and the ability to transfer the images electronically. The medical assistant is responsible for using the medical office computer to access, display (Fig. 14.1), and permanently save digital radiographs.

CONTRAST MEDIA

Radiography relies on differences in density between various body structures to produce shadows of varying intensity on the radiograph. There is a difference in density between bone and soft tissue and organs; bone is denser than soft tissue and organs. Bone absorbs more x-rays and does not allow them to reach the radiosensitive receptor device. This leaves that part of the radiograph unexposed and causes white areas to appear on the radiograph. If the x-rays penetrate structures that have a low density (soft tissue and organs), a black area appears on the radiograph. For example, the lungs are filled with air giving them a low density; therefore, x-rays are able to penetrate them easily. As a result, the lungs appear black on the radiograph while the ribs absorb the x-rays and appear as white shadows on the radiograph (Fig. 14.2). A structure such as the lungs that permits the passage of x-rays is termed **radiolucent**. A structure such as bone that obstructs the passage of x-rays and causes an image to be cast on the radiograph is termed **radiopaque**.

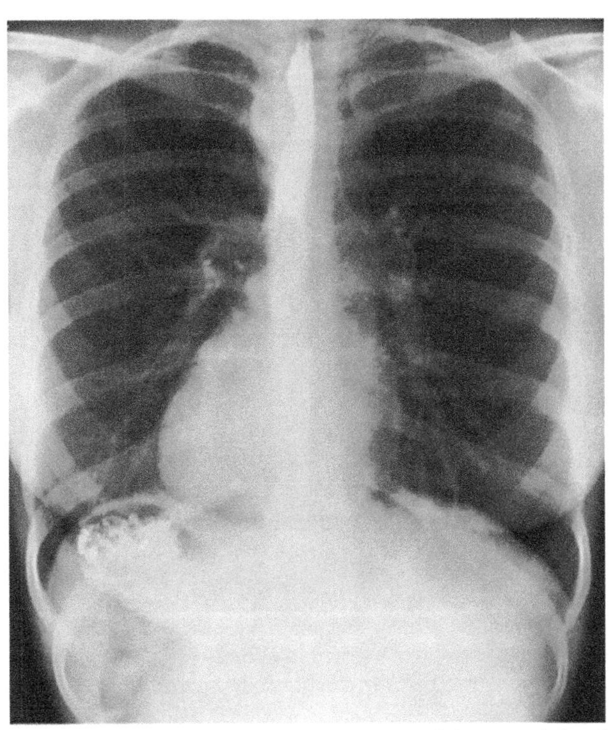

Fig. 14.2 Chest radiograph. The lungs are radiolucent and the rib bones are radiopaque. (From Meschan I: *Synopsis of radiologic anatomy with computed tomography*, Philadelphia: WB Saunders; 1980.)

In many cases, the natural densities of two adjacent structures are similar. In this instance, a **contrast medium** must be used to make a particular structure, such as an organ, visible on the radiograph. Contrast media are typically radiopaque chemical compounds that cause a body structure to absorb more radiation resulting in a contrast in density between the body structure and the surrounding area. The structure becomes visible and appears white on the radiograph. Substances used as contrast media must be able to be ingested or injected into the body without causing harm to the patient. Contrast media are administered to the patient through various routes. Some are administered orally; others are injected into a vein or are delivered through an intravenous (IV) line or an enema.

Barium sulfate and inorganic iodine compounds are commonly used radiopaque contrast media. Barium sulfate is a chalky compound that is water insoluble and does not allow penetration by x-rays. It is frequently used for examination of the GI tract because barium is not absorbed into the body through the GI tract and does not alter its normal function. Iodine salts are radiopaque and are combined with other compounds for radiographic examination of structures such as the urinary tract and blood vessels. Iodine sometimes produces an allergic reaction, and before administration, patients should be asked whether they have an allergy to iodine. Patients with known allergies may be given an iodine sensitivity test as a precautionary measure.

What Would You Do? What Would You *Not* Do?

Case Study 1

Jose Ramirez is a 10-year-old boy with episodes of unexplained abdominal pain and vomiting during the past 6 months. The medical office has scheduled an upper GI radiographic study at the local hospital. Mrs. Ramirez wants to know how best to prepare Jose for the procedure so that he will not be so afraid of the x-ray room and equipment. She asks what she can do so that he will drink the barium solution. She says he will not drink milk, and if the barium tastes anything like milk, it will be hard to get him to drink the barium. Mrs. Ramirez wants to know whether Jose can hold his favorite toy (a metal truck) during the procedure to comfort him. She also wants to know whether the barium solution has any side effects. ■

FLUOROSCOPY

A **fluoroscope** is an instrument used to view internal organs and structures of the body directly in real time on a display screen. The procedure for viewing internal organs and structures directly in real time is known as **fluoroscopy**. A radiopaque contrast medium is often used with fluoroscopy to outline various parts of the body. The patient is positioned between the radiographic tube and a fluorescent screen composed of cesium iodide crystals. When the x-rays pass through the body and strike the crystals, visible light is emitted so that the radiologist can view the action of body structures (e.g., stomach and intestines) on the screen of a monitor. During fluoroscopy, the radiologist can take radiographs that permit the study of the structures in detail and serve as a permanent record.

POSITIONING THE PATIENT

The position of the patient is determined by the purpose of the examination and the area examined. The patient is typically placed in several different positions so that different views can be obtained to provide a complete three-dimensional picture of the part examined. Articles such as jewelry and hairpins must be removed so the image on the radiograph is not obscured. To prevent blurring of the image on the radiograph, patients must maintain the position in which they are placed and not move during the radiographic examination. Blurring prevents good visualization of the part and may warrant retaking of the radiograph.

Putting It All Into Practice

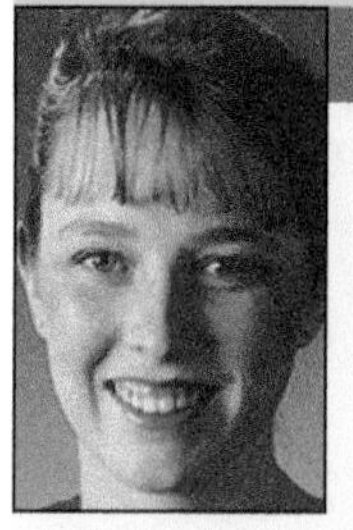

My name is Michelle, and I work for an orthopedic surgeon in a private practice. I assist the provider in minor office surgery, dressing changes, joint injections, and cast applications. When the provider performs surgery, I schedule the patients and do their preauthorizations. I have the opportunity to see a variety of problems, from sprains and strains to surgical conditions.

When our patients come to our orthopedic office, they are usually in a lot of pain. Pain plays a big part in how our patients feel on that specific day. We see patients with chronic problems that may never get better. Some patients come to our office in pain, but when their visits are over, they feel like they are on top of the world. Seeing a patient go from being unable to walk to being able to run a marathon is the best experience you can encounter. ■

RADIOGRAPHIC EXAMINATIONS

The medical assistant should understand the purpose of commonly performed radiographic examinations and should be able to instruct a patient on the proper preparation for each (Fig. 14.3). Frequently performed radiographic examinations, and the advance preparation necessary for each, are described.

MAMMOGRAPHY

Mammography is a radiographic examination of the breasts used to detect many forms of breast disease, such as benign breast masses, breast calcifications, fibrocystic breast disease,

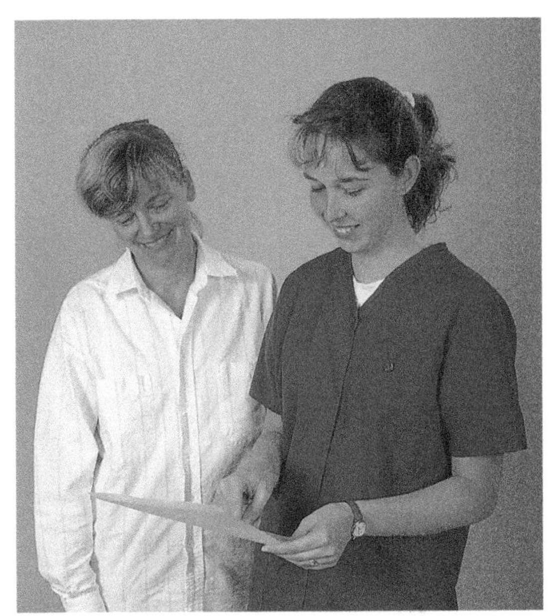

Fig. 14.3 Michelle instructs a patient in proper preparation for a radiographic examination.

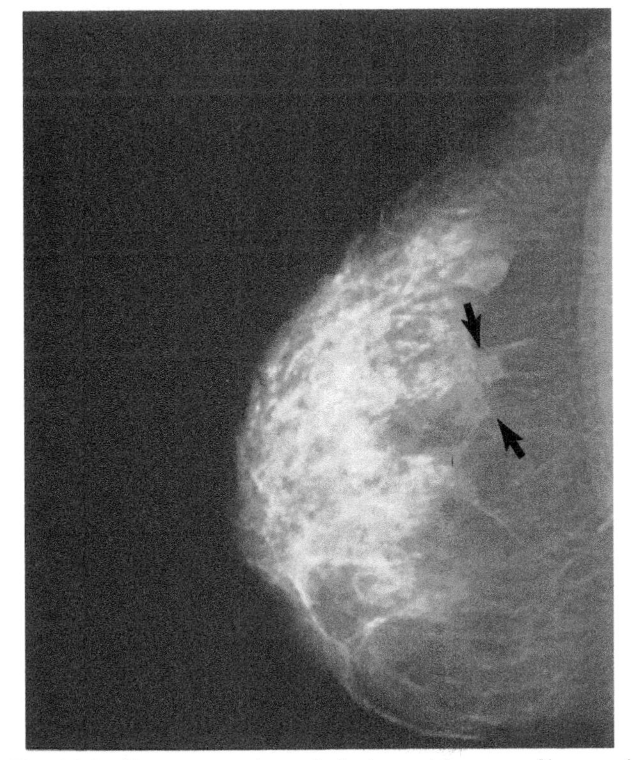

Fig. 14.4 Mammogram. *Arrows* indicate suspicious area of increased density that needs further evaluation. (From Prue L: *Atlas of mammographic positioning*, Philadelphia: WB Saunders; 1994.)

and particularly breast cancer. It is also used to monitor the effects of surgery and radiation therapy on breast tumors.

Mammography uses low doses of x-rays that pass through the breast and act on a radiosensitive receptor device to create a permanent image of each breast (Fig. 14.4). On the mammogram, an abnormal area appears noticeably different from normal breast tissue. Mammography can be used to detect a breast tumor when the growth is less than 1 cm in diameter (about the size of a pea) and before it is clinically palpable. This permits a malignant tumor to be removed at an early stage which usually results in conservative treatment with less disfigurement and a high survival rate. With early diagnosis and treatment, breast cancer survival rates for women can reach as high as 94%.

Very little preparation is required for mammography. The patient should not wear any lotions, powders, or deodorants because they may contain small amounts of metal that can be seen on the radiograph and may interfere with interpretation. For the mammogram, the patient must remove clothing from the waist up and put on an upper-body wrap; the patient should be told to wear a two-piece outfit so that the procedure is easier and more comfortable.

A radiology technician generally performs the mammogram which takes approximately 20 minutes. The patient's breast is positioned on the mammography platform, and pressure is applied with a plastic compression paddle that flattens the breast (Fig. 14.5). Compression of the breasts is necessary to obtain a clear radiograph and to lower the radiation dosage as much as possible. During the procedure, the patient must hold her breath and remain still momentarily because any type of motion, even breathing, can blur the image and make a repeat radiograph necessary.

Two radiographs are taken of each breast—one from above and one from the side. A radiologist then checks the mammogram and occasionally orders additional images to obtain a more complete view of the breast tissue. After the procedure, the radiologist studies the mammogram for any signs of breast cancer or other breast problems and sends a written report of the findings to the patient 's provider.

BONE DENSITY SCAN

A bone density scan is an enhanced form of x-ray technology that measures the bone mineral density of the human skeleton to detect bone loss. As individuals age, their bones may become less dense, causing them to become brittle and weak which may lead to a bone fracture. Factors that cause bones to lose density include osteoporosis, thyroid and parathyroid conditions, and certain medications (e.g., corticosteroids). Postmenopausal women are at particular risk for osteoporosis. *Osteoporosis* is a condition in which a gradual loss of calcium causes the bones to become thinner, more fragile, and more likely to break. It is recommended that women 65 years of age and older and men 70 years of age and older have a bone density scan.

Dual-energy x-ray absorptiometry (DXA) scanning is the most widely used bone density testing method. DXA (pronounced "dexa") uses x-rays to determine the amount of bone in the human skeleton. During a DXA scan, bone density measurements are taken at different parts of the body. The bone density measurements indicate if the patient has lost bone density. They also assist in detecting the presence of osteoporosis and can be used to predict the patient's risk of bone fracture. Patients on medication therapy for osteoporosis (e.g., Fosamax, Boniva, and Actonel) may also undergo DXA to determine if the medication is working.

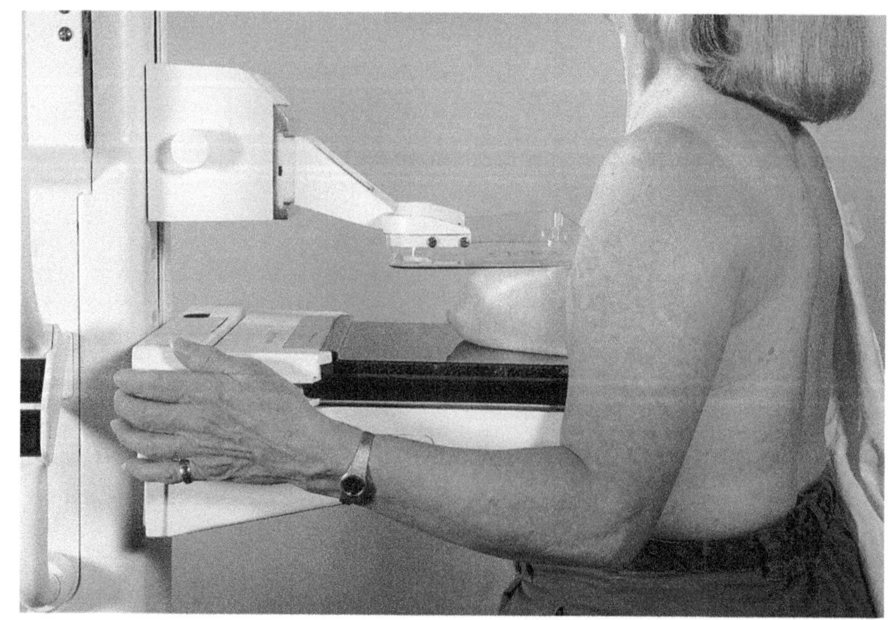

Fig. 14.5 Patient positioning for mammography. (From Ballinger PW, Frank ED, editors: *Merrill 's atlas of radiographic positions and radiologic procedures*, vol 2, ed 12, St Louis: Elsevier; 2012.)

The patient should be instructed to abstain from taking a calcium supplement or medication containing calcium (e.g., Rolaids and Tums) for 24 hours prior to the scan. These substances interfere with obtaining an accurate bone density measurement. For the examination, the patient is positioned on an x-ray table and instructed to remain as still as possible during the test. The radiologic technician then scans one or more areas of bone with the DXA equipment. Areas that are typically scanned include the lower spine and head of the femur because the bone in these areas is more likely to fracture from osteoporosis.

Test results are in the form of two scores (a T-score and a Z-score), which are sent to the patient's provider. These scores assist the provider in diagnosing and treating the patient. The *T-score* is derived by comparing the patient's measurements with those of healthy young normal adults with peak bone density of the same gender as the patient. A T-score of −1.0 or above indicates normal bone density. A T-score between −1.0 and −2.5 indicates low bone density or *osteopenia*. A T-score of −2.5 or below indicates the presence of osteoporosis. The T-score is used to estimate the patient's risk of developing a fracture. The *Z-score* is derived by comparing the patient's measurements with an established database of healthy individuals of the same age and gender as the patient. An unusually high or low Z-score may indicate the need for further testing.

PATIENT COACHING Mammography

Answer questions patients may have about mammography.

What is the purpose of mammography?

Mammography is a safe, low-dose radiographic examination used to screen for abnormal changes in the breasts. Mammography allows the provider to detect small lumps in the breast long before they can be felt. Although most breast lumps are not cancerous, breast cancer can be removed at an early stage when detected early, which usually results in treatment that is less deforming and has a much higher survival rate.

Who should have a mammogram?

The American Cancer Society recommendations for mammography for women of average breast cancer risk are as follows:

- Women between 40 and 44 should have the choice to start annual breast cancer screening with mammograms if they wish to do so.
- Women 45–54 should get mammograms every year.
- Women 55 and older should switch to a mammogram every other year, or they can choose to continue yearly mammograms.
- Screening should continue as long as a woman is in good health and is expected to live 10 more years or longer.
- All women should be familiar with how their breasts normally look and feel and report any changes to a health care provider right away.

Women at high risk for breast cancer such as a family or personal history of breast cancer or a known *BRCA1* or *BRCA2* gene mutation should follow the advice of their provider regarding mammography; age guidelines do not apply because these women undergo examination on a more frequent basis.

What occurs during the mammography procedure?

During mammography, the breast is positioned on a special platform table and is flattened with a compression paddle. Breast compression may be uncomfortable for some women. The discomfort can be reduced with avoidance of caffeine several days before the procedure and by scheduling the mammography the week after a menstrual period when the breasts are less tender. Each breast is radiographed from above and from the side. A radiologist studies the resulting mammogram to detect any abnormalities. The results are reported to the provider.

- Encourage the patient to have a mammogram according to the schedule recommended by the American Cancer Society.
- Provide the patient with educational materials on mammography. ■

GASTROINTESTINAL SERIES

Upper Gastrointestinal Radiography

An upper GI study is an examination of the upper digestive tract using fluoroscopy and radiography. The examination is helpful in the diagnosis of disorders of the esophagus, stomach, and duodenum. These disorders include gastroesophageal reflux disease (GERD), hiatal hernias, ulcers, inflammation or blockages of the upper GI tract, and benign and malignant tumors. The procedure may be ordered when the patient complains of difficulty in swallowing, vomiting, abdominal pain, gastric reflux (burping up food), severe indigestion, and blood in the stool.

Proper patient preparation is important for this procedure. The patient's stomach must be empty at the beginning of the study so food does not obscure the radiographic image. To prepare for the examination, the patient must eat a light evening meal and then not eat or drink anything, including water and medications, after midnight on the day before the examination. Food and fluid in the GI tract have a degree of density and could cause confusing shadows on the radiograph.

The upper GI tract varies little in density from the structures around it, and to make it show up on a radiograph, a contrast medium must be used. The patient drinks a suspension of barium mixed with water and flavoring, which resembles a milkshake and has a chalky taste. Before drinking the barium, the patient may be asked to drink a carbonated solution that puts air into the upper GI tract, causing it to expand. The combination of air and barium, known as a double-contrast *study*, allows the radiologist to view the esophagus, stomach, and duodenum in greater detail.

As the patient swallows the barium mixture, the radiologist observes its passage down the esophagus and into the stomach and duodenum with fluoroscopy. The barium coats the lining of the upper GI tract, making it visible on the screen of the fluoroscope. Radiographs are taken periodically during the examination to allow a detailed study of the upper GI tract and to provide a permanent record. The patient's position is changed at various times so that the upper GI tract can be visualized from different profiles. After the procedure, the radiologist prepares a report of the findings, which is sent to the patient's provider.

The medical assistant should explain to the patient that the barium suspension will appear in the stool for 1 to 3 days following the procedure and will cause the stool to have a whitish color. The barium mixture may cause constipation and the need for a laxative. To help prevent constipation, the patient should be instructed to increase fiber and fluid intake for several days following the procedure.

Lower Gastrointestinal Radiography

A lower GI examination involves filling the colon with a barium sulfate mixture with a catheter (tube) inserted into the rectum through the anus. Because of this, the procedure is sometimes called a *barium enema*. The examination uses fluoroscopy and radiography to observe and obtain permanent pictures of the colon, sigmoid colon, and rectum (Fig. 14.6). A lower GI assists in the diagnosis of disorders of the lower GI tract, such as polyps, cancerous tumors, diverticulosis, and the extent of inflammatory bowel disease (e.g., ulcerative colitis, Crohn disease). The procedures may be ordered when the patient complains of chronic diarrhea, blood in the stool, constipation, irritable bowel syndrome, unexplained weight loss, and changes in bowel habits.

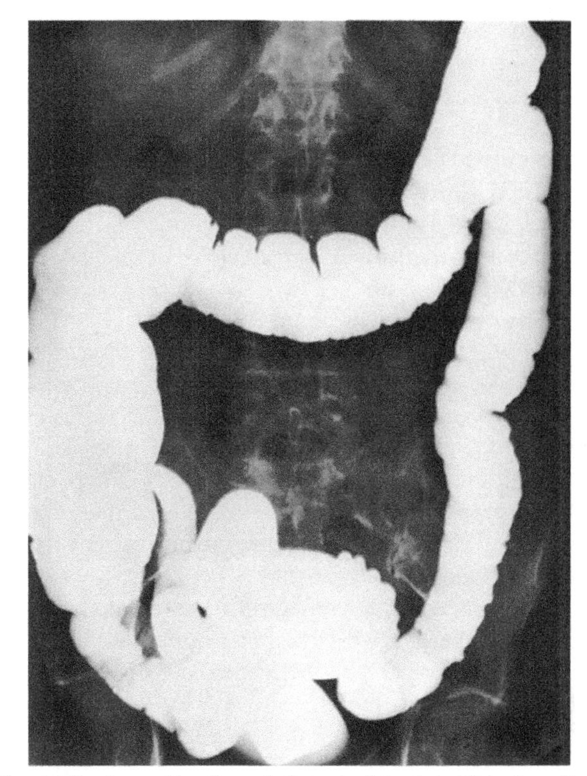

Fig. 14.6 Lower GI radiograph. Colon is distended with barium. (From Meschan I: *Synopsis of radiologic anatomy with computed tomography*, Philadelphia: WB Saunders; 1980.)

The colon must be thoroughly cleansed in advance to remove gas and fecal material. Gas has a certain degree of density and shows up as confusing shadows on the radiograph. If fecal material appears on the radiograph, the image of the colon is obscured. Instructions for cleansing the colon may vary from one medical office to another, but in general, the patient is instructed to consume only clear liquids the day before the examination, such as water, plain coffee and tea, clear broth, and strained fruit juice. A laxative should be taken on the day before the scheduled examination; an enema also may be necessary. An **enema** is an injection of fluid into the rectum to aid in the elimination of feces from the colon. The patient should not drink anything (except water) after midnight on the day before the examination. On the morning of the examination, the patient may be required to perform a warm water cleansing enema until the returns are clear.

The patient reports at the scheduled time and is instructed to relax on one side while the rectal catheter is inserted. As the barium enters the colon, the radiologist watches it on the fluoroscopic screen and periodically takes radiographs.

The patient has a sensation of fullness and the urge to defecate as the barium enters the colon. The patient is moved into various positions to allow the barium to fill the colon completely and to obtain better visualization of the colon. The tip of the enema tube is specially designed to hold in the barium in the lower GI tract. Once the examination is completed, most of the barium is emptied through the rectal catheter. The patient is then allowed to evacuate the remainder of the barium.

A *double-contrast study* of the lower GI tract is similar to a lower GI study; however (in addition to the barium), it also employs the use of air that is inserted into the colon through the same catheter as the barium. The air distends the wall of the colon and allows the radiologist to view the colon in greater detail, making it easier to detect polyps and small cancerous tumors. After the procedure, the radiologist prepares a report of the findings, which is sent to the patient's provider.

The medical assistant should explain to the patient that the barium suspension will appear in the stool for 1 to 2 days following the procedure and will cause the stool to have a whitish color. The barium mixture may cause constipation and the need for a laxative. To help prevent constipation, the patient should be instructed to increase fiber and fluid intake for several days following the procedure.

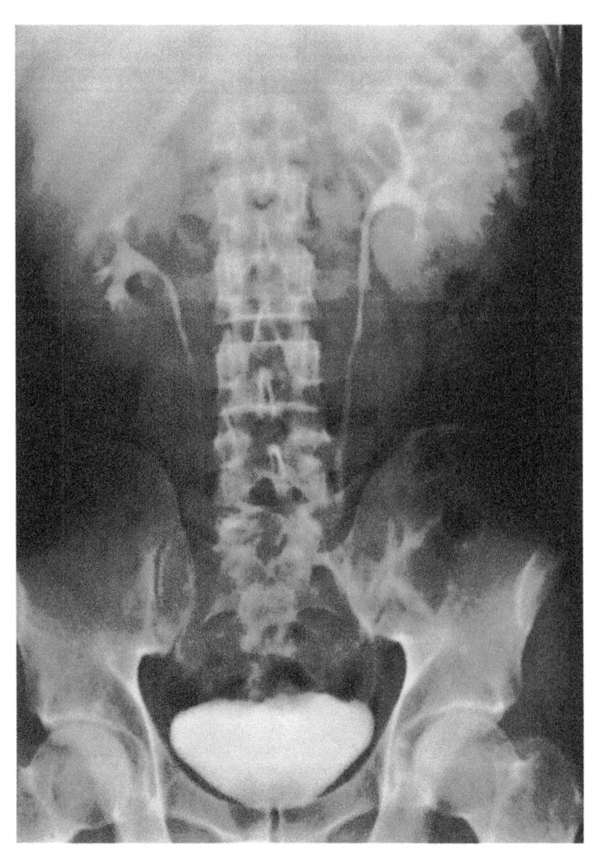

Fig. 14.7 Intravenous pyelogram. (From Meschan I: *Synopsis of radiologic anatomy with computed tomography,* Philadelphia: WB Saunders; 1980.)

INTRAVENOUS PYELOGRAPHY

An intravenous pyelogram (IVP) is a radiograph of the kidneys, ureters, and urinary bladder (Fig. 14.7). An IVP is used to assist in the diagnosis of kidney stones, kidney cysts, an enlarged prostate gland, blockage or narrowing of the urinary tract, and tumors of the urinary tract.

The patient should consume only clear liquids on the day before the examination. The evening before the examination, the patient must take a laxative to remove gas and fecal material from the intestines to permit proper visualization of the urinary tract. Starting at midnight the day before the examination, the patient should not eat, drink, smoke, or chew gum. Unless the patient is allergic to iodine, a contrast medium containing iodine is used and is administered intravenously to the patient. As the iodine enters the bloodstream, the patient may feel warm and flushed, have a mild itching sensation, and have a metallic or salty taste in the mouth. This reaction is normal and lasts for only a few minutes. If the patient is allergic to iodine, a different type of contrast medium must be used. After the procedure, the radiologist prepares a report of the findings, which is sent to the patient 's provider.

OTHER TYPES OF RADIOGRAPHS

Other types of radiographs that the medical assistant may encounter include the following:

Angiocardiogram. Radiograph of the valves and blood vessels of the heart using a contrast medium and fluoroscopy to determine if there is a restriction in the blood flow going to the heart.

Bronchogram. Radiograph of the lungs using a contrast medium to assist in the diagnosis of lung cancer, tuberculosis, and pneumonia.

Cerebral angiogram. Radiograph of the major arteries of the brain using a contrast medium to detect blockages or other abnormalities in the blood vessels of the head and neck.

Chest radiograph. Radiograph of the chest to assist in diagnosing conditions affecting the chest, its contents, and nearby structures to detect conditions such as pneumonia, heart failure, and emphysema (n o contrast medium is required).

Cholangiogram. Radiograph of the bile ducts after administration of a contrast medium to detect bile duct blockages.

Coronary angiogram. Radiograph of the coronary arteries using a contrast medium to detect a restriction in blood flow to the heart.

Cystogram. Radiograph of the urinary bladder using a contrast medium to assist in diagnosing problems of the urinary bladder.

Hysterosalpingogram. Radiograph of the uterus and fallopian tubes using a contrast medium to evaluate the shape of the uterus and determine if the fallopian tubes are patent (open and unobstructed).

Myelogram. Radiograph of the spinal canal using a contrast medium to detect conditions affecting the spinal cord and nerves within the spinal canal.

Retrograde pyelogram. Radiograph of the kidneys and urinary tract using a contrast medium injected directly into the ureter through a ureteral catheter. The dye flows to the kidneys through the ureters to detect abnormalities of the urinary tract.

Introduction to Diagnostic Imaging

Diagnostic imaging procedures allow for the visualization of internal body structures in great detail. The most common diagnostic imaging procedures are ultrasonography, computed tomography, magnetic resonance imaging, and nuclear medicine imaging. Diagnostic imaging procedures are usually performed in a hospital or a large clinic on an outpatient basis. The medical assistant may need to relay information to a patient scheduled for such a procedure, including what to expect during the procedure and any patient preparation that may be required. The medical assistant should have a basic knowledge of diagnostic imaging procedures and the preparation necessary for each.

ULTRASONOGRAPHY

Ultrasonography, also called ultrasound (US) is the oldest of the diagnostic imaging procedures. Ultrasound uses high-frequency sound waves for the study of soft tissue structures. Advances have been made in ultrasound technology. These include three-dimensional (3-D) ultrasound, in which sound waves are formatted into 3-D images (Fig. 14.8). Four-dimensional (4-D) ultrasound is another new technology that consists of 3-D ultrasound but in motion.

Ultrasound is frequently used in the diagnosis of conditions of the abdominal and pelvic organs, particularly the breasts, gallbladder, liver, spleen, pancreas, kidneys, uterus, ovaries, and abdominal aorta. Some examples of conditions that can be detected using ultrasound include breast cysts, gallstones, kidney stones, uterine polyps, and abdominal aorta aneurysms . An ultrasound examination of the heart is known as an **echocardiogram** and is used to determine the size, shape, and position of the heart and the movement of the heart valves and chambers. Ultrasonography is also used for guiding a needle or other device during a minimally invasive procedure, such as amniocentesis, a needle biopsy, cortisone injection into a joint, and needle aspiration of fluid in a joint.

Ultrasonography offers many advantages as a diagnostic imaging procedure. It shows movement, allows continuous viewing of a structure, uses sound waves rather than radiation, and is less expensive than other imaging procedures. Ultrasound does have some minor limitations. Because sound waves are unable to penetrate bone and air or gas-filled cavities such as the lungs, stomach, and intestines, ultrasound cannot be used in the evaluation of these structures. In addition, ultrasound may be difficult to use with obese patients because adipose tissue can interfere with sound wave transmission.

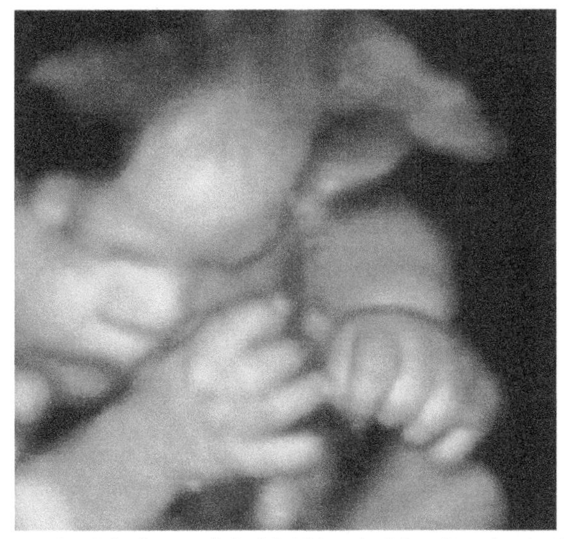

Fig. 14.8 3-D ultrasound of a third-trimester fetus. (From Leonard PC: *Building a medical vocabulary: with Spanish translations*, ed 8, St Louis: Elsevier; 2011.)

Before performing an ultrasound examination, a warm ultrasound gel must first be spread on the area to be examined. The purpose of the gel is to increase the conductivity of the sound waves between the skin and the transducer. During the ultrasound examination, the ultrasound technician places a probe containing a transducer firmly on the patient's skin and moves it over the body areas to be examined. The transducer generates sound waves that are directed into the patient's tissues and reflected back to the transducer, similar to an echo. The transducer converts the waves into electrical signals. A computer then converts these signals into digital images. The size, shape, and consistency of the images are displayed on a video display screen; this image is known as a **sonogram** (Fig. 14.9). The patient is often permitted to view the sonogram on the screen of the monitor as the procedure is performed. The digital images can be permanently stored on a computerized storage medium. A radiologist reviews and interprets the images and prepares a report of the findings that is sent to the patient 's provider.

Although ultrasound is commonly used for a wide variety of noninvasive imaging procedures, individuals are most familiar with its use in obstetrics. Obstetric ultrasound is most frequently used to confirm a pregnancy, determine the gestational age of a fetus and to confirm the due date; to detect congenital abnormalities, ectopic pregnancy, and multiple pregnancy; and to determine the fetus's position and size late in pregnancy. If the fetus is old enough and is positioned correctly, it is usually possible to determine its gender. Because the ultrasound machine is a compact unit, most obstetricians perform this procedure in their medical offices. Ultrasound is also used by gynecologists to evaluate and treat infertility problems.

Doppler ultrasound is a special application of ultrasound. It measures the direction and speed of blood as it flows through blood vessels, such as major arteries and veins in the

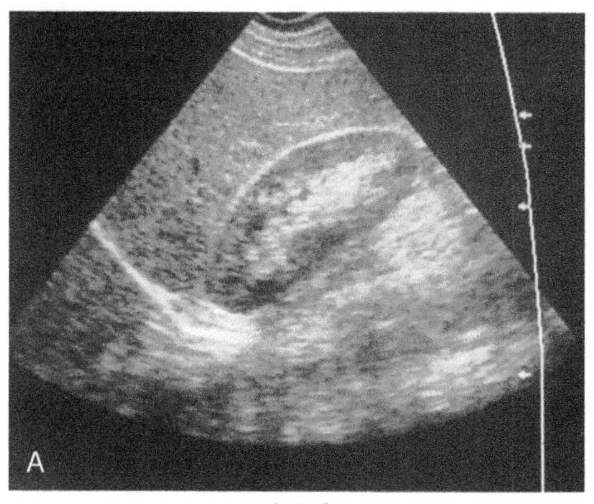

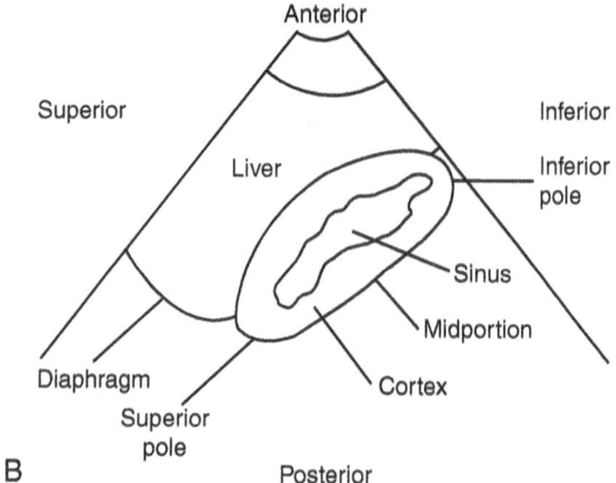

Fig. 14.9 Sonogram of the right kidney. (From Tempkin BB: *Ultrasound scanning: principles and protocols*, ed 3, St Louis: Elsevier; 2009.)

abdomen, arms, legs, and neck. Doppler ultrasound images can assist the provider in diagnosing blood flow blockages, narrowing of blood vessels due to atherosclerosis, and congenital malformations.

PATIENT GUIDELINES

The medical assistant should tell the patient what to expect during an ultrasound examination and instruct the patient in the preparation required for the procedure, as follows:

1. Ultrasound is a safe and painless procedure that takes approximately 15 to 45 minutes to complete, depending on the body part examined.
2. The patient may need to prepare for the procedure, depending on the part of the body examined. An ultrasound of the gallbladder, liver, spleen, and pancreas necessitates that the patient fast for 8 to 12 hours. For an obstetric ultrasound, the patient needs to have a full bladder. The patient should be instructed to consume approximately 32 ounces of fluid about 1 hour before the procedure.
3. The patient must remain still when requested during the procedure because movement can interfere with accurate results. In addition, the patient may be asked to change positions so that the organs can be seen at different angles.

What Would You Do? What Would You *Not* Do?

Case Study 2

Sara-Jayne Monterey has been having heart palpitations. The provider ordered an electrocardiogram, and the results did not show any abnormalities. The physician then ordered a Holter monitor. Results showed the patient was having premature ventricular contractions, especially in the evening. The physician suspects that Sara-Jayne has a prolapsed mitral valve and has scheduled an echocardiogram at the local hospital. Sara-Jayne wants to know whether this procedure involves injecting a dye into her veins. She also wants to know whether the procedure will hurt. Two days before the appointment for the echocardiogram, Sara-Jayne calls the medical office to say that she just found out that she is pregnant and wants to know whether the procedure will have to be canceled. ■

COMPUTED TOMOGRAPHY

Computed tomography (also known as a *CT scan*) is a diagnostic imaging procedure that uses x-ray technology to produce detailed images of the inside of the body. The CT machine, known as the *CT scanner*, takes a series of images of a body part, permitting the imaging of structures that cannot be visualized with conventional radiographic procedures. The series of images is processed with a computer to produce 3-D cross-sectional images of a body part similar to the slices of bread in a loaf (Fig. 14.10). Newer CT scanners take continuous pictures of a body part in a spiral fashion; a spiral CT scanner is faster and produces better quality images of areas inside the body compared with a conventional scanner.

CT scans are used primarily to detect and evaluate tumors and other abnormalities and to monitor the effects of surgery, radiation therapy, or chemotherapy on tumors. CT is particularly well suited to quickly examine individuals who may have internal injuries and bleeding from automobile accidents or other types of trauma. CT scans are used to detect tumors or lesions within the abdomen. A CT scan of the heart may be ordered when various types of heart disease or abnormalities are suspected. CT is also used to image the head in order to locate injuries, tumors, or clots that may lead to a stroke, brain hemorrhage, and other conditions. It can image the lungs in order to reveal the presence of tumors, pulmonary embolisms (blood clots), excess fluid, and other conditions such as emphysema or pneumonia. A CT scan is often used to image complex bone fractures, severely eroded joints, or bone tumors since it usually produces more detail than would be possible with a conventional x-ray.

Some CT examinations require the use of a contrast medium. The contrast medium may be given by mouth, injected into a vein, or given by enema. The contrast medium allows for a sharper image of the internal structures of the body.

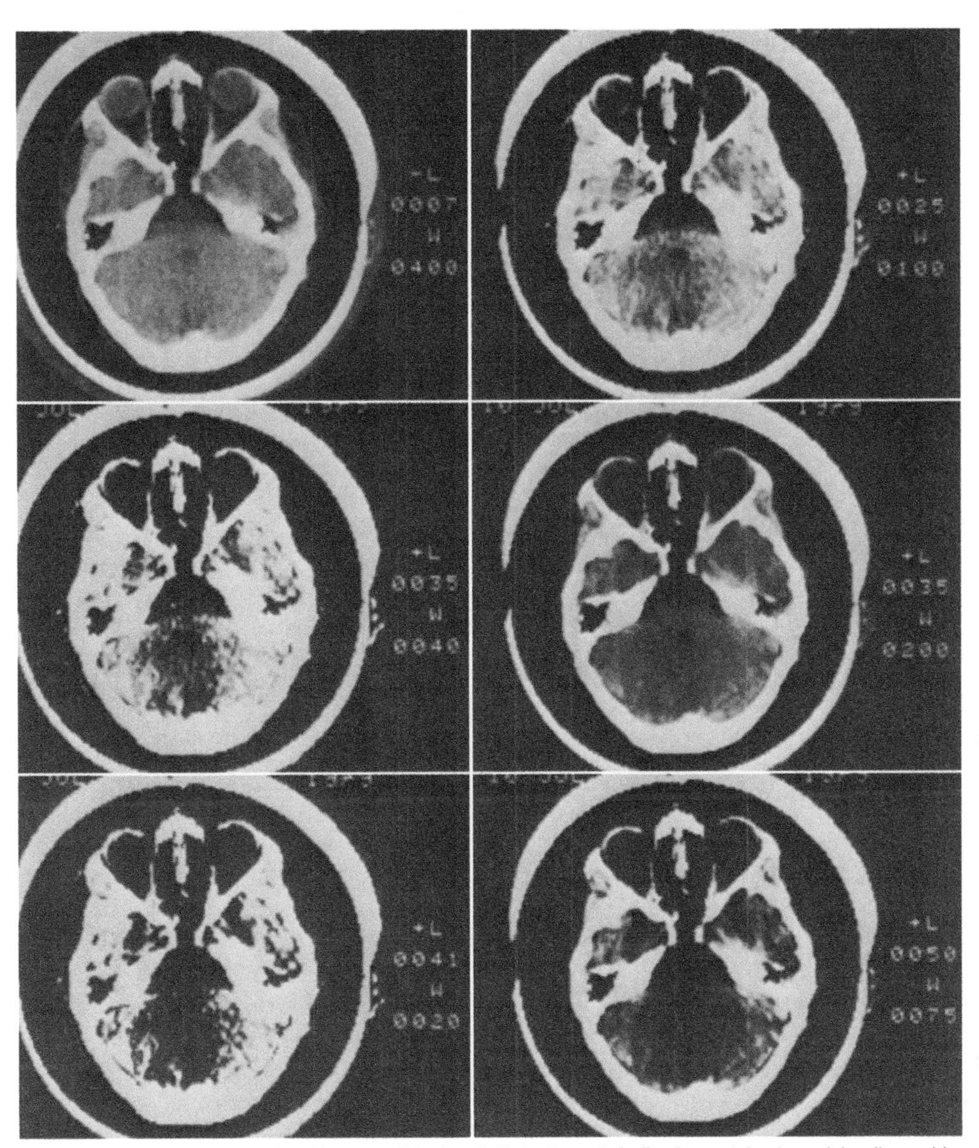

Fig. 14.10 CT cross-sectional images of the head. (From Snopek A: *Fundamentals of special radiographic procedures*, ed 5, Philadelphia: Elsevier; 2007.)

A CT scan is conducted by a diagnostic imaging technician. The patient is positioned on a narrow motorized table (Fig. 14.11). From an adjoining room, the technician mechanically moves the table into the large doughnut-shaped CT scanner. The x-ray tube within the CT scanner rotates around the patient taking multiple images as the table is slowly moved through the scanner. The images are processed with a computer to produce 3-D cross-sectional digital images of a body part which are stored digitally on electronic media for evaluation by a radiologist. The radiologist reviews and interprets the images and prepares a report of the findings, which is sent to the patient 's provider (Fig. 14.12).

PATIENT GUIDELINES

The medical assistant should tell the patient what to expect during the CT scan and should instruct the patient on the preparation required for the procedure, as follows:

1. If a contrast medium is to be used, the patient may need to fast for several hours before the procedure. It is important to ask the patient whether he or she is allergic to radiographic contrast media to avoid an adverse reaction.
2. Before the procedure, the patient must remove all radiopaque objects, such as dentures, eyeglasses, and jewelry, because they interfere with a clear image of the body part examined.
3. The technician will be in an adjacent room where the scanner controls are located. The patient is in constant sight of the technician and speakers inside the scanner enable communication with the technician.
4. The patient should lie motionless and breathe normally during the procedure. When a radiograph is being taken, the patient is usually asked to hold his or her breath to prevent blurring of the images. The patient hears slight buzzing, clicking and whirring sounds from the scanner as pictures are taken.

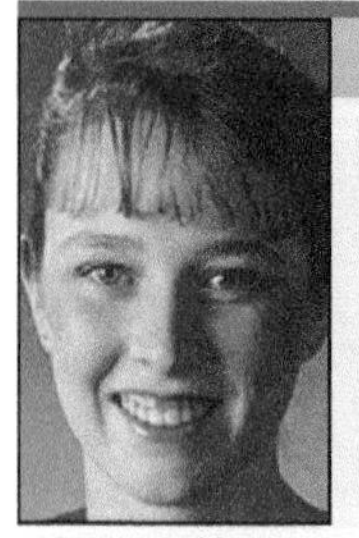

Memories *from* Practicum

Michelle: My first practicum was terrifying at first, but at the same time I was overwhelmed with excitement. I remember worrying how I was going to remember all my clinical and administrative skills. I was worried that I would hurt someone or forget to do something important.

One day a patient came into our office upset and crying. The examination rooms were full, so I took her into our staff lounge. I sat her down, fixed her a cup of coffee, and asked her if I could help. She told me that her son had drowned 2 years ago on that day, her mother had cancer, and her husband had passed away 8 months previously. I listened to everything she had to say, and I comforted her until the physician was ready to see her. She walked over to me, hugged me, and said my smile and people skills were the best treatment for her depression that she had ever had. Her telling me that made me feel good about my career choice, and it made me realize how fulfilling it was. It did not take me long to realize that all the hands-on skills that I had learned in the classroom were not forgotten. I also realized that a smile and listening to people are just as important as my skills. ■

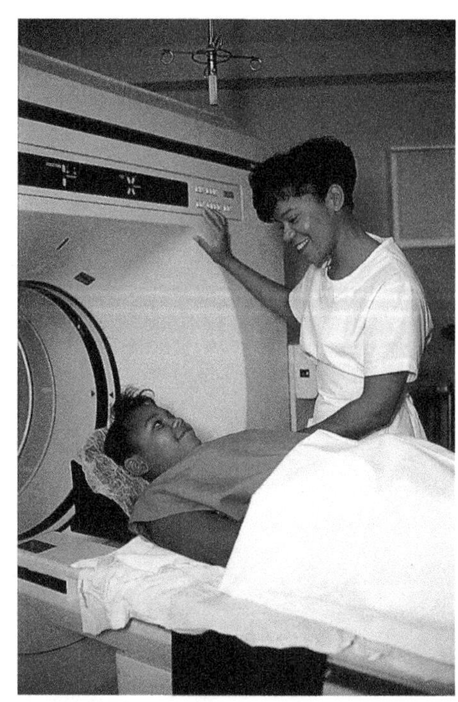

Fig. 14.11 Positioning a patient for a CT scan. (From Kowalczyk N, Donnett K: *Integrated patient care for the imaging professional,* St Louis: Mosby; 1996.)

5. The entire procedure, which includes set-up, the scan itself, checking the images, and removing the IV (if needed), takes 15 to 45 minutes depending on what part of the body is being scanned.

MAGNETIC RESONANCE IMAGING

Magnetic resonance imaging (MRI) is a diagnostic imaging procedure that uses a strong magnetic field, radio waves, and a computer to produce detailed 3-D cross-sectional images of internal body structures. Because MRI does not involve radiation, the US Food and Drug Administration has classified the MRI machine as a low-risk device.

MRI is used for imaging tissues of high fat and water content that cannot be seen with other radiologic techniques. MRI assists in the diagnosis of intracranial and spinal lesions and cardiovascular and soft tissue abnormalities, such as herniated discs, torn ligaments, and joint diseases. MRI allows the examiner to see through bone and view fluid-filled soft tissue in great detail. The brain, spinal cord, and nerves, along with muscles, ligaments, and tendons are seen much more clearly with MRI than with regular x-rays and CT.

An MRI is conducted by a diagnostic imaging technician. The patient lies on a table that is moved to the inside of the cylindrical MRI machine while a diagnostic imaging technician in an adjoining room monitors the procedure (Fig. 14.13). Because of the closed space, some patients may have difficulty with claustrophobia. The provider may order a sedative for these patients. Open MRI machines are less confining than traditional MRI machines and are helpful for examining obese patients and patients with claustrophobia; however, they are a newer technology and may not be available at some facilities.

The 3-D cross-sectional images are electronically stored on a computer for evaluation by a radiologist. The radiologist reviews and interprets the images and prepares a report of the findings, which is sent to the patient's provider.

What Would You Do? What Would You *Not* Do?

Case Study 3

Michael Wendl is an 18-year-old high school varsity football player. For the past 3 months, he has had pain and swelling in his left shoulder. The provider schedules an MRI to assist in determining the cause of the problem. Michael has had several radiographs over the past 2 years and is worried about radiation exposure to his body. He wants to know how much radiation will be involved with the procedure. Michael has problems with claustrophobia and wants to know whether he can play a game on his cellphone during the procedure to distract him. He also wants to know whether he is allowed to eat anything before the procedure. ■

PATIENT GUIDELINES

The medical assistant should tell the patient what to expect during the MRI and instruct the patient in the preparation required for the procedure, as follows:

1. MRI is a safe and painless procedure that typically takes between 20 and 60 minutes depending on the size of the area being scanned and the number of images being taken.

CT Diagnostic Imaging Report

Patient: Regina Bach
Gender: F
DOB: 10/22/xx

Ordering Physician: Brian Mendelssohn
Exam Date: 7/28/xx
Radiologist Reviewer: Daniel Baldwin

Type of Exam: CT scan of the abdomen and pelvis with intravenous and oral contrast media.

Clinical History: This is a 66-year-old female with a history of breast cancer and new onset abdominal pain.

Comparison: Comparison is made to a CT scan of the abdomen and pelvis performed 10/1/xx.

Technique: 5 mm axial images from the lung bases through the pubic symphysis following the administration of intravenous and oral contrast media.

Findings:
- Lung bases: No pulmonary nodules or evidence of pneumonia.
- Cardiac: Base of heart if within normal limits. No pericardial effusion.
- Liver: Normal size and contour. There is a new 2 cm hypoattenuating focus in segment 8. Gallbladder is surgically absent.
- Spleen: No splenomegaly.
- Pancreas: No mass or ductal dilation
- Kidneys and adrenals: No masses, stones or hydronephrosis. No adrenal nodules.
- Bladder: Within normal limits
- Uterus and adnexa: The uterus and bilateral ovaries are within normal limits for age.
- Lymph nodes: No lymphadenopathy
- Bones: No aggressive osseous lesions. Degenerative changes are present in the spine.

Impression:
1. No findings on the current CT to account for the patient's clinical complaint of abdominal pain.
2. There is a new 2 cm lesion in the liver which is indeterminate and cannot be definitely diagnosed by the study.

Recommendation:
Given the patient's personal history of breast cancer, an MRI of the liver is recommended to better characterize the indeterminate liver lesion to exclude the possibility of cancer metastases.

Fig. 14.12 CT diagnostic imaging report.

2. A contrast medium may be used for the procedure. It improves the resolution of the image by increasing the brightness in various parts of the body.
3. No special preparation is necessary for the MRI examination. The patient may eat or drink before the examination and take any prescribed medication.
4. Because the procedure involves a strong magnet, the patient should remove any metal or magnetic-sensitive items, such as coins, cell phones, eyeglasses, hearing aids, dentures, watches, rings, and keys. Avoid wearing cosmetics, as certain types of cosmetic preparations contain small amounts of metal. Individuals with a pacemaker or cochlear implant may not be able to undergo an MRI.
5. The patient must remain completely still for 15- to 20-minute intervals during the procedure. The patient hears a metallic clacking sound like a muffled drumbeat during the procedure. Earplugs or headphones are available for use if the patient desires.

NUCLEAR MEDICINE IMAGING

Nuclear medicine imaging is an advanced diagnostic procedure in which a tiny amount of radioactive material (known as a *radiopharmaceutical*) is introduced into the patient using one of the following methods: intravenously, by ingestion, or by inhalation. Most radiopharmaceuticals are chemically bound to a complex known as a *tracer*. A tracer is designed to be attracted to specific areas of the body or, in some cases, to types of diseased tissue.

A nuclear imaging technician positions the patient on a scanning table that works in association with a specialized piece of equipment known as a *gamma camera*. The gamma camera is positioned above or below the scanning table and is able to detect the radiation being given off by the body part that has been targeted by the radiation. The resulting information is displayed as still images or functional animations of body parts and organs. Because it can show the actual function of organs, nuclear medicine imaging provides more detailed information for certain conditions than is provided by other diagnostic imaging examinations (e.g., CT scan, MRI).

The most common nuclear medicine imaging procedures include bone scans and nuclear cardiac stress tests, which are described in more detail in the next section. Other types of nuclear medicine imaging procedures that may be performed include gallbladder procedures, thyroid studies, brain scans, and lung scans.

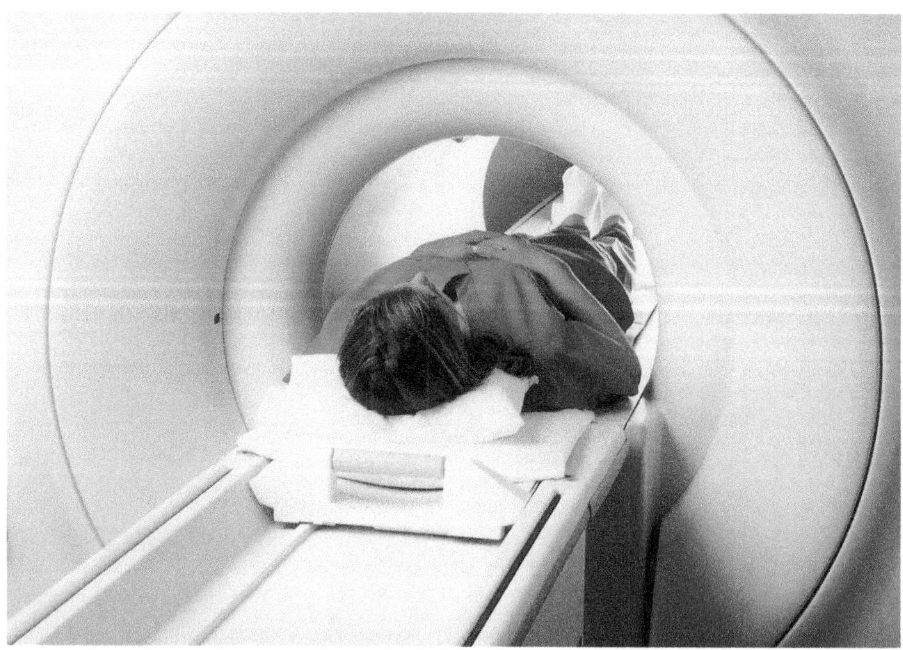

Fig. 14.13 Magnetic resonance imaging (MRI). The patient lies on a table inside the cylindrical MRI machine while an MRI technician in an adjoining room monitors the procedure. (From Ballinger PW, Frank ED, editors: *Merrill 's atlas of radiographic positions and radiologic procedures,* vol 3, ed 12, St Louis: Elsevier; 2012.)

BONE SCAN

A bone scan is performed to detect bone fractures that are difficult to locate (e.g., stress fractures and hip fractures), osteomyelitis, arthritis, bone tumors, and metastatic bone cancer. When a bone scan is performed, the patient is intravenously injected with a radiopharmaceutical. The patient must then wait at the facility for a predetermined period of time, based on the area being examined. The purpose of the waiting period is to allow the radiopharmaceutical to be absorbed sufficiently so that an accurate diagnosis can be made. The gamma camera detects radiation given off by a bone abnormality and shows up as a "hot" spot on the nuclear images (Fig. 14.14). The radiologist reviews the nuclear images and prepares a bone scan report, which is sent to the patient's provider.

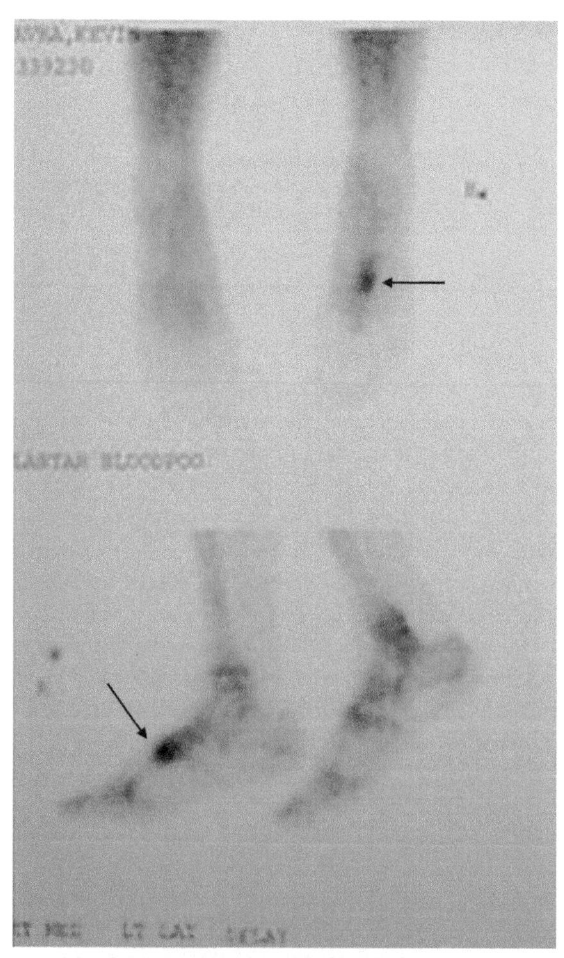

Fig. 14.14 Bone scans of the feet. *Arrows* show the hot spot that indicates a stress fracture. (From Donatelli RA: *Sports-specific rehabilitation,* St Louis: Elsevier; 2007.)

NUCLEAR CARDIAC STRESS TEST

A nuclear cardiac stress test is a diagnostic procedure used to evaluate the cardiovascular health of individuals with known heart disease or individuals at high risk for developing heart disease, particularly coronary artery disease (CAD). Although a nuclear stress test is more time-consuming and expensive to perform than a simple stress test (described in Chapter 12), it provides more accuracy in diagnosing CAD.

The radiopharmaceutical used for a nuclear stress test is administered intravenously and targets the heart. Nuclear images included in the stress test are taken by the gamma camera during two phases: a *resting phase* and a *stress phase* (which is a functional study). The resting phase is performed with the heart at a normal rate, whereas the stress phase is performed immediately after the patient exercises at his or her maximal (target) heart rate. The two sets of nuclear images—the resting images and the images taken under cardiac stress—are then compared with each other. These images assist the radiologist in determining which parts of the heart are healthy and functioning normally. The images also identify areas of the heart that exhibit decreased blood flow during exercise, meaning that a portion of the heart muscle is not receiving enough oxygen. A decreased oxygen supply to a portion of the heart is known as cardiac ischemia and is typically due to the presence of coronary artery disease. The radiologist reviews and interprets the images and prepares a report of the findings, which is sent to the patient's provider.

POSITRON EMISSION TOMOGRAPHY SCAN

A positron emission tomography (PET) scan is a special type of nuclear imaging procedure. PET uses a special camera and computer to construct a 3-D image of the area being scanned. This procedure is particularly useful in diagnosing conditions of the brain and heart, such as brain cancer and heart disease.

What Would You Do? What Would You *Not* Do? RESPONSES

Case Study 1
Page 516

What Did Michelle Do?

- ❑ Told Mrs. Ramirez that a role-playing game with Jose might help. Suggested that she play the "doctor" and pretend she is taking an x-ray of Jose.
- ❑ Told Mrs. Ramirez that the barium will have a flavoring in it but that it does taste chalky. Suggested that she explain to Jose why he needs to drink the barium—to help the doctor find what is wrong with him so that he will not get sick anymore.
- ❑ Told Mrs. Ramirez that Jose's metal truck would interfere with a good radiograph. Suggested that she bring the truck and tell Jose he can have it after the procedure.
- ❑ Explained that the barium might cause constipation and would cause Jose's next bowel movement to be white. Told her that she should encourage Jose to drink a lot of water after the procedure to help prevent constipation.

What Did Michelle Not Do?

- ❑ Did not tell Mrs. Ramirez that the barium solution would taste good and that she should not have any trouble getting Jose to drink it.

Case Study 2
Page 522

What Did Michelle Do?

- ❑ Told Sara-Jayne that the procedure uses sound waves to visualize the heart. Explained that the procedure does not use a dye injected into the veins. Gave her an educational brochure on ultrasound imaging.
- ❑ Reassured Sara-Jayne that no pain is involved with an echocardiogram.
- ❑ Told Sara-Jayne that an ultrasound exam is normally safe during pregnancy because radiation is not used. The physician would be informed that she is pregnant, however, and if there is a change in his order, Sara-Jayne would be notified.

What Did Michelle Not Do?

- ❑ Did not allow Sara-Jayne to go ahead with the procedure without checking with the physician.

Case Study 3
Page 524

What Did Michelle Do?

- ❑ Explained to Michael that an MRI does not use radiation, so he would not be exposed to any radiation during the procedure.
- ❑ Told Michael that he would not be able to play a game on his cellphone during the procedure. Explained that the MRI works with a strong magnet that might damage his cellphone and also interfere with a good image of the shoulder. Told Michael that he would need to lie still during the procedure.
- ❑ Told Michael the physician would be informed of his problem with claustrophobia. Explained that the physician may want to give him something to help him relax during the procedure.
- ❑ Told Michael that it was fine to eat before the procedure.

What Did Michelle Not Do?

- ❑ Did not overlook or minimize Michael's concern about claustrophobia. ■

TERMINOLOGY REVIEW

Medical Term	Word Parts	Definition
Contrast medium		A substance used to make a particular structure visible on a radiograph.
Echocardiogram	*ech/o-:* sound *cardi/o-:* heart *-gram:* record	An ultrasound examination of the heart.
Enema		An injection of fluid into the rectum to aid in the elimination of feces from the colon.
Fluoroscope	*fluor/o-:* fluorescence *-scope:* instrument used for visual examination	An instrument used to view internal organs and structures directly in real time.
Fluoroscopy	*fluor/o-:* fluorescence *-scopy:* visual examination	An x-ray procedure for viewing internal organs and structures directly in real time.
Radiograph	*radi/o-:* radiation *-graph:* instrument used to record, x-ray film	The permanent image produced by x-rays acting on a radiosensitive receptor device such as a digital detector or radiographic film.
Radiography	*radi/o-:* radiation *-graphy:* process of recording, x-ray filming	The taking of permanent images (radiographs) of internal body organs and structures by passing x-rays through the body to act on a radiosensitive receptor device.
Radiologist	*radi/o-:* radiation *-ologist:* one who studies and practices (specialist)	A provider who specializes in the diagnosis and treatment of disease using radiation and other imaging techniques.
Radiology	*radi/o-:* radiation *-ology:* study of	The branch of medicine that uses radiation and other imaging techniques to diagnose and treat disease.
Radiolucent	*radi/o-:* radiation *-lucent:* transparent	Describing a structure that permits the passage of x-rays.
Radiopaque	*radi/o-:* radiation *-opaque:* opaque	Describing a structure that obstructs the passage of x-rays.
Sonogram	*son/o-:* sound *-gram:* record	The image obtained with ultrasonography.
Ultrasonography	*ultra-:* beyond, excess *sono-:* sound *-graphy:* process of recording	The use of high-frequency sound waves to produce an image of an organ or tissue.

Introduction to the Clinical Laboratory

Check out the Evolve site at http://evolve.elsevier.com/Bonewit/today/ to access additional interactive activities and exercises to help you study and prepare for success.

LEARNING OUTCOMES

Clinical Laboratory

1. Identify the use of laboratory test results.
2. Explain what occurs when the body is not in homeostasis.
3. Explain the purpose of a physician's office laboratory (POL).
4. List and describe the components of a POL.
5. Identify the purpose of an emergency eyewash station.
6. Describe an outside laboratory.
7. List and describe the information included in a laboratory test directory.

Laboratory Tests

8. Explain the purpose of laboratory testing.
9. List examples specimens collected for laboratory analysis.
10. Identify the eight categories of laboratory tests based on function.
11. Explain the meaning of a reference range.
12. Explain the difference between a specific panel and a general panel.
13. Explain the use of laboratory test results.

Laboratory Forms

14. Identify the purpose of a laboratory request.
15. List and describe the information included on a laboratory request.
16. Explain the difference between a preprinted and a computer-generated laboratory request.
17. Identify the purpose of a laboratory report.
18. List and describe the information included on a laboratory report.
19. Identify methods for transmitting laboratory reports to the medical office.
20. Describe ways in which laboratory test results can be accessed and manipulated by the computer.

Patient Instructions

21. Explain the purpose of patient preparation for a laboratory test.
22. Explain the purpose of fasting for a laboratory test.

Specimen Collection for Transport to an Outside Laboratory

23. Identify the guidelines to follow when collecting a specimen for transport to an outside laboratory.
24. Explain the procedure for proper identification of the patient.
25. Describe two methods for labeling a specimen.
26. Describe the guidelines to follow when handling and storing specimens for transport to an outside laboratory.

PROCEDURES

Operate an emergency eyewash station.
Inspect an emergency eyewash station.
Use a laboratory test directory.

Complete a laboratory request.
Review a laboratory report.

Instruct a patient in the preparation necessary for a laboratory test that requires fasting.

Collect a specimen for transport to an outside laboratory.
Handle and store a specimen for transport to an outside laboratory.

CLIA–Waived Laboratory Tests

27. Describe the following CLIA test categories: waived, moderate complexity, and high complexity.
28. List and describe the information included in a package insert that accompanies a CLIA-waived test kit.
29. List the advantages of a CLIA-waived automated analyzer.
30. Explain the purpose of quality control in the laboratory.
31. Describe the guidelines to follow for CLIA-waived tests.
32. Explain the difference between an internal control and an external control.
33. Explain the difference between a qualitative and a quantitative test result.
34. List the laboratory safety guidelines to follow to prevent accidents in the POL.

Perform quality control procedures on a quality control test system.
Perform a CLIA-waived laboratory test.
Practice laboratory safety.

CHAPTER OUTLINE

Introduction to the Clinical Laboratory
- Physician's Office Laboratory
- Outside Laboratory
- Laboratory Test Directory

Laboratory Tests
- Reference Range
- Panels
- Use of Laboratory Test Results

Laboratory Documents
- Laboratory Request
- Laboratory Report
- Specimen Labels

Patient Instructions
- Patient Preparation
- Medication Restrictions

Specimen Collection for Transport to an Outside Laboratory
- Causes for Rejection of a Specimen
- Guidelines for Specimen Collection and Handling

Clinical Laboratory Improvement Amendments
- Categories of Tests

CLIA-Waived Tests in the POL

CLIA-Waived Test Systems
- CLIA-Waived Test Kits
- CLIA-Waived Automated Analyzers

POL Laboratory Testing
- Quality Control
- Storage of Test Components
- Stability of Test Components
- Calibration Procedure
- Control Procedure
- Collecting the Specimen
- Testing the Specimen
- Interpreting and Reading the Test Results
- Documenting the Test Results

Laboratory Safety
- Specimen Collection and Testing
- Hazardous Chemicals

KEY TERMS

analyte
calibration
CLIA nonwaived test
CLIA waived test
clinical diagnosis
clinical laboratory
control
critical value
fasting
homeostasis (hoe-mee-oh-STAY-sis)
laboratory test
package insert
panel
qualitative test
quality control
quantitative test
reagent
reference ranger
screening test
serum (SERE-um)
specimen (SPES-i-men)
test system
unique identifier

INTRODUCTION TO THE CLINICAL LABORATORY

A **clinical laboratory** is a facility in which laboratory tests are performed on biologic specimens to obtain valuable information regarding the health of a patient. Laboratory test results are used, along with the health history, physical examination, and diagnostic procedures to obtain essential data needed by the provider for the diagnosis, treatment, and management of a patient's condition.

When the body is healthy, its systems function normally and a state of equilibrium of the internal environment is said to exist; this is termed **homeostasis.** When the body is in a state of homeostasis, the physical and chemical characteristics of body substances are within an acceptable range.

When a pathologic condition exists, changes occur which alter the normal functioning of the body, resulting in an imbalance; in other words, the body is no longer in homeostasis. These changes cause the patient to experience the symptoms of a particular pathologic condition. For example, iron deficiency anemia may cause the patient to experience weakness, fatigue, pallor, irritability, and shortness of breath. These changes may also cause an alteration in the characteristics of body substances leading to abnormal laboratory test results. Iron-deficiency anemia may cause an alteration in normal red blood cell morphology and decreased hemoglobin, hematocrit, and ferritin levels.

This chapter serves as an introduction to the clinical laboratory by providing an overview of clinical laboratory methods and techniques. It is important that the medical assistant have knowledge of the laboratory tests that are performed most often, including the purpose and normal range of these tests, any substances that might interfere with accurate test results, and factors that may cause abnormal test results.

PHYSICIAN'S OFFICE LABORATORY

A medical office may house its own laboratory for performing laboratory tests known as a *physician's office laboratory (POL).* There are several advantages to performing laboratory tests in a POL. The test results are available while patients are still at the medical office, which may allow the provider to diagnose or monitor their conditions immediately. The provider is also able to initiate or adjust the course of treatment for patients before they leave the office, rather than delaying treatment until test results are received from the laboratory.

The laboratory tests performed in a POL are usually CLIA-waived tests. CLIA is an abbreviation for the *Clinical Laboratory Improvement Amendments,* which consist of regulations that have been developed by the federal government to improve the quality of laboratory testing in the United States to ensure accurate and reliable test results.

A **CLIA-waived test** is a laboratory test that has been determined to be a simple procedure that is easy to perform and has a low risk of erroneous test results such as urinalysis using a reagent strip (Fig. 15.1). CLIA-waived tests are exempt from most of the CLIA regulations. Medical assistants trained in the proper collection and testing procedures are qualified to perform CLIA-waived tests in the POL.

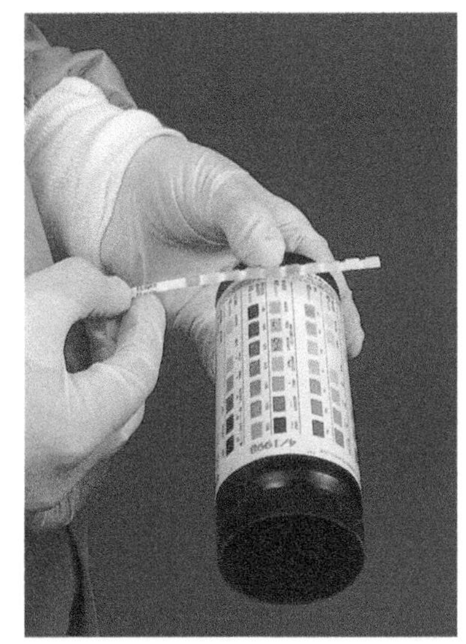

Fig. 15.1 Urinalysis using a reagent strip is a CLIA–waived test.

A **CLIA-nonwaived test** is a laboratory test that does not meet the criteria for waiver and is subject to the CLIA regulations. Nonwaived tests require a complex testing method and are usually performed in an outside laboratory by certified medical laboratory personnel. Additional information on CLIA is presented later in this chapter.

Components of a POL

The components of a POL should meet certain requirements to provide a safe and effective working environment, outlined as follows.

Physical Structure

The POL should be a separate room or work area in the medical office. Laboratory work counters should be large enough to provide ample space for testing specimens. Cabinets should be available for storing equipment and supplies. The medical assistant should check the supply inventory periodically and reorder as needed.

Room Temperature and Lighting

The temperature of the POL should be maintained at room temperature (RT), which is a temperature between 59°F and 86°F (15°C to 30°C). This temperature range is conducive to storing test components requiring RT storage. Temperatures outside of this range may cause deterioration of the test components, such as controls and test reagents.

Temperature requirements are also important when using an automated analyzer. When a specimen is tested using an automated analyzer, a chemical reaction occurs between the specimen and the test reagents to produce the test results. With some analyzers, the chemical reaction can occur only at RT. If the temperature is outside of RT, the analyzer cannot perform the test, resulting in an error message appearing on the screen of the analyzer. The temperature of the POL should be checked daily to ensure that it is at RT.

Adequate lighting is essential for the proper collection, handling, and testing of specimens. Good lighting is also needed for the proper interpretation of test results that use color comparison to determine test results, such as urinalysis using a reagent strip.

Refrigerator

A refrigerator should be available in a POL for the storage of specimens and test components requiring refrigeration. The temperature of the refrigerator must be maintained between 36 °F and 46 °F (2 °C to 8 °C) to retard alterations in the physical and chemical composition of specimens and to prevent deterioration of test components. The temperature of the refrigerator should be checked at least once each day and documented in a refrigerator temperature log. As required by the Occupational Safety and Health Administration (OSHA) Standard, food and beverages must not be stored in the laboratory refrigerator, and a biohazard warning label must be attached to the refrigerator to alert employees to the presence of potentially infectious materials.

Protective Equipment and Supplies

Laboratory testing involves the collection and handling of specimens that may contain pathogens. Protective equipment and supplies necessary to comply with the OSHA Standard should be readily accessible in the POL. This includes handwashing facilities, alcohol-based hand sanitizers, gloves, safety goggles and masks, laboratory coats, and safety-engineered syringes and needles. Biohazard sharps containers and bags must be available for disposal of medical waste such as contaminated needles and syringes and used collection supplies.

Emergency Eyewash Station

An emergency eyewash station should be available in a POL in the event of an accidental exposure incident to the eyes. An *emergency eyewash station* (Fig. 15.2) is a device that is used to flush the eyes with tepid water when substances such as blood or hazardous chemicals enter the eye. *Tepid* water consists of water with a temperature between 60 °F and 100 °F (16 °C to 38 °C). An eyewash station flushes both eyes simultaneously with water at a velocity low enough not to injure the eyes of the user.

The eyewash station is activated by pressing a lever attached to the station; the lever must be clearly identified and operate with a single easy motion. Once activated, the nozzle covers pop off the nozzle heads and each of the nozzles begins discharging water. The eyes should be flushed for a full 15 minutes, which is considered the minimum amount of time needed to clear the eyes of hazardous substances. Following activation, the eyewash station remains

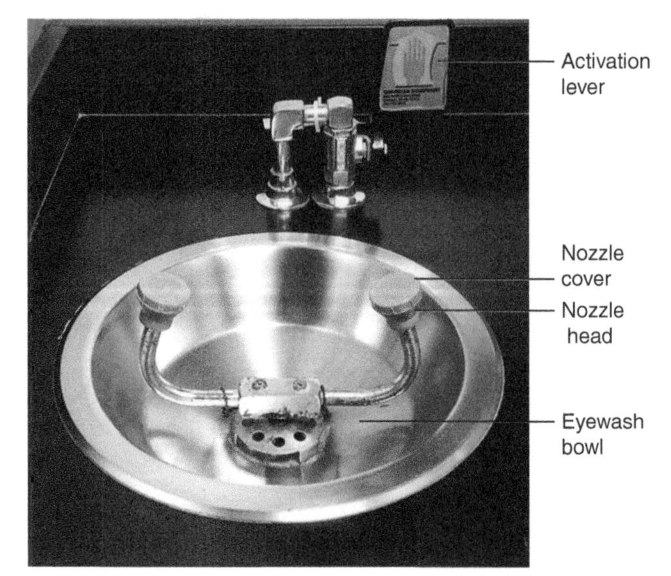

Fig. 15.2 Emergency eyewash station.

operational without requiring the user's hands for 15 minutes (or until it is manually turned off).

The eyewash station should be easily accessible and located within a 10-second walking distance (approximately 55 feet) of potential hazards. The first 10 to 15 seconds after exposure of the eye to a hazardous substance are critical, especially if it is a corrosive chemical. A delay in treatment could result in permanent damage to the eye.

It is important that the medical assistant inspect and activate the eyewash station each week to ensure that it is operating properly and to flush out the water supply lines. A more detailed inspection should be performed on an annual basis by a qualified service technician. The procedure for operating an eyewash station and performing a weekly eyewash inspection is outlined Procedure 15.1.

Maintenance of the POL

The medical assistant is responsible for making sure the POL is clean and free of clutter. Biohazard sharps containers and bags should be replaced as needed and not be allowed to overfill. An approved disinfectant should be readily available for disinfecting laboratory work surfaces each day. The medical assistant should know how to care for each piece of laboratory equipment; this information is included in the operating manual that accompanies the equipment.

OUTSIDE LABORATORY

Outside laboratories use highly sophisticated automated analyzers for performing tests which provide the medical office with fast and reliable test results. Medical offices typically use a combination of a POL and an outside laboratory to fulfill their laboratory testing requirements.

Outside laboratories include hospital and privately owned independent laboratories. Independent laboratories range from large, national corporations (e.g., *LabCorp* and *Quest Diagnostics*) to small, local independent laboratories.

Because the medical assistant works closely with an outside laboratory, knowledge of the relationship between the medical office and an outside laboratory is important.

A specimen can be collected at the medical office and transported to an outside laboratory for testing, or it can be collected (and tested) at the outside laboratory. If the specimen is collected at the medical office, the laboratory usually provides the medical office with the supplies necessary to collect and handle the specimen. The medical assistant is responsible for checking these supplies periodically and reordering them as needed.

LABORATORY TEST DIRECTORY

Most outside laboratories publish a *laboratory test directory* which serves as a valuable reference source for the medical office. It is usually in the form of an online directory to provide for quick and easy access of laboratory information. The directory includes a *test menu* which consists of an alphabetic listing of all the tests performed by the outside laboratory. Information is provided for each test in the test menu and includes patient preparation requirements, specimen collection and processing requirements, and proper preparation and storage of the specimen for transport to the outside laboratory (Fig. 15.3). If the medical assistant has a question regarding any aspect of the procedure, the laboratory should be contacted before proceeding.

The following information is typically included in the laboratory test directory for each test performed by the laboratory:

- Name and CPT code of the test.
- Synonyms for the test name.
- Type and amount of specimen required.
- Collection container(s) required.
- Patient preparation.
- Collection and processing requirements.
- Specimen storage and transport requirements.
- Specimen stability.
- Causes for rejection of the specimen by the laboratory.
- Reference range of the test.
- Uses and limitations of the test.
- Form requirements.
- Methodology used to perform the test.

LABORATORY TESTS

A **laboratory test** is defined as the clinical analysis and study of a body substance to obtain objective data for the diagnosis, treatment, and management of a patient's condition. Laboratory tests are performed on specimens collected from the body. A **specimen** is a small sample taken from the body to represent the nature of the whole. Most laboratory tests are performed on specimens that are easily obtained from the body, such as blood and urine. Other examples of specimens collected for laboratory analysis and study include stool, sputum, cervical and vaginal scrapings of cells, and secretions and discharges from various parts of the body. The medical assistant is usually responsible for the collection of most patient specimens. Certain specimens must be collected by the provider, such as a specimen for a Pap test, a sample of vaginal or urethral discharge, and a tissue specimen for biopsy. In these cases, the medical assistant assists with the collection.

Laboratory tests can be classified by function into categories. Use of these categories makes it easier to refer to laboratory tests. Table 15.1 lists and describes each of these categories and provides examples of commonly performed tests in each category.

The number of laboratory tests ordered for a patient depends on the provider's clinical diagnosis. A **clinical diagnosis** is defined as a tentative diagnosis of a patient's condition obtained through the evaluation of the health history and the physical examination, without the benefit of laboratory tests or diagnostic procedures. A clinical diagnosis of strep throat usually requires only a strep test for confirmation. However, most diseases cause more than one alteration in the physical and chemical characteristics of body substances, and a series of laboratory tests is necessary to arrive at a diagnosis.

There are some pathologic conditions that do not require the use of laboratory test results to determine a diagnosis. In some cases, the information obtained from the patient's clinical signs and symptoms is sufficient enough for the diagnosis of a condition. In these instances, the provider is so certain of the diagnosis that treatment can be instituted without laboratory confirmation. For example, most providers diagnose otitis media (middle ear infection) with the information obtained from patient symptoms (earache, fever, and feeling of fullness in the ear) and from an otoscopic examination of the tympanic membrane (the tympanic membrane is red and bulging). Information obtained through these clinical signs and symptoms is sufficiently specific to otitis media to allow the provider to make a diagnosis and to prescribe treatment.

REFERENCE RANGE

A **reference range** is defined as a certain established and acceptable range within which the laboratory test results of a healthy individual are expected to fall. A range, rather than a single value, is necessary because of individual differences within a general population caused by factors such as age, gender, race, and geographic location. The reference range for each test varies slightly from one laboratory to another, depending on the test method, equipment, and reagents used to perform the test. It is essential that test results be compared with the reference ranges supplied by the laboratory performing the test rather than with a laboratory reference source.

A test result falling outside of the reference range for a particular test may be seen with more than one pathologic condition. A decrease in the hemoglobin level may occur with iron-deficiency anemia, leukemia, cirrhosis, chronic kidney failure, and certain autoimmune diseases. In this

LABORATORY TEST DIRECTORY
Triglycerides

CPT Code:	84478
Synonyms:	Trig, Tg
Type of Specimen:	Serum
Amount of Specimen:	2 mL
Collection Container:	SST (send entire tube)
Patient Preparation:	Fasting for 9–12 h prior to collection. No alcohol consumption for 24 h prior to collection.
Collection and Processing:	1. Collect and label specimen. 2. Gently invert tube 5 times immediately after collection. 3. Place specimen in a vertical position and allow to clot for a minimum of 30 min and a maximum of 2 h. 4. Centrifuge specimen for 10 min.
Storage and Transport:	Store at RT or refrigerate until pickup by lab courier.
Specimen Stability:	RT (15°C–30°C): 5 days Refrigerated (2°C–8°C): 7 days
Causes for Rejection:	Nonfasting specimen Specimen other than serum Improper labeling of specimen Improper storage temperature
Reference Range:	Desirable: Less than 150 mg/dL Borderline high: 150–199 mg/dL High: 200–499 mg/dL Very high: 500 mg/dL or greater

Uses:

Measurement of triglycerides levels assist with the diagnosis and treatment of diabetes mellitus, nephrosis, liver obstruction, and other diseases involving lipid metabolism. In conjunction with HDL cholesterol and total cholesterol, a triglycerides determination assists in the assessment of the risk for developing coronary artery disease. Elevated levels may occur with liver disease, nephritic syndrome, hypothyroidism, increased alcohol consumption, poorly controlled diabetes, and pancreatitis.

Limitations: Pregnancy and women on estrogens may cause an increase in triglycerides level.

Forms: Order electronically or print the lab request form and submit with specimen.

Methodology: Quantitative enzymatic

Fig. 15.3 Laboratory Test Directory indicating triglycerides specimen requirements.

Table 15.1 Categories of Laboratory Tests[a]

Category	Definition and Commonly Performed Tests	Category	Definition and Commonly Performed Tests
Hematology	Hematology is the science of the study of blood and blood-forming tissues. Laboratory analysis in hematology involves the examination of blood for detection of abnormalities including blood cell counts, cellular morphology, clotting ability of blood, and identification of cell types. Tests include: White blood cell (WBC) count Red blood cell (RBC) count Differential WBC count (Diff) Hemoglobin (Hgb) Hematocrit (Hct) Platelet count Reticulocyte count Prothrombin time (PT) Sedimentation rate	**Immunology and Blood Banking**	Laboratory analysis in immunology and blood banking involves studying antigen-antibody reactions to assess the presence of a substance or to determine the presence of disease. Tests include: *Immunology* Allergy blood tests Antinuclear antibody (ANA) Antistreptolysin O (ASO) C-Reactive protein (CRP) COVID-19 test *H. pylori* test Hepatitis tests HIV tests Mononucleosis test Pregnancy test PSA test Rheumatoid factor (RF) Syphilis test (VDRL, RPR) TB blood test Thyroid function tests *Blood Banking* ABO blood typing Rh typing Rh antibody test
Clinical Chemistry	Laboratory analysis in clinical chemistry determines the amount of chemical substances present in blood, body fluids, excreta, and tissues. The largest area in clinical chemistry is blood chemistry. Tests include: Albumin ALP ALT AST Bilirubin Blood alcohol Blood lead BUN Calcium Carbon dioxide Chloride Cholesterol Cortisol Creatine kinase (CK) Creatinine Glucose Inorganic phosphorus LD Potassium Protein (total) Sodium T_3 and T_4 Triglycerides Uric acid	**Urinalysis**	The physical, chemical, and microscopic analyses of urine to detect deviations from normal. A. Tests included in physical analysis of urine: Color Appearance Specific gravity B. Tests included in chemical analysis of urine: Glucose Bilirubin Blood Ketones Leukocytes Nitrite pH Protein Urobilinogen C. A microscopic analysis of urine looks for the following structures: RBCs WBCs Bacteria Yeast Epithelial cells Casts Crystals

Continued

Table 15.1 Categories of Laboratory Tests[a]—cont'd

Category	Definition and Commonly Performed Tests	Category	Definition and Commonly Performed Tests
Microbiology	Microbiology is the scientific study of microorganisms and their activities. Laboratory analysis in microbiology involves identification of pathogens present in body specimens (e.g., urine, blood, throat, sputum, wound, urethra, vagina, cerebrospinal fluid). Tests include: Throat culture Urine culture Genital cultures Blood culture Stool culture Wound culture Sputum cultures Nasopharyngeal culture Eye and ear culture	**Cytology**	Laboratory analysis in cytology deals with detection of the presence of abnormal cells: Chromosome studies Pap test
Parasitology	Laboratory analysis in parasitology involves detection of disease-producing human parasites or eggs present in body specimens (e.g., stool, vagina, blood). Human diseases caused by parasites include the following: Amebiasis Ascariasis Hookworms Malaria Pinworms Scabies Tapeworms Toxoplasmosis Trichinosis Trichomoniasis	**Histology**	Histology is the microscopic study of the form and structure of various tissues making up living organisms. Laboratory analysis in histology involves the detection of diseased tissues. Tests include: Biopsy studies Tissue analyses

[a]Categories of laboratory tests are listed, including definitions of each and commonly performed tests or pathologic conditions in each category. Tests commonly known by their abbreviations are listed this way.

regard, the provider cannot rely solely on a low hemoglobin level to make a diagnosis but must acquire data from additional sources such as the health history, physical examination, diagnostic imaging, and further laboratory testing.

PANELS

A **panel** (also known as a *profile*) consists of a combination of laboratory tests that have been determined to be the most sensitive and specific means of identifying a disease state or evaluating a particular organ or organ system. The panels performed by an outside laboratory and the tests included in each are listed in the laboratory test directory.

A panel may be *specific* in nature (i.e., all tests included in the panel relate to a specific organ of the body or a particular disease state). A specific panel is usually ordered when the provider does not have a definite clinical diagnosis but has a good idea of the patient's condition or what organ or organs are involved in the patient's condition. The provider orders a panel of the condition or organ in question. An example of a panel used to identify a disease state is the rheumatoid panel, which assists in the diagnosis of rheumatoid arthritis. An example of a panel used to evaluate an organ is the *hepatic function panel*, which is used to assess liver function and assist in the diagnosis of pathologic conditions that affect the liver.

A panel may be *general* in nature. A general metabolic panel contains a number of routine laboratory tests. It is used primarily for a routine health evaluation of a patient to screen for any changes in the body that may be present, even though there are no symptoms to indicate these changes have occurred. A general metabolic panel is also used when the patient's symptoms are so vague that the provider does not have enough concrete evidence to support a clinical diagnosis. An example of a general panel is a *comprehensive metabolic panel*; refer to Table 15.2 for a list of the tests included in this panel. The medical assistant should know the names of common panels and the tests included in each, which are listed in Table 15.2.

USE OF LABORATORY TEST RESULTS

The most frequent use of laboratory test results is to assist in the diagnosis of a patient's condition. Laboratory test results

Table 15.2 Laboratory Panels

Panel	Tests Included	Use
Comprehensive Metabolic Panel	Albumin ALP ALT AST Bilirubin (total) BUN Calcium Carbon dioxide Chloride Creatinine Glucose Potassium Total protein Sodium	• General health screen that provides information on kidneys, liver, acid-base balance, blood glucose level, and blood proteins. • Evaluation of organ function and to check for conditions such as diabetes, liver disease, and kidney disease. • Routinely ordered as part of blood work-up for physical or medical examination (particularly when patient's symptoms are vague). • Abnormal test results are usually followed up with more specific tests before a diagnosis is made.
Electrolyte Panel	Carbon dioxide Chloride Potassium Sodium	• Screens for electrolyte or acid-base imbalance. • Monitors effect of treatment on disease or condition that causes electrolyte imbalance. • Evaluation of patients taking medication that can cause electrolyte imbalance.
Hepatic Panel	Albumin ALP ALT AST Bilirubin (direct) Bilirubin (total) Total protein	• Detection of pathologic conditions affecting the liver. • Monitor liver function of an individual with liver disease or a condition known to affect the liver. • Monitor the effectiveness of treatment of the liver. • May be ordered when an individual has been exposed to hepatitis, has a family history of liver disease, has excessive alcohol consumption, or is taking medication that can result in liver damage.
Hepatitis Panel	Hepatitis A antibody, IgM Hepatitis B core antibody, total Hepatitis B surface antigen Hepatitis C antibody	• Detection of viral hepatitis.
Lipid Panel	Total cholesterol LDL cholesterol HDL cholesterol Triglycerides VLDL cholesterol (calculation) Total cholesterol/HDL ratio (calculation)	• Determination of the risk of coronary artery disease.
Prenatal Panel	ABO grouping and Rh typing CBC w/diff and w/plt Hepatitis B surface antigen RBC antibody screen Rubella antibody Syphilis serology (RPR)	• Establish health status of prenatal patients early in the pregnancy. • Screening of prenatal patients for disease or potential problems.
Renal Function Panel	Albumin BUN Calcium Carbon dioxide Chloride Creatinine Glucose Phosphorus Potassium Sodium	• Detection of kidney problems. • Provides information on how well the kidneys are functioning to remove excess fluid and waste. • When a problem is detected, diagnostic imaging tests may be used for further evaluation and diagnosis.

Continued

Table 15.2 Laboratory Panels—cont'd

Panel	Tests Included	Use
Rheumatoid Arthritis Panel	Rheumatoid factor (RF) Cyclic citrullinated peptide (CCP) Antinuclear antibody (ANA) C-reactive protein (CRP) Erythrocyte sedimentation rate (ESR)	• Assists in diagnosis of rheumatoid arthritis and helps distinguish it from other forms of arthritis and conditions with similar symptoms. • Evaluation of the severity of rheumatoid arthritis. • Monitors rheumatoid arthritis and its complications, and assesses response to treatment.
Thyroid Panel	Thyroxine (T_4) Triiodothyronine (T_3) Uptake Thyroid-stimulating hormone (TSH) Free thyroxine intake (FTI)	• Evaluate thyroid function. • Detection of disorders affecting the thyroid gland.

ALP, Alkaline phosphatase; *ALT,* alanine aminotransferase; *AST,* aspartate aminotransferase; *BUN,* blood urea nitrogen; *CBC,* complete blood count; *CRP,* C-reactive protein; *FTI,* free thyroxine index; *HDL,* high-density lipoprotein; IgM, immunoglobulin M; *LDL,* low-density lipoprotein; *VLDL,* very-low-density lipoprotein; *w/diff,* with differential; *w/plt,* with platelet count.

also have other significant medical uses. A summary of the use of laboratory test results follows.

1. ***To assist in the diagnosis of pathologic conditions.*** Laboratory test results are most frequently used to assist in the diagnosis of pathologic conditions. Along with the health history and the physical examination, test results provide essential data needed by the provider to arrive at a diagnosis and prescribe treatment. After obtaining the health history and performing the physical examination, the provider may order laboratory tests for these reasons:
   - ***To confirm a clinical diagnosis.*** The patient's signs and symptoms may provide a strong clinical diagnosis of a particular condition, and the provider may use laboratory test results to confirm that diagnosis. For example, the patient may have the typical signs and symptoms of diabetes mellitus, which would give the provider a fairly certain clinical diagnosis. In this instance, a hemoglobin A_{1c} test or an oral glucose tolerance test (OGTT) may be ordered to confirm the diagnosis and to institute therapy.
   - ***To assist in the differential diagnosis of a patient's condition.*** Two or more diseases may have similar signs and symptoms, and the provider must use laboratory test results to assist in the differential diagnosis of the patient's condition. A diagnosis of strep throat must be made with a laboratory test to differentiate it from other pathologic conditions with similar signs and symptoms, such as pharyngitis and mononucleosis.
   - ***To obtain information regarding a patient's condition*** when not enough concrete evidence exists to support a clinical diagnosis. The patient sometimes may have vague signs and symptoms, and laboratory tests are ordered to obtain information on what may be causing the patient's problems. For example, the patient may have nonspecific abdominal pain, and the physical examination may not yield enough information to support a clinical diagnosis. In this case, the provider may order a laboratory panel to assist in pinpointing the cause of the patient's problems.
2. ***To evaluate the patient's progress and to regulate treatment.*** When a diagnosis has been made, laboratory testing may be performed to monitor the patient's progress and to regulate treatment. On the basis of the laboratory test results, the therapy may need to be adjusted or further treatment prescribed. A patient undergoing iron therapy for iron deficiency anemia should have a complete blood count (CBC) performed every month to assess the response to treatment and to ensure that the condition is improving. A patient with diabetes who measures his or her blood glucose level each day to regulate insulin dosage is an example of using laboratory test results to regulate treatment.
3. ***To establish a baseline level.*** On the basis of such factors as age, gender, race, and geographic location, individuals have different normal levels within the established reference range for a particular test. In this respect, laboratory test results can establish each patient's baseline level with which future results can be compared. A patient who is going to receive warfarin (Coumadin) therapy should have a blood specimen drawn for a prothrombin time test before administration of this anticoagulant. The results serve as a baseline recording for that particular patient against which future prothrombin time test results can be compared.
4. ***To prevent or reduce the severity of disease.*** Laboratory test results can help to prevent or reduce the severity of disease through the early detection of abnormal findings. Certain conditions, such as anemia and diabetes, are relatively common disorders and sometimes may exist without symptoms, especially early in the development of the disease. Laboratory tests known as **screening tests** are performed on a routine basis on apparently healthy individuals to assist in the early detection of disease. Screening tests are relatively easy to perform and present a minimal hazard to the patient; the most commonly performed laboratory screening tests include urinalysis, CBC, and a comprehensive metabolic panel.
5. ***To comply with state laws.*** Another reason for a laboratory test is its requirement by state law. The statutes of

most states require a syphilis test be performed on pregnant women. The purpose of this test is to protect the mother and fetus from harm in the event of a positive test result.

LABORATORY DOCUMENTS

The most common laboratory documents include laboratory requests, laboratory reports, and specimen labels, which are described as follows.

LABORATORY REQUEST

A laboratory request serves as a means of communication between the medical office and the outside laboratory to designate the test(s) ordered by the provider. The request provides the outside laboratory with essential information necessary for accurate testing, reporting of results, and billing. It is required when the specimen is collected at the medical office and transported to an outside laboratory for testing or when the specimen is collected and tested at an outside laboratory.

Once completed, the laboratory request must be transmitted to the outside laboratory. The medical assistant should realize the significance of this simple but important step. Without the request the laboratory does not have the information it needs to carry out the provider's orders, causing delays in completing the tests and reporting results. The most common methods used to transmit laboratory requests to an outside laboratory include:

- Electronic transmission
- Faxed
- Hand-delivered (along with the specimen) by a laboratory courier
- Hand-delivered by a patient having a specimen collected and tested at an outside laboratory.

Parts of a Laboratory Request

Specific information that is required on the laboratory request includes:

1. **Name and address of the laboratory.** The name and address of the laboratory performing the test must appear on the laboratory request.
2. **Medical office name, address, and account number.** This information must appear on the laboratory request to facilitate the reporting of test results to the provider.
3. **Name, identification number, and signature of the ordering provider.** This information must be included on the request in order for the tests to be performed.
4. **Patient's name, address, telephone number, identification (ID) number, and social security number.** The patient's full legal name must be entered on the request in the following format: last name, first name, and middle initial. The patient's name and address are needed for billing purposes and must include the city, state, and zip code.
5. **Patient's date of birth and gender.** The reference ranges for some tests vary depending on the patient's age and gender. The reference range for hemoglobin concentration varies according to gender (12 to 16 g/dL for a female; 14 to 18 g/dL for a male).
6. **Date and time of collection of the specimen.** The date and time of specimen collection must be documented on the request. The date of collection indicates to the laboratory the number of days that have passed since the collection, providing the laboratory with information regarding the freshness of the specimen. A time lapse that is too long between collection and testing of a specimen may affect the accuracy of some test results. The time of collection is significant with respect to certain laboratory tests. The reference range for serum cortisol varies depending on whether the specimen is collected in the morning or in the afternoon.
7. **Fasting or nonfasting.** The laboratory request must specify if the patient was in a fasting or nonfasting state when the specimen was collected. The composition of the blood is altered by the consumption of food and fluid, which can affect the results of certain laboratory tests.
8. **Name of Responsible Party.** The responsible party is the individual assuming the financial responsibility for payment of the tests.
9. **Third-party billing information.** Third-party billing information must be indicated on the request to provide the necessary information to bill the patient's insurance company for the tests performed.
10. **Laboratory tests ordered.** The test(s) ordered by the provider must be indicated on the request. The laboratory test directory contains a complete listing of all the laboratory tests and panels performed by the laboratory.
11. **Source of the microbiologic specimen.** Microbiologic tests require that the source of the specimen (e.g., throat swab, wound swab, and vaginal swab) be documented on the laboratory request. This is done for identification of the origin of the specimen for the laboratory because this information is not available by looking at the specimen. In many instances, the source dictates the test method used by the laboratory to evaluate the specimen for the presence of pathogens.
12. **Clinical diagnosis in ICD format.** ICD (International Classification of Disease) diagnosis codes must be used to indicate the patient's clinical diagnosis. This assists the laboratory in correlating clinical laboratory data with the needs of the provider. In some instances, further testing is performed by the laboratory if one test method proves inconclusive to confirm or reject the clinical diagnosis. Another function of the clinical diagnosis is to assure laboratory personnel that the

test results are within the framework of the diagnosis. When the results of a test disagree with the clinical diagnosis, the laboratory may repeat the test on the same or another specimen. The clinical diagnosis also alerts laboratory personnel to the possibility of the presence of a dangerous pathogen, such as the hepatitis virus. In addition, ICD codes are necessary for third-party billing by the laboratory. If the laboratory bills the patient's insurance company for the tests, the ICD codes for the clinical diagnosis must be indicated on the insurance form.

13. **Medications.** Certain medications may interfere with the accuracy and validity of test results and are specified in the laboratory test directory. The medical assistant should document any medications being taken by the patient that could affect the accuracy of the test results. For example, antibiotics being taken by a patient may cause a false-negative test result on a strep test.
14. **STAT.** The provider may want the laboratory test results reported as soon as possible. In this case "STAT" must be indicated on the laboratory request. Requests that are marked STAT are performed as soon as possible after receipt by the laboratory, and the results are telephoned or faxed to the provider as soon as they are available. STAT testing is available for only a limited number of tests in the test menu and requires additional fees for the expedited service.

Types of Laboratory Requests

There are two types of laboratory requests—the preprinted request and the electronic request—which are described in more detail as follows.

Preprinted Laboratory Request

A preprinted laboratory request is completed by writing in the required information on a preprinted form (Fig. 15.4). The request form includes spaces for indicating patient demographic and insurance information and includes a list of the most frequently ordered laboratory tests. The tests ordered by the provider are indicated by marking a box adjacent to those tests (and their corresponding CPT codes). A space designated as "other tests" is provided on the request form for specifying the name and CPT code of a test that is desired but not listed on the preprinted request form.

Electronic Laboratory Request

An electronic laboratory request (e-request) is completed by entering the required information into a computer using drop-down lists, radio buttons, check-boxes, and fill-in boxes (Fig. 15.5). The patient's demographic and insurance information is automatically entered by the computer, which eliminates errors in reentering this information. Once the request is completed, barcode specimen labels are automatically generated and printed out by the computer.

An electronic laboratory request can be transmitted electronically to the outside laboratory. For this to occur, the medical office computer system must be interfaced with the computer system in the outside laboratory. An electronic request can also be printed out by the computer and placed with the specimen for pickup by a laboratory courier.

What Would You Do? What Would You *Not* Do?

Case Study 1

Hans Volkman, age 28, is getting ready to leave the medical office after being seen by the physician. The physician gave him a laboratory request for a CBC and a lipid panel to take to the hospital laboratory. Hans notices that the clinical diagnosis on the form indicates iron deficiency anemia and wants to know why the physician did not prescribe any medication for him if he thought he had anemia. Hans says that he told the physician he has never had a cholesterol test and asked the physician if he would order one for him. Hans says the physician must have forgotten because the test was not included on the request. Hans has been instructed to fast for the laboratory tests. He says that he stops every morning at the Coffee Cup restaurant and has coffee with cream and sugar, orange juice, and doughnuts. He would like to know whether he could just have the coffee with cream and sugar before the tests. Hans says he has a hard time functioning in the morning without coffee. ■

LABORATORY REPORT

The purpose of a laboratory report is to relay laboratory test results to the provider. The report is usually generated by a computer. It may consist of a preprinted form with the test results printed in the appropriate spaces on the form by a computer (as illustrated in Fig. 15.6), or the entire report may be electronically generated by the computer as illustrated in Fig. 15.7.

Most laboratory computer systems automatically flag abnormal results on the laboratory report, as shown in Fig. 15.7. For example, an "H" next to a test result means the result is higher than the reference range and an "L" means it is lower than the reference range.

STAT test results and tests results with critical values are telephoned to the medical office as soon as possible, with the entire report transmitted immediately thereafter. A **critical value** is a test result that is dangerously abnormal and must be reported immediately to the ordering provider. Critical values are considered life-threatening and require immediate attention.

Laboratory reports can be transmitted to the medical office by one or more of the following methods: electronic transmission, fax, mail, or hand delivery by a laboratory courier. Once received, the provider reviews each laboratory report and the data obtained are correlated with information obtained from the health history and physical examination. The provider indicates that he or she is finished with the report by signing the report.

The medical assistant may be responsible for reviewing laboratory reports as they are received. The medical assistant

LABORATORY REQUEST

Biomedical Laboratories, Inc.
100 Main Street
Athens, Georgia 45760

Patient's Name (Last) (First) (MI) | Sex | Date of Birth MO DAY YEAR | Collection Time : AM PM | Fasting YES NO | Collection Date MO DAY YEAR

NPI/UPIN | Physician's ID # | Patient's SS # | Patient's ID # | Urine hrs/vol hrs_____ vol_____

Physician's Name (Last, First) | Physician's Signature

Medicare # (Include prefix/suffix) ☐ Primary ☐ Secondary

Medicaid # | State | Physician's Provider #

Diagnosis/Signs/Symptoms in ICD-10 Format (Highest Specificity)

REQUIRED

PATIENT: Patient's Address | Phone

City | State | ZIP

RESP. PARTY: Name of Responsible Party (if different from patient)

Address of Responsible Party (if different from patient) | APT #

City | State | ZIP

Patient's Relationship to Responsible Party ☐ 1–Self ☐ 2–Spouse ☐ 3–Child ☐ 4–Other

Performance Lab ☐ | Carrier | Group # | Employee # | Mem

INSURANCE:

Insurance Company Name | Plan | Carrier Code

Subscriber/Member # | Location | Group #

Insurance Address | Physician's Provider #

City | State | ZIP

Employer's Name or Number | Insured SS # (If not patient) | Worker's Comp ☐ Yes ☐ No

I hereby authorize the release of medical information related to the service subscribed herein and authorize payment directed to LabCorp.

X ______________________ Patient's Signature ______________ Date

MEDICARE ADVANCE BENEFICIARY NOTICE

I have read the ABN on the reverse. If Medicare denies payment, I agree to pay for the identified test(s).

X ______________________ Patient's Signature ______________ Date

NOTE: WHEN ORDERING TESTS FOR WHICH MEDICARE OR MEDICAID REIMBURSEMENT WILL BE SOUGHT, PHYSICIANS SHOULD ONLY ORDER TESTS THAT ARE MEDICALLY NECESSARY FOR THE DIAGNOSIS OR TREATMENT OF THE PATIENT. COMPONENTS OF THE ORGAN OR DISEASE PANELS/COMBINATIONS PRINTED BELOW ARE SHOWN ON THE REVERSE SIDE AND MAY ALSO BE ORDERED INDIVIDUALLY BELOW. COMPONENTS MAY BE BILLED SEPARATELY PER CARRIER POLICY.

PANELS (See reverse for components)

Code	Test	Container
80049	Basic Metabolic Panel	SST
80054	Comp Metabolic Panel	SST
80051	Electrolyte Panel	SST
80058	Hepatic Panel	SST
80059	Hepatitis Panel	SST
80061	Lipid Panel	SST
80091	Thyroid Panel	SST
80055	Prenatal Panel	RED LAV
80072	Rheumatoid Panel	SST

HEMATOLOGY

Code	Test	Container
85025	CBC w Diff	LAV
85027	CBC w/o Diff	LAV
85014	Hematocrit	LAV
85018	Hemoglobin	LAV
85595	Platelet Count	LAV
85041	RBC Count	LAV
85048	WBC Count	LAV
85007	WBC Differential	LAV
89190	Nasal Smear, Eosin	Nasal Smear
85060	Pathologist Consult–Peripheral Smear	LAV

ALPHABETICAL/COMBINATION TESTS

Code	Test	Container
86900 86901	ABO and Rh	LAV
82040	Albumin	SST
84075	Alkaline Phosphatase	SST
84460	ALT (SGPT)	SST
82150	Amylase, Serum	SST
86038	Antinuclear Antibodies	SST
84450	AST (SGOT)	SST
82607 82746	B_{12} and Folate	SST
82250	Bilirubin, Total	SST

ALPHABETICAL TESTS CON'T

Code	Test	Container
84520	BUN	SST
82310	Calcium	SST
80156	Carbamazepine (Tegretol®)	SER
82378	CEA	SST
82465	Cholesterol, Total	SST
82565	Creatinine	SST
80162	Digoxin	SER
82670	Estradiol	SST
82728	Ferritin, Serum	SST
82985	Fructosamine	SST
83001	FSH	SST
83001 83002	FSH and LH	SST
82977	GGT	SST
82947	Glucose, Plasma	GRY
82947	Glucose, Serum	SST
82950	Glucose, 2-hr. PP	SST
83036	Glycohemoglobin, Total	LAV
84703	hCG, Beta Subunit, Qual	SST
84702	hCG, Beta Subunit, Quant	SST
83718	HDL Cholesterol	SST
86677	*Helicobacter pylori*, IgG	SST
86706	Hep B Surface Antibody	SST
87340	Hep B Surface Antigen	SST
86803	Hep C Antibody	SST
83036	Hemoglobin A_{1C}	LAV
86701	HIV Antibodies	SST
83540	Iron, Total	SST
83540 83550	Iron and IBC	SST
83615	LDH	SST

ALPHABETICAL TESTS CON'T

Code	Test	Container
83002	LH	SST
83690	Lipase	SER
80178	Lithium (Eskalith®)	SER
83735	Magnesium, Serum	SST
80184	Phenobarbital (Luminal®)	SER
80185	Phenytoin (Dilantin®)	SER
84132	Potassium	SST
84146	Prolactin, Serum	SST
84153	Prostate-Specific Antigen	SST
84066	Prostatic Acid Phos	SST
84155	Protein, Total	SST
85610	Prothrombin Time (PT)	BLU
85610 85730	PT and PTT Activated	BLU
85730	PTT Activated	BLU
86431	Rheumatoid Arthritis Factor	SST
86592	RPR	SST
86762	Rubella Antibodies, IgG	SST
85651	Sed Rate	LAV
84295	Sodium	SST
84403	Testosterone	SST
80198	Theophylline	SER
84436	Thyroxine (T_4)	SST
84478	Triglycerides	SST
84480	Triiodothyronine (T_3)	SST
84443	TSH, High Sensitivity	SST
84550	Uric Acid	SST
81003	Urinalysis Microscopic on Positives	URN
81001	Urinalysis with Microscopic	URN
80164	Valproic Acid (Depakene®)	SER

MICROBIOLOGY See Reverse Side

■ENDOCERVICAL ■THROAT ■URINE ■STOOL ■URETHRAL INDICATE SOURCE

Code	Test	Container
87070	Aerobic Bacterial Culture	Bact Trnspt
87490 87590	*Chlamydia/GC* DNA Probe w/ Confirmation on Positives	Probe Trnspt
87490 87590	*Chlamydia/GC* DNA Probe Without Confirmation	Probe Trnspt
87490	*Chlamydia* DNA Probe	Probe Trnspt
87081	Genital, *Beta-Hemolytic Strep Cult, Group B*	Bact Trnspt
87070	Genital Culture, Routine	Bact Trnspt
87070	Lower Respiratory Culture	Steril Trnspt
87590	*N. gonorrhoeae* DNA Probe	Probe Trnspt
87015 87211	Ova and Parasites	O & P Kit
87081 X2 87045	Stool Culture	Fecal Trnspt
87081	Throat, *Beta-Hemolytic Strep Cult, Group A*	Bact Trnspt
87060	Upper Respiratory Culture, Routine	Bact Trnspt
87086	Urine Culture, Routine	Urn Cul Trnspt

Clinical Information/Medications

OTHER TESTS/INDIVIDUAL COMPONENTS

TEST # | TEST NAMES

LAB USE ONLY

STAT	VENIPUNCTURE	TRAVEL	NON LABCORP	VERBAL ORDER	CHART ORDER	HANDWRITTEN	24 HR TUV	PST/PSC #
☐998074	☐998085	☐998096	☐998239	☐998250	☐998261	☐998272	☐998283	

CONTAINERS RECEIVED: SST SPUN | USST UNSPUN | SER SERUM TRNSPT | FRZ FRZ TRNS | RED RED | LAV LAVENDER | SLD SLIDE | BLU LT. BLUE | GRY GREY | GRN GREEN | RYB RYL BLU | YEL ACD | PLS PLASMA | URN URINE | 24U 24 HR URINE | TA-U TART. ACID | FL FLUID | OT OTHER | BACT TRNSP | O & P KIT | PROBE TRNSP | URN CULT TRNSP | STERIL TRNSP | FECAL TRNSP | VIRAL TRNSP

300-0384

Fig. 15.4 Preprinted laboratory request form.

Assignment Name: Document Lab Results, Preventative Services, and Order for Walter Biller

Back to Assignment | View Assignment Description

Front Office | Clinical Care | Coding & Billing | TruCode

Form Repository

Calendar | Correspondence | Patient Demographics | Find Patient | Form Repository

INFO PANEL

Patient Forms

Advance Directive
Certificate to Return to Work or School
Disclosure Authorization
Doctor's First Report
General Procedure Consent
Insurance Claim Tracer
Medical Records Release
Neurological Status Exam
Notice of Privacy Practice
Patient Bill of Rights
Patient Information
Patient Records Access Request
Patient Statement
Prior Authorization Request
Referral
Requisition
School Physical
Vaccine Authorization

Office Forms

Requisition

Please perform a patient search to find a specific patient

Requisition Type: Laboratory

C-Reactive Protein	Ferritin	HIV 1 & 2 Single Assay
Carbamazepine/Tegretol/	Folate	Iron
CBC	FSH	Iron Binding (TIBC)
CBC with Differential	Gamma GT	LD (LDH)
CEA	✔ Hgb A 1C (Glycohemo)	Lead
LH Luteinizing Hormone	Prolactin	T3 Uptake
Lithium	PSA	T4 Free
Magnesium	PSA Complexed	T4 Total
Mono	PSA Screen	Testosterone Total
Phenobarbital	PT with INR	Theophylline
Phenytoin/Dilantin	PTT	TSH
Platelet Count	Reticulocyte	WBC
Pregnancy, Qual.	RPR	Urinalysis w/Micro, auto
Beta HCG Quant	T3 Free	Urinalysis w/o Micro, auto

Arthritis Panel
- Fluor Ab Scr
- ESR (Sed Rate)
- RA (Rheumatoid Factor)
- Uric Acid

Other
- Test Name

History of Kidney Problems: Yes No | Contrast Allergy: Yes No

Exam is: Routine Stat Call Report | Is the patient on anticoagulants? Yes No

Patient Preparation (if any): Due in one month, fasting

Patient Search | Print | Save to Patient Record | Cancel

Fig. 15.5 Electronic laboratory request computer entry screen. (Modified from *SimChart for the medical office: learning the medical office workflow.* St. Louis: Elsevier; 2021.)

should compare the patient's test results with the reference ranges supplied by the laboratory and notify the provider of any abnormal test results.

Parts of a Laboratory Report

A laboratory report includes the following information:

1. Name and address of the laboratory.
2. Name and address of the medical office.
3. Name of the provider ordering the test(s).
4. Patient's name, address, phone number, and ID number.
5. Patient's date of birth and gender.
6. Laboratory accession number.
7. Date and time of specimen collection.
8. Fasting or nonfasting specimen.
9. Date and time the specimen was received by the laboratory.
10. Date and time the results were reported by the laboratory.
11. Name of the laboratory test(s).
12. Test results.
13. Reference range for each test performed.
14. Identification of test results outside of the reference range.

Electronic Transmission of Laboratory Reports

Computer-generated laboratory reports are often transmitted electronically from the laboratory computer system to the medical office computer system. The laboratory report is placed in the provider's "electronic review box" for his or her review. After reviewing the report, the provider signs it with his or her electronic signature. The report is then automatically filed in the patient's electronic health record (EHR).

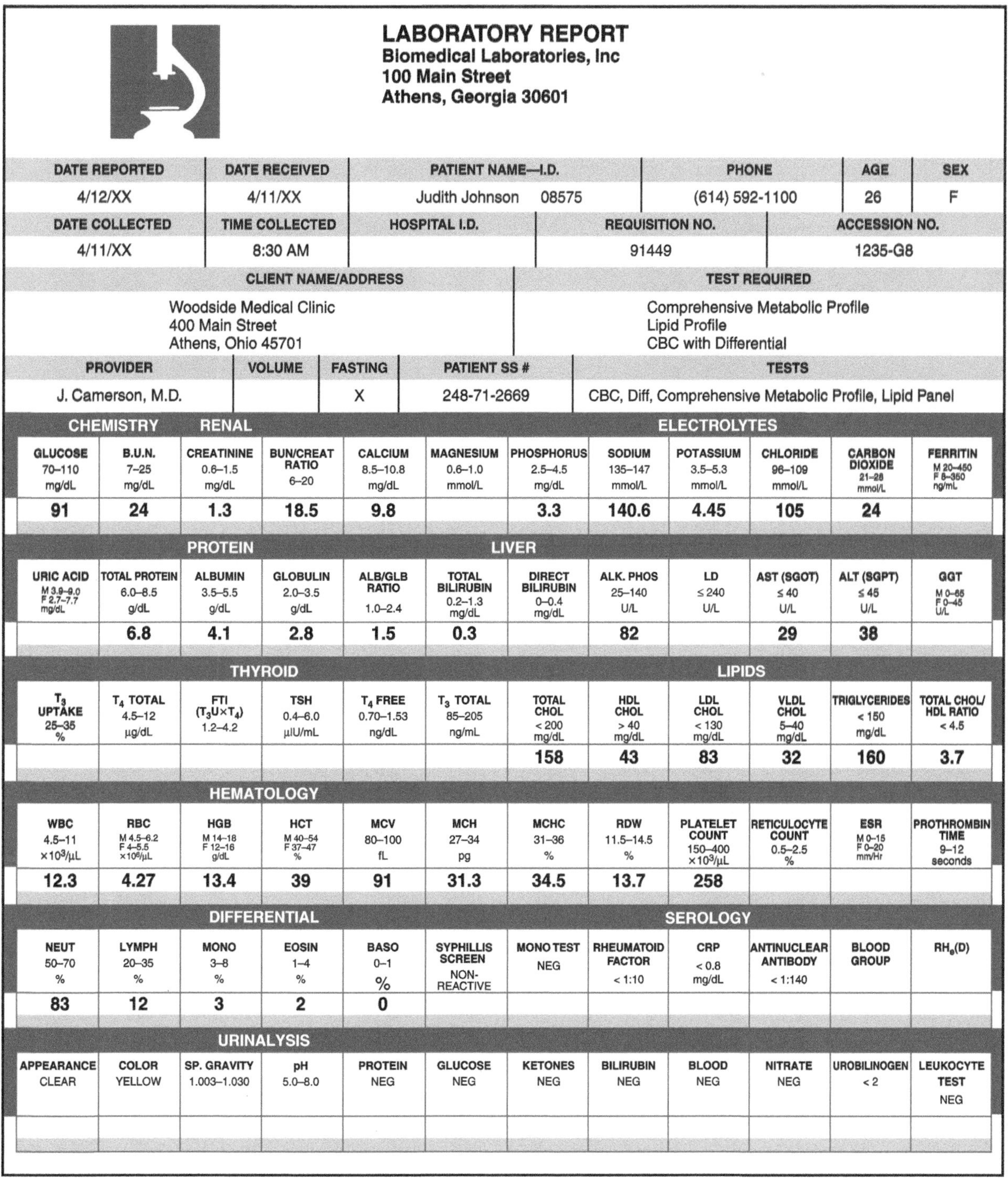

LABORATORY REPORT
Biomedical Laboratories, Inc
100 Main Street
Athens, Georgia 30601

DATE REPORTED	DATE RECEIVED	PATIENT NAME—I.D.	PHONE	AGE	SEX
4/12/XX	4/11/XX	Judith Johnson 08575	(614) 592-1100	26	F

DATE COLLECTED	TIME COLLECTED	HOSPITAL I.D.	REQUISITION NO.	ACCESSION NO.
4/11/XX	8:30 AM		91449	1235-G8

CLIENT NAME/ADDRESS	TEST REQUIRED
Woodside Medical Clinic 400 Main Street Athens, Ohio 45701	Comprehensive Metabolic Profile Lipid Profile CBC with Differential

PROVIDER	VOLUME	FASTING	PATIENT SS #	TESTS
J. Camerson, M.D.		X	248-71-2669	CBC, Diff, Comprehensive Metabolic Profile, Lipid Panel

CHEMISTRY — RENAL — ELECTROLYTES

GLUCOSE 70–110 mg/dL	B.U.N. 7–25 mg/dL	CREATININE 0.6–1.5 mg/dL	BUN/CREAT RATIO 6–20	CALCIUM 8.5–10.8 mg/dL	MAGNESIUM 0.6–1.0 mmol/L	PHOSPHORUS 2.5–4.5 mg/dL	SODIUM 135–147 mmol/L	POTASSIUM 3.5–5.3 mmol/L	CHLORIDE 96–109 mmol/L	CARBON DIOXIDE 21–28 mmol/L	FERRITIN M 20–450 F 8–350 ng/mL
91	24	1.3	18.5	9.8		3.3	140.6	4.45	105	24	

PROTEIN — LIVER

URIC ACID M 3.9–9.0 F 2.7–7.7 mg/dL	TOTAL PROTEIN 6.0–8.5 g/dL	ALBUMIN 3.5–5.5 g/dL	GLOBULIN 2.0–3.5 g/dL	ALB/GLB RATIO 1.0–2.4	TOTAL BILIRUBIN 0.2–1.3 mg/dL	DIRECT BILIRUBIN 0–0.4 mg/dL	ALK. PHOS 25–140 U/L	LD ≤ 240 U/L	AST (SGOT) ≤ 40 U/L	ALT (SGPT) ≤ 45 U/L	GGT M 0–65 F 0–45 U/L
	6.8	4.1	2.8	1.5	0.3		82		29	38	

THYROID — LIPIDS

T_3 UPTAKE 25–35 %	T_4 TOTAL 4.5–12 µg/dL	FTI ($T_3U \times T_4$) 1.2–4.2	TSH 0.4–6.0 µIU/mL	T_4 FREE 0.70–1.53 ng/dL	T_3 TOTAL 85–205 ng/mL	TOTAL CHOL < 200 mg/dL	HDL CHOL > 40 mg/dL	LDL CHOL < 130 mg/dL	VLDL CHOL 5–40 mg/dL	TRIGLYCERIDES < 150 mg/dL	TOTAL CHOL/HDL RATIO < 4.5
						158	43	83	32	160	3.7

HEMATOLOGY

WBC 4.5–11 $\times 10^3/\mu L$	RBC M 4.5–6.2 F 4–5.5 $\times 10^6/\mu L$	HGB M 14–18 F 12–16 g/dL	HCT M 40–54 F 37–47 %	MCV 80–100 fL	MCH 27–34 pg	MCHC 31–36 %	RDW 11.5–14.5 %	PLATELET COUNT 150–400 $\times 10^3/\mu L$	RETICULOCYTE COUNT 0.5–2.5 %	ESR M 0–15 F 0–20 mm/Hr	PROTHROMBIN TIME 9–12 seconds
12.3	4.27	13.4	39	91	31.3	34.5	13.7	258			

DIFFERENTIAL — SEROLOGY

NEUT 50–70 %	LYMPH 20–35 %	MONO 3–8 %	EOSIN 1–4 %	BASO 0–1 %	SYPHILLIS SCREEN NON-REACTIVE	MONO TEST NEG	RHEUMATOID FACTOR < 1:10	CRP < 0.8 mg/dL	ANTINUCLEAR ANTIBODY < 1:140	BLOOD GROUP	$RH_o(D)$
83	12	3	2	0							

URINALYSIS

APPEARANCE CLEAR	COLOR YELLOW	SP. GRAVITY 1.003–1.030	pH 5.0–8.0	PROTEIN NEG	GLUCOSE NEG	KETONES NEG	BILIRUBIN NEG	BLOOD NEG	NITRATE NEG	UROBILINOGEN < 2	LEUKOCYTE TEST NEG

Fig. 15.6 Laboratory report form.

Computer-generated laboratory reports stored in an EHR can be accessed by the computer and manipulated according to the needs of the provider. Examples include the following:

a. Laboratory reports can be displayed in chronologic order or reverse-chronologic order.
b. Current and previous results for a specific test (or tests) can be accessed by the computer and displayed in chronologic order. This permits the provider to compare changes in test results over a period of time.
c. Current and previous test results can be accessed by the computer and plotted graphically on a flowsheet in chronologic order. This permits an abnormal trend to be visually identified, so that appropriate action can be taken. Fig. 15.8 illustrates a flow sheet of hemoglobin test results.

Laboratory Report Comprehensive Metabolic Profile			
PATIENT		ORDERED BY	RESULTS PROVIDED BY
Colbert, Jason K. 2963 Flint Dr. S Clearwater, FL 33759 PH: 740-541-3575	ID #: 336879 DOB: 4/28/1970 AGE: 53 GENDER: M	Thomas Murphy, MD Pinellas Medical Office 3477 Arrowhead Ave Clearwater, FL 33759	Medical Center Laboratory 33 West Main St Clearwater, FL 33759
SPECIMEN COLL. DATE	11/25/20XX	FASTING/NONFASTING	Fasting
SPECIMEN COLL. TIME	08:00 am	ACCESSION NUMBER	3380837
SPECIMEN RECEIVED DATE/TIME	11/25/20XX 05:30 pm	LAB ID NUMBER	773978
RESULTS REPORTED DATE/TIME	11/26/20XX 10:00 am	TEST(S) ORDERED	CPT: 80053 Comprehensive Metabolic Panel

TEST	RESULT	REFERENCE RANGE	UNITS	FLAG
Albumin	**3.1**	**3.5-5.2**	**g/dL**	**L**
Alanine Aminotransferase (ALT)	16	0-45	u/L	
Alkaline Phosphastase (ALP)	81	25-140	u/L	
Aspartate Aminotransferase (AST)	9	0-40	u/L	
Bilirubin, Total	0.6	0.3-1.2	mg/dL	
Urea Nitrogen (BUN)	**28**	**7-25**	**mg/dL**	**H**
Calcium	9.3	8.5-10.2	mg/dL	
Carbon Dioxide	29.6	21.0-32.0	mEq/L	
Chloride	102.9	98.0-107.0	mmol/L	
Creatinine	**1.35**	**0.60-1.10**	**mg/dL**	**H**
Glucose	90	70-99	mg/dL	
Potassium	4.12	3.50-5.10	mmol/L	
Protein, Total	6.6	6.4-8.3	g/dL	
Sodium	139.1	136.0-145.0	mmol/L	

Fig. 15.7 Computer-generated laboratory report.

If the medical office is not networked through computers with an outside laboratory, the laboratory reports received by the office through other means (e.g., faxed) must be scanned into the computer. A scanned report has some limitations. The computer can display the report, but the data on the report cannot be accessed or manipulated by the computer. Because of this, laboratory data cannot be used for many of the functions previously described. For example, the data on scanned reports cannot be accessed and incorporated into a flowsheet for trend analysis.

SPECIMEN LABELS

Each specimen must be properly identified with a label before it is transported to an outside laboratory. Specimen labeling errors that are not discovered may cause misinterpretation of test results leading to an incorrect diagnosis and unnecessary treatment.

Two unique identifiers must be used to label each specimen. A **unique identifier** is information directly associated with an individual that reliably identifies the individual as the person for whom the service or treatment is intended. The most common identifiers used to label specimens are the patient's full legal name and date of birth. It is important to label the specimen container itself and not the lid of the container or the biohazard specimen bag used to transport the specimen.

Handwritten Label

A specimen can be labeled by handwriting the information on the label using a ball point pen (do not use a felt-tipped pen). The label information should include the patient's full

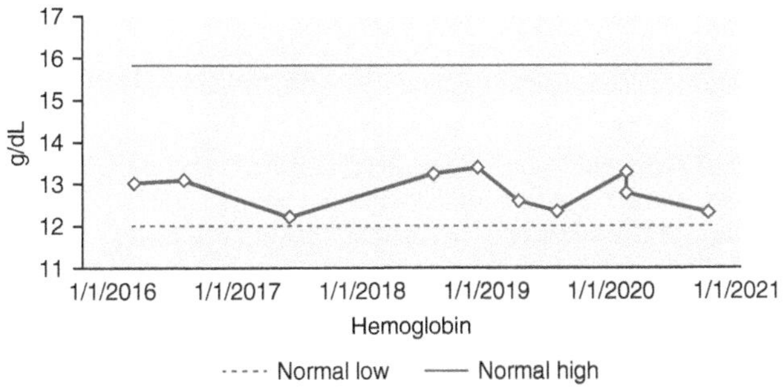

Fig. 15.8 Hemoglobin flowsheet generated by a computer.

legal name and date of birth, the date and time of collection, the initials of the individual collecting the specimen, and any other information required by the laboratory (e.g., the source of a microbiologic specimen). It is important to print legibly and to make certain that the information is accurate (Fig. 15.9A).

Barcode Label

As part of the electronic laboratory request process, the medical office computer also prints out custom barcode labels. The specimen is identified by properly attaching the adhesive barcode label to the specimen container (see Fig. 15.9B). Laboratory analyzers incorporate a barcode reader that is able to read the information on the barcode necessary for testing the specimen and generating test results. To enable the barcode reader to read the label, it must be aligned in a straight (not diagonal) position on the specimen container with no wrinkles, folds, or tears. Barcode labels result in faster processing of the specimen once it arrives at the outside laboratory leading to a faster turnaround time for test results.

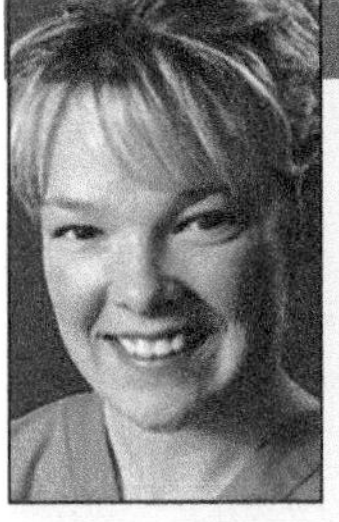

Putting It All Into Practice

My name is Korey, and I am employed by a group of physicians in a family practice medical office. Some of my duties include showing patients to examining rooms, taking vital signs, administering medication, and performing CLIA–waived laboratory tests. I have found that being a medical assistant has been challenging and rewarding, and I wish you the best of luck in reaching your goals.

When I first started working as a practicing medical assistant, I had a challenging venipuncture experience. The patient was a kind and personable 74-year-old man with hardening of the arteries. I tried to obtain the blood specimen from his arm but was not successful. The patient was calm and was not bothered at all by the unsuccessful stick. He said that it was hard to draw blood on him and to go ahead and try again. I decided to try taking the blood from a vein on the back of his hand with a butterfly setup. To my relief, I obtained the blood specimen. I think that I was more nervous about this experience than the patient was. It is important to remain calm on the outside around patients even if you are nervous on the inside. ■

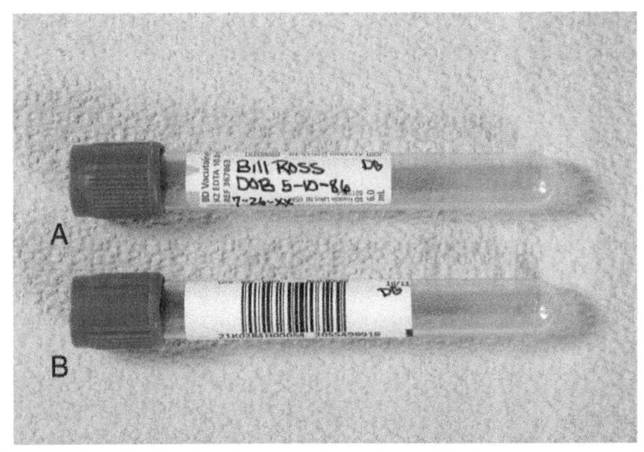

Fig. 15.9 (A) Handwritten specimen label. (B) Computer-generated barcode specimen label.

PATIENT INSTRUCTIONS

The medical assistant is often responsible for providing instructions to a patient for a laboratory test ordered for that patient. The medical assistant should inform the patient of the name and purpose of the test, how to prepare for the test, and how and when to expect the test results. After the instructions have been explained, the medical assistant should verify that the patient understands them and offer to answer any questions. It also is advisable to provide the patient with a written information sheet (Fig. 15.10) to serve as a reference, should the patient forget some of the information after leaving the medical office.

Some laboratory tests require that the patient remain at the collection site for a specified period of time; an example of this is the OGTT, which requires several hours for the collection of multiple, timed specimens. The patient should be told in advance of the time requirement, so that any necessary arrangements can be made with an employer or child care provider.

There are some specimens that need to be collected at home by the patient. For example, if a first-voided morning urine specimen is necessary for a laboratory test, the medical assistant must provide the patient with the appropriate specimen container and instruct the patient in the proper collection, handling, and storage of the specimen until it reaches the medical office. It also is advisable to provide the patient with a written information sheet to serve as a reference, should the patient forget some of the information after leaving the medical office. The instructions should be available in the languages used in the community served by the medical office.

PATIENT PREPARATION

Advance patient preparation is necessary for some laboratory tests to obtain a high-quality specimen suitable for testing. Factors such as food and fluid consumption, medication, activity, alcohol consumption, and time of day may affect the results of certain tests. The medical assistant should

ORAL GLUCOSE TOLERANCE TEST
Patient Information Sheet

General information
Your provider has ordered an oral glucose tolerance test (OGTT) for you. The purpose of this test is to see how well your body processes glucose (sugar). Glucose is the primary source of energy for your body. The OGTT is primarily used for diagnosis of prediabetes and diabetes and to screen pregnant women for gestational diabetes.

Preparation for the Test
It is very important that you prepare properly to ensure accurate test results.
1. For 3 days prior to the test you should consume a high-carbohydrate diet consisting of at least 150 grams of carbohydrate each day. High carbohydrate foods include: bread, pasta, cereal, rice, potatoes, and crackers.
2. Do NOT drink or eat anything except water for 9 –12 h before the test
3. Your test is performed in the morning because of the overnight fast.
4. Your provider will discuss what medication (if any) to discontinue before the test.
5. You will need to stay at the testing facility for the duration of the collection procedure which is approximately 2–3 h.
6. You may want to bring something to read or work on during your wait at the facility.

Collection Procedure
The collection procedure includes the following:
1. After arrival, a fasting blood specimen will be collected.
2. Following this, you will be given a very sweet glucose solution to drink. You must drink all of the glucose solution within a 5-min period of time. Some people experience a brief period of nausea after consuming the solution.
3. A blood specimen will be collected 60 min after drinking the glucose solution.
4. Another specimen will be collected 120 min (2 h) after drinking the glucose solution.
5. Another specimen may be collected 180 min (3 h) after drinking the glucose solution.

Testing Information
It is important to adhere to the following guidelines to ensure accurate test results.
1. Remain quietly seated during the testing period and do not leave the testing facility. Any form of exercise should be avoided because it can affect the test results.
2. Do not eat or drink anything except small sips of water during the collection procedure.
3. Do not smoke or chew gum during the collection procedure.
4. Following the procedure, you can eat and drink as usual and resume your normal activities.

Normal Side Effects
During the procedure, you may experience some normal side effects such as weakness, a feeling of faintness, or perspiration. They are caused by a decrease in your body's glucose level as insulin is secreted in response to the glucose solution.

Fig. 15.10 Patient information sheet for an oral glucose tolerance test.

make sure to explain the reason for the advance preparation, so the patient will be more likely to comply with the necessary preparation. A specimen obtained from a patient who has not prepared properly may invalidate the test results and necessitate calling the patient back to collect the specimen again.

The type of preparation necessary for a particular test depends on the test ordered. If an outside laboratory is performing the test, the patient preparation can be found in the laboratory test directory. If the test is performed in the POL, the medical assistant should consult the manufacturer's instructions that accompany the laboratory test to obtain this information. Advance patient preparation usually consists of fasting and medication restrictions which are described as follows in more detail.

Fasting

Some blood specimens require the patient to fast before collection. The composition of blood is altered by the consumption of food and fluid because digested food and fluid are absorbed into the circulatory system, changing the results of certain laboratory tests. Food intake causes fasting blood glucose (FBG) and triglycerides tests to yield falsely high results. Any panel including the test (e.g., comprehensive metabolic panel) requires the patient to fast before the specimen is collected.

Fasting involves abstaining from food and fluids (except water) for a specified period of time before the collection of the specimen (usually 8 to 12 hours) to allow food and fluid from the previous meal to be completely digested and absorbed. Fasting specimens are usually collected in the morning, which causes the least amount of inconvenience to the patient in terms of abstaining from food and fluid.

The medical assistant must give detailed instructions to the patient, ensuring that the patient understands that fasting includes abstaining from food and fluid for the specified period of time. However, the patient should be told that it is permissible—in fact, advisable—to drink water because dehydration caused by water abstinence can alter certain test results.

MEDICATION RESTRICTIONS

Medication may affect the physical and chemical characteristics of body substances and lead to inaccurate test results. The provider may want the patient to stop taking a medication that might interfere with the test results for a certain period of time before the collection of the specimen. The medical assistant should instruct the patient in the name of the medication to discontinue, the period of time to discontinue it, and the reason for discontinuing it.

What Would You Do? What Would You *Not* Do?

Case Study 2

Kathleen O'Leary is coming to the medical office today for a follow-up appointment. She was seen last week complaining of fatigue, shortness of breath, weight loss, insomnia, and joint pain. The provider gives Kathleen a laboratory request to have her blood drawn and tested at an outside laboratory. The provider ordered a CBC with differential and a comprehensive metabolic panel. A review of Kathleen's electronic health record shows that she did not get her lab testing done. Kathleen is contacted by phone; she says she knows she should have gone to the laboratory to have her blood drawn, but she is afraid of needles and panics at the sight of blood. She says that the last time she had her blood drawn she started feeling warm and lightheaded and had to lie down and was embarrassed by that. Kathleen says she also is worried the laboratory results might show something is wrong with her. She is thinking of not coming for her appointment today with the hope that she starts feeling better on her own. ■

SPECIMEN COLLECTION FOR TRANSPORT TO AN OUTSIDE LABORATORY

There are a number of steps involved in the collection and handling of a specimen for transport to an outside laboratory. These steps include patient preparation, collecting and processing the specimen, and preparing and storing the specimen for transport to the laboratory. The most important goal of specimen collection is to provide the laboratory with a sample that is as biologically representative as possible of the body substance collected. If the specimen is collected or handled improperly, the integrity of the specimen may be adversely affected. This may cause inaccurate test results and interfere with the accurate diagnosis and treatment of the patient's condition.

Once the specimen arrives at the outside laboratory, it is assigned an accession number. The purpose of an accession number is to provide positive identification of each specimen within the laboratory and to allow easy access to laboratory records should a test result need to be located again. If the provider desires to have the laboratory test repeated, the accession number (printed on the laboratory report) must be entered on the laboratory request.

CAUSES FOR REJECTION OF A SPECIMEN

It may not be possible to test a specimen if the specimen requirements have not been met; in these cases, the outside laboratory rejects the specimen. Sometimes the situation can be rectified, such as when a laboratory request is missing and the medical office is able to quickly supply it to the laboratory. When the situation cannot be rectified, another specimen must be collected from the patient, such as when an insufficient amount of specimen was submitted. Causes of specimen rejection by an outside laboratory include the following:

- No label on the specimen container or incorrect information on the specimen label.
- Specimen label information and information on the lab request do not match.
- Specimen is received without a laboratory request.
- Specimen is collected in the wrong container or in a container past its expiration date.
- Insufficient type or amount of specimen is submitted for the test requested.
- Hemolyzed serum or plasma specimen is submitted.
- Leakage of the specimen container.
- Damaged specimen container (broken, chipped, or cracked).
- Improper storage of the specimen.
- Significant time delay between specimen collection and receipt of the specimen by the laboratory.

GUIDELINES FOR SPECIMEN COLLECTION AND HANDLING

Specific guidelines must be followed when collecting a specimen for transport to an outside laboratory. The medical assistant is responsible for performing the following:

1. **Provide patient instructions.** Explain the patient instructions thoroughly (e.g., patient preparation), and provide the patient with written instructions to take home as a reference. Notify the patient of the time to report to the medical office for the specimen collection.
2. **Review the collection and handling requirements.** Review the collection and handling requirements in the laboratory test directory for the test(s) ordered by the provider. A review of the requirements beforehand prevents errors in collection and handling of the specimen. Contact the outside laboratory if you have any questions regarding any aspect of collection procedure. Specimen requirements include the following:

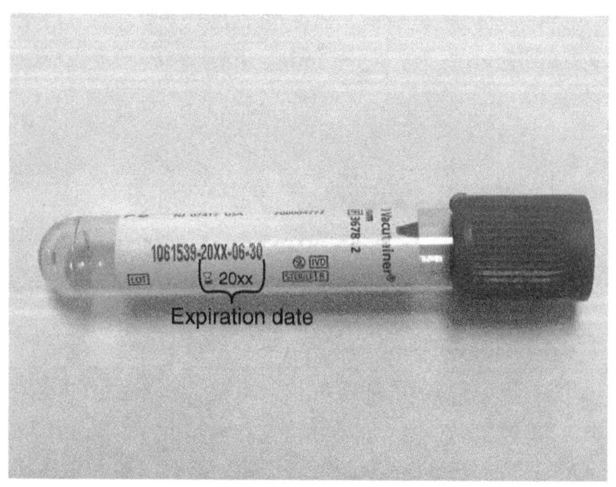

Fig. 15.11 Blood tube showing expiration date.

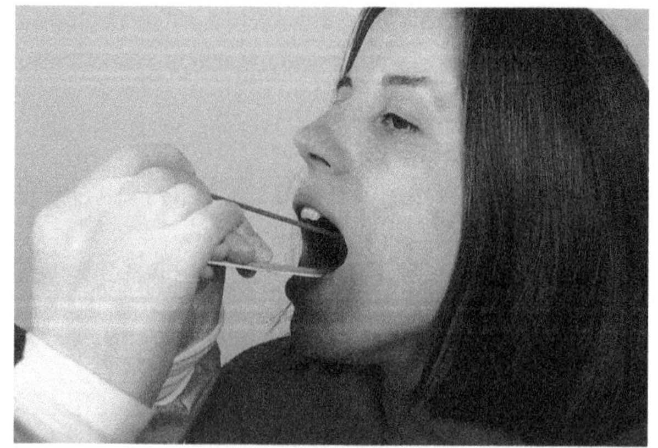

Fig. 15.12 The Occupational Safety and Health Administration Standard must be followed during specimen collection.

a. Collection materials required
b. Type of specimen to be collected (e.g., whole blood, serum, urine)
c. Amount of the specimen needed to perform the laboratory test
d. Procedure to follow to collect the specimen
e. Proper handling and storage of the specimen awaiting transport.

3. **Identify the patient.** Identify the patient by asking the patient to state his or her full name and date of birth. Compare this information with the demographic data in the patient's medical record. The patient should *not* be asked whether he or she is a certain patient. For example, the patient should not be asked, "Are you Brad Thompson?" The patient may not hear this information correctly or may not be paying attention and may answer in the affirmative even if he is not that patient. Collecting a specimen on the wrong patient by mistake may lead to an inaccurate diagnosis and the wrong treatment.
4. **Determine whether the patient has prepared properly.** If the patient was required to prepare for the test, determine whether this was performed properly. If the patient has not prepared properly, inform the provider. The provider may want the patient to prepare properly and return to the medical office. If the provider wants to go ahead with the collection, indicate this information on the laboratory request. For example, if the patient did not fast for an FBG, indicate "nonfasting specimen" on the laboratory request.
5. **Assemble the equipment and supplies.** Sanitize hands and assemble the appropriate equipment and supplies specified in the laboratory test directory. Substituting collection containers may not yield the proper type of specimen required, which can affect the test results. Check each container before use to ensure it is not broken, chipped, cracked, or otherwise damaged. Damaged containers are unsuitable for specimen collection and should be discarded. Check the expiration date on the container (Fig. 15.11). Outdated specimen containers may affect the accuracy of the test results.
6. **Complete a laboratory request.** The request may be a preprinted request or an electronic request. The completed request provides the outside laboratory with the information necessary to test the specimen.
7. **Label the specimen container.** Properly label each specimen container to prevent a mix-up of specimens. At a minimum, the label should include the patient's full legal name, date of birth, and the date and time of collection of the specimen. (*Note:* The medical assistant should follow the medical office policy as to when the container should be labeled. Some offices prefer that the container be labeled *before* the specimen is collected; other offices want the container to be labeled *after* the specimen is collected.)
8. **Collect the specimen.** Proper collection of the specimen provides the outside laboratory with a biologically representative sample of the body substance collected. The specimen should be collected according to the following guidelines:
   a. Adhere to the OSHA Bloodborne Pathogens Standards (see Chapter 2) when collecting and handling the specimen to prevent an exposure incident (Fig. 15.12).
   b. Collect the specimen according to the requirements specified in the laboratory directory.
   c. Collect the proper type of specimen (e.g., whole blood, serum, plasma, and urine).
   d. Collect the proper amount of specimen. It is critical that an adequate amount of specimen be submitted for analysis. If the amount of the specimen is insufficient to perform the test(s), a report is sent to the medical office indicating quantity not sufficient (QNS). This situation warrants calling the patient back for the collection of another specimen.
   e. Securely tighten the lids on specimen containers to prevent leakage of the specimen during storage and transport.
   f. Properly discard used collection materials in a biohazard waste container.
9. **Process the specimen.** Process the specimen according to the requirements specified in the laboratory

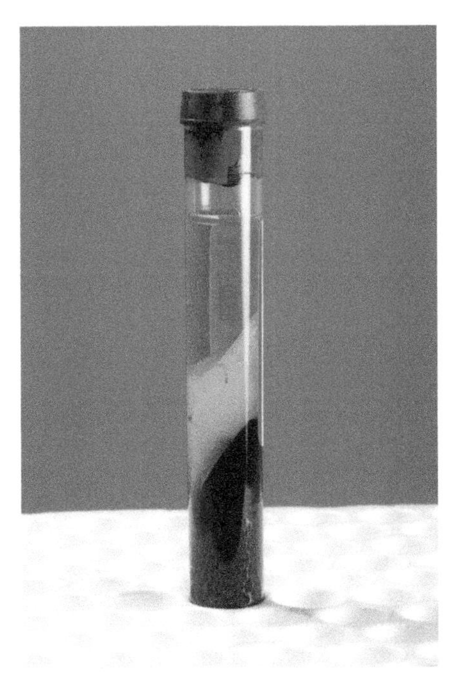

Fig. 15.13 Serum specimen in a serum separator tube that has been centrifuged.

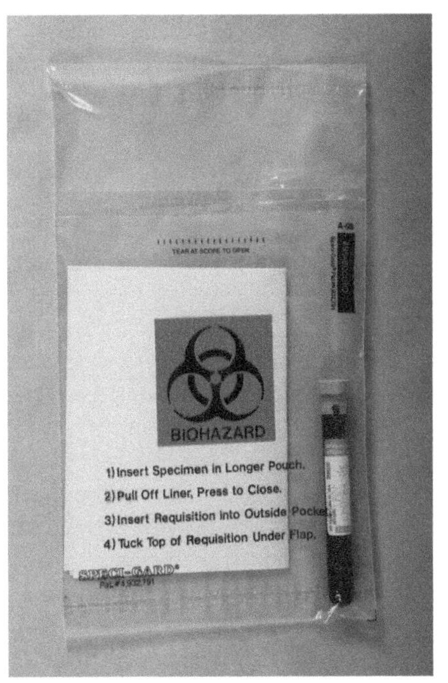

Fig. 15.14 Biohazard specimen bag.

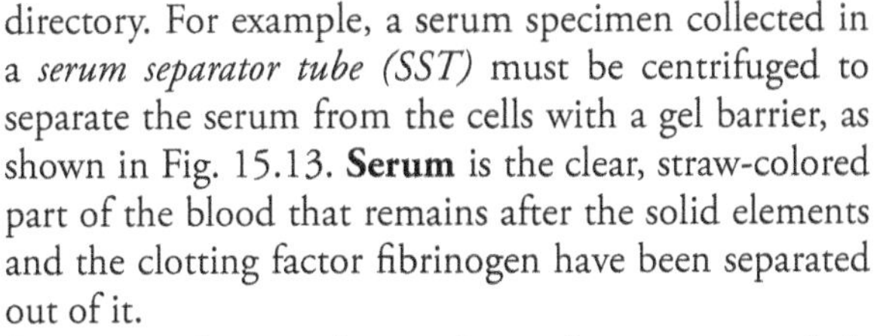

directory. For example, a serum specimen collected in a *serum separator tube (SST)* must be centrifuged to separate the serum from the cells with a gel barrier, as shown in Fig. 15.13. **Serum** is the clear, straw-colored part of the blood that remains after the solid elements and the clotting factor fibrinogen have been separated out of it.

10. **Prepare and store the specimen for transport.** It is important to store the specimen under environmental conditions that will not affect the integrity of the specimen and to transport the specimen to an outside laboratory in a timely manner as follows:
    a. Place the specimen in a biohazard specimen bag, and seal the bag (Fig. 15.14). Biohazard bags prevent contamination of the specimen and protect health care workers and laboratory couriers from the possibility of an exposure incident.
    b. Depending on the policy of the outside laboratory, transmit the laboratory request electronically and/or place the request in the outside pocket of the biohazard specimen bag.
    c. Properly store specimens awaiting pickup following the storage requirements in the laboratory directory. Many specimens can be stored at RT, whereas others may need to be refrigerated or frozen. Definitions of storage temperatures are outlined in Box 15.1. An outside laboratory may provide the medical office with a large lockable container, known as a *lockbox*, for storing specimens awaiting pickup. The laboratory provides instructions on the proper placement and storage of specimens in the lockbox.

BOX 15.1 Specimen Storage Temperatures

Storage Temperature	Temperature Range	
	Fahrenheit	Celsius
Room temperature (RT)	59 °F–86 °F	15 °C–30 °C
Refrigerated	36 °F–46 °F	2 °C–8 °C
Frozen	−4 °F or less	−20 °C or less

CLINICAL LABORATORY IMPROVEMENT AMENDMENTS

As previously discussed, the CLIA regulations were developed by the federal government to improve the quality of laboratory testing in the United States to ensure accurate and reliable test results. The CLIA regulations govern all facilities that perform laboratory tests for health assessment or for the diagnosis, prevention, or treatment of disease such as hospital and independent laboratories, medical offices, health departments, and nursing homes.

The Centers for Medicare and Medicaid Services (CMS) is a division of the US Department of Health and Human Services (HHS). The CMS is responsible for regulating and operating the CLIA program. In addition to following CLIA regulations, a clinical laboratory must also be in compliance with all other federal, state, and local legislation such as the OSHA Standard.

CATEGORIES OF TESTS

CLIA establishes three categories of laboratory tests based on the complexity of the test method: basically, the more complex the test method, the more stringent the CLIA regulations. These three categories include waived tests, moderate complexity tests, and high complexity tests which are described as follows.

CLIA-Waived Tests

A **CLIA-waived test** is a laboratory test that has been determined to be a simple procedure that is easy to perform and has a low risk of erroneous test results. Waived tests also include tests that have been approved for use by patients at home (e.g., urine pregnancy test). POLs that perform only waived tests must apply for a CLIA certificate of waiver (CW) from CMS which must be renewed every 2 years. POLs holding a CW are exempt from most of the CLIA regulations but are still expected to adhere to good laboratory practices. CLIA requires that the manufacturer's instructions that accompany the test system be followed *exactly,* which includes the following:

- Proper storage of the test system.
- Adherence to expiration dates.
- Proper collection and handling of the specimen.
- Performance of quality control procedures.
- Proper testing of the specimen.
- Correct interpretation of test results.
- Accurate documentation of test results.

CLIA-Nonwaived Tests

Laboratories performing nonwaived tests must be certified by CLIA and adhere to the CLIA regulations. These regulations include the following: proper educational and training qualifications for laboratory personnel; participation in a proficiency testing program; procedures to ensure proper test performance and accurate test results; an overall plan to monitor the quality of the laboratory's operation; and unannounced on-site inspections by CMS every 2 years. Nonwaived tests include moderate complexity and high complexity tests described as follows.

Moderate Complexity Tests

Moderate complexity tests account for 75% of the estimated 7 to 10 billion laboratory tests performed in the United States each year. Most of these tests are performed by hospital and independent laboratories. Moderate complexity tests include electrolyte profiles, chemistry profiles, CBC, drug screens, and automated immunoassays performed by highly sophisticated automated analyzers. Some medical office providers perform moderate complexity tests known as *provider-performed microscopy* (PPM) procedures, which involve the examination of a specimen under the microscope. An example of a PPM procedure is the microscopic analysis of urine sediment. PPM procedures are a subcategory of the moderately complexity test category and must be performed by an individual with the proper training and skill qualifications, such as a medical office provider. A CLIA certificate is required for PPM procedures, and the CLIA regulations must be followed; however, the POL is exempt from on-site inspections.

High Complexity Tests

High complexity tests are those that require the expertise of a clinical laboratory professional such as a pathologist. Examples include cytology (e.g., Pap test), immunohistochemistry, peripheral blood smears, flow cytometry, gel electrophoresis, and most molecular diagnostic tests.

Memories *From* Practicum

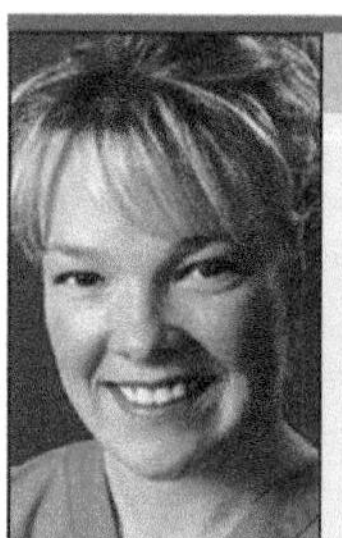

Korey: One of my most difficult situations as a medical assisting student was taking the temperature of a patient who started to have a seizure. I was scared because I was only a student, and I had never been in a situation like that before. I knew I had to act immediately, and luckily one of the certified medical assistants (CMAs [American Association of Medical Assistants (AAMA)]) was nearby. We immediately put the patient on the floor and moved things away from him to keep him from hurting himself. We then notified the physician, who was with a patient in another examining room. The seizure lasted only about 4 minutes, and the patient was fine. The CMA (AAMA) told me that the patient had a history of seizures and that I did a good job of staying calm. That surely was a difficult but valuable learning experience for me. ■

CLIA-WAIVED TESTS IN THE POL

Approximately 1400 CLIA-waived tests are commercially available that test for 120 different analytes. An **analyte** is a body substance that is being identified or measured by a laboratory test, such as glucose, hemoglobin, and group A streptococci. The number of waived tests is expected to increase as new technology becomes available.

CLIA-waived tests that are performed most frequently in the POL include the following:

- **Urine and Fecal Tests**
  - Urinalysis test (using a reagent strip or a CLIA-waived urine chemistry analyzer)
  - CLIA-waived urine drug test
  - Urine pregnancy test with visual color comparisons
  - Fecal occult blood test
- **Hematology Tests**
  - Hemoglobin test (using a CLIA-waived analyzer)
  - Spun microhematocrit test
  - Prothrombin time test (using a CLIA-waived analyzer)
- **Blood Chemistry and Immunologic Tests**
  - Blood glucose test (using CLIA-waived analyzer)
  - Hemoglobin A_{1C} test (using a CLIA-waived analyzer)
  - Cholesterol test (using a CLIA-waived analyzer)
  - Triglycerides test (using a CLIA-waived analyzer)
  - Rapid COVID test
  - Rapid human immunodeficiency virus (HIV) test
  - Rapid mononucleosis test
- **Microbiologic Tests**

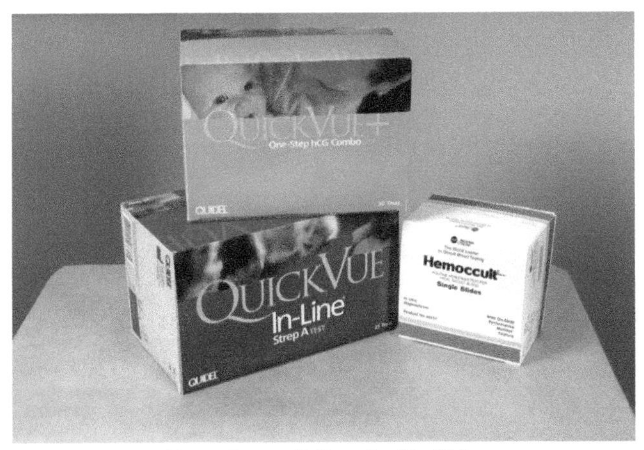

Fig. 15.15 CLIA–waived test kits.

- Group A rapid *Streptococcus* test
- Rapid influenza A and B test.

CLIA-WAIVED TEST SYSTEMS

A **test system** is defined as a setup that includes all of the test components, such as testing devices, controls, and test reagents, required to perform a laboratory test. A **reagent** is a chemical that reacts with a specimen to allow the detection or measurement of an analyte. CLIA-waived test systems include CLIA-waived test kits and CLIA-waived automated analyzers, described as follows.

CLIA-WAIVED TEST KITS

A CLIA-waived test kit consists of a box packaged with the items needed to perform the test (Fig. 15.15). Each kit contains enough supplies to perform a specific number of tests as indicated on the package label. Examples of CLIA-waived test kits include:

- Hemoccult fecal occult blood test (SmithKline Diagnostics, Palo Alto, CA).
- QuickVue HCG urine pregnancy test (Quidel, San Diego, CA).
- QuickVue In-Line Strep A test (Quidel, San Diego, CA).

Each test kit includes a package insert. A **package insert** is a printed document developed by the manufacturer of a laboratory test that provides detailed information on the use of the test and how to perform the test. The information included in a package insert is listed and described in Table 15.3. The medical assistant should carefully read the package insert and follow the instructions *exactly* to ensure accurate and reliable test results. The test kit often includes a *procedure reference card*, which is a condensed version of the steps in the testing procedure, and can be used as a quick reference guide when performing the test. Because the procedure reference card is a summary of the testing procedure, it should never be substituted for the package insert when first learning about the test.

Test kits often use a *unitized test device* to perform the test. A unitized test device is a self-contained device, such as a cassette, to which a specimen is added directly and in which all of the steps of the testing procedure occur (Fig. 15.16). A unitized device is used to perform one laboratory test (e.g., urine pregnancy test) and is discarded after testing.

Many of the test kits rely on a color change for interpretation of results. A color chart or diagram is provided with the kit for making a visual comparison and interpreting results. When the test results are documented, the brand name and lot number of the test kit should be indicated.

CLIA-WAIVED AUTOMATED ANALYZERS

CLIA-waived automated analyzers have been developed for performing laboratory tests in the POL; they are continually increasing in number as new technology becomes available. These analyzers consist of compact or handheld devices that permit the processing of a specimen in a short time with accurate test results. Reagent strips or test cassettes are often used with CLIA-waived analyzers. Test results are obtained through a direct (digital display or printed) readout (Fig. 15.17).

The ease of operating automated analyzers should not lead to a false sense of security because they have limitations which must be recognized—the most critical one being the failure of the equipment. One of the most important aspects of use of an automated analyzer is the ability to recognize signs that indicate it is malfunctioning, because this can lead to inaccurate test results.

The manufacturer of each automated analyzer provides an operating manual that includes information needed to perform quality control procedures, collect and handle the specimen, and test the specimen. Medical assistants should be completely familiar with all aspects of automated analyzers used to perform laboratory tests in their POLs.

When a CLIA-waived automated analyzer is purchased, the test components (e.g., controls, test reagents) are usually purchased separately. The medical assistant is responsible for checking the supplies periodically and reordering them as needed. Each test component comes with a package insert, which indicates its use, and proper storage and stability requirements.

Some examples of brand names of CLIA-waived automated analyzers (Fig. 15.18) include:

- Cholestech LDX (Cholestech, Hayward, CA).
- STAT-Site Hemoglobin Meter (Stanbio Laboratory, Boerne, TX).
- CoaguChek system and Accu-Chek (Roche Diagnostics, Branchburg, NJ).
- A1C Now (Bayer Corporation, Morrisville, NJ).
- Clinitek urine analyzer (Siemens Corporation, New York, NY).

Table 15.3 Information Included in the Package Insert of a Test Kit

Section	Information Included
Intended Use	A description of the purpose of the test and the reason for performing the test.
Summary and Explanation	Provides a brief overview of the condition being detected by the test, including the symptoms, prevalence, and complications of the condition.
Principles of the Procedure	A detailed explanation of how the test works to detect the substance in the patient's specimen.
Precautions and Warnings	Outlines precautions that must be taken when running the test to ensure accurate and reliable test results. Also includes guidelines for safe handling, use, and disposal of chemical reagents included in the test kit.
Reagents and Materials Provided	A list of the collection devices, controls, reagents, and other supplies included in the test kit. Describes each component in detail, including the number of tests in the kit and the types and amounts of reagents and supplies.
Materials Not Provided	A list of the materials needed to perform the test but not included in the test kit.
Storage and Stability	A description of the proper storage requirements of the test kit such as temperature range. Also identifies how long each testing component is stable for both unopened and opened components.
Specimen Collection and Handling	Type of specimen required and procedures that must be followed when collecting, handling, and storing the specimen to ensure a high-quality and reliable specimen. Also includes safety precautions to take when handling the specimen.
Test Procedure	Presents a step-by-step procedure that must be followed to test the specimen. Diagrams and illustrations of the procedural steps are often included in this section.
Interpretation and Reading Results	Guidelines for reading and interpreting the test results. If a color change is involved in reading the results, a color comparison chart or color diagram is included with the test kit. Also explains the action to take if the test results are invalid.
Quality Control	An explanation of the quality control procedures that must be performed to ensure accurate and reliable test results. Includes instructions for performing control procedures. Also includes information on how often and when controls should be run and the expected results. Describes what should be done if the controls do not produce expected results.
Limitations of the Procedure	A test system works only within certain prescribed conditions and situations. Identifies conditions or situations that might prevent the test from performing correctly and influence the test results, such as medications or the presence of certain medical conditions. Also identifies any supplemental testing needed to confirm a waived test.
Expected Values	Identifies the test result(s) that should be expected by the user.
Performance Characteristics	Presents the results of research studies that have been conducted to evaluate test performance.

What Would You Do? What Would You *Not* Do?

Case Study 3

Zachary Tyler, 21 years of age, comes to the medical office complaining of fever, sore throat, painful swallowing, and red, swollen tonsils with white patches. The physician examines Zachary and orders a CLIA-waived rapid strep test, to make a differential diagnosis of his condition. As Korey is preparing the supplies to collect a throat specimen, Zachary wants to know why the physician was not able to tell if he has strep throat from looking at his throat. He also says that he thought lab testing could only be done at a clinical laboratory by medical laboratory technologists. Zachary says that he has an overly sensitive gag reflex and wants to know if Korey could run the test using a blood sample. After Korey collects the throat specimen, Zachary says he forgot to tell the physician that he took an antibiotic this morning hoping it would help with his throat pain. The test results indicate that Zachary has group A strep, and the physician electronically orders amoxicillin from Zachary's preferred pharmacy. When leaving the office, Zachary asks Korey for his antibiotic prescription. ■

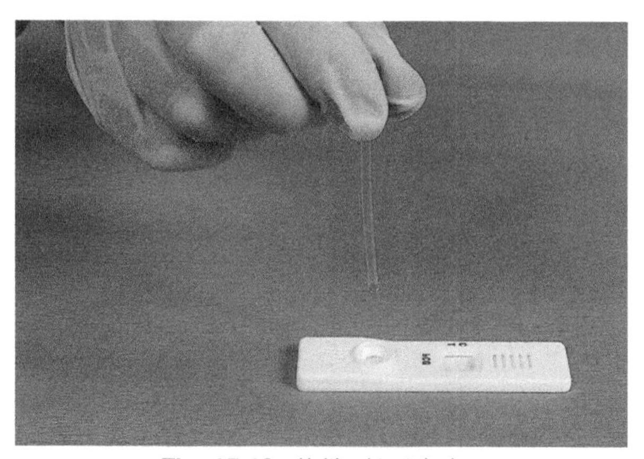

Fig. 15.16 Unitized test device.

POL LABORATORY TESTING

Testing a specimen in a POL involves a series of steps to determine the presence of a specific analyte in the specimen. The remainder of this chapter focuses on guidelines

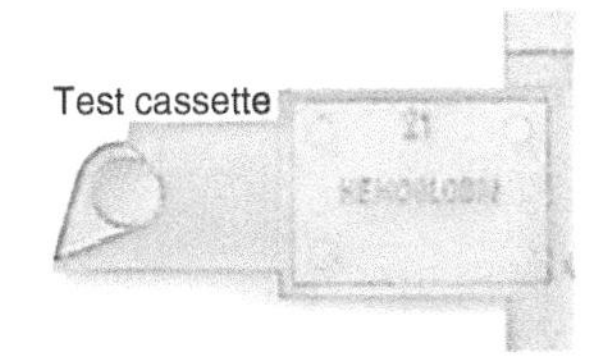

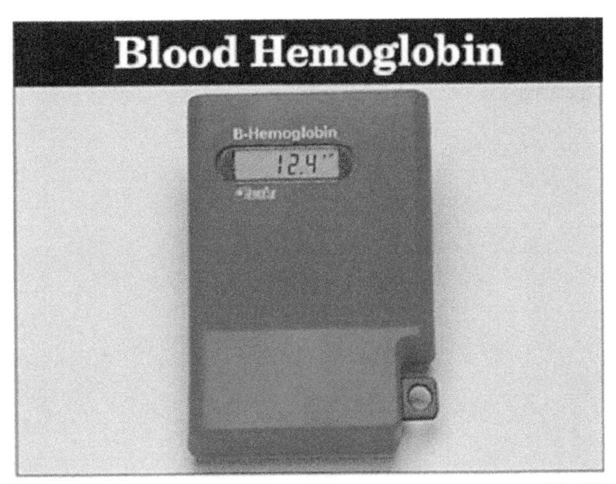

Fig. 15.17 Digital readout of test results on a CLIA-waived automated hemoglobin analyzer. (Modified from Garrels M: *Laboratory & diagnostic testing in ambulatory care*, ed 4, St Louis: Elsevier; 2019.)

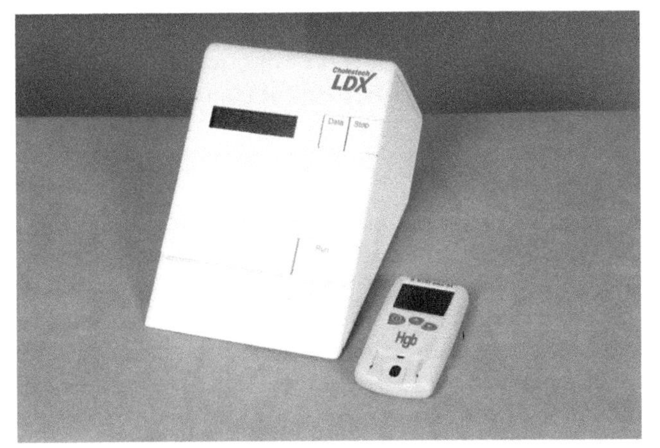

Fig. 15.18 CLIA–waived automated analyzers. Cholesterol analyzer *(left)* and hemoglobin analyzer *(right).*

that should be followed when performing a CLIA-waived test in a POL.

QUALITY CONTROL

It is important to ensure that a laboratory test accurately measures what it is supposed to measure; this involves practicing and maintaining a quality control program. **Quality control** is defined as the application of methods and means to ensure that test results are reliable and valid and that errors are detected and eliminated. Quality control methods ensure reliable information that enables the provider to make an accurate diagnosis leading to the correct treatment. Quality control is an ongoing process that encompasses every aspect of test storage, patient preparation and specimen collection, handling, and testing.

STORAGE OF TEST COMPONENTS

Test components are used to perform laboratory tests and include controls and test reagents. Test components have specific storage requirements that must be carefully followed, as outlined next.

1. Store the test components according to the information in the package insert. Improper storage can cause deterioration of the test components. Most test components need to be stored at RT in a cool, dry area away from sources of heat and sunlight because these conditions can alter their effectiveness.
2. Some test components may need to be stored in the refrigerator (e.g., controls and test reagents). Allow time for a refrigerated test component to reach RT before using it which usually takes approximately 15 to 30 minutes.
3. If indicated, gently shake the control bottle to mix it.
4. Do not transfer test components from one test kit to another.
5. Make sure environmental conditions (e.g., RT) are appropriate for running the test as specified in the package insert.

STABILITY OF TEST COMPONENTS

Stability refers to the reliability of test components to perform as expected. Guidelines to ensure the stability of test components include the following:

1. Check the expiration date of each test component before using it. Do not use a test component if it is past its expiration date. Outdated components can lead to inaccurate test results.
2. An unopened control is stable until the manufacturer's expiration date stamped on the label is reached. Once opened, some controls are stable only for a certain period of time (e.g., 30 days). For these controls, the date the control is opened *and* the date it should be discarded (expiration date) must be written on the label of the control after it has been opened. An opened control is stable until it reaches the manufacturer's expiration date or the hand-written expiration, whichever comes first.
3. Discard outdated test components as soon as they reach their expiration dates.

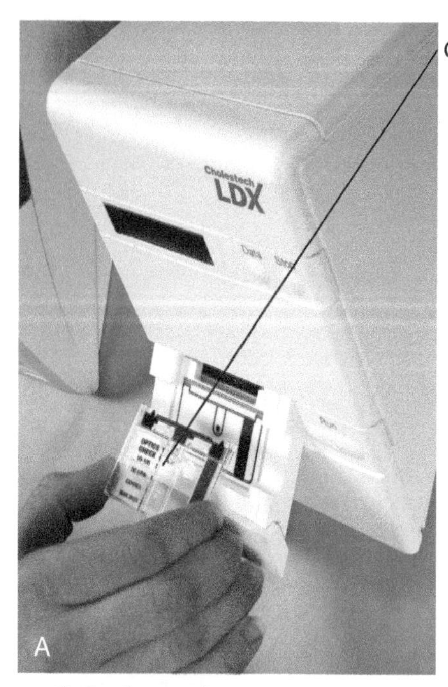

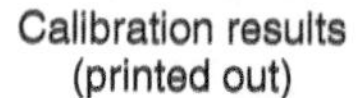

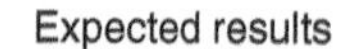

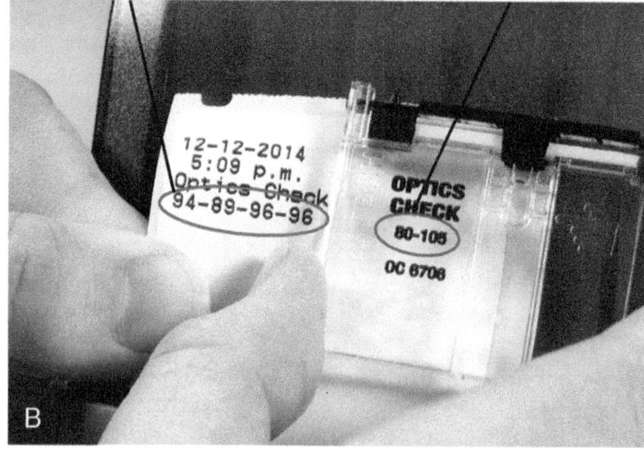

Fig. 15.19 (A) Calibration of an analyzer using a calibration standard. (B) Calibration results are compared with expected results shown on the calibration standard.

CALIBRATION PROCEDURE

Calibration is a mechanism used to check the precision and accuracy of an automated analyzer to determine if it is providing accurate test results. A calibration check detects errors caused by an analyzer that is not working properly. Calibration is typically performed using a device known as a *calibration standard.* The calibration standard may come in the form of a calibration strip or cassette. The calibration standard is inserted into the analyzer (Fig. 15.19A), and the calibration results are displayed on the screen of the analyzer or printed out by the analyzer. The calibration results are then compared with the expected results provided in the package insert or shown on the calibration standard (see Fig. 15.19B). Calibration guidelines include the following:

1. Perform the calibration check following the instructions in the operating manual accompanying the analyzer. The instructions include information on the type of calibration standard to use, how to perform the calibration procedure, and what action should be taken if the calibration procedure does not perform as expected.
2. Document calibration results in a quality control log. (This is a CLIA recommendation for waived tests and not a requirement.)
3. If the calibration procedure does not perform as expected, patient testing should not be conducted until the problem has been identified and resolved.
4. The frequency of performing the calibration procedure is indicated in the operating manual. At a minimum, a calibration check should be performed when using a new lot number of test reagents.

CONTROL PROCEDURE

A **control** is a solution used to monitor a test system to ensure reliable and accurate test results. Controls come with a package insert, which lists the expected ranges for control results. There are two categories of controls: external controls and internal controls.

Internal Controls

An internal control is built into a test device (Fig. 15.20). It evaluates whether certain aspects of the testing procedure are working properly. An internal control is performed at the same time that the testing procedure is performed. It checks for one or more of the following: whether a sufficient amount of the specimen was added, whether a sufficient amount of test reagent was added, and whether the test reagent migrated through the test device properly. If the internal control does not perform as expected, the test result is invalid and the specimen must be retested. If the test result continues to be invalid, the manufacturer of the test system should be contacted.

External Controls

External controls are used to determine if the test reagents are performing properly and to detect any errors in technique used to perform the test. External controls consist of commercially available solutions with known values. They may be included with the test system or may need to be purchased separately. In general, two levels of controls must be performed on a test system. A *low-level control* (also known as a *level 1 control*) produces results that are less than the reference range for the test; a *high-level control* (also known as a *level 2 control*) produces results that are greater than the reference range for the test (Fig. 15.21). The control procedure is performed using the same procedure for performing the test on a patient. However, instead of adding the patient specimen to the testing device, the control is added to it. Control results are compared with expected results provided on the control container or in the package insert accompanying the control. Failure of a control to produce expected results may be caused by outdated controls or test reagents, improper storage of test components, improper

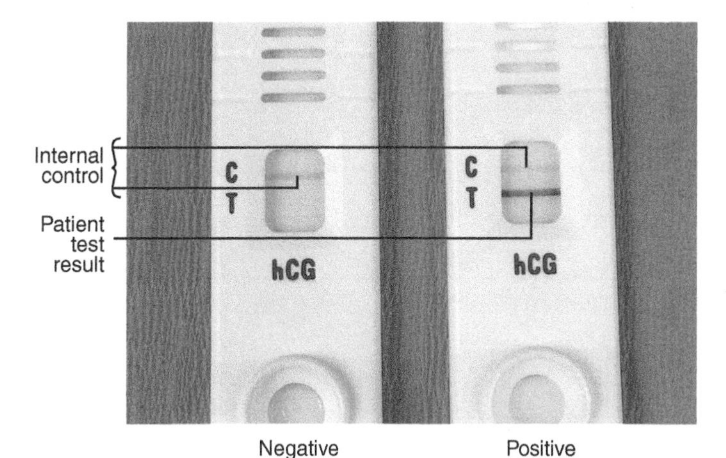

Fig. 15.20 Internal control. The blue line next to the letter *C* indicates that the internal control has performed as expected.

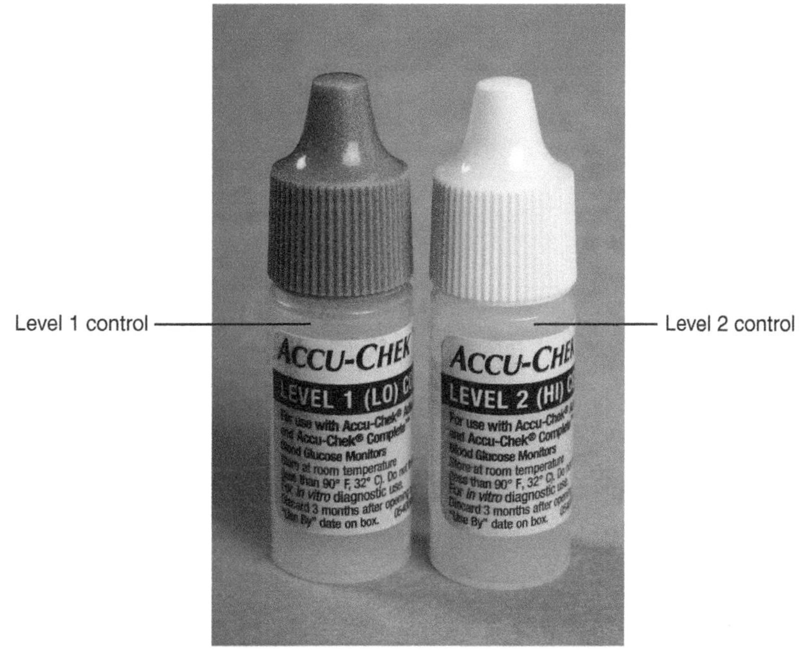

Fig. 15.21 External controls. Low or level 1 control *(left)* and high or level 2 control *(right)*.

environmental testing conditions, and an error in the technique used to perform the procedure.

External control guidelines include the following:

1. Perform the control check following the information in the package insert, which includes instructions on how to perform the control procedure and what action should be taken if the control does not perform as expected.
2. Document control results in a quality control log (Fig. 15.22). (This is a CLIA recommendation for waived tests and not a requirement.)
3. If the control procedure does not perform as expected, patient testing should not be conducted until the problem is identified and resolved. If the problem cannot be resolved, the manufacturer of the test system should be contacted.
4. The frequency of performing the external control procedure is specified in the manufacturer's instructions accompanying the test system and usually includes:
   - When first receiving the test system
   - For periodic routine checking of analyzers, test strips, and reagents.
   - When a new lot number of test strips or reagents are used
   - When the test system does not seem to be working properly
   - When the test results do not seem to be accurate.
   - When the test components have been improperly stored
   - When an analyzer has been dropped or damaged.

COLLECTING THE SPECIMEN

The collection and handling requirements necessary for CLIA-waived testing are presented in the manufacturer's instructions that accompany the test system. General

ACCU-CHEK QUALITY CONTROL LOG High/low Level Controls			
Control Level	Lot Number	Expiration Date	Expected Range (mg/dL)
High Level Control	63330	11/29/XX	270 to 324
Low Level Control	42693	11/29/XX	18 to 64

Date	High Level Results (mg/dL)	Accept	Reject	Low Level Results (mg/dL)	Accept	Reject	Technician
2/9/XX	300	X		25	X		K. McGrew
2/10/XX	290	X		30	X		K. McGrew
2/11/XX	295	X		29	X		K. McGrew
2/12/XX	302	X		32	X		K. McGrew
2/13/XX	298	X		33	X		K. McGrew

Fig. 15.22 Quality control log.

guidelines for collecting and handling specimens include the following:

1. Use the appropriate collection device to collect the specimen. Do not substitute other devices.
2. Follow the manufacturer's instructions *exactly* for collecting and handling the specimen.
3. If a specimen (e.g., urine) cannot be tested immediately, the specimen should be stored according to the information provided in the manufacturer's instructions.

TESTING THE SPECIMEN

Guidelines for performing a CLIA-waived laboratory test include the following:

1. If more than one patient is being tested at a time, label each test device with the patient's name to prevent mix-up of specimens.
2. Follow the procedure in the manufacturer's instructions *exactly* for testing the specimen. Specific requirements may include the following:
   - Adding the proper amounts of reagents.
   - Adding reagents in the proper order.
   - Adhering to proper time intervals for various steps in the procedure.
   - Reading results within the proper time frame.

INTERPRETING AND READING THE TEST RESULTS

A laboratory tests can be either a qualitative test or a quantitative test. A **qualitative test** indicates whether or not a particular analyte is present in a specimen and also may provide an approximate indication of the amount of the analyte present. Most CLIA-waived test kits are qualitative tests. Qualitative tests are useful for screening purposes because they are easy to perform and can be used to screen large numbers of individuals—a procedure that otherwise might be too expensive and time-consuming.

Interpretation and reading of qualitative tests usually involve the use of a color comparison chart or a color diagram (Fig. 15.23). Qualitative test results are expressed in descriptive terms such as positive or negative; 1+, 2+, or 3+; reactive, weakly reactive, or nonreactive; and invalid. An invalid test result means there was a problem with the collection or testing of the specimen. In this case, the problem must be identified and resolved before the specimen can be retested. If the problem cannot be resolved, the manufacturer of the test should be contacted.

A **quantitative test** measures the exact amount of an analyte present in a specimen with the test results expressed in measurable units (e.g., mg/dL). CLIA-waived automated analyzers provide quantitative test results and the results are

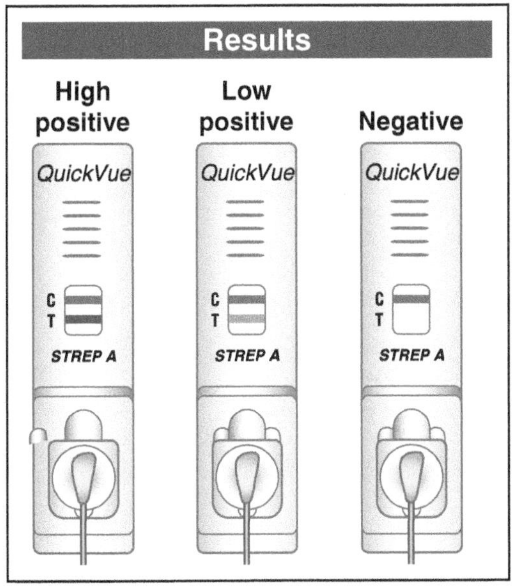

Fig. 15.23 Color diagram used to interpret test results.

printed out or displayed on the screen of the analyzer. No interpretation is required to read quantitative test results.

DOCUMENTING THE TEST RESULTS

Careful documentation is essential to avoid errors, which could affect the patient's diagnosis. Documentation of test results should include the following: the date and time, name of the test, and test results. Qualitative test results should be documented using words or abbreviations (e.g., positive, negative) and not symbols (e.g., +, −) because symbols can be accidentally changed or misinterpreted. Quantitative test results should be documented using the unit of measurement of the test system (e.g., mg/dL). The office may maintain a log of patient test results for each test performed in the POL. The log includes the name and reference range of the test, the date the test was performed, the patient's name and ID number, the test results with abnormal values flagged, and the name of the individual performing the test (Fig. 15.24).

ACCU-CHEK GLUCOSE TEST
Patient Test Results Log

Test Name: *Fasting blood glucose*

Reference Range: *70 to 110 mg/dL*

Date	Patient Name	Patient ID	FBG Test Results (mg/dL)	Flag	Technician
2/11/XX	Edward Stanton	1341	98		K. McGrew
2/11/XX	Danella Baldwin	3744	74		K. McGrew
2/12/XX	Tristen Westfall	6497	115	H	K. McGrew
2/12/XX	Amy Longstreet	5310	78		K. McGrew
2/12/XX	Andrew Johnson	2333	85		K. McGrew
2/13/XX	Benjamin Harris	1466	65	L	K. McGrew
2/13/XX	Thomas Jeffers	5399	102		K. McGrew
2/14/XX	John Adams	2512	92		K. McGrew
2/15/XX	James Grant	1788	88		K. McGrew
2/15/XX	John Tyler	3903	120	H	K. McGrew
2/16/XX	Franklin Hoover	4559	102		K. McGrew

Fig. 15.24 Patient test results log.

LABORATORY SAFETY

Laboratory safety is an important aspect of laboratory testing in the POL. Many of the laboratory tests performed in the POL involve the use of hazardous chemical reagents, the handling of specimens that may contain pathogens, and the use of laboratory equipment. Practicing good technique in testing specimens and recognizing potential hazards help to reduce accidents in the laboratory. Guidelines for laboratory safety in the POL are outlined here.

SPECIMEN COLLECTION AND TESTING

Follow the OSHA Bloodborne Pathogens Standard during the collection, handling, and testing of specimens. In the event of an exposure incident, perform first aid measures immediately and then report the incident to the provider so that medical treatment and postexposure prophylaxis (if needed) can be initiated.

1. Tie back or pin up long hair when working with specimens.
2. Cover any break in the skin, such as a cut or scratch, with a bandage.
3. Disinfect work counters before and after performing a laboratory test.
4. Wash hands immediately if any of the specimen is accidentally touched.
5. Avoid hand-to-mouth contact when working with specimens (e.g., eating, drinking, handling contact lenses, applying cosmetics).
6. Immediately clean up a specimen spilled on the work counter or floor, and thoroughly disinfect the area with an approved disinfectant.
7. Ensure that all specimen containers are tightly capped to prevent leakage.
8. Do not store food or beverages in refrigerators, freezers, and cabinets where specimens and testing supplies are stored.
9. Properly handle all laboratory equipment and supplies as indicated in the manufacturer's instructions. For example, wait until a centrifuge comes to a complete stop before opening it.
10. Properly dispose of medical waste in biohazard containers such as contaminated needles and syringes; used collection devices; and infectious waste.

HAZARDOUS CHEMICALS

Review the safety data sheet (SDS) before using a laboratory chemical reagent, to become familiar with its health hazards and measure to take to prevent injury and illness when handling the chemical reagent. The first aid measures to be taken if exposed to a hazardous chemical should also be reviewed.

1. Ensure that all reagent containers are clearly and properly labeled.
2. If a label is loose, reattach it immediately.
3. Recap reagent containers immediately after use to prevent spills.

What Would You Do? What Would You *Not* Do? RESPONSES

Case Study 1
Page 540

What Did Korey Do?

- ❑ Told Hans that the term *clinical diagnosis* means what the physician "thinks" is wrong before the laboratory tests are performed.
- ❑ Explained that when the test results are returned, the physician would be able to make a diagnosis, and then he would determine what treatment is needed.
- ❑ Told Hans that a lipid panel includes several tests, and one of those tests is a cholesterol test. Explained that the tests in a lipid panel all help to determine whether someone is at risk for heart disease.
- ❑ Told Hans that he could not have any coffee with cream and sugar until after his blood was drawn because it would affect the test results. Told him that his test could be scheduled first thing in the morning if that would help.

What Did Korey Not Do?

- ❑ Did not tell Hans he could have a cup of coffee before his blood was drawn.
- ❑ Did not tell Hans that he should not be eating doughnuts if he is concerned about his heart.

Case Study 2
Page 547

What Did Korey Do?

- ❑ Stressed to Kathleen that if the laboratory test results are abnormal, it is better to know so that the physician can help make her better.
- ❑ Told Kathleen that many patients feel the same way about having blood drawn, so she is not alone. Relayed to her that her fear is normal, and she has no reason to be embarrassed.
- ❑ Told Kathleen that she should tell the laboratory about her last experience so they can make it easier for her. Explained that they would probably put her in a reclining position to draw her blood so that she would not get lightheaded.
- ❑ Gave Kathleen some suggestions on how to relax during the venipuncture. Told her to breathe deeply and to turn her head when the blood is drawn.
- ❑ Asked Kathleen whether she had any additional symptoms.
- ❑ Checked with the physician to see whether he wanted to keep her appointment for today or have her appointment rescheduled after the laboratory tests are completed.

What Did Korey Not Do?

- ❑ Did not ignore or minimize Kathleen's concerns and fears.
- ❑ Did not tell Kathleen that her test results would probably be fine.

What Would You Do? What Would You *Not* Do? RESPONSES—cont'd

Case Study 3
Page 552

What Did Korey Do?

- ❑ Explained to Zachary that the physician cannot tell if he has strep throat by looking at his throat because there are other conditions that resemble strep throat and the only way to know for sure is to run a laboratory test.
- ❑ Told Zachary that there are certain tests that the federal government allows medical offices to perform without having to follow strict regulations and the rapid strep test is one of those tests.
- ❑ Explained to Zachary that the manufacturer's instructions for the strep test require that the test be performed on a specimen swabbed from the throat and using a different specimen would invalidate the test results.
- ❑ Explained to Zachary that it is important to first check with the physician before taking a prescription medication.
- ❑ Informed the physician that Zachary took an antibiotic before coming to the medical office, and documented this information in Zachary's medical record.
- ❑ Told Zachary that he does not need a paper prescription because the physician sent the prescription directly to his pharmacy using a computer.

What Did Korey Not Do?

- ❑ Did not scold Zachary for taking a "leftover" antibiotic that might possibly be outdated.
- ❑ Did not tell Zachary that he asks a lot of questions.

TERMINOLOGY REVIEW

Key Term	Definition
Analyte	A body substance that is being identified or measured by a laboratory test.
Calibration	A mechanism to check the precision and accuracy of an automated analyzer to determine if it is providing accurate test results. Calibration is typically performed using a calibration device, often called a *standard.*
CLIA-nonwaived test	A complex laboratory test that does not meet the criteria for waiver and is subject to the CLIA regulations.
CLIA-waived test	A laboratory test that meets the criteria for being a simple procedure that is easy to perform and has a low risk of erroneous test results.
Clinical diagnosis	A tentative diagnosis of a patient's condition obtained through an evaluation of the health history and the physical examination, without the benefit of laboratory or diagnostic tests.
Clinical laboratory	A facility in which tests are performed on biologic specimens to obtain information regarding the health of a patient.
Control	A solution that is used to monitor a test system to ensure reliable and accurate test results.
Critical value	A patient test result that is dangerously abnormal and is life-threating requiring immediate attention.
Fasting	Abstaining from food or fluids (except water) for a specified amount of time before the collection of a specimen.
Homeostasis	The state in which body systems are functioning normally and the internal environment of the body is in equilibrium; the body is in a healthy state.
Laboratory test	The clinical analysis and study of a body substance to obtain objective data for the diagnosis, treatment, and management of a patient's condition.
Package insert (laboratory test)	A printed document developed by the manufacturer of a laboratory test that provides detailed information on the use of the test and how to perform the test.
Panel	A combination of laboratory tests that have been determined to be the most sensitive and specific means of identifying a disease state or evaluating a particular organ or organ system.
Qualitative test	A test that indicates whether or not a particular analyte is present in a specimen and may also provide an approximate indication of the amount of the analyte present.
Quality control	The application of methods and means to ensure that test results are reliable and valid and that errors are detected and eliminated.
Quantitative test	A test that indicates the exact amount of an analyte that is present in a specimen, with the results being reported in measurable units.
Reagent	A chemical that reacts with a specimen to allow the detection or measurement of an analyte.

Continued

TERMINOLOGY REVIEW—cont'd

Key Term	Definition
Reference range	A certain established and acceptable range within which the laboratory test results of a healthy individual are expected to be.
Screening test (laboratory)	A laboratory test performed routinely on apparently healthy individuals to assist in the early detection of disease.
Serum	The clear, straw-colored part of the blood that remains after the solid elements and the clotting factor fibrinogen have been separated out of it.
Specimen (body)	A small sample taken from the body to represent the nature of the whole.
Test system	A setup that includes all of the test components required to perform a laboratory test such as testing devices, controls, and test reagents.
Unique identifier	Information directly associated with an individual that reliably identifies the individual as the person for whom the service or treatment is intended.

PROCEDURE 15.1 Operating an Emergency Eyewash Station

Outcome Operate and inspect an emergency eyewash station.

Equipment/Supplies

- Emergency eyewash station
- Disinfectant

Operate an Emergency Eyewash Station

1. **Procedural Step.** Immediately proceed to the emergency eyewash station after the eye(s) come in contact with a hazardous substance. Ask for assistance if needed.
2. **Procedural Step.** Activate the eyewash station using the activation lever. Once activated, the protective nozzle covers will automatically pop off the nozzle heads and water will begin to flow out of the nozzles. Once activated, the eyewash station remains operational for 15 min without requiring the use of the user's hands (or until it is manually turned off).
   Principle. The nozzle covers protect the nozzle heads from airborne contaminants.
3. **Procedural Step.** Hold both eyelids apart with your thumbs and forefingers to keep the eyes open.
   Principle. Most individuals respond to foreign substances in the eyes by closing their eyes tightly; therefore the eyes must be forcibly held open.

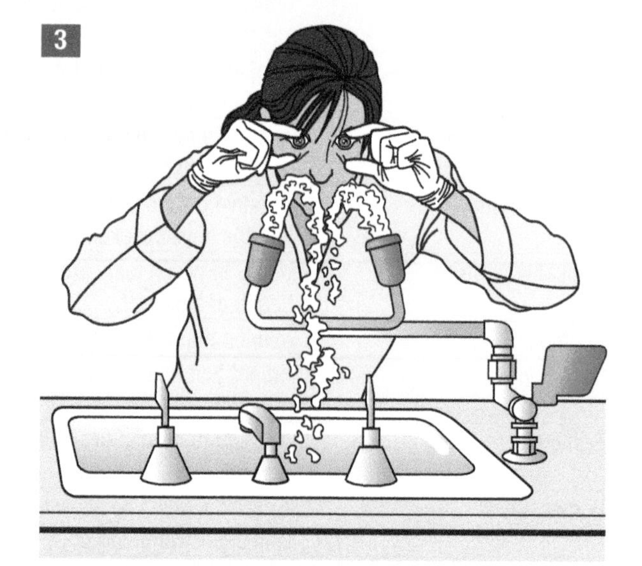

4. **Procedural Step.** Lower your eyes into the stream of water coming from the nozzles, and flush both eyes simultaneously.
5. **Procedural Step.** If necessary, gently remove contact lenses once the flushing process has begun. Flushing the eyes should not be delayed by removing the lenses before activating the eyewash station. However, in most cases, contact lenses are flushed out of the eyes by the water flow and do not need to be removed manually.

PROCEDURE 15.1 Operating an Emergency Eyewash Station—cont'd

Principle. Removing contact lenses prevents the hazardous substance from becoming trapped under the lens.

6. **Procedural Step.** Continue to hold the eyelids apart, and gently roll your eyeballs from left to right and up and down.
   Principle. Rolling the eyeballs makes sure the water is reaching all areas of the eye.
7. **Procedural Step.** Continue flushing for a full 15 min. If the irritation persists, repeat the flushing procedure.
   Principle: Fifteen minutes is the minimum amount of time it takes to sufficiently clear the eyes of harmful substances. Not flushing the eyes for the full 15 min may result in permanent damage to the eyes.
8. **Procedural Step.** Return the activation lever to its resting position to turn off the flow of water.
9. **Procedural Step.** Seek medical attention immediately to determine if further treatment is required.
10. **Procedural Step.** A staff member should clean, disinfect, rinse, and completely dry the eyewash device.

Inspect and Activate an Eyewash Station

Inspect and activate the eyewash station each week to ensure that it is operating properly and to flush out the water supply lines.

1. **Procedural Step.** Make sure the access route to the eyewash station is well-lit and free of obstructions.
2. **Procedural Step.** Make sure the eyewash station is well-lit and the area around the eyewash station is free of clutter.
   Principle. This avoids unnecessary delay in activating the eyewash station.
3. **Procedural Step.** Make sure the protective nozzle covers are in place and in good condition.
   Principle. The covers protect the nozzle heads from airborne contaminants.
4. **Procedural Step.** Make sure the eyewash bowl is clean and free of debris.
5. **Procedural Step.** Activate the eyewash device using the activation lever. The water flow from the nozzles should occur in one second or less following activation of the eyewash.
6. **Procedural Step.** Make sure the protective nozzle covers come off automatically when the eyewash device is activated.
7. **Procedural Step.** Activate the eyewash station for at least 3 min.
   Principle. Activation of the eyewash station flushes out sediment, debris, or bacteria from the water supply lines.
8. **Procedural Step.** Make sure the water flows continuously (once activated) without the use of the hands.
9. **Procedural Step.** Make sure that the nozzle heads are not clogged and that water flows equally from both nozzle heads.
10. **Procedural Step.** Return the activation lever to its resting position to turn off the flow of water.
11. **Procedural Step.** Clean, disinfect, rinse, and completely dry the eyewash device, including the nozzle heads and protective covers.
12. **Procedural Step.** Replace the nozzle covers on the nozzle heads.
13. **Procedural Step.** Report any problems to the appropriate personnel.
14. **Procedural Step.** Document the inspection date and your initials on either an eyewash inspection log sheet or an eyewash inspection tag that is attached to the device

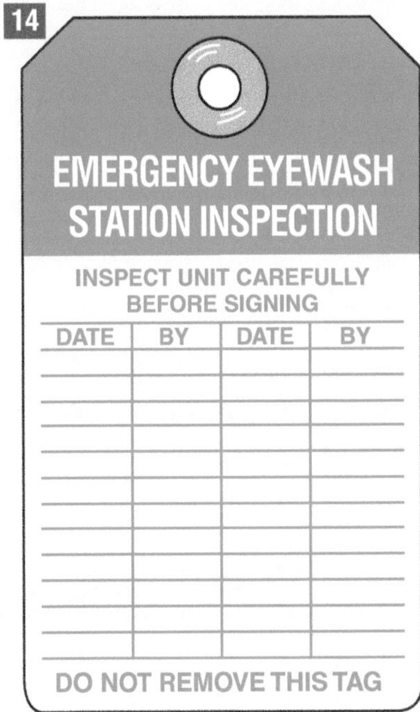

Emergency eyewash station inspection tag.

Urinalysis

 Check out the Evolve site at http://evolve.elsevier.com/Bonewit/today/ to access additional interactive activities and exercises to help you study and prepare for success.

LEARNING OUTCOMES	PROCEDURES
Urinary System	
1. Describe the structures that make up the urinary system, and state the function of each.	
2. List conditions that may cause polyuria and oliguria.	
3. List and define the terms used to describe symptoms of the urinary system.	
Collection of Urine	
4. Explain why a first-voided morning specimen is often preferred for urinalysis.	Instruct a patient in the collection of a clean-catch midstream urine specimen.
5. Explain the purpose of collecting a clean-catch midstream specimen and a first-catch urine specimen.	Instruct a patient in the collection of a 24-hour urine specimen.
6. Explain the purpose of a 24-hour urine specimen.	
7. List changes that may occur if urine is allowed to remain standing for longer than 1 hour.	
Urinalysis	
8. List factors that may cause urine to have an unusual color or become cloudy.	Assess the color and appearance of a urine specimen. Perform a chemical assessment of a urine specimen using a Clinical Laboratory Improvement Amendments (CLIA)-waived reagent strip.
9. Identify the various tests that are included in the physical and chemical examination of urine.	Prepare a urine specimen for microscopic examination by the provider.
10. List the structures that may be found in a microscopic examination of urine.	
Urine Pregnancy Testing	
11. Explain the basis for urine pregnancy tests.	Perform a CLIA-waived urine pregnancy test.
12. List the guidelines that must be followed in a urine pregnancy test to ensure accurate test results.	

CHAPTER OUTLINE

KEY TERMS

anuria (ah-NOOR-ee-ah)
bilirubinuria (bill-ih-roo-bin-YUR-ee-ah)
bladder catheterization
diuresis (di-ah-REE-sis)
dysuria (dis-YUR-ee-ah)
frequency
glycosuria (glie-koe-SOO-ree-ah)
hematuria (hem-ah-TOOR-ee-ah)
ketonuria (kee-toe-NOO-ree-ah)
ketosis (kee-TOE-sis)
micturition (mik-tur-ISH-un)
nephron (NEF-ron)
nocturia (nok-TOOR-ee-ah)
nocturnal enuresis (nok-TOOR-nal en-YUR-ee-sis)
oliguria (oh-lig-YUR-ee-ah)
pH (PEE-AYCH)
polyuria (pol-ee-YUR-ee-ah)
proteinuria (proe-teen-YUR-ee-ah)
pyuria (pi-YUR-ee-ah)
renal threshold (REE-nul THRESH-hold)
retention
specific gravity
supernatant (soo-per-NAY-tent)
suprapubic aspiration
urgency
urinalysis (yur-in-AL-ih-sis)
urinary incontinence

STRUCTURE AND FUNCTION OF THE URINARY SYSTEM

The function of the urinary system is to regulate the fluid and electrolyte balance of the body and to remove waste products. The urinary system consists of the kidneys, ureters, urinary bladder, and urethra (Fig. 16.1). The *kidneys* are bean-shaped organs approximately 4.5 inches (11.5 cm) long and 2 to 3 inches (5 to 8 cm) wide; they are located in the lumbar region of the body. Urine drains from the kidneys into the urinary bladder through two tubes known as *ureters.* Each ureter is approximately 10 to 12 inches long and (½) inch in diameter. The urine produced by the kidneys is propelled into the urinary bladder by the force of gravity and the peristaltic waves of the ureters. The *urinary bladder* is a hollow, muscular sac that can hold approximately 500 mL of urine. Its function is to store and expel urine. The *urethra* is a tube that extends from the urinary bladder to the outside of the body. The *urinary meatus* is the external opening of the urethra. In males, the urethra functions in transporting urine and reproductive secretions. In females, the urethra functions in urination only.

Each kidney contains approximately 1 million smaller units known as **nephrons** (Fig. 16.2). The nephron is the functional unit of the kidney. It filters waste substances from the blood and dilutes them with water to produce urine. Another function of the nephron is reabsorption. Some substances filtered by the nephron, such as water, glucose, and electrolytes, are needed by the body and are reabsorbed or returned to the body for future use.

COMPOSITION OF URINE

A physiologic change in the body caused by disease may create a disturbance in one or more of the functions of the kidney. Detection of such a disturbance can be made with the examination of urine and other body fluids such as blood.

Urine is composed of 95% water and 5% organic and inorganic waste products. Organic waste products consist of urea, uric acid, ammonia, and creatinine. Urea is present in the greatest amounts and is derived from the breakdown of proteins. Inorganic waste products include chloride, sodium, potassium, calcium, magnesium, phosphate, and sulfate.

A normal adult excretes approximately 750 to 2000 mL of urine per day. This amount varies according to the amount of fluid consumed and the amount of fluid lost through other means, such as perspiration, feces, and water vapor from the lungs. An excessive increase in urine output is known as **polyuria,** with the urine volume exceeding 2000 mL in 24 hours. Polyuria may be caused by the excessive intake of fluids or the intake of fluids that contain caffeine (e.g., coffee, tea, cola), which is a mild diuretic. Certain drugs, such as diuretics, and the pathologic conditions of diabetes mellitus, diabetes insipidus, and renal disease also may result in polyuria. Decreased or scanty urine output is known as **oliguria.** In the case of oliguria, the urine volume is less than 400 mL in 24 hours. Oliguria may occur with decreased fluid intake, dehydration, profuse perspiration, vomiting, diarrhea, or kidney disease. The normal act of voiding urine is known as **micturition.**

TERMS RELATED TO THE URINARY SYSTEM

The medical assistant should have a thorough knowledge of the following terms used to describe symptoms associated with the urinary system:

Anuria Failure of the kidneys to produce urine
Diuresis Secretion and passage of large amounts of urine
Dysuria Difficult or painful urination
Frequency The condition of having to urinate often
Hematuria Blood present in the urine
Nocturia Excessive (voluntary) urination during the night

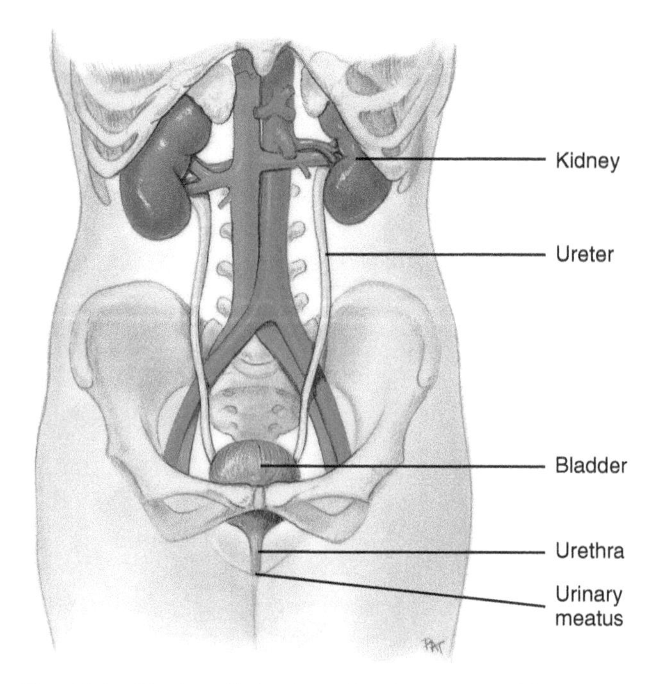

Fig. 16.1 Structures that make up the urinary system. (Modified from Applegate EJ: *The anatomy and physiology learning system*, ed 4, St Louis: Elsevier; 2011.)

Nocturnal enuresis Inability of an individual to control urination at night during sleep (bedwetting)
Oliguria Decreased output of urine
Polyuria Increased output of urine
Pyuria Pus present in the urine
Retention The inability to empty the bladder. The urine is being produced normally but is not being voided
Urgency The immediate need to urinate
Urinary incontinence The inability to retain urine

COLLECTION OF URINE

The advantages of urine testing are that urine is readily available and obtaining it does not require an invasive procedure or the use of special equipment. For accurate test results, the medical assistant must adhere to proper urine collection procedures to obtain the correct specimen for the type of test being performed.

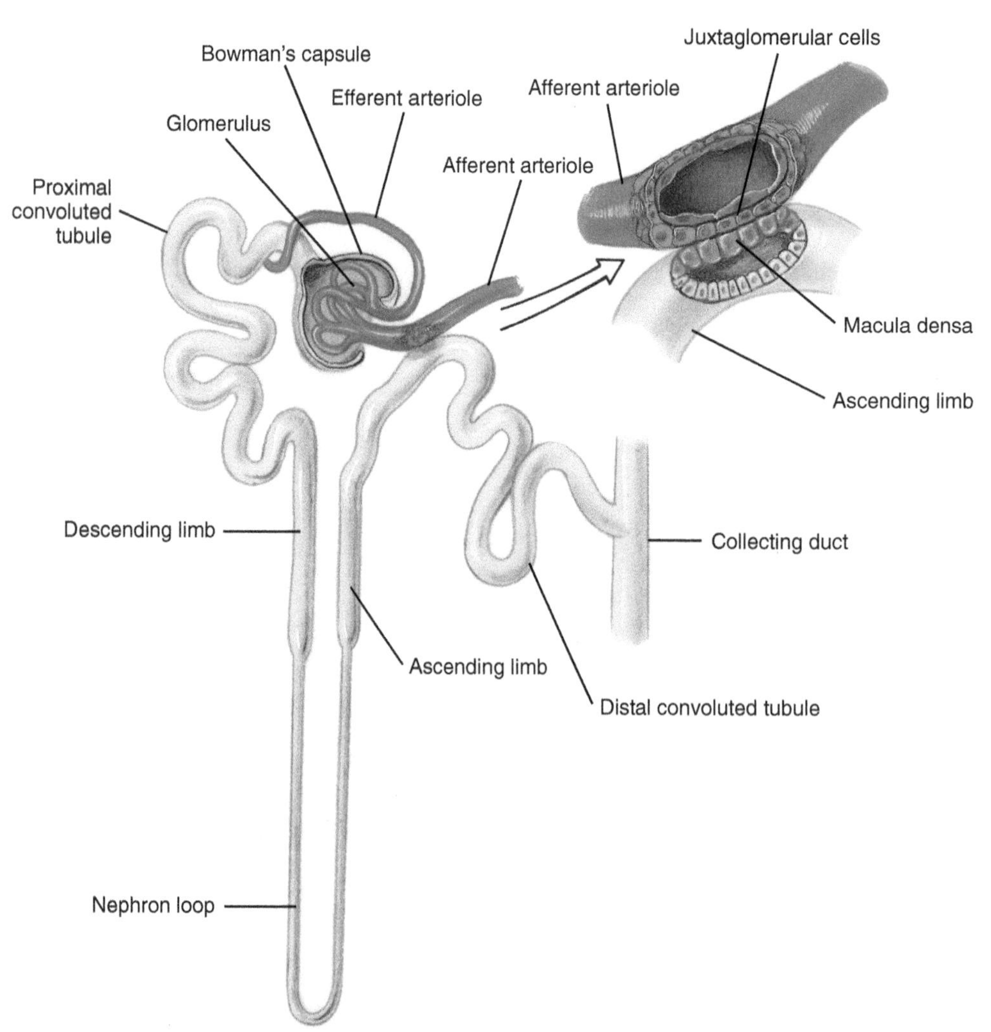

Fig. 16.2 Nephron. (From Applegate EJ: *The anatomy and physiology learning system*, ed 4, St Louis: Elsevier; 2011.)

GUIDELINES FOR URINE COLLECTION

The following guidelines should be followed in the collection of a urine specimen:

1. Make sure to obtain an adequate volume of urine as necessary for the type of test being performed (usually 30 to 50 mL of urine).
2. Each specimen must be labeled properly with the patient's full name and date of birth, the date and time of collection, and the type of specimen (i.e., urine).
3. Medications being taken by the patient that may affect the test results should be documented on the laboratory request and in the patient's medical record.
4. If possible, the collection of a urine specimen should be avoided in women during menstruation and for several days thereafter because the specimen may become contaminated with blood. This results in a false-positive test result for blood in the urine.
5. Take into consideration that voiding may be difficult for patients under stress and anxiety. In these instances, understanding and patience should be conveyed to the patient.
6. A urine specimen may be difficult to obtain from a child, even with the assistance of a parent. In this case, the provider should be informed because another collection method may be used, such as a urine collection bag, suprapubic aspiration, or catheterization of the patient.

COLLECTION METHODS

The type of test to be performed on the urine dictates the method used to collect the urine specimen. A first-voided morning specimen is recommended for pregnancy testing, and a clean-catch midstream specimen is necessary for identification of the presence of a urinary tract infection (UTI).

What Would You Do? What Would You *Not* Do?

Case Study 1

Yusuke Urameshi is at the office with fever and chills, urinary frequency, and painful and difficult urination. The physician suspects that Mr. Urameshi has prostatitis and orders a clean-catch urine specimen for a complete urinalysis, including a microscopic examination of the urine sediment. Mr. Urameshi tries to collect the specimen but is able to collect only 5 mL of urine. He says that he is worried about what is wrong with him and he thinks his nervousness is making it hard to get a specimen. Mr. Urameshi says that it is probably just as well because he did not understand how to cleanse himself, and he is not sure that he did it correctly. ■

Most offices use disposable plastic urine specimen containers. These containers are available in different sizes and come with screw-on lids to prevent spillage and to reduce bacterial and other types of contamination.

Random Specimen

Urine testing in the medical office is often performed on freshly voided, random specimens. The medical assistant instructs the patient to void into a clean, dry, wide-mouthed container, and the urine is tested immediately at the medical office.

First-Voided Morning Specimen

In many cases a first-voided morning specimen may be desired for testing because it contains the greatest concentration of dissolved substances, and a small amount of an abnormal substance that is present would be more easily detected. The patient should be instructed to collect the first specimen of the morning after rising and to preserve the specimen by refrigerating it until it is brought to the medical office. It is important to provide the patient with a specimen container to prevent the patient's use of a container from home that might harbor contaminants and affect the test results.

Clean-Catch Midstream Specimen

The urinary bladder and most of the urethra are normally free of microorganisms, whereas the distal urethra and the urinary meatus normally harbor microorganisms. If the urine is being cultured and examined for bacteria, a clean-catch midstream specimen is necessary to prevent contamination of the specimen with these normally present microorganisms. Only microorganisms that may be causing the patient's condition are desired in the urine specimen. A clean-catch midstream collection may be ordered for the detection of a UTI or for the evaluation of the effectiveness of drug therapy in a patient undergoing treatment for such an infection.

The purpose of a clean-catch midstream collection is to remove microorganisms from the urinary meatus and the distal urethra. This is accomplished by instructing the patient to thoroughly cleanse the area surrounding the meatus and to void a small amount of urine into the toilet, which flushes out microorganisms in the distal urethra. The urine specimen is collected in a sterile container using medically aseptic techniques. A properly collected specimen reduces the possibility of having to perform a bladder catheterization or a suprapubic aspiration of the bladder. **Bladder catheterization** involves the passing of a sterile tube (the catheter) through the urethra and into the bladder to remove urine. **Suprapubic aspiration** involves the passing of a sterile needle through the abdominal wall into the bladder to remove urine. Both of these procedures must be performed using sterile technique.

Guidelines

Guidelines that should be followed when collecting a clean-catch midstream specimen are as follows:

1. A clean-catch midstream specimen is collected by the patient at the medical office. The medical assistant must provide complete instructions for collection of this specimen. Failure to instruct the patient adequately may necessitate a return to the medical office for the collection of another specimen because of bacterial contamination. Patient instructions for obtaining a clean-catch midstream specimen are presented in Procedure 16.1.
2. If the specimen is to be tested at an outside laboratory, a laboratory request must be completed.
3. The container must be labeled with the patient's name and date of birth, the date, the time of collection, and the type of specimen (clean-catch midstream urine specimen).
4. For reliable test results, the specimen should be tested immediately and should not be allowed to stand. If this is not possible, the specimen should be refrigerated or a preservative should be added to it.
5. The procedure should be documented in the patient's medical record. The information to be documented for a specimen tested at the medical office includes the date and time, the type of specimen collected, and the laboratory test results. If the specimen is being transported to an outside laboratory for testing, document the date and time of the specimen collection, the type of specimen collected, and the date the specimen was transported to the laboratory.

FIRST-CATCH URINE SPECIMEN

A first-catch urine specimen can be used to test for the presence of chlamydia and gonorrhea using a nucleic acid amplification (NAA) test. (Refer to Chapter 8 for more information on chlamydia and gonorrhea and the NAA test.) To obtain a first-catch urine specimen, the patient should not urinate for at least 1 hour prior to the collection of the urine specimen. The patient should not cleanse the genital area before collecting the specimen because this results in the removal of pathogens from the area, which could lead to false-negative test results. The patient should be instructed to collect only 15 to 30 mL (1 to 2 tablespoons) of the initial urine stream in the specimen container. If more than 30 mL of urine is collected, the patient must start the procedure over again. The first 15 to 30 mL of urine voided by the patient contains the greatest concentration of chlamydia and/or gonorrhea bacteria, resulting in a greater likelihood that the NAA test will detect the presence of these pathogens. Collection of more than 30 mL of urine results in dilution of the specimen, which may affect the accuracy of the test results.

Following collection of the specimen, the medical assistant is responsible for transferring 2 mL of the urine specimen to a transport tube using a disposable pipette. The specimen should then be placed in a biohazard specimen bag and stored in the refrigerator for pick-up by a courier from an outside laboratory.

TWENTY-FOUR–HOUR URINE SPECIMEN

A 24-hour urine specimen is used for the quantitative measurement of specific urinary components. Collecting urine over a 24-hour period provides greater accuracy in the measurement of urinary components than with a random specimen. This is because body metabolism, exercise, and hydration can affect the excretion rate of substances in the urine. Examples of substances measured in a 24-hour specimen include calcium, cortisol, lead, potassium, protein, and urea nitrogen. A 24-hour specimen is often used in the diagnosis of the cause of kidney stone formation and in the control and prevention of new stone formation. It may also be used to perform a creatinine clearance test, which provides information on kidney function.

A large wide-mouthed container (3000 mL) is used to store the urine collected over the 24-hour period. To prevent changes in the quality of the urine specimen, the specimen must be kept refrigerated or placed in an ice chest. Some containers also contain a chemical preservative (in the form of crystals, tablets, or a liquid) to assist in maintaining the quality of the specimen. Examples of urine preservatives include hydrochloric acid, boric acid, acetic acid, and toluene. A hazardous chemical warning label should be attached to a specimen container with a preservative, and the patient should be instructed not to discard or touch the preservative in the container.

The patient is provided with a smaller container to collect each urine specimen. A female patient may be given a urine "hat," which is placed under the seat of the commode, and a male patient is often provided with a collection cup. After collection, the urine is poured into the large specimen container. This method makes collection easier and safer for the patient. If the patient voids urine directly into a specimen container that holds a preservative, the preservative could splash onto the patient's skin, resulting in a chemical burn.

The medical assistant should provide the patient with verbal and written instructions for collection of the urine specimen. The patient should be advised to drink a normal amount of fluid during the collection period and to avoid alcohol intake for 24 hours before and during the collection period. The patient should be instructed to choose a 24-hour period when he or she will be at home, so that the urine container will not have to be transported. The test should not be performed when the patient is menstruating. Because certain medications, such as thiazides, phosphorus-binding antacids, allopurinol, and vitamin C, can alter the test results, the provider usually requires the patient to discontinue any of these medications being taken by the patient for 1 week before the test. The procedure for instructing a patient in the collection of a 24-hour urine specimen is presented in Procedure 16.2.

URINALYSIS

Urinalysis is the analysis of urine and is the laboratory test most commonly performed in the medical office because a urine specimen is readily obtainable and can be easily tested. Urinalysis consists of a *physical, chemical,* and *microscopic examination* of urine. Deviation from normal in any of the three areas assists the provider in the diagnosis and treatment of pathologic conditions, not only of the urinary system but also of other body systems. Urinalysis may be performed as a screening measure as part of a routine health examination or to assist in the diagnosis of a pathologic condition. It also may assist in the evaluation of effectiveness of therapy after treatment has been initiated for a pathologic condition.

Urinalysis should be performed on a fresh or preserved specimen. If a specimen cannot be examined within 1 hour of voiding, it should be preserved at once in the refrigerator in a closed container and later returned to room temperature and mixed before testing. Chemical additives can be used to preserve urine specimens but are typically only used with specimens that require prolonged storage.

If the urine is allowed to stand at room temperature for longer than 1 hour, the following changes may occur:

1. Bacteria in the environment that get into the specimen work on urea present in the urine, converting it to ammonia. Because ammonia is alkaline, acid urine becomes alkaline which increases the pH of the urine. An alkaline pH may result in a false-positive result on the protein test.
2. Bacteria multiply rapidly in the urine, resulting in a cloudy specimen and an increase in the nitrite.
3. If glucose is present in the specimen, it decreases in amount because microorganisms use the glucose as a source of food.
4. Any red or white blood cells present in the urine may break down.
5. Casts decompose after several hours.

PHYSICAL EXAMINATION OF URINE

The physical examination of urine includes a determination of the color, appearance, and specific gravity of the urine. The color and appearance of the urine specimen may be evaluated during the preparation of the urine for another test, such as the chemical testing of the urine. For an accurate evaluation of the color and appearance, the urine specimen must be collected in a clear plastic container.

Color

The normal color of urine ranges from almost colorless to dark yellow. Dilute urine tends to be lighter yellow in color, whereas concentrated urine contains more dissolved substances causing it to be a darker yellow. A first-voided morning specimen is usually the most concentrated because consumption of fluids is decreased during the night. Urine becomes more dilute as the day progresses as more fluids are consumed.

The color of the urine is the result of the presence of a yellow pigment known as *urochrome,* produced by the breakdown of hemoglobin. It is common for the color of urine to vary among different shades of yellow within the course of a day. Classifications that can be used to describe the color of urine include light yellow, yellow, dark yellow, amber, and dark amber (Fig. 16.3).

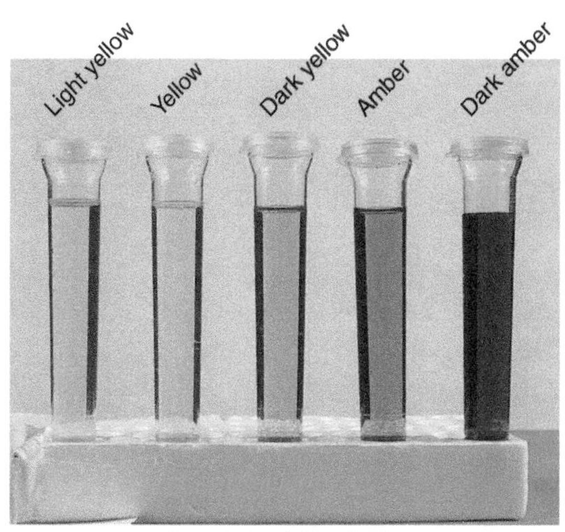

Fig. 16.3 Color of urine.

An abnormal urine color assists in determining additional tests that may be necessary. Abnormal colors may be caused by the presence of hemoglobin or blood (resulting in a red or reddish color), bile pigments (resulting in a yellow-brown or greenish color), and fat droplets or pus (resulting in a milky color). Some foods and medications also may cause the urine to change to an abnormal color. Phenazopyridine (Pyridium), a urinary tract analgesic, causes the urine to change to an orange to red color.

Appearance

Evaluation of the appearance of urine is usually performed at the same time as the color evaluation. Fresh urine is usually clear, or transparent, but becomes cloudy if left standing out too long. Cloudiness in a freshly voided specimen may be the result of the presence of bacteria, pus, blood, fat, yeast, sperm, mucous threads, or fecal contaminants. A microscopic examination of the urine sediment is usually performed on all cloudy specimens to determine the cause of the cloudiness. Cloudiness resulting from bacteria may be caused by a UTI.

Classifications used to describe the appearance of urine include clear, slightly cloudy, cloudy, and very cloudy (Fig. 16.4). The medical assistant should develop skill in recognizing the varying degrees of urine clarity.

Odor

Freshly voided urine normally should have a slightly aromatic odor. Urine left standing out for a long time develops an ammonia odor from the breakdown of urea by bacteria in the specimen. The urine of a patient with diabetes mellitus may have a fruity odor from the presence of ketone. The urine of a patient with a UTI is usually foul smelling, and the odor becomes worse on standing. Certain foods, such as asparagus, can cause the urine to have a musty smell. Although urine may have many characteristic odors, as a rule the odor of urine is not typically used in the diagnosis of a patient's condition.

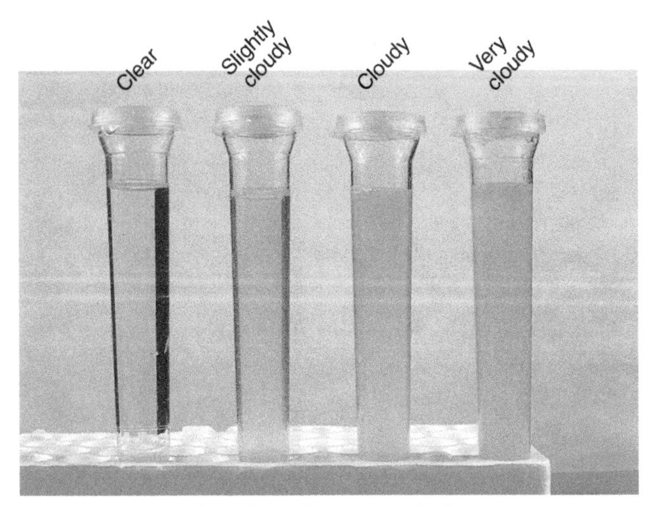

Fig. 16.4 Appearance of urine.

Specific Gravity

The **specific gravity** of urine measures the weight of the urine compared with the weight of an equal volume of distilled water. Specific gravity indicates the amount of dissolved substances present in the urine, providing information on the ability of the kidneys to dilute or concentrate the urine. Specific gravity is decreased in conditions in which the kidneys cannot concentrate the urine, such as chronic renal insufficiency, diabetes insipidus, and malignant hypertension. The specific gravity is increased in patients with adrenal insufficiency, congestive heart failure, hepatic disease, diabetes mellitus with glycosuria, and conditions that cause dehydration, such as fever, vomiting, and diarrhea.

The normal specific gravity of urine ranges from 1.005 to 1.030 but is usually between 1.010 and 1.025 (the specific gravity of distilled water is 1.000). Specific gravity varies greatly with fluid intake and the state of hydration of an individual. Dilute urine contains fewer dissolved substances and has a lower specific gravity. Concentrated urine has a higher specific gravity because of the increased amount of dissolved substances. In general, a urine specimen is more concentrated in the morning and becomes more dilute after fluid consumption.

In the medical office, specific gravity is most commonly measured using a reagent strip. This involves a color comparison determination with a reagent strip that includes a reagent pad for specific gravity. The reagent strip is dipped into the urine specimen, and the results are compared with a color chart (Procedure 16.3).

What Would You Do? What Would You *Not* Do?

Case Study 2

Nora Sheridan is at the clinic complaining of urinary frequency, urgency, dysuria, and blood in her urine. During the past 6 months, Nora has been having problems with UTIs. She wants to know why these infections continue to occur and whether she can do anything to prevent them. Nora says that she has a lot of deadlines at work and that it is difficult to find time to come to the medical office. She says that her drugstore sells urine testing strips. Nora wants to know whether she could get a container of the strips and test her urine at home when she is having problems. That way she could just contact the office when she has positive test results, and the physician could call in a prescription for an antibiotic for her. ■

Putting It All Into Practice

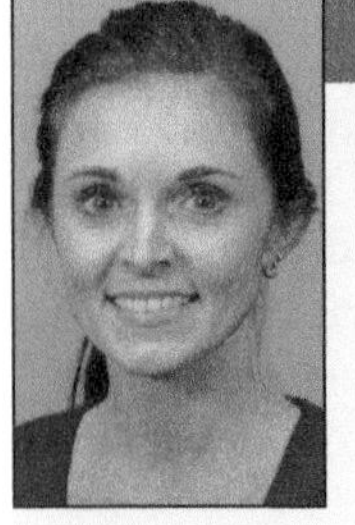

My name is Kayla, and I work for a urologist and his wife, who is a pediatrician. I work primarily in the urology practice and only occasionally in pediatrics. I am responsible for having the medical records ready when the patients are seen and for doing their urinalysis. Another one of my responsibilities is to assist with special procedures, such as catheter insertions, male and female dilations, ultrasound examinations of the bladder, and prostate examinations.

When I first started working in the urology office, I had to learn to assist with transrectal ultrasounds of the prostate in case the ultrasound technician was sick. When she retired, I inherited the position. At first, I dreaded doing the procedures and would be so nervous that I would get the shakes and forget the order in which things were supposed to be done. My physician was understanding and would help by talking me through it. I think the reason I was so nervous was that sometimes patients have trouble and we have to administer oxygen and run intravenous lines. One time, a patient had a reaction to the sedative we gave before the procedure. Time, practice, and confidence in myself have improved my nerves, even with the occasional emergency situation. ■

HIGHLIGHT on Drug Testing in the Workplace

Statistics

Statistics suggest that the problem of drug abuse is growing in the workplace. On any 1 day, 8.9–16 million employees are estimated to be working under the influence of drugs. The effects of on-the-job drug use extend into every segment of the population and touch every business and industry. The US Department of Labor estimates that 65% of all work-related accidents can be traced to substance abuse. According to the National Council on Alcoholism

HIGHLIGHT on Drug Testing in the Workplace—cont'd

and Drug Dependence (NCADD), drug abuse costs industry $81 billion annually because of accidents, high employee turnover, absenteeism, lost productivity, workplace theft, and higher health care costs.

Drug Testing Programs

Because of these economic and safety factors, businesses across the United States are adopting a less permissive attitude toward drug use and are requiring compulsory drug testing in the workplace. Approximately one half of US employers have implemented drug-testing programs in the workplace. These employers include utility companies, transportation operations, construction companies, sports associations, and governmental agencies. Currently, many companies test blue-collar and white-collar employees for drug use. Companies with drug-testing programs report a significant reduction in employee accidents, fewer sick days, and healthier employees.

A comprehensive drug-testing program includes the detection of drug use in the workplace, policies to discourage further abuse, and the referral of employees for treatment and rehabilitation. Drug testing may be performed for one or more of the following purposes: (1) preemployment drug screening, (2) testing for probable cause after unexplained behavior or an incident (e.g., an accident on the job), and (3) random sample testing of the workforce to detect use of controlled substances by employees on the job.

Drug Testing Methods

Blood testing is the best means for determining precise information concerning the amount of drug used and when the drug was taken. However, blood tests are costly and time-consuming to perform. Urine drug testing offers the next best alternative; it is noninvasive and technically easier and less expensive to perform. Current urine screening tests target the most common drugs of abuse: alcohol, amphetamines, barbiturates, benzodiazepines, cocaine, marijuana, opioids, phencyclidine (PCP), and methadone. Clinical Laboratory Improvement Amendments (CLIA)-waived urine drug-testing kits are available for testing the specimen in the medical office. These kits provide immediate results and take only a few minutes to perform.

Chain of Custody

The usual procedure for urine drug testing involves screening the specimen and confirming positive results with more-specific urine tests. The specimen may be collected at the workplace, at the medical office, or at an outside laboratory. To help ensure reliable and valid drug-testing results, a security system or "chain of custody" must be followed in the collection and handling of the specimen. This includes ensuring the identification of the individual undergoing drug testing, taking precautions to avoid falsification of or tampering with specimens, properly labeling the urine specimen, sealing the specimen container after collection, and immediately sending the specimen to an outside laboratory for analysis or refrigerating it if there is a delay in transport.

Disadvantages

The main disadvantage of urine drug testing is that a positive test result indicates only the presence of a drug in the urine; it does not provide any information as to when the drug was taken. Drugs that are detected in the urine may or may not still be present in the blood, where they can affect an individual's behavior and impair performance. A positive urine test result does not reveal whether an individual is impaired by drugs. In addition, the initial urine screening tests are sometimes unreliable; unless positive results are confirmed with a more specific test, an individual may be unjustly accused of drug use. These factors and the violation of an individual's right to privacy are the main areas of dispute for individuals who oppose drug testing in the workplace.

Intervention

Companies with drug-testing programs have various options when results are positive, such as recommendations for drug treatment programs or disciplinary action. Many companies have established in-house employee assistance programs that include counseling and drug withdrawal therapy for employees who desire help. Most companies prefer to help current employees with rehabilitation instead of discharging them and hiring and training new employees. Studies show a 35%–60% recovery rate for employees enrolled in drug treatment programs. ■

CHEMICAL EXAMINATION OF URINE

The chemical examination of urine is used to assist in the evaluation and diagnosis of kidney function, UTI, carbohydrate metabolism (diabetes mellitus), and liver function. Substances present in excessive (abnormal) amounts in the blood are usually removed by the urine. For example, glucose is normally present in the blood, but if it exceeds a certain level or threshold, the excess amount is excreted in the urine. Chemical testing of urine is an indirect means of detecting abnormal amounts of chemicals in the body, indicating a pathologic condition. The chemical examination of urine also can be used to detect the presence of substances that, in the absence of disease, do not normally appear in the urine, such as blood and nitrite.

Chemical tests that are routinely performed during a urinalysis include testing for pH, glucose, protein, and ketone. Other chemical tests that may be performed include testing for blood, bilirubin, urobilinogen, nitrite, and leukocytes. The urine chemical test parameters and the diagnoses they assist with are outlined in Table 16.1. A computer-generated laboratory report for a complete urinalysis is illustrated in Fig. 16.5.

pH

The **pH** is the unit that indicates the acidity or alkalinity of a solution. The pH scale ranges from 0.0 to 14.0. The lower the number, the greater the acidity; the higher the number, the greater the alkalinity. A pH reading of 7.0 is neutral; a

Table 16.1 Urine Chemical Parameters and the Diagnoses They Assist

System/ Source	Leukocytes	Nitrite	Urine pH	Protein	Glucose	Ketone	Urobilinogen	Bilirubin	Blood, Erythrocytes (Hematuria)	Hemoglobin
Genitourinary	Renal infection or inflammation • Acute/chronic pyelonephritis • Glomerulonephritis • Urolithiasis • Tumors • Lower urinary tract infection (cystitis, urethritis, prostatitis)	Bacteriuria • Urinary tract infection (cystitis, urethritis, prostatitis, pyelonephritis)	Up (greater than 6) in: • Renal failure • Bacterial infection (e.g., *Proteus* bacteriuria) • Renal tubular acidosis	Renal, glomerular, or tubular disease • Glomerulonephritis • Glomerulosclerosis (e.g., in diabetes) • Nephrotic syndrome • Pyelonephritis • Renal tuberculosis	Renal glycosuria (e.g., during pregnancy) Renal tubular disease (e.g., in Fanconi syndrome) Decreased renal glucose threshold (e.g., in old age)				Renal infection, inflammation, or injury • Renal tuberculosis • Renal infarction • Calculi (urethral, renal) • Polycystic kidneys • Tumors (bladder, renal pelvis, prostate) • Salpingitis • Cystitis	Renal intravascular Hemolysis Acute glomerulonephritis
Hepatobiliary							Liver cell damage Chronic liver stasis Cirrhosis Dubin-Johnson syndrome ***Note:*** May be 0 or down in biliary obstruction	Biliary dysfunction • Gallstones Obstructive jaundice Hepatitis (viral toxic) Dubin-Johnson syndrome	Cirrhosis	
Gastrointestinal			Up in: • Pyloric obstruction			Vomiting Diarrhea	***Note:*** May be negative with inhibition of intestinal flora by antimicrobial agents		Colon tumor Diverticulitis	
Cardiovascular				Congestive heart failure	Myocardial infarction				Bacterial endocarditis	
Hormonal, metabolic, and other systems			Up in: • Alkalosis (metabolic, respiratory)	Gout Hypokalemia Preeclampsia Severe febrile infection	Diabetes mellitus Hemochromatosis Hyperthyroidism Cushing's syndrome Pheochromocytomas	Diabetic ketosis Glycogen storage disease Preeclampsia Acute fever	Sickle cell anemia Hemolytic disease • Pernicious anemia Leptospirosis	Hemolytic disease Leptospirosis	Blood dyscrasias • Hemophilia • Thrombocytopenia • Sickle cell anemia Disseminated lupus erythematosus Malignant hypertension	Hemolytic disease Plasmodium (malaria) Clostridium (tetanus)
Environmental (diet, drugs, stress)	Phenacetin-induced nephritis		Up in: • Diet high in vegetables, citrus fruits • Alkalizing drug use (sodium bicarbonate, acetazolamide)	Nephrotoxic drugs	Sudden shock or pain Steroid therapy	Weight-reducing diet Ketogenic diet (e.g., in anticonvulsant therapy) Starvation			Hemorrhagic drugs (e.g., anticoagulant, salicylate) Nephrotoxic agents Internal injury or foreign body Vitamin C or K deficiency	Overexertion Exposure to cold Incompatible blood transfusion Drug-induced hemolysis

Note: Reagent strip detection of abnormal urine constituent or concentration characteristic of disease (e.g., glycosuria in diabetes mellitus) may provide useful screen or monitor but requires confirmation with other laboratory and clinical evidence.

Courtesy Boehringer-Mannheim Diagnostics, Indianapolis, IN.

Data from Conn HF, Conn RB, editors: *Current diagnosis*, ed 5, Philadelphia, 1977, WB Saunders; Davidson I, Henry JB, editors: *Todd-Stanford clinical diagnosis by laboratory methods*, ed 15, Philadelphia, 1974, WB Saunders; Rap[illegible] SS, et al: *Lynch's medical laboratory* [illegible]*logy*, ed 3, Philadelphia: WB Saunders; 1976; Wallach J: *Interpretation of diagnostic tests*, ed 2, Bo[illegible]ittle, Brown; 1974; Widmann FK: *Goodale's clinical interpretation of laboratory tests*, ed 7, Philadelp[illegible]avis; 1973.

Laboratory Report Complete Urinalysis			
PATIENT		ORDERED BY	RESULTS PROVIDED BY
Colbert, Evelyn K. 2963 Flint Dr. S Clearwater, FL 33759 PH: 727-541-3575	ID #: 336879 DOB: 4/28/1990 AGE: 34 GENDER: F	Thomas Murphy, MD Pinellas Medical Office 3477 Arrowhead Ave Clearwater, FL 33759	Medical Center Laboratory 33 West Main St Clearwater, FL 33759
SPECIMEN COLL. DATE	6/25/20XX	FASTING/NONFASTING	Nonfasting
SPECIMEN COLL. TIME	02:53 pm	LAB ACCESSION NUMBER	33804237
SPECIMEN RECEIVED DATE/TIME	6/25/20XX 05:30 pm	LAB ID NUMBER	373978
RESULTS REPORTED DATE/TIME	6/26/20XX 10:00 am	TEST(S) ORDERED	CPT: 81001 Complete Urinalysis

TEST	RESULT	REFERENCE RANGE	UNITS	FLAG
PHYSICAL EXAMINATION				
Color	Yellow	Yellow		
Appearance	**Cloudy**	**Clear**		**Abnormal**
Specific gravity	1.020	1.005-1.030		
CHEMICAL EXAMINATION				
Glucose	Negative	Negative		
Bilirubin	Negative	Negative		
Ketone	Negative	Negative		
Blood	Negative	Negative		
pH	6.5	5-7.5		
Protein	Trace	Negative/Trace		
Urobilinogen	0.6	0.2-1.0	mg/dL	
Nitrite	**Positive**	**Negative**		**Abnormal**
Leukocytes	**2+**	**Negative**		**Abnormal**
MICROSCOPIC EXAMINATION				
WBC	**8-10**	**0-5**	**/HPF**	**Abnormal**
RBC	0-2	0-3	/HPF	
Epithelial Cells	0-8	0-10	/HPF	
Casts	None seen	None	/LPF	
Mucus Threads	Present	Not Established		
Bacteria	**Moderate**	**None Seen/ Few**	**/HPF**	**Abnormal**

Fig. 16.5 Urinalysis laboratory report. *HPF*, High-power field.

reading less than 7.0 indicates acidity; and a reading greater than 7.0 indicates alkalinity.

The kidneys help to regulate the acid-base balance of the body. For an accurate pH reading of the urine, the measurement should be performed on freshly voided urine. If the urine is allowed to remain standing, it becomes more alkaline as urea is converted to ammonia by bacterial action.

Although the pH of urine can normally range from 5 to 7.5, the pH of a freshly voided specimen of a patient on a normal diet is usually acidic and has a pH reading of approximately 6.0. An abnormally high pH reading on a fresh specimen (i.e., alkaline urine) may indicate a bacterial infection of the urinary tract.

Glucose

Normally, no glucose should be detectable in the urine. Glucose in the blood is filtered through the nephrons and is reabsorbed into the body. If the glucose concentration in the blood becomes too high, the kidneys are unable to reabsorb all of it back into the blood, the renal threshold is exceeded, and glucose is spilled into the urine—a condition known as **glycosuria.** (The **renal threshold** is the concentration at which a substance in the blood that is not normally excreted by the kidneys begins to appear in the urine.) The renal threshold for glucose is typically 160 to 180 mg/dL (100 mL of blood), but this number may vary among individuals. Diabetes mellitus is the most common cause of glycosuria. Some individuals have a low renal threshold, and glucose may appear in their urine after the consumption of a large quantity of foods containing sugar. This condition is known as *alimentary glycosuria.*

Protein

The presence of protein in the urine is known as **proteinuria.** Protein in the urine usually indicates a pathologic condition if found in several samples over a period of time. A temporary increase in urine protein may be caused by stress or strenuous exercise. Some of the conditions that may cause proteinuria include glomerular filtration problems, renal disease, and bacterial infection of the urinary tract. If proteinuria occurs, the provider usually requests an examination of the sediment to determine, through visual observation, what is causing protein to be in the urine.

Ketone

Ketones are the normal products of fat metabolism and can be used by muscle tissue as a source of energy. There are three types of ketone bodies: β-hydroxybutyric acid, acetoacetic acid, and acetone. When more than normal amounts of fat are metabolized by the body, the muscles cannot handle all of the ketones that result. Large amounts of ketone accumulate in the tissues and body fluids; this condition is known as **ketosis.** The body rids itself of these excess ketones by excreting them in the urine. **Ketonuria** is the term that refers to the presence of ketone bodies in the urine. Conditions that can cause increased fat metabolism resulting in ketonuria include uncontrolled diabetes mellitus, starvation, and a diet composed almost entirely of fat.

Bilirubin

The average life span of a red blood cell is 120 days. When a red blood cell breaks down, one of the substances released from the breakdown of hemoglobin is a vivid yellow pigment known as *bilirubin.* Normally, bilirubin is transported to the liver by the blood and excreted into the bile, and it eventually leaves the body through the intestines in the feces, giving the stool its brown color. If damaged, the liver is unable to remove bilirubin from the blood. The bilirubin builds up in the blood and is excreted in the urine. Certain liver conditions and gallbladder problems, such as gallstones, hepatitis, and cirrhosis, may result in the presence of bilirubin in the urine, or **bilirubinuria.** The urine becomes yellow-brown or greenish, and a yellow foam appears when the urine is shaken.

Urobilinogen

Normally, bilirubin is excreted by the liver into the intestinal tract. Bacteria present in the intestines convert it to urobilinogen. Approximately 50% of the urobilinogen is reabsorbed into the body for reexcretion by the liver. Small amounts may appear in the urine, but most of the urobilinogen is excreted in the feces. An increase in the production of bilirubin increases the amount of urobilinogen excreted in the urine. Conditions such as excessive hemolysis of red blood cells, infectious hepatitis, cirrhosis, congestive heart failure, and infectious mononucleosis may increase the level of urobilinogen in the urine.

Blood

Blood is considered an abnormal constituent of urine, unless it is present as a contaminant during menstruation. The condition in which blood is found in the urine is termed *hematuria.* Hematuria may be the result of injury or disorders such as cystitis, tumors of the bladder, urethritis, kidney stones, and certain kidney disorders.

Nitrite

Nitrite in the urine indicates the presence of a pathogen in the (normally sterile) urinary tract, which results in a UTI. The pathogen possesses the ability to convert nitrate, which normally occurs in the urine, to nitrite, which is normally absent. The nitrite test must be performed with urine that has been in the bladder for at least 4 to 6 hours to ensure that bacteria have converted nitrate to nitrite. Therefore use of a first-voided morning specimen is recommended. The test should *not* be performed on specimens that have been left standing out, because a false-positive result may occur from bacterial contamination from the environment. The nitrite test is a screening test and is usually followed by a quantitative urine culture and identification of the invading pathogen.

Leukocytes

The presence of leukocytes in the urine is known as *leukocyturia* and accompanies inflammation of the kidneys and the lower urinary tract. Examples of specific conditions include acute and chronic pyelonephritis, cystitis, and urethritis. Urine reagent strips are available that contain a reagent pad that permits the chemical detection of intact and lysed leukocytes in the urine. The advantage of detecting lysed leukocytes is that these cells cannot be observed during a microscopic examination of urine sediment and would otherwise remain undetected. The recommended urine specimen, particularly for women, is a clean-catch midstream collection to prevent contamination of the specimen with leukocytes from vaginal secretions, leading to a false-positive test result.

CLIA-Waived Reagent Strips

CLIA-waived reagent strips are frequently used in the medical office for the chemical testing of urine. Reagent strips consist of disposable plastic strips on which separate reagent pads are affixed for testing specific chemicals that may be present in the urine during pathologic conditions.

The number and type of reagent pads included on the reagent strip depend on the particular brand of reagent strips. Multistix 10 SG (Siemens Medical Solutions, Malvern, PA). is a CLIA-waived test that contains 10 reagent pads for testing pH, protein, glucose, ketone, bilirubin, blood, urobilinogen, nitrite, specific gravity, and leukocytes. The procedure for performing urinalysis using a Multistix 10 SG reagent strip is presented in Procedure 16.3.

Test results are qualitative results, and a positive result may indicate the need for further testing. *Qualitative test results* indicate whether a substance is present in the urine and also may provide an approximate indication of the amount of the substance present. Interpretation of reagent strip results involves the use of a color comparison chart, with results documented in terms of positive or negative; 1+, 2+, or 3+; trace, and small, moderate, or large.

The reagent strip test results provide information to assist in diagnosis of the following:

- Conditions affecting kidney function (e.g., kidney stones)
- UTIs
- Conditions affecting carbohydrate metabolism (e.g., diabetes mellitus)
- Conditions affecting liver function (e.g., hepatitis)

Test results also provide information related to the status of the patient's acid-base balance and urine concentration.

Guidelines

Testing urine with a reagent strip is a relatively easy procedure to perform. However, specific guidelines must be followed to ensure accurate test results.

1. *Type of specimen.* The best results are obtained with a freshly voided and thoroughly mixed urine specimen. If the medical assistant is unable to test the specimen within 1 hour of voiding, the specimen should be refrigerated immediately and then allowed to return to room temperature before testing.
2. *Type of collection.* Most reagent strips are designed to be used with a random specimen collection; however, clean-catch midstream and first-voided morning specimens are suggested for specific tests. The nitrite test results are optimized with a first-voided morning specimen, whereas a clean-catch midstream collection is recommended for the leukocyte test.
3. *Urine specimen container.* The specimen container used must be thoroughly clean and free from any detergent or disinfectant residue because cleansing agents contain oxidants that react with the chemicals on the reagent strip, leading to inaccurate test results. The container should be large enough to allow for complete immersion of all of the reagent strip pads.
4. *Time intervals.* Read the test results at the exact time intervals specified on the color chart. Do not read any test results after 2 minutes.
5. *Interpretation and reading of results.* Of particular importance is the comparison of the reagent strip with the color chart on the strip container. The reagent strip must be compared with the color chart in good lighting to obtain a good visual match to ensure accurate test results.
6. *Storage of reagent strips.* The reagents on the strips are sensitive to light, heat, and moisture, and the container of strips must be stored in a cool, dry area away from direct sunlight, with the cap tightly closed to maintain reactivity of the reagent. Most reagent strips are packaged in opaque containers to protect them from light. The container may include a desiccant that should not be removed because its purpose is to promote dryness by absorbing moisture. The container of reagent strips must be stored at a temperature between 59°F (15°C) and 86°F (30°C). The strips should not be stored in the refrigerator or freezer. The reagent strips must never be transferred from their original container to another, because the other container may harbor traces of moisture, dirt, or chemicals that could affect the test results. A tan-to-brown discoloration or darkening on the reagent pads indicates deterioration of the reagent strips, in which case the strips should not be used because the test results would be inaccurate.

Quality Control Test

A quality control test should be performed when testing urine with reagent strips. Quality control testing ensures the reliability of test results by (1) determining whether the reagent strips are reacting properly, and (2) confirming that the test is being properly performed and accurately interpreted.

To check the reliability of Multistix reagent strips, a Chek-Stix control (Siemens Medical Solutions Diagnostics) should be used. A Chek-Stix control consists of a firm plastic strip to which are affixed synthetic ingredients (Fig. 16.6). The control strip is reconstituted by immersing it in distilled water for 30 minutes, which allows the ingredients on the strip to dissolve in the water. After reconstitution, the resulting solution is tested in the same manner as a urine specimen. The values to be expected are outlined in the package insert that accompanies the control strips. The results of the control test should be documented in a quality control log. If the expected values are not obtained, the cause of the problem must be determined and corrected. Factors that can cause a problem include outdated reagent strips, improper storage of the strips, and an error in testing technique. The quality control test should be performed when each new container of strips is opened for the first time or when a question of reliability arises regarding the test strips.

Urine Analyzer

CLIA-waived urine analyzers are used to perform an automatic chemical examination of urine with reagent strips.

They offer the advantage of the ability to perform the chemical analysis quickly and to interpret results automatically. These analyzers are used most often in medical offices that perform moderate-volume to large-volume urine testing.

The Clinitek Analyzer (Siemens Medical Solutions Diagnostics) is an example of a CLIA-waived urine analyzer that automatically reads Multistix SG and other (Siemens) urine reagent strips (Fig. 16.7A). The results are printed out, and abnormal results are flagged to call attention to them (see Fig. 16.7B).

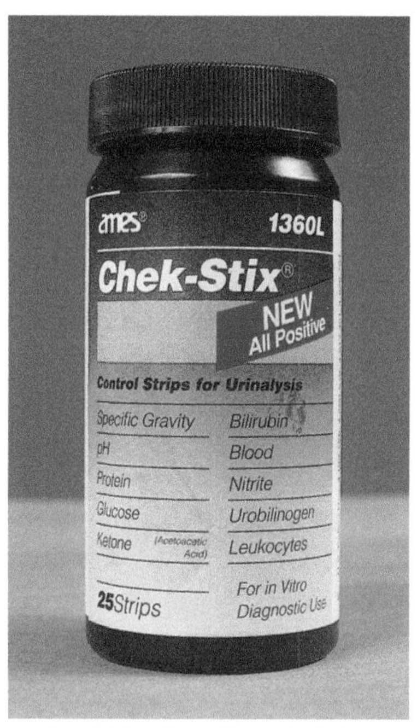

Fig. 16.6 Chek-Stix control strips.

MICROSCOPIC EXAMINATION OF URINE

As discussed in Chapter 15, some medical offices perform moderate complexity tests known as *provider-performed microscopy* (PPM) procedures, which involve the examination of a specimen under the microscope. The microscopic examination of urine sediment is a PPM procedure and must be performed by an individual with the proper training and skill qualifications, such as a medical office provider. A CLIA certificate for PPM procedures is required, and the CLIA regulations must be followed; however, the physician's office laboratory (POL) is exempt from on-site inspections.

Urine sediment is the solid material contained in the urine. A microscopic examination of the urine sediment helps to clarify the results of the physical and chemical examination of urine. A first-voided morning specimen is preferred because it is more concentrated and contains more dissolved substances; small amounts of abnormal substances are more likely to be detected. A fresh urine specimen should be used to perform the examination because of the changes that occur in a specimen left standing out. These changes can affect the reliability of the results. The medical assistant is responsible for preparing the urine specimen for microscopic examination by the provider, as presented in Procedure 16.4.

RED BLOOD CELLS

Red blood cells appear as round, colorless, biconcave discs that are highly refractive (Table 16.2). The presence of zero to three per high-power field (HPF) is considered normal. More than this number may indicate bleeding somewhere along the urinary tract. Table 16.2 lists the possible causes of an abnormal number of red blood cells in the urine. Concentrated urine causes the red blood cells to become shrunken

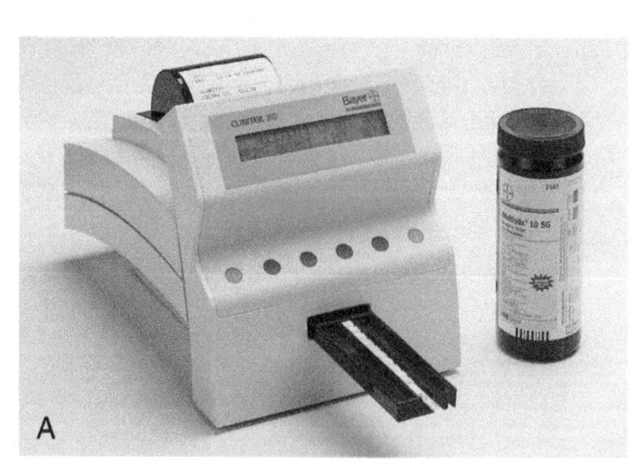

B

ID: Erika Seager
11-16-XX 5:37 PM

CLARITY: Clear
COLOR: YELLOW

MULTISTIX 10 SG

GLU	NEGATIVE
BIL	NEGATIVE
KET	NEGATIVE
SG	1.025
BLO*	TRACE-LYSED
pH	5.5
PRO	NEGATIVE
URO	0.2 E.U./dl
NIT	NEGATIVE
LEU	NEGATIVE

Fig. 16.7 (A) Clinitek urine analyzer. (B) Clinitek printout of test results.

Table 16.2 Structures in Urine Sediment

Structure	Possible Causes	Microscopic Appearance
Red blood cells	Inflammatory diseases Acute glomerulonephritis Pyelonephritis Hypertension Renal infarction Trauma Stones Tumor Bleeding diseases Use of anticoagulants	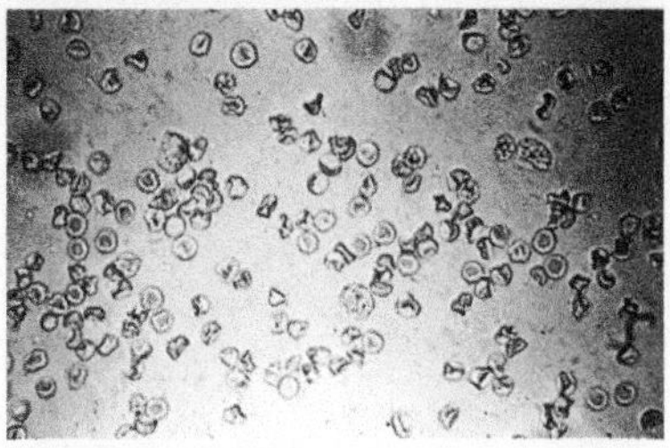 Red blood cells[a]
White blood cells	Pyelonephritis Cystitis Urethritis Prostatitis Transplant rejection (manifested by lymphocytes in urine) Tissue injury accompanied by severe inflammation (manifested by monocytes in urine) Inflammation, immune mechanisms, and other host defense mechanisms (manifested by histiocytes in urine)	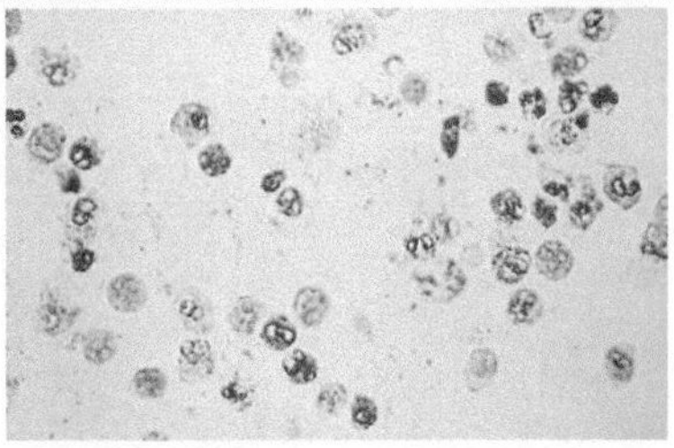 White blood cells[a]
Squamous epithelial cells	Vaginal contamination	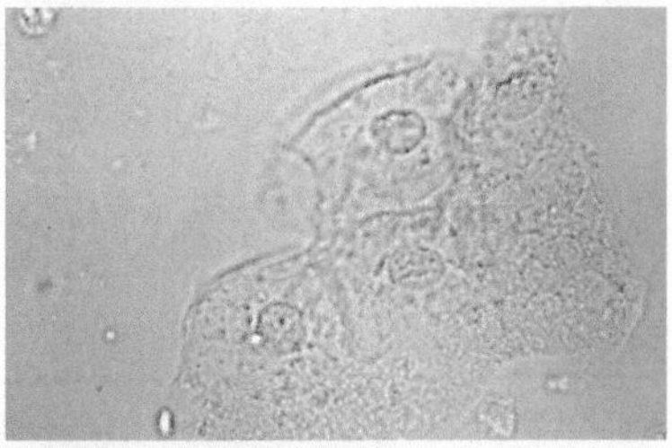 Squamous epithelial cells[a]
Renal tubular epithelial cells	Acute tubular necrosis Glomerulonephritis Acute infection Renal toxicity Viral infection	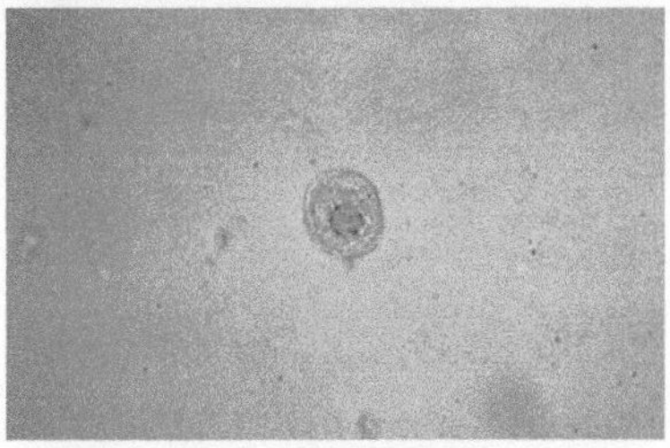 Renal tubular epithelial cells[a]
Hyaline casts	Normal urine Strenuous exercise Acute glomerulonephritis Acute pyelonephritis Malignant hypertension Chronic renal disease	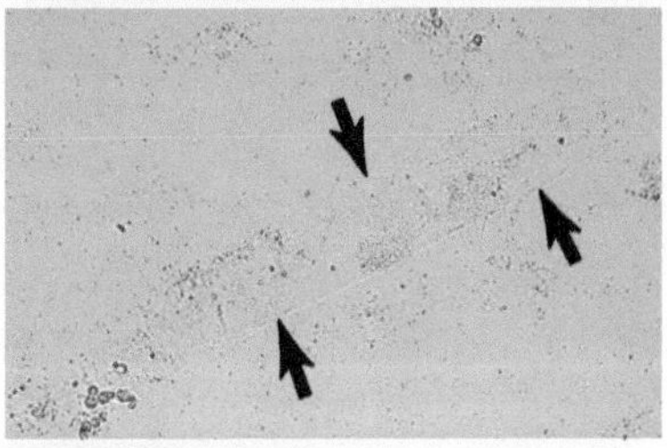 Hyaline cast[b]
Amorphous urate	Nonpathologic	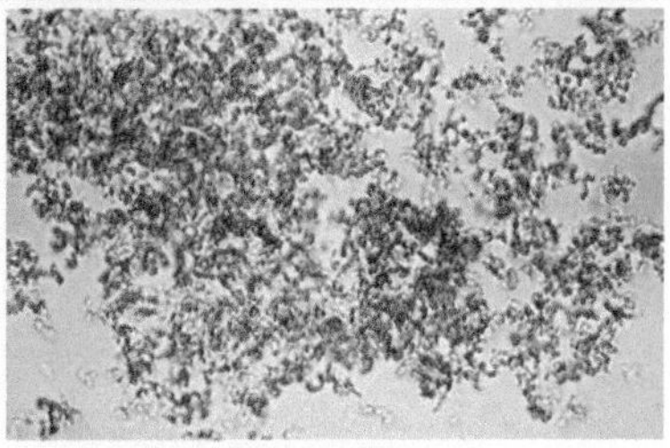 Amorphous urate crystals[a]

Continued

Table 16.2 Structures in Urine Sediment—cont'd

Structure	Possible Causes	Microscopic Appearance
Uric acid	Usually nonpathologic; in large numbers, may indicate gout	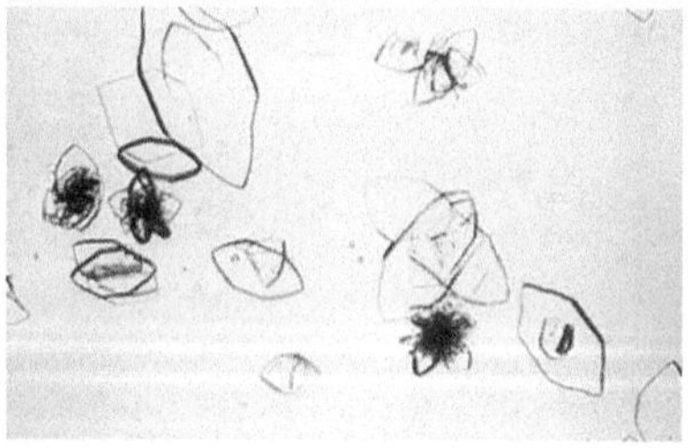 Uric acid crystals[a]
Calcium oxalate	Usually nonpathologic; may be associated with stone formation	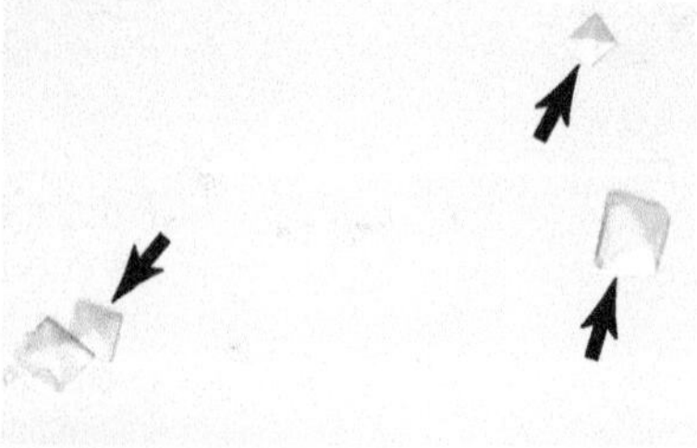 Calcium oxalate crystals[b]
Bacteria	More than 100,000 bacteria per mL indicates urinary tract infection 10,000–100,000 bacteria per mL indicates that tests should be repeated Less than 10,000 bacteria per mL may signify urine in which any bacteria are urethral organisms or the result of contamination Bacteria accompanied by white blood cells or white blood cell or mixed casts may indicate acute pyelonephritis	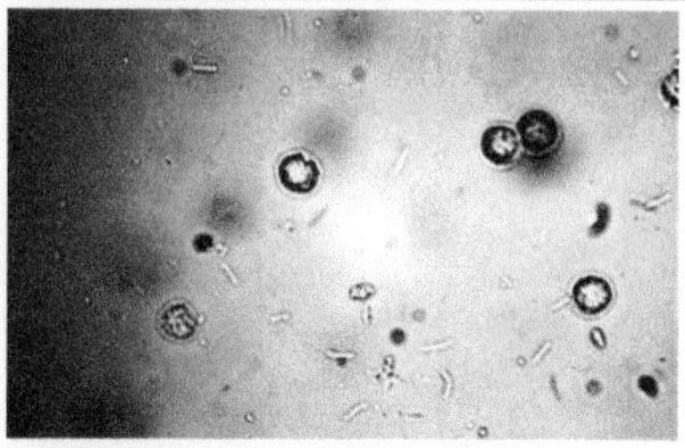 Bacteria (small rod structures)[a]
Yeast	May indicate contamination by yeasts from skin or hair May indicate diabetes mellitus or urinary tract infection *Candida albicans* may occur in patients with diabetes mellitus or in the contaminated urine of female patients with candidal vaginitis	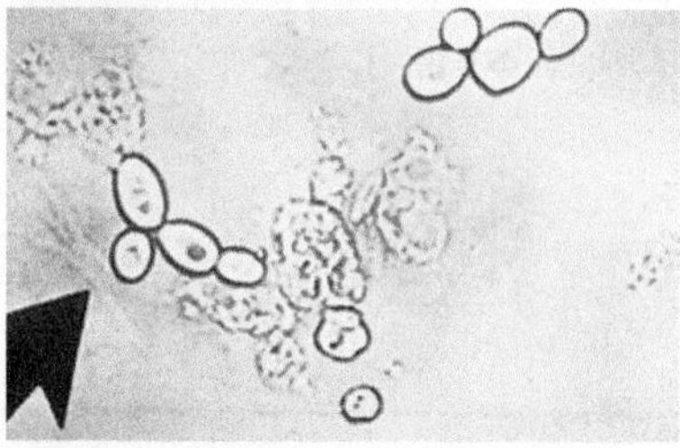 *Candida albicans* (yeast)[a]
Parasites and parasitic ova	Usually indicate fecal or vaginal contamination and should be reported *Trichomonas* may be found in patients with urethritis and in contaminated urine of women with *Trichomonas* vaginitis Pinworm is a common contaminant and should be reported	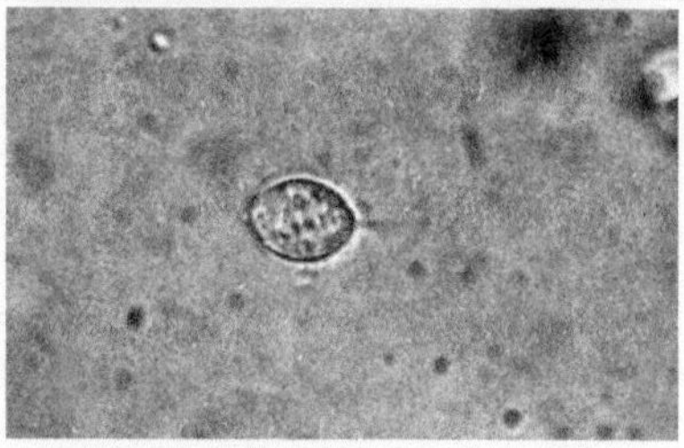 *Trichomonas* (parasite)[a]
Spermatozoa	Nonpathologic	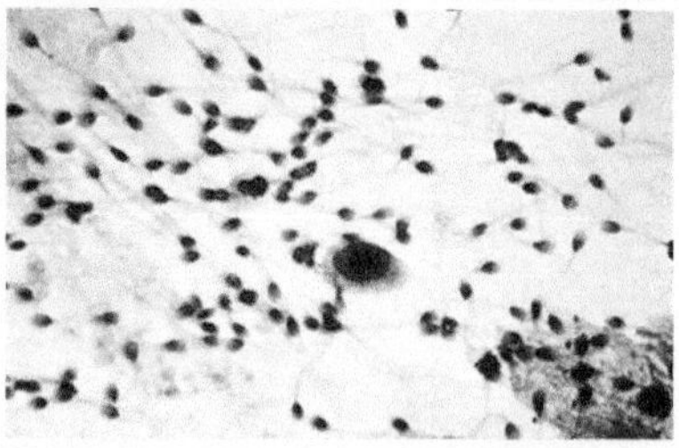 Spermatozoa[a]

Table 16.2 Structures in Urine Sediment—cont'd

Structure	Possible Causes	Microscopic Appearance
Urinary artifacts Hair (a) Pollen grains Bubbles Oil droplets Fibers (b) Powder (c) Dust Mucous threads (d) Glass particles	Nonpathologic May result from improper urine collection, improper slide preparation, or outside contamination	(a) Hair[c] (b) Fiber[a] (c) Powder[a] (d) Mucous threads[b]

[a]Photomicrographs courtesy Bayer Corporation, Diagnostics Division, Elkhart, IN.
[b]Photomicrographs from Stepp CA, Woods M: *Laboratory procedures for medical office personnel,* Philadelphia: WB Saunders; 1998.
[c]Photomicrograph from Lehman CA: *Saunders manual of clinical laboratory science,* Philadelphia: WB Saunders; 1998.
Text courtesy Boehringer Mannheim Diagnostics, Indianapolis, Ind.

or *crenated,* whereas dilute urine causes them to swell and become rounded, which may cause them to hemolyze. If the red blood cells have hemolyzed, they cannot be seen under the microscope. However, the presence of blood in the urine still can be identified with a reagent strip, such as Multistix, which is designed to detect free hemoglobin.

WHITE BLOOD CELLS

White blood cells are round and granular and have a nucleus (see Table 16.2). They are approximately 1.5 times as large as red blood cells. The presence of 0 to 5 per HPF is considered normal. More than this amount may indicate inflammation of the genitourinary tract. Table 16.2 lists the possible causes of an abnormal number of white blood cells in the urine.

EPITHELIAL CELLS

Most structures that make up the urinary system are composed of several layers of epithelial cells. The outer layer is constantly sloughed off and replaced by the cells underneath it. *Squamous epithelial cells* are large, clear, flat cells with an irregular shape. They contain a small nucleus and come from the urethra, bladder, and vagina. Squamous epithelial cells are normally present in small amounts in the urine. *Renal epithelial cells* are round and contain a large nucleus. They come from the deeper layers of the urinary tract, and their presence in the urine is considered abnormal. Table 16.2 lists the types of epithelial cells and possible causes of the presence of abnormal amounts in the urine.

CASTS

Casts are cylindric structures formed in the lumen of the tubules that make up the nephron. Materials in the tubules harden, are flushed out, and appear in the urine in the form of casts. Various types of casts may be present in the urine. In general, their presence indicates a diseased condition.

Casts are named according to what they contain. *Hyaline casts* are pale, colorless cylinders with rounded edges that vary in size (see Table 16.2). *Granular casts* are hyaline casts that contain granules and are described as "coarsely granular" or "finely granular," depending on the size of the granules. *Fatty casts* are hyaline casts that contain fat droplets. *Waxy casts* are light yellow and have serrated edges; their name is derived from the fact that they appear to be made of wax. *Cellular casts* contain organized structures and are named according to what they contain. Examples include red blood cell casts, which are hyaline casts containing red blood cells; white blood cell casts, which are hyaline casts containing white blood cells; epithelial casts, which are hyaline casts containing epithelial cells; and bacterial casts, which are hyaline casts containing bacteria.

CRYSTALS

A variety of crystals may be found in the urine. The type and number vary with the pH of the urine. Abnormal crystals include leucine, tyrosine, cystine, and cholesterol. Crystals that commonly appear in acid urine include amorphous urates, uric acid, and calcium oxalate (see Table 16.2). Crystals that commonly appear in alkaline urine include amorphous phosphate, triple phosphate, calcium phosphate, and ammonium urate crystals.

MISCELLANEOUS STRUCTURES

Miscellaneous structures are illustrated in Table 16.2 and include the following:

Mucous threads are normally present in small amounts in the urine. They appear as long, wavy, threadlike structures with pointed ends.

Bacteria should not normally exist in the urinary tract. The presence of more than a few bacteria may indicate either contamination of the specimen during collection or a UTI. Bacteria are small structures that may be rod-shaped or round.

Yeast cells are smooth, refractile bodies with an oval shape. A distinguishing feature of yeast cells is small buds that project from the cells involved with reproduction. Yeast cells in the urine of female patients are usually a vaginal contaminant caused by the yeast *Candida albicans* and produce the vaginal infection known as *vulvovaginal candidiasis.* Yeast cells also may be present in the urine of patients with diabetes mellitus.

Parasites may be present in the urine sediment as a contaminant from fecal or vaginal material. *Trichomonas vaginalis* is a parasite that causes trichomoniasis vaginitis.

Spermatozoa may be present in the urine of a man or woman after intercourse. The spermatozoa have round heads and long, slender, hairlike tails.

Fig. 16.5 is an example of a laboratory report that includes a microscopic examination of urine.

Memories *from* Practicum

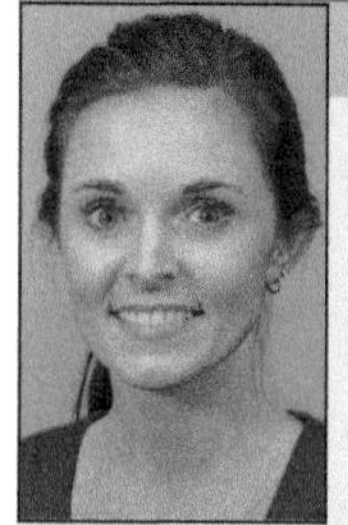

Kayla: My main problem as a student on practicum was that I was a little shy. I learned that when your patient is relaxed, he or she is more likely to give you additional and important information about what is wrong. If your patient tenses up during a procedure, this can cause pain for the patient and make the procedure more difficult. When I started to make myself talk more to the patients and staff, things went more smoothly. ■

PATIENT COACHING Urinary Tract Infections

Answer questions that patients may have about urinary tract infections (UTIs).

What is a UTI?

Urinary tract infection (UTI) is a general term for the presence of bacteria in any portion of the urinary tract. UTIs, particularly those involving the bladder (cystitis) and urethra (urethritis), are common and treatable. A UTI is usually treated with an antibiotic. Use of all of the antibiotic for the total number of days prescribed is important, even if the symptoms disappear. If the medication is stopped too soon, the infection may recur and may be more difficult to treat than the original infection.

What are the symptoms of a UTI?

The symptoms of a simple UTI (cystitis) commonly include the frequent need to urinate, urgency (meaning the immediate need to urinate), a burning sensation during urination, and sometimes blood in the urine. Symptoms of a more complicated UTI involving the kidneys (pyelonephritis) include the aforementioned symptoms as well as lower abdominal discomfort, low back pain, fever, cloudy or foul-smelling urine, and blood in the urine.

Why do women have UTIs more frequently than men?

Women are more prone than men to the type of UTI called *cystitis* because the urethra of a woman is shorter than that of a man, which

PATIENT COACHING **Urinary Tract Infections—cont'd**

makes travel up the urethra and into the bladder easier for bacteria. The most common source of infection is bacteria *(Escherichia coli)*. *E. coli* organisms are normally found in the large intestine but can travel from the anal area to the urinary bladder, often as the result of poor hygienic practices. Cystitis occurs if *E. coli* organisms are able to overcome the body's natural defenses when the bacteria reach the urinary bladder and set up an infection.

What can women do to prevent a UTI?

Women prone to development of UTIs should practice the following prevention measures:

- Practice good hygienic measures by always cleaning the genital area from front to back after a bowel movement.
- Avoid possible irritants, such as bubble baths, perfumed soaps, feminine hygiene sprays, and the use of strong powders and bleaches for washing underclothes.
- Avoid clothing that traps moisture and encourages the growth of microorganisms, such as tight, constricting clothing; nylon panties; and pantyhose.
- Avoid activities that can contribute to irritation of the urinary meatus, such as prolonged bicycling, motorcycling, horseback riding, and travel that involves prolonged sitting.
- Urinate as soon as possible when you feel the urge. Holding urine in the bladder gives the bacteria more time to grow, which can cause a more severe infection. The more often you urinate, the more quickly the bacteria are removed from the bladder.
- Seek prompt treatment if you experience any of the symptoms of a UTI.

Encourage the patient with a UTI to drink plenty of water to help flush the bacteria out of the urinary tract.

Emphasize to the patient the importance of taking all of the antibiotic for the duration of time prescribed.

Emphasize the importance of practicing preventive measures to prevent the occurrence of UTIs.

Provide the patient with educational materials on UTIs. ■

Urine Pregnancy Testing

The diagnosis of pregnancy can be accomplished several ways. By the eighth week after conception, pregnancy can be confirmed with the medical history and physical examination. However, the provider may desire an earlier diagnosis with a pregnancy test, to initiate early prenatal care. A pregnancy test also may be necessary before certain medications are ordered or procedures are performed that may cause injury to a fetus.

In the medical office, immunologic tests are often used for pregnancy testing. These tests are performed on a concentrated urine specimen and rely on the presence of a hormone known as *human chorionic gonadotropin* (HCG) for a positive reaction.

HUMAN CHORIONIC GONADOTROPIN

HCG is produced by the developing fertilized egg, and small amounts of it are secreted into the urine and blood. Immediately after conception and implantation of the fertilized egg, the plasma level of HCG increases rapidly and can be used to detect pregnancy with a serum pregnancy test as early as 6 days before the first missed menstrual period. The highest plasma levels of HCG occur at approximately 8 weeks after conception. After this time, the production of HCG declines and remains at a lower level for the duration of the pregnancy. Within 72 hours of delivery, HCG disappears entirely from the plasma. As a result, pregnancy tests are more sensitive during the first trimester and may show a negative reaction when the level of HCG begins to decline during the second and third trimesters.

IMMUNOASSAY URINE PREGNANCY TEST

CLIA-waived immunoassay urine tests are used in the medical office for the detection of pregnancy. These tests are convenient to perform and provide immediate test results. Positive and negative reactions are evidenced by a specific visible reaction that is observed and interpreted by the individual performing the test.

Immunoassay pregnancy tests are commercially available in test kits that contain the required reagents and supplies to perform the test. Each kit can be used to perform a specific number of tests, ranging from 25 to 50. The instructions in the package insert accompanying the test kit should be followed *exactly* to prevent inaccurate test results. When performed correctly, most urine pregnancy tests are 99% accurate with low occurrences of false-positive test results.

Immunoassay pregnancy tests provide for the rapid, qualitative detection of HCG in a urine specimen; brand names include QuickVue HCG Urine Test (Quidel, San Diego, CA), OSOM HCG Urine Test (Genzyme Diagnostics, Cambridge, MA), and ICON HCG Pregnancy Test (Beckman Coulter, Brea, CA). Early prediction pregnancy tests may be able to detect pregnancy as early as 2 to 3 days before a first missed menstrual period. However, urine pregnancy tests performed this early may show a false-negative result and should be repeated later to confirm the results. Accurate results are much more probable if the urine is tested 1 week after a missed period.

Immunoassay tests take approximately 5 minutes to perform, and the test results are easily observed as a color change. Specific instructions for interpreting the test results are included in the package insert. The procedure for performing an immunoassay with the QuickVue HCG Urine Test (Quidel) is outlined in Procedure 16.5.

GUIDELINES FOR URINE PREGNANCY TESTING

Specific guidelines must be followed for urine pregnancy testing to ensure accurate test results:

1. Use clean, preferably disposable, urine containers to collect the specimen. Traces of detergent in the specimen container may cause inaccurate test results.
2. The preferred specimen for a urine pregnancy test is a first-voided morning specimen because it contains the highest concentration of HCG; however, a random urine specimen can also be used. If the urine specimen cannot be tested immediately after voiding, it should be preserved in the refrigerator. A patient who collects the specimen at home should be given instructions on preserving the specimen.
3. The specific gravity of the urine specimen should be determined before the test is performed. A specific gravity of less than 1.007 is considered too dilute for pregnancy testing because it may lead to a false-negative test result.
4. The urine specimen should be at room temperature before the procedure is performed.
5. The urine pregnancy test kit should be stored according to the information in the package insert. Most test kits are stored at a room temperature between 59°F (15°C) and 86°F (30°C) and away from direct sunlight.
6. Test kits past their expiration dates should not be used.
7. If more than one patient is being tested at a time, label each test device with the patient's name to prevent a mix-up of specimens.
8. Most urine pregnancy test kits include a built-in internal control to evaluate whether certain aspects of the testing procedure are working properly. The internal control is performed at the same time that the testing procedure is performed. It determines whether a sufficient amount of the specimen was added to the test cassette and if the correct procedural technique was followed. If the internal control does not perform as expected, the test result is invalid and the specimen must be retested. It is recommended that the internal control results be documented in a quality control log for the first pregnancy test run each day.
9. It is recommended that a positive and a negative external control be performed with each new lot of test kits. External controls are used to determine if the test reagents are performing properly and to detect any errors in technique of the individual performing the test. External controls consist of commercially available solutions and may be included with the test system or may need to be purchased separately. The control procedure is performed using the same procedure for performing the test on a patient. However, instead of adding the patient specimen to the test device, the control is added to it. The positive control should produce a positive result, and the negative control should produce a negative result. The results should be documented in a quality control log (Fig. 16.8). Failure of an external control to produce expected results may be caused by outdated controls or test reagents, improper storage of test components, improper environmental testing conditions and an error in the technique used to perform the procedure.
10. Conditions other than a normal pregnancy that can result in a positive result include ectopic pregnancy and molar pregnancy.

What Would You Do? What Would You *Not* Do?

Case Study 3

Rita Lavelle is (8½) months pregnant and is at the clinic for a prenatal appointment. Lately, she has been having difficulty obtaining a urine specimen at the medical office because of her enlarged abdomen. At her last appointment, the office provided her with a urine specimen container so that she could obtain her specimen more easily at home. Rita brings in a first-voided urine specimen in a glass jar. She says her dog chewed up the specimen container from the office, so she used an empty peanut butter jar. The urine test results from her specimen show that her glucose level is normal, but her protein level is 4+. Until this time, her urine test results all have been normal. Rita is concerned about her baby. She says that she was cleaning her bathroom cabinet yesterday and came across a pregnancy test; just for the fun of it, she decided to run the test. The results were negative, and now she is worried that something is wrong. Rita says that she has not been sleeping as well at night and that she has noticed more Braxton-Hicks contractions, but the baby has been kicking and moving as usual. ■

SERUM PREGNANCY TEST

The radioimmunoassay (RIA) for HCG is a (nonwaived) quantitative test used to detect HCG in the serum of the blood. This test can detect pregnancy earlier and with greater accuracy than a urine pregnancy test. A serum pregnancy test can usually detect pregnancy at approximately the eighth day after fertilization, which is 6 days before the first missed menstrual period. This test uses a radioisotope technique and is capable of detecting minute amounts of HCG in the blood. This test is usually used to diagnose abnormalities, such as ectopic pregnancy; to follow the course of early pregnancy when abnormalities of embryonic development are suspected; and to provide an early diagnosis of pregnancy in individuals at high risk, such as patients with diabetes.

QUALITY CONTROL LOG

URINE PREGNANCY TEST

	Date	Name of test	Control lot #	Control expiration date	External positive control	External negative control	Technician
1	3/25 20XX	QuickVue One Step HCG	140400	3/16/XX	+	–	L.Proffit CMA (AAMA)
2	4/22 20XX	QuickVue One Step HCG	140400	3/16/XX	+	–	L.Proffit CMA (AAMA)
3	5/27 20XX	QuickVue One Step HCG	140400	3/16/XX	+	–	L.Proffit CMA (AAMA)
4							
5							
6							
7							
8							
9							
10							

Fig. 16.8 Quality control log for urine pregnancy testing.

What Would You Do? What Would You *Not* Do? RESPONSES

Case Study 1

Page 565

What Did Kayla Do?

- ❑ Took some time to try to calm and relax Mr. Urameshi. Reassured him that the physician would do everything he could to make Mr. Urameshi better.
- ❑ Offered Mr. Urameshi something to drink and told him it might help him obtain a specimen.
- ❑ Went over the directions again with Mr. Urameshi.
- ❑ Asked Mr. Urameshi if he would try again to obtain a specimen.

What Did Kayla Not Do?

- ❑ Did not tell Mr. Urameshi that he was not trying hard enough.

Case Study 2

Page 568

What Did Kayla Do?

- ❑ Asked Nora whether she takes all of the antibiotic she is prescribed when she has a UTI.
- ❑ Explained to Nora in terms she can understand why women seem to be more prone to development of UTIs.
- ❑ Explained to Nora what she could do to help prevent UTIs. Gave her a patient education brochure on UTIs to take home.
- ❑ Told Nora that the physician is not legally or ethically permitted to call in a prescription for her without seeing her. Also explained that it is in the best interests of her health care to be seen by the physician.

What Did Kayla Not Do?

- ❑ Did not tell Nora that she could not test her urine at home.

Case Study 3

Page 580

What Did Kayla Do?

- ❑ Told Rita that some peanut butter residue might have been left in the jar she used and might have affected the test results. Asked her to try to collect another specimen at the office so that the urine could be tested again.
- ❑ Told Rita that if something happens to the specimen container again, she should come to the office and get another one.
- ❑ Told Rita that several things could have caused her pregnancy test result to be negative. Explained to her that the test could have been outdated or not stored properly. Also explained that, as a pregnancy gets farther along, less of the hormone that causes the test to be positive is secreted, so negative test results at the end of a pregnancy are not unusual.
- ❑ Reassured Rita that many women have trouble sleeping during the last month of pregnancy and that it is normal to have more Braxton-Hicks contractions as she gets closer to delivery.
- ❑ Told Rita that she would inform the physician of her symptoms so that he could discuss them in more detail with her.

What Did Kayla Not Do?

- ❑ Did not criticize Rita for collecting her specimen in a peanut butter jar.
- ❑ Did not ignore or minimize Rita's concerns.

TERMINOLOGY REVIEW

Key Term	Word Parts	Definition
Anuria	*an-:* without, absence of *ur/o:* urine *-ia:* condition of disease or abnormal state	Failure of the kidneys to produce urine.
Bilirubinuria	*bilirubino/o:* bilirubin *ur/o-:* urine *-ia:* condition of disease or abnormal state	The presence of bilirubin in the urine.
Bladder catheterization		The passing of a sterile catheter through the urethra and into the bladder to remove urine.
Diuresis		Secretion and passage of large amounts of urine.
Dysuria	*dys-:* difficult, labored, painful *ur/o:* urine *-ia:* condition of disease or abnormal state	Difficult or painful urination.
Frequency		The condition of having to urinate often.
Glycosuria	*glyc/o:* sugar *ur/o:* urine *-ia:* condition of disease or abnormal state	The presence of glucose in the urine.
Hematuria	*hemato/o:* blood *ur/o:* urine *-ia:* condition of disease or abnormal state	Blood present in the urine.
Ketonuria	*keton/o:* ketone *ur/o:* urine *-ia:* condition of disease or abnormal state	The presence of ketone bodies in the urine.
Ketosis	*keton/o:* ketone *-osis:* abnormal condition	An accumulation of large amounts of ketone bodies in the tissues and body fluids.
Micturition		The act of voiding urine.
Nephron		The functional unit of the kidney that filters waste substances from the blood and dilutes them with water to produce urine.
Nocturia	*noct/i:* night *ur/o:* urine *-ia:* condition of disease or abnormal state	Excessive (voluntary) urination during the night.
Nocturnal enuresis		Inability of an individual to control urination at night during sleep (bedwetting).
Oliguria	*olig/o:* scanty, few *ur/o:* urine *-ia:* condition of disease or abnormal state	Decreased or scanty output of urine.
pH		The unit that describes the acidity or alkalinity of a solution.
Polyuria	*poly-:* many *ur/o:* urine *-ia:* condition of disease or abnormal state	Increased output of urine.
Proteinuria	*protein-:* protein *ur/o:* urine *-ia:* condition of disease or abnormal state	The presence of protein in the urine.
Pyuria	*py/o:* pus *ur/o:* urine *-ia:* condition of disease or abnormal state	The presence of pus in the urine.

TERMINOLOGY REVIEW—cont'd

Key Term	Word Parts	Definition
Renal threshold		The concentration at which a substance in the blood that is not normally excreted by the kidneys begins to appear in the urine.
Retention		The inability to empty the bladder. The urine is being produced normally but is not being voided.
Specific gravity (urine)		The weight of a substance compared with the weight of an equal volume of distilled water. In urinalysis, the *specific gravity* refers to the measurement of the amount of dissolved substances present in the urine compared with the same amount of distilled water.
Supernatant	*super:* over, above	The clear liquid that remains at the top after a precipitate has settled.
Suprapubic aspiration	*supra-:* above *pub/o:* pubis *-ic:* pertaining to	The passing of a sterile needle through the abdominal wall into the bladder to remove urine.
Urgency		The immediate need to urinate.
Urinalysis	*urin/o:* urine	The physical, chemical, and microscopic analyses of urine.
Urinary incontinence		The inability to retain urine.

PROCEDURE 16.1 Collection of a Clean-Catch Midstream Urine Specimen

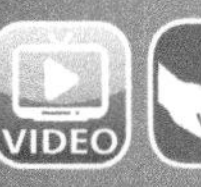

Outcome Instruct a patient in the collection of a clean-catch midstream urine specimen.

Equipment/Supplies

- Sterile specimen container and label
- Personal antiseptic towelettes
- Tissues

1. **Procedural Step.** Sanitize your hands. Greet the patient, and introduce yourself. Identify the patient, and explain the procedure.

2. **Procedural Step.** Assemble equipment. Label the specimen container with the patient's name and date of birth, the date, the type of specimen (clean-catch midstream), and your initials.

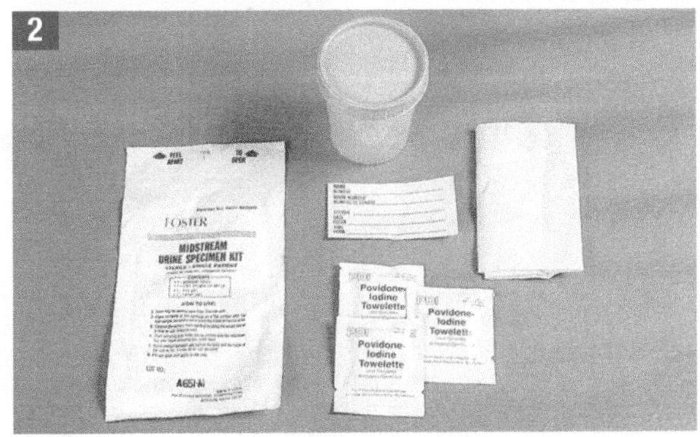

Assemble the equipment.

3. **Procedural Step.** Instruct a female patient on collection of the specimen as follows:
   a. Wash the hands, open the package of towelettes, and place them on their wrapper.
   b. Remove the lid from the specimen container and place it on a paper towel with the opening of the lid facing upward. Do not touch the inside of the lid or the inside of the specimen container.
   c. Pull undergarments down and sit on the toilet. Expose the urinary meatus by spreading apart the labia with one hand.
   d. Cleanse each side of the urinary meatus with an antiseptic towelette using a front-to-back motion (from pubis to anus). Use a separate antiseptic towelette for each side of the meatus. After use, discard each towelette in the toilet.

Continued

PROCEDURE 16.1 Collection of a Clean-Catch Midstream Urine Specimen—cont'd

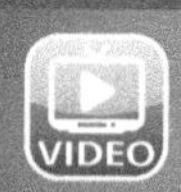

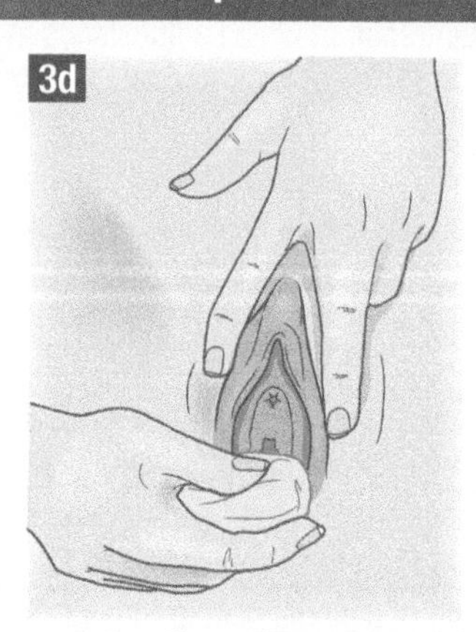

Cleanse the urinary meatus. (From Niedzwiecki B, Pepper J, Weaver P: *Kinn's the medical assistant*, ed 14, St Louis: Elsevier; 2020.)

e. Cleanse directly across the meatus (front to back) with a third antiseptic towelette. Discard the towelette.

f. Continue to hold the labia apart, and void a small amount of urine into the toilet.

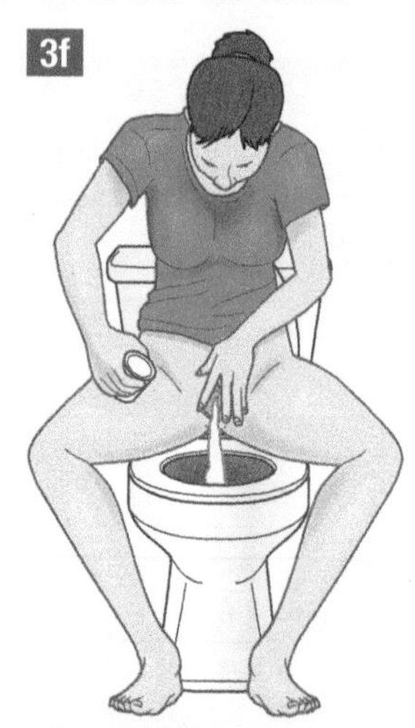

Void a small amount of urine into the toilet. (From Niedzwiecki B, Pepper J, Weaver P: *Kinn's the medical assistant*, ed 14, St Louis: Elsevier; 2020.)

g. Without stopping the urine flow, collect the next amount of urine (midstream flow of urine) by voiding into the sterile container. Do not touch the inside of the sterile container. Fill the specimen container about half full with urine.

h. Void the last amount of urine into the toilet. This means that the first and last portions of the urine flow are not included in the specimen. Replace the lid of the specimen container.

i. Wipe the area dry with a tissue, and discard it in the toilet. Flush the toilet and wash the hands.

Principle. Cleansing removes microorganisms from the urinary meatus. A front-to-back motion must be used for cleansing to avoid drawing microorganisms from the anal region into the area that is being cleansed. Voiding a small amount flushes microorganisms out of the distal urethra. Touching the inside of the container contaminates it with microorganisms that normally reside on the skin.

4. **Procedural Step.** Instruct a male patient as follows:

a. Wash the hands, open the towelettes, remove the lid from the specimen container, and remove undergarments.

b. Stand in front of the toilet. Retract the foreskin of the penis (if uncircumcised).

c. Cleanse the area around the meatus (glans penis) and the urethral opening (meatal orifice) by wiping each side of the meatus with a separate antiseptic towelette.

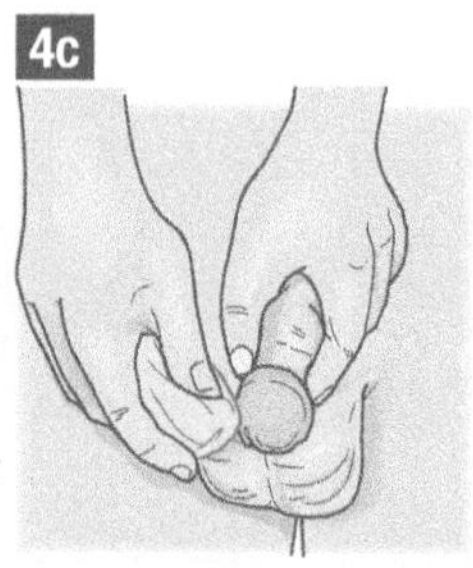

Cleanse the area around the meatus. (From Niedzwiecki B, Pepper J, Weaver P: *Kinn's the medical assistant*, ed 14, St Louis: Elsevier; 2020.)

d. Cleanse directly across the meatus with a third antiseptic towelette. After use, discard each towelette in the toilet.

e. Void a small amount of urine into the toilet.

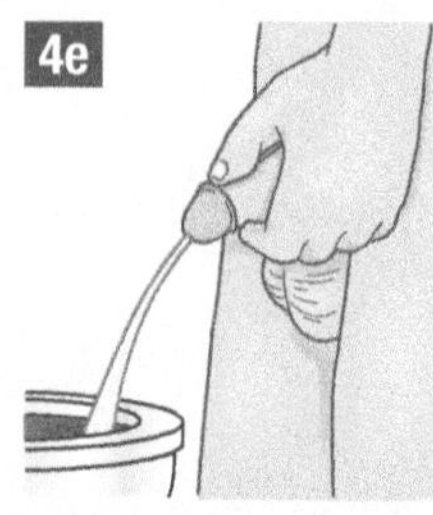

Void a small amount of urine into the toilet. (From Niedzwiecki B, Pepper J, Weaver P: *Kinn's the medical assistant*, ed 14, St Louis: Elsevier; 2020.)

f. Collect the next amount of urine by voiding into the sterile container without touching the inside of the container with the hands or penis. Fill the container about half full with urine.

PROCEDURE 16.1 Collection of a Clean-Catch Midstream Urine Specimen—cont'd

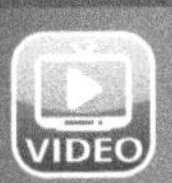

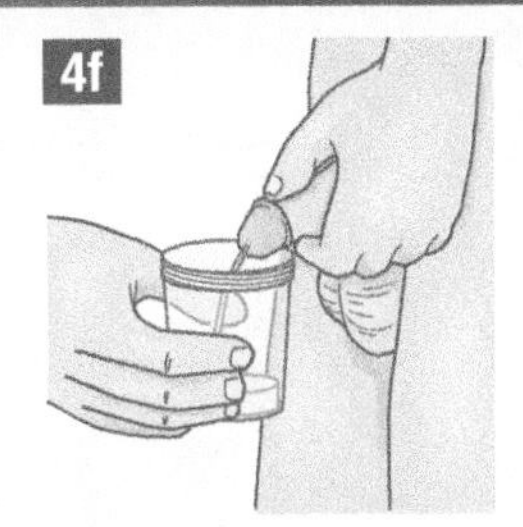

Void into the sterile container. (From Niedzwiecki B, Pepper J, Weaver P: *Kinn's the medical assistant*, ed 14, St Louis: Elsevier; 2020.)

g. Void the last amount of urine into the toilet, and replace the lid on the container.
h. Wipe the area dry with a tissue, and discard it in the toilet. Flush the toilet, and wash the hands.

5. **Procedural Step.** Provide the patient with instructions about what to do with the specimen after it has been collected (e.g., placing it in a designated area, directly handing it to the medical assistant).
6. **Procedural Step.** Test the specimen at the office, or prepare the specimen for transport to an outside laboratory for testing. If the specimen is to be transported to an outside laboratory, do the following:
   a. Place the specimen container in a biohazard specimen bag.
   b. Place the laboratory request in the outside pocket of the specimen bag.
   c. Properly preserve the specimen while awaiting pickup by a laboratory courier by placing it in a refrigerator.
7. **Procedural Step.** Document the procedure in the patient's medical record.
   a. *Electronic health record:* Document the type of specimen collected (clean-catch specimen, midstream collection) and the test results or the date the specimen was transported to the laboratory, using the appropriate radio buttons, drop-down menus, and free text fields.
   b. *Paper-based patient record (PPR):* Document the date and time and the type of specimen collected (clean-catch midstream collection). Document either the test results or the date the specimen was transported to the laboratory. Refer to the PPR documentation example.

PPR Documentation Example

Date	
3/24/XX	10:15 a.m. Clean-catch midstream collected
	by pt. Sent to Medical Center Laboratory for
	C&S on 3/24/XX. ——K. Smith, CMA (AAMA)

PROCEDURE 16.2 Collection of a 24-hour Urine Specimen

Outcome Instruct a patient in the collection of a 24-hour urine specimen.

Equipment/Supplies

- Large urine collection container and label
- Collecting container
- Written instructions
- Laboratory requisition

1. **Procedural Step.** Sanitize your hands. Greet the patient, and introduce yourself. Identify the patient, and explain the procedure.
2. **Procedural Step.** Assemble the equipment. Label the large specimen container with the patient's name and date of birth, the date, the type of specimen (24-h urine specimen), and your initials.
   Instruct the patient on collection of the specimen as follows.

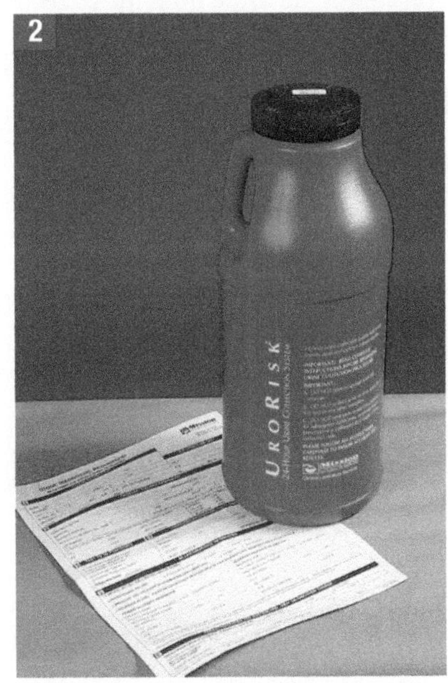

Assemble the equipment.

Continued

PROCEDURE 16.2 Collection of a 24-hour Urine Specimen—cont'd

3. **Procedural Step.** When you get up in the morning, empty your bladder into the toilet just as you normally do. In other words, this urine is not to be saved. Make a note of what time it is, and write the date and start time in the appropriate space on the label of the container.
   Principle. This urine was produced before the collection period began and should not be included in the collection.
4. **Procedural Step.** The next time you need to urinate, void in the collecting container and then pour the urine into the large wide-mouthed specimen container.
5. **Procedural Step.** Tightly screw the lid onto the 24-h specimen container, and put the container in your refrigerator or into an ice chest.
6. **Procedural Step.** Repeat procedural steps 4 and 5 each time you urinate.
7. **Procedural Step.** Emphasize the importance of the following to the patient:
   a. The urine must be stored only in the designated container.
   b. Collect all of the urine during the 24-h period, including urine that you void if you get up during the night. The information this test provides would be inaccurate if any urine from the 24-h period does not go into the container.
   c. Urinate into the collection container before having a bowel movement to avoid losing urine you might pass during the bowel movement.
   d. The collection must be started again from the beginning if any of the following occurs:
   - You forget to collect the urine when you void.
   - You spill some urine from the collection container.
   - Your urine becomes contaminated with stool from a bowel movement.
   - The child wets the bed (if the specimen is being obtained from a child).
   - You go beyond the 24-h collection period and collect too much urine.

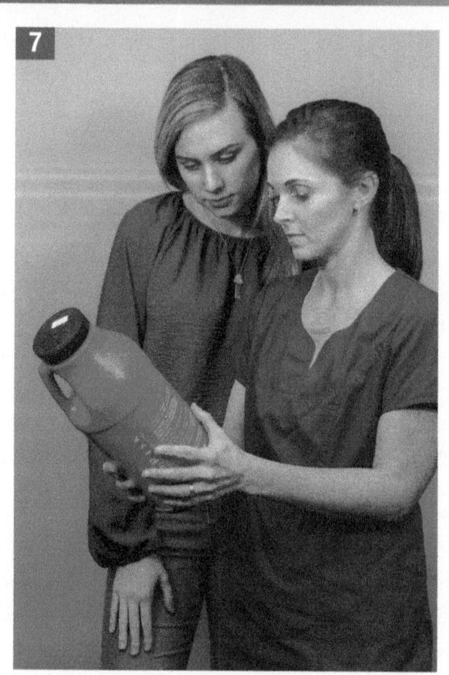

Explain the procedure.

8. **Procedural Step.** On the following morning, get up and void at the same time (exactly 24 h after beginning the test). Void into the collection container for the last time, and pour the urine into the large specimen container.
9. **Procedural Step.** Put the lid on the specimen container tightly, and write the date and time the test ended on the label in the appropriate space. Return the 24-h specimen container to the office the same morning you complete the urine collection.
10. **Procedural Step.** Provide the patient with the 24-h specimen container, a collection container, and written instructions. If the specimen container contains a chemical preservative, provide the patient with a Material Safety Data Sheet (MSDS) so that the patient has information regarding the chemical, its hazards, and measures to take to prevent injury and illness when handling the chemical. Document this information in the patient's medical record.
11. **Procedural Step.** When the patient returns the 24-h urine specimen container, ask the patient whether he or she encountered any difficulty in following the instructions for the 24-h collection. If any problems occurred that resulted in undercollection or overcollection of urine, the entire collection process must be repeated.
12. **Procedural Step.** Prepare the specimen for transport to the laboratory. Complete a laboratory request form.
13. **Procedural Step.** Document this information in the patient's medical record.

PROCEDURE 16.2 Collection of a 24-hour Urine Specimen—cont'd

a. *Electronic health record (EHR):* Document the type of specimen collected (24-h specimen) and information on sending the specimen to the laboratory, using the appropriate radio buttons, drop-down menus, and free text fields.

b. *Paper-based patient record (PPR):* Document the date and time, the type of specimen collected (24-h specimen), and information on sending the specimen to the laboratory (refer to the PPR documentation example).

PPR Documentation Example

Date	
3/26/XX	3:30 p.m. Container and verbal/written
	instructions provided on 24-hour specimen
	collection. ________ L. Proffitt, CMA (AAMA)
3/28/XX	10:00 a.m. 24-hour urine specimen sent to
	Medical Center Laboratory for kidney stone
	risk analysis. ________ K. Smith, CMA (AAMA)

PROCEDURE 16.3 Chemical Assessment of a Urine Specimen Using a Reagent Strip

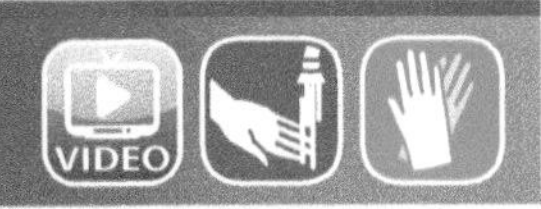

Outcome Perform a chemical assessment of a urine specimen using a reagent strip.

Equipment/Supplies

- Disposable gloves
- Container of Multistix 10 SG reagent strips
- Urine container
- Timer
- Laboratory report form

1. **Procedural Step.** Perform the quality control procedure if using a new container of test strips.
   Principle. Performing the quality control procedure ensures the reliability of test results.
2. **Procedural Step.** Obtain a freshly voided urine specimen from the patient in a clean, dry container. The specimen should be uncentrifuged and at room temperature.
   Principle. The best results are obtained with a freshly voided specimen. The urine container should be clean because contaminants could affect the results. Uncentrifuged specimens ensure a homogeneous sample.
3. **Procedural Step.** Sanitize your hands.
4. **Procedural Step.** Assemble the equipment. Check the expiration date of the reagent strips.
   Principle. Outdated reagent strips may lead to inaccurate test results.
5. **Procedural Step.** Apply gloves. Remove a reagent strip from its container, and recap the container immediately. Do not touch the test reagent pads with your fingers or lay the strip on the table. However, it is permissible to lay the reagent strip on a clean, dry paper towel.
   Principle. Recapping the container is necessary to prevent exposing the strips to environmental moisture, light, and heat, which cause altered reagent reactivity. Contamination of test pads by the hands or table surface may affect the accuracy of test results.
6. **Procedural Step.** Thoroughly mix the urine specimen, and remove the lid from the urine container. Using the dominant hand, completely immerse the reagent strip in the urine specimen to moisten all the test pads. Remove the strip immediately. While removing, run the edge of the strip against the rim of the urine container to remove excess urine.
   Principle. The strip should be completely immersed to ensure that all test pads are moistened for accurate test results. Prolonged immersion of the reagent strip and failure to remove excess urine may cause the reagents to dissolve and leach onto adjacent test pads, affecting the accuracy of the test results.

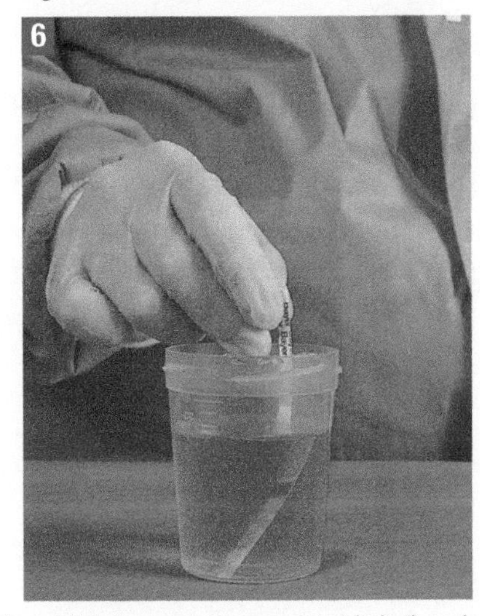

Completely immerse the reagent strip in the urine.

Continued

PROCEDURE 16.3 Chemical Assessment of a Urine Specimen Using a Reagent Strip—cont'd

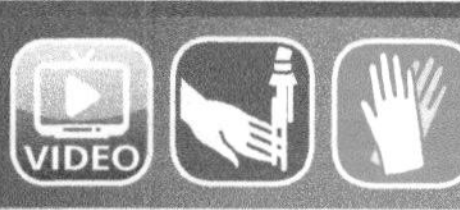

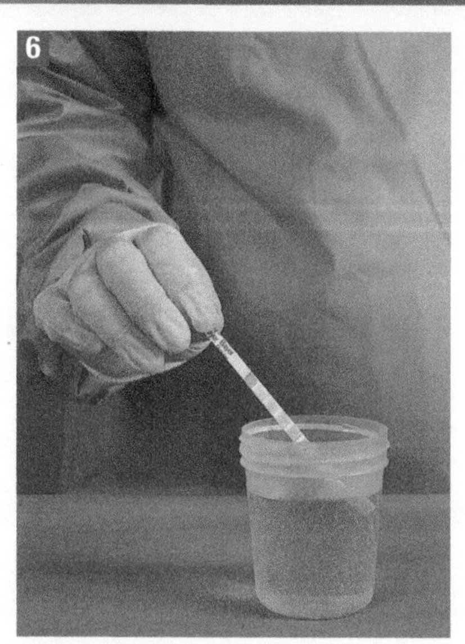

Run the edge of the strip against the urine container.

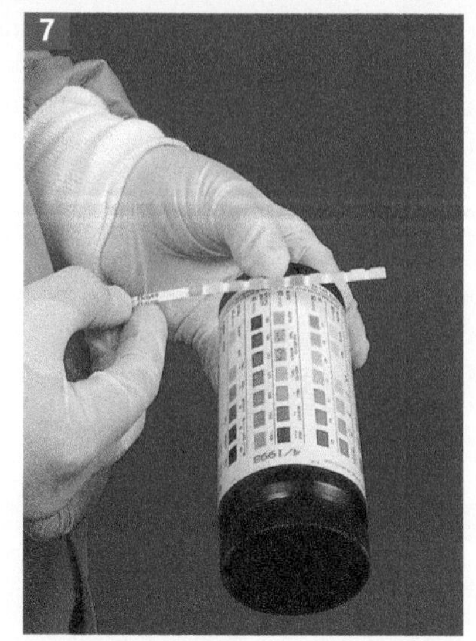

Hold the strip horizontally and read the results.

7. **Procedural Step.** With the nondominant hand, start the timer, pick up the reagent strip container, and rotate it to the color chart. Hold the reagent strip in a horizontal position, and place it as close as possible to the corresponding color blocks on the color chart. Do not lay the strip directly on the color chart because this will result in soiling of the chart by the urine. Compare each test pad to the corresponding row of color blocks on the container label. Read the results carefully and at the exact reading times, starting with the shortest time specified on the color chart and as indicated here:

Glucose: 30 s	pH: 60 s
Bilirubin: 30 s	Protein: 60 s
Ketone: 40 s	Urobilinogen: 60 s
Specific gravity: 45 s	Nitrite: 60 s
Blood: 60 s	Leukocytes, 2 min

Principle. Holding the strip in a horizontal position avoids soiling your gloves with urine and prevents reagents from running over into adjacent test pads, causing inaccurate test results. The strip must be read at the proper time interval to avoid dissolving out reagents, leading to inaccurate test results.

8. **Procedural Step.** Dispose of the strip in a regular waste container.
9. **Procedural Step.** Remove gloves, and sanitize your hands.
10. **Procedural Step.** Document the results in the patient's medical record. The results should be documented by following the interpretation guide provided above each color block on the color chart.
    a. *Electronic health record (EHR):* Document the brand name of the test used (Multistix 10 SG) and the results, using the appropriate radio buttons, drop-down menus, and free text fields.
    b. *Paper-based patient record (PPR):* Most offices use a preprinted reporting form to make it easier to document results. The documentation should include the date and time, the brand name of the test used (Multistix 10 SG), and the results (refer to the PPR documentation example).

PROCEDURE 16.3 Chemical Assessment of a Urine Specimen Using a Reagent Strip—cont'd

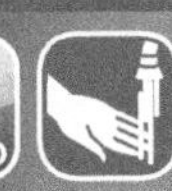

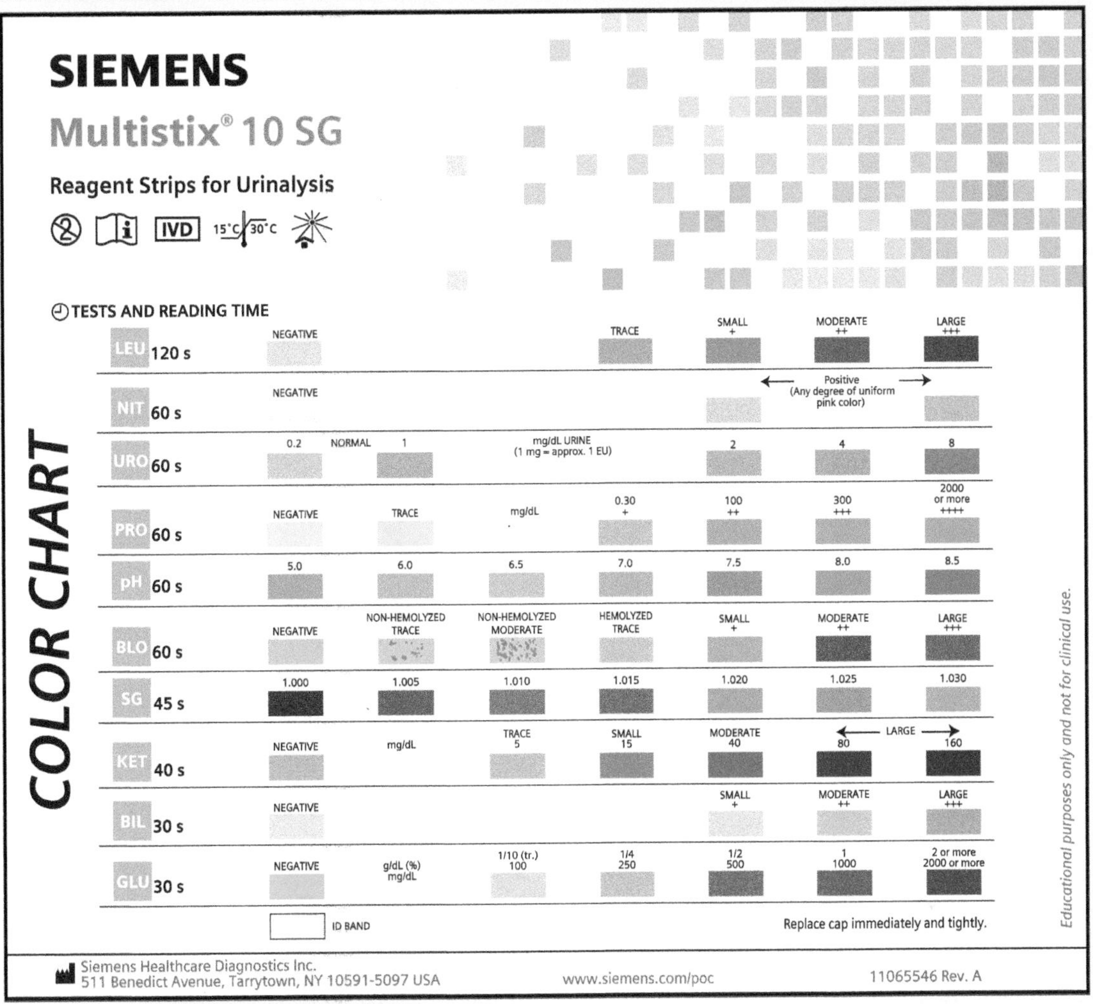

(Multistix Color Chart modified and printed by permission of Siemens Medical Solutions Diagnostics, Tarrytown, NY.)

PPR Documentation Example

***Multistix®* 10 SG** Reagent Strips for Urinalysis

PATIENT *Annette Ross*

DATE *3/22/XX* TIME *9:45 a.m.*

LEUKOCYTES	NEGATIVE ☑		TRACE ☐	SMALL + ☐	MODERATE ++ ☐	LARGE +++ ☐	
NITRITE	NEGATIVE ☑		POSITIVE ☐	POSITIVE ☐	(Any degree of uniform pink color is found)		
UROBILINOGEN	NORMAL 0.2 ☑	NORMAL 1 ☐	mg/dL 2 ☐	4 ☐	8 ☐ (1mg = approx. 1 BU)		
PROTEIN	NEGATIVE ☐	TRACE ☑	mg/dL 30 + ☐	100 ++ ☐	300 +++ ☐	2000 OR MORE ☐	
pH	5.0 ☑	6.0 ☐	6.5 ☐	7.0 ☐	7.5 ☐	8.0 ☐	8.5 ☐
BLOOD	NEGATIVE ☑	NON-HEMOLYZED TRACE ☐	NON-HEMOLYZED MODERATE ☐	HEMOLYZED TRACE ☐	SMALL + ☐	MODERATE ++ ☐	LARGE +++ ☐
SPECIFIC GRAVITY	1.000 ☐	1.005 ☐	1.010 ☐	1.015 ☑	1.020 ☐	1.025 ☐	1.030 ☐
KETONE	NEGATIVE ☑	mg/dL	TRACE 5 ☐	SMALL 15 ☐	MODERATE 40 ☐	LARGE 80 ☐	LARGE 160 ☐
BILIRUBIN	NEGATIVE ☑		SMALL + ☐	MODERATE ++ ☐	LARGE +++ ☐		
GLUCOSE	NEGATIVE ☑	g/L (%) mg/dL	1/10 tr.) 100 ☐	1/6 250 ☐	1/2 500 ☐	1 1000 ☐	2 or more 2000 or more ☐

PROCEDURE 16.4 Prepare a Urine Specimen for Microscopic Examination: Kova Method

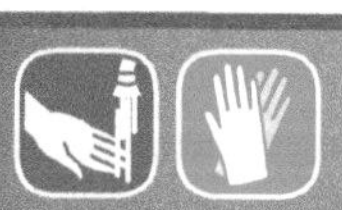

Outcome Prepare a urine specimen for microscopic examination by the provider.

Equipment/Supplies

- Disposable gloves
- Urine specimen (first-voided morning specimen)
- Kova urine centrifuge tube
- Kova cap
- Kova pipet
- Kova slide
- Kova stain
- Test tube rack
- Urine centrifuge
- Mechanical stage microscope

1. Procedural Step. Sanitize the hands, and assemble the equipment.

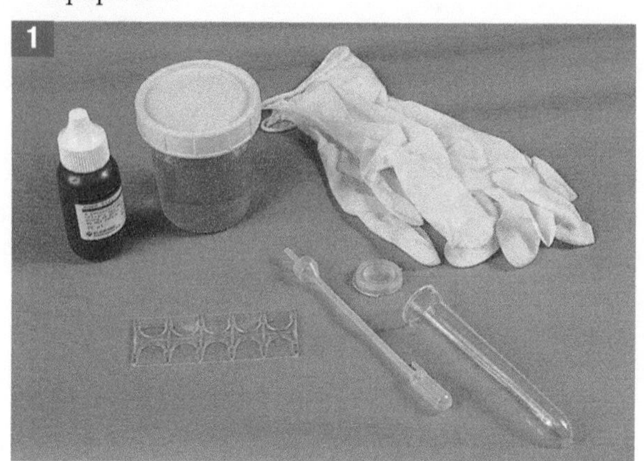

Assemble the equipment.

2. Procedural Step. Apply gloves. Mix the urine specimen with the Kova pipet.
Principle. The specimen must be well mixed to ensure accurate test results.

3. Procedural Step. Pour the urine specimen into the urine centrifuge tube. Fill it to the 12-mL graduation mark, and cap the tube.

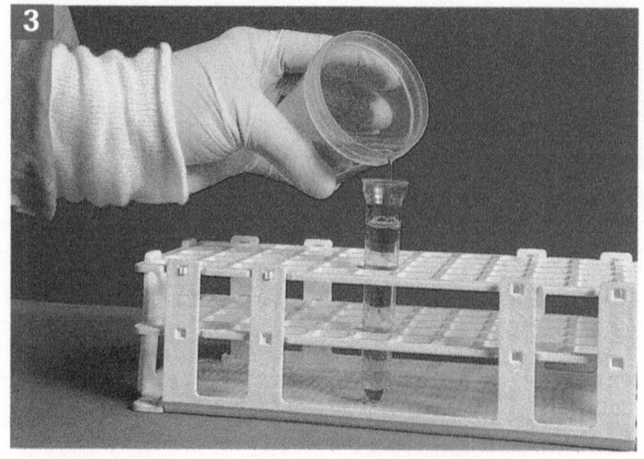

Pour the specimen into the urine tube.

4. Procedural Step. Centrifuge the tube for 5 min at approximately 1500 revolutions per minute (rpm).
Principle. Centrifuging the specimen causes the solid elements in the urine to settle to the bottom of the tube.

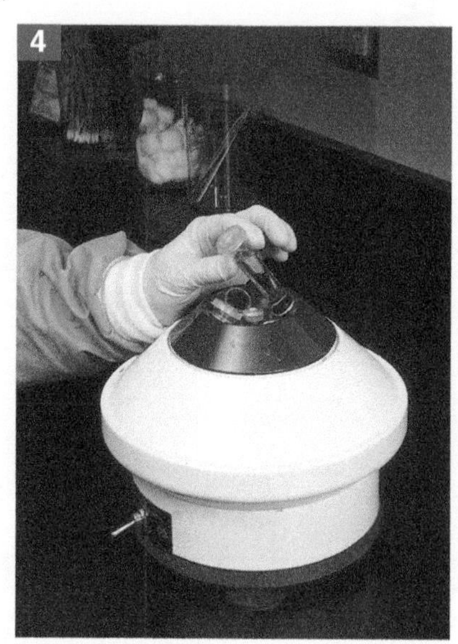

Centrifuge the specimen.

5. Procedural Step. Remove the urine tube from the centrifuge; do not disturb or dislodge the sediment.

6. Procedural Step. Remove the cap. Insert the Kova pipet into the urine tube, and push it to the bottom of the tube until it seats firmly. Ensure that the clip on the bulb is hooked over the outside edge of the tube.

PROCEDURE 16.4 Prepare a Urine Specimen for Microscopic Examination: Kova Method—cont'd

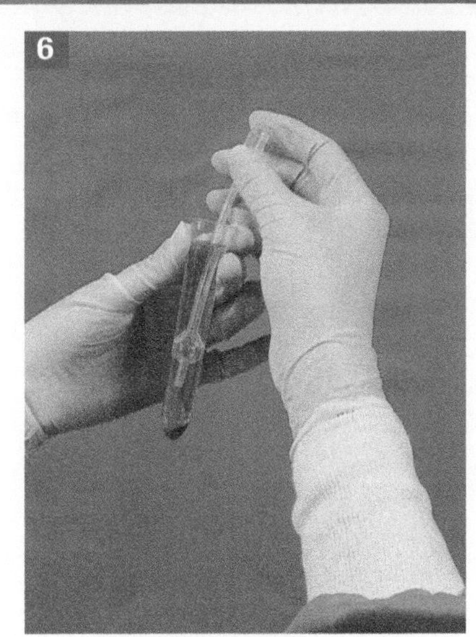

Insert the pipet until it seats firmly.

7. Procedural Step. Decant the specimen by inverting the tube and pouring off the **supernatant** fluid. Approximately 1 mL of sediment is retained in the bottom of the tube.

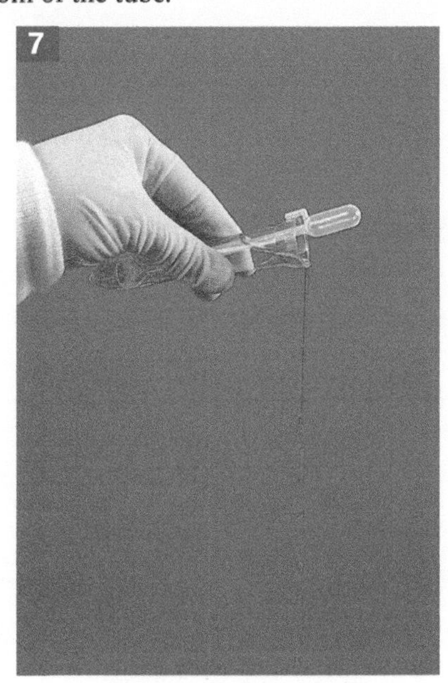

Pour the supernatant fluid.

8. Procedural Step. Remove the pipet from the tube. Add 1 drop of Kova stain to the tube. Place the pipet back in the tube, and mix the sediment and stain together vigorously with the pipet. Ensure that the sediment and the stain are well mixed. Place the urine tube in a test tube rack.

Principle. Kova stain improves the detail of the sediment for better visualization of structures under the microscope.

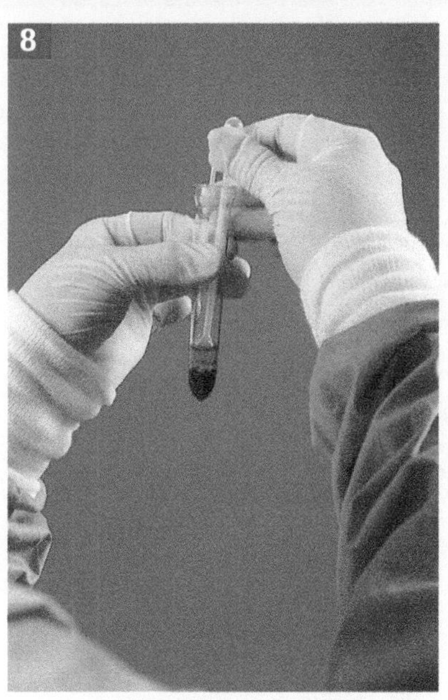

Mix the sediment and stain.

9. Procedural Step. Transfer a sample of the sediment to the Kova slide as follows:

a. Place the Kova slide on a flat surface with the open "envelope" areas facing upward.
b. Squeeze the bulb of the pipet to draw a sample of the sediment into the tip of the pipet.
c. Place the tip of the pipet so that it just touches the notched corner edge of the slide.
d. Gently squeeze the bulb to allow the specimen to fill the well. Do not overfill or underfill the well.
e. Place the pipet in the urine tube.

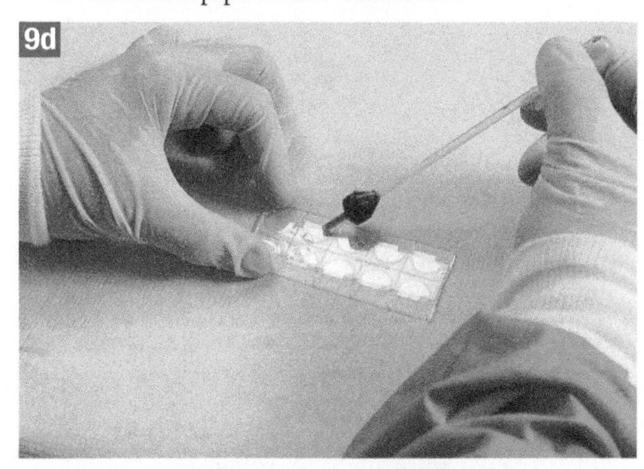

Fill the well with the specimen.

10. Procedural Step. Allow the specimen to sit for 1 min to permit the sediment to settle in the well.

Principle. Allowing the sediment to settle prevents structures from moving when the slide is viewed under the microscope.

11. Procedural Step. Place the slide on the stage of the microscope. Focus the specimen for the provider

Continued

PROCEDURE 16.4 Prepare a Urine Specimen for Microscopic Examination: Kova Method—cont'd

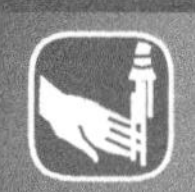

under the microscope by following the procedure presented in Procedure 20.1: Using the Microscope.

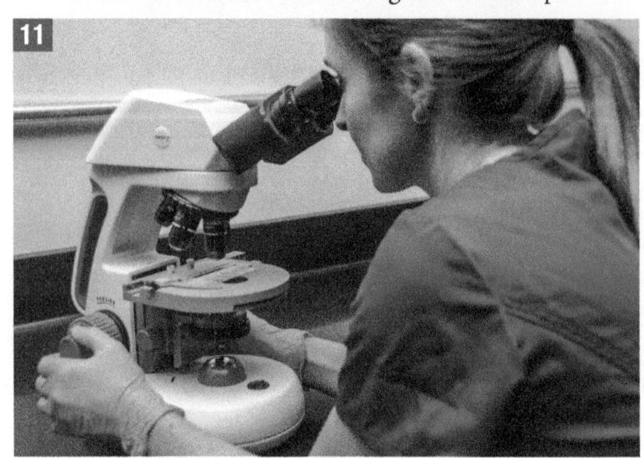

Focus the specimen for the provider.

12. **Procedural Step.** When the provider is finished examining the urine sediment and documenting results (refer to the laboratory report), remove the slide from the stage.
13. **Procedural Step.** Dispose of the plastic slide and pipet in a regular waste container. Rinse the remaining urine down the sink. Cap the empty plastic urine tube, and dispose of it in a regular waste container.
14. **Procedural Step.** Remove gloves, and sanitize your hands.

LAB REPORT

Date	Time	Name	
3/18/XX	10:00 a.m.	Tanya Howe	
	MICROSCOPIC		
	WBCs		20/HPF
	RBCs		3/HPF
	CASTS (Hyaline)		0/LPF
	CASTS (Granular)		0/LPF
	CASTS (Cellular)		0/LPF
	CASTS (Waxy)		0/LPF
	EPITHELIAL CELLS		0/LPF
	BACTERIA		Freq
	MUCUS		Occ
	CRYSTALS		0
			T. Bach, MD

PROCEDURE 16.5 Perform a Clinical Laboratory Improvement Amendments (CLIA)-Waived Urine Pregnancy Test

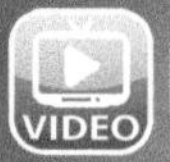

Outcome Perform a CLIA-waived urine pregnancy test.

Equipment/Supplies

- Disposable gloves
- Urine pregnancy test kit (QuickVue HCG Urine Test by Quidel)
- Urine specimen (first-voided morning specimen)

1. **Procedural Step.** Sanitize the hands, and assemble the equipment. Check the expiration date on the urine pregnancy test kit. It should not be used if the expiration date has passed. When a new test kit is opened (and thereafter on a monthly basis), external positive and negative controls should be performed according to the instructions in the package insert accompanying the controls. Document the control results in a quality control log. If the controls do not perform as expected, patient testing should not be conducted until the problem has been identified and resolved.

   Principle. An expired pregnancy test may produce inaccurate test results. Running positive and negative external controls ensures that the test results are valid and reliable. Factors that can cause abnormal control results include outdated controls or test reagents, improper storage of test components, and an error in the technique used to perform the procedure.

PROCEDURE 16.5 Perform a Clinical Laboratory Improvement Amendments (CLIA)-Waived Urine Pregnancy Test—cont'd

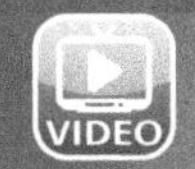

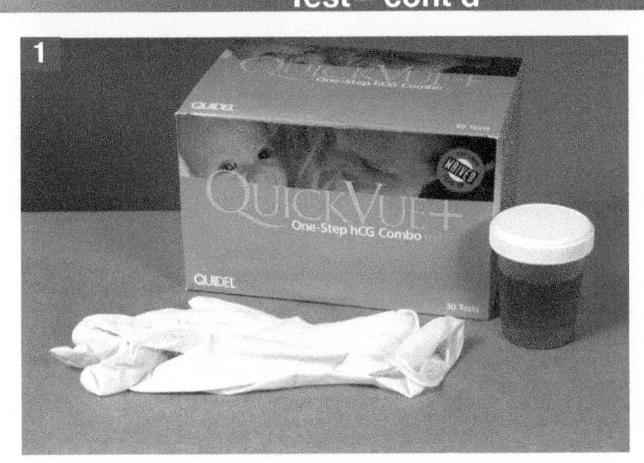

Assemble the equipment.

2. **Procedural Step.** Apply gloves. Rotate the urine specimen cup to mix the urine. Inspect the foil pouch containing the cassette. If it is torn or punctured, discard the test and obtain another one from the test kit. Remove the test cassette from its foil pouch, and place it on a clean, dry, level surface.
   Principle. The foil pouch should not be opened until it is time to perform the test.
3. **Procedural Step.** Add 3 drops of urine to the round sample well on the test cassette with a disposable pipet supplied with the kit. The test cassette should not be handled or moved again until the test is ready for interpretation. Dispose of the pipet in a regular waste container.

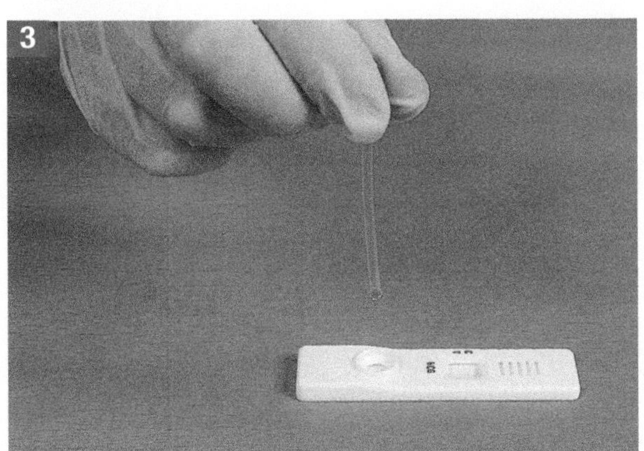

Add 3 drops of urine to the test well.

4. **Procedural Step.** Wait 3 min, and read the results by observing the test result window.
5. **Procedural Step.** Interpret the test results as follows:
   Negative: The appearance of the blue internal control line next to the letter *C* only and no pink to purple test line next to the letter *T* in the test result window. In addition, the background of the test window should be clear and not interfere with the ability to read the test results. (*Note:* If the test result is negative and pregnancy is suspected, another specimen should be collected and tested 48 to 72 h later.)
   Positive: The appearance of any pink to purple line next to the letter *T* along with a blue internal control line next to the letter *C* in the test result window. In addition, the background of the test window should be clear and should not interfere with the ability to read test results.
   Invalid result: If no blue internal control line appears within 3 min or if the background of the test window interferes with reading the results, the test result is invalid, and the specimen must be retested with a new cassette.
   Principle. The blue control line is a positive internal control indicator designating that a sufficient urine sample was added to the cassette well and that the test is working properly. A background in the test window that is clear and does not interfere with reading the test results is a negative internal quality control indicator and also indicates that the test is working properly.

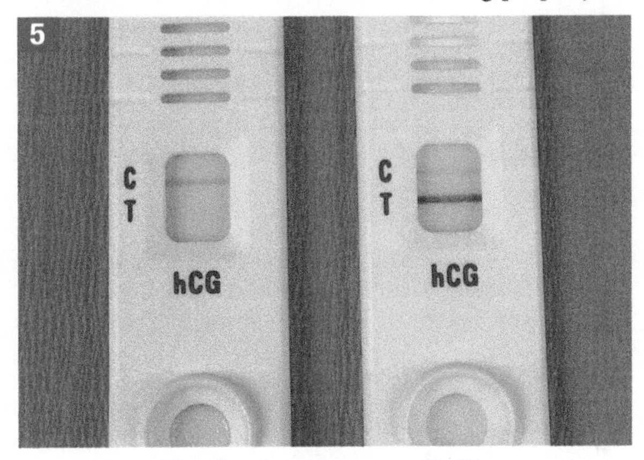

Interpret the results.

6. **Procedural Step.** Dispose of the test cassette in a regular waste container. Remove gloves, and sanitize your hands.
7. **Procedural Step.** Document the results in the patient's medical record.
   a. *Electronic health record:* Document the date of the patient's last menstrual period (LMP), the name of the test, and the results documented as either positive or negative, using the appropriate radio buttons, drop-down menus, and free text fields.
   b. *Paper-based patient record (PPR):* Document the date and time, the date of the patient's LMP, the name of the test, and the results documented as either positive or negative (refer to the PPR documentation example).

PPR Documentation Example

Date	
3/25/XX	10:30 a.m. LMP: 2/20/XX.
	QuickVue preg test: Positive.
	K. Smith, CMA (AAMA)

PROCEDURE 16.5

17 Phlebotomy

 Check out the Evolve site at http://evolve.elsevier.com/Bonewit/today/ to access additional interactive activities and exercises to help you study and prepare for success.

LEARNING OUTCOMES

Venipuncture

1. List and describe the guidelines that should be followed when performing a venipuncture.
2. Explain how each of the following blood specimens is obtained:
   - Clotted blood
   - Serum
   - Whole blood
   - Plasma
3. List the layers into which the blood separates when an anticoagulant is added to the specimen.
4. List the layers into which the blood separates when an anticoagulant is not added to the specimen.
5. List the OSHA safety precautions that must be followed during venipuncture.
6. State the additive content of each of the following evacuated collection tubes, and list the types of blood specimens that can be obtained from each: red, lavender, gray, light blue, green, royal blue.
7. Identify and explain the order of draw for the Vacutainer and butterfly methods of venipuncture.
8. List and describe guidelines for use of blood collection tubes.
9. Identify problems that may occur during a venipuncture.
10. List four ways to prevent a blood specimen from becoming hemolyzed.
11. Explain how a serum separator tube functions in the collection of a serum specimen.

Skin Puncture

12. Explain when a skin puncture is preferred over a venipuncture.
13. Identify skin puncture sites for adults and infants.
14. List and describe guidelines for performing a finger puncture.

PROCEDURES

Perform a venipuncture using the Vacutainer method.

Perform a venipuncture using the butterfly method.

Collect a capillary blood specimen using a disposable lancet.

CHAPTER OUTLINE

KEY TERMS

antecubital space (an-tih-KYOO-bih-tul SPAYS)
anticoagulant (an-tih-koe-AG-yoo-lent)
buffy coat
evacuated collection tube
hematoma (hee-mah-TOE-mah)
hemoconcentration (hee-moe-kon-sen-TRAY-shun)
hemolysis (hee-MOL-ih-sis)
osteochondritis (OS-tee-oh-kon-DRY-tis)
osteomyelitis (OS-tee-oh-mie-LIE-tis)
phlebotomist (fleh-BOT-oe-mist)
phlebotomy (fleh-BOT-oe-mee)
plasma
serum
venipuncture (VEN-ih-punk-chur)
venous reflux (VEEN-us REE-fluks)
venous stasis (VEEN-us STAE-sis)

Introduction to Phlebotomy

The purpose of phlebotomy is to collect a blood specimen for laboratory analysis. The word *phlebotomy* is derived from the Greek words for "vein" *(phlebos)* and "incision" *(otomy)* and literally means "making an incision into a vein." As used in the clinical laboratory sciences, **phlebotomy** is defined as the collection of blood. An individual who collects a blood sample is a **phlebotomist**. Phlebotomy encompasses three major areas of blood collection:

- ***Arterial puncture*** for the collection of an arterial blood specimen
- ***Venipuncture*** for the collection of a venous blood specimen
- ***Skin puncture*** for the collection of a capillary blood specimen

An arterial puncture is typically performed in a hospital to assess the oxygen level, carbon dioxide level, and acid-base balance of arterial blood; medical assistants do not perform arterial punctures. In the medical office, medical assistants perform venipunctures and skin punctures which are described in detail in this chapter.

Capillary blood specimens are usually tested in the medical office while venous blood specimens are transported to an outside laboratory for testing. Specimens for transport must be placed in a biohazard specimen bag to protect healthcare workers and laboratory couriers from an exposure incident (Fig. 17.1). A laboratory request must be completed for specimens being transported to an outside laboratory. The purpose of the request is to provide the outside laboratory with information necessary for accurate testing, reporting of results, and billing.

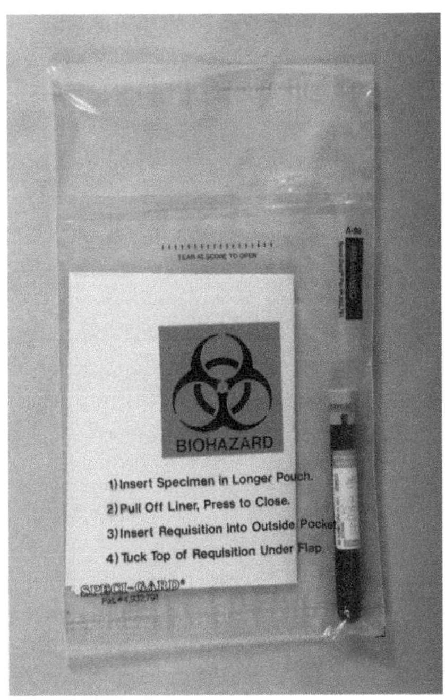

Fig. 17.1 Specimen in a biohazard specimen bag along with the laboratory request form.

Venipuncture

Venipuncture means the puncturing of a vein for the removal of a venous blood specimen. Venipuncture is usually performed in the medical office using the following methods:

- Vacutainer method
- Butterfly method

The Vacutainer method is the fastest and most convenient method and is used most often. This method relies on the use of Vacutainer blood collection system (commercially available from Becton Dickinson, Franklin Lakes, NJ). The Vacutainer setup consists of a blood collection needle, a plastic tube holder, and an evacuated collection tube. An **evacuated collection tube** is a sterile plastic or glass blood collection tube with a color-coded closure that contains a vacuum. The butterfly method is used for difficult draws, such as when a vein is small or sclerosed (hardened). The butterfly method also uses evacuated collection tubes and a tube holder; however, the collection needle is different than the one used with the Vacutainer method. This chapter presents the theory and procedure for both of these methods.

GUIDELINES FOR VENIPUNCTURE

General guidelines that should be followed for venipuncture are listed and described below.

PATIENT PREPARATION

If advance preparation is required for a laboratory test, the patient should be given instructions an appropriate number of days before the specimen collection. Information on the preparation required is specified in the laboratory test directory provided by the outside laboratory. Although most tests require no preparation, some tests require fasting or the avoidance of certain medications. *Fasting* involves abstaining from food and fluids (except water) for a specified period of time before the collection of the specimen (usually 8 to 12 hours) to allow food and fluid from the previous meal to be completely digested and absorbed.

When a laboratory test requires advance preparation, the medical assistant must verify that the patient has prepared properly before performing the venipuncture. If the patient has not properly prepared, do not collect the specimen unless directed otherwise by the provider. If the venipuncture is to be rescheduled, carefully review the preparation requirements with the patient.

REVIEW COLLECTION AND HANDLING REQUIREMENTS

The medical assistant should carefully review the collection and handling requirements in the laboratory test directory for the test(s) ordered by the provider. These include the collection supplies necessary, the type of specimen to be collected, the amount of the specimen needed to perform the laboratory test, the procedure to follow to collect the specimen, and the proper handling and storage of the specimen awaiting transport to an outside laboratory.

A review of the requirements beforehand prevents errors in collection and handling of the specimen. The medical assistant should contact the outside laboratory if there are any questions regarding any aspect of collection procedure. Fig. 17.2 shows an example of the collection and handling requirements for a complete blood count (CBC) as it is presented in a laboratory test directory.

IDENTIFICATION OF THE PATIENT

The patient must be identified using two unique identifiers (e.g., full, legal name and date of birth) before performing the venipuncture. Proper patient identification is essential to avoid collecting a specimen from the wrong patient by mistake, which could lead to an inaccurate diagnosis and the wrong treatment. After greeting the patient, the medical assistant should ask the patient to state his or her full name and date of birth. This information should be compared with the demographic data indicated in the patient's medical record.

ASSEMBLE THE EQUIPMENT AND SUPPLIES

The medical assistant must make sure to use the appropriate blood collection tube for each test ordered by the provider as specified in the laboratory test directory. Substituting one collection tube for another will not yield the proper type of specimen required for the test, as shown by the following example. If a serum specimen is required and a tube containing an anticoagulant is used (instead of a tube without an anticoagulant), the blood separates into plasma and cells rather than serum and cells, and the wrong type of blood specimen is obtained. This is a cause for rejection of the specimen by the outside laboratory and necessitates obtaining another specimen from the patient.

The medical assistant should check each blood collection tube before use to ensure that it is not broken, chipped, cracked, or otherwise damaged. Damaged collection tubes are unsuitable for specimen collection and should be discarded. Collection tubes also have an expiration date (Fig. 17.3). The medical assistant should make sure to check the expiration date on the tube to avoid using an outdated collection tube, which is also a cause for rejection of the blood specimen by the outside laboratory.

COMPLETE A LABORATORY REQUEST

The laboratory request may be a preprinted request form or a computer-generated electronic request. The completed request provides the outside laboratory with the information necessary to test the specimen.

LABEL THE BLOOD SPECIMEN TUBE(S)

The medical assistant must make sure to properly label each collection tube. At a minimum, the label should include the patient's full legal name, date of birth, and the date and time of collection of the specimen. (*Note:* The medical assistant should follow the medical office policy as to when the collection tube should be labeled. Some offices prefer that the tube be labeled *before* the specimen is collected; other offices want the tube to be labeled *after* the specimen is collected.)

LABORATORY TEST DIRECTORY CBC with Differential	
CPT Code:	85025
Tests Included:	WBC, RBC, Hemoglobin, Hematocrit, MCV, MCH, MCHC, RDW, Platelet Count, MPV and Differential (Absolute and Percent - Neutrophils, Lymphocytes, Monocytes, Eosinophils, and Basophils). If abnormal cells are noted on a manual review of the peripheral blood smear or if the automated differential information meets specific criteria, a full manual differential will be performed.
Alternative Names:	Complete blood count
Type of Specimen:	Whole blood
Amount of Specimen:	7 mL
Collection Container:	7-mL lavender-top tube
Patient Preparation:	None
Collection and Processing:	1. Red and SST tubes should be drawn before the lavender tube. 2. Completely fill tube to the exhaustion of the vacuum to ensure a proper blood-to-anticoagulant ratio. 3. Gently invert tube 8 to 10 times immediately after collection to mix the anticoagulant with the blood. 4. Traumatic draw can introduce thromboplastin and trap WBC and platelets. 5. Refrigeration can precipitate fibrin and trap WBC and platelets.
Storage and Transport:	Store at RT. Do not refrigerate.
Specimen Stability:	RT (15°-35° C): 48 hours
Causes for Rejection:	Hemolyzed or clotted specimen Underfilled tube Specimen collected in any tube other than an EDTA tube Improper labeling of specimen Improper storage temperature Specimen is more than 48 hours old
Reference Range:	Values given with laboratory report.
Use:	The CBC is used as a screening test to assess the overall health of an individual and to detect a wide range of hematologic conditions such as anemia, leukemia, infection, bleeding disorders, and inflammation. The CBC is also used to assist in managing medication and chemotherapeutic decisions.
Limitations:	A manual differential can identify cells that may be misidentified by an automated analyzer.
Forms:	Order electronically or print lab request and submit with specimen.
Methodology:	Automated cell counter and microscopy

Fig. 17.2 CBC specimen requirements from a laboratory directory.

Barcode Label: A specimen can be labeled by attaching an adhesive barcode label to the collection tube. Laboratory analyzers incorporate a barcode reader that is able to read the information on the barcode necessary for testing the specimen and generating test results. Along with the barcode, additional printed information is included on a barcode label (Fig. 17.4). It is important to properly attach the barcode label to the correct collection tube. Inspect the label for information indicating the color of the tube closure (e.g., LV for lavender) to which the label must be attached. For example, the barcode label illustrated in Fig. 17.4 must be placed on a lavender (LV) tube for a specimen that is being collected to perform a CBC. The barcode label must be properly attached to the tube. The label should be placed lengthwise on the tube and aligned with the top of the manufacturer's label and no higher. To enable the barcode reader to read the label, it must be placed in a straight (not diagonal) position on the collection tube with no wrinkles, folds, or tears (Fig. 17.5A).

Handwritten Label: A blood specimen can also be labeled by handwriting the required information on the label (patient's full legal name and date of birth, the date and time of collection, the medical assistant's initials, and any other information required by the laboratory) (Fig. 17.5B). The information should be printed legibly with a ball point pen, and the medical assistant should be certain that the information is accurate to avoid a mix-up of specimens.

REASSURE THE PATIENT

Venipuncture is often a frightening experience for the patient. For many patients, the anticipation of the procedure is worse than the actual drawing of the blood. The medical assistant should take time to explain the procedure to the patient in an unhurried and confident manner. This helps to alleviate the patient's fears, which relaxes the patient's veins. Relaxed veins make venipuncture easier to perform and result in less pain for the patient.

Instruct the patient to remain still during the procedure. Explain to the patient that a small amount of pain is associated with a venipuncture, but it is brief. Never tell the patient that the venipuncture will not hurt. Just before inserting the needle, tell the patient that he or she will "feel a small stick." This prevents startling the patient, which could cause the patient to move. Movement causes pain for the patient, and it may damage tissue at the venipuncture site.

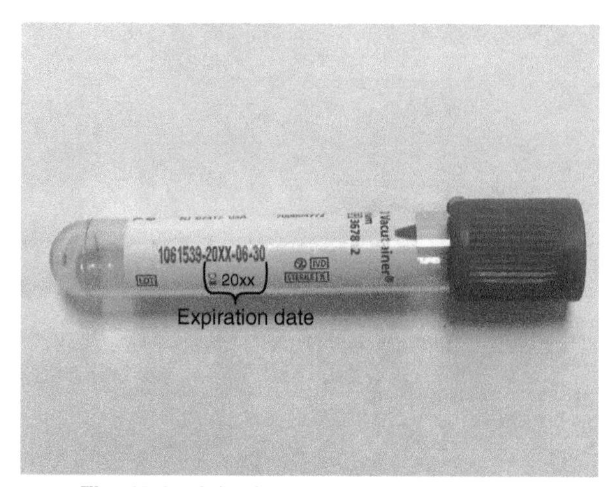

Fig. 17.3 Collection tube showing expiration date.

PATIENT POSITION FOR VENIPUNCTURE

The patient position for venipuncture is especially important to the successful collection of a blood specimen. Proper positioning allows easy access to the vein and is more comfortable for the patient. The patient position depends on the vein to be used. The most common site for venipuncture is the **antecubital space**, which is the surface of the arm in front of the elbow. Information on positioning the patient presented next refers to the antecubital venipuncture site.

The patient should be seated comfortably in a phlebotomy chair. The arm should be extended downward to form a straight line from the shoulder to the wrist with the palm facing up; the arm should not bend at the elbow (Fig. 17.6). The arm can be supported on the armrest by a rolled towel or by having the patient place the fist of the other hand under the elbow.

A venipuncture should never be performed with the patient sitting on a stool or standing. The patient may faint and become injured. If the patient appears nervous or has fainted in the past from a venipuncture, it is best to place the patient in a semi-reclining position (semi-Fowler position) on the examining table.

Although unusual, it is possible for blood to flow from the collection tube back into the patient's vein during the procedure. This condition is known as **venous reflux**. Venous

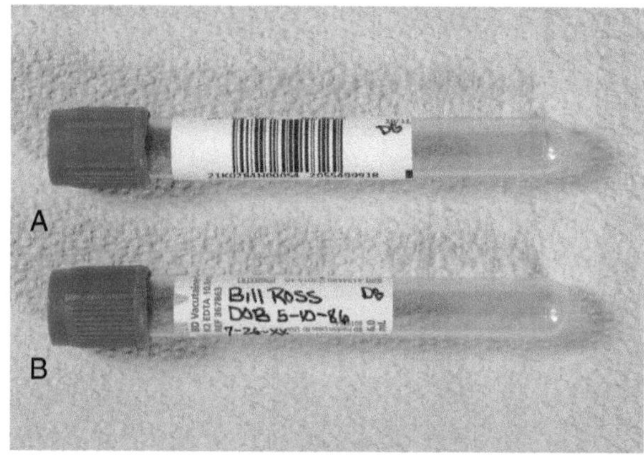

Fig. 17.5 (A) Barcode label. (B) Handwritten label.

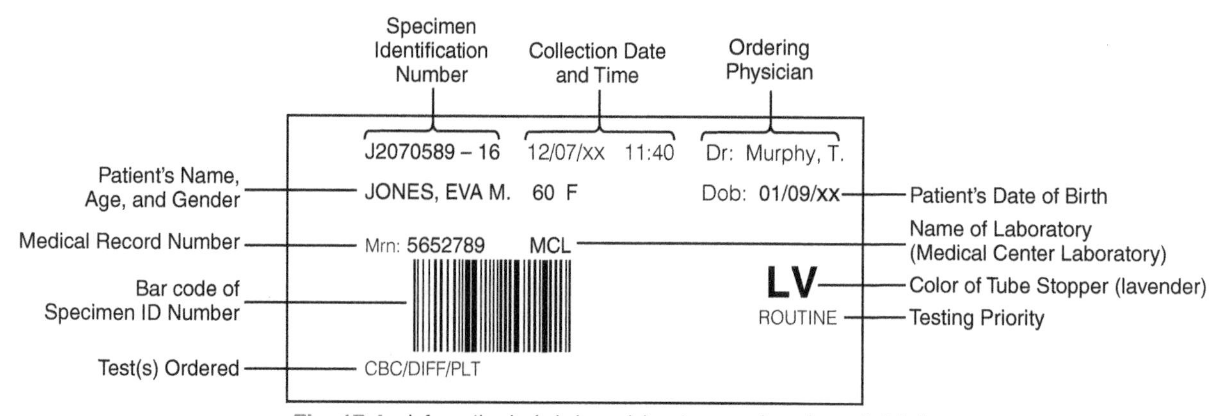

Fig. 17.4 Information included on a laboratory specimen barcode label.

reflux could cause the patient to have an adverse reaction to a tube additive, particularly if the additive in the tube is ethylenediaminetetraacetic acid (EDTA). Venous reflux can occur only if the contents of the collection tube are in contact with the tube stopper while the specimen is being drawn. Venous reflux is prevented by keeping the patient's arm in a downward position so that the collection tube remains below the venipuncture site and fills from the bottom up.

Putting It All Into Practice

My name is Dori, and I work in a very busy, fast-paced family practice office for two physicians. I love my job. The physicians are great, with very different styles; the pace is fast; and the time flies by. I am constantly challenged, learning new things, meeting and helping people, and being a part of a team that works well together.

While performing a venipuncture for a routine blood chemistry panel (a procedure I have performed many times), I accidentally stuck myself after collecting the specimen. I could see the blood inside my glove, and I could see the patient's blood clinging to the point of the needle—my heart sank. I activated the safety shield and placed the needle and holder in the sharps container and tried to keep my cool and not alarm the patient. I mentally assessed the patient. He was an older man from a rural community, but I know you cannot always judge a book by its cover.

I excused myself and immediately proceeded to wash my hands thoroughly with soap and water and rinse, rinse, rinse! I then notified the physician. The physician questioned the patient regarding operations he had had in the previous year. He had undergone bypass surgery and had received two units of blood. Although blood is effectively screened, I thought about that one-in-a-zillion chance that it could have been contaminated. Thankfully, I had received the hepatitis B immunization series, but there was still concern regarding hepatitis C and, of course, HIV.

The patient was gracious and complied with our request to be tested for hepatitis and HIV. The physician and I discussed the situation, and we determined the risk to be low, but he nonetheless offered me the option of getting the HIV postexposure prophylactic treatment. I decided not to get the treatment and proceeded to wait in agony for the patient's test results. The word *relief* hardly describes how I felt when the patient's laboratory results came back negative!

This incident confirmed the importance of getting the hepatitis B immunization and paying attention to good technique when performing procedures involving blood. ■

APPLICATION OF A TOURNIQUET

An important step in the venipuncture procedure is the application of the tourniquet. A tourniquet consists of a flat, soft band of rubber approximately 1 inch (2.5 cm) wide and 15 to 18 inches (38 to 45 cm) long. Most offices use latex-free tourniquets which consist of synthetic rubber. This protects both health care workers and patients with a hypersensitivity to latex.

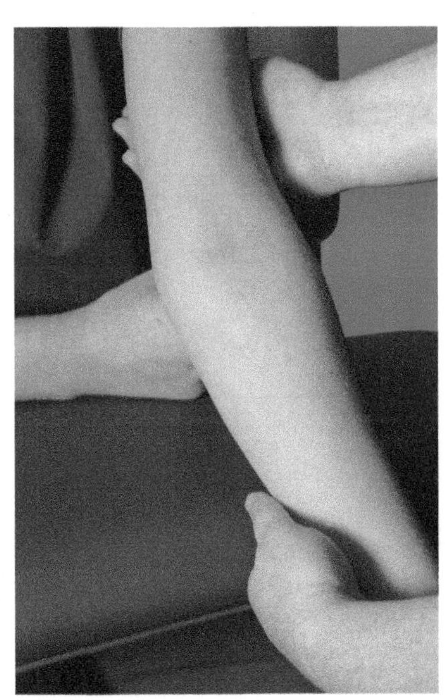

Fig. 17.6 Patient position for obtaining a blood specimen from the antecubital veins.

The tourniquet makes the patient's veins stand out so that they are easier to palpate. The tourniquet acts as a "dam" that causes the venous blood to slow down and pool in the veins in front of the tourniquet. This pooling of blood makes the veins more prominent so that they are more visible and can be palpated.

When applying a tourniquet, it is important to obtain the correct tourniquet tension. The tourniquet should be applied with enough tension to slow the venous flow without affecting the arterial flow. A tourniquet that is too tight is uncomfortable for the patient; it also obstructs both venous blood flow and arterial flow, which may result in a specimen that produces inaccurate test results. A tourniquet that is too loose fails to cause the veins to stand out enough to be palpated. A correctly applied tourniquet should fit snugly and not pinch the patient's skin.

Guidelines for Applying a Tourniquet

The following guidelines help to ensure successful application of the tourniquet:

1. Do not apply the tourniquet over sores or burned skin.
2. Hold each end of the tourniquet with one hand. Position the tourniquet 3 to 4 inches (7.5 to 10 cm) above the bend in the elbow. This allows adequate room for cleansing the site and performing the venipuncture without the tourniquet getting in the way. Make sure the tourniquet lies flat against the patient's skin. Pull the ends away from each other to create tension (Fig. 17.7A).
3. Bring the ends of the tourniquet toward each other and cross one over the other at the point of your grasp, with enough tension that the tourniquet is snug but is not pinching the patient's skin or is otherwise painful to the patient (see Fig. 17.7B).
4. Tuck a portion of the top length into the bottom length, forming a loop between the tourniquet and the patient's

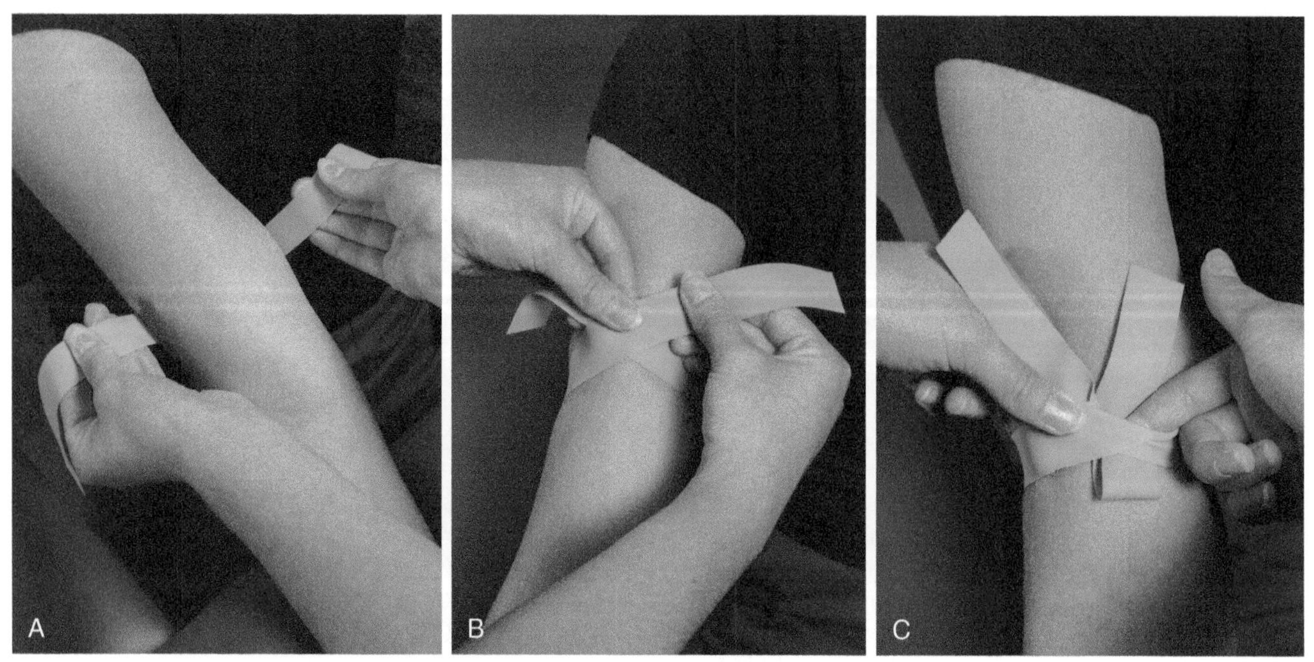

Fig. 17.7 Application of a latex-free tourniquet. (A) Create tension by pulling the ends of the tourniquet away from each other. (B) With tension, cross one flap over the other at the point of your grasp. (C), Form a loop by tucking a portion of the top length into the bottom length.

arm. This allows for a one-handed release of the tourniquet when pulled on one end. Make sure the flaps are directed upward so that they do not dangle into the working area (see Fig. 17.7C).

5. Never leave the tourniquet on for longer than 1 minute because this would be uncomfortable for the patient. In addition, prolonged application of the tourniquet causes the venous blood to stagnate, or pool in one place too long—a condition known as **venous stasis**. When venous stasis occurs, the plasma portion of the blood filters into the tissues, causing hemoconcentration. **Hemoconcentration** is an increase in the concentration of nonfilterable blood components in the blood vessels, such as red blood cells, enzymes, iron, and calcium, as a result of a decrease in the fluid content of the blood. This can result in inaccurate results for a variety of laboratory tests.
6. Remove the tourniquet as soon as a good blood flow is established; however, this may not be practical when you are first learning the venipuncture procedure. Removing the tourniquet may cause the needle to move such that no more blood can be obtained, and the blood has to be redrawn. When first learning the venipuncture procedure, it is better to wait until just before the needle is removed to remove the tourniquet.
7. *Always* remove the tourniquet before removing the needle from the patient's arm. If the needle is removed first, the pressure of the tourniquet causes blood to be forced out of the puncture site and into the surrounding tissue, resulting in a hematoma. A **hematoma** is defined as a swelling or mass of coagulated blood caused by a break in a blood vessel.

SITE SELECTION FOR VENIPUNCTURE

For most patients, the best site to use is the veins in the antecubital space (Fig. 17.8). If the patient has large, visible antecubital veins, drawing blood is easy. If the patient has small veins or veins that cannot be palpated, obtaining a blood specimen can be quite a challenge, even for the most experienced medical assistant.

The antecubital veins typically have a wide lumen and are close to the surface of the skin, which makes them easily accessible. In addition, these veins typically have thick walls, making them less likely to collapse. Using the antecubital space spares the patient unnecessary pain because the skin is less sensitive there than at other sites, such as the back of the hand. The medical assistant should not be misled by the presence in some patients of many small, very blue "spidery" veins that lie close to the surface of the skin. These veins are not suitable for performing a venipuncture. The antecubital veins lie beneath these veins.

The best vein to use in the antecubital space is the *median cubital.* The median cubital is a prominent vein in the middle of the antecubital space and does not roll (see Fig. 17.8). At times, however, the median cubital vein cannot be used—for example, when it lies deep in the tissues and cannot be palpated or is scarred from repeated venipunctures.

The *cephalic* and *basilic* veins are located on opposite sides of the antecubital space and provide an alternative site when the median cubital vein is unavailable. The cephalic vein is located on the thumb side of the antecubital space, and the basilic vein is located on the little finger side of the antecubital space. The disadvantage of these "side" veins is that they tend to roll or move away from the needle, escaping puncture. To

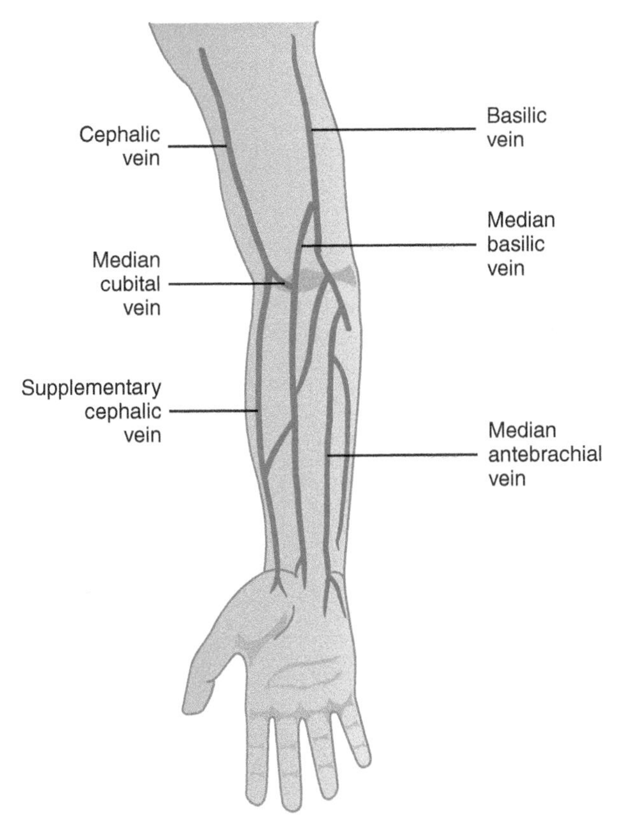

Fig. 17.8 Antecubital veins.

prevent rolling, firm pressure should be applied below and to the side of the vein to stabilize it as the needle is inserted.

The brachial artery also is located in the antecubital space, but it lies deeper in the tissues. This is the artery that is used to measure blood pressure. Before performing a venipuncture, palpate for the presence of this artery. In contrast to a vein, an artery pulsates, is more elastic, and has a thicker wall than a vein. If the brachial artery is inadvertently punctured, the patient feels more than the usual amount of pain, and the blood is bright red and comes out in pulsing movements. If this situation occurs, the tourniquet should be removed and then the needle. Pressure with a gauze pad should be applied for 4 to 5 minutes.

Guidelines for Site Selection

Specific guidelines should be followed to facilitate the selection of a good vein:

1. *Ensure that the lighting is adequate.* Good lighting facilitates inspection of the veins.
2. *Ensure that the veins "stand out" as much as possible.* Before locating a venipuncture site, always apply the tourniquet. When the tourniquet is in place, ask the patient to clench his or her fist. This pushes blood from the lower arm into the veins making them more prominent and easier to palpate. You can ask the patient to clench and unclench the fist a few times; however, vigorous pumping should be avoided because it could lead to hemoconcentration, which could produce inaccurate test results.
3. *Examine the antecubital veins of both arms.* The best site to perform a venipuncture varies with each individual. The patient may have larger veins in one arm than in the other. It is advisable to ask the patient whether he or she has had a venipuncture before. Most adults have had previous venipunctures and know which of their veins are best to use and which should be avoided. Listen to and evaluate information offered by the patient.
4. *Use inspection and particularly palpation to select a vein.* A vein does not have to be seen to be a good selection. If you cannot see a vein, palpation alone can be used to locate it. A vein feels like an elastic tube that "gives" under the pressure of the fingertips.
5. *Always palpate for the median cubital vein (middle vein) first.* It usually is bigger, is anchored better, bruises less, and poses the smallest risk of injuring underlying structures (e.g., nerves and arteries) than the other veins. Because of this, if the patient's median cubital vein cannot be seen but still can be palpated, it should be used as the first choice when selecting a vein. If the median cubital vein is good in both arms, select the one that appears the fullest. The cephalic vein located on the thumb side is the next best vein choice because it does not roll and bruise as easily as the basilic vein. The basilic vein, located on the little finger side of the antecubital space, is the least desirable venipuncture site in the antecubital space. Branches of the median nerve may lie close to this vein in some individuals. In addition, the basilic vein lies in close proximity to the brachial artery. Both of these conditions pose a risk of injury to underlying structures when blood is drawn from the basilic vein.
6. *Thoroughly assess the patient's veins.* To assess a vein as a possible site for venipuncture, place one or two fingertips (index and middle fingers) over it and press lightly, then release pressure. Do not use your thumb to palpate the vein because it is not as sensitive as the index finger. To be suitable for a venipuncture, the vein should feel round, firm, elastic, and engorged. When you depress and release an engorged vein, it should spring back in a rounded, filled state.
7. *Determine the size, depth, and direction of the vein.* When a suitable vein has been located, it should be palpated thoroughly and carefully to determine the direction of the vein and to estimate the size and depth of the vein. Palpate and trace the path of the vein several times by rolling your index finger back and forth over the vein to determine its size. Inspect and palpate the vein for problems. Some veins that appear suitable at first sight feel small, hard, bumpy, or flat when palpated.
8. *Map the location of the site.* After locating an acceptable vein, mentally "map" the location of the puncture site on the patient's arm with "skin marks." This technique is particularly helpful if the vein cannot be seen, but only palpated. The puncture site may be located on or next to a skin mark, such as a freckle, skin crease, or a

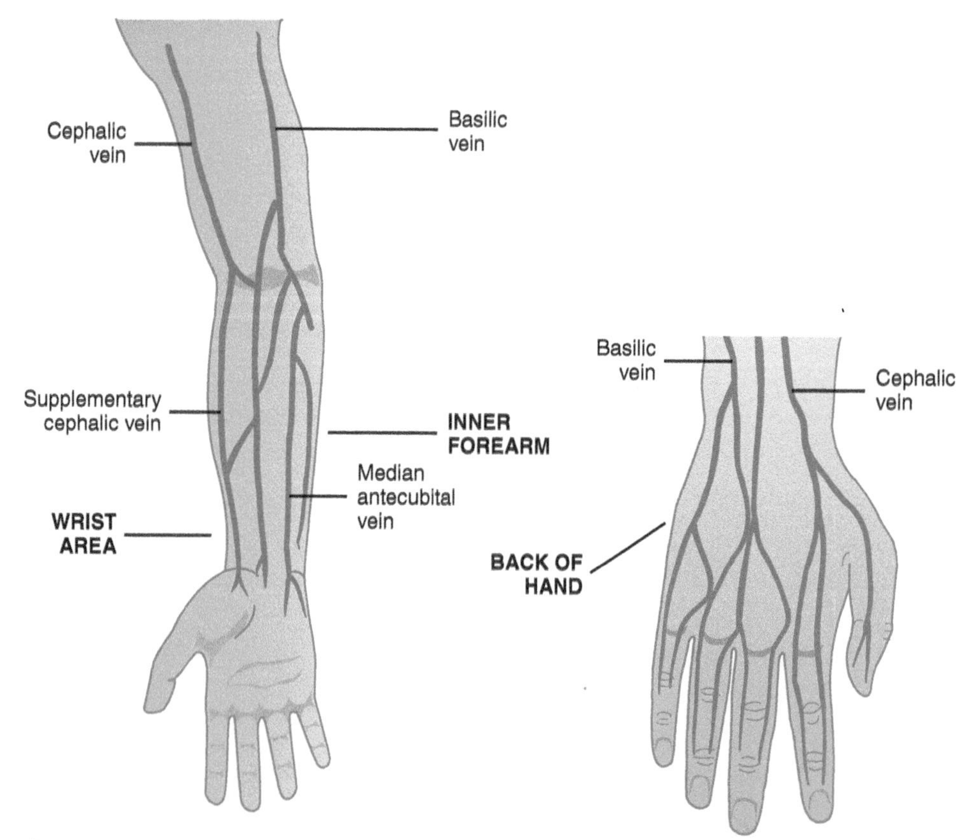

Fig. 17.9 Alternative venipuncture sites: the inner forearm, the wrist area above the thumb, and the back of the hand.

pigmented area. Do not mark the site with a pen as this contaminates the site.

9. *Do not leave the tourniquet on for longer than 1 minute.* When first learning the venipuncture procedure, you may need to perform numerous assessments of the patient's arms to locate the best vein. After each assessment, remove the tourniquet for approximately 2 minutes to allow normal circulation of the blood to occur. This prevents patient discomfort and hemoconcentration, which can lead to inaccurate results for a variety of laboratory tests.
10. *If a suitable vein cannot be found*, the following techniques can be employed to make the veins more prominent:
    - Remove the tourniquet, and have the patient dangle the arm over the side of the chair for 1 to 2 minutes.
    - Tap the vein site sharply a few times with your index finger and second finger.
    - Gently massage the arm from the wrist to the elbow.
    - Apply a warm, moist washcloth to the area for 5 minutes.

ALTERNATIVE VENIPUNCTURE SITES

If it is impossible to locate a suitable vein in the antecubital space, alternative sites are available, including the inner forearm, the wrist area above the thumb, and the back of the hand (Fig. 17.9). These alternative veins are smaller and have thinner walls than the antecubital veins and should be used for venipuncture only when all possibilities for obtaining the blood specimen at the antecubital site have been considered. If the medical assistant is able to palpate a small vein in the antecubital space, it may be possible to obtain blood there using the butterfly method of venipuncture.

The hand veins, in particular, should be used only as a last resort. The veins of the hand have a tendency to roll because they are not supported by much tissue and are close to the surface of the skin. This makes them more difficult to stick. In addition, an abundant supply of nerves is present in the hands, which makes this procedure more uncomfortable for the patient. Hand veins tend to have thin walls, which makes them more susceptible to collapsing, bruising, and phlebitis. In some patients, however, especially the obese and the elderly, the hand veins may be the only accessible site.

TYPES OF BLOOD SPECIMENS

The type of blood specimen required depends on the type of test to be performed. Serum is required for most blood chemistry tests, whereas whole blood is required for a CBC. The various types of blood specimens that can be obtained through the venipuncture procedure are as follows:

1. *Clotted blood.* Clotted blood is obtained from a tube that does not contain an anticoagulant. A tube without an anticoagulant causes the blood cells to clot.

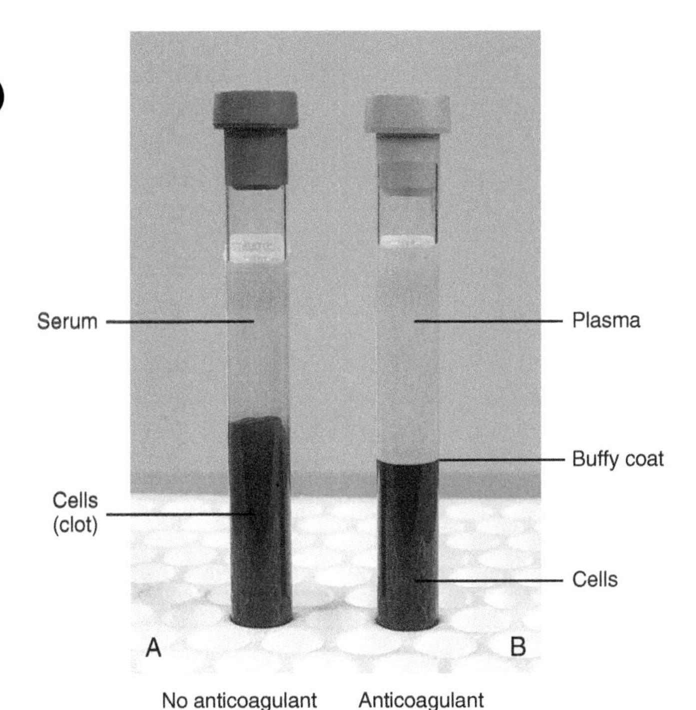

Fig. 17.10 (A) Layers into which the blood separates when there is no anticoagulant and (B) when an anticoagulant is present.

2. *Serum.* **Serum** is plasma from which the clotting factor fibrinogen has been removed. Serum is obtained from clotted blood by allowing the specimen to stand and then centrifuging it. Centrifuging a blood specimen that does not contain an anticoagulant causes the blood to separate into the following layers (Fig. 17.10A):
   - Top layer—serum
   - Bottom layer—clotted blood cells
3. *Whole blood.* Whole blood is obtained by using a tube that contains an **anticoagulant**. An anticoagulant is a substance that inhibits blood clotting. It is important to mix the anticoagulant with the blood by gently inverting the tube back and forth 8 to 10 times after collection.
4. *Plasma.* **Plasma** is the liquid part of the blood consisting of a clear, straw-colored fluid that comprises approximately 55% of the blood volume. Plasma is obtained from whole blood that has been centrifuged. Centrifuging a blood specimen that contains an anticoagulant causes the blood to separate into the following layers (see Fig. 17.10B):
   - Top layer—plasma
   - Middle layer—**buffy coat** (contains white blood cells and platelets)
   - Bottom layer—red blood cells

OCCUPATIONAL SAFETY AND HEALTH ADMINISTRATION (OSHA) SAFETY PRECAUTIONS

The OSHA Bloodborne Pathogens Standard presented in Chapter 2 must be carefully followed during the venipuncture procedure to avoid exposure to bloodborne pathogens. The following OSHA requirements apply specifically to the venipuncture procedure and to separation of serum from whole blood (see later):

1. Wear gloves when it is reasonably anticipated that you will have hand contact with blood.
2. Avoid hand-to-mouth contact, such as eating, drinking, handling contact lenses, and applying cosmetics while working with blood specimens.
3. Wear a face shield or mask in combination with an eye protection device whenever splashes, spray, splatter, or droplets of blood may be generated.
4. Perform all procedures involving blood in a manner so as to minimize splashing, spraying, splattering, and generating droplets of blood.
5. If your hands or other skin surfaces come in contact with blood, wash the area as soon as possible with soap and water.
6. If your mucous membranes (e.g., eyes, nose, and mouth) come in contact with blood, flush them with water as soon as possible.
7. Do not bend, break, or shear contaminated venipuncture needles.
8. Do not recap a contaminated venipuncture needle.
9. Locate the sharps container as close as possible to the area of use. Immediately after use, place the contaminated blood collection needle (and tube holder) in the biohazard sharps container.
10. Handle all laboratory equipment and supplies properly and with care as indicated by the manufacturer. For example, wait until the centrifuge comes to a complete stop before opening it.
11. Do not store food in refrigerators where testing supplies or specimens are stored.
12. Sanitize hands as soon as possible after removing gloves.
13. If you are exposed to blood, report the incident immediately to your provider-employer.

What Would You Do? What Would You *Not* Do?

Case Study 1

Camila Hernadez is 21 years old and comes to the office at 9:00 AM to have her blood drawn for a CBC and a thyroid panel. She has brought a friend along with her. Camila seems nervous, and her voice is shaking. She says this is the first venipuncture she has ever had. Camila asks whether her friend can stay with her to give her moral support while her blood is being drawn. Camila says that the blood has to be taken out of her left arm. She says she is right-handed and has a softball game this evening. When the veins of Camila's left arm are examined, a suitable vein cannot be located; however, she has a good median cubital vein in her right arm. Camila then wants to know whether the blood could be drawn from her left hand like they do on hospital television shows. ■

VACUTAINER METHOD OF VENIPUNCTURE

The Vacutainer method is frequently used to collect venous blood specimens. This method is considered ideal for collecting blood from normal healthy antecubital veins that are adequate in size to withstand the pressure of the vacuum in the collection tube. The Vacutainer system consists of a blood collection needle, a plastic tube holder, and a collection tube (Fig. 17.11). Procedure 17.1 outlines the venipuncture Vacutainer method.

BLOOD COLLECTION NEEDLE

The safety-engineered needle used with the Vacutainer method consists of a double-pointed stainless steel needle with a threaded hub near its center and a safety shield (Fig. 17.12). The needle is coated with silicon, enabling it to penetrate the skin smoothly. The threaded hub of the needle screws into the tube holder. Blood collection needles are packaged in sealed twist-apart plastic containers. The needle gauge and length are printed on the paper seal on the container (see Fig. 17.12). A needle should not be used if the seal has been broken.

The double-pointed needle consists of an anterior needle and a posterior needle. The *anterior needle* is longer and has a beveled point designed to facilitate entry into the skin and the vein. The *posterior needle* is shorter, and its purpose is to pierce the rubber stopper of the collection tube. The posterior needle has a rubber sleeve that functions as a valve which permits the collection of multiple blood specimens. Pushing the tube stopper of a collection tube onto the posterior needle compresses this rubber sleeve and exposes the opening of the needle, allowing blood to enter the tube. When a tube is removed, the sleeve slides back over the needle opening and stops the flow of blood.

Blood collection needles are available in two gauges: 21 G and 22 G. A 21-G needle is used most often for a routine venipuncture. A 22-G needle is recommended for children and adults with small veins. Manufacturers often color-code the needle guard by gauge for easier identification—for example, Becton Dickinson uses the following color-coding system: green for 21-G needles (see Fig. 17.12), and black for 22-G needles. Blood collection needles come in three lengths: 1 inch, 1.25 inches, and 1.5 inches. The length used is based on individual preference; most medical assistants prefer the 1- or 1.25-inch needle for routine venipunctures; they are less intimidating to the patient and tend to offer greater control because they allow the medical assistant to rest the fourth and fifth fingers on the patient's arm for stability. A 1.5-inch needle allows more room for stabilizing the vein.

OSHA stipulates requirements to reduce needlestick and other sharps injuries among health care workers. As discussed in Chapter 2, employers are required to evaluate and implement commercially available safer medical devices that reduce occupational exposure to the lowest extent feasible. Safer medical devices include safety-engineered blood collection needles which incorporate a built-in safety feature

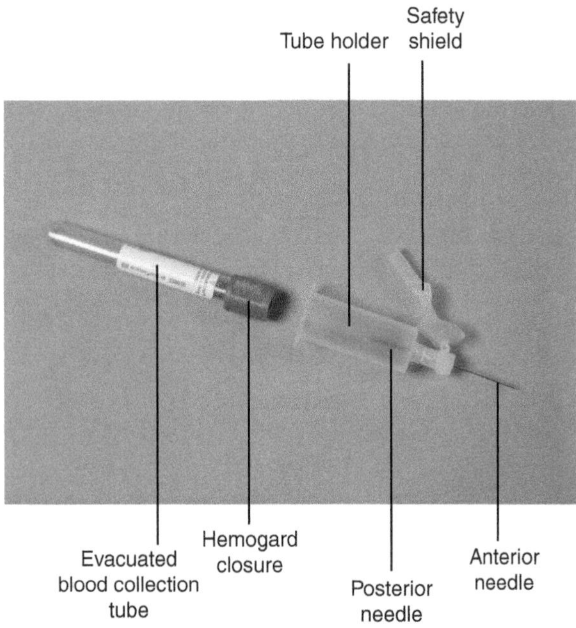

Fig. 17.11 Vacutainer system.

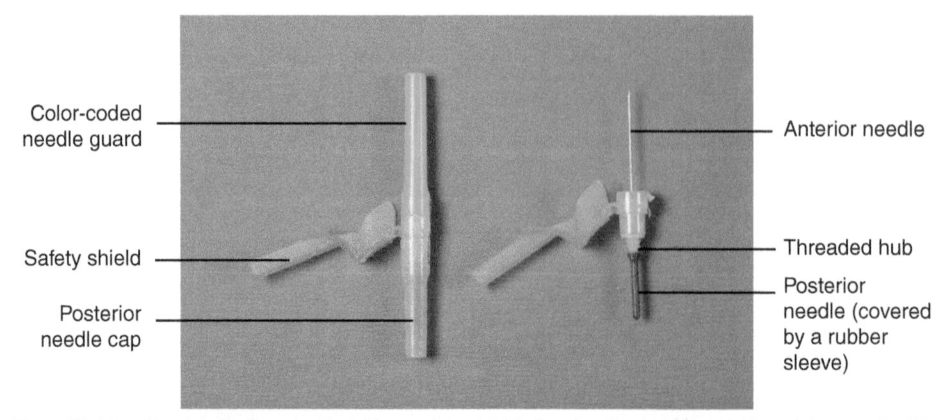

Fig. 17.12 Blood collection needle with a safety shield showing the gauge and size of the needle. The gauge of this needle is 21 G, and the size is 1 inch.

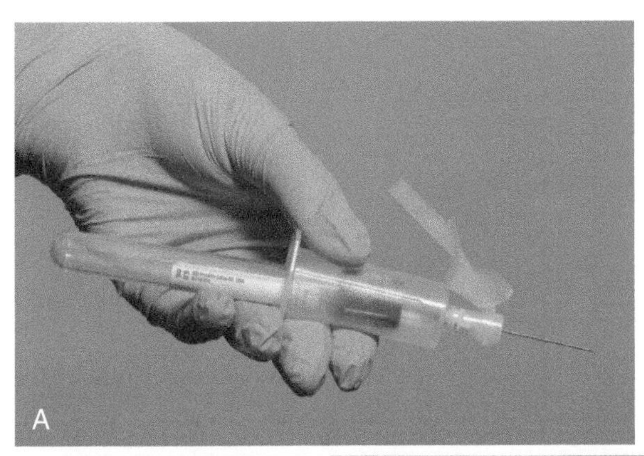

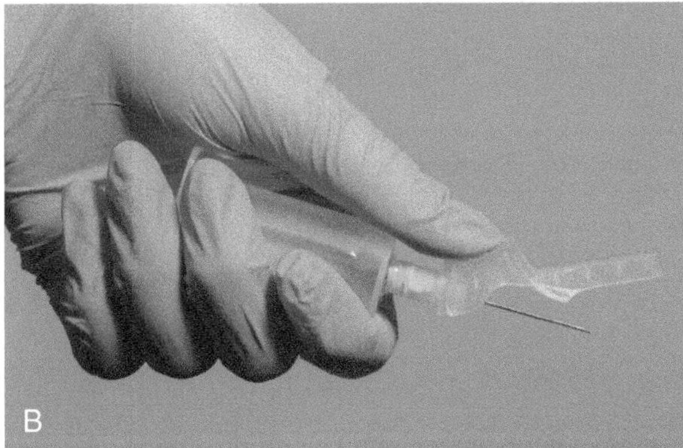

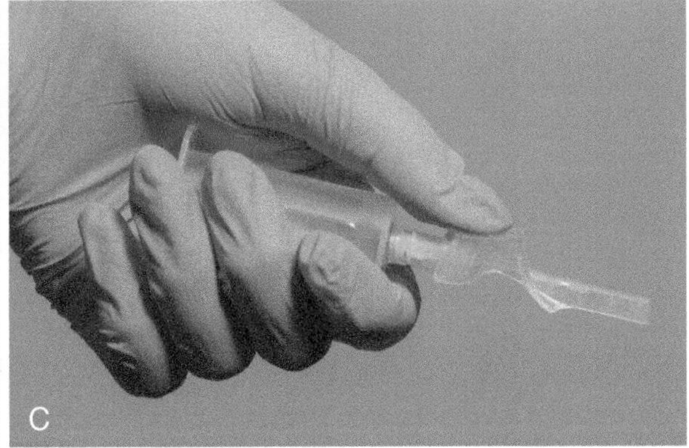

Fig. 17.13 Activation of the safety shield on a blood collection needle. (A) Perform the venipuncture with the shield straight back toward the holder. (B) After performing the venipuncture, place the thumb on the safety shield thumb pad and push the safety shield forward. (C) Continue pushing the safety shield forward with your thumb until an audible click is heard, which indicates the shield has locked into place Discard the needle and holder in a biohazard sharps container.

to reduce the risk of a needlestick injury. Fig. 17.13 illustrates a safety-engineered blood collection needle and the method for activating it.

PLASTIC TUBE HOLDER

The plastic tube holder consists of a plastic cylinder with two openings. The small opening is used to secure the double-pointed needle, and the large opening is used to hold the collection tube. The large opening has a plastic extension known as the *flange*. The flange assists in the insertion and removal of collection tubes and prevents the tube holder from rolling when it is placed on a flat surface.

The tube holder has an indentation about .5 inch from the hub of the needle. This marks the point at which the posterior needle starts to enter the rubber stopper of the tube. If a tube stopper is inserted past this point before the vein is entered, the tube fills with air, which prevents blood from entering the tube.

EVACUATED COLLECTION TUBES

Evacuated collection tubes consist of a sterile plastic or glass tube with either a *Hemogard closure* (Fig. 17.14) or a *conventional rubber stopper closure* (Fig. 17.15). A collection tube contains a vacuum that creates suction to pull the blood specimen into the tube. The tube has a label affixed to it indicating the additive content, expiration date, and tube capacity. Collection tubes are available in varying capacities that range from 2 to 10 mL. The capacity of the tube used depends on the amount of the specimen required for the test.

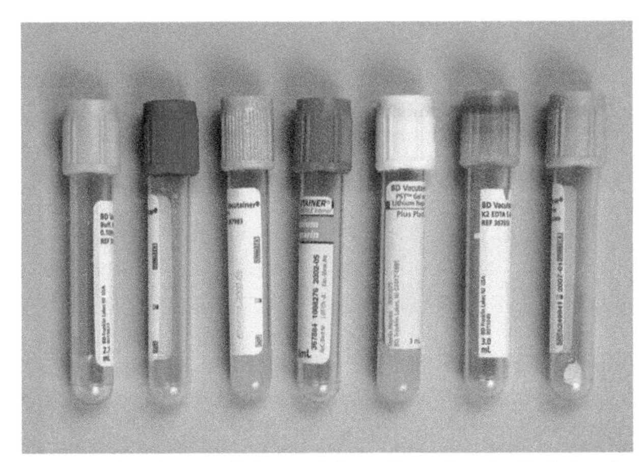

Fig. 17.14 Hemogard closure tubes. (From Garrels M: *Laboratory and diagnostic testing in ambulatory care*, ed 4, St Louis: Elsevier; 2019. Photo by Zack Bent.)

A *Hemogard closure* consists of a special rubber stopper and a plastic safety-engineered closure that overhangs the

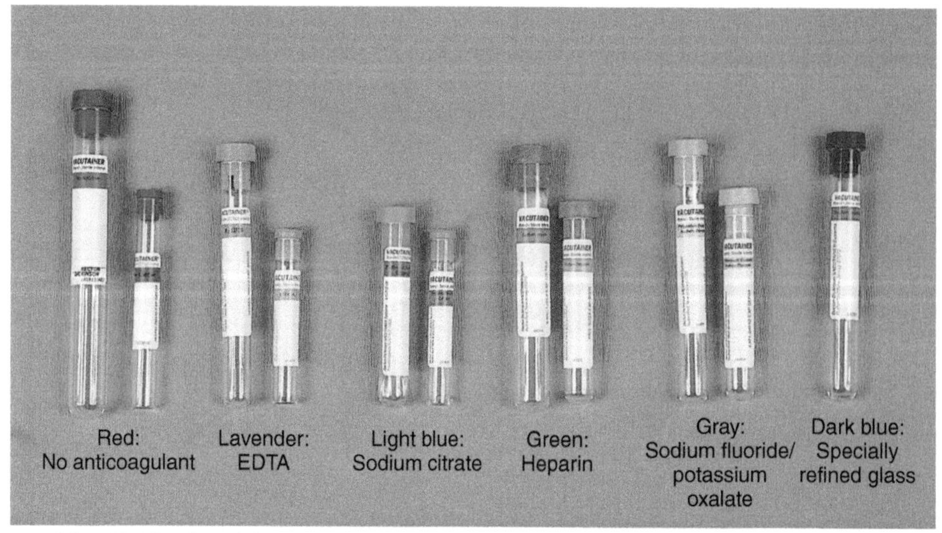

Fig. 17.15 Conventional rubber stopper closure tubes. *EDTA*, Ethylenediaminetetraacetic acid.

outside of the tube. Together, these components act as a single unit to reduce the likelihood of coming in contact with the contents of the tube. After collecting a blood specimen, the medical assistant may need to gain access to the blood in the tube for further processing, such as when separating serum from whole blood. A conventional rubber stopper tube "pops" as the stopper is removed, which may result in splattering of blood. The design of the Hemogard closure works to prevent splattering of blood when the top is removed.

ADDITIVE CONTENT OF COLLECTION TUBES

Collection tubes use a color-coded system for ease in identifying the additive content of each tube (Table 17.1). A tube additive must not alter the blood components or affect the laboratory test to be performed. The medical assistant must determine the correct closure color to use for each test ordered by the provider as specified in the laboratory test directory. Substituting one collection tube for another may not yield the proper type of specimen required for the test. If a CBC has been ordered by the provider, a lavender-closure tube must be used, and a tube with a different colored closure cannot be substituted for it.

The most frequently used collection tubes in the medical office are classified here according to the color of the closure and the additive content:

1. *Red.* A tube with a red closure does not contain an anticoagulant and is used to obtain clotted blood or serum. Clotted blood is used for blood banking. Serum is required for serologic tests and blood chemistry tests.
2. *Gold and marbled red/gray (often called a "tiger top" tube) closures.* These tubes are used to obtain serum. They do not contain an anticoagulant; however, they do contain an additive known as a *clot activator.* A clot activator consists of a substance that makes the red blood cells in the tube clot more quickly to yield serum. Tubes with a gold or marbled red/gray closure are known as serum separator tubes (SSTs) because they contain a gel that separates the cells from the serum when the tube is centrifuged. A tube with a clot activator must be inverted five times after the blood has been drawn to mix the clot activator with the blood specimen. The most common use of these tubes is to collect a specimen for blood chemistry testing.
3. *Lavender.* A tube with a lavender closure contains the anticoagulant EDTA and is used to obtain whole blood or plasma. The most common use is to collect a blood specimen for a CBC.
4. *Light blue.* A tube with a light blue closure contains the anticoagulant sodium citrate and is used to obtain whole blood or plasma; the most common use is for coagulation tests, such as prothrombin time.
5. *Green.* A tube with a green closure contains the anticoagulant heparin and is used to collect a blood specimen to perform a blood gas determination or pH assay.
6. *Gray.* A tube with a gray closure contains sodium fluoride (a preservative) and potassium oxalate (an anticoagulant) and is used to obtain whole blood or plasma; the most common use is to collect a blood specimen to perform a blood alcohol test, a drug test, or an oral glucose tolerance test (OGTT).
7. *Royal blue.* A tube with a royal blue closure contains either EDTA or no additive at all. This type of tube is made of a specially refined glass and rubber stopper and is used for the detection of trace elements, such as lead, zinc, arsenic, and copper, which are contracted through occupational or environmental exposure.

ORDER OF DRAW FOR MULTIPLE TUBES

When multiple tubes of blood need to be drawn, the following order of draw (see Table 17.1) is recommended by the *Clinical and Laboratory Standards Institute (CLSI).*

Table 17.1 Order of Draw for Collection of Multiple Evacuated Tubes

BD Hemogard Plastic Colors	Rubber Stopper Colors	Additive or Anticoagulant	Number of Inversions to Mix During Blood Draw	Laboratory Use
Yellow, Sterile	Yellow, Sterile	Sodium polyanetholsulfonate (SPS)	8–10	Blood cultures
Light blue	Light blue	Sodium citrate	3–4	Coagulation tests
Red	Red	Glass: no additive Plastic: clot activator	0 5	Chemistries Serology Blood bank
Gold	Marbled red and gray[a]	Serum separator Gel and clot activator	5	Most chemistry testing
Light green	Marbled green and gray[a]	Plasma separator gel and lithium heparin	8–10	Potassium determinations
Green	Green	Sodium heparin, or lithium heparin, or ammonium heparin	8–10	Blood gas determination and pH assays
Lavender	Lavender	EDTA	8–10	Whole blood hematology cell count, CBC
Gray	Gray	Sodium fluoride and potassium oxalate	8–10	Oral glucose tolerance test Blood alcohol test

[a]Note the mixing requirements.

CBC, Complete blood count; *EDTA,* ethylenediaminetetraacetic acid.

BD Hemogard plastic covers and rubber stopper colors from BD Diagnostics, Preanalytical Systems, 1 Becton Drive, Franklin Lakes, NJ 07417, USA. www.bd.com/vacutainer. BD, BD Logo and all other trademarks are property of Becton, Dickinson, and Company. © 2014.

Modified from Garrels M: *Laboratory and diagnostic testing in ambulatory care,* ed 3, St Louis: Mosby; 2014.

Following the order of draw avoids cross-contamination of the specimen by additives found in different tubes.

Blood culture tube: Yellow-closure glass tube that contains the anticoagulant sodium polyanethol sulfonate (SPS), which is used for blood cultures and other tests that require sterile specimens.

Rationale: To prevent contamination of the specimen by other tubes, which may lead to inaccurate test results.

1. *Coagulation tube:* Light blue–closure tube for coagulation tests.
   Rationale: To prevent additives from other tubes from getting into the tube.
   (*Note for Butterfly Setup:* The tubing of the butterfly setup contains 0.3 to 0.5 mL of air. If a light blue–closure tube is the first or only tube to be drawn, a 5-mL red-closure tube must be drawn first and discarded. This is because some of the tube's vacuum is exhausted by the air in the tubing (rather than blood), resulting in underfilling of the tube. If the light blue–closure tube is filled first, the underfilled tube results in an incorrect anticoagulant-to-blood ratio. An incorrect ratio when performing a coagulation test leads to inaccurate coagulation test results. It is also important to completely fill coagulation tubes to the exhaustion of the vacuum; failure to do so leads to erroneous coagulation test results.)
2. *Serum tubes:* Tubes with or without a clot activator, and tubes with or without a gel barrier (e.g., red-closure tube; marbled red/gray or gold-closure tubes)
   Rationale: To prevent contamination of serum tubes by tubes with an anticoagulant.
3. *Anticoagulant tubes* in this order of closure color: green, lavender, royal blue (tube that contains EDTA), and gray
   Rationale: To prevent cross-contamination among different types of anticoagulants, which may lead to inaccurate test results.

What Would You Do? What Would You *Not* Do?

Case Study 2

Buzz Braydon had a heart attack 4 weeks ago and is taking the anticoagulant warfarin (Coumadin). He is at the office for a checkup and to have his prothrombin time tested. Blood is collected from a small vein in Buzz's left arm using the butterfly method. After the specimen has been collected, Buzz wants to know why a red-stoppered tube was used to draw blood from him and then thrown away. Buzz says that he is going on vacation in North Carolina for 2 weeks. He says that they explained to him at the hospital why he should have his blood tested every week, but he's not sure where to go to get his blood tested while he's on vacation. Buzz wants to know if, as long as he takes his medication exactly as he should, it would be all right to skip his weekly prothrombin test during that time. ■

COLLECTION TUBE GUIDELINES

Certain guidelines should be followed when using evacuated blood collection tubes:

1. Select the proper collection tubes according to the type and amount of specimen required.
2. Check to ensure that the tube is not cracked. A cracked tube no longer has a vacuum.
3. Check the expiration date on each tube. Outdated tubes may no longer contain a vacuum, and as a result they would not be able to draw blood into the tube.
4. Make sure each tube is properly labeled. Proper labeling avoids mixing up specimens.
5. Before using tubes that contain powdered additives (e.g., gray-closure tube), gently tap the tube just below the stopper so that all of the additive is dislodged from the stopper. If an additive remains trapped in the stopper, erroneous test results may occur.
6. Take precautions to avoid premature loss of the tube's vacuum. Premature loss of vacuum can occur from the following:
   - Dropping the tube
   - Pushing the posterior needle through the tube closure before puncturing the vein
   - Partially pulling the needle out of the vein after penetrating the patient's vein
7. Use a continuous, steady motion to make the puncture. Performing the puncture with a slow, timid motion or a rapid, jabbing motion is painful for the patient. In addition, a rapid motion could cause the needle to go completely through the vein, resulting in failure to obtain blood and possibly a hematoma.
8. When multiple tubes are to be drawn, follow the proper *order of draw.* This prevents contamination of nonadditive tubes by additive tubes and cross-contamination among different types of additive tubes, which could lead to inaccurate test results.
9. Fill collection tubes until the vacuum is exhausted, as evidenced by cessation of blood flow into the tube. The tube is almost but not quite full when the vacuum is exhausted. If the collection tube is removed before the vacuum is exhausted, a rush of air enters the tube, damaging the red blood cells. A tube that contains an anticoagulant must be filled completely to ensure the proper ratio of anticoagulant to the blood specimen.
10. Remove the last tube from the tube holder before removing the needle from the patient's vein. This prevents blood from dripping out of the tip of the needle after it has been withdrawn from the patient's skin.
11. Mix tubes that contain a clot activator or an anticoagulant immediately after drawing by gently inverting them. Gentle inversion provides adequate mixing without causing **hemolysis**, or breakdown of blood cells. One inversion consists of one complete turn of the wrist (180 degrees) and then back again. Tubes with a clot activator should be inverted 5 times, and tubes with an anticoagulant (with the exception of sodium

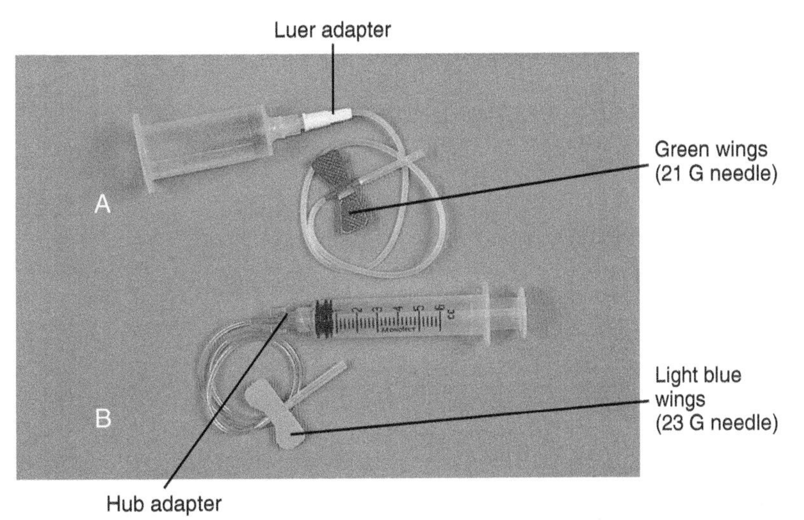

Fig. 17.16 Winged infusion set. (A) Luer adapter with collection tube. (B) Hub adapter with syringe.

citrate tubes) should be inverted 8 to 10 times. Tubes containing sodium citrate (light-blue stopper) should be gently inverted three or four times (see Table 17.1). Inadequate mixing or not mixing tubes with an anticoagulant immediately after drawing the specimen may result in clotting of the blood, leading to inaccurate test results.

12. After the venipuncture, the top of a conventional rubber stopper tube may contain residual blood. Take precautions by following the OSHA Standard when handling these tubes.

BUTTERFLY METHOD OF VENIPUNCTURE

The butterfly method of venipuncture is also called the *winged infusion method.* This is because a winged infusion set is used to perform the procedure. The term *butterfly* is derived from the plastic "wings" located between the needle and the tubing of the winged infusion set (Fig. 17.16).

The butterfly method is used to collect blood from patients who are difficult to stick by conventional methods because it provides better control when making the puncture, and less pressure is exerted on the vein wall from the collection tube. The butterfly method is recommended for adults with small antecubital veins and children, who typically have small antecubital veins.

The butterfly method also is used when the antecubital veins are unavailable and veins in the forearm, wrist area, or back of the hand are used, as may occur with elderly and obese patients. These alternative veins are usually smaller and sometimes have a thin wall (e.g., hand veins), making them more likely to collapse with the Vacutainer method of venipuncture. With the Vacutainer method, the "sucking action" exerted on the vein when the pressure in the vacuum is released causes the vein to collapse, blocking the flow of blood into the tube. The butterfly method results in less pressure on the vein wall because the pressure exerted by the collection tube must travel through a length of tubing before reaching the vein. Because the pressure against the vein wall is minimized, the vein is less likely to collapse with the butterfly method. Procedure 17.2 describes the venipuncture procedure with the butterfly method.

The gauge of the butterfly needle used to collect a blood specimen ranges from 21 G to 23 G, and the length of the needle ranges from .5 to .75 inch. The needle is short and sharp, making it easier to stick difficult veins. For extremely small veins, a 23-G needle should be used to prevent rupture of the vein by a larger needle. In this case, it is preferable to use smaller-volume tubes (e.g., 2-mL collection tubes) because large collection tubes may put too much vacuum pressure on the vein, causing it to collapse. Manufacturers often color-code the wings of the infusion setup by gauge for easier identification—for example, Becton Dickinson uses the following color-coding system: green for 21-G needles and light blue for 23-G needles (see Fig. 17.16).

The butterfly needle is attached to a 7- or 12-inch (18- or 30.5-cm) length of tubing and a *Luer adapter,* which is attached to a (posterior) needle with a rubber sleeve. A plastic tube holder is screwed onto the Luer adapter, which allows it to be used with collection tubes (see Fig. 17.16A). Winged infusion sets also are available with a hub adapter that allows them to be used with a syringe (see Fig.17.16B). Safety needles are available with a shield that covers the contaminated needle after it has been withdrawn from the patient's vein (Fig. 17.17).

GUIDELINES FOR THE BUTTERFLY METHOD

Certain guidelines should be followed when performing the butterfly method of venipuncture:

1. Position the patient according to the site selected for the venipuncture as follows:

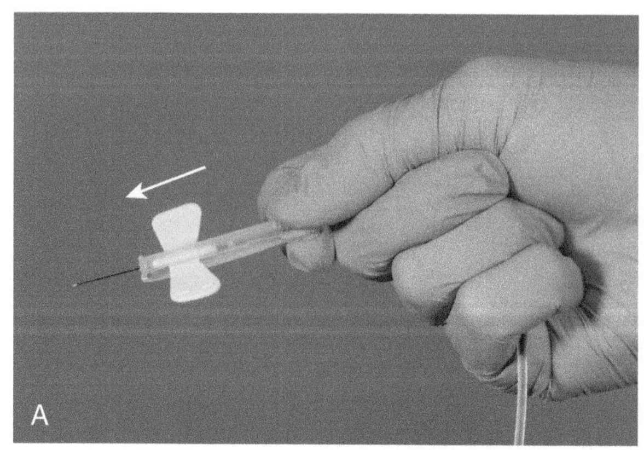

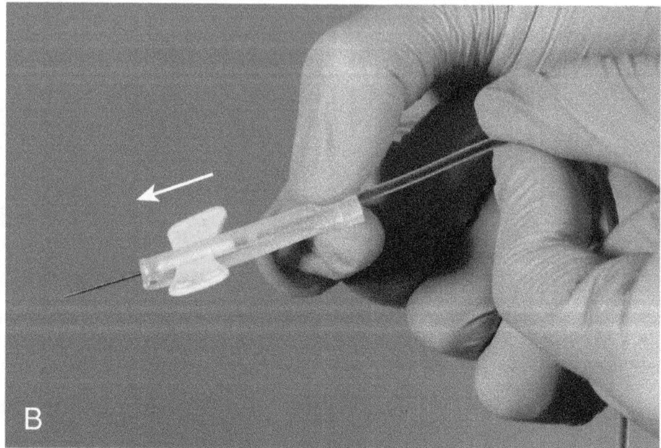

Fig. 17.17 Activation of the safety shield on a butterfly set. (A) ***One-Handed Technique:*** *A,* Grasp the yellow safety shield grip area with your thumb and index finger and at the same time grasp the tubing with your hand. *B,* Push the safety shield forward with the thumb and index finger until a click is heard indicating the needle is completely retracted and the safety shield is locked in place. (B) ***Two-Handed Technique:*** *A,* Grasp the yellow safety shield grip area with your thumb and index finger. With your opposite hand, grasp the tubing with the thumb and index finger. *B,* Push the safety shield forward with the thumb and index finger until a click is heard indicating the needle is completely retracted and the safety shield is locked in place.

- *Antecubital, wrist, and forearm veins.* Position the arm in a straight line from the shoulder to the wrist as described for the Vacutainer method of venipuncture.
- *Hand veins.* Position the patient's hand on the armrest and ask the patient to make a loose fist or to grasp a rolled towel. This combination causes the hand veins to stand out so that accurate selection of a puncture site can be made. Locate a suitable vein between the knuckles and the wrist bones. Hand veins are usually visible and easy to locate.

2. Position the tourniquet according to the venipuncture site as follows:
   - If the antecubital space is used, position the tourniquet 3 to 4 inches above the bend in the elbow. If the veins of the forearm or wrist are used, apply the tourniquet to the forearm, approximately 3 inches above the puncture site (Fig. 17.18A and B). For hand veins, position the tourniquet on the arm just above the wrist bone (see Fig. 17.18C).
3. Grasp the needle by compressing the plastic wings together. Insert the needle with the bevel facing up at a 15-degree angle to the skin. When the vein has been entered, decrease the angle to 5 degrees.
4. After decreasing the needle angle to 5 degrees, slowly thread the needle inside the vein an additional 1/4 inch. This anchors or seats the needle in the center of the vein and allows the medical assistant to use both hands to change tubes.
5. To prevent venous reflux, keep the collection tube and holder in a downward position as in the Vacutainer venipuncture procedure. This technique ensures that the blood fills from the bottom up and not near the rubber stopper.
6. When multiple tubes are to be drawn, follow the proper order of draw. Following the order of draw avoids cross-contamination of the specimen by additives found in different tubes.

Memories *from* Practicum

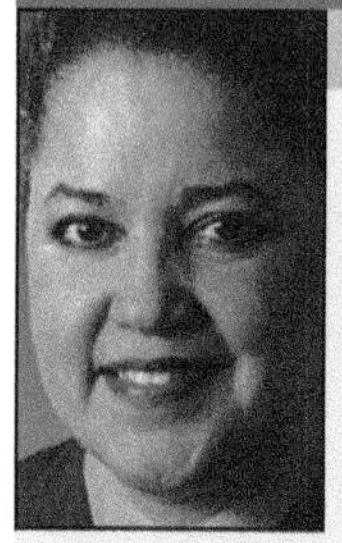

Dori: One of the most terrifying things for me as a student was learning venipuncture. Even though I would practice during classroom laboratory hours and felt comfortable with it, it still scared me to know I would have to draw on a real person one day. When the day arrived to draw on my laboratory partner, I became sick to my stomach. In the end, we both got through it just fine and walked away without hurting each other. I spent days trying to prepare myself for that first experience, but after it was over, I felt more confident and relaxed that I could do this. At my practicum site, I was able to perform several venipunctures a day, which raised my confidence level. Today venipuncture is my favorite responsibility of all. I would draw blood all day if I could. I know I could even draw with my eyes closed, but never would, of course! ■

What Would You Do? What Would You *Not* Do?

Case Study 3

Porsha Coleman is at the office complaining of persistent headaches and abdominal pain over the past 3 months. The physician gives Mrs. Coleman a laboratory requisition to have her blood collected and tested at an outside laboratory. Mrs. Coleman says that her daughter who lives with her works as a phlebotomist at the local hospital. Mrs. Coleman wants to know whether her daughter can draw her blood at home and then drop it off at the laboratory. She says that the last time she had her blood drawn, they had to stick her two times and then she got a big bruise on her arm afterward. She says the laboratory technician kept digging around in her arm to find the vein and that it was quite painful. ■

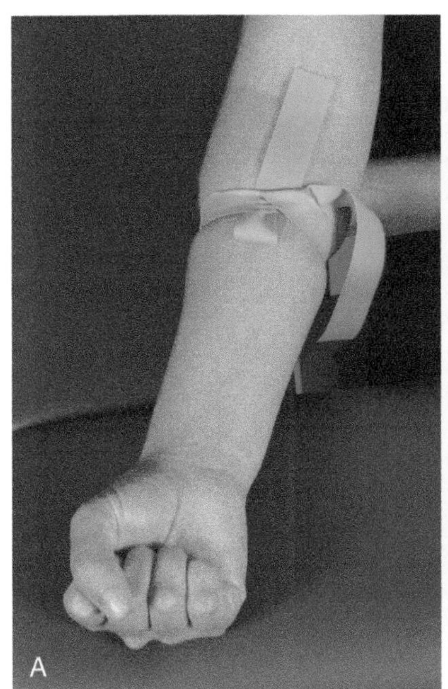

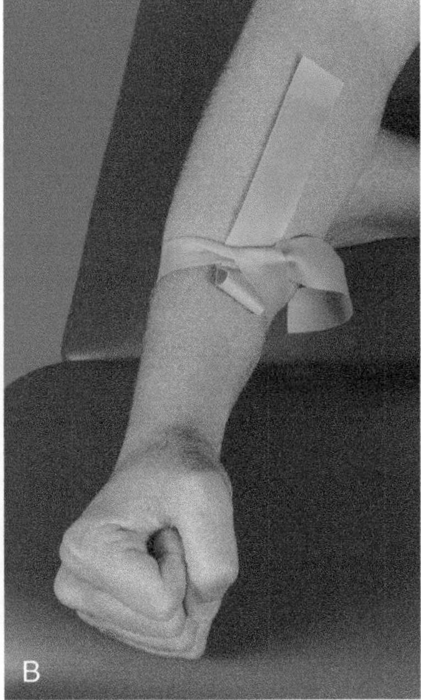

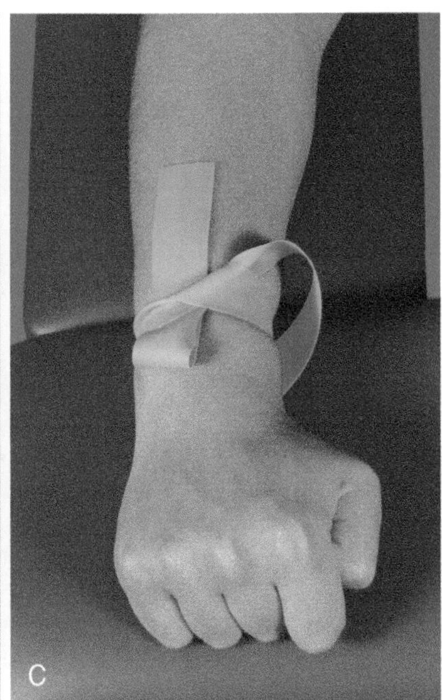

Fig. 17.18 Application of the tourniquet for alternative venipuncture sites. (A) Forearm site. (B) Wrist site. (C) Hand site.

PROBLEMS ENCOUNTERED WITH VENIPUNCTURE

Sometimes the medical assistant encounters problems when attempting to draw blood from a patient. The appropriate response depends on the type of problem.

FAILURE TO OBTAIN BLOOD

Periodically, even individuals highly skilled at performing venipuncture have difficulty obtaining blood. Although large and prominent veins make it easier to collect the blood specimen, conditions often exist that make the procedure more difficult (Fig. 17.19).

It is often difficult to draw blood from obese patients who have small, superficial veins and whose veins suitable for venipuncture are buried in adipose tissue. Elderly patients with arteriosclerosis may have veins that are thick and hard, making them difficult to puncture. Other patients have veins that are small or have a thin wall, making the veins likely to collapse. After two unsuccessful attempts at venipuncture, the medical assistant should seek assistance in obtaining the blood specimen.

Factors that result in failure to obtain blood after the needle has been inserted include not inserting the needle far enough, preventing it from entering the vein (see Fig. 17.19B); insertion of the needle too far, causing it to go through the vein (see Fig. 17.19C); and the bevel opening becoming lodged against the wall of the vein. In these instances, most authorities recommend removing the needle rather than trying to probe the vein. Probing is often uncomfortable for the patient and can affect the integrity of the blood specimen, leading to inaccurate test results. Occasionally, a collection tube loses its vacuum because of a manufacturing defect or through improper handling of the tube. If suspected, this problem can be corrected by removing the defective tube and inserting another collection tube.

INAPPROPRIATE PUNCTURE SITES

If a patient complains of pain or soreness at a potential venipuncture site, this area should be avoided. In addition, any skin areas that are scarred, bruised, burned, or adjacent to areas of infection should not be used. A venipuncture should not be performed on an arm with edema. Swelling makes it more difficult to locate a vein and increases healing time of the puncture site. Other sites to avoid include an arm that has a cast applied to it and an arm on the same side as a radical mastectomy.

SCARRED AND SCLEROSED VEINS

An individual who has had many venipunctures over a period of years often develops scar tissue in the wall of the vein. Elderly patients may have veins that have become thickened from arteriosclerosis. In both cases, the veins feel stiff and hard when palpated. A scarred or sclerosed vein is difficult to stick, and the blood return may be poor owing to a narrowed lumen; it is recommended that another vein be used for the venipuncture. If this is impossible, the needle should be inserted with careful pressure to avoid going completely through the vein.

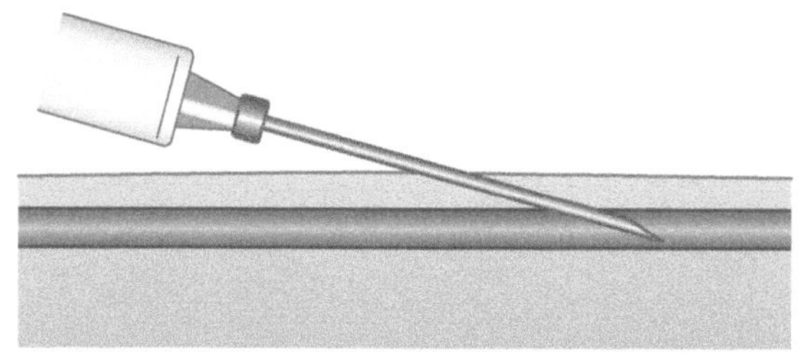

A. Correct insertion of the needle into the vein.

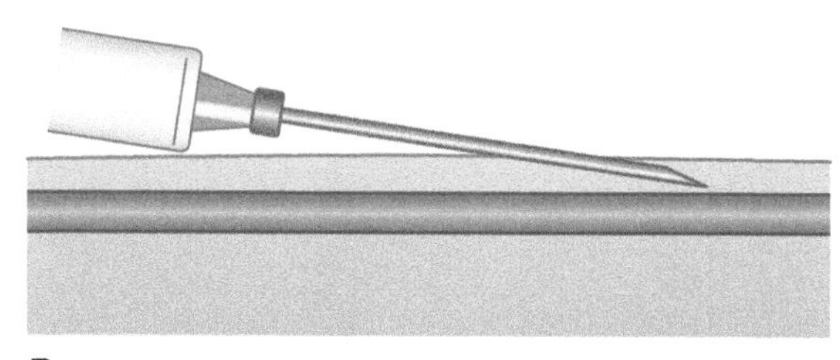

B. Improper angle of insertion (<15°), causing the needle to enter above the vein.

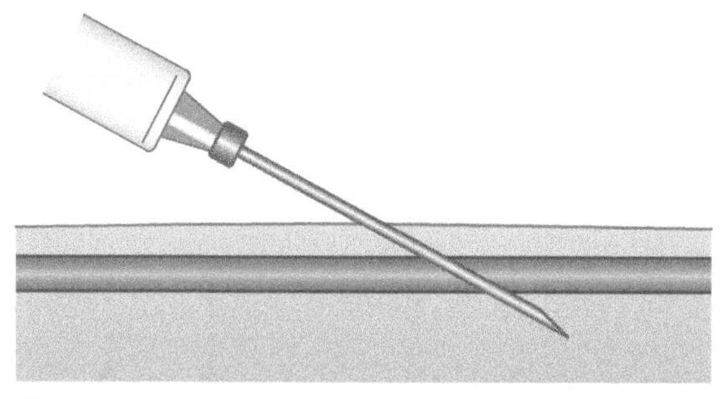

C. Improper angle of insertion (>15°), causing the needle to go through the vein.

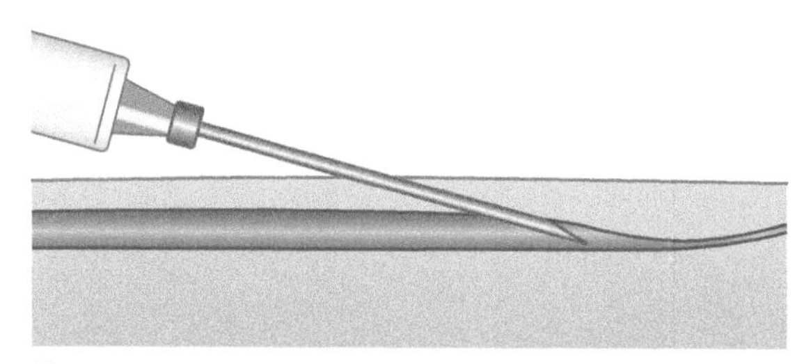

D. Collapsed vein (most likely to occur in persons with small veins).

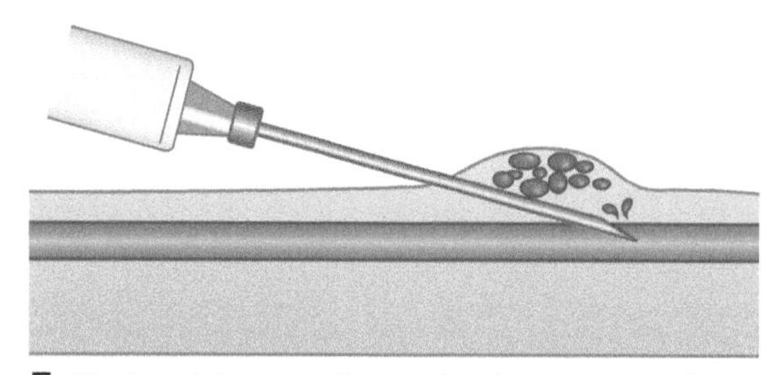

E. The beveled opening is partially within and partially outside of the vein, causing a hematoma.

Fig. 17.19 Problems encountered with venipuncture.

ROLLING VEINS

The median cubital vein, located in the center of the antecubital space, is considered the best vein for a venipuncture. Sometimes it is impossible to use this vein, however, such as when it lies deep in the tissues and cannot be palpated or is scarred from repeated venipunctures. The veins on either side of the median cubital (cephalic or basilic) can be used, but they have a tendency to "roll," or move away from the needle, escaping puncture. To prevent rolling, firm pressure should be applied below and to the side of the vein to stabilize it as the needle is inserted.

COLLAPSING VEINS

Veins are most likely to collapse in individuals who have small veins or veins with thin walls. This is particularly true when the Vacutainer method is used. The "sucking action" exerted on the vein when the pressure in the vacuum is released causes the vein to collapse, blocking the flow of blood into the tube (see Fig. 17.19D). The typical result observed is that a small amount of blood enters the tube and then stops. Because better control and less pressure on the vein are possible, the butterfly method of venipuncture is recommended to obtain the specimen in patients with small veins.

PREMATURE NEEDLE WITHDRAWAL

Patient movement or improper venipuncture technique can cause the needle to come out of the vein prematurely. Because of the pressure exerted by the tourniquet, blood may be forced out of the puncture site, and immediate action is required to prevent a hematoma. The tourniquet should be removed at once, a gauze pad placed on the puncture site, and pressure applied until the bleeding has stopped.

HEMATOMA

A hematoma is caused by blood leaking from the puncture site of the vein and into the surrounding tissues, resulting in a bruise. A hematoma is caused by a needle that is inserted too far and goes through the vein, a bevel opening that is partially in the vein and partially out of the vein (see Fig. 17.19E), and insufficient pressure applied to the puncture site after removal of the needle. The first sign of a hematoma is a sudden swelling around the puncture site. If this occurs when the needle is in the patient's vein, first the tourniquet and then the needle should be removed immediately, and pressure should be applied to the puncture site until the bleeding stops.

HEMOLYSIS

The blood specimen should be handled carefully at all times. Blood cells are fragile, and rough handling may cause hemolysis, or breakdown of the blood cells. Hemolyzed blood specimens produce inaccurate test results. To prevent hemolysis, these guidelines should be followed:

1. Store the collection tubes at room temperature because chilled tubes can result in hemolysis.
2. Allow the alcohol to air-dry completely before performing the venipuncture. Alcohol entering a blood specimen can cause hemolysis.
3. Use an appropriate-gauge needle to collect the specimen. Using a small-gauge needle (e.g., 25 G) can cause the blood cells to rupture as they pass through the lumen of the needle.
4. Practice good technique in collecting the specimen; excessive trauma (e.g., probing) to the blood vessel can result in hemolysis.
5. Leaving the tourniquet on for an extended period of time (more than 1 minute)
6. Always handle the collection tube carefully; do not shake it or handle it roughly.

FAINTING

Occasionally a patient experiences dizziness or fainting during or after a venipuncture. Should this occur, the most immediate concern is to protect the patient from injury—for example, by preventing the patient from falling. The patient should be placed in a position that promotes blood flow to the brain, and the provider should be notified for further treatment; see the box *Highlight on Vasovagal Syncope (Fainting).*

HIGHLIGHT on Vasovagal Syncope (Fainting)

Most people experience no change in their sense of well-being when they have blood taken. A very small percentage of individuals experience a type of fainting, however, known as *vasovagal syncope.*

Cause and Symptoms

Vasovagal syncope is caused by unpleasant physical or emotional stimuli, such as pain, fright, and the sight of blood. A sudden pooling of blood occurs, which results in a sudden decrease in blood pressure. This momentarily deprives the brain of blood, causing a temporary loss of consciousness, usually lasting only 1–2 min. Vasovagal syncope usually occurs when an individual is in an upright position, as in standing or sitting. Before fainting, the patient usually experiences some warning signals, such as sudden lightheadedness, nausea, weakness, yawning, paleness, blurred vision, a feeling of warmth, and sweating followed by drooping eyelids; a weak, rapid pulse; and finally, unconsciousness.

Treatment

A person who is about to faint should be placed in a position that facilitates blood flow to the brain and told to breathe deeply. The preferred position is lying down (supine) with the legs elevated and the collar and clothing loosened. This position may not always be possible, such as when a patient is seated and the venipuncture needle has already been inserted. In this case, the tourniquet and then the needle should be removed, and the patient's head should be lowered between the legs. An individual who has fainted should be protected from injury from falling and should be placed in a position that facilitates blood flow to the brain, as just described.

Prevention

Fainting during or after venipuncture is more likely in the following individuals: patients having a venipuncture for the first time, young patients, thin patients, patients with a low diastolic or high systolic blood pressure, patients with a history of fainting, nervous and apprehensive patients, and patients who are very quiet or very talkative. Fainting often can be prevented by identifying and closely observing individuals who are more likely to faint (as described). Talking to the patient often helps relax the patient and divert attention from the venipuncture procedure. If a patient has a history of fainting, he or she should be in a semi-reclining position for the venipuncture procedure because people rarely faint in this position. Other factors that contribute to fainting and that should be avoided include fatigue, lack of sleep, hunger, and environmental factors, such as a noisy, crowded, or overheated room. ■

OBTAINING A SERUM SPECIMEN

SERUM

Serum is plasma from which the clotting factor fibrinogen has been removed. Serum is normally clear in appearance and light-yellow to yellow in color. Serum contains many dissolved substances, such as glucose, cholesterol, sodium, potassium, chloride, antibodies, hormones, and enzymes. As a result, many laboratory tests require a serum specimen to determine whether levels of these substances are within normal limits and to detect substances that should not normally be in the serum and that if present indicate a pathologic condition.

COLLECTION TUBE SELECTION

A tube without an anticoagulant (e.g., SST or red closure) must be used to collect the blood specimen, to allow the specimen to separate into serum and clotted blood cells. Because the amount of serum recovered is only a portion of the specimen, a blood specimen must be drawn that is 2.5 times the amount required for the test. If 2 mL of serum is required, a 5-mL tube of blood must be collected; if 3 mL of serum is required, an 8-mL tube of blood is collected; and if 4 mL of serum is required, a 10-mL tube of blood is collected.

PROCESSING THE SPECIMEN

After the blood specimen has been collected, the red-closure tube or SST must be allowed to stand upright at room temperature for 30 to 45 minutes before being centrifuged. This allows clot formation of the blood cells, which yields more serum from the specimen. If the specimen is centrifuged too soon after collection of the blood specimen, the clotting factors do not have an opportunity to settle down into the cell layer to form a whole blood clot. The result of this is the formation of a *fibrin clot* in the serum layer. A fibrin clot is a spongy substance that occupies space, interfering with adequate serum collection (Fig. 17.20). The blood specimen should not be allowed to stand for longer than 1 hour, however, because leaching of substances from the cell layer into the serum may occur. This leaching of substances changes the integrity of the serum, leading to inaccurate test results. After the specimen has been allowed to stand and the blood cells have clotted, the specimen is centrifuged for 10 minutes to separate the serum from the blood cells.

SERUM SEPARATOR TUBES

An SST, also known as a *gel barrier tube,* is a collection tube specially designed to facilitate the collection of a serum specimen. The SST is identified by a gold or marbled red/gray closure and is used for collection and separation of blood. The SST contains a thixotropic gel, which is in a solid state at the bottom of the unused tube (Fig. 17.21A).

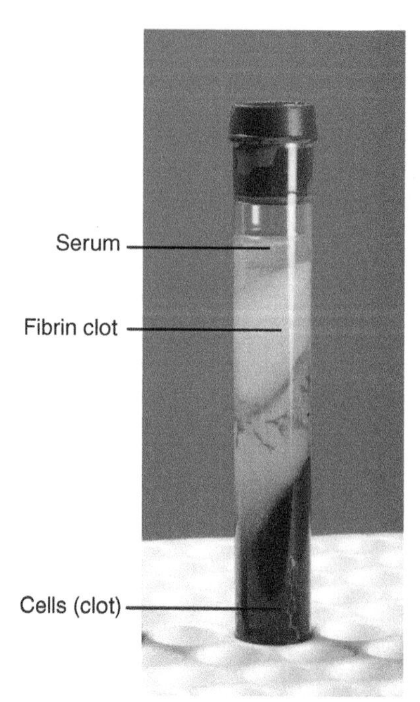

Fig. 17.20 A fibrin clot may interfere with adequate collection of serum.

The blood specimen is collected following the appropriate venipuncture method (Vacutainer or butterfly). The specimen must then be allowed to stand in an upright position for 30 to 45 minutes for proper clot formation of the blood cells and must be centrifuged as previously described. During centrifugation, the gel temporarily becomes fluid and moves to the dividing point between the serum and clotted cells, where it re-forms into a solid gel, serving as a physical barrier between the serum and the clot (see Fig. 17.21B). It is important to centrifuge the specimen for the proper length of time (i.e., 10 minutes). Centrifuging the specimen for less than 10 minutes can result in an incomplete gel barrier between the serum and the clot.

The serum can be transported to an outside laboratory in the serum separator tube. The medical assistant must first inspect the tube carefully to ensure that the gel barrier is firmly attached to the glass wall. If a complete barrier has not formed, the serum specimen must be removed and placed in a transfer tube to prevent leaching of substances from the cell layer into the serum, affecting the accuracy of the test results.

RED-CLOSURE TUBES

If a red-closure tube has been used to collect the specimen, the serum must be removed from the clot to prevent leaching of substances from the cell layer into the serum which affects the accuracy of the test results. The serum is removed using a pipet and placed in a separate transfer tube. It is important that proper technique be employed in removing the serum, to avoid disturbing the cell layer of the clot and drawing red blood cells into the serum layer. If cells do enter the serum, the entire specimen must be recentrifuged.

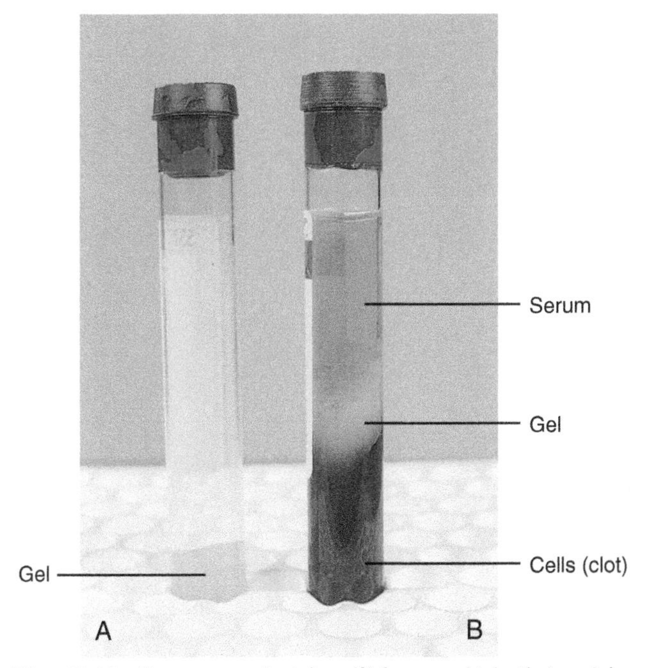

Fig. 17.21 Serum separator tubes. (A) An unused tube that contains the thixotropic gel in the bottom of the tube. (B) A tube that has been used to collect a blood specimen. During centrifugation, the gel temporarily becomes fluid and moves to the dividing point between the serum and blood cells in a fibrin clot.

When the serum has been removed from the blood specimen, the medical assistant should hold the specimen in the transfer tube up to good light. The serum specimen should be inspected for the presence of intact red blood cells or hemolyzed blood; in both cases, the specimen has a reddish appearance. A specimen that has a reddish appearance must be recentrifuged. If the specimen contains intact red blood cells, they settle to the bottom of the tube, and the serum can be removed. If the blood is hemolyzed, re-centrifugation would not make the red color disappear because the red blood cells have ruptured and released hemoglobin into the serum. Hemolyzed serum is unsuitable for laboratory tests because the results would be inaccurate; another blood specimen must be collected. Procedure 17.3 presents the method for separating serum from whole blood using a red-closure tube.

Skin Puncture

A skin puncture is used to obtain a capillary blood specimen and is also called a *capillary puncture.* Laboratory testing of a capillary blood specimen is usually performed in the medical office. Examples of such tests are hemoglobin, hematocrit, blood glucose, mononucleosis, and prothrombin time.

A skin puncture is performed when a test requires only a small blood specimen. Skin puncture is the method preferred for obtaining blood from infants and young children. Collecting blood from patients in this age group by venipuncture is often difficult and may damage veins and surrounding tissues.

PUNCTURE SITES

The puncture site varies depending on the age of the patient. The lateral part of the tip of the third or fourth finger is the preferred site for a skin puncture in an adult. In an infant (up to 1 year old), the skin puncture should be performed on the lateral or medical plantar surface of the heel. A finger puncture should *never* be performed on infants. The amount of tissue between skin surface and bone is so small that an injury to the bone is likely. After a child has begun to walk, the skin puncture can be performed on the fingertip.

DISPOSABLE RETRACTABLE LANCET

According to OSHA, a skin puncture should be performed in the medical office using a disposable retractable lancet which consists of a spring-loaded plastic holder with a metal blade inside the holder. OSHA does not recommend the use of lancets that are not retractable. Non-retractable lancets increase the possibility that the medical assistant will stick himself or herself accidentally, resulting in an exposure incident. In addition, some patients may become apprehensive and flinch when they see the point of a lancet. Children might pull their hands out of the medical assistant's grasp.

The skin puncture must not penetrate deeper than 3.1 mm in adults (finger) and 2.0 mm in infants (plantar surface of the heel) and children. If the puncture is deeper than this, the bone may be penetrated, which could result in the painful and serious conditions of osteochondritis or osteomyelitis. **Osteochondritis** is inflammation of bone and cartilage, and **osteomyelitis** is inflammation of the bone or bone marrow caused by bacterial infection. To avoid these complications, lancets are available in different blade lengths to control the depth of puncture. Adults with thin fingers and children require a shorter blade to avoid penetration of the bone.

The gauge of the lancet used to perform the skin puncture is based on the amount of blood specimen required. The gauge refers to the diameter of the lancet needle; needles are available in sizes ranging from 18 G to 30 G. As the size of the gauge increases, the diameter of the lancet needle decreases. For example, a needle with a gauge of 23 has a smaller diameter than a needle with a gauge of 19. A smaller gauge lancet must be used to obtain enough blood to fill a microcollection device, whereas a larger gauge and shorter blade can be used if only a drop of blood is needed.

The plastic holder of a disposable lancet may be color-coded by the manufacturer for ease in identifying the blade length of the lancet—for example, Surgilance Safety Lancet (Surgilance, Norcross, GA) (Fig. 17.22A). The plastic holder conceals the blade so the patient cannot see it during the puncture, as with the CoaguChek Lancet (Roche Diagnostics, Branchburg, NJ) (see Fig. 17.22B). Another example is the Quikheel Infant Lancet (Becton Dickinson), which is used for heel punctures in infants.

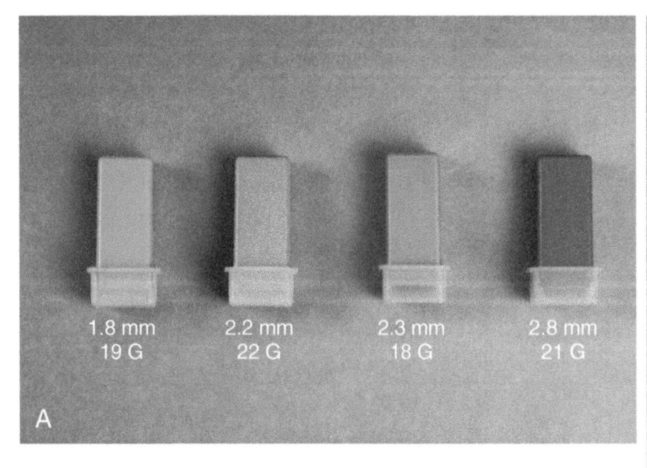

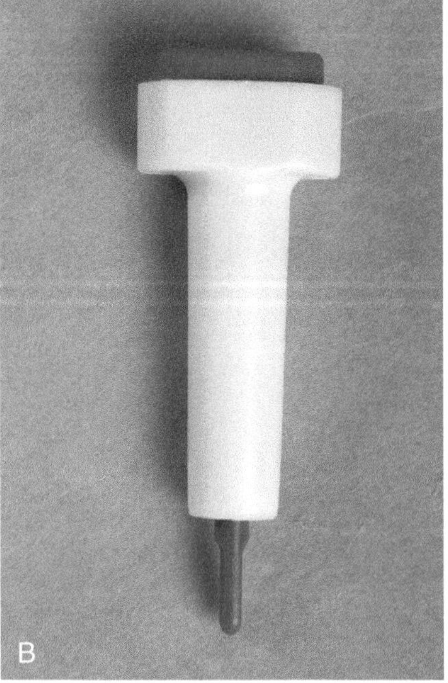

Fig. 17.22 (A) Surgilance color-coded lancets indicating length and gauge of the lancet. (B) CoaguChek Lancet.

When performing a finger puncture, use the lateral part of the tip of the third or fourth finger (middle or ring finger) of the nondominant hand for the puncture site. The capillary beds in these fingers are large, and the skin is easy to penetrate. The puncture site should be free of lesions, scars, bruises, and edema. The index finger is not recommended as a puncture site. The index finger is more calloused, which makes it harder to penetrate than the other fingers. Also, the patient uses that finger more and would notice the pain longer. The little finger also should not be used as a puncture site. The amount of tissue between the skin surface and the bone is so small that using this finger as a puncture site could result in injury to the bone.

To perform the skin puncture, the retractable lancet is placed on the patient's skin and activated. Depending on the brand, this is accomplished by one of the following methods:

- Depressing an activation button located on the top of the lancet until an audible click is heard (e.g., CoaguChek Lancet)
- Pushing the lancet firmly onto the puncture site until an audible click is heard (e.g., Surgilance Safety Lancet)

When the lancet is activated, the spring forces the blade into the skin and retracts the blade into the holder. The concealed blade and automatic puncture tend to result in less patient apprehension. After the puncture, the entire lancet is discarded in a biohazard sharps container. Procedure 17.4 describes the skin puncture procedure for use of a disposable retractable lancet.

MICROCOLLECTION DEVICES

After the skin has been punctured, a capillary blood specimen must be collected. The blood specimen can be collected directly onto a reagent strip, such as occurs with blood glucose monitors. It also can be collected in a small container known as a *microcollection device.* The device depends on the laboratory equipment running the test. Common microcollection devices are capillary tubes and microcollection tubes.

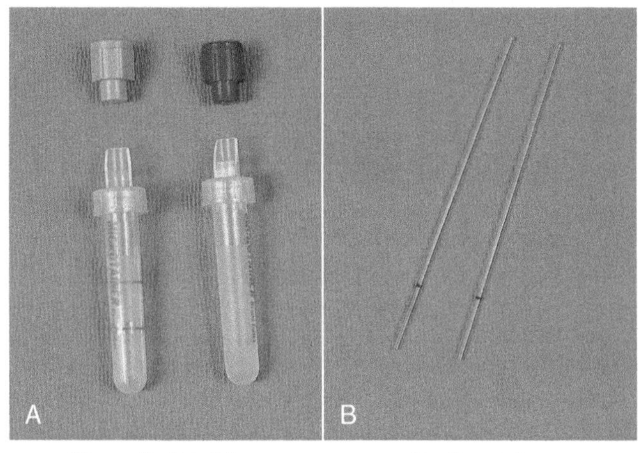

Fig. 17.23 Microcollection devices. (A) Microcollection tubes. (B) Capillary tubes.

Microcollection Tubes: A microcollection tube consists of a small plastic tube with a removable blood collector tip. The tip is designed to collect capillary blood from a skin puncture, which results in a relatively large blood specimen. After the specimen has been collected, the collector tip is removed, discarded, and replaced by a plastic plug. Microcollection tubes are available with or without an anticoagulant. The plugs are color-coded and correspond to the color-coded collection tube system used in venipuncture. One such device is the Microtainer (Becton Dickinson) (Fig. 17.23A).

Capillary Tubes: A capillary tube consists of a disposable glass or plastic tube (see Fig. 17.23B). Depending on the size of the tube, it can hold 5 to 75 μL of blood. In the medical office, a capillary tube is used to collect a blood specimen for a hematocrit determination. This procedure is presented in Chapter 18.

What Would You Do? What Would You *Not* Do? RESPONSES

Case Study 1
Page 603

What Did Dori Do?
- ❑ Told Camila that it was fine to have her friend there while she gets her blood drawn.
- ❑ Told Camila that she could not have the blood drawn out of her left arm because a good vein could not be located in that arm.
- ❑ Told Camila that using the hand veins is always the last choice when drawing blood. Explained to Camila that there will just be a small stick and that it will heal quickly, and there should be no reason it would affect her softball game this evening.
- ❑ Tried to relax and reassure Camila before the venipuncture. Carefully explained the procedure to her because it was her first one.
- ❑ Because Camila is nervous, took precautions to prevent her from fainting by placing her in a semi-Fowler position on the examining table.
- ❑ Had Camila's friend stand near the head of the table to help calm her down.

What Did Dori Not Do?
- ❑ Did not try to draw Camila's blood from her left arm or hand.
- ❑ Did not ignore the fact that Camila was nervous about the venipuncture.

Case Study 2
Page 608

What Did Dori Do?
- ❑ Told Buzz that when a butterfly setup is used, the air in the tubing alters the test results. Explained that the red tube is used to get rid of the air, and because it is not needed for testing, it is thrown away.
- ❑ Stressed to Buzz how important it is to have his blood tested every week, which helps the physician determine if there is too much or too little Coumadin in his body. Explained to him again what might occur if his Coumadin were at the wrong level.
- ❑ Told Buzz that the office would help him locate a medical laboratory where he will be vacationing, so he can have his test done.
- ❑ Made sure that Buzz had a laboratory requisition so that he could have his test done while he was on vacation.

What Did Dori Not Do?
- ❑ Did not tell Buzz that it would be all right to skip his prothrombin test during his vacation.

Case Study 3
Page 610

What Did Dori Do?
- ❑ Told Mrs. Coleman that the laboratory can accept only specimens drawn at the laboratory or at the medical office.
- ❑ Told Mrs. Coleman that if it would make her feel more comfortable, the laboratory could drop off the blood-drawing supplies at the office, and her blood could be drawn tomorrow at the office.
- ❑ Informed the physician about Mrs. Coleman's experience at the laboratory.

What Did Dori Not Do?
- ❑ Did not tell Mrs. Coleman that probing a vein could cause the test results to be inaccurate. ■

TERMINOLOGY REVIEW

Key Term	Word Parts	Definition
Antecubital space	*ante-:* before	The surface of the arm in front of the elbow.
Anticoagulant	*anti-:* against	A substance that inhibits blood clotting.
Buffy coat		A thin, light-colored layer of white blood cells and platelets that lies between a top layer of plasma and a bottom layer of red blood cells when an anticoagulant has been added to a blood specimen.
Evacuated collection tube		A sterile glass or plastic blood collection tube with a color-coded closure that contains a vacuum.
Hematoma	*hemat/o:* blood *-oma:* tumor or swelling	A swelling or mass of coagulated blood caused by a break in a blood vessel.
Hemoconcentration	*hem/o:* blood	An increase in the concentration of the nonfilterable blood components in the blood vessels, such as red blood cells, enzymes, iron, and calcium, as a result of a decrease in the fluid content of the blood.
Hemolysis	*hem/o:* blood *-lysis:* breakdown	The breakdown of blood cells.
Osteochondritis	*oste/o:* bone *myel/o:* bone marrow *-itis:* inflammation	Inflammation of bone and cartilage.

Continued

TERMINOLOGY REVIEW—cont'd

Key Term	Word Parts	Definition
Osteomyelitis	*oste/o:* bone *myel/o:* bone marrow *-itis:* inflammation	Inflammation of the bone or bone marrow as a result of bacterial infection.
Phlebotomist	*phleb/o:* vein *tomist:* specialist	A health care professional trained in the collection of blood specimens.
Phlebotomy	*phleb/o:* vein *-otomy:* incision	Incision of a vein for the removal of blood; the collection of blood.
Plasma		The liquid part of the blood consisting of a clear, straw-colored fluid that comprises approximately 55% of the blood volume.
Serum		Plasma from which the clotting factor fibrinogen has been removed.
Venipuncture	*ven/o:* vein	Puncturing of a vein.
Venous reflux	*ven/o:* vein *-ous:* pertaining to	The backflow of blood (from a collection tube) into the patient's vein.
Venous stasis	*ven/o:* vein *stasis:* control, stop	The temporary cessation or slowing of the venous blood flow.

PROCEDURE 17.1 Venipuncture—Vacutainer Method

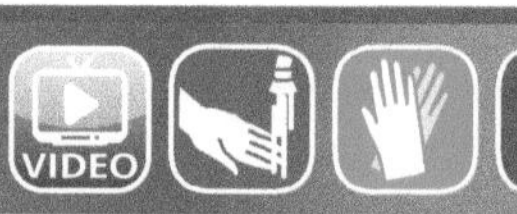

Outcome Perform a venipuncture using the Vacutainer method

Equipment/Supplies

- Disposable gloves
- Tourniquet
- Antiseptic wipe
- Blood collection needle with a safety shield
- Plastic tube holder
- Collection tubes
- Sterile 2 × 2 gauze pad
- Adhesive bandage
- Biohazard sharps container
- Biohazard specimen bag

1. **Procedural Step.** Review the collection and handling requirements for the tests ordered by the provider in the laboratory test directory.
2. **Procedural Step.** Sanitize your hands. Greet the patient and introduce yourself. Identify the patient by asking the patient to state his or her full name and date of birth. Compare this information with the demographic data in the patient's medical record. Seat the patient comfortably in a phlebotomy chair.
   Principle. It is important to confirm that you have the correct patient to avoid collecting a specimen from the wrong patient.
3. **Procedural Step.** If the patient was required to prepare for the test (e.g., fasting, medication restriction), determine whether he or she has prepared properly. If the patient has not followed the patient preparation requirements, notify the provider for instructions on handling this situation.
   Principle. The patient must prepare properly so the medical assistant can obtain a high-quality specimen that will yield accurate test results.
4. **Procedural Step.** Assemble the equipment.
   a. Select the proper collection tubes for the tests ordered by the provider and check the expiration date on the tubes.
   b. Complete a laboratory request by writing in the information on a preprinted form or by entering the required information into a computer.
   c. Label each tube using one of the following methods: attaching a computer barcode label to each tube, or manually labeling each tube with the patient's name and date of birth, the date, and your initials. (*Note:* Follow the medical office policy as to when the tubes should be labeled. Some offices prefer that tubes be labeled *before* the specimen is drawn; other offices want the tubes to be labeled right *after* the specimen has been drawn.)
   Principle. Outdated tubes may no longer contain a vacuum, and as a result they may not be able to draw blood into the tube. Proper labeling of blood specimens avoids a mix-up of specimens.

PROCEDURE **17.1** Venipuncture—Vacutainer Method—cont'd

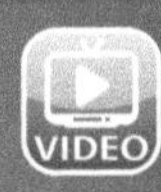

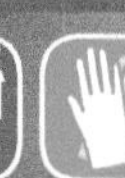

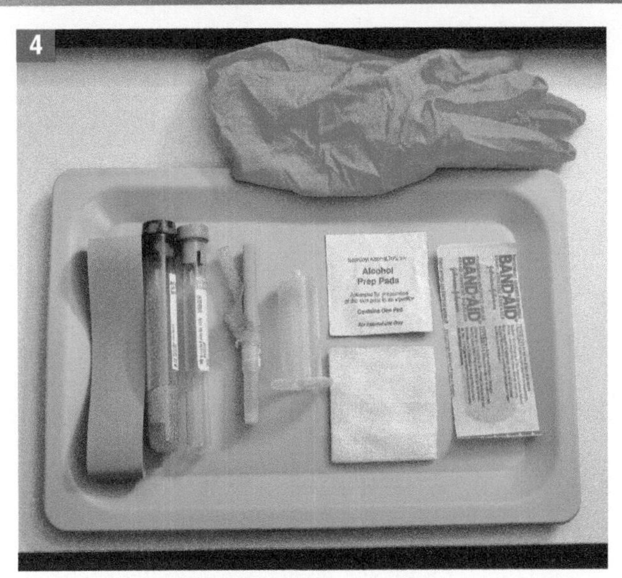

Assemble the equipment.

5. **Procedural Step.** Prepare the Vacutainer system. Remove the cap from the posterior needle using a twisting and pulling motion. Insert the posterior needle into the small opening on the tube holder. Screw the tube holder onto the Luer adapter and tighten it securely.
   Principle. An unsecured needle can fall out of its tube holder.

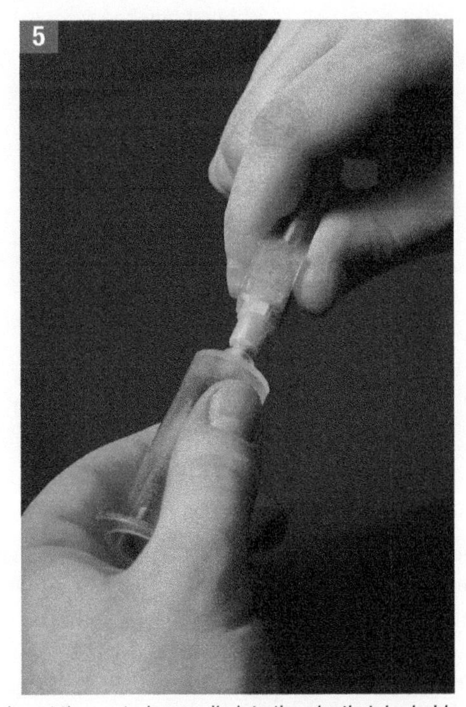

Insert the posterior needle into the plastic tube holder.

6. **Procedural Step.** Open the sterile gauze packet and lay it flat to allow the gauze pad to rest on the inside of its wrapper. Position the collection tubes in the correct order of draw. If the collection tube contains a powdered additive, tap the tube just below the stopper to release any additive adhering to the stopper.
   Principle. If an additive remains trapped in the stopper, erroneous test results may occur.
7. **Procedural Step.** Place the first tube loosely in the tube holder.
8. **Procedural Step.** Explain the procedure to the patient and reassure the patient. Perform a preliminary assessment of both arms to determine the best vein to use. It also is helpful to ask the patient which arm has been used in the past to obtain blood.
   Principle. Venipuncture is often a frightening experience for the patient, and reassurance should be offered to reduce apprehension.
9. **Procedural Step.** Apply the tourniquet. Position the tourniquet 3–4 inches above the bend in the elbow. The tourniquet should be snug but not tight. Ask the patient to clench the fist of the arm to which the tourniquet has been applied.
   Principle. The combined effect of the pressure of the tourniquet and the clenched fist should cause the antecubital veins to stand out so that accurate selection of a puncture site can be made.

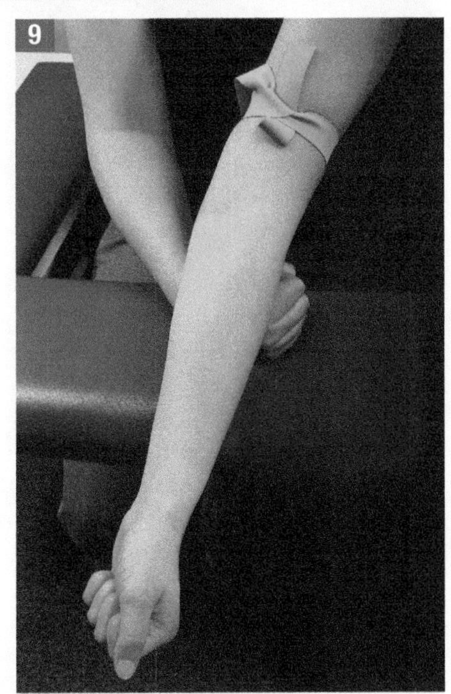

Apply the tourniquet.

10. **Procedural Step.** With a tourniquet in place, thoroughly assess the veins of first one arm and then the other to determine the best vein to use.
11. **Procedural Step.** Position the patient's arm. The arm with the vein selected for the venipuncture should be extended and placed in a straight line from the shoulder to the wrist with the antecubital veins facing

Continued

PROCEDURE 17.1 Venipuncture—Vacutainer Method—cont'd

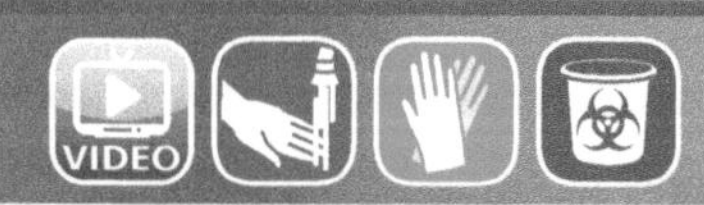

anteriorly. The arm can be supported on the armrest by a rolled towel or by having the patient place the first of the other hand under the elbow.

Principle. This position allows easy access to the antecubital veins.

12. Procedural Step. Thoroughly palpate the selected vein. Gently palpate the vein with the fingertips to determine the direction of the vein and to estimate its size and depth. Never leave the tourniquet on an arm for longer than 1 minute at a time. (*Note:* If you need to perform several assessments to locate the best vein, the tourniquet must be removed and reapplied after a 2-minute waiting period.)

Principle. Leaving the tourniquet on for longer than 1 minute is uncomfortable for the patient and may alter the test results.

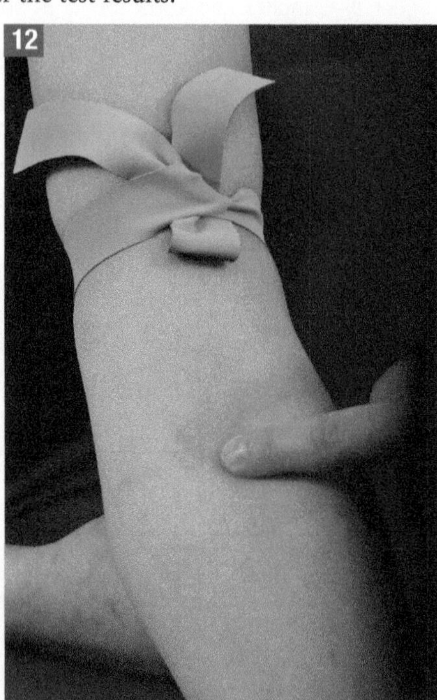

Palpate the vein.

13. Procedural Step. Remove the tourniquet (if more than 1 minute has elapsed) and cleanse the site with an antiseptic wipe. Cleansing should be done in a circular motion, starting from the inside, and moving away from the puncture site. Allow the site to air-dry; after cleansing, *do not touch the area*, wipe the area with gauze, or fan the area with your hand. Place the remaining supplies within comfortable reach of your nondominant hand.

Principle. Using a circular motion helps carry foreign particles away from the puncture site. The site must be allowed to air-dry to allow the alcohol enough time to destroy microorganisms on the patient's skin. Residual alcohol entering the blood specimen can cause hemolysis, leading to inaccurate test results. In addition, residual alcohol causes the patient to experience a stinging sensation when the puncture is made. Touching or fanning the area causes contamination of the puncture site, and the cleansing process must be repeated. Items used during the procedure should be positioned so that you do not have to reach over the patient and possibly move the needle, resulting in pain, injury, or both.

14. Procedural Step. Reapply the tourniquet. Apply gloves. Gently position the pink safety shield straight back toward the holder (refer to Fig. 17.13A). Remove the needle guard from the needle using a twisting and pulling motion. Hold the Vacutainer system by placing the thumb of the dominant hand on top of the tube holder and the pads of the first three fingers underneath the holder and collection tube. The needle bevel is in the correct position (bevel facing up) when the pink safety shield is facing up. Position the collection tube so that the label is facing down.

Principle. Gloves provide a barrier against bloodborne pathogens. A bevel up position allows easier entry of the needle into the skin and the vein, resulting in less pain for the patient. With the label facing down, you can observe the blood as it fills the tube, which allows you to know when the tube is full.

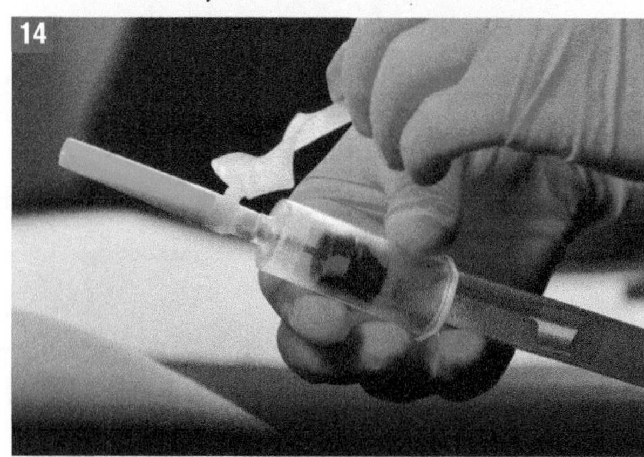

Position the safety shield straight back towards the holder.

15. Procedural Step. Anchor the vein. Grasp the patient's arm with the nondominant hand. Your thumb should be placed 1–2 inches below and to the side of the puncture site. Using your thumb, draw the skin taut over the vein in the direction of the patient's hand.

Principle. The thumb helps hold the skin taut for easier entry and helps stabilize the vein to be punctured. Placing the thumb to the side keeps it out of the way of the Vacutainer setup, so that you can maintain a 15-degree angle when entering the vein.

PROCEDURE 17.1 Venipuncture—Vacutainer Method—cont'd

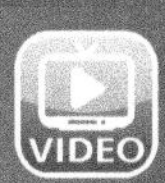
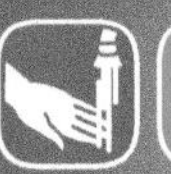
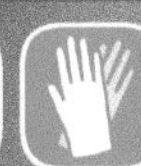
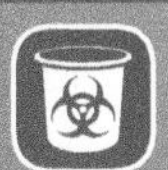

16. **Procedural Step.** Position the needle at a 15-degree angle to the arm. Rest the backs of the fingers on the patient's forearm. Ensure that the needle points in the same direction as the vein to be entered. The needle should be positioned so that it enters the vein approximately 1/8-inch below the place where the vein is to be entered.

Principle. An angle of less than 15 degrees may cause the needle to enter above the vein, preventing puncture. An angle of more than 15 degrees may cause the needle to go through the vein by puncturing the posterior wall. This could result in a hematoma.

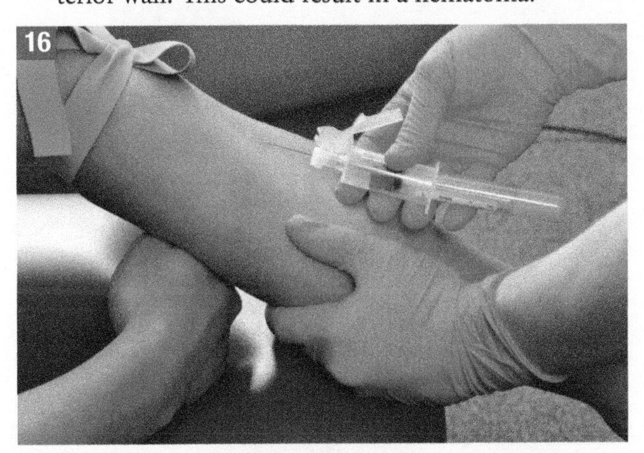

Position the needle.

17. **Procedural Step.** Tell the patient that he or she will "feel a small stick," and with one continuous steady motion, enter the skin and then the vein. You will feel a sensation of resistance followed by a "release" as the vein is entered. When the "release" is felt, you have entered the vein and should not advance the needle any farther.

Principle. Alerting the patient to the stick prevents startling the patient, which could cause the patient to move. Movement causes pain for the patient, and it may damage tissue at the venipuncture site. Using one continuous steady motion helps to prevent tissue damage.

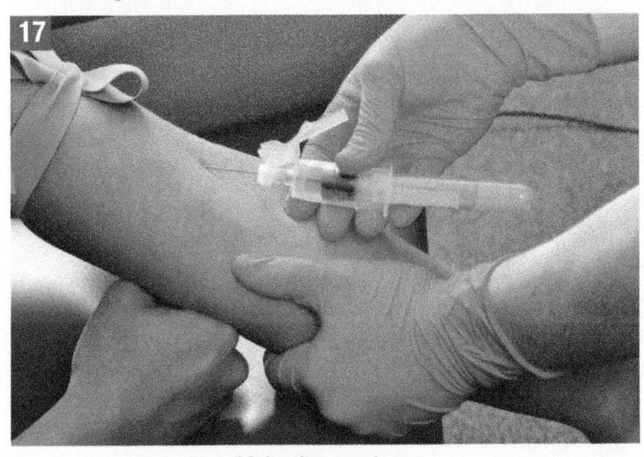

Make the puncture.

18. **Procedural Step.** Stabilize the Vacutainer setup by firmly grasping the holder between the thumb and the underlying fingers to prevent the needle from moving. Do *not* change hands during the procedure.

Principle. Stabilizing the holder helps prevent the needle from moving when a tube is inserted or removed. Changing hands may cause the needle to move, which is painful for the patient.

19. **Procedural Step.** With the nondominant hand, place the first two fingers on the underside of the flange on the tube holder, and with the thumb, slowly push the tube forward to the end of the holder. This allows the posterior needle to puncture the rubber stopper. Blood begins flowing into the tube if the (anterior) needle is in a vein.

Principle. Not using the flange may cause the needle to advance forward and go completely through the vein, resulting in failure to obtain blood; internal bleeding also may occur, resulting in a hematoma.

20. **Procedural Step.** Allow the collection tube to fill to the exhaustion of the vacuum, as indicated by cessation of the blood flow into the tube. The suction of the collection tube automatically draws the blood into the tube.

Principle. If the collection tube is removed before the vacuum is exhausted, a rush of air enters the tube, damaging the red blood cells. Also, a tube containing an additive, such as an anticoagulant, must be filled completely to ensure accurate test results.

21. **Procedural Step.** Remove the tube from the holder by grasping the tube with the fingers, placing the thumb or index finger against the flange, and pulling the tube off the posterior needle. Do not change the position of the needle in the vein. If the tube contains a clot activator, gently invert the tube back and forth 5 times before laying it down. If the tube contains an anticoagulant, gently invert the tube 8–10 times.

Principle. The rubber sheath covers the point of the needle, stopping the flow of blood until the next tube is inserted. Not using the flange to remove the tube can cause the needle to come out of the vein prematurely, resulting in blood being forced out of the puncture site. A tube containing an anticoagulant must be inverted immediately to prevent the blood from clotting. Gentle inversion of a tube with a clot activator or an anticoagulant prevents hemolysis.

Continued

PROCEDURE 17.1 Venipuncture—Vacutainer Method—cont'd

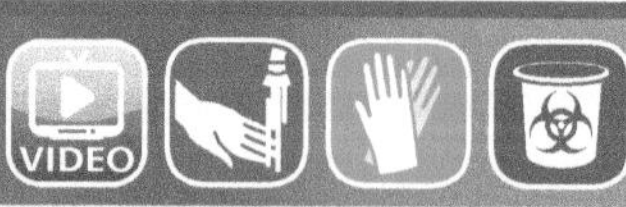

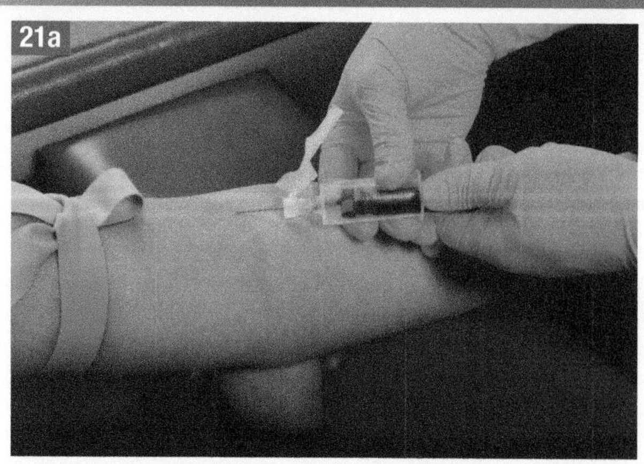

Remove the tube from the holder.

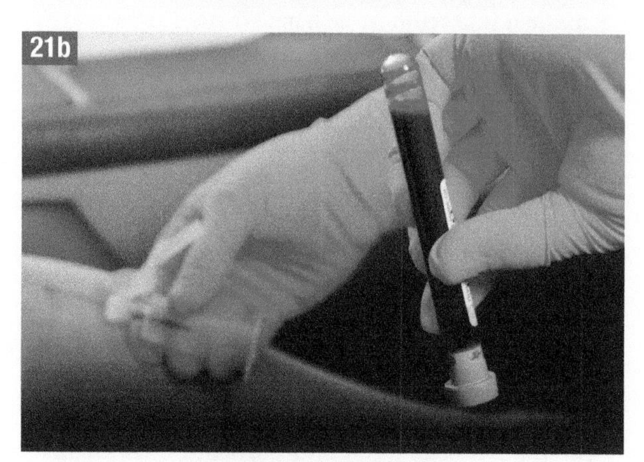

Invert the tube 8 to 10 times.

22. **Procedural Step.** Using the flange, carefully insert the next tube into the holder. Continue in this manner until the last tube has been filled.
23. **Procedural Step.** Remove the tension from the tourniquet by pulling upward on one of the flaps of the tourniquet. Ask the patient to unclench the fist.
    Principle. The tourniquet tension must be removed before the needle. Otherwise, the pressure on the vein from the tourniquet could cause internal and external bleeding around the puncture site resulting in a hematoma.
24. **Procedural Step.** Remove the last tube from the holder. Immediately invert the tube back and forth 5 times if it contains a clot activator and 8–10 times if it contains an anticoagulant.
    Principle. Removing the last tube prevents blood from dripping out of the tip of the needle after it has been removed from the patient's arm.
25. **Procedural Step.** Place a sterile gauze pad slightly above the puncture site, and carefully withdraw the needle at the same angle as for penetration. Immediately move the gauze over the puncture site, and apply firm pressure. (Do not apply any pressure to the puncture site until the needle has been completely removed.) Activate the safety shield away from yourself and the patient and as illustrated in Fig. 17.13.
    Principle. Placing the gauze pad above the puncture helps prevent tissue movement as the needle is withdrawn and reduces patient discomfort. Careful withdrawal prevents further tissue damage.

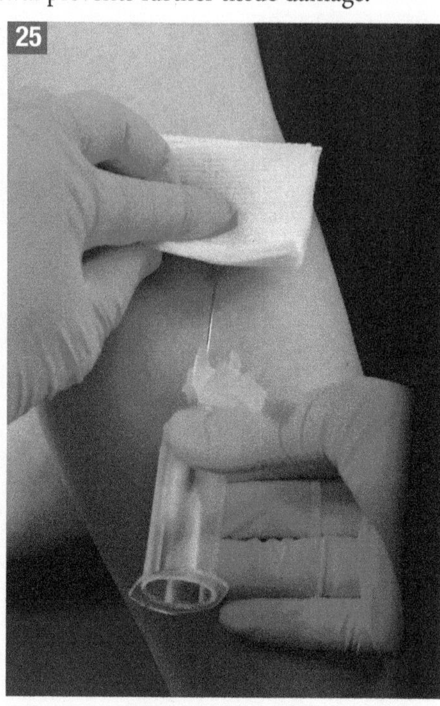

Withdraw the needle.

26. **Procedural Step.** Immediately discard the tube holder and attached needle as one unit in a biohazard sharps container. Do not remove the needle from the holder; the holder must be discarded and not reused.
    Principle. Immediate disposal of the needle and holder unit is required by the OSHA Standard to prevent a needlestick injury; even though the safety shield encases the anterior needle, a needlestick injury can still occur from the posterior needle, which is covered only with a rubber sleeve. Tube holders are often contaminated with blood and must not be reused.
27. **Procedural Step.** Continue to apply pressure with the gauze pad. Cooperative patients can be asked to assist by applying pressure with the gauze pad for 1–2 min. The arm can be elevated to facilitate clot formation. Do not allow the patient to bend the arm at the elbow because this increases blood loss from the puncture site.
    Principle. Applying pressure reduces the leakage of blood from the puncture site externally or internally. Internal leakage of blood into the tissues could result in a hematoma.

PROCEDURE 17.1 Venipuncture—Vacutainer Method—cont'd

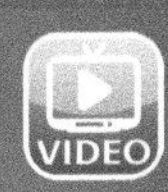
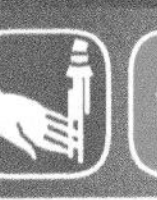
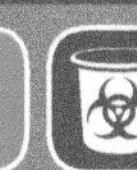

28. **Procedural Step.** Stay with the patient until the bleeding has stopped. Remove the gauze and inspect the puncture site to ensure that the opening is sealed with a clot. Apply an adhesive bandage to the puncture site. As an alternative, the gauze pad can be folded into quarters and taped on the puncture site to be used as a pressure bandage. Instruct the patient not to pick up anything heavy for about an hour. (*Note:* If swelling or discoloration occurs, apply an ice pack to the site after bandaging it.)
    Principle. Lifting a heavy object causes pressure on the puncture site, which could result in bleeding.
29. **Procedural Step.** Place the tubes in an upright position in a test tube rack. Remove the gloves and sanitize your hands.
30. **Procedural Step.** Document the procedure in the patient's medical record.
    a. *Electronic health record (EHR):* Document which arm and vein were used, as well as any unusual patient reactions, using the appropriate radio buttons, drop-down menus, and free text fields.
    b. *Paper-based patient record:* Document the date and time, which arm and vein were used, unusual patient reaction, and your initials (refer to the PPR documentation example).
31. **Procedural Step.** If needed, process the specimen by letting it stand for 30–45 min and then centrifuging it to separate serum from the cells. Prepare the specimen for transport to an outside laboratory as follows:
    a. Place the specimen tube in a biohazard specimen bag.
    b. Place the laboratory request in the outside pocket of the specimen bag (or transmit it electronically).
    c. Properly handle and store the specimen while awaiting pickup by a laboratory courier.
    d. Document the date the specimen was transported to the laboratory in the patient's medical record.

Principle. The biohazard bag protects the laboratory courier from the possibility of an exposure incident. The outside laboratory must have the completed request form to know which laboratory tests have been ordered by the provider. The specimen must be handled and stored properly to maintain the in vivo characteristics of the specimen.

PPR Documentation Example

Date	
4/5/XX	9:00 a.m. Venous blood specimen collected
	from (L) arm. Picked up by Medical Center
	Laboratory on 4/5/xx. ________________
	________________ D. Glover, CMA (AAMA)

PROCEDURE 17.2

PROCEDURE 17.2 Venipuncture—Butterfly Method

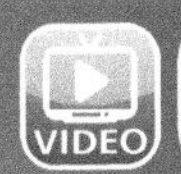
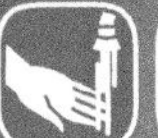

Outcome Perform a venipuncture using the butterfly method

Equipment/Supplies

- Disposable gloves
- Tourniquet
- Antiseptic wipe
- Winged infusion set with a Luer adapter and safety shield
- Plastic tube holder
- Collection tubes
- Sterile 2 × 2 gauze pad
- Adhesive bandage
- Biohazard sharps container
- Biohazard specimen bag

1. **Procedural Step.** Review the collection and handling requirements in the laboratory test directory for the tests ordered by the provider.
2. **Procedural Step.** Sanitize your hands. Greet the patient and introduce yourself. Identify the patient by asking the patient to state his or her full name and date of birth. Compare this information with the demographic data in the patient's medical record. Seat the patient comfortably in a phlebotomy chair.
3. **Procedural Step.** If the patient was required to prepare for the test (e.g., fasting, medication restriction), determine whether he or she has prepared properly. If the patient has not followed the patient preparation requirements, notify the provider for instructions on handling this situation.
4. **Procedural Step.** Assemble the equipment.
    a. Select the proper collection tubes for the tests ordered by the provider and check the expiration date on the tubes.
    b. Complete a laboratory request by writing in the information on a preprinted form or by entering the required information into a computer.

Continued

PROCEDURE 17.2 Venipuncture—Butterfly Method—cont'd

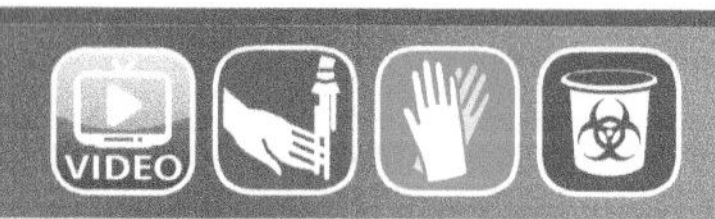

c. Label each tube using one of the following methods: attaching a computer barcode label to each tube, or manually labeling each tube with the patient's name and date of birth, the date, and your initials. (*Note:* Follow the medical office policy as to when the tubes should be labeled. Some offices prefer that tubes be labeled *before* the specimen is drawn; other offices want the tubes to be labeled right *after* the specimen has been drawn.)

Principle. Outdated tubes may no longer contain a vacuum, and as a result they may not be able to draw blood into the tube. Proper labeling of blood specimens avoids the mix-up of specimens.

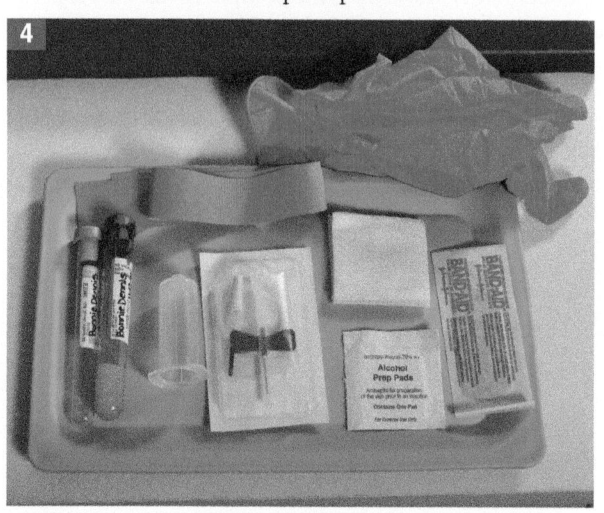

Assemble the equipment.

5. Procedural Step. Prepare the winged infusion set. Remove the winged infusion set from its package. Extend the tubing to its full length and stretch it slightly to prevent it from recoiling. Insert the posterior needle into the small opening on the tube holder. Screw the tube holder onto the Luer adapter and tighten it securely.

Principle. Extending the tubing straightens it to permit a free flow of blood in the tubing. An unsecured needle can fall out of its tube holder.

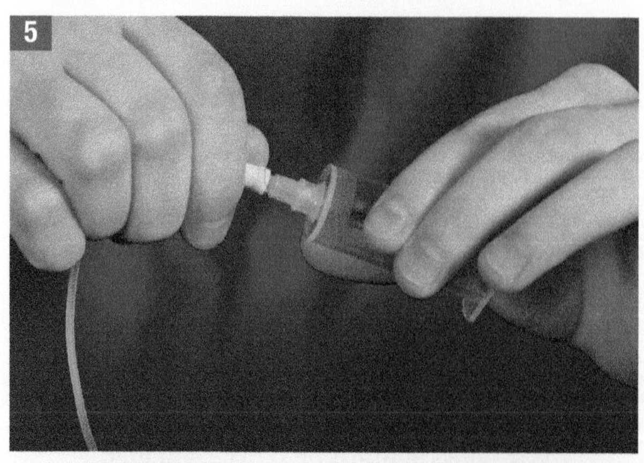

Screw the plastic tube holder onto the Luer adapter.

6. Procedural Step. Open the sterile gauze packet and lay it flat to allow the gauze pad to rest on the inside of its wrapper. Position the collection tubes in the correct order of draw. If the collection tube contains a powdered additive, tap the tube just below the stopper to release any additive adhering to the stopper.

Principle. If an additive remains trapped in the stopper, erroneous test results may occur.

7. Procedural Step. Place the first tube loosely in the tube holder with the label facing down.

Principle. With the label facing down, you can observe the blood as it fills the tube, which allows you to know when the tube is full.

8. Procedural Step. Explain the procedure to the patient, and reassure the patient. Perform a preliminary assessment of both arms to determine the best vein to use. It also is helpful to ask the patient which arm has been used in the past to obtain blood.

Principle. Venipuncture is often a frightening experience for the patient, and reassurance should be offered to reduce apprehension.

9. Procedural Step. Apply the tourniquet. Position the tourniquet 3–4 inches above the bend in the elbow. The tourniquet should be snug but not tight. Ask the patient to clench the fist of the arm to which the tourniquet has been applied.

Principle. The combined effect of the pressure of the tourniquet and the clenched fist should cause the antecubital veins to stand out so that accurate selection of a puncture site can be made.

10. Procedural Step. With a tourniquet in place, thoroughly assess the veins of first one arm and then the other to determine the best vein to use.

11. Procedural Step. Position the patient's arm. The arm with the vein selected for the venipuncture should be extended and placed in a straight line from the shoulder to the wrist with the antecubital veins facing anteriorly. The arm should be supported on the armrest by a rolled towel or by having the patient place the fist of the other hand under the elbow.

Principle. This position allows easy access to the antecubital veins.

12. Procedural Step. Thoroughly palpate the selected vein. Gently palpate the vein with the fingertips to determine the direction of the vein and to estimate its size and depth. Never leave the tourniquet on an arm for longer than 1 minute at a time. (*Note:* If you need to perform several assessments to locate the best vein, the tourniquet must be removed and reapplied after a 2-minute waiting period.)

Principle. Leaving the tourniquet on for longer than 1 minute is uncomfortable for the patient and may alter the test results.

PROCEDURE 17.2 Venipuncture—Butterfly Method—cont'd

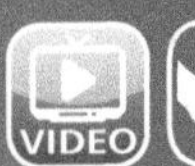
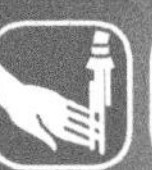

13. **Procedural Step.** Remove the tourniquet (if more than 1 minute has elapsed) and cleanse the site with an antiseptic. Cleansing should be done in a circular motion, starting from the inside and moving away from the puncture site. Allow the site to air-dry; after cleansing, *do not touch the area*, wipe the area with gauze, or fan the area with your hand. Place your remaining supplies within comfortable reach.
    Principle. Using a circular motion helps carry foreign particles away from the puncture site. The site must be allowed to air-dry to allow the alcohol enough time to destroy microorganisms on the patient's skin. Residual alcohol entering the blood specimen can cause hemolysis, leading to inaccurate test results. In addition, residual alcohol causes the patient to experience a stinging sensation when the puncture is made. Touching or fanning the area causes contamination of the puncture site, and the cleansing process must be repeated. Items used during the procedure should be positioned so that you do not have to reach over the patient and possibly move the needle, resulting in patient pain, injury, or both.
14. **Procedural Step.** Reapply the tourniquet. Apply gloves. With the dominant hand, grasp the winged infusion set by pressing the butterfly tips together. Remove the protective sheath from the needle of the infusion set. The needle should be positioned with the bevel facing up.
    Principle. Gloves provide a barrier against bloodborne pathogens. Positioning the needle with the bevel up allows easier entry into the skin and the vein, resulting in less pain for the patient.

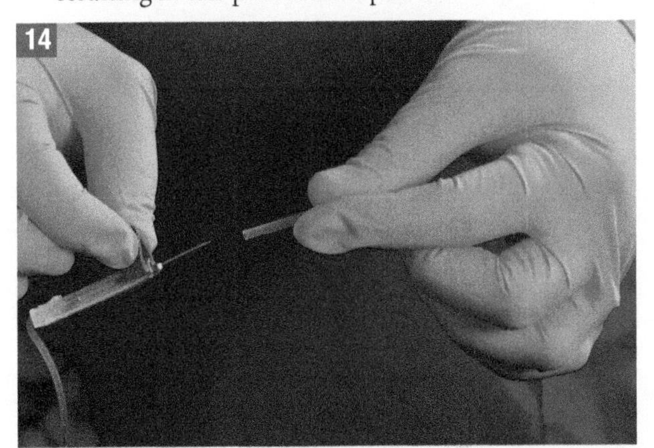

Remove the protective shield from the needle.

15. **Procedural Step.** Anchor the vein. Grasp the patient's arm with the nondominant hand. The thumb should be placed 1–2 inches below and to the side of the puncture site. Using the thumb, draw the skin taut over the vein in the direction of the patient's hand.
    Principle. The thumb helps hold the skin taut for easier entry and helps stabilize the vein to be punctured. Placing the thumb to the side keeps it out of the way of the winged infusion setup so that you can maintain a 15-degree angle when entering the vein.
16. **Procedural Step.** Position the needle at a 15-degree angle to the arm. Rest the backs of the fingertips on the patient's skin. Make sure the needle points in the same direction as the vein to be entered. The needle should be positioned so that it enters the vein approximately 1/8-inch below the place where the vein is to be entered.
    Principle. An angle of less than 15 degrees may cause the needle to enter above the vein, preventing puncture. An angle of more than 15 degrees may cause the needle to go through the vein by puncturing the posterior wall. This could result in a hematoma.
17. **Procedural Step.** Tell the patient that he or she will "feel a small stick," and with one continuous steady motion, enter the skin and then the vein. You will feel a sensation of resistance followed by a "release" as the vein is entered. After penetrating the vein, decrease the angle of the needle to 5 degrees. If the needle is in the vein, a flash of blood appears at the top of the tubing.
    Principle. Using one continuous motion reduces tissue damage.

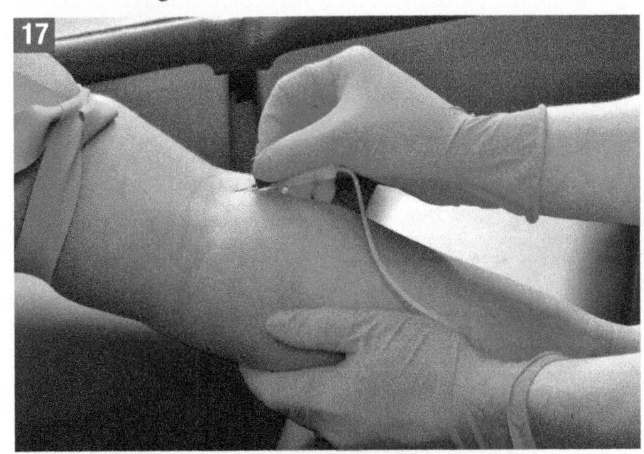

Make the puncture.

18. **Procedural Step.** Seat the needle by threading it forward an additional 1/4-inch inside the center of the vein so that it does not twist out of the vein, even if you let go of it. Open the butterfly wings and securely rest the wings flat against the skin. Ensure that the needle does not move.
    Principle. Seating the needle anchors the needle in the center of the vein and allows the use of both hands for changing tubes. Moving the needle is painful for the patient.

Continued

PROCEDURE 17.2 Venipuncture—Butterfly Method—cont'd

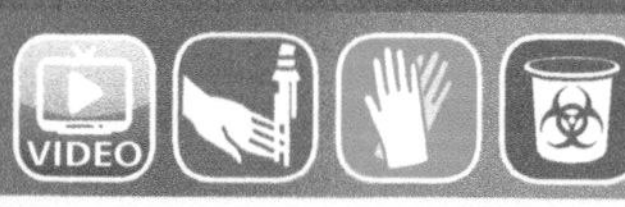

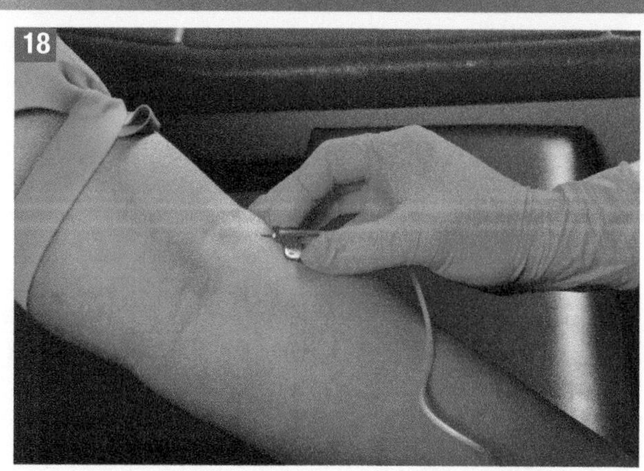

Rest the butterfly wings flat against the patient's skin.

19. Procedural Step. Keep the tube and holder in a downward position so that the tube fills from the bottom up and not near the rubber stopper. Slowly push the tube forward to the end of the holder. This allows the needle to puncture the rubber stopper. Blood begins to flow into the tube. Allow the collection tube to fill to the exhaustion of the vacuum, as indicated by cessation of the blood flow into the tube. The suction of the collection tube automatically draws the blood into the tube.

Principle. The tube must fill from the bottom up to prevent venous reflux. If the collection tube is removed before the vacuum is exhausted, a rush of air enters the tube, damaging the red blood cells. Also, a tube containing an anticoagulant must be filled completely to ensure accurate test results.

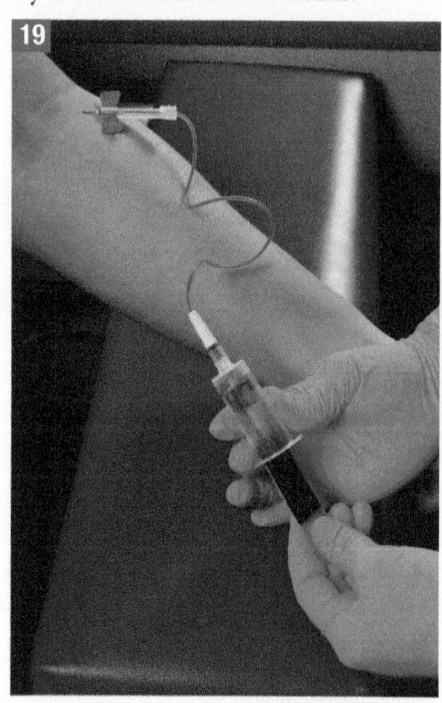

Fill the tube in a downward position.

20. Procedural Step. Remove the tube from the tube holder. If the tube contains a clot activator, gently invert the tube back and forth 5 times before laying it down. If the tube contains an anticoagulant, gently invert the tube 8–10 times.

Principle. The rubber sheath covers the point of the needle, stopping the flow of blood until the next tube is inserted. You must invert a tube containing an anticoagulant before laying it down, to prevent the blood from clotting. Gentle inversion of a tube with a clot activator or an anticoagulant prevents hemolysis.

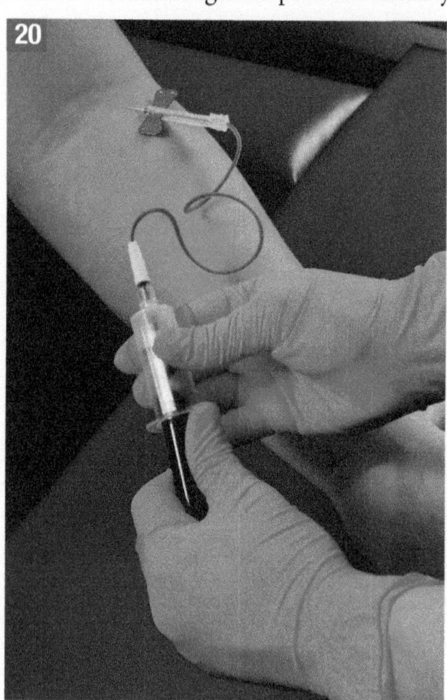

Remove the tube from the holder.

21. **Procedural Step.** Using the flange, carefully insert the next tube into the holder. Continue in this manner until the last tube has been filled.
22. **Procedural Step.** Remove the tension from the tourniquet by pulling upward on one of the flaps of the tourniquet. Ask the patient to unclench the fist.

    Principle. The tourniquet tension must be removed before the needle. Otherwise, pressure on the vein from the tourniquet could cause internal and external bleeding around the puncture.
23. **Procedural Step.** Remove the last tube from the holder. Immediately invert the tube back and forth 5 times if it contains a clot activator and 8–10 times if it contains an anticoagulant.

    Principle. Removing the last tube from the holder prevents blood from dripping out of the tip of the needle after it has been removed from the patient's arm.

PROCEDURE 17.2 Venipuncture—Butterfly Method—cont'd

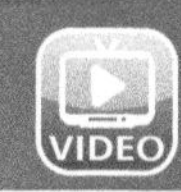
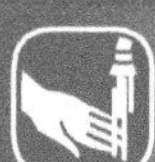

24. Procedural Step. Place a sterile gauze pad slightly above the puncture site. Grasp the setup just below the wings, and slowly withdraw the needle at the same angle as for penetration. Immediately move the gauze over the puncture site, and apply firm pressure. (*Note:* Do not apply pressure to the puncture site until the needle has been completely removed.) Cooperative patients can be asked to assist by applying pressure with the gauze pad. Activate the safety shield away from yourself and the patient and as illustrated in Fig. 17.18.

Principle. Placing the gauze pad above the puncture site helps prevent tissue movement as the needle is withdrawn and reduces patient discomfort. Careful withdrawal prevents further tissue damage.

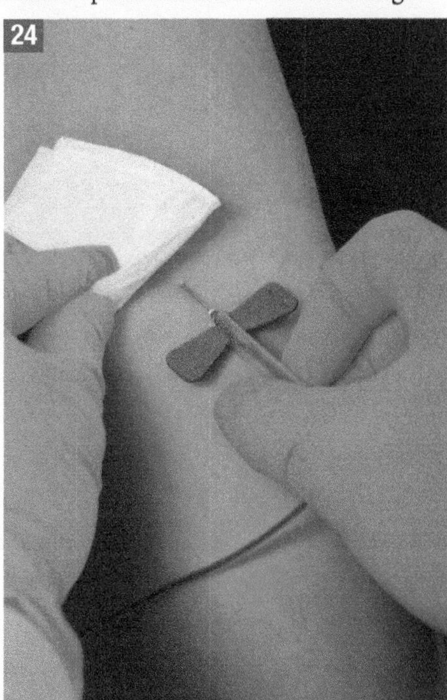

Release the tourniquet and remove the needle.

25. Procedural Step. Immediately discard the winged infusion set and attached tube holder. Holding onto the tube holder, first drop the needle into a biohazard sharps container, followed by the tubing and holder. Do not remove the tube holder from the setup; the tube holder must be discarded and not reused.

Principle. Proper disposal is required by the OSHA Standard to prevent a needlestick injury; even though the safety shield has been activated to encase the butterfly needle, a needlestick injury can still result from the posterior needle, which is covered with only a rubber sleeve. Tube holders are often contaminated with blood and must not be reused.

26. Procedural Step. Continue to apply pressure with the gauze pad. The arm can be elevated to facilitate clot formation. Do not allow the patient to bend the arm at the elbow because this increases blood loss from the puncture site.

Principle. Applying pressure reduces the leakage of blood from the puncture site externally or internally. Internal leakage into the tissues could result in a hematoma.

27. Procedural Step. Stay with the patient until the bleeding has stopped. Remove pressure, and inspect the puncture site to ensure that the opening is sealed with a clot. Apply an adhesive bandage to the puncture site. As an alternative, the gauze pad can be folded into quarters and taped onto the puncture site to be used as a pressure bandage. Instruct the patient not to pick up anything heavy for about an hour. (*Note:* If swelling or discoloration occurs, apply an ice pack to the site after bandaging it.)

Principle. Lifting a heavy object causes pressure on the puncture site, which could result in bleeding.

28. Procedural Step. Place the tubes in an upright position in a test tube rack. Remove the gloves, and sanitize your hands.

29. Procedural Step. Document the procedure in the patient's medical record.

a. *Electronic health record (EHR):* Document which arm and vein were used and any unusual patient reactions using the appropriate radio buttons, drop-down menus, and free text fields.

b. *Paper-based patient record:* Document the date and time, which arm and vein were used, unusual patient reactions, and your initials (refer to the PPR documentation example).

30. Procedural Step. If needed, process the specimen. Prepare the specimen for transport to an outside laboratory as follows:

a. Place the specimen tube in a biohazard specimen bag.

b. Place the laboratory request in the outside pocket of the specimen bag (or transmit it electronically).

c. Properly handle and store the specimen while awaiting pickup by a laboratory courier.

d. Document the date the specimen was transported to the laboratory in the patient's medical record.

Principle. The biohazard bag protects the laboratory courier from the possibility of an exposure incident. The outside laboratory must have the completed request form to know which laboratory tests have been ordered by the provider. The specimen must be handled and stored properly to maintain the in vivo characteristics of the specimen.

PPR Documentation Example

Date	
4/10/XX	10:30 a.m. Venous blood specimen collected
	from (L) arm. Picked up by Medical Center
	Laboratory on 4/10/xx.
	D. Glover, CMA (AAMA)

Continued

PROCEDURE 17.3 Separating Serum From a Blood Specimen

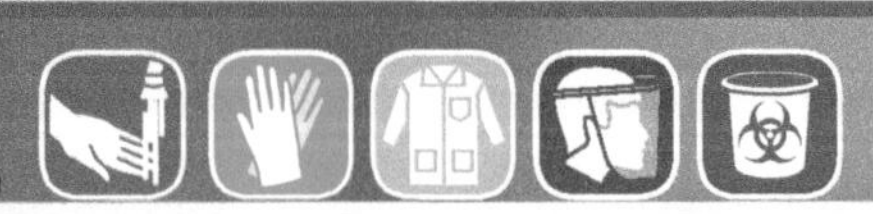

Outcome Separate serum from a blood specimen.

Equipment/Supplies:

- Red collection tube setup
- Test tube rack
- Disposable pipet
- Transfer tube
- Disposable gloves
- Face shield or mask and an eye protection device
- Protective laboratory coat
- Centrifuge
- Biohazard sharps container

1. Procedural Step. Collect the blood specimen by following the venipuncture procedure. Use a tube containing no anticoagulants (red closure) to collect the specimen. The tube selected should have a capacity of 2.5 times the amount of serum required. Label the red-closure tube and the transfer tube with the patient's name and date of birth, the date, and your initials. In addition, the transfer tube should bear the word "serum." Allow the tube to fill until the vacuum is exhausted.

Principle. To obtain serum, a tube containing no additives must be used. The tube must be allowed to fill completely to obtain the proper amount of serum. Several types of specimen, such as serum, plasma, and urine, are straw-colored; the transfer tube containing serum must be labeled as such to avoid confusion and mix-up among these specimens.

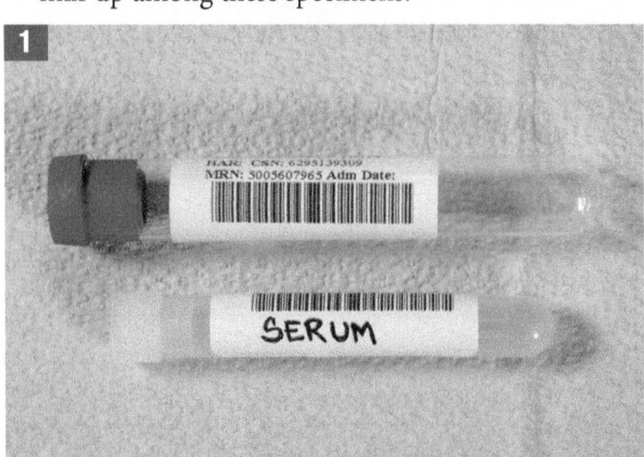

Label the tubes.

2. Procedural Step. Place the blood specimen tube in an upright position in a test tube rack for 30–45 min at room temperature. To prevent evaporation of the serum sample, do not remove the tube's stopper.

Principle. Specimens must be placed in an upright position and allowed to stand to permit clot formation of the blood cells and avoid the formation of a fibrin clot in the serum, which yields more serum from the specimen. Evaporation of the sample leads to falsely elevated test results.

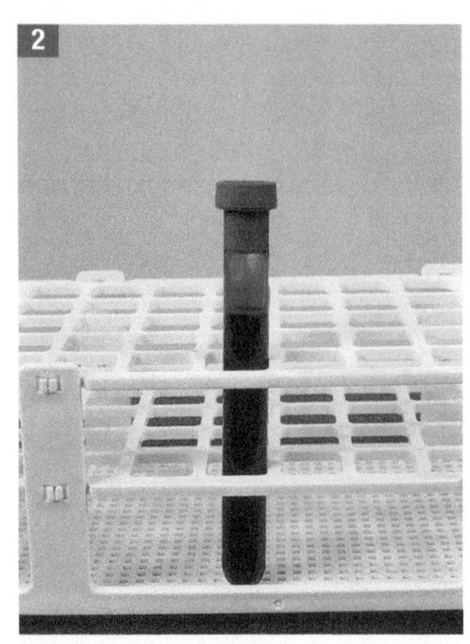

Allow the specimen to stand for 30 to 45 minutes.

3. Procedural Step. Centrifuge the specimen as follows:

a. Place the specimen in the centrifuge, closure end up.

b. Balance the specimen with another specimen tube or a water tube of the same type and weight as the specimen tube.

c. Centrifuge the specimen for 10 min.

d. Allow the centrifuge to come to a complete stop after the timer goes off. Do not open the lid or try to stop the centrifuge with your hand.

Principle. Centrifuging packs the cells and causes them to settle at the bottom of the tube, yielding more serum. If the centrifuge is not balanced, it may vibrate and move across the tabletop. An unbalanced centrifuge also can cause specimen tubes to break. Centrifuging the specimen for longer than 10 min can result in hemolysis of blood cells.

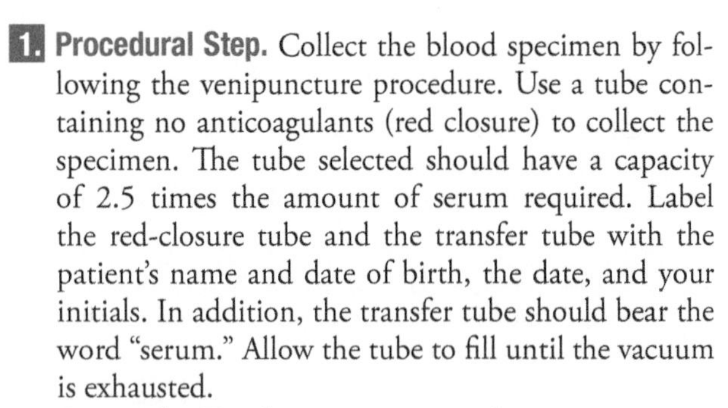

PROCEDURE 17.3 Separating Serum From a Blood Specimen—cont'd

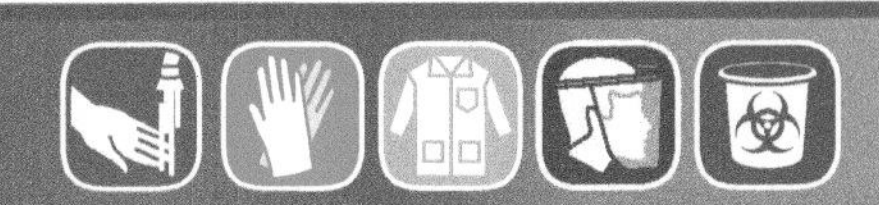

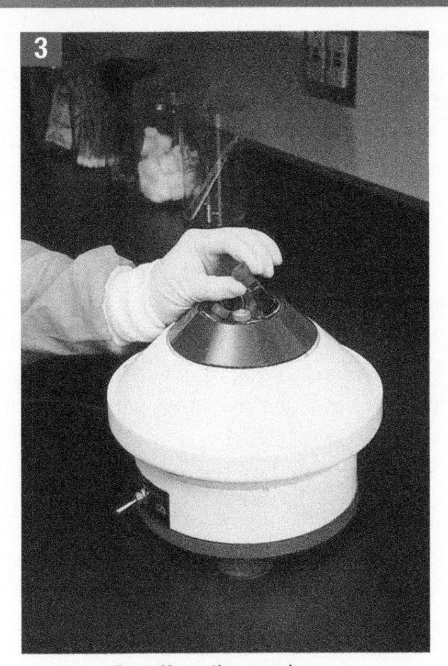

Centrifuge the specimen.

4. **Procedural Step.** Put on a face shield or a mask and an eye protection device such as goggles or glasses with solid side shields. Apply gloves. Carefully remove the tube from the centrifuge without disturbing the contents.
   Principle. The OSHA Standard requires the use of personal protective equipment whenever spraying or splashing of blood might be generated. Disturbing the contents may cause the cells to enter the serum, and the specimen will need to be recentrifuged.
5. **Procedural Step.** Remove the closure from the tube as follows:
   - *Hemogard closure tube:*
     a. Grasp the tube with one hand placing the thumb under the plastic closure.
     b. With the other hand, twist the plastic closure while simultaneously pushing up with the thumb of the other hand.
     c. Move the thumb away before lifting the closure. (Do not use the thumb to push the closure off the tube).
     d. Lift the closure off the tube.

     Principle. A glass tube has the potential to break or crack. To help prevent injury during closure removal, the thumb used to push upward on the closure should be removed from contact with the tube as soon as the closure is loosened.
   - *Rubber stopper closure tube:*
     a. Point the rubber stopper closure away from you.
     b. Using a twisting and pulling motion, carefully remove the stopper.

     Principle. Pointing the stopper away prevents accidental spraying or splashing of the specimen onto the medical assistant.
6. **Procedural Step.** Remove the serum from the tube as follows:
   a. Squeeze the bulb of the pipet to push the air out, and then insert it into the serum.
   b. Place the tip of the pipet against the side of the tube approximately 1/4 inch above the cell layer.
   c. Release the bulb to suction serum into the pipet. Do not allow the tip of the pipet to touch the cell layer.
   d. Transfer the serum in the pipet to the transfer tube.
   e. Continue pipetting until as much serum as possible is removed without disturbing the cell layer.
   f. Tightly cap the transfer tube to prevent sample evaporation.
   g. Replace the closure on the collection tube.

   Principle. The air must be removed from the bulb before inserting the pipet into the serum to prevent disturbance of the cell layer. If the cell layer is disturbed, red blood cells would enter the serum, and the specimen would need to be recentrifuged.

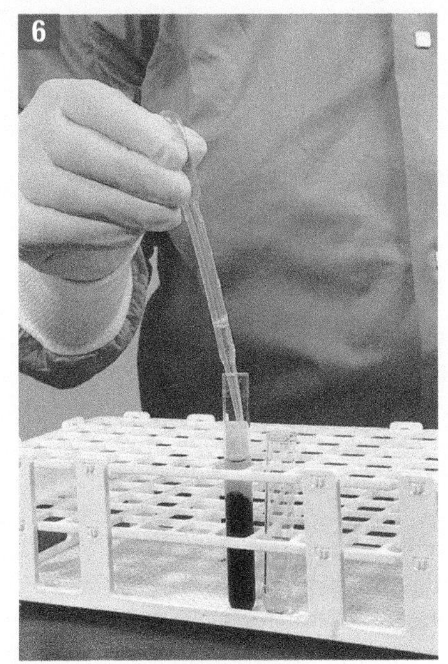

Pipet the serum.

7. **Procedural Step.** Hold the serum specimen up to the light and examine it for the presence of hemolysis. Ensure that the proper amount of serum has been obtained.
   Principle. Hemolyzed serum is unsuitable for laboratory testing.

Continued

PROCEDURE 17.3 Separating Serum From a Blood Specimen—cont'd

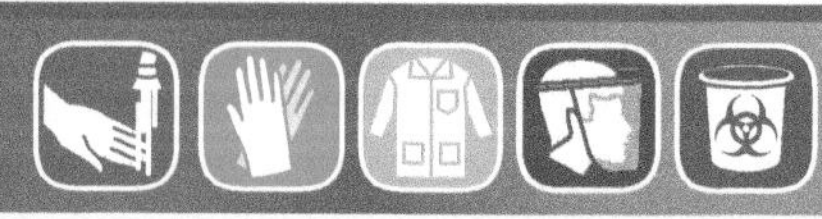

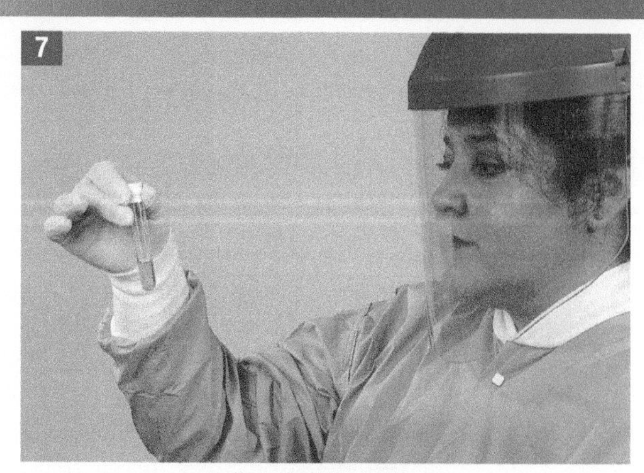

Examine the serum.

8. **Procedural Step.** Properly dispose of equipment. Following the OSHA Standard, the collection tube (containing the blood specimen) and the disposable pipet must be discarded in a biohazard sharps container.
9. **Procedural Step.** Remove your gloves and sanitize your hands.
10. **Procedural Step.** Prepare the specimen for transport to an outside laboratory as follows:
    a. Place the specimen tube in a biohazard specimen bag.
    b. Place the laboratory request in the outside pocket of the biohazard bag (or electronically transmit it).
    c. Properly store the specimen while awaiting pickup by a laboratory courier.
    d. Document the date the specimen was transported to the laboratory in the patient's medical record.

PROCEDURE 17.4 Skin Puncture—Disposable Lancet

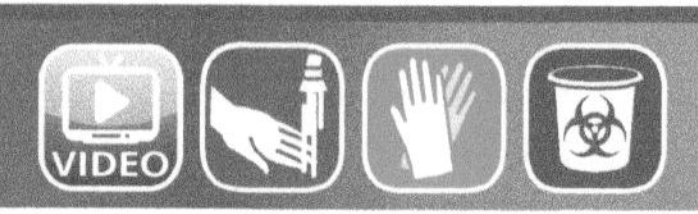

Outcome Obtain a capillary blood specimen

Equipment/Supplies

- Disposable gloves
- Antiseptic wipe
- CoaguChek lancet
- Sterile 2 × 2 gauze pad
- Adhesive bandage
- Biohazard sharps container

1. **Procedural Step.** Sanitize your hands.
2. **Procedural Step.** Greet the patient and introduce yourself. Identify the patient by asking the patient to state his or her full name and date of birth. Compare this information with the demographic data in the patient's medical record. If the patient was required to prepare for the test (e.g., fasting, medication restriction), determine whether he or she has prepared properly. If the patient has not followed the patient preparation requirements, notify the provider for instructions on handling this situation.
3. **Procedural Step.** Assemble the equipment. Open the sterile gauze packet and lay it flat to allow the gauze pad to rest on the inside of its wrapper.

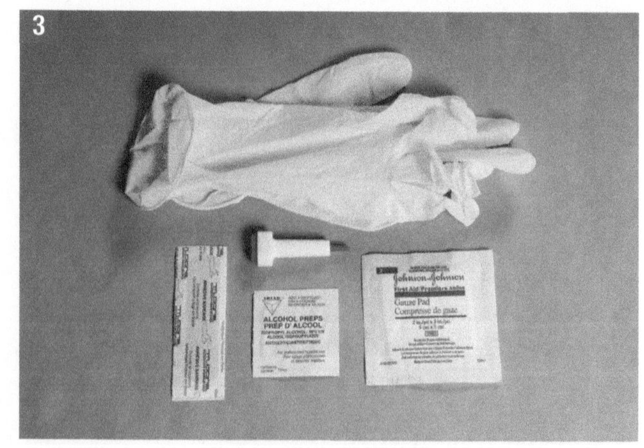

Assemble the equipment.

PROCEDURE 17.4 Skin Puncture—Disposable Lancet—cont'd

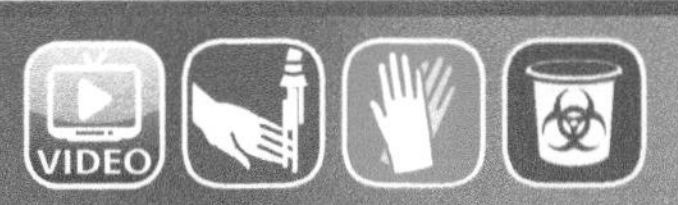

4. **Procedural Step.** Explain the procedure and reassure the patient. Explain to the patient that the procedure should be relatively quick and only slightly uncomfortable.
   Principle. Reassurance should be offered to reduce apprehension.
5. **Procedural Step.** Seat the patient comfortably in a chair. The patient's arm should be firmly supported and extended with the palmar surface of the hand facing up.
6. **Procedural Step.** Select an appropriate puncture site. Use the lateral part of the tip of the third or fourth finger of the nondominant hand to make the puncture. If the patient's finger is cold, you can warm it by gently massaging the finger five or six times from base to tip, or by placing the hand in warm water for a few minutes.
   Principle. Warming the site increases the blood flow to the area and promotes bleeding from the puncture site.
7. **Procedural Step.** Cleanse the site with an antiseptic wipe. Allow the site to air-dry, and after cleansing it do not touch the area, wipe the area with gauze, or fan the area with your hand.
   Principle. The site must be allowed to air-dry to allow enough time for the alcohol to destroy microorganisms on the patient's skin. If the site is dry, a round drop of blood forms on the finger, making it easy to collect the specimen. If the site is not dry, the blood leaches out and runs down the finger, making it difficult to collect. Residual alcohol entering the blood specimen can cause hemolysis, leading to inaccurate test results. In addition, residual alcohol causes the patient to experience a stinging sensation when the puncture is made. Touching or fanning the area causes contamination, and the cleansing process has to be repeated.
8. **Procedural Step.** Apply gloves. Using a twisting motion, remove the plastic post from the lancet.
   Principle. Gloves provide a barrier precaution against bloodborne pathogens.
9. **Procedural Step.** Without touching the puncture site, firmly grasp the patient's finger in front of the most distal knuckle joint. Apply enough pressure to cause the fingertip to become hard and red. Position the blade of the lancet perpendicular to the lines of the fingerprint on the fleshy portion of the fingertip, slightly to the side of center. This facilitates the formation of a well-formed drop of blood that is easy to collect.
   Principle. The site must be grasped with enough pressure so that adequate penetration and depth of puncture can occur. Punctures that are not perpendicular cause the blood to run down the finger, making it difficult to collect. Puncturing the side or tip of the finger may cause the lancet to penetrate the bone.

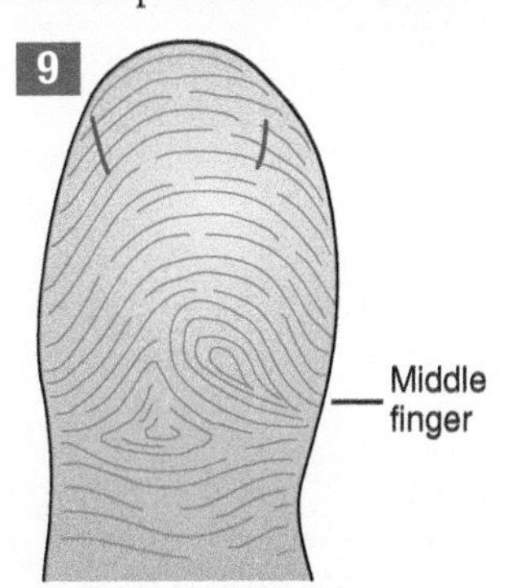

Recommended sites for a finger puncture.

10. **Procedural Step.** Just before making the puncture, tell the patient that he or she will "feel a small stick." Firmly depress the activation button, without moving the lancet or finger, until an audible click is heard. Pressing the activation button causes the lancet to puncture the skin and then retract into its plastic casing. A well-made puncture results in a free-flowing wound that needs only slight pressure to make it bleed.
    Principle. Alerting the patient to the stick prevents startling the patient, which could cause the patient to move. Moving the lancet or finger before the process is complete can result in an inadequate puncture and poor blood flow.

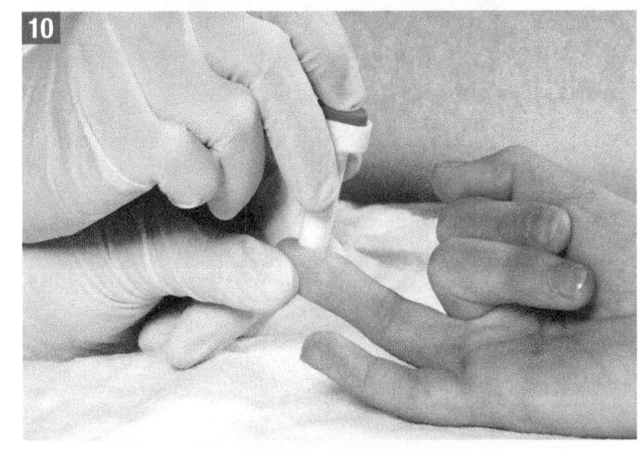

Make the puncture.

11. **Procedural Step.** Immediately dispose of the lancet in a biohazard sharps container.
    Principle. Proper disposal of contaminated sharps is required by the OSHA Standard to prevent exposure to bloodborne pathogens.

Continued

PROCEDURE 17.4

PROCEDURE 17.4 Skin Puncture—Disposable Lancet—cont'd

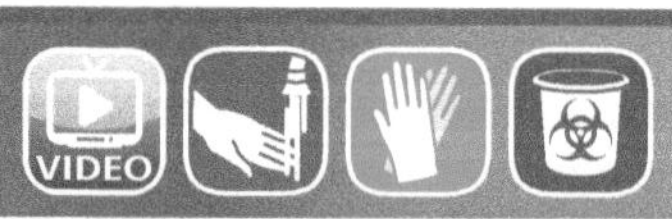

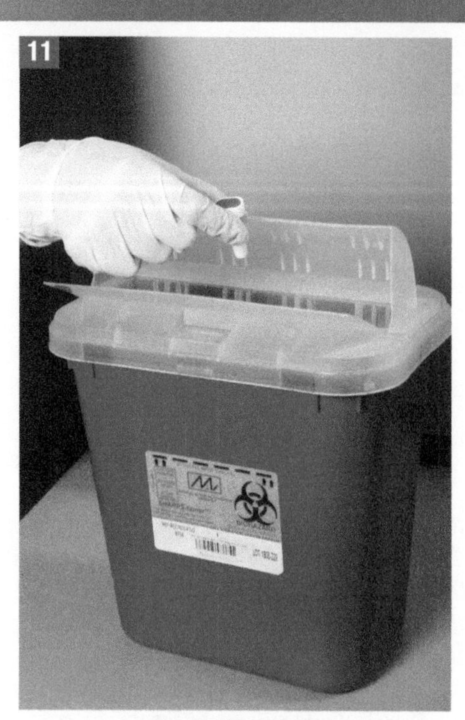

Discard the lancet.

12. Procedural Step. Wait a few seconds to allow blood flow to begin. Wipe away the first drop of blood with a gauze pad.
Principle. The first drop of blood is diluted with alcohol and tissue fluid and is not a suitable specimen.

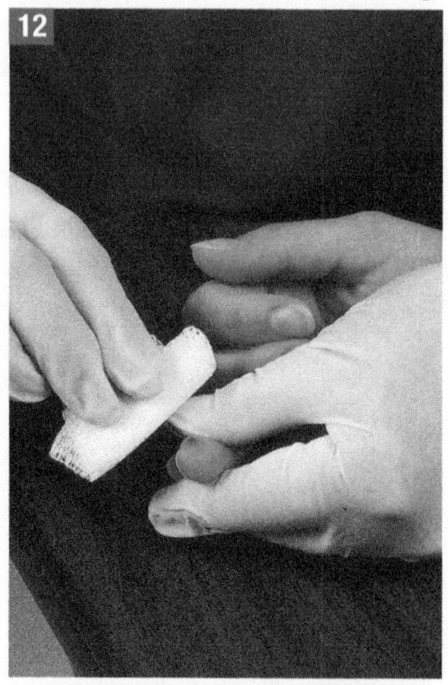

Wipe away the first drop of blood.

13. Procedural Step. Use the second drop of blood for the test. Allow a large well-rounded drop of blood to form by holding the hand in a downward position and applying gentle continuous pressure without squeezing the finger. You can massage the tissue surrounding the puncture firmly but gently to encourage blood flow.
Principle. Squeezing or massaging the site excessively causes dilution of the blood sample with tissue fluid, leading to inaccurate test results.

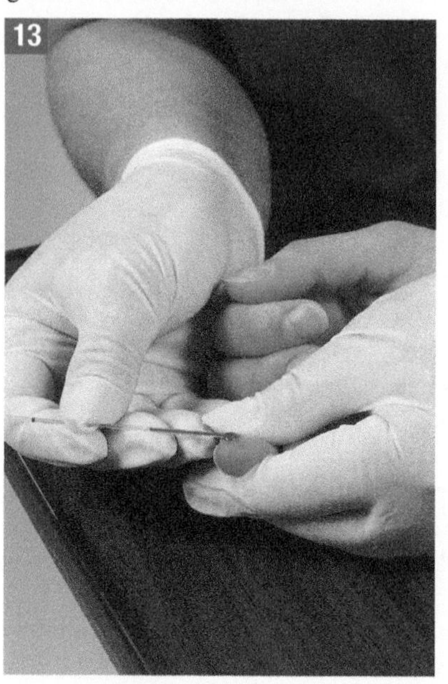

Collect the specimen.

14. **Procedural Step.** Collect the blood specimen on a test strip or in the appropriate microcollection device.
15. **Procedural Step.** Have the patient hold a gauze pad over the puncture and apply pressure until the bleeding stops. As a safety precaution, remain with the patient until the bleeding stops. If needed, apply an adhesive bandage. A bandage is not recommended for children younger than 2 years.
    Principle. A bandage may irritate the skin of a young child, and the child might put the bandage in his or her mouth, aspirate it, and choke.
16. **Procedural Step.** Test the blood specimen by following the manufacturer's instructions that accompany the blood analyzer or test kit.
17. **Procedural Step.** Remove the gloves and sanitize your hands.

Hematology

Check out the Evolve site at http://evolve.elsevier.com/Bonewit/today/ to access additional interactive activities and exercises to help you study and prepare for success.

LEARNING OUTCOMES

Composition and Function of Blood

1. Identify the components of blood.
2. Describe the function of red blood cells (RBCs).
3. Explain the purpose of the biconcave shape of an erythrocyte.
4. Describe the composition of hemoglobin and explain its function.
5. Explain the function of leukocytes.
6. Explain how leukocytes move from the circulatory system and into the tissues.
7. Explain the difference between granulocytes and agranulocytes.
8. Describe the normal appearance of the five types of white blood cells (WBCs).
9. Identify the function of each of the five types of WBCs.

Complete Blood Count

10. List the tests included in a complete blood count (CBC).
11. State the reference range for each test included in a CBC:
12. Identify conditions that can cause an increase or decrease in the hemoglobin level.
13. State the purpose of the hematocrit and list the layers into which the blood separates after it has been centrifuged.
14. Identify conditions that cause an increase or decrease in the RBC count.
15. Identify conditions that cause an increase and decrease of the WBC count.
16. Explain how the RBC indices can help diagnose the various types of anemia.
17. Explain the purpose of the WBC differential count.
18. Explain the difference between an automated and manual WBC differential count.

Coagulation Tests

19. State the purpose of a platelet count.
20. Identify conditions that cause an increase or decrease in the platelet count.
21. State the purpose of the prothrombin time (PT) test.
22. Identify the symptoms of a bleeding disorder.
23. Identify the symptoms of a clotting disorder.
24. Explain why the sodium citrate tube for a PT test must be filled completely.
25. Explain what to do if a winged infusion set is used to collect a PT specimen.
26. Explain why a PT/INR test is performed on patients on long-term warfarin therapy.
27. Identify conditions for which warfarin therapy may be prescribed.
28. List the advantages of prothrombin time home testing.

PROCEDURES

Perform a CLIA-waived hemoglobin test.

Perform a CLIA-waived hematocrit test.

Prepare a blood smear for transport to an outside laboratory.

Collect a specimen for a prothrombin time test for transport to an outside laboratory.

Perform a CLIA-waived prothrombin time test.

CHAPTER OUTLINE

Hemoglobin
Hematocrit
Red Blood Cell Count
White Blood Cell Count

Coagulation Tests
Platelet Count
Prothrombin Time Test
PT/INR Test

KEY TERMS

ameboid movement (ah-MEE-boid-MOVE-ment)
anemia (ah-NEE-mee-ah)
anisocytosis
anticoagulant (an-tih-koe-AG-yoo-lent)
bilirubin (bill-ih-ROO-bin)
diapedesis (die-ah-pah-DEE-sis)
erythrocyte
hematology (hee-mah-TOL-oe-jee)
hematopoiesis
hemoglobin (HEE-moe-gloe-bin)
hemolysis (hee-MOL-oe-sis)
hypochromic (hahy-puh-KROH-mik)
leukocyte
leukocytosis (loo-koe-sie-TOE-sis)
leukopenia (loo-koe-PEE-nee-ah)
macrocytic (mak-ruh-SIT-ik)
microcytic (mahy-kruh-SIT-ik)
morphology
normochromic (NAWR-muh-kroh-mik)
normocytic (NAWR-muh-sahyt-ik)
oxyhemoglobin (ok-see-HEE-moe-gloe-bin)
phagocytosis (fay-goe-sie-TOE-sis)
polycythemia (pol-ee-sie-THEE-mee-ah)
thrombocyte
thrombocytopenia
thrombocytosis

INTRODUCTION TO HEMATOLOGY

Hematology is the study of blood, including the morphologic appearance and function of blood cells and diseases of the blood and blood-forming tissues. Laboratory analysis in hematology is concerned with the testing of a blood specimen for the purpose of detecting pathologic conditions. It includes performing blood cell counts, evaluating the clotting ability of the blood, and identifying blood cell types. These tests are valuable tools that allow the provider to determine whether each blood component falls within its reference range.

Examples of hematologic tests that are frequently ordered on patients include:

- Red blood cell (RBC) count
- White blood cell (WBC) count
- Hemoglobin
- Hematocrit
- WBC differential count
- Platelet count
- Erythrocyte sedimentation rate
- Prothrombin time

Several of these hematologic tests may be performed in the medical office using CLIA-waived instruments. Each CLIA-waived instrument is accompanied by a detailed operating manual that explains its operation, test parameters, care, and maintenance. CLIA-waived instruments permit testing of the specimen in a short time with accurate and reliable test results. This allows the provider to evaluate the test results while the patient is still at the medical office without a delay in waiting for test results to be transmitted from an outside laboratory.

This chapter presents information on hematology including the components and function of blood with an emphasis on CLIA-waived testing in the medical office.

COMPOSITION AND FUNCTION OF BLOOD

The average adult body contains 10 to 12 pints (5 to 6 L) of blood which makes up about 8% of the total body weight. Blood consists of two parts—*plasma* and *formed elements* (Fig. 18.1). Plasma, the liquid part of the blood, consists of a clear yellowish fluid that makes up approximately 55% of the total blood volume. Most of the plasma (90%) is made up of water and the remaining 10% consists of solutes such as plasma proteins (albumin, globulins, and fibrinogen). Plasma transports nutrients to the tissues of the body to nourish and sustain them. Plasma picks up wastes from the tissues which are then eliminated through the kidneys. The plasma also transports antibodies, enzymes, and hormones to help regulate normal body functioning.

The formed elements consist of three types of cells: erythrocytes, leukocytes, and thrombocytes. The formed elements make up approximately 45% of the total blood volume. The formed elements are produced in the red bone marrow and the process of blood cell formation is known as **hematopoiesis.** All blood cells are derived from *hematopoietic stem* cells that are able to differentiate into the various types of blood cells in the bone marrow. Hematopoietic stem cells are responsible for the constant renewal of blood cells in the body. Each day the bone marrow produces more than 200 billion new blood cells.

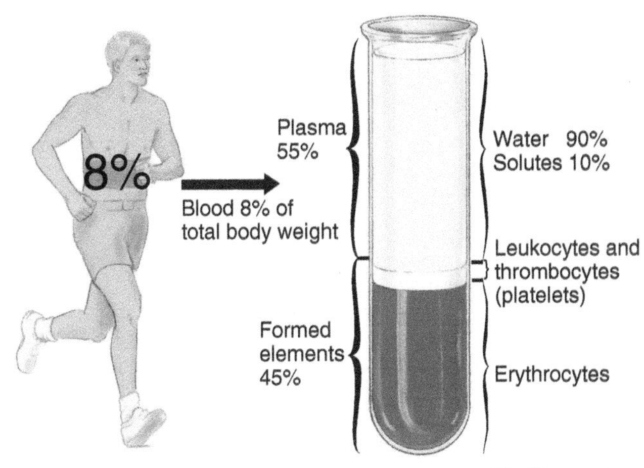

Fig. 18.1 Composition of blood. (From Applegate EJ: *The anatomy and physiology learning system*, ed 4, St Louis: Elsevier; 2011.)

RED BLOOD CELLS

RBCs, or **erythrocytes,** are the most numerous blood cells in the circulating blood. An erythrocyte is approximately 7 to 8 μm in diameter. The primary function of RBCs is transporting oxygen and carbon dioxide in the body (which is directly related to hemoglobin). The number of RBCs in a healthy adult ranges from 4 to 5.5 million per cubic millimeter of blood in a woman, and from 4.5 to 6.2 million per cubic millimeter of blood in a man.

In an adult, erythrocytes are produced in the red bone marrow of the ribs, sternum, skull, and pelvic bone and the ends of the long bones of the limbs. The immature form of an erythrocyte contains a nucleus. As the cell develops and matures, however, it loses its nucleus and acquires the shape of a biconcave disc, thin in the middle and thicker around the rim. This shape provides the erythrocyte with a greater surface area for the exchange of gases (oxygen and carbon dioxide) between the blood and tissues. The shape of the erythrocyte also provides the cell with the flexibility to bend and squeeze through tiny capillaries.

A major portion of the erythrocyte consists of hemoglobin. **Hemoglobin** is a complex compound that carries oxygen to the tissues and is responsible for the red color of the erythrocyte. The amount of hemoglobin in the blood averages 12 to 16 g/dL for a female and 14 to 18 g/dL for a male. A decrease in the number of erythrocytes or amount of hemoglobin in the blood is known as **anemia** and an increase in the number of erythrocytes or amount of hemoglobin is known as **polycythemia.**

A hemoglobin molecule consists of a globin or protein, and an iron-containing pigment called *heme.* One hemoglobin molecule loosely combines with four oxygen molecules in the lungs to form a substance called **oxyhemoglobin.** Oxyhemoglobin is transported by the circulatory system and distributed to the tissues, where oxygen is easily released from the hemoglobin. The blood then picks up carbon dioxide (a waste product) from the tissues and transports it back to the lungs to be expelled. When oxygen combines with hemoglobin, a bright red color results characteristic of arterial blood. Venous blood is darker red owing to its lower oxygen content.

The average life span of a RBC is 120 days. Toward the end of this time, the membrane of the RBC becomes more and more fragile and eventually ruptures and breaks down; this process is known as **hemolysis.** Hemolyzed RBCs are replaced by an equal number of new RBCs. Under typical conditions, more than 2 million RBCs are destroyed and replaced every second. Hemoglobin molecules are liberated from the breakdown of RBCs. The molecules release iron which is stored and then later reused to make new hemoglobin molecules. **Bilirubin** is an orange-colored bile pigment that is a by-product of heme destruction from the hemoglobin molecule. It is transported to the liver, where it is excreted as a waste product into the bile and then it eventually leaves the body in the stool.

WHITE BLOOD CELLS

WBCs, or **leukocytes,** are clear, colorless cells that contain a nucleus. They make up 1% of the total blood volume making them much less numerous than erythrocytes. The number of leukocytes in a healthy adult ranges from 4500 to 11,000 per cubic millimeter of blood. **Leukocytosis** is the condition of having an abnormal increase in the number of leukocytes ($>11,000/mm^3$), and **leukopenia** is the condition of having an abnormal decrease in the number of leukocytes ($<4500/mm^3$).

The function of leukocytes is to defend the body against infection and foreign materials. The bone marrow stores an estimated 80% to 90% of the WBCs. When an infection or inflammatory response occurs, the bone marrow releases WBCs to fight the infection.

Pathogens can gain entrance into the body in a variety of ways (review the infection process cycle in Chapter 2). Leukocytes attempt to destroy invading pathogens and remove them from the body. In contrast to erythrocytes, leukocytes do their work in the tissues; they are transported to the site of infection by the circulatory system.

During inflammation, the capillaries in the infected area dilate, resulting in an increased blood supply. More oxygen, nutrients, and WBCs can be delivered to the infected area to aid in the healing process. The cells in the capillary walls spread apart, enlarging the pores between the cells. WBCs squeeze through these pores by **ameboid movement** and move out into the tissues to fight the infection. This movement of the leukocytes through the pores of the capillaries and out into the tissues is known as **diapedesis.**

TYPES OF WHITE BLOOD CELLS

There are five types of WBCs, or leukocytes, each having a certain size, shape, appearance, and function (Fig. 18.2).

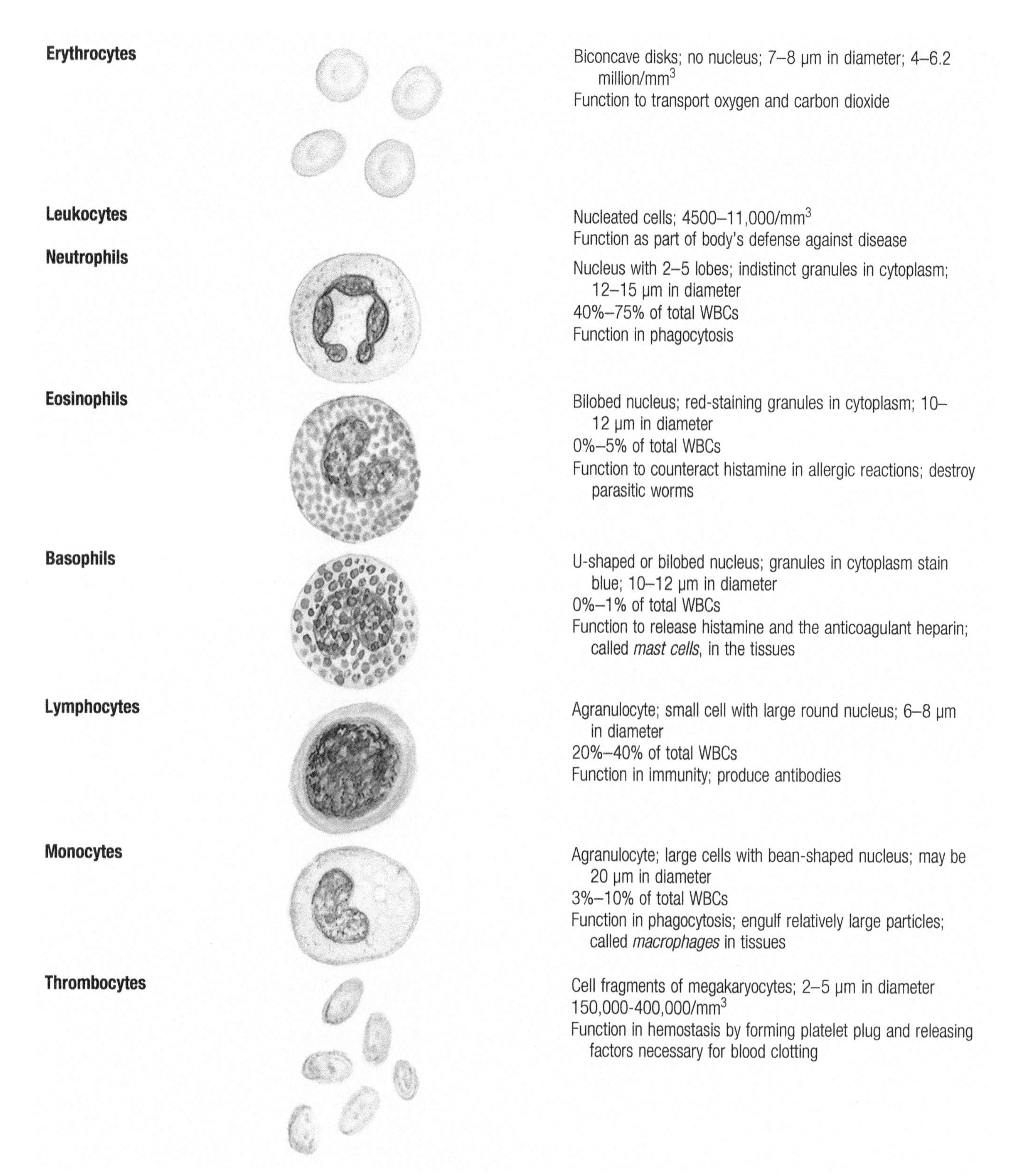

Fig. 18.2 Types of blood cells. (From Applegate EJ: *The anatomy and physiology learning system*, ed 4, St Louis: Elsevier; 2011.)

Leukocytes are classified into two major categories—granulocytes and agranulocytes.

Granulocytes have a multilobed nucleus and contain distinct granules in the cytoplasm; they include neutrophils, eosinophils, and basophils. The granules contain enzymes that damage and digest pathogens; these enzymes also trigger the inflammatory response. The *inflammatory response* is a protective response of the body to the entrance of pathogens into the body. The purpose of inflammation is to destroy invading pathogens and to remove damaged tissue debris from the area so that proper healing can occur. Symptoms of inflammation include pain, swelling, redness, and warmth at the infection site. *Agranulocytes* have a single round nucleus and contain few or no granules in the cytoplasm; they include lymphocytes and monocytes. They play an important role in the immune system such as the production of antibodies.

Leukocytes (especially granulocytes) are phagocytic, and when they arrive at the site of infection, they begin the process of phagocytosis. **Phagocytosis** is the engulfing and destruction of foreign particles such as pathogens and damaged cells. In some conditions, pus forms in the infected area; pus contains dead leukocytes, dead bacteria, and dead tissue cells.

Each type of leukocyte has a specific function in defending the body against infection which is described as follows.

Neutrophils

Neutrophils are the most numerous of the WBCs and are also known as "segs" because of their segmented nucleus. Neutrophils defend the body against bacterial and fungal infections and are the first type of WBC to respond to an invader. Because of this, they are considered the body's first line of defense against infection. Neutrophils also send out signals to alert other WBCs to respond to the infection. They exhibit a high degree of ameboid movement allowing them to move from the circulatory system to the site of the infection. Neutrophils engulf and destroy invaders through phagocytosis. The granules in neutrophils contain lysosomes which then digests the invaders. Neutrophils do not live very long. After digesting several invaders, the neutrophil can no longer survive and dies.

Immature forms of neutrophils known as *bands* can be identified by their curved, nonsegmented nuclei. Normally, 0% to 5% of the neutrophils present are in the immature band form. When the percentage of band forms increases, this condition is referred to as a "shift to the left." An increase in the number of neutrophils, including band forms, is usually seen during an acute bacterial infection.

Eosinophils

Eosinophils are not seen very often in the circulating blood but are numerous in the connective tissue of the stomach and intestines. Eosinophils function as part of the allergic response by counteracting the effect of histamine in an allergic reaction. Eosinophils also play an important role in responding to parasitic infections by secreting a chemical that destroys parasitic worms, such as hookworms and tapeworms. An increase in eosinophils is often seen in allergic reactions and parasitic infestations. Eosinophils also play a role in the inflammatory response of the body.

Basophils

Basophils are the least numerous of the WBCs and are about the same size as eosinophils. The granules in basophils release histamine and heparin into the tissues. Histamine dilates capillaries in the infected area which increases the flow of blood to the damaged tissue. This allows more oxygen, nutrients, and WBCs to be delivered to the infected area to aid in the healing process. Histamine also makes capillaries more permeable, allowing WBCs to squeeze through the pores of the capillaries (diapedesis) to fight infection in the tissues. The heparin released by basophils inhibits blood clotting to facilitate the movement of WBCs into the infected area.

Lymphocytes

Lymphocytes are the smallest WBCs. They function in immunity by producing antibodies to destroy foreign invaders. An increase in lymphocytes generally occurs with certain viral diseases, including infectious mononucleosis, mumps, chickenpox, rubella, and viral hepatitis. Lymphocytes can be classified as B cells, T cells, and natural killer cells. *B cells* produce and secrete antibodies to help the immune system mount a response to infection. *T cells* search out and destroy targeted cells. *Natural killer cells* are responsible for attacking and killing viral cells, as well as cancer cells.

Monocytes

Monocytes are the largest WBCs and live longer than neutrophils. They are considered the body's second line of defense against infection. Monocytes migrate from the circulatory system to the site of the infection and differentiate into *macrophages*. Macrophages function as "scavengers" to clean up the infection site through phagocytosis by engulfing dead tissue cells, dead neutrophils, and any remaining pathogens which eventually become pus.

PLATELETS

Platelets, also known as **thrombocytes,** are tiny irregularly shaped cell fragments. They lack a nucleus and are formed in the red bone marrow from giant cells known as *megakaryocytes*. The number of platelets in a healthy adult ranges from 150,000 to 400,000 per cubic millimeter of blood. An increase in the number of platelets is known as **thrombocytosis** and a decrease in the number of platelets is known as **thrombocytopenia.**

Platelets function by participating in the blood-clotting mechanism in the body. When the lining of a blood vessel breaks, platelets accumulate at the site of the injury and become sticky. This stickiness causes them to attach to one another as well as to the blood vessel wall. This results in a *platelet plug* that seals the opening in the blood vessel wall and stops the flow of blood. A fibrin network forms next which attaches to the platelet plug to hold it in place and to trap more platelets as well as RBCs. This results in the platelet plug becoming harder and more durable. The platelet plug is now known as a *thrombus* or blood clot (Fig. 18.3). The blood clot eventually becomes the scab and remains in place until the wound heals.

Platelets survive in the circulatory system for approximately 8 to 10 days. The bone marrow must continuously produce new platelets that break down, are used up during the clotting process, or are lost through bleeding.

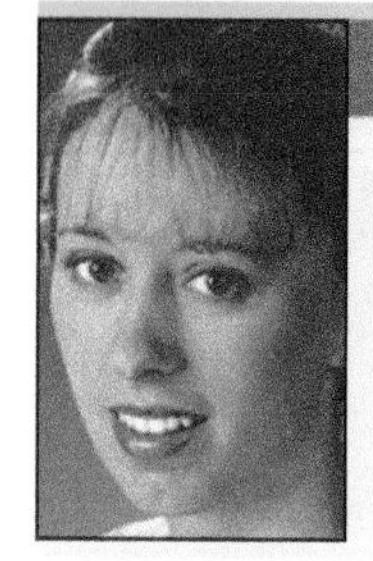

Putting It All Into Practice

My name is Latisha, and I work in a multi-physician office as a laboratory technician in our POL. I have worked in this office for 3 years and I really enjoy my job. My responsibilities mostly include venipuncture, preparing blood specimens for pickup by the lab courier, and performing CLIA-waived laboratory tests. One day, a frail older lady came in who had just been diagnosed with atrial fibrillation and was placed on Coumadin therapy. I needed to draw a blood specimen on her for a PT/INR test—a procedure I had done many times before. I looked up information on the test in the laboratory test directory. I next checked the veins in the lady's arms and couldn't find any veins that could be used. I knew that I would have to draw the blood from her hand and I really hated to do that to her because I know that a stick can hurt a lot more in the hand. I got out a blue-topped tube and the butterfly setup. I was just about ready to make the stick when I suddenly realized that I first needed to draw a discard tube with a butterfly setup. I broke into a sweat thinking of what could have happened if I had forgotten the discarded tube. I would have had stuck that sweet lady's hand again causing her more pain. To this day, I always read the information in the test directory more than one time. ■

COMPLETE BLOOD COUNT

The most frequently performed hematologic laboratory test is the complete blood count (CBC). A CBC includes a group of tests that determine the number of RBCs, WBCs and platelets in the circulatory system along with a determination of the hemoglobin and hematocrit levels.

A CBC is used as a screening test to assess the overall health of an individual and to detect a wide range of hematologic conditions such as anemia, leukemia, infection, bleeding disorders, and inflammation. The CBC is also used to monitor patients undergoing chemotherapy or radiation therapy for cancer because these treatments suppress the production of blood cells in the bone marrow. Test results from a CBC provide valuable information to assist the provider in making a diagnosis, evaluating the patient's progress, and regulating treatment. The tests included in a CBC and the reference range for each test are summarized in Table 18.1.

A CBC is usually performed by an outside laboratory since many of the tests included in a CBC are moderate complexity tests. Guidelines for collecting a specimen for a CBC to be transported to an outside laboratory are presented below.

There are two tests included in a CBC that can be performed using CLIA-waived equipment: these tests include hemoglobin and hematocrit. These tests are presented first in this section followed by the moderate complexity tests included in a CBC (WBC, RBC, platelet count, WBC differential count, and the RBC indices).

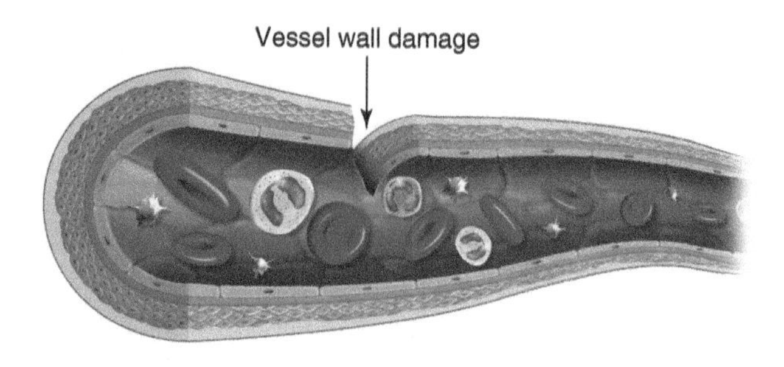

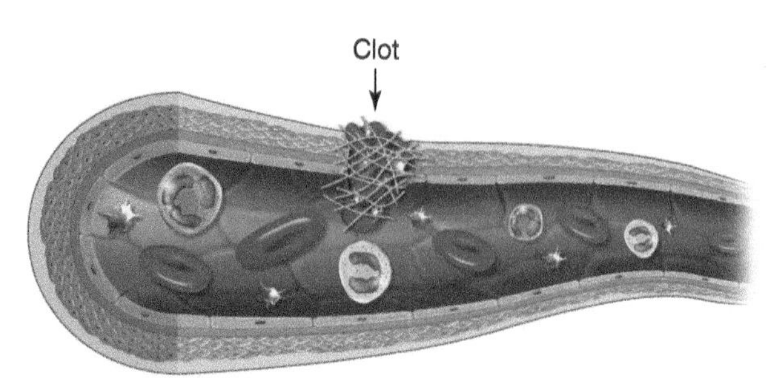

Fig. 18.3 Blood clotting. (From Yoost B, Crawford L: *Fundamentals of nursing: active learning for collaborative practice*, ed 2, St Louis: Elsevier; 2020.)

SPECIMEN COLLECTION FOR A COMPLETE BLOOD COUNT

The medical assistant is often required to collect a blood specimen for a CBC for transport to an outside laboratory for testing. The guidelines listed below should be followed when collecting the specimen:

1. Collect the blood specimen in a lavender closure tube. A whole blood specimen is required for a CBC.
2. Completely fill the collection tube to the exhaustion of the vacuum to ensure a proper blood-to-anticoagulant ratio.
3. Gently invert the tube 8 to 10 times following collection to mix the anticoagulant with the blood. This prevents the formation of blood clots which can affect the accuracy of the test results.
4. Store the specimen at room temperature (RT) while awaiting pickup by a laboratory courier. The specimen is stable for 48 hours at RT. The specimen should not be refrigerated because refrigeration can precipitate the formation of a fibrin clot which traps WBCs and platelets affecting the accuracy of the test results.

After testing the specimen, the outside laboratory transmits the results to the medical office. An example of a computer-generated laboratory report indicating the results of a CBC is presented in Fig. 18.4.

HEMOGLOBIN

As previously discussed, hemoglobin (Hgb) is a major component of an RBC. It carries oxygen to the tissues of the body and is responsible for the red color of the erythrocyte. A Hgb determination is a measurement of the Hgb

Table 18.1 Complete Blood Count Purpose and Reference Ranges

COMPLETE BLOOD COUNT			
Test	**Purpose**	**Reference Range**	**Units**
RBC Count	Measurement of the number of RBCs in the circulating blood	F: 4–5.5 M: 4.5–6.2	$\times 10^6/mm^3$
WBC Count	Measurement of the number of WBCs in the circulating blood.	4.5–11.0	$\times 10^3/mm^3$
Hemoglobin	Measurement of the hemoglobin level to assess the oxygen-carrying capacity of the blood	F: 12–16 M: 14–18	g/dL
Hematocrit	To measure the percentage by volume of the packed RBCs in whole blood.	F: 37–47 M: 40–54	%
Platelet Count	Measurement of the number of platelets in the circulating blood to assess the clotting ability of the blood	150–400	$\times 10^3/mm^3$
RED BLOOD CELL INDICES			
Test	**Purpose**	**Reference Range**	**Units**
MCV	Measurement of the average size of an RBC	80–100	f/L
MCH	Measurement of the average amount of hemoglobin in an RBC	27–31	pg
MCHC	Measurement of the average concentration of hemoglobin within an RBC	32–36	mg/dL
RDW	Measurement of any variation in size of the RBCs	11.5–14.5	%
WHITE BLOOD CELL DIFFERENTIAL COUNT			
Cell Type	**Function**	**Reference Range**	**Unit**
Neutrophils	Destruction of invaders through phagocytosis	40–75	%
Eosinophils	Destruction of parasitic worms Counteracts the effects of histamine in an allergic reaction	0–5	%
Basophils	Release of histamine and heparin	0–1	%
Lymphocytes	Production of antibodies to destroy foreign invaders	20–40	%
Monocytes	Clean up the infection site through phagocytosis	3–10	%

MCH, Mean corpuscular hemoglobin; *MCHC,* mean cell hemoglobin concentration; *MCV,* mean corpuscular volume; *RBC,* red blood cell; *RDW,* red cell distribution width; *WBC,* white blood cell.

level in the body to assess the oxygen-carrying capacity of the blood. A Hgb test is used to screen for anemia, determine its severity, and monitor the response to treatment. The reference range for Hgb for a healthy woman is 12 to 16 g/dL and the reference range for a healthy man is 14 to 18 g/dL.

A decreased Hgb level reduces the oxygen-carrying capacity of the blood. This can occur with anemia (especially iron-deficiency anemia), hyperthyroidism, cirrhosis of the liver, severe hemorrhaging, hemolytic reactions, and certain systemic diseases, such as leukemia and Hodgkin's disease. Increased levels of Hgb are present with chronic obstructive pulmonary disease, and congestive heart failure.

CLIA-Waived Hemoglobin Test

A CLIA-waived Hgb test is often performed in the medical office as a routine screening test on individuals who are at risk for developing iron-deficiency anemia, such as children younger than 2 years, adolescent girls, and pregnant women; all of whom have an increased demand for iron in the body. The Hgb test is a quantitative test that measures the specific amount of Hgb present in the body with the results being reported in grams per deciliter (g/dL).

There are several advantages of using a CLIA-waived Hgb analyzer. The analyzer only requires a capillary specimen collected through a finger or heel puncture to perform the test, rather than a venous blood specimen collected through venipuncture. The Hgb analyzer permits testing of the specimen in a short time with accurate and reliable results, allowing the provider to evaluate the patient while still at the medical office.

The manufacturer of the Hgb analyzer provides an operating manual that includes information needed to perform quality control procedures, collect the specimen, test the specimen, and properly store the test devices (e.g., microcuvettes or testing cards) and control reagents. It is important that the medical assistant become familiar with all aspects of the Hgb analyzer. Quality control procedures are of particular importance to ensure that the analyzer is functioning properly and that test results are reliable and accurate. Examples of CLIA-waived Hgb analyzers include the HemoPoint H2 Meter (Stanbio Laboratory, Boerne, TX), Hgb Hb 201+ Analyzer (HemoCue, Lake Forest, CA).

Laboratory Report Complete Blood Count with Diff/Platelets			
PATIENT		ORDERED BY	RESULTS PROVIDED BY
Yang, Hu 2963 Flint Dr. Clearwater, FL 33759 PH: 740-541-3575	ID #: 336879 DOB: 4/28/1970 AGE: 53 GENDER: M	Thomas Murphy, MD Pinellas Medical Office 3477 Arrowhead Ave Clearwater, FL 33759	Medical Center Laboratory 33 West Main St Clearwater, FL 33759
SPECIMEN COLL. DATE	11/25/20XX	FASTING/NONFASTING	Nonfasting
SPECIMEN COLL. TIME	02:53 pm	ACCESSION NUMBER	3380837
SPECIMEN RECEIVED DATE/TIME	11/25/20XX 05:30 pm	LAB ID NUMBER	773978
RESULTS REPORTED DATE/TIME	11/26/20XX 10:00 am	TEST(S) ORDERED	CPT: 85025 CBC with Diff/Platelets

TEST	RESULT	REFERENCE RANGE	UNITS	FLAG
RBC	**3.57**	**4.5-6.2**	**$\times10^6$/mm^3**	**L**
WBC	4.6	4.5-11.0	$\times10^3$/mm^3	
Hemoglobin	**12.2**	**14.0-18.0**	**g/dL**	**L**
Hematocrit	**35.6**	**40.0-54.0**	**%**	**L**
MCV	92	80-100	f/L	
MCH	31.4	27.0-31.0	pg	
MCHC	34	32.0-36.0	mg/dL	
RDW	**17.6**	**11.5-14.5**	**%**	**H**
Platelets	308	150-400	$\times10^3$/mm^3	
Neutrophils	73	40-75	%	
Eosinophils	1	0%-5%	%	
Basophils	1	0%-1%	%	
Lymphoytes	14	20-40	%	
Monocytes	11	3-10	%	

Fig. 18.4 Complete blood cell laboratory report (computer-generated).

Procedure for the CLIA-Waived Hemoglobin Hb 201+ Analyzer

The medical assistant must follow the Hgb collection and testing procedure *exactly* as presented in the operating manual. An overview of the procedure for performing a CLIA-waived Hgb test using the Hgb Hb 201+ Analyzer is outlined here:

1. Pull out the cuvette tray from the front of the analyzer.
2. Perform a finger puncture to obtain a capillary blood specimen and wipe away the first 2 or 3 drops of blood.
3. Touch the open end of the microcuvette to the drop of blood and fill the microcuvette in one continuous process (Fig. 18.5).
4. Wipe off excess blood from the outside of the microcuvette and place it in the cuvette holder on the analyzer (Fig. 18.6).
5. When three dashes appear on the liquid crystal display (LCD) screen of the analyzer, push the tray back into the analyzer.
6. After a countdown, the Hgb test result is displayed on the LCD screen of the analyzer. The Hgb result for this test is 14.2 g/dL which is a normal result for both a male and a female (Fig. 18.7).
7. Document the results in the patient's medical record, including the date and time, the name of the test (Hgb), and the test result measured in g/dL.

HEMATOCRIT

The hematocrit (Hct) is a simple, reliable, and informative test that is frequently performed in the medical office. The word *Hct* means "to separate blood." The formed elements

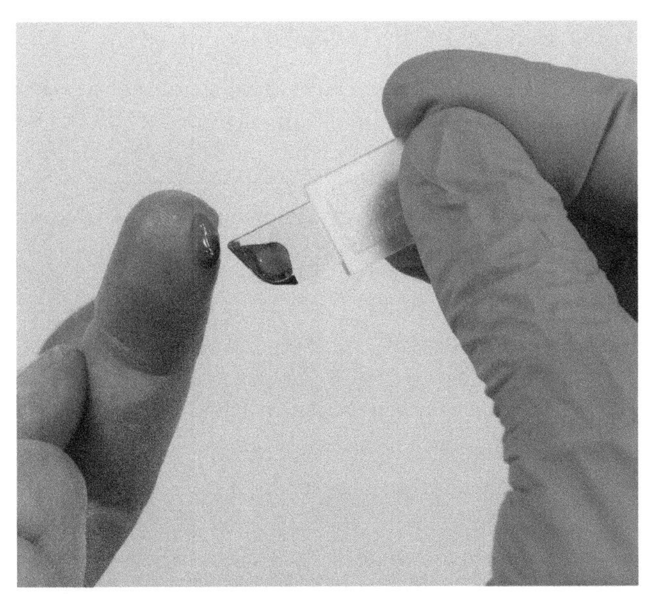

Fig. 18.5 The microcuvette is filled with blood. (From Garrels M: *Laboratory and diagnostic testing in ambulatory care*, ed 4, St Louis: Elsevier; 2019.)

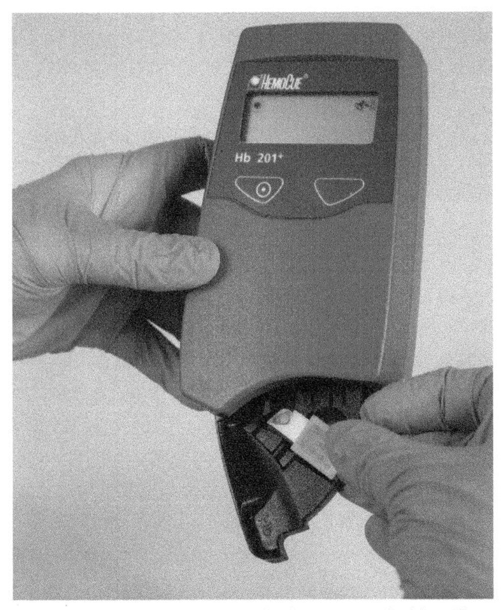

Fig. 18.6 Place the microcuvette in the cuvette holder. (From Garrels M: *Laboratory and diagnostic testing in ambulatory care*, ed 4, St Louis: Elsevier; 2019.)

are separated from the plasma by centrifuging an anticoagulated blood specimen. The heavier RBCs become packed and settle to the bottom of a tube. The top layer contains the clear, straw-colored plasma. Between the plasma and the packed RBCs is a small, thin, yellowish-gray layer known as the *buffy coat,* which contains the platelets and WBCs (Fig. 18.8).

The purpose of the Hct is to measure the percentage by volume of packed RBCs in whole blood. The Hct is used as a screening measure for the early detection of anemia and is often included as part of a general health examination. The Hct reference range for a healthy woman is 37% to 47% and the reference range for a healthy man is 40% to 54%. A low Hct reading may indicate anemia, and a high reading may indicate polycythemia.

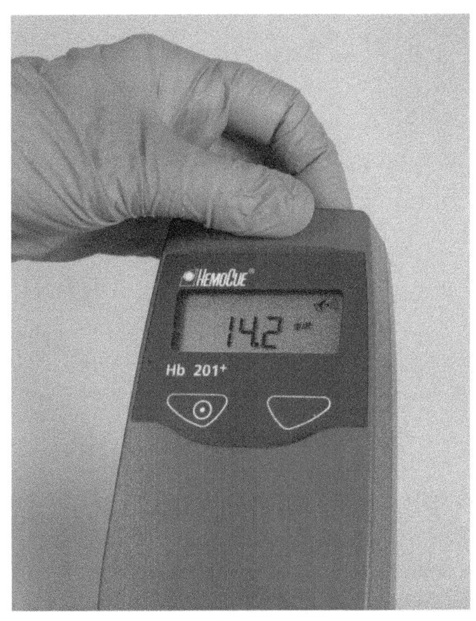

Fig. 18.7 Test results are displayed on the LCD screen. (From Garrels M: *Laboratory and diagnostic testing in ambulatory care*, ed 4, St Louis: Elsevier; 2019.)

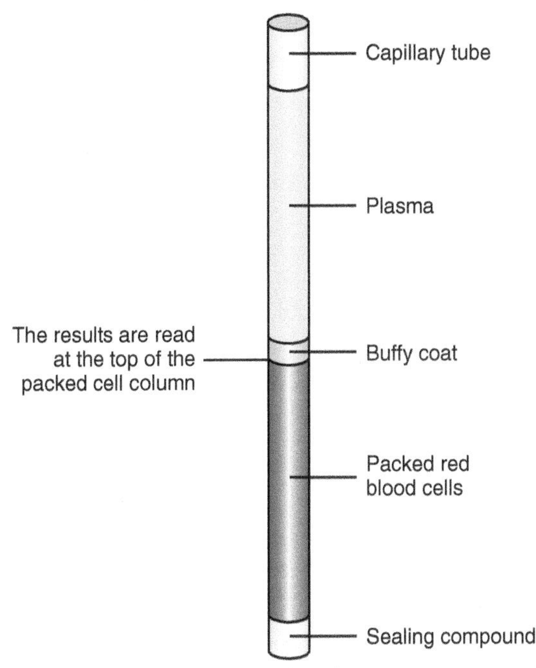

Fig. 18.8 Hematocrit test results. The blood cells are separated from the plasma by centrifuging an anticoagulated blood specimen, and the results are read at the top of the packed cell column.

CLIA-Waived Hematocrit Test

The CLIA-waived *microhematocrit method* is used in the medical office to perform a Hct determination. Through capillary action, blood is drawn directly from a free-flowing skin puncture into a disposable capillary tube. After the specimen has been collected, one end of the capillary tube is sealed with a sealing compound and placed in a microhematocrit centrifuge. The centrifuge spins the blood at an extremely high speed for 3 to 5 minutes to pack the RBCs at the bottom of the tube. The results are read at the top of the packed cell column. Procedure 18.1 describes how to perform a Hct test.

What Would You Do? What Would You *Not* Do?

Case Study 1

Theodore Pascal is at the office for a general health examination. The physician orders a CBC and CMP (comprehensive metabolic panel) on Theodore. Theodore says he has been feeling fine and wants to know why lab tests have been ordered for him. When Theodore realizes that the tests require a venipuncture, he says that he gets nervous about having blood drawn and wants to know if a finger stick could be done instead so it will not hurt so much. He also wants to know why two tubes of blood have to be drawn from him and why one tube of blood can't be used for the tests. ■

RED BLOOD CELL COUNT

The RBC count is a measurement of the number of RBCs in the circulating blood. The reference range for the RBC count in a healthy woman is 4 to 5.5 million RBCs per cubic millimeter of blood, expressed in laboratory reports as 4 to 5.5 ($\times 10^6/mm^3$). The reference range for a healthy man is 4.5 to 6.2 million RBCs per cubic millimeter of blood, expressed in a laboratory report as 4.5 to 6.2 ($\times 10^6/mm^3$). In the medical office, the RBC is performed using a nonwaived blood cell counter.

A decrease in the RBC count can be caused by blood loss, production of defective red RBCs, decreased production of RBCs and increased destruction of RBCs. An increase in

PATIENT COACHING Iron-Deficiency Anemia

Answer questions that patients have about iron-deficiency anemia.

What is anemia?

Anemia is a decrease in the number of RBCs or the amount Hgb in the body. Hgb, the part of the blood that gives RBCs their red color, carries oxygen to all the cells in the body. There are many types of anemia, of which iron-deficiency anemia is the most common. Other types of anemia include pernicious anemia, sickle cell anemia, hemolytic anemia, and aplastic anemia.

What causes iron-deficiency anemia?

In general, iron-deficiency anemia is caused by conditions that deplete the iron stored in the body; it can result from an increased need for iron by the body or an increased loss of iron from the body. Iron-deficiency anemia may occur in children younger than 2 years if their diet does not include enough iron to meet the demands of rapid growth. This is especially true in children whose main source of nutrition during these years is breast milk or bottled milk, because milk contains very little iron. Adolescent girls are prone to iron-deficiency anemia because of growth spurts during puberty and blood loss through menstruation. Pregnant women also are at increased risk because of the demands of the growing fetus. In adults, the most common cause of anemia is chronic blood loss, such as from a bleeding ulcer or bleeding hemorrhoids and heavy menstrual bleeding.

What can be done for individuals at risk for iron-deficiency anemia?

Individuals prone to developing iron-deficiency anemia are encouraged to increase foods in their diet that contain iron such as beef, liver, spinach, eggs, and iron-fortified bread and cereals. As a preventive measure, the provider usually prescribes vitamin supplements containing iron for individuals who are at increased risk for developing iron-deficiency anemia, such as pregnant women, infants, and young children. Infant formulas and cereals that have been supplemented with iron are also available.

What are the symptoms of anemia?

All types of anemia have the same general symptoms. Often these symptoms do not develop right away; when they do develop, feeling tired and run down may be the only sign of anemia. Other symptoms that may occur, particularly as the anemia becomes worse, are paleness of the skin, fingernail beds, and mucous membranes; shortness of breath, especially during physical activity; dizziness; headache; irritability; and inability to concentrate. These symptoms result from the diminished ability of the blood to carry oxygen to the cells of the body. Blood tests are necessary to diagnose anemia and to determine the specific type of anemia present.

How is iron-deficiency anemia treated?

The most important part of treating anemia is to determine its cause, such as not enough iron consumed in the diet or chronic blood loss, and to correct that condition. The provider usually prescribes an iron supplement to replace the iron that has been depleted from the body. It is typically prescribed in oral form, but it is given through an injection if the patient cannot take iron by mouth because of the side effects. Iron may also be given through an injection if the iron content in the blood is so low that oral supplements would be too slow in increasing the iron level. An oral iron supplement causes the stool to turn a black, tarlike color. This is normal and should not be a cause for concern. Also, an effort should be made to consume foods high in iron content.

- For patients who have had a vitamin supplement prescribed to *prevent* iron-deficiency anemia, such as children younger than 2 years and pregnant women, emphasize to the patient (or parent) the importance of taking the vitamin supplement every day to prevent the development of iron-deficiency anemia.
- For patients who have had an iron supplement prescribed to *treat* iron-deficiency anemia, emphasize to the patient the importance of taking the iron supplement for the period of time prescribed by the provider, because replacement of iron takes time.
- Explain to patients that there are some side effects that may occur when taking oral iron which include stomach upset and pain, constipation or diarrhea, nausea, and vomiting. Explain that taking an iron supplement with food may reduce some of these side effects.
- Instruct patients to keep iron supplements out of the reach of children to prevent iron poisoning.
- Provide patients with written educational materials on iron-deficiency anemia. ■

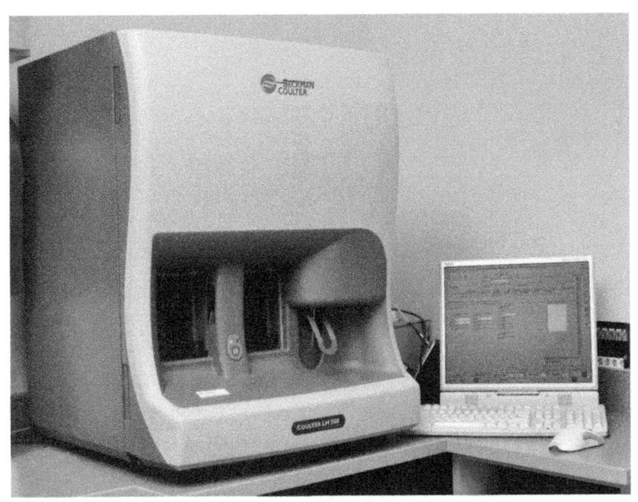

Fig. 18.9 Coulter blood cell counter. (Courtesy of Holzer Health Systems, Athens, OH.)

the RBC count can be caused by the production of RBCs to compensate for chronically low oxygen levels in conditions such as lung or heart disease.

An RBC count is a moderate complexity test and is performed on an automated (nonwaived) blood cell counter. Blood cell counters are also able to perform a WBC count, platelet count, Hgb, Hct, and WBC differential count, as well as a calculation of the RBC indices. Examples of nonwaived blood cell counters include the QBC Autoread Plus (Becton, Dickinson), the Cell-Dyn (Abbott, Santa Clara, CA), and the Beckman Coulter Counter (Beckman Coulter, Brea, CA) (Fig. 18.9).

Red Blood Cell Indices

The RBC indices help to determine the cause of anemia. They are measurements that are reported as part of the CBC. RBC indices provide information about the size and Hgb content of a patient's RBCs. The RBC indices include the MCV (mean corpuscular volume), MCH (mean corpuscular hemoglobin), MCHC (mean cell hemoglobin concentration), and RDW (red cell distribution width). Most of the RBC indices are obtained from calculations performed on certain test results included in a CBC—specifically, the RBC count, Hgb, and Hct. The calculation is automatically performed by the automated blood cell analyzer that performs the CBC. Refer to Table 18.1 for the purpose and reference ranges of the red blood cell indices.

More than 400 types of anemia have been identified, but many of them are rare conditions. Each of the various forms of anemia (e.g., iron-deficiency anemia, pernicious anemia) may alter one or more of the RBC indices in a particular way. This information is used by the provider to assist in the diagnosis of the type of anemia a patient has and in the determination of its cause.

Mean Corpuscular Volume

The MCV is a measurement of the average size of a single RBC. The MCV is the index used most often to assist in the diagnosis of a particular type of anemia. The MCV results are expressed in femtoliters (fL). The MCV reference range for a normal-sized RBC is 80 to 100 fL, and the cell is described as being **normocytic.**

An MCV result below 80 means that the patient's RBCs are smaller than normal and are described as being **microcytic.** The most common cause of microcytic anemia (low MCV) is a lack of iron in the diet, known as iron-deficiency anemia. Microcytic anemia may also be due to *thalassemia,* which is a hereditary type of anemia. An MCV result greater than 100 fL means that the cells are larger than normal, or **macrocytic.** The most common causes of macrocytic anemia (high MCV) are a folic acid deficiency and a lack of vitamin B_{12} in the body, known as *pernicious anemia.*

Mean Corpuscular Hemoglobin

The MCH measures the average amount of Hgb within a RBC. The results are expressed in pictograms (pg). The reference range for an MCH is 27 to 31 pg. The cause of MCH values outside of the reference range are the same as those for MCV values outside of the reference range. For example, iron-deficiency anemia is associated with both a decreased MCV and a decreased MCH.

Mean Cell Hemoglobin Concentration

The MCHC measures the average concentration of Hgb within RBCs. The MCHC reference range for a RBC with a normal concentration of Hgb is 32% to 36%, and the cell is described as being **normochromic.** An example of a type of anemia that exhibits normochromia is pernicious anemia, which is caused by a lack of vitamin B_{12} in the body. An MCHC result below 32% means that the patient's RBCs contain less than the normal concentration of Hgb or are **hypochromic,** a condition that occurs with iron-deficiency anemia and thalassemia. Because there is a physical limit to the amount of Hgb that can fit into an RBC, an MCHC level above 36% does not occur (and therefore, RBCs cannot be *hyperchromic*).

Red Cell Distribution Width

The RDW measures any variation in the size of the RBCs in a patient's specimen. Normally, all the RBCs in a patient's specimen should be the same size, with very little variation. The RDW reference range is 11.5% to 14.5%. Certain anemias, such as iron-deficiency anemia, can change the size of some of the RBCs, resulting in an increase in the RDW. **Anisocytosis** is the term used to describe a variation in the size of RBCs.

WHITE BLOOD CELL COUNT

The WBC count is used to assist in the diagnosis and management of pathologic conditions that affect the defense mechanism of the body that protects against infection and foreign materials. The WBC count is a measurement of the number of WBCs in the circulating blood. The reference range for a WBC count for a healthy adult is 4500 to 11,000 WBCs per cubic millimeter of blood, which is expressed as 4.5 to 11 ($\times 10^3/mm^3$) on laboratory reports. Conditions that result in an increase in leukocytes (leukocytosis) include acute infections such as appendicitis, chickenpox, diphtheria, infectious mononucleosis, meningitis, and rheumatic fever. Normal elevation of the WBC count can occur with pregnancy, strenuous exercise, stress, and treatment with corticosteroids. Conditions that result in a decrease in leukocytes (leukopenia) include viral infections, bone marrow damage, chemotherapy, and radiation therapy.

What Would You Do? What Would You *Not* Do?

Case Study 2

Paulina Torres brings in her 6-month-old son, Juan, for a well-child visit. Mrs. Torres has been breastfeeding Juan since he was born, and he is not yet on solid food. She says that Juan has been doing just fine, but he did not like his liquid vitamins, so she stopped giving them to him. Mrs. Torres says that she is eating a well-balanced diet and takes a multivitamin every day, so she didn't think it would be a problem. Juan's Hgb level is tested during the visit, and it is 9 g/dL. The physician prescribes ferrous sulfate drops for Juan. After the physician leaves the room, Mrs. Torres becomes quite upset. She says she does not understand why Juan's Hgb is low. She says that she thought that breast milk provided the best nutrition possible for infants. ■

White Blood Cell Differential Count

The purpose of the WBC differential count (Diff) is to identify and count the five types of WBCs in a representative blood sample. The results are expressed as a percentage. The reference ranges for a WBC differential count for an adult is presented in Table 18.1. The results of a differential count assist the provider in diagnosing conditions that affect one or more types of WBCs and in monitoring individuals undergoing treatment for these conditions.

The WBC differential count is a moderate complexity test that can be performed by an automated blood cell counter or manually through the examination of a blood smear. An automated differential count is faster and more convenient and permits the identification of many more WBCs than a manual differential count. A manual differential count; however, allows for closer inspection of abnormal WBCs.

Automated Differential Count

An automated differential count involves the use of a sophisticated automated blood cell counter, such as the Sysmex XE2100 hematology analyzer (Sysmex Corp) or the Coulter cell counter (see Fig. 18.9). The specimen required is an EDTA–anticoagulated blood specimen obtained through venipuncture using a lavender-closure tube. The blood specimen is loaded into the automated analyzer which measures the various properties of WBCs (size, shape, and electrical properties) to determine which type of WBC it is. If abnormal features are present in the WBCs that the analyzer is unable to identify, the results are flagged, and a manual differential count is performed by the outside laboratory. Between 10% and 25% of specimens are flagged by the analyzer for a manual review.

Manual Differential Count

If the provider orders a manual differential count on a blood specimen, the medical assistant may need to prepare two blood smears using fresh whole blood for transport to an outside laboratory. The preparation of a blood smear is outlined in Procedure 18.2. Fresh whole blood is preferred for blood smears; however, a satisfactory smear can be made at the outside laboratory from an EDTA-anticoagulated blood specimen, provided that the smear is made within 24 hours after collection. Other anticoagulants should not be used because they could alter the morphology of the WBCs. Blood cell **morphology** refers to the size, shape, and structure of a blood cell. After preparing the blood smear, the medical assistant must place the slides into a protective slide container for transport to an outside laboratory.

The blood smear is evaluated by a medical laboratory technologist at the outside laboratory. Because WBCs are clear and colorless, they must be stained with an appropriate dye (usually Wright's stain) before they can be identified. The nucleus, the cytoplasm, and any granules in the cytoplasm take on the characteristic colors of their cell type which aids in proper identification. A minimum of 100 WBCs are identified under a microscope based on the size, color, and structure of the nucleus and the color and texture of the cytoplasm. Each cell is assigned to its appropriate category: neutrophil, eosinophil, basophil, lymphocyte, or monocyte (Fig. 18.10). The number of each type of leukocyte is documented as a percentage and reflects the overall distribution of WBCs in the patient's bloodstream. During the manual evaluation of the blood smear, the laboratory technologist will also examine the morphology of RBCs and platelets including their size, shape, and structure. If immature or abnormal blood cells are observed on the slide, it is referred to a hematomorphologist and/or a pathologist for further evaluation and interpretation.

Memories *from* Practicum

Latisha: My practicum was at a cardiology office. A lot of venipunctures were performed at this office. Most of the blood specimens were picked up by Labcorp and taken to their laboratory for testing. I felt lucky I was able to get so much experience in drawing blood at this office. When I first started my practicum, the patients were apprehensive about someone new drawing their blood. This made me nervous because it seemed they were questioning my ability to perform the procedure. I explained to the patients that I had received the proper training for drawing blood and that I had successfully drawn blood on several of my classmates. Before drawing blood, I would go over the procedure many times in my head and I tried to be relaxed and confident performing the venipuncture. By doing this, I gained their trust and before long, they were requesting that I draw their blood. This taught me that if you believe in yourself and have confidence you can succeed at anything. ■

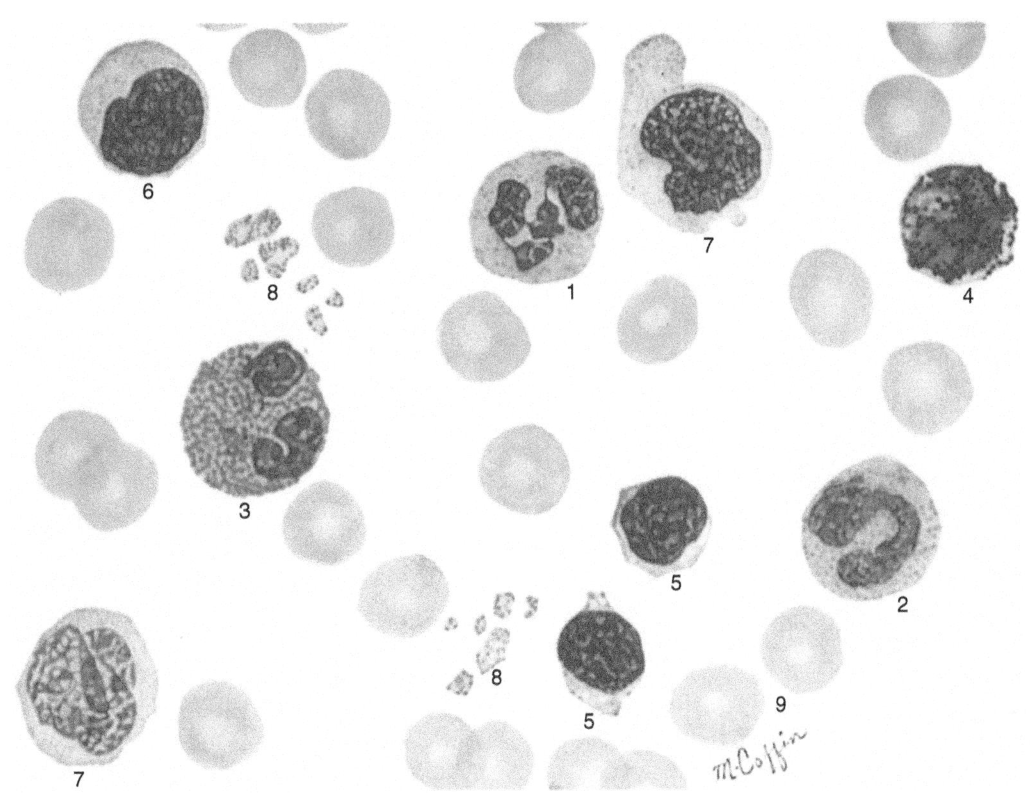

Fig. 18.10 Types of blood cells in a blood smear. *1* to *7*, White blood cells (leukocytes) stained as they are in the laboratory to show the many types. They play an active role in immune response or defense against disease. *1*, Neutrophil; *2*, neutrophilic band; *3*, eosinophil; *4*, basophil; *5*, lymphocyte; *6*, (large) lymphocyte; *7*, monocyte; *8*, platelets (thrombocytes), which are responsible for clotting; and *9*, red blood cells (erythrocytes), which carry oxygen. (From Custer RP: *An atlas of the blood and bone marrow*, ed 2, Philadelphia: WB Saunders; 1974.)

What Would You Do? What Would You *Not* Do?

Case Study 3

Marjorie Merrick comes to the office for a follow-up visit to discuss her laboratory results with the physician. Marjorie is in perimenopause and has been having problems with heavy menstrual periods, bleeding between periods, hot flashes, insomnia, fatigue, and shortness of breath. Marjorie's laboratory tests indicate that she has iron-deficiency anemia. Because Marjorie's hemoglobin level is extremely low, the physician orders an injection of iron dextran, Z-track technique, and instructs Marjorie to increase foods in her diet that contain iron. Marjorie says she has heard that an iron injection can stain the skin and wants to know whether that is true. She wants to know what foods contain iron. Marjorie says she has a friend who has received a vitamin B_{12} injection every 2 weeks. Marjorie wants to know whether she will have to do that, too. Marjorie signed up to donate blood this week at her church's Red Cross blood drive. She wants to know whether it is all right for her to donate. ■

COAGULATION TESTS

Most coagulation tests are moderate complexity tests and are performed at an outside laboratory. Examples of coagulation tests include prothrombin time (PT), partial thromboplastin time (PTT), platelet count, fibrinogen level, factor V assay, and thrombin time. Commonly performed coagulation tests include the platelet count and the PT test which are described in more detail below.

PLATELET COUNT

The platelet (PLT) count is included in a CBC; however, since it is a coagulation test, it is discussed in this section. A PLT count is a moderate complexity test performed on an automated blood cell counter. The PLT count is a measurement of the number of platelets in the circulating blood. The reference for a PLT count in a healthy adult is 150,000 to 400,000 platelets per cubic millimeter of blood, which is expressed as 150 to 400 ($\times 10^3/mm^3$) on a laboratory report.

The PLT count is used to assist in the diagnosis and management of conditions that affect the clotting mechanism of the body. A PLT count may be ordered when a patient has signs and symptoms associated with thrombocytopenia (decreased platelets) such as unexplained bruising, prolonged bleeding from a cut or wound, nosebleeds, heavy menstrual bleeding, small red spots on the skin known as *petechiae*, and small purplish spots on the skin known as *purpura* caused by bleeding under the skin. Conditions that can cause thrombocytopenia include iron-deficiency anemia, cancer, splenectomy, acute blood loss, and hemolytic anemia.

A PLT count may also be ordered when a patient has signs and symptoms associated with thrombocytosis (increased platelets) such as excessive clotting. Thrombocytosis is less common than thrombocytopenia and can be caused by the following conditions: viral infections (e.g., mononucleosis, hepatitis, HIV, and measles), leukemia, lymphoma, sepsis, cirrhosis, aplastic anemia, and autoimmune disorders.

PROTHROMBIN TIME TEST

Prothrombin is a protein produced by your liver. It is one of many factors in the blood that help it clot appropriately. Vitamin K is needed for the production of prothrombin. A PT test measures the time it takes for the blood to form a clot. A PT test helps to detect bleeding and clotting disorders in patients exhibiting symptoms of these disorders. Their reference range for a PT test for a healthy adult is 9 to 12 seconds.

If the PT result is more than 12 seconds, the blood is clotting slower than normal which could result in excessive bleeding. Symptoms of a bleeding disorder that may warrant a PT test include unexplained nosebleeds, excessive bleeding from the gums, easy bruising, heavy menstrual periods, and unexplained blood in the stool or urine. Conditions that can cause a prolonged PT include liver disease, vitamin K deficiency, or a deficiency of a clotting factor.

If the PT result is less than 9 seconds, the blood is clotting faster than normal which could result in excessive clot formation in arteries or veins. Symptoms of a clotting disorder that may warrant a PT test include swelling, redness, tenderness or warmth in a leg; redness or red streaks on the legs; shortness of breath, cough, and chest pain. The conditions causing these symptoms are those associated with the presence of a blood clot such as thrombophlebitis (usually in a leg) and a pulmonary embolism (PE).

PT/INR TEST

A PT/INR (prothrombin time with INR) test is a combination of a PT test and a mathematical calculation performed on the PT test result to arrive at a standardized value known as an *INR (International Normalized Ratio).*

The PT/INR test is most commonly used to monitor patients on long-term warfarin anticoagulant therapy to determine how well the warfarin is working to prevent blood clots. An **anticoagulant** inhibits the formation of blood clots by interfering with the blood clotting mechanism in the body. This causes the blood to take longer to clot. Warfarin works by reducing the available vitamin K in the liver responsible for producing some of the clotting factors including prothrombin; brand names for warfarin include Coumadin and Jantoven.

Purpose of the PT/INR Test

A PT/INR test is recommended for patients on long-term warfarin therapy. Patients on warfarin therapy have to have their blood tested every 2 to 4 weeks for as long as they are on warfarin which may be for the rest of their lives. Reagents used to perform the test vary from one laboratory to another and sometimes even within the same laboratory over time. The INR is a calculation performed by the automated coagulation analyzer on the PT result that adjusts for changes in the reagents and allows results from different laboratories to be compared. The INR is expressed as a ratio and provides a good comparison of test results for patients on long-term warfarin therapy.

The INR is a standardized measurement of the rate at which the blood clots. It is expressed as a number, and because the value is a ratio, the result does not have a unit of measurement attached to it. A healthy individual with a normal clotting ability (and not on warfarin therapy) should have an INR result that falls between 0.9 and 1.2. Most laboratories report both the PT and INR values when a PT/INR test is performed.

A low INR means there is an increased risk of blood clot formation in an artery or vein. An elevated INR means that there is an increased risk of bleeding; the higher the number, the longer it takes for the blood to clot. For example, an individual with an INR of 3.0 would have blood that takes longer to clot than an individual with an INR of 1.0. The risk of spontaneous bleeding begins to rise as the INR reaches a level of 4.0 or higher.

Long-Term Warfarin Therapy

Conditions for which long-term warfarin therapy is prescribed include the following:

1. Patients who experience recurrent atrial fibrillation. *Arial fibrillation* is an irregular heartbeat, which can cause blood to pool in the atrium of the heart; the pooled blood may cause the formation of a blood clot, which can travel to the brain, resulting in a stroke.
2. Patients who have experienced a PE or thrombophlebitis (also known as *deep vein thrombosis* [DVT]) to prevent the formation of another clot.
3. Patients who have had a heart valve replaced with a mechanical valve because of the increased risk that a clot may form on the mechanical valve, causing heart blockage.

The goal of warfarin therapy is to increase the clotting time to a level that prevents the formation of blood clots in an individual with one of the conditions listed above, without causing excessive bleeding or bruising. The ideal INR range for a patient on warfarin therapy depends on the condition being treated. The ideal INR range for a patient on moderate-intensity warfarin therapy following a DVT or PE; or a patient with recurring atrial fibrillation is between 2.0 and 3.0. The ideal INR range for a patient with a mechanical valve replacement is between 2.5 and 3.5.

PT/INR Testing Schedule

To ensure that patients on long-term warfarin therapy remain within their ideal INR range, they must undergo periodic PT/INR testing. When patients are first placed

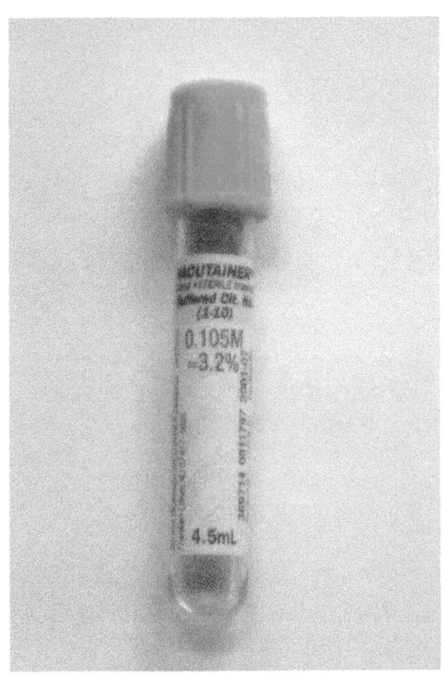

Fig. 18.11 A light-blue closure tube used to collect a specimen for a PT/INR test.

on warfarin therapy, a PT/INR test is performed once or twice a week to assess their response to the warfarin. Based on the INR results, the dose of warfarin is adjusted so that the results become stable and consistently fall within their ideal INR range. Once the test results become stabilized, the patient should have a PT/INR test performed every 2 to 4 weeks.

PT/INR Specimen Collection for Transport

The medical assistant may be responsible for collecting the specimen for a PT/INR test for transport to an outside laboratory for testing. The PT/INR test requires only a small collection tube (usually 4 to 5 mL). The blood must be collected in a tube containing sodium citrate, which is a light-blue closure tube (Fig. 18.11). The sodium citrate prevents the specimen from clotting without affecting the test results.

When collecting the specimen, it is very important to fill the light-blue closure tube to the exhaustion of the vacuum to provide for the correct anticoagulant-to-blood ratio. Failure to completely fill the tube is a cause for rejection of the specimen by the outside laboratory because it leads to inaccurate test results. Some light-blue tubes have a fill indicator so that the medical assistant can verify visually that the tube is completely filled.

If the butterfly method is used to collect the specimen, a modification in the collection procedure is required under the following circumstances. If the light-blue closure tube is the first or only tube to be drawn, a 5-mL red closure tube must be drawn first and discarded. This must be done to remove the air in the butterfly tubing and replace it with blood. If the light-blue closure tube is filled without drawing a discard tube, some of the tube's vacuum is exhausted by the air in the butterfly tubing (rather than blood), resulting in underfilling of the tube. An underfilled tube results in an incorrect anticoagulant-to-blood ratio which is a cause for rejection of the specimen by the outside laboratory.

Once the tube has been drawn, it should be immediately and gently inverted three or four times to mix the anticoagulant with the blood to prevent the formation of clots. The tube should then be placed in a biohazard specimen bag for transport to an outside laboratory. A laboratory request form must be placed with the specimen or transmitted electronically to the laboratory. Information on the collection and handling of a specimen for a PT/INR test as presented in a laboratory test directory is outlined in Fig. 18.12.

CLIA-Waived PT/INR Test

A PT/INR test can be performed in the medical office using a CLIA-waived automated coagulation analyzer. One of the advantages of CLIA-waived coagulation analyzers is that they only require a capillary specimen to perform the test. The manufacturer of each coagulation analyzer provides an operating manual that includes information needed to perform quality control procedures, collect and test the specimen, and properly store the test strips. It is important that the medical assistant become familiar with all aspects of the coagulation analyzer used to perform a PT/INR test. Quality control procedures are of particular importance to ensure that the analyzer is functioning properly and that the test results are reliable and accurate. Brand names of coagulation analyzers include HemoSense InRatio 2 (Hemosense Inc., San Diego, CA) and CoaguChek XS (Roche Diagnostics, Branchburg, NJ).

Procedure for the CLIA-Waived CoaguChek XS Test

The medical assistant must follow the PT/INR collection and testing procedure *exactly* as presented in the operating manual. An overview of the procedure for performing a PR/INR test using the CLIA-waived CoaguChek XS is outlined here:

1. Perform a finger puncture to obtain a capillary blood specimen.
2. Apply the first drop of blood to the test strip (Fig. 18.13).
3. Read the results after a countdown period in which the analyzer determines the PT test results and then calculates the INR. The INR on this meter is 0.9, which is within the reference range for a healthy adult not on warfarin therapy (Fig. 18.14).
4. Document the results in the patient's medical record, including the date and time, the name of the test (PT/INR), and the INR ratio value.

Home Testing

Patients on long-term warfarin therapy are able to test their blood at home with a CLIA-waived coagulation analyzer (Fig. 18.15). Home PT/INR testing with a coagulation analyzer is covered by Medicare and most private insurance companies. Home testing provides patients with the convenience of not having to make periodic visits to a laboratory or medical office to have a PT/INR test performed. Patients can check their PT/INR when conditions occur that might

Test Directory
Prothrombin Time with INR

CPT Code:	85610
Synonyms:	PT/INR, PT, Protime
Type of Specimen:	Whole blood or plasma
Amount of Specimen:	4.5 mL
Collection Container:	Light-blue top tube
Patient Preparation:	None
Collection and Processing:	1. Collect and label specimen. 2. With a winged-infusion setup, draw a 5 mL discard tube first to account for air in the tubing to prevent underfilling the tube. 3. Fill the light-blue top tube completely. 4. Gently invert tube 3-4 times immediately after collection.
Storage and Transport:	Store at RT
Specimen Stability:	RT (15°-35° C): 24 hours If testing cannot be performed within 24 hours, centrifuge the specimen for 15 minutes and remove the plasma using a plastic pipet being careful not to disturb the buffy coat. Place the plasma in a labeled transfer tube freeze immediately at –20° C for pickup by a courier.
Causes for Rejection:	Specimen collected in any tube other than a sodium citrate tube Hemolyzed or clotted specimen. Underfilled tube (less than 90%) Collection tube past its expiration date Improper labeling of tube
Reference Range:	**INR:** *For patients with normal clotting ability:* 0.9-1.2 *For patients taking warfarin:* Moderate intensity warfarin therapy 2.0-3.0 Higher intensity warfarin therapy 2.5-3.5 **PT:** 9–12 seconds

Uses:
Detection of bleeding and clotting disorders.
Screening for congenital and acquired deficiencies of factors II, V, VII, X, and fibrinogen.
Therapeutic monitoring of warfarin (Coumadin®) anticoagulant therapy.

Limitations:	Consumption of food containing rich in Vitamin K can decrease the PT/INR Barbiturates, oral contraceptives, and HRT can decrease the PT/INR
Forms:	Order electronically or print the lab request form and submit with specimen.
Methodology:	Photo-optical clot detection analyzer.

Fig. 18.12 PT/INR test specimen requirements from a laboratory test directory.

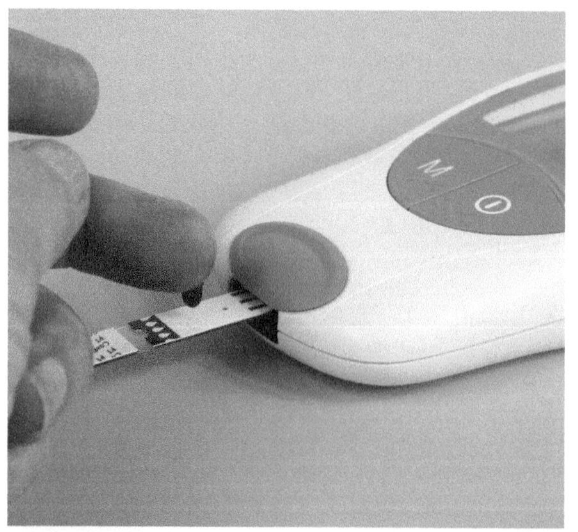

Fig. 18.13 A drop of blood is placed on the test strip. (From Garrels M: *Laboratory and diagnostic testing in ambulatory care*, ed 4, St Louis: Elsevier; 2019.)

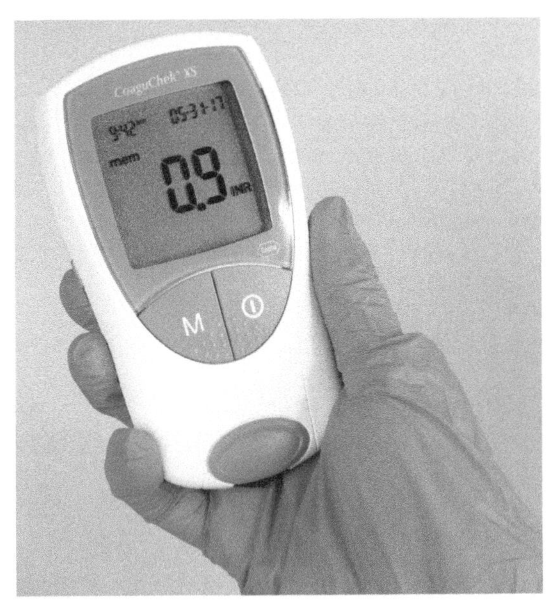

Fig. 18.14 Test results are displayed on the LCD screen. (From Garrels M: *Laboratory and diagnostic testing in ambulatory care*, ed 4, St Louis: Elsevier; 2019.)

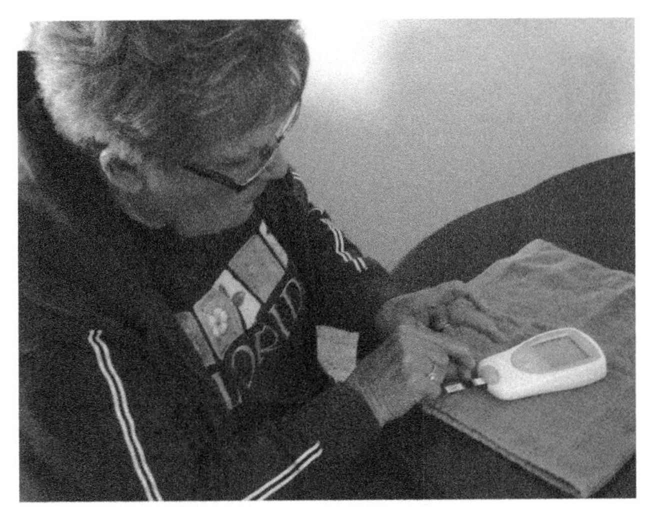

Fig. 18.15 PT/INR home testing.

indicate a problem, such as nosebleeds, bleeding gums, or unexplained bruising. In these situations, treatment can be instituted immediately to prevent the problem from getting worse.

Factors that can affect INR results and cause them to be outside of a patient's ideal range include the following: a change in diet; use of prescription or over-the-counter medications that interact with warfarin; vitamins and herbal preparations; a change in the level of exercise; illness; smoking; and alcohol consumption. It is important that the patient keep his or her provider informed of any factors that may alter the body's response to warfarin.

What Would You Do? What Would You *Not* Do? RESPONSES

Case Study 1

Page 642

What Did Latisha Do?

- ❑ Told Theodore that the tests are routine screening tests that are being run to make sure he is in good health.
- ❑ Told Theodore that it is not possible to obtain the specimen from his finger because it would not provide enough blood to perform the tests.
- ❑ Explained to Theodore that a small amount of pain is associated with a blood draw, but it would be brief.
- ❑ Explained to Theodore that two different tests are being run on him and they each require a certain type of tube.
- ❑ Placed Theodore in a semi-reclining position for the venipuncture as a safety precaution.
- ❑ Helped Theodore to relax during the venipuncture by telling him to breathe deeply.
- ❑ Just before inserting the needle, told Theodore that he would feel a "small stick" to prevent startling him when the needle is inserted.

Did Latisha Not Do?

- ❑ Did not tell Theodore that he is healthy and does not have anything wrong with him.
- ❑ Did not tell Theodore that he should try to be braver about having his blood drawn.
- ❑ Did not tell Theodore that the venipuncture would not hurt.

Case Study 2

Page 644

What Did Latisha Do?

- ❑ Commended Mrs. Torres on eating nutritiously.
- ❑ Told Mrs. Torres that breast milk does not contain very much iron. Explained that because of this, it is important to give Juan his liquid vitamins, which have iron in them.
- ❑ Reassured Mrs. Torres that breastfeeding does provide very good nutrition for Juan.
- ❑ Explained to Mrs. Torres that the iron supplement may cause Juan's stool to be a dark, tarlike color, and she should not be alarmed because this is normal.

What Did Latisha Not Do?

- ❑ Did not scold Mrs. Torres for not giving Juan his vitamins

Continued

What Would You Do? What Would You *Not* Do? RESPONSES—cont'd

- ❑ Did not make Mrs. Torres feel like it was her fault that Juan's hemoglobin was low.

Case Study 3

Page 645

What Did Latisha Do?

- ❑ Explained to Marjorie that the iron injection can stain the skin but that it would be given in a special way to prevent that from happening.
- ❑ Told Marjorie that the following foods contain iron: beef, liver, spinach, eggs, and iron-fortified breads and cereals.
- ❑ Told Marjorie that she wouldn't be getting a vitamin B_{12} injection because vitamin B_{12} is not used to treat iron-deficiency anemia.
- ❑ Told Marjorie that the Red Cross requires that a blood donor's hemoglobin level be within the normal range to donate blood. Explained that she could not donate this time, but that when her hemoglobin is back to normal, she will be able to donate.
- ❑ Explained to Marjorie that the iron supplement may cause her stool to be a dark, tarlike color, and she should not be alarmed because this is normal.
- ❑ Gave Marjorie a patient education brochure on iron-deficiency anemia to take home with her.

What Did Latisha Not Do?

- ❑ Did not tell Marjorie that her hemoglobin level was really low and should be a cause for concern.
- ❑ Did not tell Marjorie that her friend has pernicious anemia because there is no way of knowing this.

TERMINOLOGY REVIEW

Medical Term	Word Parts	Definition
Ameboid movement		The movement used by leukocytes that permits them to propel themselves from the capillaries into the tissues.
Anemia	*an-:* without or absence of *-emia:* blood condition	A condition in which there is a decrease in the number of erythrocytes or the amount of hemoglobin in the blood.
Anisocytosis	*anis/o-:* unequal, dissimilar *cyt/o:* cell *-osis:* abnormal condition	A variation in the size of RBCs.
Anticoagulant	*anti-:* against *-coagulant:* clotting	A substance that inhibits blood clotting.
Bilirubin	*bili-:* bile	An orange-colored bile pigment that is a by-product of heme destruction from the hemoglobin molecule.
Diapedesis	*dia-:* through	The ameboid movement of blood cells (especially leukocytes) through the wall of a capillary and out into the tissues.
Erythrocyte	*erythro-: red* *cyte: cell*	RBCs. RBCs are responsible for transporting oxygen and carbon dioxide in the body.
Hematology	*hemat/o-:* blood *-ology:* study of	The study of blood and blood-forming tissues.
Hamatopoiesis	*hemato/o: blood* *-poiesis: formation of*	The process of blood cell formation.
Hemoglobin	*hem/o-:* blood *-globin:* protein	The protein- and iron-containing pigment of erythrocytes that carries oxygen to the tissues of the body.
Hemolysis	*hem/o-:* blood *-lysis:* breakdown	The breakdown of erythrocytes with the release of hemoglobin into the plasma.
Hypochromic	*hypo-:* below, deficient *chrom/o:* color *-ic:* pertaining to	A RBC with a decreased concentration of hemoglobin.
Leukocyte	*leuk/o-:* white *cyt/o:* cell	WBC. WBCs function in defending the body against infection and foreign materials.

TERMINOLOGY REVIEW—cont'd

Medical Term	Word Parts	Definition
Leukocytosis	*leuk/o-:* white *cyt/o:* cell *-osis:* abnormal condition (means increased when used with blood cell word parts)	An abnormal increase in the number of leukocytes (>11,000 per cubic millimeter of blood).
Leukopenia	*leuk/o-:* white *-penia:* abnormal reduction in number	An abnormal decrease in the number of leukocytes (<4500 per cubic millimeter of blood).
Macrocytic	*macr/o-:* abnormally large *cyt/o:* cell *-ic:* pertaining to	An abnormally large RBC.
Microcytic	*micro-:* small *cyt/o:* cell *-ic:* pertaining to	An abnormally small RBC.
Morphology (blood cells)	*morpho-: form and structure* *-ology:* study of	The study of the size, shape, and structure of a blood cell.
Normochromic	*norm/o-:* normal *chrom/o:* color *-ic:* pertaining to	An RBC with a normal concentration of hemoglobin.
Normocytic	*norm/o:* normal *cyt/o:* cell *-ic:* pertaining to	A normal-sized RBC.
Oxyhemoglobin	*oxy/i-:* oxygen *hem/o:* blood *-globin:* protein	Hemoglobin that has combined with oxygen.
Phagocytosis	*phag/o-:* eat, swallow *cyt/o:* cell *-osis:* abnormal condition	The engulfing and destruction of foreign particles, such as pathogens and damaged cells by certain cells in the body.
Polycythemia	*poly-:* many *cyt/o:* cell *hem/o:* blood *-ia:* condition of diseased or abnormal state	A disorder in which there is an increase in the number of RBCs or the amount of hemoglobin.
Thrombocyte	*thrombo-: clot* *cyt/o:* cell	Platelets. Thrombocytes function by participating in the blood clotting mechanism of the body.
Thrombocytopenia	*thrombo-: clot* *cyt/o:* cell *-penia:* abnormal reduction in number	An abnormal decrease in the number of thrombocytes (< 150,000 per cubic millimeter of blood).
Thrombocytosis	*thrombo-: clot* *cyt/o:* cell *-osis:* abnormal condition (means increased when used	An abnormal increase in the number of thrombocytes (greater than 150,000 per cubic millimeter of blood).

PROCEDURE 18.1 Perform a CLIA-Waived Hematocrit Test

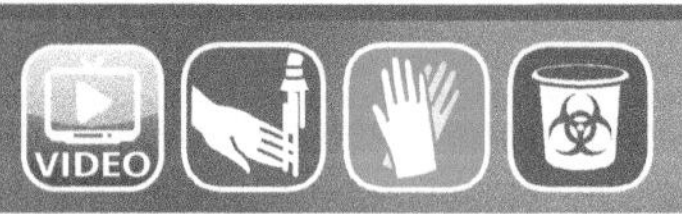

Outcome Perform a hematocrit test.

Equipment/Supplies

- CLIA-waived microhematocrit centrifuge
- Disposable gloves
- Lancet
- Antiseptic wipe
- Gauze pads
- Capillary tubes
- Sealing compound
- Adhesive bandage
- Biohazard sharps container

1. **Procedural Step.** Sanitize your hands. Greet the patient and introduce yourself. Identify the patient by full name and date of birth, and explain the procedure.
2. **Procedural Step.** Assemble equipment. Open the gauze packet. Cleanse the puncture site with an antiseptic wipe, and allow it to air-dry. Apply gloves and perform a finger puncture, then dispose of the lancet in a biohazard sharps container.
   Principle. Personal protective equipment and proper disposal of the lancet are required by the OSHA standard to prevent exposure to bloodborne pathogens.
3. **Procedural Step.** Wipe away the first drop of blood with a gauze pad. Fill the first capillary tube by holding one end of it horizontally, but slightly downward, next to the free-flowing puncture. Keep the tip of the capillary tube in the blood, but do not allow it to press against the patient's skin. Calibrated tubes are filled to the calibration line; uncalibrated tubes are filled approximately three quarters (within 10–20 mm of the end of the tube). The blood is drawn into the tube through capillary action. Fill a second tube using the method just described. Place a gauze pad over the puncture site and apply pressure.
   Principle. Not keeping the tip of the capillary tube in the blood can cause air bubbles in the stem of the tube, which leads to inaccurate test results. Allowing the capillary tube to press against the skin closes the opening of the capillary tubes and does not allow blood to enter. The type of tube (calibrated or uncalibrated) is based on the method used to read the test results. The hematocrit should be performed in duplicate to ensure accurate and reliable test results.

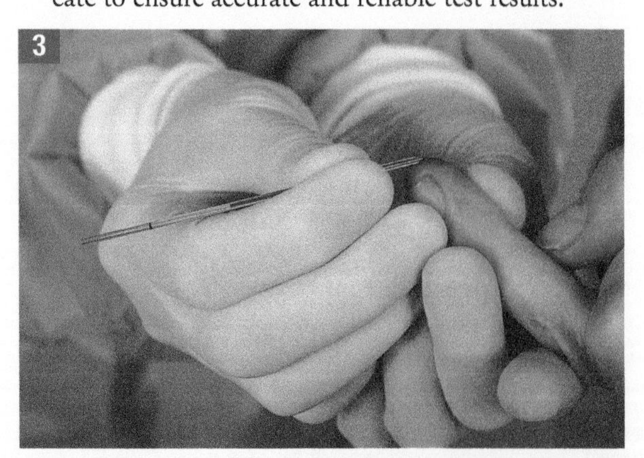

Fill the capillary tube.

4. **Procedural Step.** Push the dry end of the tube (end opposite the filling end that does not contain blood) down into the sealing compound. This seals the end of the capillary tube. The sealing compound can be used to hold the capillary tubes until they are ready to be placed in the microhematocrit centrifuge. To do this, place the sealing compound on a flat surface with the tubes in a vertical position. Before removing a capillary tube from the sealing compound, rotate the tube between the thumb and index finger to prevent the sealing compound from pulling out when the tube is lifted out of the sealing compound.
   Principle. Capillary tubes must be sealed properly to prevent leakage of the blood specimen during centrifugation

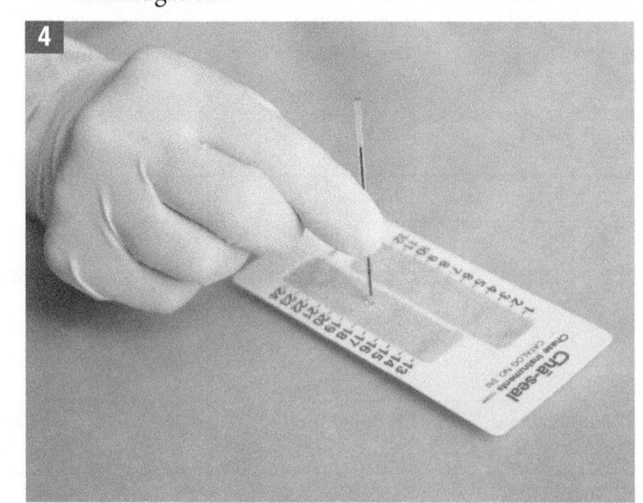

Seal the end of the tube.

5. **Procedural Step.** Check the patient's puncture site for bleeding and apply an adhesive bandage, if needed.
6. **Procedural Step.** Place the capillary tubes in the microhematocrit centrifuge with the sealed end facing out. Balance one tube with the other capillary tube placed on the opposite side of the centrifuge.
   Principle. Placing the sealed end toward the outside prevents the blood specimen from spinning out of the capillary tube when the centrifuge is in operation.

PROCEDURE 18.1 Perform a CLIA-Waived Hematocrit Test—cont'd

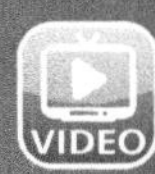

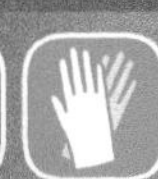

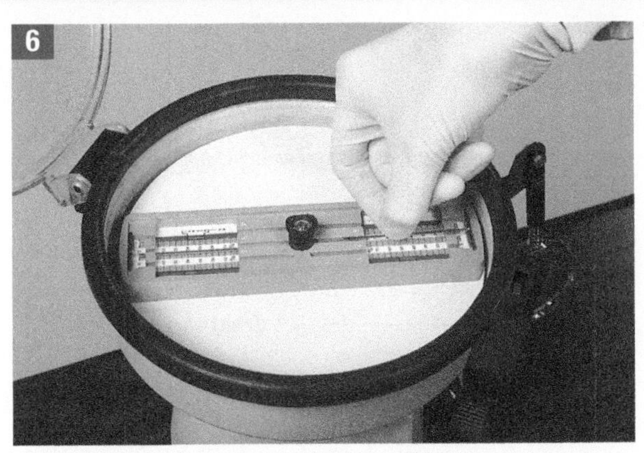

Place the tube in the centrifuge.

7. **Procedural Step.** Place the cover on the centrifuge, and lock it securely. Centrifuge the blood specimen for 3 to 5 minutes at a speed of 10,000 rpm.
   Principle. Centrifuging the blood specimen causes the red blood cells (RBCs) to become packed and settle on the bottom of the tube.
8. **Procedural Step.** Allow the centrifuge to come to a complete stop. Read the results, as follows:
   Calibrated tube. If a capillary tube with a calibration line was used, read the results using the special graphic reading device that is part of the centrifuge. Adjust the capillary tube so that the bottom of the RBC column (just above the sealing compound) is placed on the 0 line. With a magnifying glass, read the results at the top of the packed RBC column, and you will see a percentage on the reading device.
   Uncalibrated tube. If an uncalibrated tube was used, you must use a microhematocrit reader card to determine the results; place the top of the plasma column on the 100% mark and the bottom of the cell column on the 0 line. Read the results on the scale, which corresponds to the top of the packed cell column.
   In both cases, the buffy coat should not be included in the reading. The answer represents the percentage of blood volume occupied by the RBCs. (The hematocrit test on this reading device is 38.)
   Principle. Stopping the centrifuge with your hands can injure you and can damage the machine.

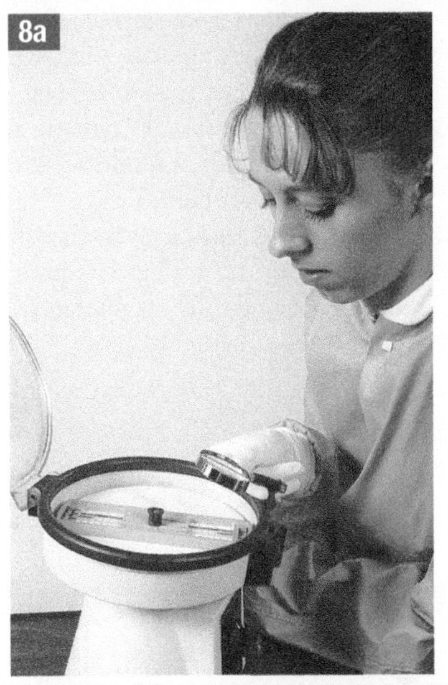

Align the bottom of the red cell column with the 0 line.

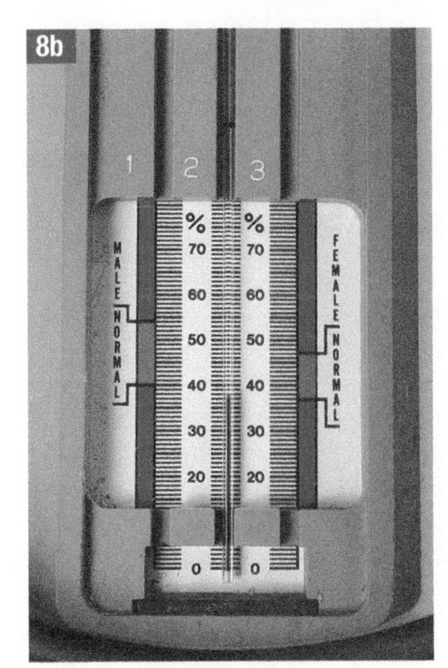

Read the results.

9. **Procedural Step.** Read the second tube in the manner just described; the results of the tubes should agree within 4 percentage points. If not, the hematocrit procedure must be repeated. If they are within 4 percentage points, the two values are averaged to derive the test results.
10. **Procedural Step.** Properly dispose of the capillary tubes in a biohazard sharps container. Remove gloves and sanitize your hands.
11. **Procedural Step.** Document the results in the patient's medical record.

Continued

PROCEDURE 18.1 Perform a CLIA-Waived Hematocrit Test—cont'd

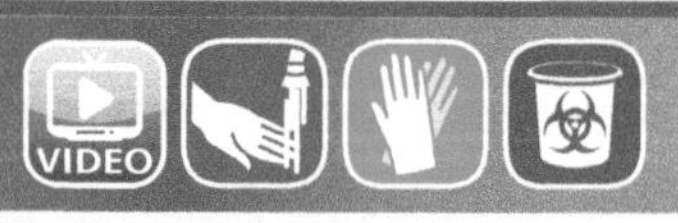

a. *Electronic health record (EHR):* Document the hematocrit results using the appropriate radio buttons, drop-down menus, and free text fields.
b. *Paper-based patient record:* Document the date and time and the hematocrit results (refer to the PPR documentation example).

12. **Procedural Step.** Return the equipment to its proper storage place. Store the sealing compound at room temperature. Exposing it to a temperature above 80°F adversely affects its consistency.

Reference Range for Hematocrit

Female: 37% to 47%
Male: 40% to 54%

PPR Documentation Example

Date	
5/5/XX	11:15 a.m. Hct: 38%.
	L. Sharpe, CMA (AAMA)

PROCEDURE 18.2 Preparation of a Blood Smear for a WBC Differential Count

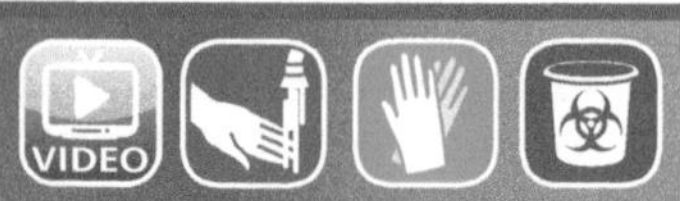

Outcome Prepare a blood smear for a WBC differential count.

Equipment/Supplies

- Disposable gloves
- Supplies to perform a finger puncture or venipuncture
- Slides with a frosted edge
- Slide container
- Biohazard specimen bag
- Laboratory request form
- Biohazard sharps container

1. **Procedural Step.** Sanitize your hands. Greet the patient and introduce yourself. Identify the patient by full name and date of birth and explain the procedure.
2. **Procedural Step.** Assemble the equipment. Complete a laboratory request by writing in the information on a preprinted form or by entering the required information into a computer.
   Using a pencil, label two slides on the frosted edge with the patient's name and date of birth, and the date.
   Principle. Laboratories request the preparation of two blood smears as a means of quality control.
3. **Procedural Step.** Open the gauze packet. Cleanse the puncture site with an antiseptic wipe. Perform a finger puncture and wipe away the first drop of blood. Place a drop of blood from the patient's finger in the middle of each slide, approximately 1/4 inch from the slide's frosted edge, by touching the slide to the drop of blood. Do not allow the patient's finger to touch the slide.
   Principle. If the patient's finger touches the slide, it will spread out the blood specimen, producing an uneven smear. In addition, moisture or oil from the patient's finger could interfere with the smear.
4. **Procedural Step.** Make the blood smear as follows:
   a. Hold a second "spreader" slide between the thumb and index finger of the dominant hand. Position a nondominant finger (or fingers) at the end of the slide (end opposite the frosted edge). Position the spreader slide in front of the drop of blood and at a 30-degree angle to the first slide.

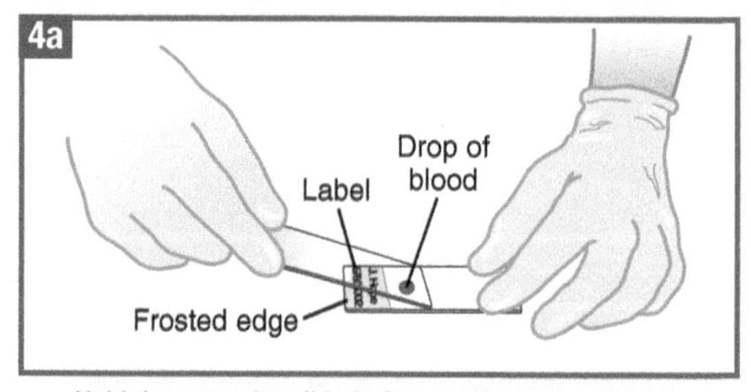

Hold the spreader slide in front of the drop of blood.

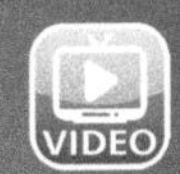

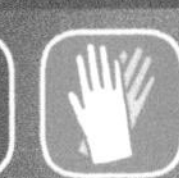
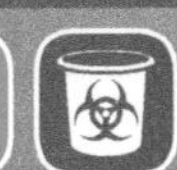

b. Move the spreader slide until it touches the drop of blood. The blood distributes itself along the edge of the spreader by capillary action.

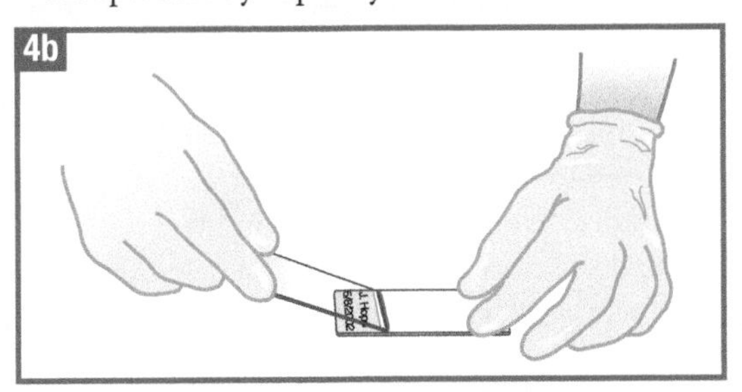

Move the spreader into the drop of blood.

c. Using a smooth, continuous motion with a light but firm pressure, spread the blood thinly and evenly across the surface of the first slide, ending the motion by lifting the spreader slide off the specimen in a smooth, low arc. The smear should be approximately 1 1/2 inches long. The blood smear is thickest at the beginning and gradually thins to a very fine "feathered" edge which is only one cell layer thick.

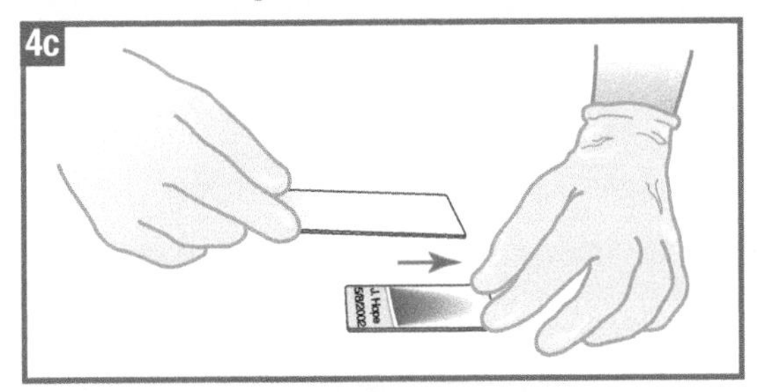

Spread the blood across the slide.

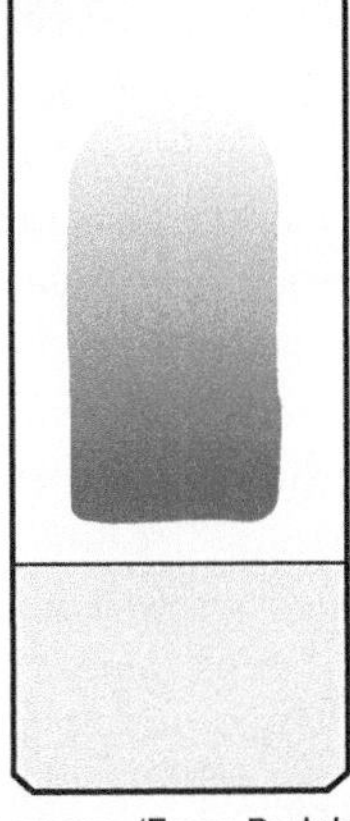

Properly prepared blood smear. (From Rodak BF: *Hematology: clinical principles and applications*, ed 4, St Louis: Elsevier; 2012.)

d. Repeat the above procedure to prepare the second blood smear. If the blood smear has been prepared correctly, it exhibits the following characteristics: (1) It is smooth and even with no ridges, holes, lines, streaks, or clumps; (2) it is not too thick or too thin; (3) a feathered edge is seen at the thin end of the smear; and (4) a margin is evident on all sides of the smear. Repeat this step with the other slide.

Principle. An angle of more than 30 degrees causes the smear to be too thick; the cells overlap, do not stain well, and are smaller than normal, making them difficult to count. If the angle is smaller than 30 degrees, the smear will be too thin, and the cells will be spread out, increasing the time needed to count them.

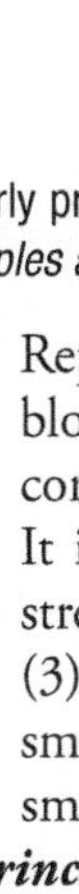

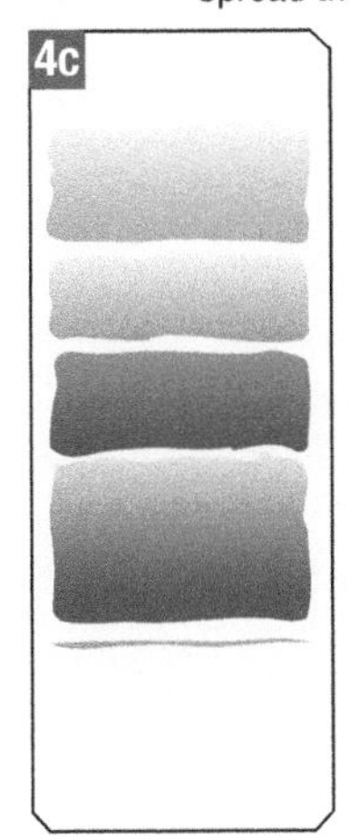

Slide contains gaps or ridges
Cause:
- Too much pressure applied to spreader slide
- Uneven pressure used to push spreader slide

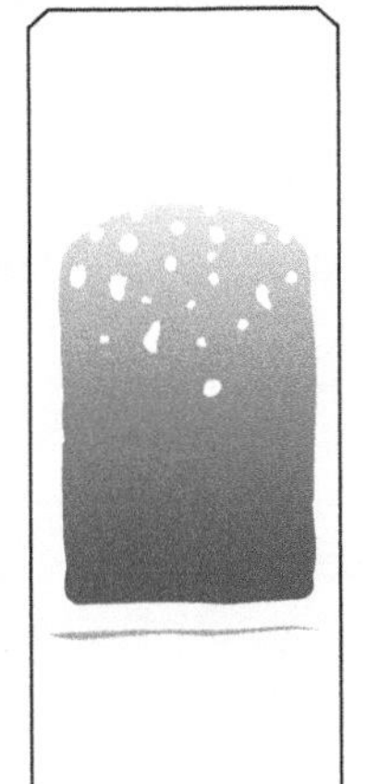

Slide contains holes
Cause:
- Dirt or fingerprints on the slide
- Fat globules or lipids in the specimen
- Blood is contaminated with powder from glove

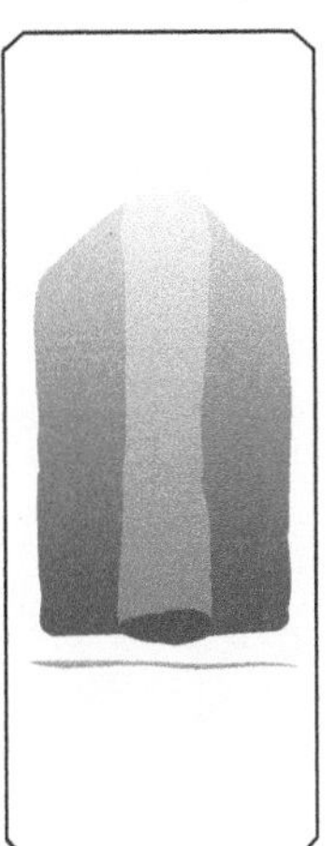

Slide contains streaks
Cause:
- Uneven pressure used to push spreader slide
- Drop of blood started to dry out

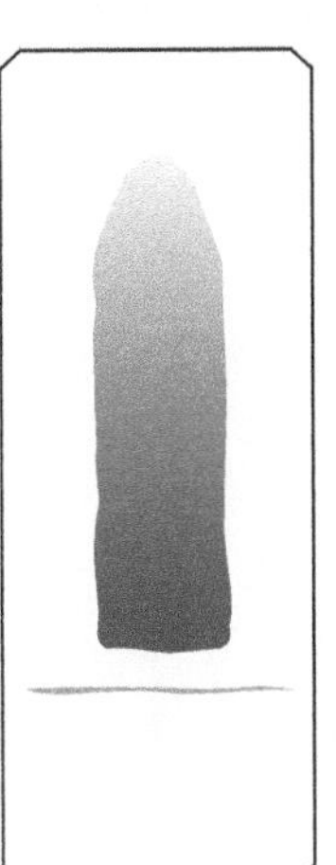

Slide is too thin
Cause:
- Blood drop is too small
- Angle of less than 30 degrees is used

Slide is too thick
Cause:
- Blood drop is too large
- Angle of less than 30 degrees is used

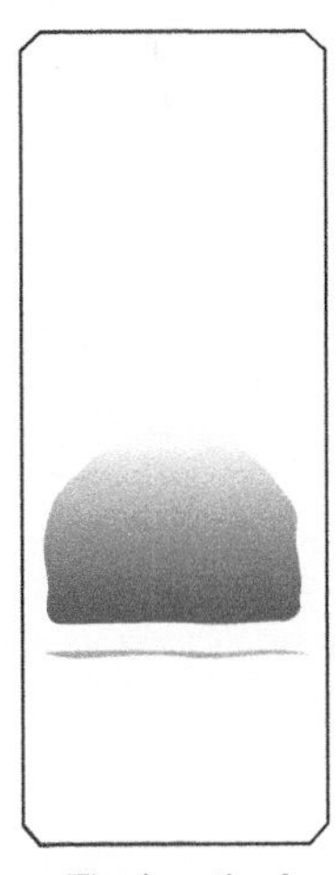

The length of the smear is too short
Cause:
- Blood drop is too small
- Angle of more than 30 degrees is used
- Spreader slide is pushed too quickly and not far enough along the slide

Improperly prepared blood smears. (Modified from Rodak BF: *Hematology: clinical principles and applications*, ed 4, St Louis: Elsevier; 2012.)

Continued

PROCEDURE 18.2 Preparation of a Blood Smear for a WBC Differential Count —cont'd

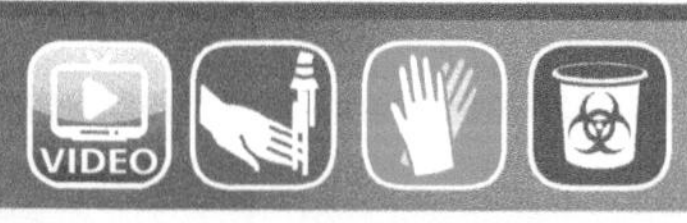

5. **Procedural Step.** Dispose of the spreader slide in a biohazard sharps container.
6. **Procedural Step.** Lay the blood smears on a flat surface and allow them to air-dry. Never blow on the slides to dry them.
   Principle. The blood smears must be dried immediately to prevent shrinkage of the blood cells, which makes them difficult to identify. Blowing on the slide might cause exhaled water droplets to make holes in the smears.
7. **Procedural Step.** Once the slides are completely dry, apply gloves and place them in a protective slide container. Prepare the slides for transport to the outside laboratory.
   a. Place slide container in a biohazard specimen bag.
   b. If a blood specimen was collected for a CBC, place the lavender closure tube in the specimen bag.
   c. Seal the bag and place the laboratory request in the outside pocket of the specimen bag (or transmit it electronically).
   d. Properly store the specimen while awaiting pickup by a laboratory courier.
8. **Procedural Step.** Remove your gloves and sanitize your hands.
9. **Procedural Step.** Document the procedure in the patient's medical record.
   a. *Electronic health record (EHR):* Document the type of collection and the date the specimen was transported to the laboratory using the appropriate radio buttons, drop-down menus, and free text fields.
   b. *Paper-based patient record:* Document the date and time, the type of collection and the date the specimen was transported to the laboratory (refer to the PPR documentation example).
10. **Procedural Step.** Place the specimen bag in the appropriate location for pickup by a laboratory courier.

PPR Documentation Example

Date	
5/05/XX	11:15 a.m. Venous blood specimen collected
	from Ⓡ arm. Capillary specimen collected
	from Ⓛ ring finger for preparation of 2 blood
	smear slides. Specimens to Medical Center
	Laboratory for CBC c̄ diff on 5/05/xx.——
	————————L. Sharpe, CMA (AAMA)

PROCEDURE 18.2

Blood Chemistry and Immunology

Check out the Evolve site at http://evolve.elsevier.com/Bonewit to access additional interactive activities and exercises to help you study and prepare for success.

LEARNING OUTCOMES

Blood Chemistry Testing

1. Explain the purpose of a blood chemistry test.
2. State the use of a comprehensive metabolic panel (CMP).
3. Describe the purpose of the test reagent area on a test strip.
4. Explain the purpose of the calibration and control procedures.
5. List factors that can result in the failure of a control to produce expected results.
6. Identify when a control procedure should be performed.
7. Explain the functions of glucose and insulin in the body.
8. State the purpose of each of the following tests: random blood glucose test, fasting blood glucose test, 2-hour postprandial glucose test, and oral glucose tolerance test.
9. State the patient preparation for a fasting blood glucose test.
10. Identify the American Diabetes Association (ADA) guidelines for interpretation of FBG test results.
11. Describe the procedure for a 2-hour postprandial blood glucose test.
12. Identify test requirements for an oral glucose tolerance test (OGTT).
13. State the restrictions that must be followed by the patient during an OGTT.
14. Explain the purpose of the hemoglobin A_{1c} test.
15. State the hemoglobin A_{1c} level for an individual without diabetes.
16. Identify the ADA guidelines for interpretation of hemoglobin A_{1c} test results
17. List advantages of self-monitoring of blood glucose by diabetic patients.
18. Describe the functions of low-density lipoprotein (LDL) cholesterol and high-density lipoprotein (HDL) cholesterol in the body.
19. State the desirable ranges for each of the following tests: total cholesterol, LDL cholesterol, and HDL cholesterol.
20. State the patient preparation for a triglycerides test.

PROCEDURES

Collect a specimen for a blood chemistry test for transport to an outside laboratory.

Perform a fasting blood glucose test using a CLIA-waived glucose meter.

Immunologic Testing

21. Explain the purpose of each of the following immunologic tests: hepatitis, HIV, syphilis, mononucleosis, rheumatoid factor, antistreptolysin O, C-reactive protein, cold agglutinins, ABO and Rh blood typing, and Rh antibody titer.
22. List the symptoms of infectious mononucleosis.
23. Identify the location of the blood antigens and the blood antibodies.
24. Explain how the blood antigen-antibody reaction is used for blood typing in vitro.
25. List the antigens and antibodies in the following blood types: A, B, AB, and O.
26. Explain the difference between Rh-positive and Rh-negative blood.

Perform a CLIA-waived rapid mononucleosis test.

CHAPTER OUTLINE

KEY TERMS

agglutination (ah-gloo-ti-NAY-shun)
antibody (AN-ti-bod-ee)
antigen (AN-ti-jen)
antiserum (AN-ti-sere-um)
cholesterol
donor
glucose
glycogen (GLIE-koe-jen)
glycosylation
HDL cholesterol
hemoglobin A_{1c}
hyperglycemia (hie-per-glie-SEE-me-ah)
hypoglycemia (hie-poe-glie-SEE-me-ah)
in vitro (in-VEE-troe)
in vivo (in-VEE-voe)
insulin
LDL cholesterol
lipoprotein (lie-poe-PROE-teen)
prediabetes
recipient (ree-SIP-ee-ent)

Introduction to Blood Chemistry and Immunology

Blood chemistry and immunologic tests are frequently ordered by the provider to assist in the diagnosis, treatment, and management of disease. There are certain blood chemistry and immunologic laboratory tests that can be performed in the medical office. Advances in CLIA-waived automated analyzers and test kits designed specifically for use in the medical office have made this possible. CLIA-waived test systems can perform these tests in a short time with accurate test results. This allows the provider to make decisions immediately regarding a patient's health care without having to wait for the results from an outside laboratory. This chapter is divided into two units. The first unit presents blood chemistry testing, and the second unit presents immunologic testing; each unit focuses on CLIA-waived tests and conditions causing abnormal test results.

Blood Chemistry Testing

Blood chemistry testing involves the quantitative measurement of chemical substances dissolved in the plasma of the blood. There are many different types of blood chemistry tests; the type of test (or tests) the provider orders depends on the patient's clinical diagnosis. Table 19.1 lists common blood chemistry tests including the purpose of the test, reference range, and conditions that cause abnormal test results.

A blood chemistry panel frequently ordered on patients is the *comprehensive metabolic panel* (CMP). A CMP contains numerous blood chemistry tests that provide information on the kidneys, liver, acid-base balance, blood glucose level, and blood proteins. It is used primarily for the routine health screening of a patient to detect any changes in the body's biologic processes that may be present, although the patient may not have had any symptoms to indicate that these changes have occurred. A CMP is also ordered when the patient's symptoms are so vague that the provider does not have enough concrete evidence to support a clinical diagnosis of a specific organ or disease state. Abnormal CMP test results are usually followed up with more specific tests before a diagnosis is made. Another important use of a CMP is to monitor and manage a variety of diseases and conditions such as kidney disease, liver disease, hypertension, and diabetes.

SPECIMEN COLLECTION FOR BLOOD CHEMISTRY TESTS

Most blood chemistry tests are moderate complexity tests and are performed by an outside laboratory. The medical assistant may be required to collect a blood specimen for blood chemistry testing following the information presented in the laboratory test directory of the outside laboratory. The specimen collection and handling requirements for a CMP as presented in a laboratory text directory are outlined in Fig. 19.1.

Blood chemistry tests usually require a serum specimen collected in an SST (serum separator tube). General guidelines for the collection of a serum specimen for transport to an outside laboratory include the following:

1. Collect the blood specimen in an SST (gold or marbled red/gray closure tube). The tube selected should have a capacity of 2½ times the amount of serum required.
2. Completely fill the collection tube to the exhaustion of the vacuum to obtain an adequate amount of serum.
3. Gently invert the tube five times immediately after collection to mix the clot activator with the blood specimen.
4. Place the blood specimen tube in an upright position in a test tube rack for 30 to 45 minutes to permit clot formation of the blood cells and avoid the formation of a fibrin clot in the serum.
5. Centrifuge the specimen for 10 minutes. During centrifugation, the gel in the SST temporarily becomes fluid and moves to the dividing point between the serum and the clotted blood cells, where it re-forms into a solid gel, serving as a physical barrier between the serum and the clot (Fig. 19.2). Inspect the tube carefully to ensure that the gel barrier is firmly attached to the glass wall. The serum can be transported to an outside laboratory in the serum separator tube.
6. Store the specimen at room temperature while awaiting pickup by a laboratory courier. The specimen is stable for 3 days at room temperature.

AUTOMATED BLOOD CHEMISTRY ANALYZERS

Automated blood chemistry analyzers are used to perform blood chemistry tests. The analyzer consists of a reflectance photometer that quantitatively measures the amount of chemical substances, or analytes, in the blood. Specifically, a reflectance photometer measures light intensity to determine the exact amount of an analyte present in a specimen.

Outside laboratories use highly sophisticated automated blood chemistry analyzers for performing blood chemistry tests (Fig. 19.3) which provide fast and reliable test results. CLIA-waived automated analyzers have been developed for performing blood chemistry tests in the POL; they are continually increasing in number as new technology becomes available. Medical offices typically use a combination of a POL and an outside laboratory to fulfill their blood chemistry testing requirements. The remainder of this section focuses on CLIA-waived analyzers used to perform blood chemistry tests in the medical office.

CLIA-WAIVED AUTOMATED ANALYZERS

CLIA-waived blood chemistry analyzers consist of compact portable devices that permit the testing of a capillary

Table 19.1 Common Blood Chemistry Tests

Name of Test	Purpose of Test	Reference Range	Increased With	Decreased With
Albumin	To monitor and treat liver and kidney disease	3.6–5.1 g/dL	Dehydration	Liver disease Nephrotic syndrome Crohn disease Thyroid disease Heart failure
Alanine aminotransferase (ALT)	To detect liver disease	45 U/L or less	Hepatocellular disease Active cirrhosis Metastatic liver tumor Obstructive jaundice Pancreatitis	
Alkaline phosphatase (ALP)	Assists in diagnosis of liver and bone diseases	25–140 U/L	Liver disease Bone disease Hyperparathyroidism Infectious mononucleosis	Hypophosphatasia Malnutrition Hypothyroidism Chronic nephritis
Aspartate aminotransferase (AST)	To detect tissue damage	40 U/L or less	Myocardial infarction Liver disease Acute pancreatitis Acute hemolytic anemia	Beriberi Uncontrolled diabetes with acidosis
Bilirubin, total (TB)	To evaluate liver functioning and hemolytic anemia	0.2–1.3 mg/dL	Liver disease Obstruction of bile ducts Hemolytic anemia	
Protein, total (TP)	To screen for diseases that alter protein balance To assess body hydration	6–8.5 g/dL	Dehydration Chronic infections Acute liver disease Multiple myeloma Lupus erythematosus	Severe hemorrhaging Hodgkin disease Sever liver disease Malabsorption
Blood urea nitrogen (BUN)	To screen for kidney disease To monitor the effectiveness of dialysis	7–25 mg/dL	Kidney disease Urinary obstruction Dehydration	Liver failure Malnutrition Impaired absorption
Calcium (Ca)	To assess parathyroid functioning and calcium metabolism To evaluate malignancies	8.5–10.8 mg/dL	Hypercalcemia Hyperparathyroidism Bone metastases Multiple myeloma Hodgkin disease Addison disease Hyperthyroidism	Hypocalcemia Hypoparathyroidism Acute pancreatitis Renal failure
Carbon dioxide (CO_2)	To diagnose and treat disorders associated with changes in acid-base balance in the body	20–32 mmol/L	Severe, prolonged vomiting and/or diarrhea Cushing syndrome Metabolic alkalosis	Addison disease Diabetic ketoacidosis Metabolic acidosis Respiratory alkalosis Chronic diarrhea
Chloride (Cl)	Assists in diagnosing disorders of acid-base and water balance	96–109 mmol/L	Dehydration Cushing syndrome Hyperventilation Preeclampsia Anemia	Severe vomiting Severe diarrhea Ulcerative colitis Pyloric obstruction Severe burns Heat exhaustion
Cholesterol (Chol)	To screen for atherosclerosis related to CVD To monitor the effectiveness of lipid-lowering medication	Less than 200 mg/dL	Atherosclerosis Cardiovascular disease Obstructive jaundice Hypothyroidism Nephrosis	Malabsorption Liver disease Hyperthyroidism Anemia

Table 19.1 Common Blood Chemistry Tests—cont'd

Name of Test	Purpose of Test	Reference Range	Increased With	Decreased With
Creatinine (Creat)	Screening test of kidney functioning	0.6–1.5 mg/dL	Impaired renal function Chronic nephritis Obstruction of urinary tract Muscle disease	Muscular dystrophy
Globulin (Glob)	To identify abnormalities in rate of protein synthesis and removal	2–3.5 g/dL	Brucellosis Chronic infections Rheumatoid arthritis Dehydration Hepatic carcinoma Hodgkin disease	Agammaglobulinemia Severe burns
Glucose	To detect disorders of glucose metabolism	*FBG:* 70–99 mg/dL *OGTT:* Less than 140 mg/dL	*Hyperglycemia* Diabetes	*Hypoglycemia* Excess insulin
Lactate dehydrogenase, 30°C (LD)	Assists in confirming myocardial or pulmonary infarction Differential diagnosis of muscular dystrophy and pernicious anemia	240 U/L or less	Acute myocardial infarction Acute leukemia Muscular dystrophy Pernicious anemia Hemolytic anemia Hepatic disease Extensive cancer	
Phosphorus (P)	To evaluate and interpret calcium levels To detect disorders of endocrine system, bone diseases, and kidney dysfunction	2.5–4.5 mg/dL	Hyperphosphatemia Renal insufficiency Severe nephritis Hypoparathyroidism Hypocalcemia Addison's disease	Hypophosphatemia Hyperparathyroidism Rickets and osteomalacia Diabetic coma Hyperinsulinism
Potassium (K)	To diagnose disorders of acid-base and water balance in the body To monitor kidney disease To monitor treatment for high BP	3.5–5.3 mmol/L	Hyperkalemia Renal failure Cell damage Acidosis Addison disease Internal bleeding	Hypokalemia Diarrhea Pyloric obstruction Starvation Malabsorption Severe vomiting Severe burns Diuretic administration Chronic stress Liver disease with ascites
Sodium (Na)	To detect changes in water and salt balance in the body	135–147 mmol/L	Hypernatremia Dehydration Conn syndrome Primary aldosteronism Coma Cushing disease Diabetes insipidus	Hyponatremia Severe burns Severe diarrhea Addison disease Severe nephritis Pyloric obstruction
Total thyroxine (Total T_4)	To assess thyroid functioning To evaluate thyroid replacement therapy	4.5–12 μg/dL	Hyperthyroidism Graves disease Thyrotoxicosis Thyroiditis	Hypothyroidism Cretinism Goiter Myxedema Hypoproteinemia
Triglycerides (Trig)	To evaluate patients with suspected atherosclerosis	*Desirable:* Less than 150 mg/dL	Liver disease Kidney disease Obesity Hypothyroidism Pancreatitis	Malnutrition Congenital lipoproteinemia Hyperthyroidism

Continued

Table 19.1 Common Blood Chemistry Tests—cont'd

Name of Test	Purpose of Test	Reference Range	Increased With	Decreased With
Uric acid (UA)	To evaluate renal failure, gout, and leukemia	*Male:* 3.9–9 mg/dL *Female:* 2.2–7.7 mg/dL	Renal failure Gout Leukemia Severe eclampsia Lymphomas	Patients undergoing treatment with uricosuric drugs

LABORATORY TEST DIRECTORY
Comprehensive Metabolic Panel

CPT Code:	80053
Synonyms:	CMP
Type of Specimen:	Serum
Amount of Specimen:	2 mL
Collection Container:	SST (send entire tube)
Tests Included:	Albumin, ALT, ALP, AST, total bilirubin, BUN, calcium, carbon dioxide, chloride, creatinine, glucose, potassium, total protein, sodium
Patient Preparation:	Fasting for 8 to 12 hours prior to collection.
Collection and Processing:	1. Collect and label specimen. 2. Gently invert tube 5 times immediately after collection. 3. Place specimen in a vertical position and allow to clot for a minimum of 30 minutes and a maximum of 2 hours. 4. Centrifuge specimen for 10 minutes.
Storage and Transport:	Store at RT or refrigerate until pickup by lab courier.
Specimen Stability:	RT (15°-35° C): 72 hours Refrigerated (2°-8° C): 72 hours Frozen: Unacceptable
Causes for Rejection:	Nonfasting specimen Specimen other than serum Improper labeling of specimen Hemolysis
Reference Range:	Values given with laboratory report.
Uses:	To determine a patient's general health status; to monitor a variety of diseases and conditions such as kidney disease, liver disease, hypertension, and diabetes; and to monitor the use of specific medications that may affect kidney or liver functioning.
Limitations:	See individual tests for limitations.
Forms:	Order electronically or print the lab request form and submit with specimen.
Methodology:	See individual tests for methodologies.

Fig. 19.1 Comprehensive metabolic panel (CMP) specimen collection and handling requirements as presented in a laboratory test directory.

blood specimen in a short time with accurate test results. Test strips, test cassettes, or test cartridges are typically used with these analyzers; the testing device contains a reagent area that contains chemicals which react with the capillary blood specimen (Fig. 19.4). The chemical reaction enables the analyzer to quantitatively measure the amount of an analyte in the blood specimen and display the results as a direct readout (Fig. 19.5).

It is important that the medical assistant become familiar with all aspects of a CLIA-waived blood chemistry analyzer. The medical assistant is required to follow the manufacturer's instructions *exactly* for each test procedure.

Instructions include information needed to perform quality control procedures, collect and handle the specimen, and test the specimen. Quality control procedures are of particular importance to ensure that the analyzer is functioning properly and that the test results are reliable and accurate. An overview of quality control procedures for CLIA-waived blood chemistry analyzers is presented next while more detailed information on quality control procedures is presented in Chapter 15.

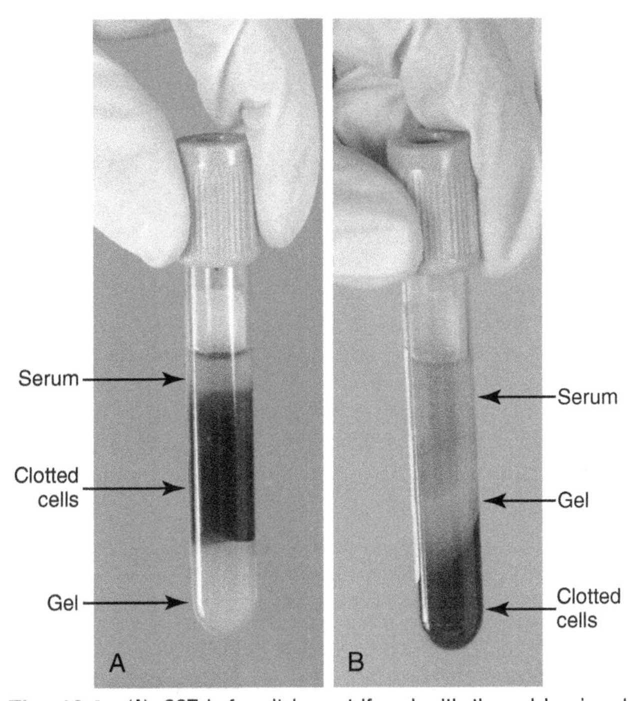

Fig. 19.2 (A), SST before it is centrifuged with the gel barrier at the bottom of the tube. (B) After centrifuging, the gel barrier provides a physical barrier between the serum and the clot. (From Garrels M. *Laboratory and diagnostic testing in ambulatory care*, ed 4, St Louis, 2019, Elsevier)

QUALITY CONTROL

The ultimate goal when performing a blood chemistry test is to ensure that the test accurately measures what it is supposed to measure; this involves practicing and maintaining a quality control program. Quality control consists of methods and means to ensure that test results are reliable and valid. Two important quality control procedures must be performed routinely when a blood chemistry analyzer is used: these procedures include a calibration procedure and a control procedure.

Calibration Procedure

Calibration is a mechanism used to check the precision and accuracy of a blood chemistry analyzer, to determine if the system is providing accurate results. Calibration detects errors caused by laboratory equipment that is not working properly. The calibration procedure is typically performed using a calibration device known as a *standard.* The standard may come in the form of a calibration strip, cassette, or code key. The standard is inserted into the analyzer (Fig. 19.6A) and the calibration results are printed out or displayed on the screen of the analyzer. The calibration results are then compared with the expected results provided in the package insert accompanying the calibration device or on

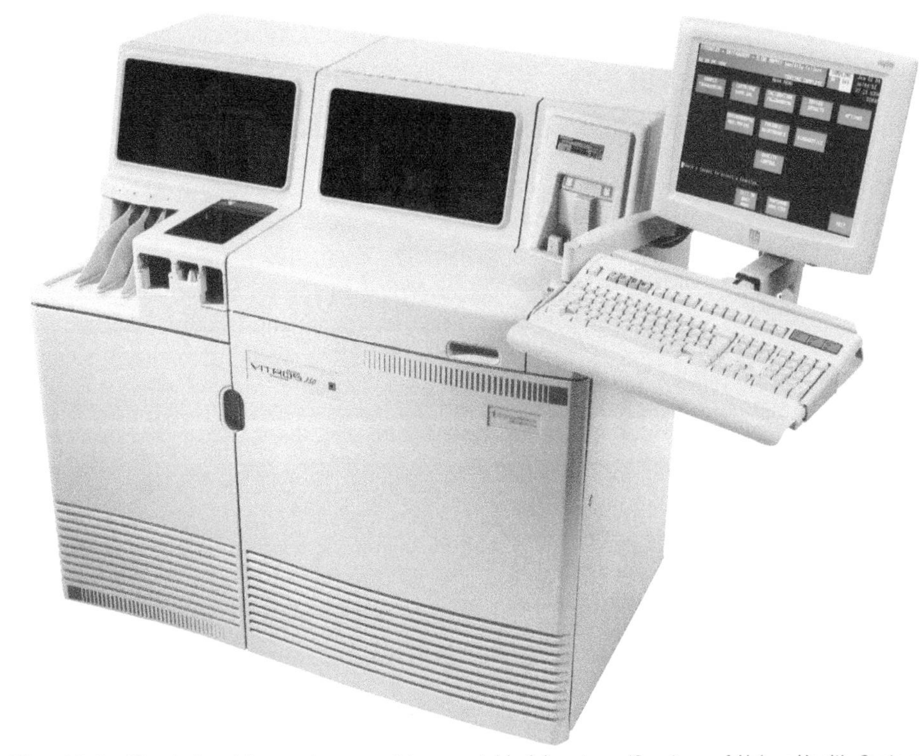

Fig. 19.3 Blood chemistry analyzer used in an outside laboratory. (Courtesy of Holzer Health Systems, Athens, OH.)

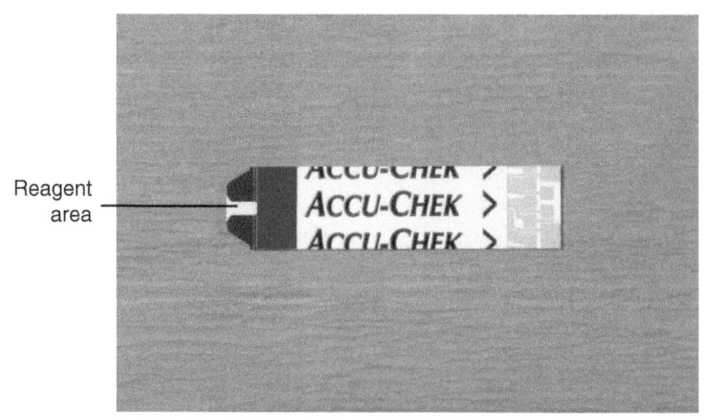

Fig. 19.4 Reagent area of a test strip.

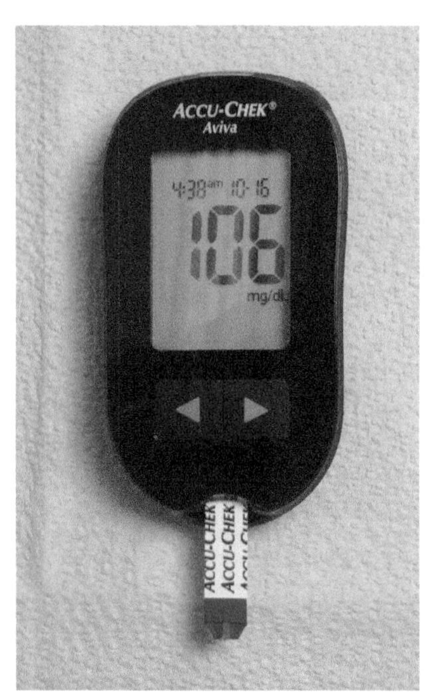

Fig. 19.5 Test results displayed on a CLIA-waived blood chemistry analyzer.

the calibration device itself (see Fig. 19.6B). If the calibration procedure does not perform as expected, patient testing should not be conducted until the problem has been identified and resolved. The frequency of performing the calibration procedure is indicated in the manufacturer's instructions. At a minimum, the calibration procedure should be performed when a new lot number of test reagents is put into use.

Some blood chemistry analyzers, such as blood glucose meters, are manufactured with *no-code* technology. This means that the glucose meter does not require calibration; the meter automatically calibrates itself when a test strip is inserted into the meter. A no-code glucose meter eliminates having to perform the calibration procedure and also eliminates errors in technique when calibrating the meter.

Control Procedure

A blood chemistry control is a solution with a known value used to monitor a blood chemistry analyzer to ensure reliable and accurate test results. It typically comes with a package insert, which lists expected ranges for control results (Fig. 19.7); however, expected ranges may sometimes be printed on the test reagent container. Controls are used to determine if the test reagents are performing properly and to detect any errors in technique by the individual performing the test.

Generally, two levels of controls must be performed on a blood chemistry analyzer. A *low-level control* (also known as a *Level 1 control*) produces results that fall below the reference range for the test, and a *high-level control* (also known as a *Level 2 control*) produces results that fall above the reference range for the test. The control procedure is performed using the same procedure for performing the test on a patient; however, instead of adding the patient specimen to the test device, the control is added to it (Fig. 19.8). The control results are compared with expected results provided in the package insert or on the test reagent container label (Fig. 19.9).

Failure of a control to produce expected results may be due to the following: expired test components, improper storage of test components, improper environmental testing conditions, and errors in the technique used to perform the procedure. If the controls do not perform as expected, patient testing should not be conducted until the problem has been identified and resolved.

The frequency of performing the control procedure is specified in the manufacturer's instructions accompanying the test system and usually includes:

- When first receiving the test system
- For periodic routine checking of analyzers and test reagents
- When a new lot number of test reagents is used
- When the test system does not seem to be working properly
- When the test results do not seem to be accurate
- When the test components have been improperly stored
- When an analyzer has been dropped or damaged.

BLOOD CHEMISTRY TESTS

The most common CLIA-waived blood chemistry tests performed in the medical office include random blood glucose,

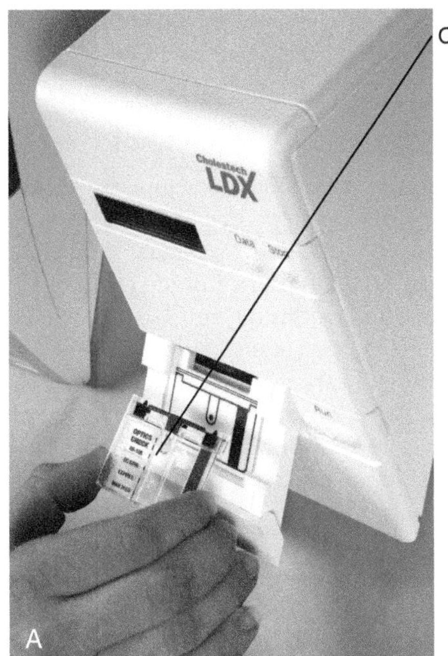

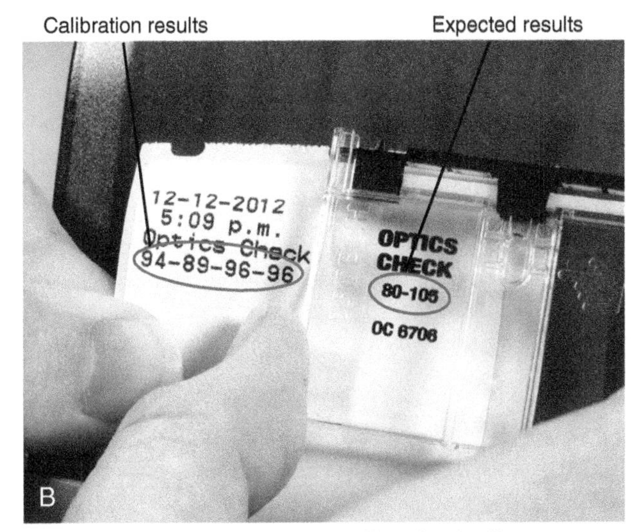

Fig. 19.6 (A), Calibrating a blood chemistry analyzer using a calibration standard. (B) The printed calibration results are compared with the expected results on the calibration standard.

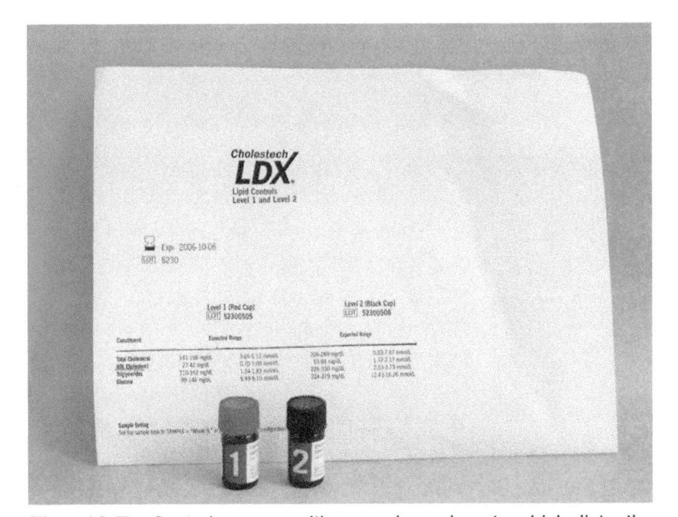

Fig. 19.7 Controls come with a package insert, which lists the expected ranges for control results.

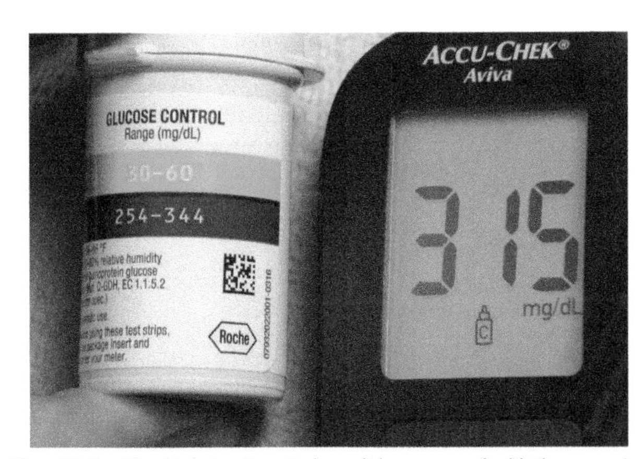

Fig. 19.9 The high-level control result is compared with the expected results.

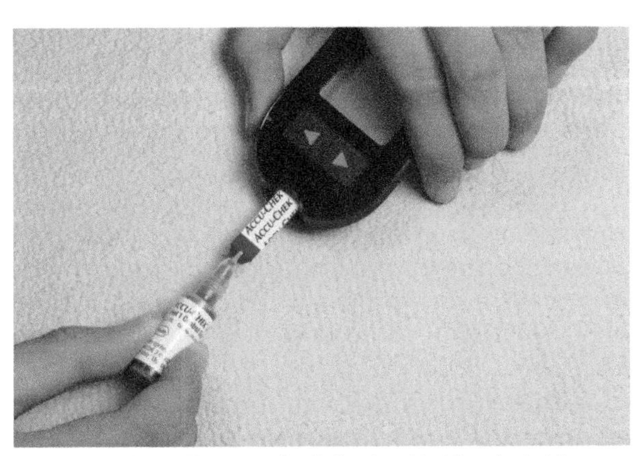

Fig. 19.8 The control solution is added to a test strip.

fasting blood glucose, hemoglobin A_{1c}, and cholesterol which are described here in more detail.

BLOOD GLUCOSE TESTS

Glucose is the end product of carbohydrate metabolism and is the chief source of energy for the body. Energy is needed for normal body functioning and for maintaining body temperature. The body maintains a constant blood glucose level to ensure a continuous source of energy for the body. Ingested glucose that is not needed for energy can be stored for later use in the form of **glycogen** in muscle and liver tissue. When no more tissue storage is possible, excess glycogen is converted to triglycerides (a form of fat) and is stored as adipose tissue.

Insulin is a hormone secreted by the beta cells of the pancreas and is required for normal utilization of glucose in the body. Insulin enables glucose to enter the body's cells and be converted to energy. Insulin also is needed for the proper storage of glycogen in liver and muscle cells.

Measuring the amount of glucose in a blood specimen is one of the most commonly performed blood chemistry tests. It is used to detect abnormalities in carbohydrate metabolism such as those that occur with prediabetes, diabetes, gestational diabetes, hypoglycemia, and liver and adrenocortical dysfunction.

Blood glucose is measured by several different types of tests. Each of these tests serves a specific role in diagnosing and evaluating abnormalities in carbohydrate metabolism. Glucose tests include the following: random blood glucose test, fasting blood glucose test, 2-hour postprandial blood glucose test, and the oral glucose tolerance test.

Random Blood Glucose Test

A random blood glucose test can be performed at any time of day on a nonfasting patient. In the medical office, this test is performed using a CLIA-waived analyzer as a screening measure to detect the presence of hyperglycemia and hypoglycemia. **Hyperglycemia** is defined as an abnormally high level of glucose in the blood. **Hypoglycemia** is defined as an abnormally low level of glucose in the blood. An elevated blood glucose level of 200 of mg/dL or higher on a random blood glucose test typically means the patient has diabetes; however, more specific tests must be performed to make a diagnosis. Random blood glucose testing is also performed by patients with diabetes as part of their diabetes management plan.

Fasting Blood Glucose Test

Blood glucose is often measured when the patient is in a fasting state. This type of test is known as a *fasting blood glucose* (FBG) test. Fasting requires that a patient not have anything to eat or drink except water for 8 to 12 hours preceding the test. Certain medications, such as oral contraceptives, antidepressants, beta-blockers, and corticosteroids, may affect the test results, and because of this, the provider may place the patient on medication restrictions for a specific period of time before the test—usually 3 days. The patient is typically scheduled for the test in the morning to minimize the inconvenience of abstaining from food and fluid. The FBG test provides more specific information as compared with a random blood glucose test.

The FBG test may be performed in the medical office using a CLIA-waived analyzer to screen patients for prediabetes and diabetes. **Prediabetes** is a condition in which glucose levels are higher than normal, but not high enough to be classified as diabetes. An individual with prediabetes has an increased risk of developing type 2 diabetes. Guidelines recommended by the American Diabetes Association (ADA) for interpretation of FBG test results are outlined in Table 19.2. A FBG test is routinely performed (along with random glucose testing) by patients diagnosed with diabetes to evaluate their progress and regulate treatment. Procedure 19.1 presents the procedure for performing a fasting blood glucose test using a CLIA-waived glucose analyzer.

Two-Hour Postprandial Blood Glucose Test

The two-hour postprandial blood glucose (2-hour PPBG) test is used to screen for diabetes and to monitor the effects of insulin dosage in patients with diabetes. The patient is required to fast, beginning at midnight preceding the test and continuing until breakfast. For breakfast, the patient must consume a prescribed meal that contains 100 g of carbohydrate, which consists of orange juice, cereal with sugar, toast, and milk. An alternative to this is the consumption of a 100 g test-load glucose solution. A blood specimen is collected from the patient exactly 2 hours after consumption of the meal or glucose solution.

In a nondiabetic patient, the glucose level returns to the fasting level within 1½ to 2 hours of glucose consumption, whereas the glucose level in a diabetic patient does not return to the fasting level. A postprandial glucose level of 140 g/dL or higher suggests diabetes and warrants further testing, such as the oral glucose tolerance test or the hemoglobin A_{1c} test. A 2-hour PPBG test may also be performed by diabetic patients at home to help regulate their insulin dosage.

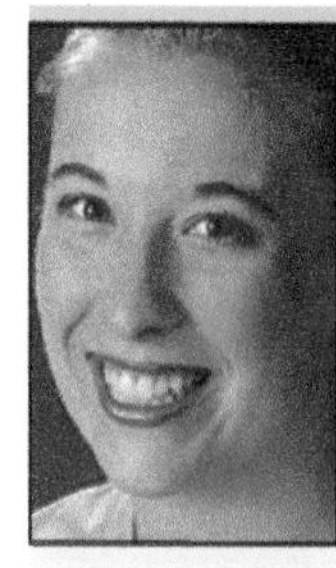

Putting It All Into Practice

My name is Michelle, and I work for a physician in an internal medicine medical office. My responsibilities include working up patients, running electrocardiograms, applying Holter monitors, and performing pulmonary function tests. I also draw blood and perform CLIA-waived laboratory tests. When performing a venipuncture, you need to make sure all the necessary supplies are on hand and ready for use. Sometimes you may have a tube that has no vacuum in it. In cases like this, it is always better to have a couple of spare tubes on hand. I recently had an experience in which I was collecting a blood specimen for a blood chemistry panel and my SST had no vacuum. Luckily, I had extra tubes within arm's reach, so I did not have to interrupt the procedure to get a new one. I have learned that you can never be too prepared. ■

Oral Glucose Tolerance Test

The oral glucose tolerance test (OGTT) provides more detailed information about the ability of the body to metabolize glucose by assessing the insulin response to a glucose load. The OGTT is used to assist in the diagnosis of prediabetes, diabetes, gestational diabetes, hypoglycemia, and liver and adrenocortical dysfunction. It provides a more thorough analysis of glucose utilization than is provided by the

Table 19.2 American Diabetes Association Guidelines for the Interpretation of Fasting Blood Glucose Test Results

FBG Test Result	Interpretation
70–99 mg/dL	Normal
100–125 mg/dL	Prediabetes (also termed *impaired fasting glucose*)
126 mg/dL or above	Diabetes (confirm by repeating the FBG test on another day)

FBG, Fasting blood glucose.

FBG test or the 2-hour PPBG test. The OGTT is usually performed at an outside laboratory; however, the medical assistant is often responsible for providing the patient with instructions regarding this test.

Test Requirements

The patient is required to consume a high-carbohydrate diet, consisting of 150 g of carbohydrate per day, for 3 days before the OGTT. High carbohydrate foods include bread, pasta, cereal, rice, potatoes, and crackers. The provider will relay to the patient what medication (if any) to discontinue before the test. The patient must be instructed not to eat or drink anything except water for 8 to 12 hours before the test.

When the patient arrives at the test site, a blood specimen is drawn from the patient for a FBG test. The patient is then instructed to drink a very sweet solution containing 75 g of glucose within a 5-minute time frame. At regular intervals (60, 120, and 180 minutes), a blood specimen is collected to determine the patient's ability to handle the increased amount of glucose. Each blood specimen is carefully labeled with the exact time of collection. The patient is permitted to eat and drink normally after completion of the test.

It is important that the patient adhere to certain restrictions during the test to ensure accurate results. Because food and fluid affect blood glucose levels, the patient must not eat or drink anything except small sips of water during the test. Smoking is not permitted during the test because tobacco is a stimulant that increases the blood glucose level. The patient must remain at the test site for 3 to 4 hours to be available for the collection of blood specimens and to minimize activity. Activity affects the test results by using up glucose; the patient should remain relatively inactive during the test. Sitting and reading is an activity that would be recommended.

Side Effects

During the test, the patient may experience some normal side effects, including weakness, a feeling of faintness, and perspiration. These are considered normal reactions of the body to a decrease in the glucose level as insulin is secreted in response to the glucose load. The patient should be reassured that this is a temporary condition. Serious symptoms of severe hypoglycemia that should be reported immediately include headache; pale, cold, and clammy skin; irrational speech or behavior; profuse perspiration; and fainting.

Interpretation of Results

As glucose is absorbed into the bloodstream, the blood glucose level of a nondiabetic individual increases to a peak level of 160 to 180 mg/dL approximately 30 to 60 minutes after the glucose solution is consumed. The pancreas secretes insulin to compensate for this rise, and the blood glucose returns to the fasting level within 2 hours of ingestion of the glucose solution.

An individual with diabetes does not exhibit the normal use of glucose just described. This is because patients with diabetes are unable to remove glucose from the bloodstream at the same rate as nondiabetic individuals. The blood glucose peaks at a much higher level. In addition, blood glucose levels are above normal throughout the test because of the lack of insulin or the inability of the body to use the insulin it does produce (insulin resistance). Two hours after the glucose solution is consumed, the test results are interpreted according to guidelines set forth by the ADA as outlined in Table 19.3.

The OGTT is also used to diagnose hypoglycemia. During the OGTT, individuals with hypoglycemia exhibit an abnormally low blood glucose level, beginning at the 2-hour interval and continuing for 4 or 5 hours. Hypoglycemia results from the removal of glucose from the blood at an excessive rate, or from an increased secretion of insulin into the blood, which can be caused by anorexia, bacterial sepsis, carcinoma of the pancreas, hepatic necrosis, or hypothyroidism.

What Would You Do? What Would You *Not* Do?

Case Study 1

Bianca Diaz previously came to the medical office complaining of symptoms that typically occur with diabetes. A random blood glucose test was performed on Bianca at the medical office and the test results indicated an elevated blood glucose level. The provider ordered an oral glucose tolerance test (OGTT) for Bianca to be performed at an outside laboratory. The instructions for the test were explained to Bianca and she was provided with an information sheet to take home. Bianca returns to the office 1 week later for her OGTT results. Bianca says that she tried to fast but got extremely hungry while driving to the test site and stopped at McDonald's for a sausage biscuit and orange juice. Bianca says she got quite upset when the test could not be performed requiring her to return to the lab a second time. She demands to know why this test takes so long and why she can't have anything to eat before the test. Bianca also wants to know why she was not allowed to go outside to take a walk and smoke during the test. She says that it's boring to sit so long at the test site and that she's a "nicotine" addict and it's hard to go very long without smoking. Bianca says that she felt weak and perspired a little during the test but did not say anything and wants to know if those symptoms were normal. ■

Table 19.3 American Diabetes Association Guidelines for the Interpretation of Oral Glucose Tolerance Test Results

OGTT Test Result	Interpretation
Less than 140 mg/dL	Normal
140–199 mg/dL	Prediabetes (also known as *impaired glucose tolerance*)
200 mg/dL or above	Diabetes (confirm by repeating the OGTT test on another day)

OGTT, Oral glucose tolerance test.

Table 19.4 American Diabetes Association Guidelines for the Interpretation of Hemoglobin A_{1c} Test Results

Hb A1c Test Result	Interpretation
Less than 5.7%	Normal
5.7% to 6.4%	Prediabetes (also known as *impaired glucose tolerance*)
6.5% or higher	Diabetes

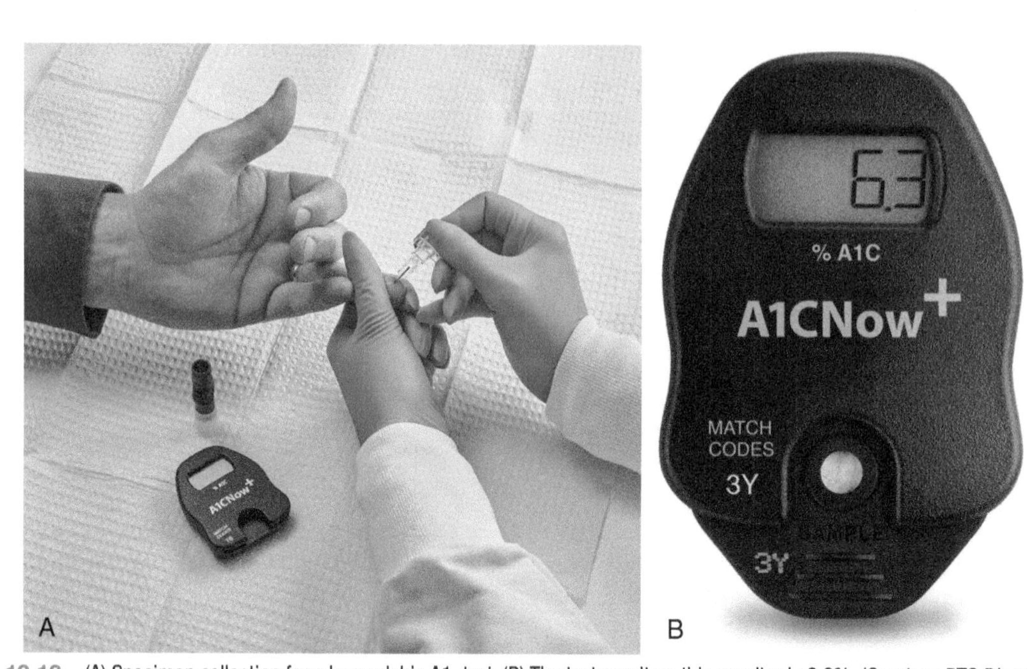

Fig. 19.10 (A) Specimen collection for a hemoglobin $A1_c$ test. (B) The test result on this monitor is 6.3%. (Courtesy PTS Diagnostics.)

HEMOGLOBIN A_{1C} TEST

The hemoglobin A_{1c} test (Hb A_{1c} test or A_{1c} test) is used to assist in the diagnosis of prediabetes and diabetes. It is also used to determine whether a diabetic patient's blood glucose level is under good control. The A_{1c} test supplies the provider with an assessment of the average amount of glucose in the blood over a 3-month period.

When an individual consumes food containing glucose, the glucose is absorbed from the digestive tract and into the circulatory system. Glucose (sugar) has a "sticky" quality to it and thus has a tendency to stick to protein in the body. One of the proteins it attaches to is the protein making up hemoglobin. Hemoglobin is found in red blood cells and functions in transporting oxygen in the body. The process of glucose attaching to hemoglobin is known as **glycosylation.**

When glucose attaches or glycosylates to the protein in hemoglobin, it forms a compound known as **hemoglobin A_{1c}**. Glycosylation occurs in all individuals—hemoglobin A_{1c} is formed in diabetic patients and healthy individuals. The amount of glucose that attaches to hemoglobin is proportional to the amount of glucose in the blood; the more glucose in the blood, the more hemoglobin becomes glycosylated and the higher the A_{1c} level. Individuals with undiagnosed or poorly controlled diabetes have a higher-than-normal blood glucose level, and more hemoglobin A_{1c} forms in these individuals. The percentage of hemoglobin A_{1c} in the blood can be measured by the A_{1c} test. The attachment of the glucose to the hemoglobin is permanent for the life of the red blood cell (90 to 120 days); because of this, the A_{1c} test result is able to provide an overall picture of the patient's blood glucose level for the past 3 months. CLIA-waived analyzers are available for performing a hemoglobin A_{1c} test in the medical office; an example is the A1c Now (Bayer Corporation) which is illustrated in Fig. 19.10.

Test Results

The Hb A_{1c} test results are reported as a percentage; the higher the percentage, the higher the blood glucose level. The ADA guidelines for the interpretation of Hb A_{1c} test results are outlined in Table 19.4.

The A_{1c} test is also used for the management of diabetes to evaluate the effectiveness of a patient's diabetes management plan. The normal A_{1c} level for an individual without diabetes is less than 5.7%. Patients with diabetes usually have a higher A_{1c} level than this. The ADA strongly recommends that patients with diabetes maintain an A_{1c} level of less than 7%. Table 19.5 shows the correlation between hemoglobin A_{1c} percentages and average blood glucose levels. A change in a patient's diabetes management plan is almost always required if the A_{1c} test result is greater than 8%. Patients who keep their hemoglobin A_{1c} levels close to 7% have a much better chance of delaying or preventing diabetic complications than do patients with A_{1c} levels that are 8% or higher.

For stable diabetic patients under good control, the A_{1c} test is typically ordered at least 2 times a year (every 6 months). The test is ordered on a more frequent basis for patients who have difficulty maintaining control of their blood glucose levels. The A_{1c} test also is ordered when the provider makes an adjustment to a patient's diabetes management plan to assess the effectiveness of the change in treatment.

Memories *from* Practicum

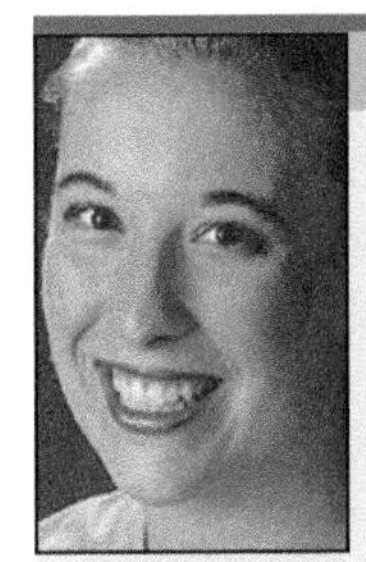

Michelle: During my practicum experience, I was assigned to a four-physician pediatric practice. The office was constantly busy with screaming children. As if I were not nervous enough, I was asked to assist in the removal of sutures. When I walked into the room with the physician, beads of sweat began to form on my forehead. A child was laying on the examining table—a little boy no more than 7 years old. He was there to have sutures removed from a recent surgery. The sutures had been tied very well, and it was difficult for the physician to remove them. The little boy lay there with tears streaming down his cheeks. I reassured him and talked to him, and his tears began to subside. "A few more minutes and it will be all over," I told him. And within those next few minutes, the physician cut the last suture. The little boy eagerly hopped down off the examining table and gave me a big hug. I learned that day how a little reassurance can make everyone involved feel better. ■

PATIENT COACHING Diabetes

Answer questions patients have about diabetes.

What is diabetes?

Diabetes is a lifelong condition that occurs when the body is not able to use glucose for energy because of a problem with insulin. Diabetes develops when the body produces little or no insulin or when the body cannot use the insulin it does produce (known as *insulin resistance*). According to the American Diabetes Association, more than 34 million Americans have diabetes (1 in 10 individuals); of these, nearly 7 million are not yet diagnosed and are unaware that they have diabetes. An additional 88 million people have prediabetes (1 in 3 individuals) which gives them an increased risk of developing type 2 diabetes.

What is the function of insulin?

Insulin is a hormone produced and secreted by the beta cells of the pancreas. The pancreas is a gland located behind and below the stomach and is about the size of a hand. Insulin is required for the normal use of glucose in the body. Through the process of digestion, carbohydrates are broken down into glucose. Shortly after a meal containing carbohydrates is consumed, glucose levels in the blood begin to increase. This sends a message to the pancreas to secrete insulin. Insulin acts like a key to "unlock" the cells of the body and allow glucose to enter the cells which lowers the glucose level in the blood. Inside the cells, glucose is converted into energy. Glucose is the main source of energy for the body and is needed to carry out normal body functions and to assist in maintaining body temperature.

What are the symptoms of diabetes?

Individuals with diabetes produce little or no insulin or cannot use the insulin they do produce (insulin resistance). Without insulin or proper insulin utilization, glucose cannot enter the cells of the body, causing it to build up in the bloodstream, resulting in a high blood glucose level or hyperglycemia. Although blood glucose levels are increased, the body is unable to use the glucose for energy because it cannot enter the cells to be converted to energy. This results in increased hunger, weight loss, and fatigue. The body attempts to get rid of the excess glucose by expelling it in the urine. To be excreted, the glucose must be diluted in large amounts of water. This results in frequent urination and increased thirst to replace the water being lost. A summary of the symptoms of diabetes include:

- Frequent urination
- Increased thirst
- Unintended weight loss
- Increased hunger
- Nausea and vomiting
- Abdominal pain
- Fatigue
- Blurred vision

What is the difference between type 1 diabetes and type 2 diabetes?

Two main categories of diabetes have been identified: type 1 diabetes and type 2 diabetes. Type 2 diabetes is the most common type; approximately 90%– 95% of individuals with diabetes have type 2 diabetes.

Type 1 Diabetes

Type 1 diabetes can occur at any age but is most apt to begin in childhood, adolescence, or early adulthood (before age 30). Type 1 diabetes is an autoimmune disease in which the body produces antibodies that attack and gradually destroy the insulin-producing beta cells of the pancreas. This results in an inability of the body to produce any insulin at all, or it may produce very little insulin. The symptoms are usually severe and occur rapidly—typically over weeks or months. Individuals with type 1 diabetes almost always require insulin therapy. The insulin is administered subcutaneously using an insulin syringe/needle or an insulin pen. An insulin pen is an insulin injection device that is either disposable or reusable. A *disposable insulin pen* contains a prefilled insulin cartridge. After use, the entire pen unit is discarded. A *reusable inulin pen* contains a replaceable

Continued

PATIENT COACHING Diabetes—cont'd

cartridge filled with insulin. Once empty, the patient discards the cartridge and replaces it with a new one. The patient must replace the disposable needle on a reusable pen after each insulin injection.

Insulin also can be administered through an insulin pump, which is a small, computerized device that is clipped to a belt or carried in a pocket (see illustration). The pump continually delivers insulin to the subcutaneous tissue of the abdomen. This is accomplished through a length of tubing leading from the pump to a thin cannula placed under the patient's skin. An insulin pump also can be programmed to deliver varying doses of insulin as a patient's need for insulin changes during the day (e.g., before exercise or meals).

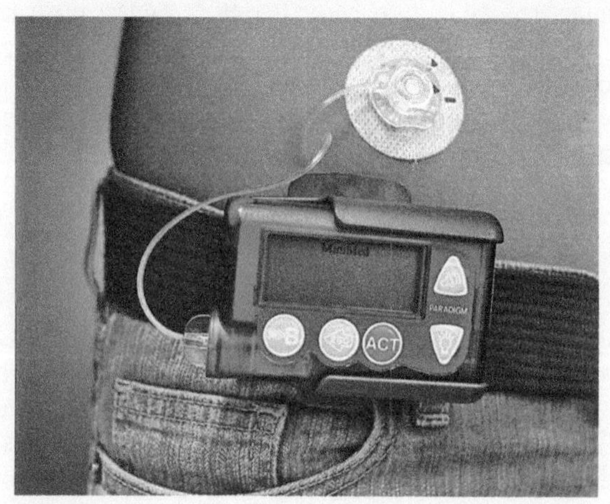

Insulin pump. (From Lewis S. *Medical-surgical nursing,* ed 9, St Louis: Mosby; 2014.)

Type 2 Diabetes

Type 2 diabetes is usually caused by insulin resistance meaning the body can produce insulin but is unable to use the insulin it produces resulting in high blood glucose levels. Type 2 diabetes can affect people at any age, but the chance of developing it increases with age, and is more likely to occur in individuals 45 years of age and older. The biggest risk factor for developing type 2 diabetes is excess body weight. As a result of the recent increase in childhood obesity combined with a sedentary lifestyle, type 2 diabetes is starting to appear in younger age groups (children, teens, and young adults). Type 2 diabetes almost always has a slow onset with mild symptoms that appear gradually over a long time (often years). Some individuals have no symptoms at all (except for elevated glucose levels). Because of this, they may be unaware that they have diabetes until a complication from prolonged hyperglycemia occurs, such as a vision problem or foot pain. Type 2 diabetes is first treated by dietary adjustments, weight reduction, and exercise. These changes sometimes can restore insulin sensitivity, even if the weight loss is modest. Approximately 20% of cases of type 2 diabetes can be managed by lifestyle changes alone. The next step, if necessary, is treatment with oral hypoglycemics, which are medications taken by mouth that stimulate the release of insulin from the pancreas or help the body use its own insulin better, or both. If this treatment is ineffective, insulin therapy becomes necessary to maintain normal or near-normal glucose levels.

What factors increase the risk of developing type 2 diabetes?

The cause of type 2 diabetes is unknown, although certain factors, known as *risk factors,* make a person more prone to developing it. The more risk factors present, the more likely it is that an individual will develop type 2 diabetes. Some of these factors can be controlled, and others cannot.

Risk Factors That Can Be Controlled

1. *Weight.* The risk factor that contributes most to the development of type 2 diabetes is excess body weight. Approximately 90% of individuals with type 2 diabetes are overweight or obese. Being overweight or obese (body mass index of 25 or greater) makes it harder for the body to use insulin. Research shows that people who followed a low-fat, low-calorie diet; lost a moderate amount of weight; and engaged in regular physical activity (five times a week for 30 min) sharply reduced their chances of developing type 2 diabetes.
2. *Fat distribution.* Storing fat primarily in the abdomen, rather than the hips and thighs, is a risk factor for diabetes. Men with a waist measurement above 40 inches (101.6 cm) and women with a waist measurement above 35 inches (88.9 cm) are at increased risk for type 2 diabetes.
3. *Smoking.* Smoking makes it harder for the body to regulate insulin levels. High levels of nicotine decrease the effectiveness of insulin, causing the body to require more insulin to regulate the blood glucose level.
4. *Lack of physical activity.* Regular exercise helps the body to use insulin normally, whereas a sedentary lifestyle contributes to insulin resistance.
5. *Prediabetes.* Left untreated, prediabetes often progresses to type 2 diabetes.
6. *High blood pressure, abnormal lipid panel, or both.* The following factors contribute to insulin resistance: a blood pressure greater than 130/80 mm Hg, HDL cholesterol less than 40 mg/dL for a man and less than 50 mg/dL for a woman, and a triglycerides level of 150 mg/dL or greater. Decreasing blood pressure also can reduce the risk of cardiovascular complications.

Risk Factors That Cannot Be Controlled

1. *Family history.* The risk of developing type 2 diabetes is increased if a close relative (parent or sibling) has type 2 diabetes.
2. *Gestational diabetes or giving birth to a large infant.* Women who have diabetes during pregnancy or gave birth to an infant weighing more than 9 lb are at greater risk for developing type 2 diabetes.
3. *Age.* Type 2 diabetes is more common in people 45 years and older.
4. *Ethnic group.* The following ethnic groups are more likely to develop type 2 diabetes: African Americans, Latinos, Hispanics, Native Americans, Asian Americans, and Pacific Islanders.

Can diabetes be cured?

There is no cure for diabetes, but the outlook for individuals with this condition is improving. This is primarily due to better patient education, advances in blood glucose monitoring, and newer methods of insulin delivery that help simplify management of the disease. Today, most individuals with diabetes under good control have life expectancies comparable with those of individuals without diabetes. ■

Table 19.5 Comparison of Hemoglobin A_{1c} Percentages With Blood Glucose Levels

Hemoglobin A_{1c} (%)	Average Daily Blood Glucose Level (mg/dL)
5	100
6	126
6.5	140
7	154
7.5	169
8	183
8.5	197
9	212
9.5	226
10	240
10.5	254

What Would You Do? What Would You *Not* Do?

Case Study 2

Jackson Williams has recently been diagnosed with type 1 diabetes and is taking insulin. He has come to the office for an FBG test. A finger puncture is performed to collect the specimen and a glucose meter is used to test the specimen. Jackson has been performing this test on himself at home now for 2 weeks and wants to know whether he can stick his own finger and have someone watch him to make sure he is doing it correctly. Jackson says that he's been having a few problems giving himself his insulin injections. He says that he has been getting some very large air bubbles in his syringe when he draws up the insulin. He says he's been having trouble getting them out and wants to know how important that is. Jackson says he is on a limited income and wants to know whether he could use his needle and syringe for more than one injection. ■

MANAGEMENT OF DIABETES

It is important that individuals with diabetes manage their condition effectively. This is best accomplished by keeping blood glucose levels as close to normal as possible. Diabetic patients who maintain good blood glucose control generally experience fewer symptoms and delay or prevent long-term complications of the disease leading to a longer and healthier life.

Two testing methods are used for the management of diabetes: self-monitoring of blood glucose and the hemoglobin A_{1c} test. Self-monitoring of blood glucose, which diabetic patients perform at home, measures day-to-day fluctuations in blood glucose levels. The hemoglobin A_{1c} test must be ordered by the provider and provides an average or overall picture of the patient's blood glucose levels over time. These testing methods assist the patient and the provider in determining whether the diabetes management plan is working or whether it needs to be adjusted. SMBG is described in more detail as follows.

SELF-MONITORING OF BLOOD GLUCOSE

Individuals with diabetes cannot usually tell by the way they feel whether or not their blood glucose levels are within normal range. The only way for them to know for certain is by self-monitoring of blood glucose (SMBG). SMBG not only provides diabetic patients with feedback for maintaining normal blood glucose levels, but it also assists them in anticipating and treating day-to-day, or even hour-to-hour, fluctuations in glucose levels brought on by food, exercise, stress, and illness.

Diabetic patients who take insulin (insulin dependent) must monitor their blood glucose levels each day. Based on the results of SMBG, decisions can be made regarding insulin and dietary adjustments that may be necessary to maintain normal glucose levels and to avoid the extremes of hypoglycemia and hyperglycemia. Satisfactory control of the blood glucose level on a day-to-day basis through SMBG reduces symptoms of the disease and helps delay or prevent long-term complications that can occur with diabetes.

Frequency of Testing

The frequency of blood glucose testing is determined by a patient's provider and depends on the following factors: the severity of the diabetes, type of treatment, diet, activity level, and special conditions such as pregnancy. Ideally, the blood glucose level for an insulin-dependent diabetic patient should be measured four times a day: in the morning (after an 8-hour fast), before lunch, before dinner, and at bedtime. The blood glucose level should also be measured if the patient is experiencing symptoms indicative of hyperglycemia or hypoglycemia. The FBG test result (obtained in the morning) is the best overall indicator of control, and the other glucose determinations provide guidance for adjusting insulin dosage, diet, and exercise.

Glucose Monitoring Devices

Blood glucose levels can be monitored by a patient with diabetes with a glucose meter or a continuous monitoring device (CMD).

- *Glucose Meter:* A glucose meter is a small, portable, battery-operated device that quantitatively measures the blood glucose level in a capillary blood specimen. The medical assistant may be responsible for instructing the patient in the procedure for using a glucose meter which is outlined in Procedure 19.1.
- *Continuous Monitoring Device:* A CMD measures a patient's blood glucose level continuously throughout the day and night using a sensor inserted under the

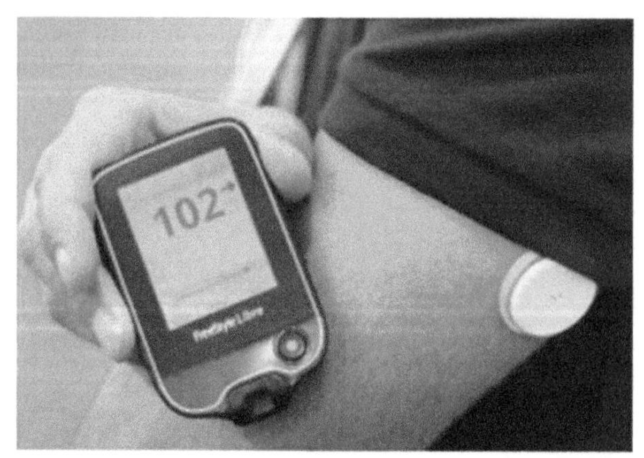

Fig. 19.11 Continuous glucose monitor. (FreeStyle Libre is a trademark of Abbott or its related companies. Reproduced with permission of Abbott, © 2022. All rights reserved.)

patient's skin; brand names include the Dexcom System (Dexcom, Inc., San Diego, CA) and the FreeStyle Libre System (Abbott, Chicago, IL). The CMD provides real-time measurements and reduces the need for a finger puncture. The CGM also sends an alert to the patient if the blood glucose level becomes high or low. Depending on the CMD brand, the sensor can last up to two weeks before needing to be replaced. The glucose readings are viewed by the patient on a special receiver device or a smart phone (Fig. 19.11).

Target Blood Glucose Levels

Target blood glucose levels for a patient with diabetes are determined by a patient's provider. The ADA recommends the following general guidelines for target blood glucose levels:

- Before meals and snacks: 80 to 130 mg/dL
- 1 to 2 hours after meals: Less than 180 mg/dL

Diabetic patients should maintain a cumulative record of their daily SMBG test results for periodic review by the provider. This record assists the provider in making decisions regarding the patient's diabetes management plan. Most glucose meters have a built-in memory system that stores test results along with the time and date and can transfer this data electronically to a computer. This provides for the tracking of blood glucose fluctuations over time.

Advantages

Research shows that SMBG is the most effective way for a diabetic patient to maintain normal blood glucose levels. Advantages of SMBG include the following:

1. *Delay or prevention of long-term complications.* High blood glucose levels (greater than 180 mg/dL) for a long period of time can cause progressive damage to the body organs. SMBG can delay or prevent long-term complications associated with diabetes which include the following: cardiovascular disease (CVD), blindness (retinopathy), hearing impairment, nerve damage (neuropathy), kidney damage (nephropathy), skin conditions, and poor circulation, which can result in amputation of a limb
2. *Prevention of hypoglycemia.* Hypoglycemia is a short-term complication of diabetes caused by too much insulin in the body which can be due to the administration of too much insulin, skipping meals, and unexpected or unusual exercise. The symptoms of hypoglycemia occur rapidly, usually over 5 to 20 minutes after the blood glucose level begins to decrease. Symptoms begin with sweating or cold, clammy skin, shakiness, dizziness, headache, and tachycardia. If not treated, the blood glucose level continues to drop and the patient may experience confusion, irritability, sleepiness, anxiety, problems with speaking (e.g., slurring words), and problems with vision (e.g., double-vision and blurred vision). Without treatment, serious life-threatening symptoms may occur which include seizures, loss of consciousness, and coma. Because the brain requires a constant supply of glucose for proper functioning, permanent brain damage or death can result from severe hypoglycemia (also known as insulin shock). Refer to Chapter 23 for a more thorough discussion of diabetic emergencies and the treatment required.
3. *Convenience of testing.* Patients are able to test their blood at any time of the day without a laboratory order from the provider. This allows patients to check their blood glucose level when a side effect common to diabetes occurs, such as hypoglycemia. In these situations, treatment can be instituted immediately to prevent the problem from getting worse.
4. *Greater involvement in self-management decisions.* The patient is able to become more involved in self-management decisions regarding insulin dosage, meal planning, and physical activity. More reliable decisions regarding insulin needs can be made during situations that affect the blood glucose level, such as illness, emotional stress, increased physical activity, and hypoglycemia. Initially some patients may lack confidence in making insulin and dietary adjustments based on the blood glucose results. The medical assistant should provide encouragement and emphasize the benefits to be derived in terms of improved regulation of the blood glucose level.

CHOLESTEROL TEST

CHOLESTEROL

Cholesterol is a white, waxy, fatlike substance (lipid) that is essential for normal functioning of the body. It is an important component of all cell membranes in the body and is used in the production of essential hormones and bile. Most of the cholesterol circulating in the blood is manufactured by the liver; however, a small portion of it comes from an individual's diet and is known as *dietary cholesterol.* Dietary cholesterol is found only in animal products, such as organ meats, egg yolk, and dairy products.

High blood cholesterol means an excessive amount of cholesterol is present in the blood. An individual's cholesterol level is determined by his or her genetic makeup and by the amounts of saturated fat and dietary cholesterol consumed. High blood cholesterol may cause fatty deposits, or plaque, to build up on the walls of the arteries, a condition known as *atherosclerosis.* As the atherosclerosis progresses, the arteries become more occluded, which eventually could lead to a heart attack or stroke. Because of this, high blood cholesterol is considered a risk factor for CVD. Refer to *Highlight on Cardiovascular Disease* for more information on CVD.

LIPOPROTEINS

Cholesterol is transported in the blood as a complex molecule known as a **lipoprotein**. Two types of lipoproteins contain cholesterol: low-density lipoprotein (LDL) and high-density lipoprotein (HDL).

LDL cholesterol picks up cholesterol from ingested fats and the liver and carries it in the blood. When there is too much cholesterol in the blood, the LDL cholesterol combines with other substances to form plaque on the walls of arteries resulting in atherosclerosis; because of this, LDL cholesterol is often referred to as "bad" cholesterol.

HDL cholesterol removes excess cholesterol from the walls of arteries and carries it to the liver for removal by the body. Because HDL removes excess cholesterol, it is protective and beneficial to the body and is often called "good" cholesterol. A high HDL cholesterol level has been shown

HIGHLIGHT on Cardiovascular Disease

The cardiovascular or circulatory system supplies the body with blood and consists of the heart, arteries, veins, and capillaries. *Cardiovascular disease (CVD)* is a general term used to refer to a variety of conditions that affect the heart and blood vessels and interfere with the flow of blood to the heart. CVD is the number one killer of adults in the United States today. Approximately 655,000 deaths occur each year due to CVD; this equates to 1 in every 4 deaths.

Types of Cardiovascular Disease

Types of cardiovascular disease include the following:

- Coronary artery disease (CAD): A condition in which there is a build-up of plaque in the arteries supplying blood to the heart which narrows the lumen of the arteries and reduces the flow of blood to the heart.
- High blood pressure: A condition in which there is an increased force of circulating blood against the walls of blood vessels which damages them and increases the risk of a heart attack or heart failure, stroke, or aneurysm.
- Heart attack: A condition in which there is a sudden blockage of the blood flow to a part of the heart. If the blood flow is cut off completely, the muscle tissue in that part of the heart dies.
- Stroke: A condition in which the blood supply to a part of the brain is cut off which could result in brain damage and possibly death.
- Heart failure: A condition in which the heart cannot pump as well as it should due to weakened heart muscle. It may be due to an injury to the heart muscle (e.g., uncontrolled high blood pressure), a heart attack, or a heart valve that does not work properly.
- Congenital heart disease: A condition in which the heart does not function properly because the heart did not develop normally before birth.
- Rheumatic heart disease: A condition in which the heart valves have been permanently damaged by rheumatic fever.
- Cardiomyopathy: A condition in which the heart enlarges and is unable to pump blood efficiently.
- Aortic aneurysm: A condition in which the aorta becomes weakened and bulges outwards. It may burst and cause life-threatening bleeding.
- Cardiac arrhythmias: Abnormal heart rhythms which may prevent the heart from pumping enough blood to meet the body's needs.
- Heart valve disease: A condition in which one or more of the heart valves does not work properly, interfering with the flow of blood through the heart.
- Peripheral artery disease: The build-up of plaque in the arteries supplying blood to the limbs (usually the legs) which interferes with the flow of blood to the limbs.
- Venous thrombosis: A condition in which a clot forms in a vein which interferes with the flow of blood. If a clot forms in the leg (DVT), part of the clot may break off and cause a pulmonary embolism.

Cardiovascular Disease Risk Factors

Not everyone is equal when it comes to CVD. Some individuals have a much higher risk of developing CVD than others. The following are risk factors for CVD:

- High total blood cholesterol (greater than 200 mg/dL)
- High blood pressure
- Cigarette smoking
- Atherosclerosis
- Family history of CVD
- Unhealthy diet
- Lack of physical activity
- Diabetes
- Being overweight or obese
- Low HDL cholesterol (less than 40 mg/dL)
- Elevated triglycerides level (above 150 mg/dL)
- Being a man older than 45 years
- Being a woman older than 55 years or postmenopausal

Some of these risk factors can be modified; others, such as age, gender, and a family history of CVD, cannot be modified or controlled. Each person's overall risk of CVD must be assessed individually by the provider, based on the type and number of risk factors present. A 47-year-old man with a total blood cholesterol level of 220 mg/dL who smokes a pack of cigarettes a day and is overweight is at greater risk than a 28-year-old man who has a normal weight, does not smoke, and exercises regularly but has a total blood cholesterol level of 250 mg/dL.

Continued

HIGHLIGHT on Cardiovascular Disease—cont'd

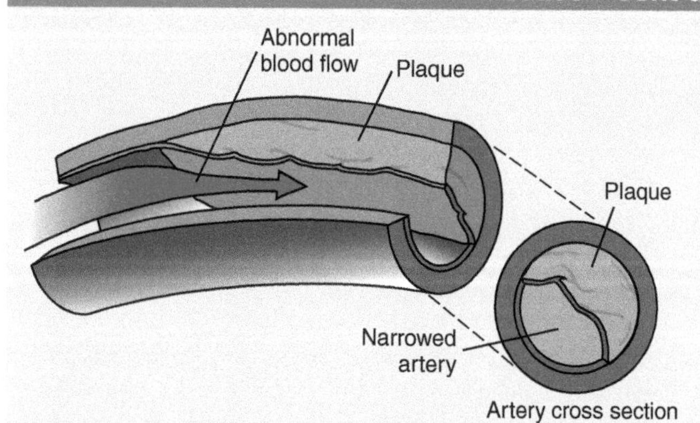

Atherosclerosis. (From Workman ML, LaCharity L. Understanding pharmacology: essentials for medication safety, ed 2, St Louis, 2018, Elsevier.)

Coronary Artery Disease

The most common type of CVD in the U.S. is coronary artery disease (CAD) which is also known as coronary heart disease. Coronary artery disease is due to atherosclerosis of the coronary arteries, which are the blood vessels that supply the heart with oxygen. *Atherosclerosis* of the coronary arteries is a condition in which fibrous plaques of fatty deposits and cholesterol build up on the inner walls of the coronary arteries. This causes narrowing and partial blockage of the lumen of these arteries, along with hardening of the arterial wall. CAD results in a reduction of oxygenated blood flow to the heart muscle. Despite the narrowing, enough oxygen may still reach the heart muscle for normal needs. More oxygen is needed, however, when situations occur that increase the workload of the heart, such as physical activity, emotional stress, a heavy meal, and exposure to cold weather. If the coronary arteries cannot deliver enough oxygen to the heart muscle during these times of increased need, angina pectoris may result. Angina pectoris occurs when the muscle tissue of the heart does not receive enough oxygenated blood, resulting in discomfort or pain under the sternum. Severe and prolonged angina pain generally suggests a myocardial infarction (heart attack) caused by complete blockage of the coronary arteries and requires immediate medical attention.

Prevention of Cardiovascular Disease

It is estimated that up to 90% of cases of CVD can be prevented by following a healthy lifestyle. This includes a healthy diet, maintaining a healthy weigh, quitting smoking, limiting alcohol consumption, and exercising regularly. Individuals who have a particularly high risk of developing CVD may be prescribed medication to reduce their risk. Depending on the patient's health status, he or she may be prescribed cholesterol-lowering medication or anti-hypertensive medication. ■

to reduce the risk of CVD whereas a low level of HDL cholesterol is a risk factor for CVD.

CHOLESTEROL TESTING

All adults older than 20 years of age should have a cholesterol test at least every 4 to 6 years. Initial testing includes a *total cholesterol* determination, which is a combined measurement of LDL cholesterol and HDL cholesterol in the blood. Cholesterol testing does not require a fasting specimen because the test results are not affected by food or beverages. If the total cholesterol level is 200 mg/dL or greater, the provider usually orders a *lipid panel,* which includes total cholesterol, HDL cholesterol, LDL cholesterol, and triglycerides. The LDL cholesterol level is usually determined as a calculation from the triglycerides and HDL cholesterol levels.

A lipid panel is often performed by an outside laboratory and the medical assistant may be responsible for collecting the blood specimen for transport to the laboratory. Most providers prefer that the patient fast for a lipid panel since the triglycerides test is affected by the consumption of food and beverages.

CLIA-waived analyzers are available for performing cholesterol testing in the medical office; an example is the Cholestech LDX Cholesterol System (Cholestech Corporation) which can perform a lipid panel and a glucose test (Fig. 19.12). It is important to follow the manufacturer's instructions *exactly* for performing the test. Quality control procedures are of particular importance to ensure that the analyzer is functioning properly, and that the test results are reliable and accurate.

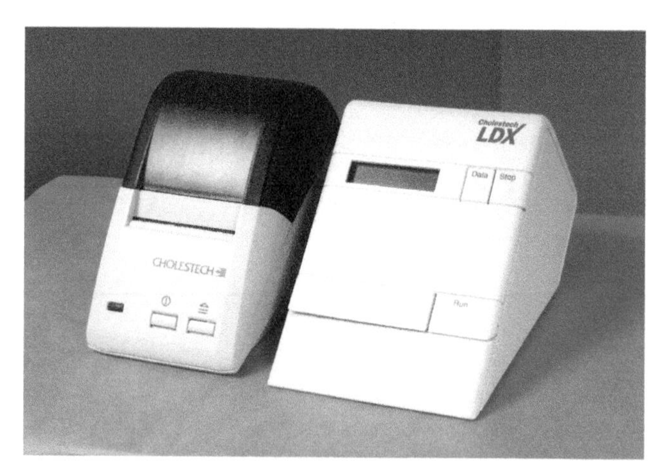

Fig. 19.12 Cholestech LDX Cholesterol System.

The results of cholesterol testing assist in determining the patient's risk for CVD. The interpretation of these results is outlined in Table 19.6. Total cholesterol test results of less than 200 mg/dL are desirable. Individuals in the high category for total cholesterol are at increased risk for CVD, and individuals in the borderline high category are at increased risk if they have other risk factors, such as being overweight or smoking. According to the American Heart Association, an HDL cholesterol level less than

What Would You Do? What Would You *Not* Do?

Case Study 3

Karen Scrimshaw is at the office. She is 20 years old and is mildly obese. Karen had her cholesterol tested at a health fair, and it was 325. The physician orders a CBC, lipid panel, and thyroid panel on Karen and tells her to return in 1 week for a follow-up visit to discuss the test results. Karen is very concerned about her cholesterol. She says that she had a candy bar and some potato chips before going to the health fair and wants to know whether that could have caused her cholesterol to be so high. She also wants to know the accuracy of machines that are used at health fairs. Karen says that if she has to go on cholesterol medication, it would be hard to decide between Lipitor and Zocor. She says she has seen them advertised on television, and they both seem pretty good to her. ■

40 mg/dL for men and less than 50 mg/dL for women is considered a risk factor for CVD. An HDL cholesterol level greater than 60 mg/dL is considered optimal and provides some protection against CVD. Refer to Fig. 19.13 for a lipid panel laboratory report.

TRIGLYCERIDES TEST

Triglycerides are the chemical form in which most fat exists in food, as well as in the body. Triglycerides are derived from two sources. The first is synthesis by the body. Ingested glucose that is not needed for energy can be stored in the form of **glycogen** in muscle and liver tissue for later use. When no more tissue storage is possible, most of the excess glycogen is synthesized by the body into triglycerides (a form of fat) and stored as adipose tissue. Excess protein not needed by the body is also converted to triglycerides and stored as adipose tissue. The second source of triglycerides is food. Excess triglycerides consumed by eating foods containing fat are also stored as adipose tissue.

Some of the triglycerides in the body are not stored as fat, but remain in the bloodstream, specifically in the plasma. Most triglycerides in the bloodstream are carried by a lipoprotein known as very-low-density lipoprotein (VLDL). In normal amounts, triglycerides are essential to good health. Triglycerides carried by the blood serve as a major source of energy for the body. An excess of blood triglycerides, however, places an individual at increased risk for CVD, particularly when the LDL cholesterol is high and the HDL cholesterol is low. Triglycerides levels in the blood are usually measured as part of a lipid panel. The interpretation of triglycerides test results are outlined in Table 19.7. Conditions that result in elevated blood triglycerides levels include obesity, type 2 diabetes, being physically inactive, excessive alcohol consumption, smoking, hypothyroidism, kidney disease, and liver disease.

BLOOD UREA NITROGEN TEST

The blood urea nitrogen (BUN) test is a kidney function test. Urea is the end product of protein metabolism and is normally present in the blood. Certain kidney diseases may interfere with the ability of the body to

Table 19.6 Interpretation of Cholesterol Test Results

Total Cholesterol Test Result (mg/dL)	Interpretation
Less than 200	Desirable
200–239	Borderline high
240 or above	High
LDL Cholesterol Test Result (mg/dL)	**Interpretation**
Less than 100	Optimal
100–129	Near optimal
130–159	Borderline high
160–189	High
190 or above	Very high
HDL Cholesterol Test Result (mg/dL)	**Interpretation**
60 or above	Optimal
Men: 40–50 Women: 50–60	Desirable
Men: Less than 40 Women: Less than 50	Increased risk for CVD

CVD, Cardiovascular disease; *HDL*, high-density lipoprotein; *LDL*, low-density lipoprotein.

LABORATORY REPORT Lipid Panel			
Patient		**Ordered by**	**Results provided by**
Elsie Mendelssohn 2963 Flint Dr. Clearwater, FL 33759 PH:740-541-3575	ID #: 336879 DOB: 4/28/1970 Age: 66 Gender: F	Thomas Murphy, MD Pinellas Medical Office 3477 Arrowhead Ave Clearwater, FL 33759	Medical Center Laboratory 33 West Main St Clearwater, FL 33759
Specimen Coll. Date	11/25/20XX	Fasting/Nonfasting	Fasting
Specimen Coll. Time	08:00 am	Accession Number	3380837
Specimen Received Date/Time	11/25/20XX 05:30 pm	Lab ID Number	773978
Results Reported Date/Time	11/26/20XX 10:00 am	Test(s) Ordered	CPT: 7600 Lipid Panel

Test	Result	Reference Range	Units	Flag
Cholesterol, Total	**230**	**<200**	**mg/dL**	**H**
HDL cholesterol	64	≥50	mg/dL	
Triglycerides	98	<150	mg/dL	
LDL Cholesterol (Calculated)	**130**	**<100**	**mg/dL**	**H**
VLDL	24	<30	mg/dL	
Cholesterol/HDL ratio	3.6	<5.0		

Fig. 19.13 Lipid panel laboratory report.

Table 19.7 Interpretation of Triglycerides Test Results

Triglycerides Test Result (mg/dL)	Interpretation
Less than 150 mg/dL	Normal
150–199 mg/dL	Borderline high
200–499 mg/dL	High
500 mg/dL or higher	Very high

excrete the urea properly, causing an increased level of urea in the blood. See Table 19.1, presented earlier, for a list of specific conditions that cause abnormal BUN test results.

Immunologic Testing

Immunology is the scientific study of antigen and antibody reactions. An **antigen** is a substance that is capable of stimulating the formation of antibodies in an individual. Antigens may consist of protein, glycoprotein, complex polysaccharides, or nucleic acid. Specific examples of antigens include bacteria and viruses, bacterial toxins, and allergen. An **antibody** is a substance that is capable of combining with an antigen, resulting in an antigen-antibody reaction.

Laboratory testing in immunology deals with studying antigen-antibody reactions to assess the presence of a substance (e.g., C-reactive protein) or to assist in the diagnosis of disease (e.g., mononucleosis). Immunologic tests are often used for the early diagnosis of disease and are used to follow the course of the disease.

IMMUNOLOGIC TESTS

Specific examples of immunologic tests are described next.

HEPATITIS TESTS

Hepatitis tests are performed to detect viral hepatitis. There are five types of viral hepatitis—A, B, C, D, and E. Hepatitis testing not only detects the presence of viral hepatitis, but it also determines the type of hepatitis present.

HIV TEST

The enzyme immune assay (EIA) test and the enzyme-linked immunosorbent assay (ELISA) test are used as screening tests for the presence of HIV. Newer rapid screening HIV test kits are also commercially available; brand names include Uni-Gold Recombigen HIV (Trinity Biotech) and

OraQuick Rapid HIV test (OraSure Technologies). Because of the possibility of a false-positive result, a second screening test is always performed if a blood specimen tests positive. If the second test also is positive, a more specific test, such as the Western blot test, is performed to confirm the test results. An individual who tests positive for HIV is seropositive.

A negative HIV test is not conclusive for the absence of HIV infection. If an individual has recently been infected with HIV, the antibodies may not have had time to develop. It generally takes 2 to 12 weeks (but possibly as long as 6 months) for the HIV antibodies to appear in the blood.

SYPHILIS TEST

Syphilis is a sexually transmitted disease (STD) caused by the microorganism *Treponema pallidum.* The most common tests used to detect the presence of syphilis are the Venereal Disease Research Laboratories (VDRL) test and the rapid plasma reagin (RPR) test. Test results are reported as nonreactive, weakly reactive, or reactive. Weakly reactive and reactive results are considered positive for the presence of syphilis antibodies. These tests are screening tests, and a positive result warrants more specific tests to arrive at a diagnosis of syphilis.

RHEUMATOID FACTOR TEST

Rheumatoid arthritis is a chronic inflammatory disease that affects the joints of the body. The blood of patients with rheumatoid arthritis contains a type of antibody called *rheumatoid factor* (RF). This test detects the presence of rheumatoid factor antibodies and assists in the diagnosis of rheumatoid arthritis.

ANTISTREPTOLYSIN O TEST

The antistreptolysin O (ASO) test is used to detect ASO antibodies in the serum; ASO antibodies are common antibodies produced by the immune system in response to a strep infection. The ASO test is the most widely used immunologic test for the detection of conditions resulting from streptococcal infections and diseases that occur secondary to a streptococcal infection. This test is useful in assisting in the diagnosis of rheumatic fever, glomerulonephritis, bacterial endocarditis, and scarlet fever.

C-REACTIVE PROTEIN TEST

During inflammation and tissue destruction, an abnormal protein called *C-reactive protein* (CRP) appears in the blood. Patients with inflammatory conditions or disorders accompanied by tissue destruction have positive results to this test. Because of this, the CRP test is used to assist in diagnosing or documenting the progress of rheumatoid arthritis, acute rheumatic fever, widespread malignancy, and bacterial infections.

COLD AGGLUTININS TEST

The cold agglutinins test is used to detect the presence of antibodies called *cold agglutinins.* This test is performed by incubating the patient's serum with erythrocytes at cold temperatures. If cold agglutinins are present, this causes agglutination of the erythrocytes. **Agglutination** refers to the clumping of red blood cells. Cold agglutinins are found in patients with infectious mononucleosis, mycoplasmal pneumonia, chronic parasitic infections, and lymphoma.

H. PYLORI TEST

Helicobacter pylori (*H. pylori*) is a bacteria that infects the digestive system. Approximately two-thirds of the world's population has *H. pylori* in their body; however, for most individuals, it does not cause a problem. In some people, the bacteria cause a variety of digestive disorders which include gastritis, ulcers of the stomach, small intestine, or esophagus, and certain types of stomach cancer. A blood test can be performed to check for the presence of antibodies to *H. pylori.* CLIA-waived rapid testing kits are available to perform this test in the medical office; brand names include Clearview *H. pylori* (Alere Inc.) and QuickVue *H. pylori* (Quidel Corporation).

MONONUCLEOSIS TEST

The mononucleosis test ("mono test") is used to detect the presence of infectious mononucleosis which is an acute infectious disease caused by the Epstein-Barr virus (EBV). Infectious mononucleosis most frequently affects children and young adults. It is transmitted through saliva by direct oral contact, and because of this, it is often called the "kissing disease." Symptoms of infectious mononucleosis include mental and physical fatigue, fever, sore throat, severe weakness, headache, and swollen lymph nodes. The mononucleosis test may be performed in the medical office using a CLIA-waived testing kit which is discussed in more detail below.

CLIA-WAIVED RAPID MONONUCLEOSIS TEST

A CLIA-waived rapid mononucleosis test is easy to perform and provides reliable results in a short time. Patients with infectious mononucleosis produce an antibody called *heterophile antibody,* usually by 6 to 10 days into the illness. Rapid mono tests detect this antibody. The presence of the heterophile antibody, along with patient symptoms, provide the basis for the diagnosis of infectious mononucleosis.

Fig. 19.14 illustrates the QuickVue+ Mononucleosis Test setup (Quidel Corporation) and Fig. 19.15 outlines

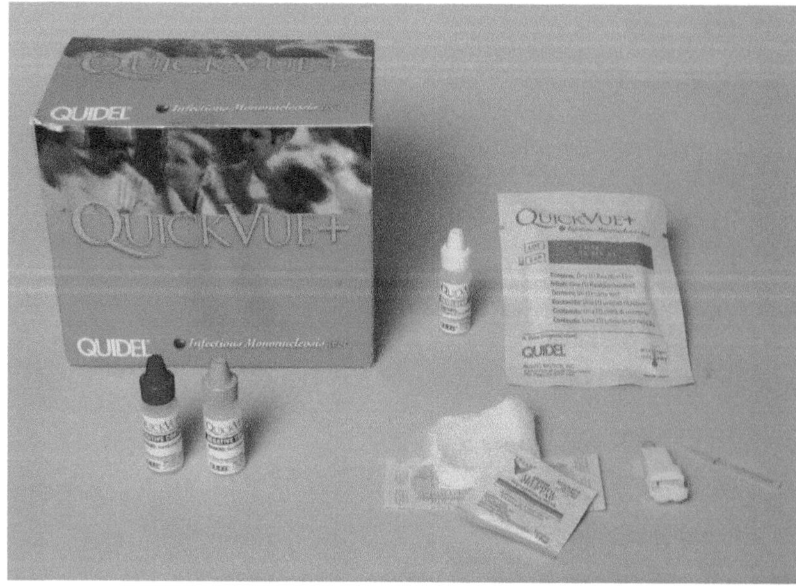

Fig. 19.14 QuickVue+ Mononucleosis Test setup. (From Garrels M, Oatis CS. *Laboratory testing for ambulatory settings*, ed 3, St Louis: Elsevier; 2015.)

the procedure for performing a rapid mono test using the QuickVue+ Mononucleosis Test. Fig. 19.16 illustrates positive and negative test results for the QuickVue+ Mononucleosis Test.

IMMUNOHEMATOLOGIC TESTS

Immunohematology is a branch of immunology and is the study of red blood cell antigens and antibodies; it is also known as blood banking. Immunohematology tests include the following:

RH ANTIBODY TITER TEST

The Rh antibody titer test detects the amount of circulating Rh antibodies in the blood. These antibodies can occur in a pregnant woman who is Rh-negative and is carrying an Rh-positive fetus. This test is most frequently used to detect the presence of an Rh incompatibility problem with a mother and her unborn child.

ABO AND *RH* BLOOD TYPING

Blood typing is performed to determine an individual's ABO and Rh blood type. Knowledge of blood type helps to prevent transfusion and transplant reactions and helps to identify problems such as hemolytic disease of the newborn.

BLOOD ANTIGENS

Each individual has a blood type. Blood type depends on the presence of certain factors, or antigens, on the surface of the red blood cells. **Blood antigens** consist of protein and are inherited through **genes,** which program the body to produce a particular antigen. If a blood antigen is present, it appears on the surface of all the red blood cells in the body.

Many types of antigens can appear on the surface of red blood cells. These antigens can be grouped into categories known as *blood group systems.* The blood group systems that are most likely to cause problems in blood transfusions and in Rh disease of the newborn are the ABO and Rh blood group systems. These are the blood group systems most commonly tested for in the medical laboratory.

Within the ABO blood group system are four main blood types—A, B, AB, and O. The blood type depends on which antigens are present on the surface of the red blood cells.

- If the A antigen is present, the blood type is A.
- If the B antigen is present, the blood type is B.
- If A and B antigens are present, the blood type is AB.
- If neither the A nor the B antigen is present, the blood type is O.

Fig. 19.17 illustrates this principle.

BLOOD ANTIBODIES

Blood antibodies are proteins that are naturally present in the plasma of the blood. An antibody is a substance that is capable of combining with an antigen. The body never produces an antibody to combine with its own blood antigen. If the blood type is A, the plasma does not contain the A antibody. The B antibody naturally occurs in that plasma, however. The B antibody cannot combine with the A antigen. If a blood antigen and its corresponding antibody combine (in this case, the A antigen combining with the A antibody), a serious antigen-antibody reaction occurs that could be life-threatening.

QuickVue + Mononucleosis Test

FOR INFORMATIONAL USE ONLY ■ FOR INFORMATIONAL USE ONLY ■ FOR INFORMATIONAL USE ONLY

Not to be used for performing assay. Refer to most current package insert accompanying your test kit.

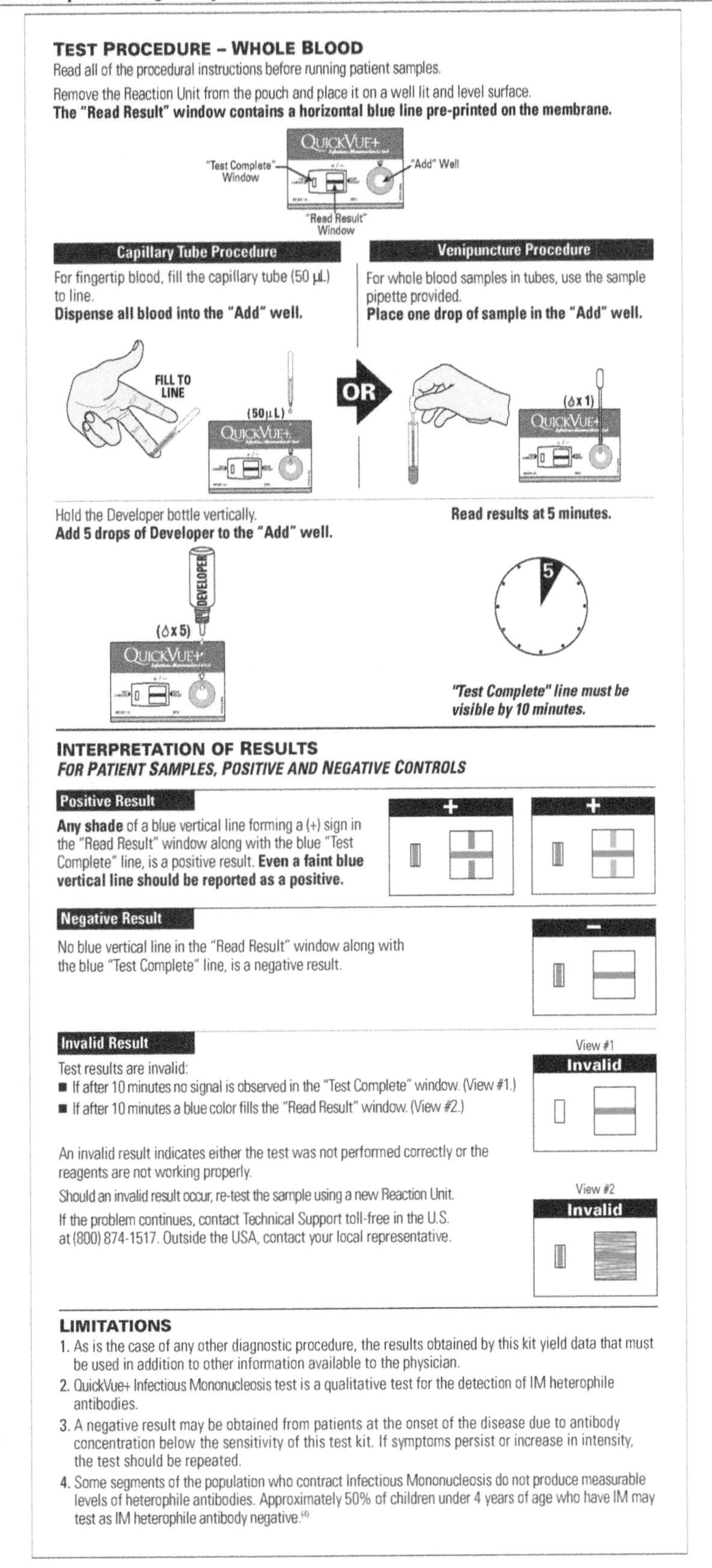

TEST PROCEDURE – WHOLE BLOOD

Read all of the procedural instructions before running patient samples.

Remove the Reaction Unit from the pouch and place it on a well lit and level surface.
The "Read Result" window contains a horizontal blue line pre-printed on the membrane.

Capillary Tube Procedure

For fingertip blood, fill the capillary tube (50 µL) to line.
Dispense all blood into the "Add" well.

Venipuncture Procedure

For whole blood samples in tubes, use the sample pipette provided.
Place one drop of sample in the "Add" well.

Hold the Developer bottle vertically.
Add 5 drops of Developer to the "Add" well.

Read results at 5 minutes.

"Test Complete" line must be visible by 10 minutes.

INTERPRETATION OF RESULTS
FOR PATIENT SAMPLES, POSITIVE AND NEGATIVE CONTROLS

Positive Result

Any shade of a blue vertical line forming a (+) sign in the "Read Result" window along with the blue "Test Complete" line, is a positive result. **Even a faint blue vertical line should be reported as a positive.**

Negative Result

No blue vertical line in the "Read Result" window along with the blue "Test Complete" line, is a negative result.

Invalid Result

Test results are invalid:
- If after 10 minutes no signal is observed in the "Test Complete" window. (View #1.)
- If after 10 minutes a blue color fills the "Read Result" window. (View #2.)

An invalid result indicates either the test was not performed correctly or the reagents are not working properly.

Should an invalid result occur, re-test the sample using a new Reaction Unit.

If the problem continues, contact Technical Support toll-free in the U.S. at (800) 874-1517. Outside the USA, contact your local representative.

LIMITATIONS

1. As is the case of any other diagnostic procedure, the results obtained by this kit yield data that must be used in addition to other information available to the physician.
2. QuickVue+ Infectious Mononucleosis test is a qualitative test for the detection of IM heterophile antibodies.
3. A negative result may be obtained from patients at the onset of the disease due to antibody concentration below the sensitivity of this test kit. If symptoms persist or increase in intensity, the test should be repeated.
4. Some segments of the population who contract Infectious Mononucleosis do not produce measurable levels of heterophile antibodies. Approximately 50% of children under 4 years of age who have IM may test as IM heterophile antibody negative.[4]

Fig. 19.15 Procedure for performing the QuickVue+ Mononucleosis test. (Courtesy of and modified from Quidel Corporation, San Diego, CA.)

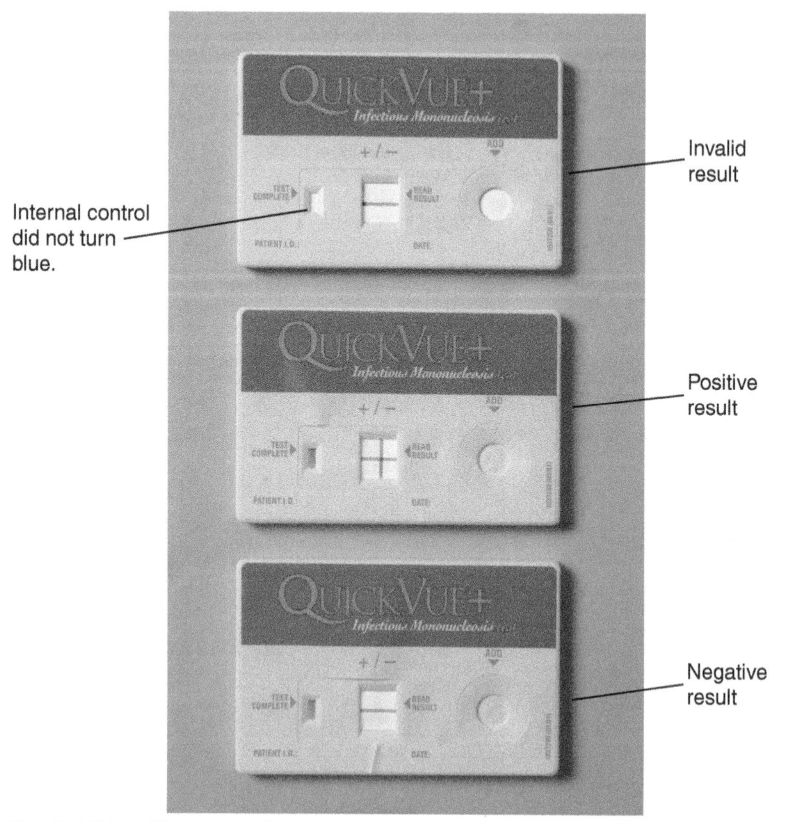

Fig. 19.16 QuickVue+ Mononucleosis test results. (Modified from Garrels M, Oatis CS. *Laboratory testing for ambulatory settings*, ed 3, St Louis: Elsevier; 2015.)

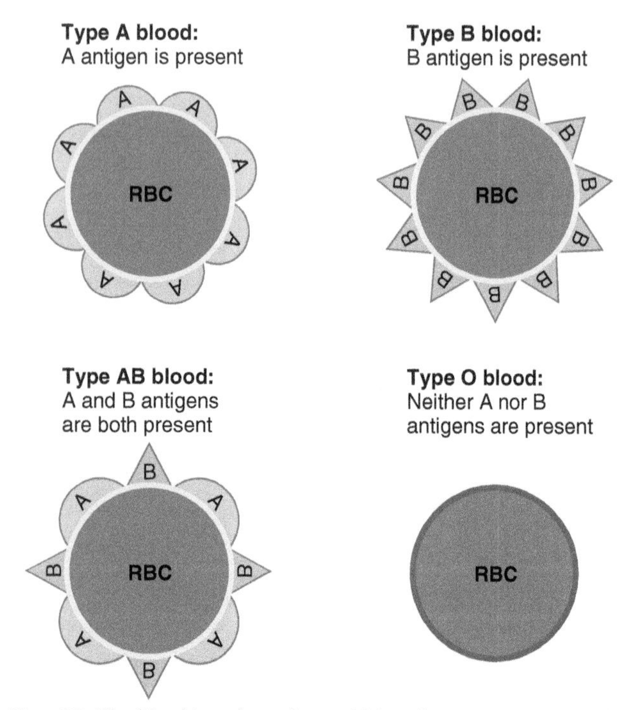

Fig. 19.17 Blood type depends on which antigens are present on the surface of the red blood cells (RBCs).

Table 19.8 ABO Blood Group System

Blood Type	Antigen Present on Red Blood Cell	Antibody Present in Plasma
A	A	B
B	B	A
AB	A, B	Neither A nor B
0	Neither A nor B	A, B

- If the blood type is A, the plasma contains the B antibody.
- If the blood type is B, the plasma contains the A antibody.
- If the blood type is AB, neither the A nor the B antibody appears in the plasma.
- If the blood type is O, the A and B antibodies appear in the plasma. Type O blood has neither the A nor the B antigen on the surface of its red blood cells. The A and B antibodies in the plasma would not have an A or B antigen to combine with them (Table 19.8).

RH BLOOD GROUP SYSTEM

In 1940, Landsteiner and Wiener discovered the Rh blood group system while working with rhesus monkeys. Most people in the United States (85%) have the Rh antigen present on the red blood cells and have type Rh-positive (Rh+) blood. The remaining 15% of the population do not have the Rh antigen present on the red blood cells and have type Rh-negative (Rh-) blood. In contrast to the A and B antibodies, the Rh antibodies do not normally occur in the plasma.

BLOOD ANTIGEN AND ANTIBODY REACTIONS

When a blood antigen and its corresponding antibody unite, the result is the clumping, or agglutination, of red blood cells. Agglutination of red blood cells can be serious and fatal if it occurs **in vivo** (in the living body). The clumped red blood cells cannot pass through the small tubules of the kidneys, and this may lead to kidney failure. Also, the clumping of the red blood cells eventually leads to hemolysis, or breakdown of the red blood cells.

Blood antigen-antibody reactions can occur if the wrong blood type is administered to a patient during a blood transfusion. If an individual with type A blood is given a transfusion of type B blood, the B antibody of the **recipient** (person receiving the blood) would combine with the B antigen of the **donor** (person donating the blood), and an antigen-antibody reaction would occur, resulting in agglutination of red blood cells. We say that type A blood is incompatible with type B blood.

HIGHLIGHT on Blood Donor Criteria

Every year, approximately 5 million Americans require blood transfusions, resulting in transfusion of 16 million units of blood. A safe, readily available blood supply is essential for lifesaving medical procedures, such as replacing blood loss from hemorrhages or surgical procedures, replacing plasma in burn and shock victims, and providing platelets to control bleeding. In an average population, 38% of the people are physically and medically eligible to donate blood, but only 10% of those eligible donate.

Basic blood donor criteria have been established on a national basis to ensure donor safety and a quality blood donation. All blood collection facilities, such as the American Red Cross, must follow these regulations. In general, blood donors must be in good health and must be of a certain age and weight.

Health History

To protect the donor and the recipient, each donor is asked to give a brief health history. The prospective donor is asked to provide information related to diseases that may be transmitted through the blood (e.g., hepatitis, AIDS) and medications being taken that could affect the quality of the blood donation. Information also is obtained related to medical conditions that might jeopardize the health of the donor if he or she were to donate.

Based on this information, a prospective donor could be *temporarily deferred* from donating blood because of the following: blood transfusion, treatment for cancer, a human bite in which the skin was broken, certain immunizations, organ transplant, pregnancy, treatment for syphilis or gonorrhea, a skin infection, certain medical conditions such as a recent heart attack or active tuberculosis, taking of certain prescription medications (e.g., anticoagulants), and travel to a malaria-prone area. Temporarily deferred donors are told how long they must wait and are encouraged to donate blood when the waiting period is over. The waiting period varies based on the condition or situation; the waiting period is at least 12 months after treatment for syphilis or gonorrhea is received, whereas only a 7-day wait is required after the potential donor has been immunized for hepatitis B.

A prospective donor is *permanently deferred* from giving blood for any of the following reasons: leukemia, a clotting disorder, hepatitis, infection with HIV, and behavior associated with the spread of HIV, and a history of IV drug use.

Age

An individual must be at least 17 years old to donate blood. With written parental consent, however, some states permit 16-year-olds to donate blood. No upper age limit has been established for blood donation, as long as the individual feels well and has no restrictions or limitations on his or her activities.

Date of Last Donation

At least 56 days (8 weeks) must elapse between donations.

Weight

The donor must weigh at least 110 lb. (In some states, the minimum weight is 105 lb.) The volume of blood collected is approximately 8% of the average adult's total blood volume. Underweight donors are not accepted because a full donation would result in a proportionately greater reduction in blood volume and might precipitate a reaction. No upper weight limit is in place as long as the individual's weight is not greater than the weight limit of the blood donor bed being used.

Temperature

Body temperature of donors may not exceed 99.5°F (37.5°C). The primary purpose of temperature measurement is to eliminate donors who are ill.

Pulse

The acceptable range for the pulse rate is 50–110 beats/min. If the pulse rate seems to be elevated because of physical exertion, the donor may be asked to remain seated for 5–10 min, with a recheck taken after the rest period.

Continued

HIGHLIGHT on Blood Donor Criteria—cont'd

Blood Pressure

The acceptable limit for blood pressure is a reading no higher than 180 mmHg for the systolic pressure and a reading no higher than 100 mmHg for the diastolic pressure.

Hemoglobin

The hemoglobin must be 12.5 g/dL or greater for men and women.

Blood-Donating Process

It takes approximately 1 h to donate blood. The process begins with the health history, followed by a mini-physical check of temperature, pulse, blood pressure, and hemoglobin level. Next, 1 unit (1 pint) of blood is collected using a sterile needle and a sterile plastic bag that contains an additive. A donor should feel no pain during the blood collection procedure, which takes approximately 8–10 min. It is not possible to contract AIDS or any other infectious disease by donating blood. After the unit of blood has been collected, the donor is encouraged to have refreshments to begin replenishing the fluids and nutrients temporarily lost during the donation.

Processing the Blood

Each blood donation is tested for HIV, hepatitis, and syphilis. Any unit of blood that tests positive is discarded and the donor is notified of the test results. Each accepted unit of blood is typed and labeled with its ABO and Rh blood type. It is then available for distribution to hospitals for transfusing purposes. ■

AGGLUTINATION AND BLOOD TYPING

Agglutination of red blood cells is the basis for the ABO and Rh blood typing procedure. The antigen-antibody reaction occurs **in vitro,** or "in glass" in the laboratory, meaning outside of the living body in an artificial environment.

To test for the ABO blood group system, a commercially prepared antiserum is used. An **antiserum** is a serum that contains antibodies. An antiserum containing the A antibody is added to an unknown blood specimen. If the A antigen is present, it combines with the A antibody, resulting in agglutination. An antiserum containing the B antibody is added to another sample of the unknown blood. If the B antigen is present, it combines with the B antibody, resulting in agglutination. If agglutination occurs in both instances, the sample is type AB. If no agglutination occurs, this indicates the absence of blood antigens, or type O blood. Agglutination that occurs in vitro is visible to the naked eye. The antigen-antibody reaction that occurs when the unknown blood sample is type A is diagrammed in Fig. 19.18.

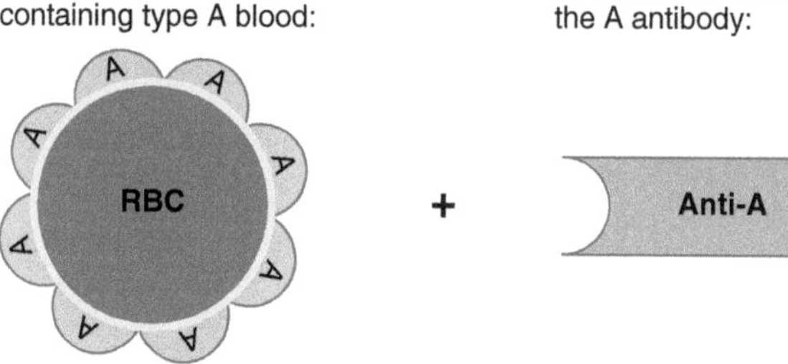

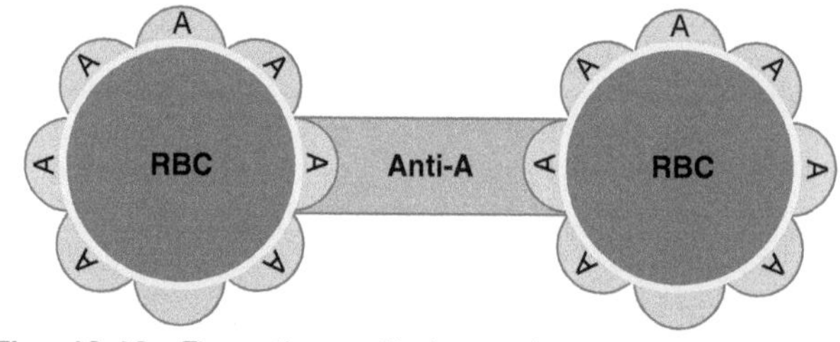

Fig. 19.18 The antigen-antibody reaction that occurs when the unknown blood sample is type A.

What Would You Do? What Would You *Not* Do? RESPONSES

Case Study 1
Page 667

What Did Michelle Do?

- ❑ Empathized with Bianca that it is hard to fast but eating and drinking causes an increase in the blood sugar level that causes the test results to be inaccurate.
- ❑ Empathized with Bianca for having to be at the test site so long. Explained to her that it takes 3–4 h to run an OGTT because several specimens must be collected over time to see how her body handles sugar.
- ❑ Told Bianca that walking burns up sugar in the body, which affects the test results.
- ❑ Explained to Bianca that smoking elevates the blood sugar level, causing the test results to be inaccurate.
- ❑ Explained to Bianca that weakness and slight perspiration are considered normal side effects of an OGTT.
- ❑ Notified the physician of the side effects experienced by Bianca during the test and documented this information in Bianca's medical record.

What Would You Do? What Would You *Not* Do? RESPONSES—cont'd

What Did Michelle Not Do?

- ❑ Did not become defensive or intimidated by Bianca's behavior but tried to understand that patients often become fearful and anxious when faced with a health concern.
- ❑ Did not scold Bianca for not paying attention to the verbal and written instructions that were given to her at the medical office.

Case Study 2

Page 671

What Did Michelle Do?

- ❑ Told Jackson that it would be fine for him to perform his own finger stick.
- ❑ Made sure that Jackson cleansed his finger with an antiseptic wipe before making the finger puncture.
- ❑ Observed the finger puncture performed by Jackson and offered suggestions if needed.
- ❑ Explained to Jackson that the air bubbles take up space that the insulin should occupy, and that if he does not get rid of them he will not get his full dose of insulin.
- ❑ Demonstrated how to remove air bubbles, and had Jackson practice it at the office.
- ❑ Told Jackson he must not reuse his needle and syringe. Explained that a used needle could cause him to get an infection.
- ❑ Asked Jackson if he had checked to see if his insurance would cover the cost of the needles and syringes.

What Did Michelle Not Do?

- ❑ Did not tell Jackson he didn't need to worry about the air bubbles in the syringe.

Case Study 3

Page 675

What Did Michelle Do?

- ❑ Tried to calm and reassure Karen.
- ❑ Explained to Karen that the cholesterol results are not affected by food, so eating before the health fair should not have affected her results.
- ❑ Told Karen that before a cholesterol analyzer is used, it is usually checked to ensure that it is working properly.
- ❑ Reassured Karen that the physician was checking her cholesterol again and was running some additional tests to determine whether she is having any problems.
- ❑ Told Karen that if she must take medication, the physician will determine what drug is best for her.

What Did Michelle Not Do?

- ❑ Did not tell Karen that her cholesterol is extremely high.
- ❑ Did not tell Karen that she should be more careful about what she eats because she is overweight.
- ❑ Did not tell Karen that there was no way to know whether the cholesterol analyzer used at the health fair was calibrated and had controls run on it. ■

TERMINOLOGY REVIEW

Medical Term	Word Parts	Definition
Agglutination (as it pertains to blood)	*agglutin-:* clumping *-ation:* action or process	Clumping of blood cells.
Antibody	*anti-:* against	A substance that is capable of combining with an antigen, resulting in an antigen-antibody reaction.
Antigen	*anti-:* against *-gen:* substance or agent that produces or causes	A substance capable of stimulating the formation of antibodies.
Antiserum (*pl.* antisera)	*anti-:* against	A serum that contains antibodies.
Cholesterol		A white, waxy, fatlike substance (lipid) that is essential for normal functioning of the body.
Donor		One who furnishes something, such as blood, tissue, or organs, to be used in another individual.
Glucose	*gluco-:* glucose *-ose:* full of	The end product of carbohydrate metabolism which serves as the chief source of energy for the body.

Continued

TERMINOLOGY REVIEW—cont'd

Medical Term	Word Parts	Definition
Glycogen	*glyco-:* sugar *-gen:* substance or agent that produces or causes	The form in which glucose is stored in the body.
Glycosylation	*glyco-:* sugar	The process of glucose attaching to hemoglobin.
HDL cholesterol		A lipoprotein, consisting of protein and cholesterol, that removes excess cholesterol from the cells and carries it to the liver to be excreted.
Hemoglobin A_{1c}	*hemo-:* blood	A compound formed when glucose attaches or glycosylates to the protein in hemoglobin.
Hyperglycemia	*hyper-:* above, excessive *glyc/o:* sugar *-emia:* blood condition	An abnormally high level of glucose in the blood.
Hypoglycemia	*hypo-:* below, deficient *glyc/o:* sugar *-emia:* blood condition	An abnormally low level of glucose in the blood.
Immunology	*Immun/o:* immune	The scientific study of antigen and antibody reactions.
In vitro	*vitro*: glass	Occurring in glass. Refers to tests performed under artificial conditions, as in the laboratory.
In vivo	*vivo*: living	Occurring in the living body or organism.
Insulin		A hormone secreted by the beta cells of the pancreas required for the normal use of glucose in the body.
LDL cholesterol		A lipoprotein, consisting of protein and cholesterol that picks up cholesterol and delivers it to blood vessels and muscles.
Lipoprotein	*lipo-:* fat	A complex molecule consisting of protein and a lipid fraction such as cholesterol. Lipoproteins function in transporting lipids in the blood.
Recipient		One who receives something, such as a blood transfusion, from a donor.

PROCEDURE 19.1

PROCEDURE 19.1 CLIA-Waived Blood Glucose Test

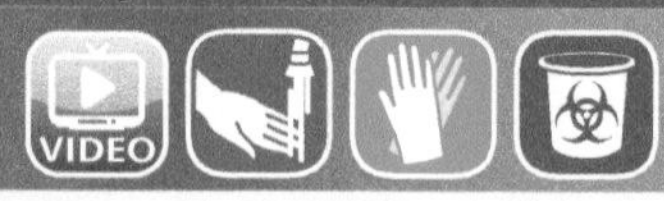

Outcome Perform a fasting blood glucose (FBG) test using an Accu-Chek Aviva glucose meter.

Equipment/Supplies

- Disposable gloves
- Accu-Chek Aviva glucose meter
- Accu-Chek Aviva test strips
- Control solutions
- Lancet
- Antiseptic wipe
- Gauze pad
- Biohazard sharps container

1. Procedural Step. Sanitize your hands. Assemble the equipment. Check the expiration date (Use By date) on the container of test strips. Check the expiration date on the control solution bottle. The control solution is effective for 3 months from the date it is opened. When opening a new bottle of control solution, write the date on the container label. The control solution can then be used for 3 months from this date or until the manufacturer's expiration date (stamped on the container) is reached, whichever comes first. Make sure the environmental room temperature falls between 57°F (14°C) and 100°F (38°C).

Principle. Test strips or controls past their expiration can cause inaccurate test results. If the environmental temperature is outside of the required range, the

PROCEDURE 19.1 CLIA-Waived Blood Glucose Test—cont'd

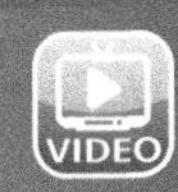
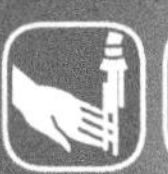

glucose meter is unable to perform the test, causing an error message to appear on the screen of the analyzer.

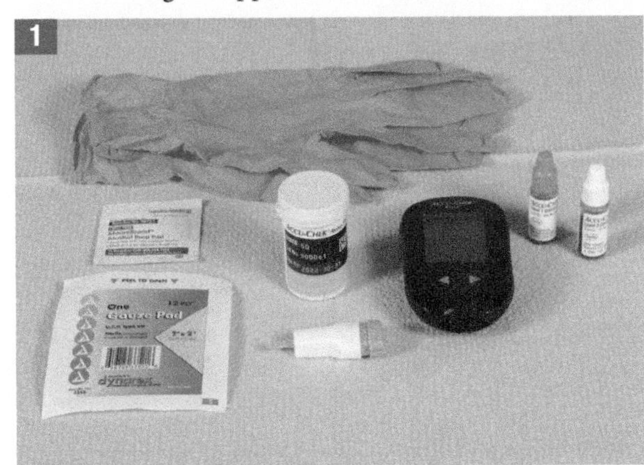
Assemble the equipment.

2. Procedural Step. Insert a test strip into the glucose meter as follows:

a. Remove a test strip from the container and immediately recap the container to prevent the strips from being exposed to moisture.
b. Insert the test strip into the meter in the direction of the arrows with the yellow window facing up. This automatically turns on the meter and a beep sounds.
c. Place the meter on a flat surface.
d. When the strip is ready to accept the control solution or a blood specimen, a symbol of a test strip and a flashing blood drop appear on the display screen.

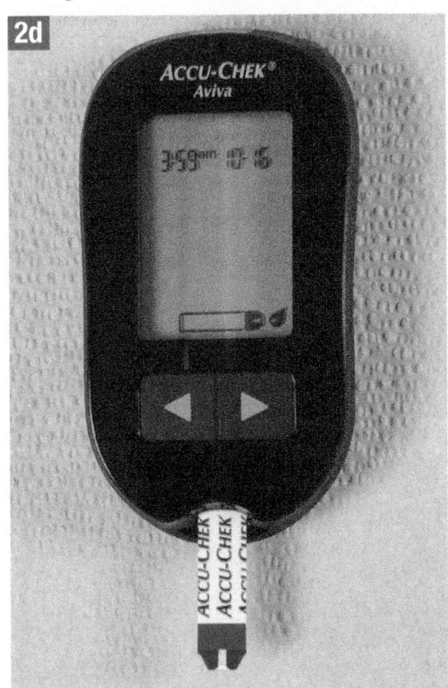

Symbol of the test strip and blood drop.

Principle. Moisture results in deterioration of the chemical reagents on the test strips leading to inaccurate test results. If the meter is tilted the control solution may drip into the meter and damage it.

3. Procedural Step. Perform a Level 1 and 2 control procedure as follows:

a. Remove the cap from the Level 1 (low) control solution bottle and wipe the tip of the bottle with a tissue.
b. Squeeze the bottle until a tiny drop forms at the tip of the bottle.
c. Touch and hold the drop of control solution to the front edge of the yellow window of the test strip. Do not put the control solution on top of the test strip. The meter will beep and an "hourglass" symbol flashes when there is enough control solution on the test strip. The meter automatically recognizes the difference between the control solution and a blood specimen.

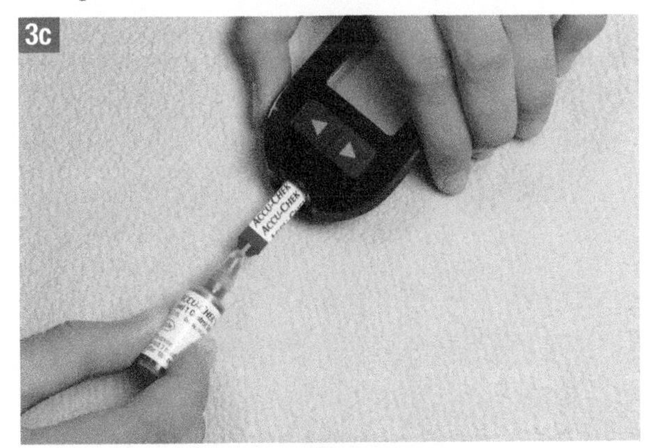
Apply the control solution.

d. Wipe the tip of the bottle with a tissue and recap the bottle tightly.
e. After a short time, the control result appears on the display screen along with a control bottle symbol and a flashing "L." Press and release the right arrow key once to mark the control result as a Level 1 control. Press the Power/Set Button (located on the top of the meter) to set the control level in the meter.
f. If the Level 1 control result is within the acceptable range, the control result will alternate with the word "OK" on the display screen. The control result can also be compared with the expected Level 1 range stamped on the test strip container label. The word "Err" and the control result will alternate on the display if the control result is not within the expected range.

Continued

PROCEDURE 19.1

PROCEDURE 19.1 CLIA-Waived Blood Glucose Test—cont'd

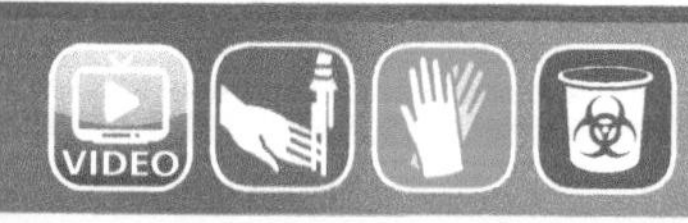

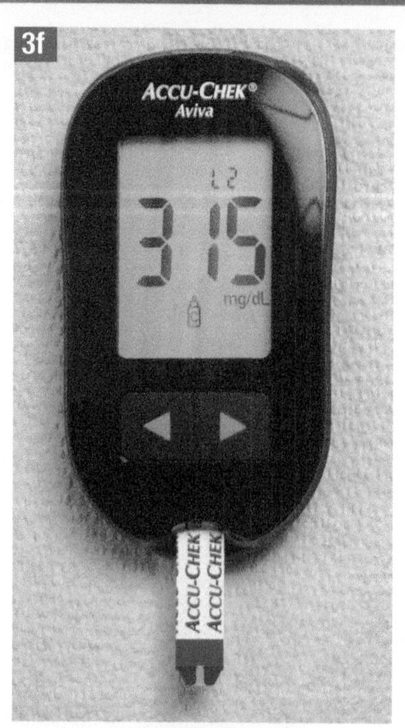

The control results alternate with the word "OK."

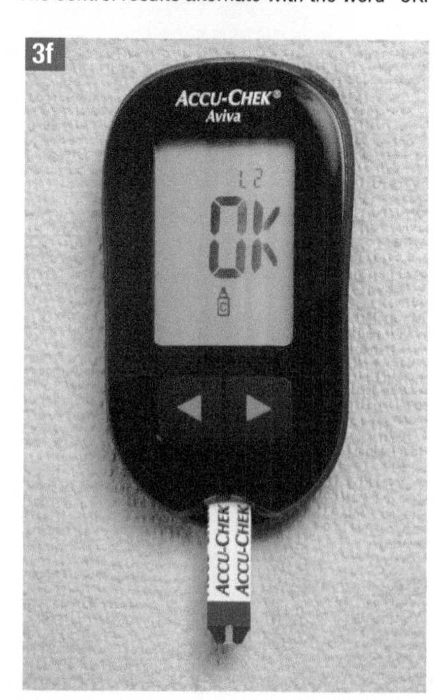

g. If the control result is not within the expected range, review the technique used to run the control to make sure it was performed correctly. Any errors should be corrected, and the control should be run again. If the results are still not within the expected range, the manufacturer of the glucose meter should be contacted.

h. Remove and discard the used test strip.

i. Repeat the control procedure outlined above using a Level 2 (high) control. When the control result and the flashing "L" appear on the display, press and release the right arrow key twice to mark the control result as a Level 2 control.

j. Document the control results in the quality control log.

Principle. Running a Level 1 and a Level 2 control procedure ensures that the test results are reliable and valid. Gloves do not need to be worn because the control consists of a glucose solution.

4. **Procedural Step.** Sanitize your hands. Greet the patient and introduce yourself. Identify the patient by full name and date of birth. Explain the procedure.

5. **Procedural Step.** Ask the patient whether he or she has had anything to eat or drink (besides water) for the past 8–12 h.

   Principle. Consumption of food or fluid increases the blood glucose level, leading to an inaccurate interpretation of the test results.

6. **Procedural Step.** Perform the blood glucose test as follows:

   a. Insert the test strip into the glucose meter (as previously presented).

   b. Cleanse the puncture site with an antiseptic wipe and allow it to air dry.

   c. Apply gloves and perform a finger puncture. Dispose of the lancet in a biohazard sharps container.

   d. Wipe away the first drop of blood with a gauze pad.

   e. Place the patient's hand in a dependent position (palm facing down), and gently massage the finger around the puncture site until a drop of blood forms.

   f. Touch and hold the drop of blood to the front edge (not the top) of the yellow window of the test strip. The meter will beep and an "hourglass" symbol flashes when there is enough blood on the test strip.

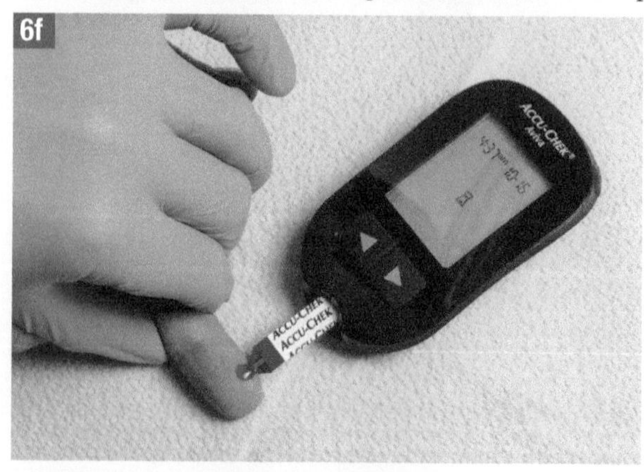

Apply a drop of blood.

PROCEDURE 19.1 CLIA-Waived Blood Glucose Test—cont'd

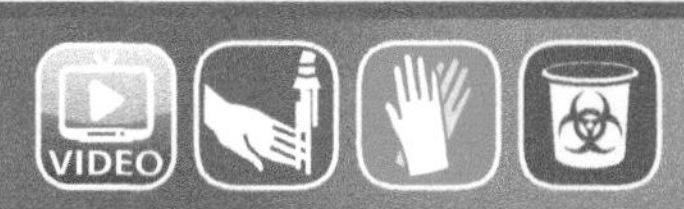

g. Have the patient hold a gauze pad over the puncture site and apply pressure until the bleeding stops.

h. An hourglass is displayed on the screen while the meter analyzes the blood specimen. After a short time, the glucose value is displayed in milligrams per deciliter (mg/dL). (The glucose result indicated on this glucose meter is 106 mg/dL.) If the glucose value is higher or lower than the measurement range of the meter, or if the screen displays something other than the glucose value (e.g., an error code), refer to the Troubleshooting Guide section of the operator's manual to obtain instructions for correcting the problem.

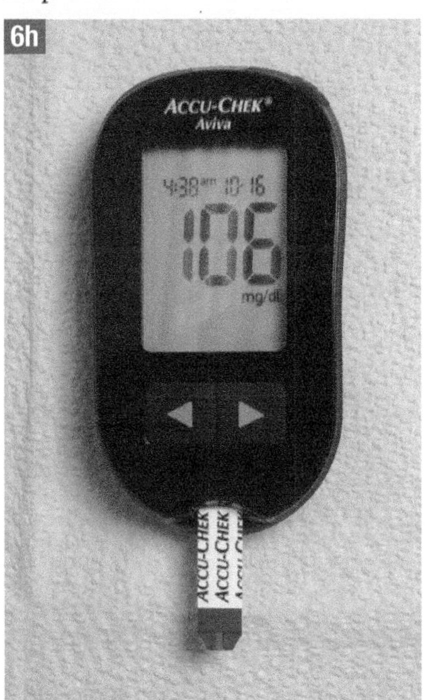

Read the glucose results.

i. Remove the test strip from the meter and discard it in a biohazard waste container. The meter automatically turns off 5 s after the test strip is removed.

j. Check the puncture site and apply an adhesive bandage to the patient's finger if needed.

Principle. The antiseptic must be allowed to dry to prevent it from reacting with the chemicals on the reagent pad, which would lead to inaccurate test results. Gloves provide a barrier against bloodborne pathogens. The first drop of blood contains a large amount of tissue fluid, which dilutes the specimen and leads to inaccurate test results.

7. **Procedural Step.** Remove gloves and sanitize your hands.
8. **Procedural Step.** Document the results in the patient's medical record.
   a. *Electronic health record (EHR):* Document the type of glucose test (i.e., FBG), the glucose test results, and when the patient last ate. If the patient has diabetes, also document the time of his or her last insulin injection or last consumption of oral hypoglycemic medication using the appropriate radio buttons, drop-down menus, and free text fields.
   b. *Paper-based patient record:* Document the date and time, the type of glucose test (i.e., FBG), the glucose test results, and when the patient last ate. If the patient has diabetes, also document the time of his or her last insulin injection or last consumption of oral hypoglycemic medication (refer to the PPR documentation example).
9. **Procedural Step.** Clean and disinfect the glucose meter according to the information in the operating manual.

PPR Documentation Example

Date	
5/18/XX	8:30 a.m. FBG: 106 mg/dL. Pt last ate on
	5/17 @ 7:00 p.m.————————
	————————M. Villers, CMA (AAMA)

PROCEDURE 19.1

Medical Microbiology

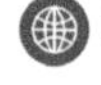 Check out the Evolve site at http://evolve.elsevier.com/Bonewit to access additional interactive activities and exercises to help you study and prepare for success.

LEARNING OUTCOMES / PROCEDURES

Microorganisms and Disease

1. List and explain the stages of an infectious disease.
2. List and describe the three classifications of bacteria based on shape.
3. Give examples of infectious diseases caused by the following types of cocci:
   - Staphylococci
   - Streptococci
   - Diplococci
4. State examples of infectious diseases caused by bacilli, spirilla, and viruses.

Microscope

5. Explain the function of each of the following parts of a compound microscope: base, arm, stage, light source, condenser, diaphragm, eyepieces, objectives, and adjustment knobs.
6. Identify the function of each of the following microscope lenses: low power, high power, and oil immersion.
7. List the guidelines for proper care of the microscope.

Procedures:

Operate a microscope.
Properly handle and care for a microscope.

Microbiologic Specimen Collection

8. Explain the purpose of obtaining a specimen and identify body areas from which a specimen can be taken for microbiologic examination.
9. List ways to prevent contamination of a specimen by extraneous microorganisms.
10. Explain the precautions a medical assistant should take to prevent infection from a pathogenic specimen.

Procedures:

Collect a throat specimen.
Collect a nasopharyngeal specimen.

CLIA-Waived Microbiologic Testing

11. Describe the symptoms of strep throat.
12. Explain the importance of the early diagnosis of streptococcal pharyngitis.
13. Explain the advantage of using a rapid strep test to diagnose group A streptococcus.
14. List and describe the three different types of influenza viruses.
15. Describe the symptoms, treatment, and potential complications of influenza.
16. Explain why a new influenza vaccine must be produced each year.

Perform CLIA–waived streptococcus test.
Perform a CLIA-waived influenza test.

Culture and Sensitivity Testing

17. State the purpose of culturing a microbiologic specimen.
18. Explain the difference between a mixed culture and a pure culture.
19. Explain the purpose of and describe the procedure for a sensitivity test.
20. Give examples of methods to prevent and control infectious diseases in the community.

CHAPTER OUTLINE

Introduction to Microbiology
Normal Flora
Infection
- Stages of an Infectious Disease

Microorganisms and Disease
- Bacteria
- Viruses

Microscope
- Support System
- Optical System
- Function of the Objective Lenses
- Care of the Microscope

Microbiologic Specimen Collection
- Handling and Transporting Microbiologic Specimens
- Collection and Transport Systems
- CLIA-Waived Microbiologic Tests

Culture and Sensitivity Testing
- Microbial Cultures
- Sensitivity Testing

Prevention and Control of Infectious Diseases

KEY TERMS

bacilli (bah-SILL-ie)
cocci (KOK-sie)
contagious (kon-TAE-jus)
culture
culture medium
false-negative result
incubate
incubation period
infection
infectious disease
inoculate
microbiology (mie-kroe-bie-OL-oe-jee)
mucous membrane (MYOO-kus MEM-brain)
normal flora
specimen (SPESS-ih-men)
spirilla (spa-RILL-ah)

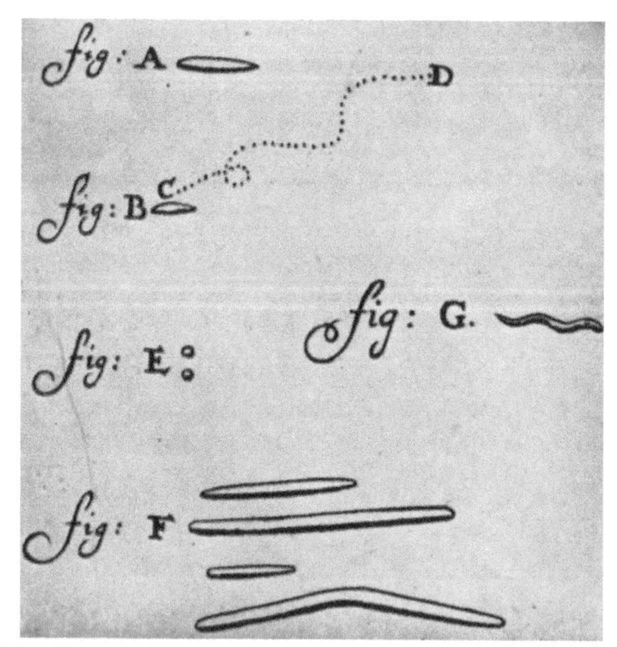

Fig. 20.1 Bacteria drawn by van Leeuwenhoek in 1684. (From Fuerst R: *Frobisher and Fuerst's microbiology in health and disease*, ed 15, Philadelphia: WB Saunders; 1983.)

If the provider is not able to diagnose the disease from the patient's clinical signs and symptoms, laboratory tests must be used to help the provider identify the pathogen. Identification of the pathogen leads to proper treatment of the disease. Laboratory analyses used to identify a pathogen include the following:

- Biochemical tests
- DNA testing (also known as PCR testing)
- Microbial culture

Although the type of laboratory analysis used to identify a pathogen is often performed at an outside laboratory, the medical assistant is frequently responsible for collecting the microbiologic specimen that will be transported to the outside laboratory.

This chapter provides an introduction to microbiology, including a description of proper microbiologic collection and handling techniques that must be followed to ensure a quality specimen. This chapter also presents CLIA-waived tests that can be performed in the medical office to identify pathogens. Before undertaking this study, the medical assistant should review Chapter 2, which discusses introductory concepts that are basic to this chapter.

INTRODUCTION TO MICROBIOLOGY

Microbiology is the scientific study of microorganisms and their activities. As described in Chapter 2, microorganisms are tiny living plants and animals that cannot be seen by the naked eye but must be viewed under a microscope. Anton van Leeuwenhoek (1632–1723) designed a magnifying glass strong enough for viewing microorganisms. He was the first individual to observe and describe protozoa and bacteria (Fig. 20.1). Leeuwenhoek's magnifying glass was the precursor of modern microscopes used today to study microorganisms. A microscope allows the observer to see individual microbial cells and to differentiate and identify microorganisms.

For the most part, microbiology deals with unicellular, or one-celled, microscopic organisms. All of the life processes necessary to sustain the microbe are performed by one cell. Among them are the ingestion of food substances and their use for energy, growth, reproduction, and excretion.

Microorganisms are ubiquitous; they are found almost everywhere—in the air, in food and water, in the soil, and in association with plants, animals, and human life. Although vast numbers of microorganisms exist, only a relatively small number are pathogenic and able to cause disease.

When a pathogen infects a host, it often produces a set of symptoms peculiar to that disease. Scarlet fever is characterized by a sore throat, swelling of the lymph nodes in the neck, a red and swollen tongue, and a bright red rash covering the body. These symptoms aid the provider in diagnosing the disease. The medical assistant must be alert to all symptoms that the patient describes and must relay this information to the provider through careful and concise documentation of these symptoms in the patient's medical record.

NORMAL FLORA

Every individual has a **normal flora**, which consists of harmless microorganisms that normally reside in many parts of the body but do not cause disease. The surface of the skin, the **mucous membrane** of the gastrointestinal tract, and parts of the respiratory and genitourinary tracts all have an abundant normal flora. Some microorganisms that make up the normal flora are beneficial to the body, such as those that inhabit the intestinal tract that feed on other potentially harmful microscopic organisms. Another example is microorganisms found in the intestinal tract that synthesize vitamin K, an essential vitamin needed by the body for proper blood clotting. In rare instances, if the opportunity arises (e.g., lowered body resistance), certain microorganisms of the normal flora can become pathogenic and cause disease.

INFECTION

Invasion of the body by pathogenic microorganisms is known as **infection.** Under conditions favorable to the pathogens, they grow and multiply, resulting in an **infectious disease** (also known as a communicable disease) that produces harmful effects on the host. Not all pathogens that enter a host are able to cause disease, however. When a pathogen enters the body, it attempts to invade the tissues so that it can grow and multiply. The body tries to stop the invasion with its second line of natural defense mechanisms,[a] which includes inflammation, phagocytosis by white blood cells, and the

[a]The first line of natural defense mechanisms, which work to prevent the entrance of pathogens into the body (e.g., coughing, sneezing), is described in Chapter 2.

production of antibodies. These defense mechanisms work to destroy pathogens and remove them from the body. If the body is successful, the pathogens are destroyed, and the individual experiences no adverse effects. If the pathogens are able to overcome the body's natural defense mechanisms, an infectious disease results.

Many infectious diseases are **contagious**, meaning that the pathogen that causes the disease can be spread from one person to another directly or indirectly. Frequently, *droplet infection* is the mode of transmission of a contagious disease.

Droplet infection refers to an infection that is indirectly transmitted by tiny, contaminated droplets of moisture expelled from the upper respiratory tract of an infected individual. When an individual exhales (as during breathing, talking, coughing, or sneezing), he or she emits a fine spray of moisture droplets from the upper respiratory tract. If the individual has a contagious disease that is transmitted by droplet infection, the pathogens are carried into the air by these tiny moisture droplets. Another individual may inhale these contaminated droplets and become infected with the disease. To help prevent the spread of droplet infections, contagious individuals should cover their mouths and noses while coughing or sneezing. See Fig. 2.1 in Chapter 2 for examples of other means of pathogen transmission.

STAGES OF AN INFECTIOUS DISEASE

When a pathogen becomes established in the host, a series of events occur in stages. The stages of an infectious disease are as follows:

1. The *infection* is the invasion and multiplication of pathogenic microorganisms in the body.
2. The *incubation period* is the interval of time between the invasion by a pathogenic microorganism and the appearance of the first symptoms of the disease. Depending on the type of disease, the **incubation period** may range from a few days to several months. During this time, the pathogen is growing and multiplying.
3. The *prodromal period* is a short period in which the first symptoms that indicate an approaching disease occur. Headache and a feeling of illness are common prodromal symptoms.
4. The *acute period* is when the disease is at its peak and symptoms are fully developed. Fever is a common symptom of many infectious diseases.
5. The *decline period* is when symptoms of the disease begin to subside.
6. The *convalescent period* is the stage in which the patient regains strength and returns to a state of good health.

MICROORGANISMS AND DISEASE

The groups of microorganisms known to contain species capable of causing human disease include bacteria, viruses, protozoa, fungi (including yeasts), and animal parasites.

What Would You Do? What Would You *Not* Do?

Case Study 1

John Seimer calls the medical office. He says that he is not a patient at the office but would like some assistance. He says that for the past 3 days he has had a headache, fever, chills, and aching muscles. He says that a week ago he pulled a tick off his lower leg, and several days later he found a red rash around the tick bite. He says that he went on the internet and looked up his symptoms, and he is sure that he has Lyme disease. The internet site recommended taking doxycycline for 3 weeks to treat Lyme disease. John says that he does not like to go to the doctor and has not been to see a doctor for more than 10 years. He wants to know whether the doctor could call in a prescription for doxycycline for him. He says that he has health insurance and the doctor could bill him for an appointment, just as long as he does not have to come in. ■

Bacteria and viruses are most frequently responsible for causing human diseases and are discussed next.

BACTERIA

Bacteria are microscopic single-celled organisms. Of the 1700 species known to dwell in humans, only approximately 100 produce human disease. The discovery of antibiotics has helped immensely in combating and controlling bacterial infections. Antibiotics are not effective against viral infections, however.

Bacteria can be classified according to their shape into three basic groups (Fig. 20.2). Round bacteria are known as **cocci**. Cocci can be categorized further as diplococci, streptococci, or staphylococci, depending on their pattern of growth. Rod-shaped bacteria are **bacilli**. Spiral and curve-shaped bacteria are **spirilla**, and they include spirochetes and vibrios.

Cocci

Staphylococci are round bacteria that grow in grapelike clusters (Fig. 20.3 A). The species *Staphylococcus epidermidis* is widely distributed and is normally present on the surface of the skin and the mucous membranes of the mouth, nose, throat, and intestines. *S. epidermidis* is usually nonpathogenic; however, cuts, abrasions, and other breaks in the skin can allow invasion of the tissues by the organism, resulting in a mild infection.

Staphylococcus aureus is commonly associated with pathologic conditions such as boils, carbuncles, pimples, impetigo, abscesses, *Staphylococcus* food poisoning, and wound infections. Infections caused by staphylococci usually cause much pus formation (suppuration) and are termed *pyogenic* infections.

Streptococci are round bacteria that grow in chains (see Fig. 20.3 B). Before the advent of antibiotics, streptococcal infections were a major cause of human death. Diseases caused by streptococci include streptococcal sore throat

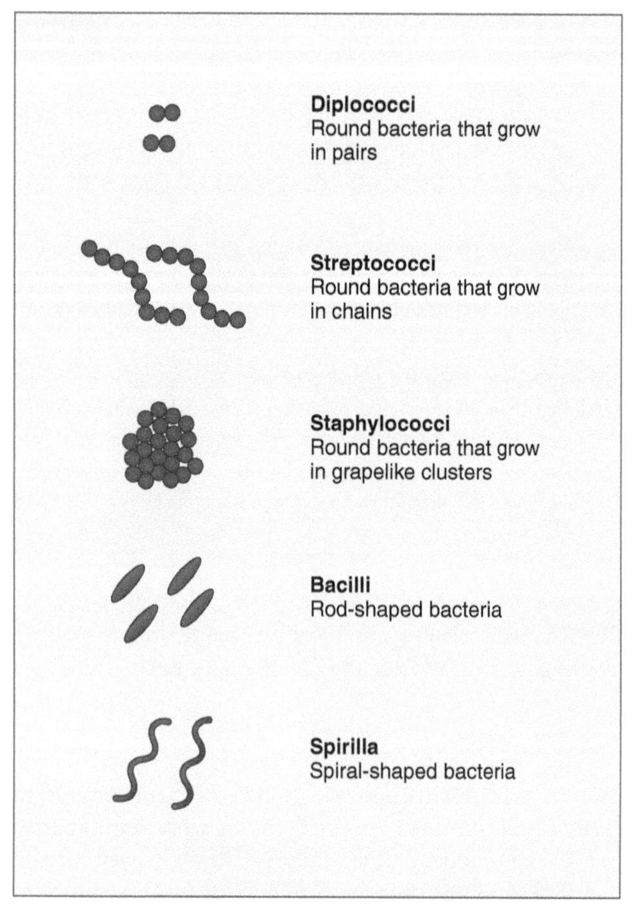

Fig. 20.2 Classification of bacteria based on shape.

("strep throat"), scarlet fever, rheumatic fever, pneumonia, puerperal sepsis, erysipelas, and skin conditions such as carbuncles and impetigo.

Diplococci are round bacteria that grow in pairs. Pneumonia, gonorrhea, and meningitis are infectious diseases caused by diplococci.

Bacilli

Bacilli are rod-shaped bacteria that are frequently found in the soil and air (see Fig. 20.3 C). Some bacilli are able to form spores, a characteristic that enables them to resist adverse conditions such as heat and disinfectants. Diseases caused by bacilli include botulism, tetanus, gas gangrene, gastroenteritis produced by *Salmonella* food poisoning, typhoid fever, pertussis (whooping cough), bacillary dysentery, diphtheria, tuberculosis, leprosy, and plague.

Escherichia coli is a species of bacillus that is found among the normal flora of the large intestine in enormous numbers (see Fig. 20.3 D). It is normally a harmless bacterium; however, if it enters the urinary tract as a result of lowered resistance, poor hygiene practices, or both, it may cause a urinary tract infection.

Spirilla

Spirilla are spiral or curve-shaped bacteria. *Treponema pallidum,* a spirochete, is the causative agent of syphilis (see Fig. 20.3 E). This microorganism cannot be grown in commonly available culture media; the diagnosis of syphilis is generally made using serologic tests. A serologic test is performed on the serum of the blood. Cholera is caused by another type of spirillum, *Vibrio cholerae.* Immunization and proper methods of sanitation and water purification have all but eliminated cholera in the United States.

VIRUSES

Viruses are the smallest living organisms. They are so small that an electron microscope must be used to view them. Viruses infect plants, animals, and humans and use nutrients inside the host's cells for their metabolic and reproductive needs. Infectious diseases caused by viruses include chickenpox, rubeola (measles), rubella (German measles), mumps, poliomyelitis, smallpox, rabies, herpes simplex, herpes zoster, yellow fever, hepatitis, the common cold, influenza, and COVID-19 (refer to the box on Patient Coaching: COVID-19).

MICROSCOPE

Many kinds of microscopes are available, but the type used most often for office laboratory work is the *compound microscope.* The compound microscope consists of a two-lens system, and the magnification of one system is increased by the other. A source of bright light is required for proper illumination of the object to be viewed. This combination of lenses and light permits visualization of structures that cannot be seen with the unaided eye, such as microorganisms and cellular forms. The compound microscope consists of two main components: the support system and the optical system. The medical assistant should be able to identify the parts of a microscope (Fig. 20.4) and should be able to operate and care for it properly. Procedure 20.1 outlines the correct operation and care of a microscope.

SUPPORT SYSTEM

Frame

The working parts of the microscope are supported by a sturdy frame consisting of a *base* for support and an *arm* for carrying it without damaging the delicate parts. The arm also is needed to support the magnifying and adjusting systems.

Stage

The *stage* of a microscope is the flat, horizontal platform on which the microscope slide is placed. It is located directly over the condenser and beneath the objective lenses. The stage has a small round opening in the center that permits light from below to pass through the object being viewed and up into the magnifying lenses above. The slide should be placed on the stage; the object to be viewed is positioned over this opening so that it is satisfactorily illuminated by the light source below.

PATIENT COACHING COVID-19

Answer questions patients have about COVID-19.

What is COVID-19?

Coronavirus disease 2019 (COVID-19) is a contagious disease caused by a novel (or new) strain of coronavirus known as *SARS-CoV-2* (severe acute respiratory syndrome coronavirus 2). The virus is considered novel because it is a new coronavirus that has not been previously identified in humans and the 19 in COVID-19 represents the year in which the virus first appeared.

While it's well known that the upper airways and lungs are primary sites of SARS-CoV-2 infection, there are clues the virus can infect cells in other parts of the body, such as the digestive system, blood vessels, kidneys, and, as this new study shows, the mouth. The potential of the virus to infect multiple areas of the body might help explain the wide-ranging symptoms experienced by COVID-19 patients.

How is COVID-19 transmitted?

COVID-19 is primarily transmitted by close contact with an infected person through breathing coughing, sneezing, singing, and speaking. An infected individual can transmit the virus for up to two days before exhibiting symptoms. An individual remains infectious for up to 10 days following the onset of symptoms in moderate cases. In severe cases, an individual remains infectious for up to 20 days.

What are the symptoms of COVID-19?

COVID-19 affects the upper and lower respiratory tracts, especially the lungs. The symptoms of COVID-19 vary among individuals and may include the following:

- Fever
- Sore throat
- Cough
- Congestion
- Headache
- Fatigue
- Muscle or body aches
- Breathing difficulties
- Loss of smell and taste
- Nausea or vomiting
- Diarrhea

Symptoms begin anywhere from 2 to 14 days following exposure to the virus and can range from mild to severe. Approximately one-third of individuals infected with COVID-19 do not develop any symptoms. Most infected individuals develop mild to moderate symptoms and get better on their own. Severe symptoms include constant trouble with breathing, blue lips or face, confusion, and persistent pain or pressure in the chest known as *acute respiratory distress syndrome* (ARDS). Older adults and individuals with chronic health conditions or compromised immune systems are more likely to become severely ill with COVID-19 and require hospitalization.

How can COVID-19 be prevented?

The following measures help prevent the spread of COVID-19:

- Get the COVID-19 vaccines
- Wear a mask to protect yourself and others from the spread of COVID-19
- Stay at least 6 feet (about 2 arm lengths) from people who do not live with you
- Avoid touching your eyes, nose, and mouth with unwashed hands
- Avoid crowds and poorly ventilated areas
- Sanitize your hands frequently, either with soap and water for 20 s or an alcohol-based hand sanitizer
- Avoid close contact with people who are ill
- Cover your mouth with your elbow when you cough or sneeze or use a tissue
- Clean and disinfect frequently touched objects and surfaces daily ■

Most microscopes have a *mechanical stage* that allows movement of the slide in a vertical or horizontal position using adjustment knobs. The mechanical stage has a slide holder that secures the slide and provides precise positioning of the slide, which is essential for performing certain procedures, such as WBC differential counts (manual method) and inspection of Gram-stained smears. *(Note: Bacteria are colorless and usually difficult to identify under a microscope unless some type of staining is used. Gram staining allows for the direct viewing of the size, shape, and growth patterns of bacteria under a microscope.)*

Standard microscope stages have metal clips attached to the stage to hold the glass slide securely in place. With this type of stage, the slide must be moved by hand for examination of various areas on it.

Light Source

The light source is at the base of the microscope and consists of a built-in illuminator, along with a switch for turning it on and off. The light is directed to the condenser above it and then through the specimen and the objective and ocular lenses to be viewed. An intensity dial is used to increase or decrease the brightness of the illuminator.

Condenser

Compound microscopes have a lens system between the light source and the specimen, known as the *substage condenser.* A popular condenser is the *Abbé condenser,* which consists of two lenses used to illuminate a specimen with transmitted light. The condenser collects and concentrates the light rays from the illuminator and directs them up, bringing them to a focus on the specimen so that it is well illuminated.

Diaphragm

The amount of light focused on the specimen also can be controlled by the *diaphragm,* located beneath the condenser. The diaphragm consists of a series of horizontally arranged

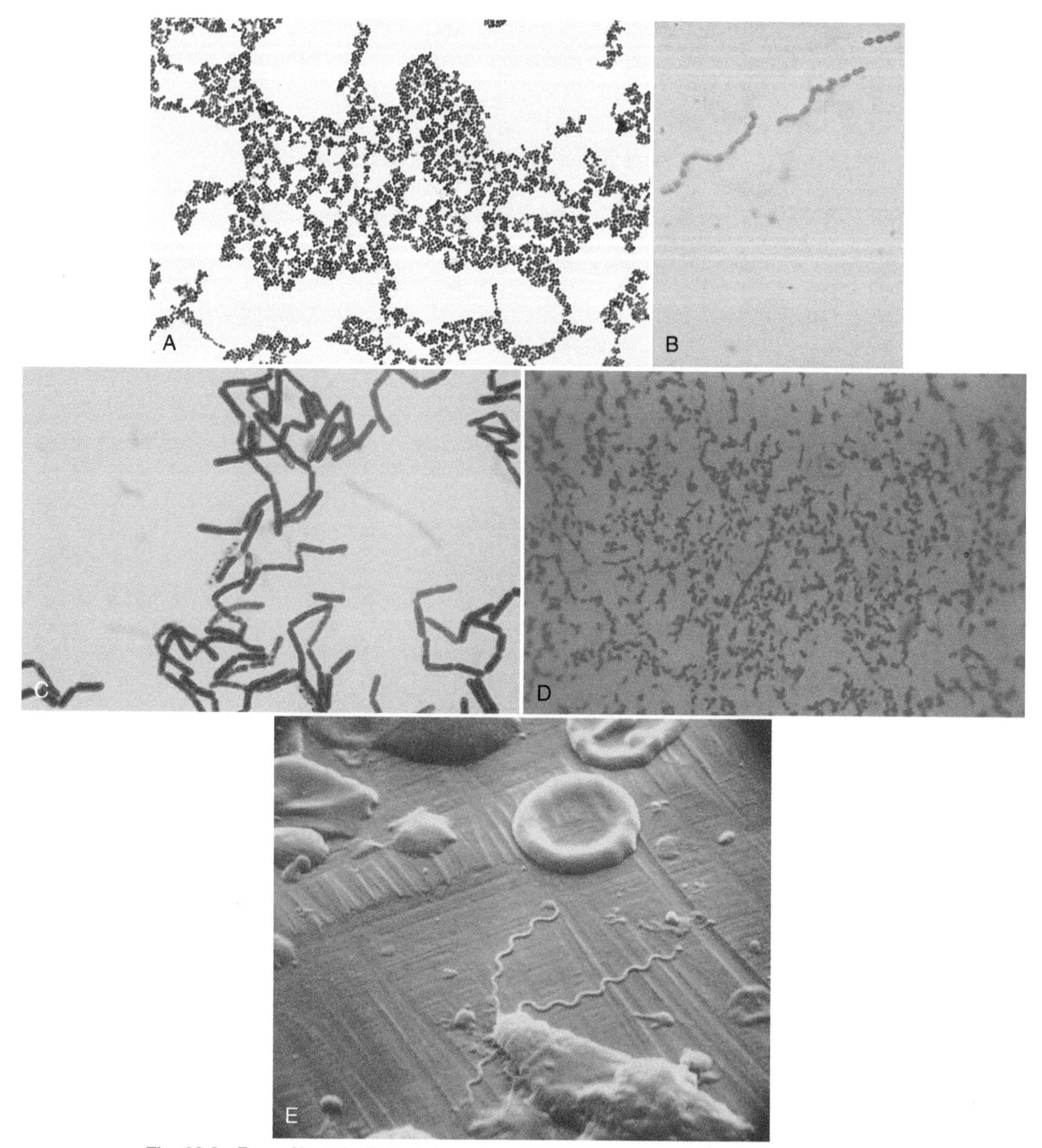

Fig. 20.3 Types of bacteria. (A) Staphylococci. (B) Streptococci. (C) Bacilli. (D) *Escherichia coli.* (E) Spirilla. (A, B, and D, From Mahon CR, Lehman DC, Manuselis G Jr.: *Textbook of diagnostic microbiology,* ed 4, Philadelphia: Elsevier; 2010; C, Courtesy Cathy Bissonette; E, Courtesy Dr. Andrew G. Smith.)

interlocking plates with a central opening, or *aperture.* The diaphragm has a lever that is used to increase or decrease the amount of light admitted by increasing or decreasing the aperture.

Appropriate light intensity is essential for proper viewing of the specimens, especially at a higher magnification. A general rule is that as the desired magnification increases, the more intense the light must be. Increased light intensity is required for good visualization of a specimen with the oil-immersion objective. With the low-power objective, the light must be diminished to produce the appropriate contrast for specimen detail and to reduce glare. The density of the specimen also influences the degree of illumination; stained structures (e.g., a Gram-stained smear of bacteria) usually require more light intensity than do unstained specimens.

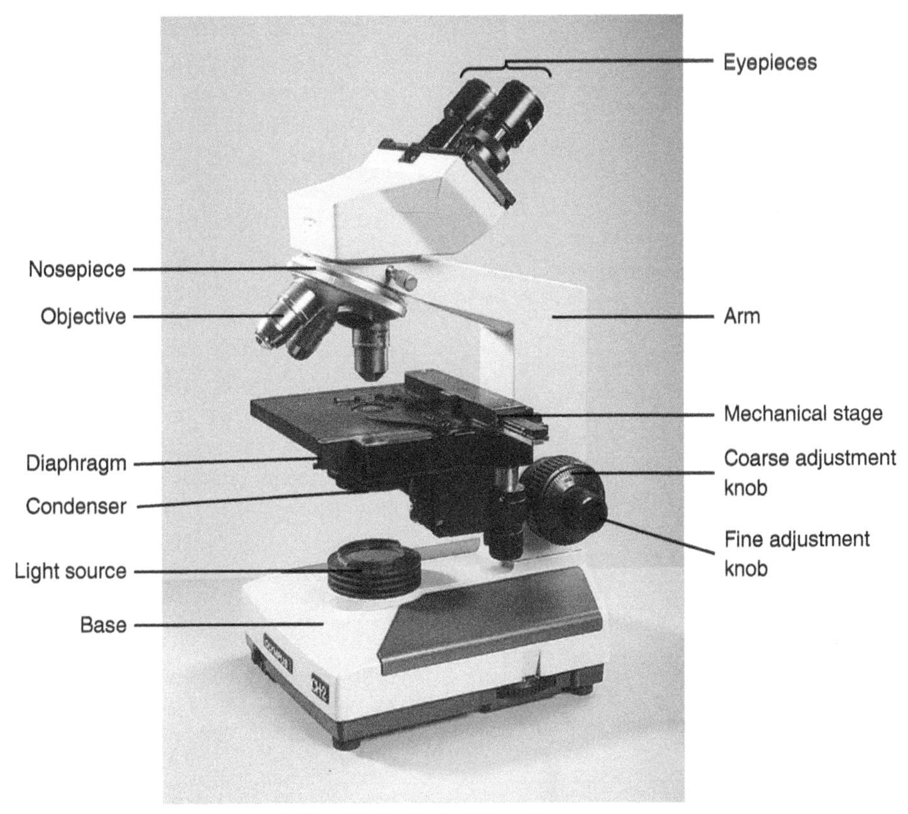

Fig. 20.4 Parts of the microscope.

OPTICAL SYSTEM

Compound microscopes have a two-lens magnification system. *Magnification* is defined as the ratio of the apparent size of an object viewed through the microscope to the actual size of the object.

Eyepiece

The first lens system is the eyepiece, or ocular lens, located at the top of the microscope and marked 10×, meaning that it magnifies 10 times. Microscopes that have one eyepiece only are called *monocular* microscopes, and microscopes with two eyepieces are called *binocular.* A binocular microscope is recommended for medical office laboratory work because it causes less eye fatigue than the monocular type. The binocular eyepieces can be adjusted to the individual by moving the eyepieces apart or together as needed.

Objective Lenses

The second lens system consists of three objective lenses located on a rotating *nosepiece,* each with a different degree of magnification. The metal shafts of the objective lenses differ in length and are identified by the power of magnification. The objective with the shortest shaft is known as the *low-power objective* and has a magnification of 10×. The objective with a mid-length shaft is the *high-power objective*; it has a magnification of 40×. The objective with the longest shaft is the *oil-immersion objective;* it has the highest power of magnification, which is 100×.

The degree of magnification is engraved onto the metal shaft of each objective. In addition, some microscope manufacturers identify each objective lens by colored rings that encircle the metal shaft of the objective. Yellow is used for low power, blue for high power, and white for oil immersion. If the objective is not color-coded , it can be identified by the length of the metal shaft.

The objective lens magnifies the specimen, and the ocular lens magnifies the image produced by the objective lens. The *total magnification* of each objective is determined by multiplying the ocular magnification by the objective magnification. The total magnification of the low-power objective is 100 times (100×) the actual size of the object being viewed (10 × 10). The total magnification of the high-power objective is 400× (10 × 40), and that of the oil-immersion magnification is 1000× (10 × 100).

Focusing System

Two adjustment knobs are used to raise and lower the stage of the microscope to bring the specimen into focus: these include the coarse adjustment knob and the fine adjustment knob. The *coarse adjustment knob* is used first to obtain an approximate focus. The *fine adjustment knob* is then used to obtain the precise focusing necessary to produce a sharp, clear image. On some microscope models, the adjustment knobs are mounted as two separate knobs; on others, they are placed together with the smaller fine adjustment knob extending from a larger coarse adjustment wheel.

Most compound microscopes are *parfocal.* This means that once the specimen is focused with the low-power objective, the nosepiece can be rotated to a higher-power objective and focused simply with the fine adjustment knob.

FUNCTION OF THE OBJECTIVE LENSES

Low and High Power Objectives

The low-power objective is used for the initial focusing and light adjustment of the microscope. The low-power objective also is used for the initial observation and scanning requirements needed for most microscopic work. Urine sediment is first examined using the low-power objective to scan the specimen for the presence of casts.

The high-power objective is used for a more thorough study, such as observing cells in greater detail. The *working distance,* defined as the distance between the tip of the lens and the slide, is short when using the high-power objective. Because of this, care must be taken in focusing this objective to prevent it from striking and breaking the slide or damaging the lens.

Oil Immersion Objective

The oil-immersion objective provides the highest magnification and is used to view very small structures or the detail of larger structures, such as microorganisms and blood cells. The oil-immersion objective has a very short working distance, and when it is in use, the lens nearly rests on the microscope slide itself. A special grade of oil, known as *immersion oil,* must be used with this lens. Oil has the advantage of not drying out when exposed to air for a long time. A drop of oil is placed on the slide and resides between the oil-immersion objective and the slide. The oil provides a path for the light to travel on between the slide and the lens and prevents the scattering of light rays, which permits clear viewing of very small structures. The oil also improves the resolution of the objective lens, that is, its ability to provide sharp detail, which is particularly necessary at high magnifications. Procedures that require oil immersion include WBC differential counts (manual method) and examination of Gram-stained smears.

CARE OF THE MICROSCOPE

The microscope is a delicate instrument and must be handled carefully. These guidelines should be followed to care for the microscope properly:

1. Always carry the microscope with two hands. Place one hand firmly on the arm and the other hand under the base for support. Place the microscope down gently to prevent jarring it, which could damage delicate parts.
2. Always handle the microscope so that your fingers do not touch the lenses and leave fingerprints on them. When using a microscope, avoid wearing mascara because it is difficult to remove from the ocular lens.
3. When it is not in use, keep the microscope covered with its plastic dust cover and stored in a case or cupboard. Store it with the nosepiece rotated to the low-power objective with the stage at its lowest position.
4. Periodically clean the microscope by washing the enameled surfaces with mild soap and water and drying them thoroughly with a soft cloth. Never use alcohol on the enameled surfaces because it might remove the finish.
5. After each use, wipe the metal stage clean with gauze or tissue. If immersion oil comes in contact with the stage, remove it with a piece of gauze that is slightly moistened with xylene.
6. The ocular, objectives, and condenser consist of hand-ground optical lenses, which must be kept spotlessly clean by using clean, dry lens paper. Optical glass is softer than ordinary glass; to prevent scratching the lens, do not use tissues or gauze. If the lenses are especially dirty, use a commercial lens cleaner or xylene in the cleaning process. Apply a small amount of cleaner to the lens paper, followed by thorough drying and polishing with a clean piece of lens paper.
7. Keep the light source free of dust, lint, and dirt by periodic polishing with lens paper.
8. A malfunctioning microscope should be repaired only by a qualified service person. Attempting to fix the microscope yourself may result in further damage.

MICROBIOLOGIC SPECIMEN COLLECTION

If the provider suspects that a particular disease is caused by a pathogen, he or she may want to obtain a specimen for analysis by an outside laboratory. This analysis identifies the pathogen causing the disease and aids in diagnosis. If a urinary tract infection is suspected, a urine specimen is obtained for bacterial examination. In this instance, a clean-catch midstream collection is required to obtain a specimen that excludes the normal flora of the urethra and urinary meatus.

A **specimen** is a small sample or part taken from the body to represent the whole. The medical assistant is often responsible for collecting specimens from certain areas of the body, such as the throat, nose, and wounds. The medical assistant may be responsible for assisting the provider in the collection of specimens from other areas, such as the cervix, vagina, urethra, and rectum. In most instances, a sterile swab is used to collect the specimen. A *swab* is a small piece of cotton wrapped around the end of a slender wooden or plastic stick. It is passed across a body surface or opening to obtain a specimen for microbiologic analysis.

To prevent inaccurate test results, good techniques of medical and surgical asepsis must be practiced when a specimen is obtained. The medical assistant must be careful not to contaminate the specimen with *extraneous microorganisms.* These are undesirable microorganisms that can enter the specimen in various ways; they grow and multiply and possibly obscure and prevent visualization and identification of pathogens that might be present. To prevent extraneous microorganisms (i.e., normal flora) from contaminating the specimen, all supplies used to obtain the specimen (e.g., swabs, specimen containers) must be sterile. In addition, the specimen should not contain microorganisms from areas surrounding the collection site. When obtaining a throat specimen, the swab should not be allowed to touch the inside of the mouth.

The OSHA Bloodborne Pathogens Standard presented in Chapter 2 should be carefully followed when collecting a microbiologic specimen. Specifically, the medical assistant must wear gloves when it is reasonably anticipated that hand contact might occur with blood or other potentially infectious materials. Eating, drinking, handling contact lenses, and applying cosmetics are strictly forbidden when one is working with microorganisms because pathogens can be transmitted to the medical assistant. If the medical assistant accidentally touches some of the material in the specimen, the area of contact should be washed immediately and thoroughly with soap and water. If the specimen comes in contact with the worktable, the table should be cleaned immediately with soap and water, followed by a suitable disinfectant, such as phenol. The worktable also should be cleaned with a disinfectant at the end of each day.

After collection, the specimen must be placed in its proper container with the lid securely fastened. The container must be clearly labeled with the patient's name and date of birth, the date, the source of the specimen, the medical assistant's initials, and any other required information. Procedure 20.2 outlines the procedure for collecting a throat specimen for transport to an outside laboratory.

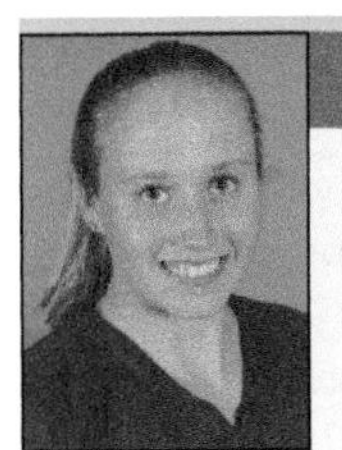

Putting It All Into Practice

My name is Alexandra, and I work for a physician who specializes in family practice. Working as a medical assistant, one can encounter many challenges. One experience that I had involved a 4-year-old boy. The little boy came into the office with a very sore throat and a high fever. He did not think that his office visit had gone too badly until he found out that the physician had ordered a rapid streptococcus test to check for strep throat. That's when he decided he did not care for me, my tongue depressor, or my swab. He decided to protest by keeping his mouth tightly shut. Rather than forcing the procedure on the child, I took my time and kept my patience. I managed to convince him that even though the procedure was uncomfortable and tasted bad, it was the only way we would know if he was really sick or not. I also explained that the test was the only way the doctor would know what kind of medicine to prescribe so he could get well and feel like playing again. It took a while, but we got our specimen. The strep test was positive and the little boy got the right antibiotic that he needed to get better. After the procedure, he gave me a smile and said "I am so glad that is over!" ■

HANDLING AND TRANSPORTING MICROBIOLOGIC SPECIMENS

After the microbiologic specimen has been collected, care should be taken in handling the specimen and preparing it for transport to an outside laboratory. Delay in processing a specimen for microbial culture may cause the death of pathogens or overgrowth of the specimen by microorganisms that are part of the normal flora usually collected along with the pathogen from the specimen site.

Specimens transported to an outside medical laboratory are often placed in a transport medium. The transport medium prevents the drying of the specimen and preserves it in its original state until it reaches its destination. Transport media are discussed in greater detail in the section on "Collection and Transport Systems."

Outside laboratories provide the medical office with specific instructions on the care and handling of specimens being transported to them. These specimens must be accompanied by a laboratory request that designates the provider's name and address; the patient's name, age, and gender; the date and time of collection; the type of microbiologic examination requested; the source of the specimen (e.g., throat, wound, urine); and the provider's clinical diagnosis. The form usually includes a space to indicate whether the patient is receiving antibiotic therapy. Antibiotics may suppress the growth of bacteria, a factor that could produce a false-negative result. A **false-negative result** denotes a condition is absent when it is actually present.

Wound Specimens

Wound specimens are collected using many of the techniques described previously. In many cases, two swabs are used to collect the specimen. The specimen is obtained by inserting the swab into the area of the wound that contains the most drainage and gently rotating the swab from side to side to allow it to absorb completely any microorganisms present. The swab is placed in the specimen container, and the process is repeated using a second swab. To obtain accurate and reliable test results, it is important to collect a specimen from within the wound, rather than from the surface.

COLLECTION AND TRANSPORT SYSTEMS

Microbiologic collection and transport systems are available to facilitate the collection of a specimen to be transported to an outside laboratory for analysis; examples include Culturette (Becton Dickinson, Franklin Lakes, NJ) and Starswab II (Starplex Scientific, Beverly, MA) (Fig. 20.5). These systems consist of a sterile swab and a plastic tube that contains a transport medium. The transport medium prevents the drying of the specimen and preserves it in its original state until it reaches its destination. The collection and transport system comes packaged in a peel-apart envelope and should be stored at room temperature. The procedure for the use of a microbiologic collection and transport system is outlined next:

1. Sanitize your hands, and apply gloves.
2. Check the expiration date on the peel-apart envelope.
3. Peel back the package, and remove the cap from the collection tube. Remove the cap/swab unit from the peel-apart package. The cap is permanently attached to the sterile swab.
4. Using the aseptic technique, collect the specimen. Do not allow the swab to touch any area other than the collection site.
5. Insert the swab into the collection tube.
6. Push the cap/swab in as far as it will go to immerse the swab completely in the transport medium. Make sure the cap is tightly in place.
7. Remove gloves and sanitize your hands.
8. Label the tube with the patient's name and date of birth, the date, the source of the specimen (e.g., throat, wound), and your initials.
9. Complete a preprinted laboratory request form or a computer-generated electronic request.
10. Place the collection tube in a biohazard specimen bag with the preprinted request form in the outside pocket. Transmit computer-generated requests electronically.
11. Document the procedure in the patient's medical record.
12. Transport the specimen to the laboratory within 24 hours.

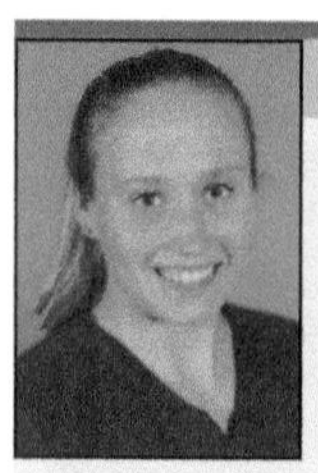

Memories *from* Practicum

Alexandra: Terrified and excited at the same time to be experiencing my first externship, I found myself in a busy pediatric office. After a few days of watching and learning, I prepared to work up an infant for a well-child examination. Before entering the room, I was told by a staff member that the HIV status of the infant's mother was questionable. Alarmed at first as to how I would feel in this situation, I immediately remembered all the precautions we had talked about in class. As I took the infant from the mother to weigh and measure him, I have to admit many thoughts ran through my mind, but again I was calmed because of all the information we had received in school regarding OSHA precautions. Faced with that situation today, after practicing wisely and safely for 5 years, I would not think twice about it because I know from my education and experience that these types of situations can be handled without alarm. ■

CLIA-WAIVED MICROBIOLOGIC TESTS

A microbiologic specimen may be collected and tested in the physician's office laboratory (POL) using CLIA-waived biochemical testing kits. The most common tests performed on microbiologic specimens in the medical office include CLIA-waived strep tests and CLIA-waived influenza tests which are described in detail as follows.

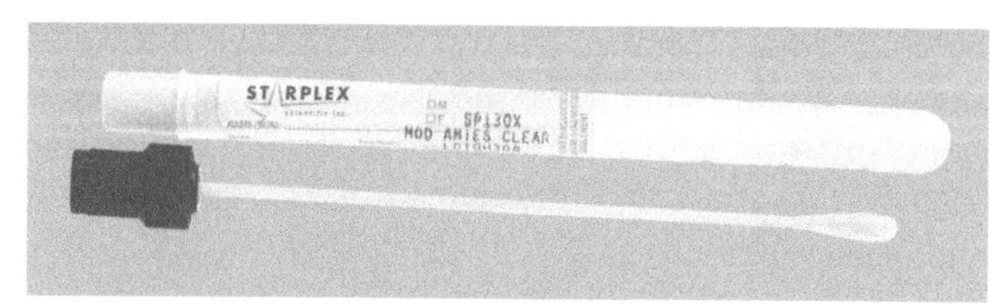

Fig. 20.5 Starswab II Collection and Transport System.

Streptococcal Pharyngitis (Strep Throat)

The most common streptococcal condition is streptococcal pharyngitis, or strep throat, which is a bacterial infection of the back of the throat and tonsils. The causative agent of strep throat is group A streptococcus, known as *Streptococcus pyogenes.* Strep throat is seasonal in nature with the highest prevalence occurring during the winter and early spring. Strep throat occurs most frequently in children ages 5 to 15 years old.

Symptoms

The symptoms of strep throat include the following:

- Severe and sudden sore throat
- Fever of 101° F (38.3° C) or higher
- Red and swollen tonsils
- White patches or streaks on the throat and tonsils
- Severe pain and difficulty upon swallowing
- Tender and swollen lymph nodes on the sides of the neck
- Tiny red spots at the back of the roof of the mouth
- Headache

Strep throat can easily be spread from one person to another through droplet infection and by sharing personal items with an infected person such as eating utensils. The incubation period for strep throat ranges from 1 to 3 days, with most patients recovering within 7 to 10 days.

Strep throat is a potentially serious condition because (although rare) some patients develop a poststreptococcal complication. A poststreptococcal complication is a morbid secondary condition that occurs as a result of a less serious primary infection. Occasionally a patient with strep throat (primary infection) develops a rheumatic fever or acute glomerulonephritis. Owing to the risk of a poststreptococcal complication, early diagnosis and treatment of strep throat with antibiotics is important.

CLIA-Waived Streptococcus Testing

In the medical office, a CLIA-waived RADT *(rapid antigen detection test)* is often used for the identification of group A streptococci. RADTs are immunoassay tests for the qualitative detection of group A streptococcus. They are biochemical tests that detect group A streptococcus from a throat specimen in a very short time. Most tests require only 4 to 10 minutes to process; diagnosis can often be made and antibiotics prescribed, if necessary, before the patient leaves the office.

A RADT confirms the presence of group A streptococcus through an antigen-antibody reaction. The test works by combining particles sensitized to the streptococcus antibody with a throat specimen collected from the patient. If group A streptococcal antigen is in the specimen, it combines with the antibody-sensitized particles to produce a color change that can be observed with the unaided eye. Rapid streptococcus tests also include an internal control that determines whether the test results are accurate and reliable.

The advantage of the RADT is that it gives the provider immediate test results rather than requiring an overnight culture. Specific instructions are included with every commercially available CLIA-waived RADT; examples of these tests include QuickVue In-Line Strep A (Quidel), OSOM Strep A Test (Sekisui Diagnostics), and BinaxNOW Strep A Test (Binax, Inc.). The procedure for performing a CLIA-waived RADT is presented in Procedure 20.3.

What Would You Do? What Would You *Not* Do?

Case Study 2

Paula Hutchinson brings her 8-year-old daughter Caitlin to the medical office. Caitlin has had a fever, sore throat, and difficulty eating for the past 2 days. The physician orders a rapid strep test. Caitlin refuses to open her mouth so that the specimen can be collected. She says that she doesn't want that "swab thing" in her mouth because she's afraid it will make her throw up. Paula wants to know why the strep test must be run. She says that Caitlin's throat is very red with white patches and wants to know why the physician doesn't just prescribe an antibiotic for her without running the test. ■

Influenza

Influenza (commonly called the flu) is a highly contagious acute infectious disease caused by viruses that infect the respiratory system (nose, throat, and lungs). According to the Centers for Disease Control (CDC), approximately 5% to 20% of the U.S. population will contract influenza each year. Influenza outbreaks are most apt to occur between the late fall and early spring (November through April). There are three different types of influenza viruses (A, B, and C), which are described as follows:

- *Influenza type A:* This type is most prevalent and is responsible for most annual influenza outbreaks. It causes moderate to severe illness, and at times it can lead to serious complications. Influenza A can be further divided into numerous subtypes; for example, H3N2 (Hong Kong flu) and H1N1 (swine flu) are subtypes of influenza type A.
- *Influenza type B:* This type can cause influenza outbreaks but is usually associated with a less severe infection than type A.
- *Influenza type C:* This type only causes a mild upper respiratory illness and occurs much less frequently than types A and B.

Transmission and Incubation Period

Influenza spreads easily from one person to another. It is transmitted primarily through droplet infection from the respiratory tract of an infected individual when they cough, sneeze, or, talk. Influenza is less frequently transmitted through indirect contact such as when a person touches an object or surface that is contaminated with the influenza virus and then touches his or her mouth, eyes, or nose. An individual usually becomes infected with either type A or type B influenza, but in rare instances, an individual may become infected with both type A and type B influenza at the same time.

The incubation period for influenza is usually two days but it can range from 1 to 4 days. An infected individual is contagious approximately 24 to 48 hours before the onset of symptoms and up to 5 to 7 days after symptoms appear.

Symptoms

In the early stages of influenza, symptoms may be difficult to distinguish from those of the common cold; however, colds usually develop slowly, whereas the flu has a more sudden onset and the symptoms are much worse. Symptoms of influenza vary by age but commonly include the following:

- Fever and chills
- Muscle aches and joint pain
- Sore throat
- Runny nose
- Nasal congestion
- Dry cough
- Headache
- Joint pain
- Anorexia
- Fatigue
- Gastrointestinal symptoms such as nausea, vomiting, and diarrhea (more common in children)

Complications

Influenza can occur among people of all ages. Most individuals with healthy immune systems recover within 7 to 14 days, with the worst symptoms lasting 3 to 4 days. There are certain factors that can increase an individual's risk of developing serious and even life-threatening complications from influenza. These risk factors can be categorized into *health-related factors* and *age-related factors* and are presented in Box 20.1.

Influenza complications range in severity and can include the following: viral pneumonia, a worsening of a chronic medical condition, and secondary bacterial infections such as bacterial pneumonia, bronchitis, sinusitis, and otitis media. Some of these complications can lead to hospitalization and even death. Because of this, individuals with risk factors should seek prompt medical attention at the first sign of flulike symptoms. Most, but not all, flu-related deaths occur in individuals 65 years of age and older.

Prevention

The primary means of preventing influenza is through an influenza vaccine and infection control measures, which are discussed in more detail as follows.

BOX 20.1 Factors That Increase the Risk of Influenza Complications

Individuals with the following health-related and age-related factors are at an increased risk of developing influenza complications and should seek prompt medical attention at the first sign of flulike symptoms.

Health-Related Factors

Chronic Medical Conditions

- Asthma
- Chronic bronchitis
- Emphysema
- Cystic fibrosis
- Diabetes
- Heart disease
- Kidney or liver disorders
- Blood disorders (e.g., sickle cell disease)
- Very severely obese (body mass index [BMI] of 40 or more)
- Diseases or treatments that weaken the immune system:
  - HIV/AIDS
  - Treatment with corticosteroids, immunosuppressants, or chemotherapy

Age-Related Factors

- Adults age 65 years and older
- Young children under 5 years of age, but especially children younger than 2 years of age

Additional Factors

- Individuals with severe influenza symptoms
- Pregnant women
- Residents of nursing homes and other long-term care facilities
- American Indians and Alaska Natives

Influenza Vaccine

The best means of preventing influenza and its complications is through an annual influenza vaccination. The vaccine is recommended for all individuals ages 6 months and older who do not have contraindications to receiving the vaccine (e.g., severe egg allergy). The vaccine provides protection against both type A and type B influenza viruses. As previously discussed, there are numerous subtypes of influenza type A. Small changes continuously take place in the genetic material of these subtype viruses resulting in new strains developing that replace the older strains. Because of this, a new vaccine must be produced each year to provide protection against the most recent strains predicted to be circulating during that year's flu season.

It takes approximately 2 weeks following vaccination for the antibodies to develop that provide protection against the virus strains included in the vaccine. The flu vaccine provides reasonable protection among healthy adults. Vaccination is most effective when the circulating virus strains are well-matched with the virus strains included in the vaccine. Even if the vaccine does not prevent the flu, however, it can reduce the severity of symptoms and decrease the risk of complications.

The influenza vaccine has only mild side effects or none at all, and it is available as an intramuscular injection (e.g., Fluvirin), an intradermal injection (e.g., Fluzone Intradermal), or a nasal spray (e.g., FluMist). Flu vaccination is offered in many locations within a community such as medical offices, health departments, pharmacies, college health centers, workplaces, and even schools. Many communities have programs that offer the vaccine free of charge or at a reduced cost.

Infection Control Measures

Infection control measures provide reasonably effective ways to prevent the transmission of influenza. These measures include the following:

1. Practice good hand hygiene such as frequent handwashing or the use of an alcohol-based hand rub.
2. Avoid close contact with infected individuals.
3. Try not to touch your eyes, nose, or mouth to prevent the influenza virus from gaining entrance into your body.
4. Always cover your nose and mouth when you cough or sneeze. To avoid contaminating the hands, cough or sneeze into a tissue or the crook of the elbow.
5. If infected with influenza, stay home from work, school, or public places for at least 24 hours after the fever has subsided.

Treatment

Treatment for influenza primarily involves home care measures to ease the symptoms but may occasionally involve the use of antiviral medication. These treatment measures are discussed in more detail as follows:

Home Care

Most people who contract influenza recover on their own without medical intervention. Home care is usually all that is necessary to treat the symptoms of influenza. These measures are outlined as follows:

- Get plenty of rest.
- Increase fluid intake to stay hydrated.
- Avoid the use of alcohol and tobacco.
- Take over-the-counter medications to relieve the symptoms of the disease.

Antiviral Medications

Antiviral medications are available through a prescription and work by limiting the multiplication of the influenza virus. Antiviral medications lessen the severity of influenza and shorten the duration of the disease by 1 to 2 days. They are not intended, however, to serve as a substitute for an annual influenza vaccine. Antiviral medications are recommended primarily for unvaccinated individuals infected with influenza who are at risk of developing complications from influenza (see Box 20.1).

There are three antiviral medications recommended by the Food and Drug Administration (FDA) for the treatment of influenza. These include oseltamivir (Tamiflu), zanamivir (Relenza), and peramivir (Rapivab). These antiviral medications are effective against both influenza virus types A and B and must be started within the first 48 hours of developing symptoms to be most effective. Because of this, individuals at risk for influenza complications are encouraged to contact their providers at the first sign of flulike symptoms.

CLIA-Waived Influenza Testing

In the medical office, a CLIA-waived RIDT *(rapid influenza diagnostic test)* may be used to assist in the diagnosis of influenza. RIDTs are immunoassay tests for the qualitative detection of the influenza virus antigen. They are biochemical tests that are easy to perform and provide results in a short period of time (15 minutes or less).

In the majority of cases, influenza is diagnosed solely on the clinical signs and symptoms exhibited by the patient. This is because flu symptoms are self-limiting and most individuals recover without requiring medical treatment. An influenza test may be ordered for a patient who is at high risk for developing influenza complications as a basis for prescribing an antiviral medication.

Rapid influenza tests vary in their ability to detect type A and type B influenza viruses. Each RIDT detects the influenza virus in one of the following ways:

1. Detects the presence of the influenza virus without identifying the type
2. Detects only influenza type A virus
3. Detects the presence of type A and B influenza virus, but does not distinguish between the two
4. Detects and distinguishes between the presence of type A and type B influenza virus

It is important to perform a rapid influenza test as close to the onset of symptoms as possible, preferably within the first 2 days after symptoms appear. As previously discussed, in order for antiviral medications to be effective, they must be administered within 48 hours following the onset of symptoms. In addition, a patient infected with the influenza virus is most apt to show a positive test result within the first 3 to 4 days after the appearance of symptoms.

The main disadvantage of RIDTs is that there is a high rate of false-negative test results. Because of this, the CDC recommends that anticipated treatment not be withheld from patients with suspected influenza even if the patient tests negative. More specific tests are available (e.g., viral culture) that can be performed by an outside laboratory; however, it can take from 2 to 10 days to perform the test and obtain the results.

The specimen required to perform the RIDT depends on the brand of test being utilized and includes one or more of the following: nasopharyngeal swab specimen, nasal swab specimen, nasal wash, nasal aspirate, and throat specimen. The influenza virus is most likely to be found in the nasopharynx; therefore, a nasopharyngeal swab specimen is considered the preferred specimen for a rapid influenza test and is discussed in more detail next.

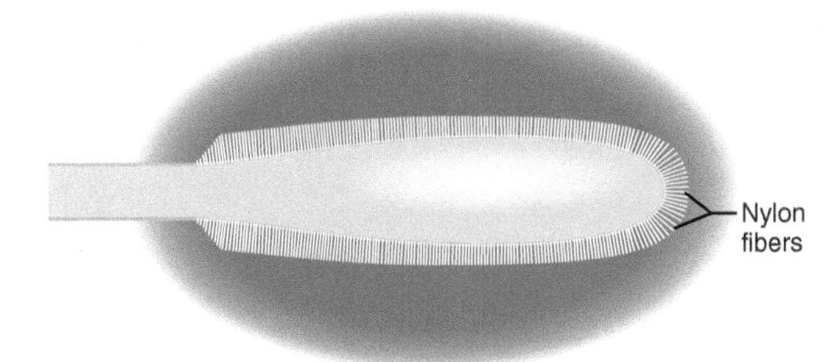

Fig. 20.6 A nasopharyngeal flocked swab consists of a flexible shaft with a small brushlike tip made of nylon fibers.

Nasopharyngeal Swab Specimen

The nasopharynx is the part of the pharynx above the soft palate that is directly continuous with the nasal passages. This is the area from which a nasopharyngeal swab specimen is collected for the detection of the influenza virus. The influenza virus invades epithelial cells in the nasopharynx; therefore a specimen obtained from this area is preferred for RIDT testing.

The preferred specimen collection device for a nasopharyngeal specimen is a flocked swab. A nasopharyngeal flocked swab consists of a flexible shaft with a small brushlike tip (Fig. 20.6). The shaft of the swab has a thicker diameter at one end (where it is held) and progressively narrows to a thinner end, culminating in the soft brush tip. The tip is coated with short nylon fibers that are arranged in a perpendicular manner. This arrangement results from a process called *flocking,* in which nylon fibers are sprayed onto the tip of the swab. Flocking results in a more abrasive swab tip than a cotton-tipped swab and leads to the removal of a greater number of epithelial cells from the nasopharynx.

The depth to which the swab should be inserted is specific to each patient. For example, in order to reach the nasopharyngeal mucosa, the swab must be inserted to a greater depth in an adult than that of a child. It is possible to determine the distance to which the swab should be inserted by visually estimating the distance between the corner of the nose and the earlobe. The swab should be inserted approximately one-half this distance (Fig. 20.7). This depth usually falls between 4 to 6 cm (approximately 1 1/2 to 2 1/2 inches). The procedure for collecting a nasopharyngeal swab specimen and performing a CLIA-waived RIDT is presented in Procedure 20.4.

CULTURE AND SENSITIVITY TESTING

MICROBIAL CULTURES

After a microbiologic specimen is collected and transported to an outside laboratory, it may be examined to determine the type of microorganisms present. Because most specimens generally contain only a few pathogens, it is often desirable to induce any pathogens that are present to grow and multiply.

What Would You Do? What Would You *Not* Do?

Case Study 3

Hollie Dolley, age 18, is at the medical office complaining of fatigue, fever, headache, muscle aching, runny nose, and a sore throat. Hollie also has severe problems with asthma, which began when she was a child. Hollie just enrolled in a medical assisting program at a local college and has been really worried about doing well in her classes. The physician orders a rapid influenza test on Hollie, and it is positive. The physician writes a prescription for an antiviral medication and advises Hollie to get plenty of rest, increase her fluid intake, and stay at home for at least 24 hours after the fever has subsided. Hollie says she doesn't know why she has the flu because she got a flu vaccine a week ago. Hollie also wants to know why the physician did not prescribe an antibiotic for her so that she could get well sooner and not have to miss many classes. ■

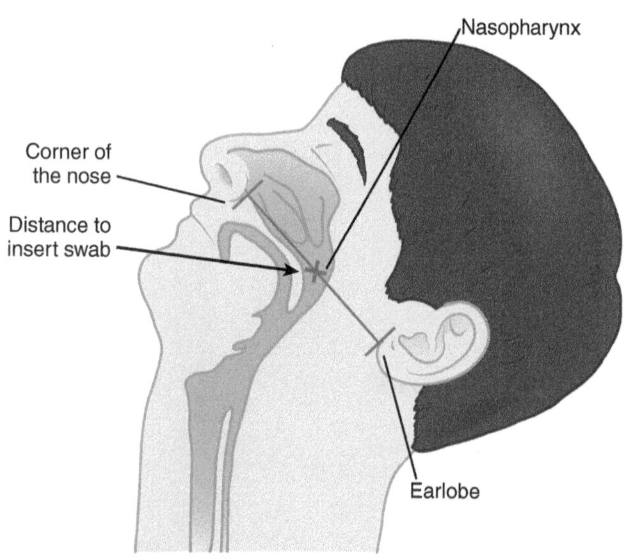

Fig. 20.7 A swab used to collect a nasopharyngeal specimen should be inserted approximately one-half the distance between the corner of the nose and the earlobe.

Most microorganisms, especially bacteria, can be grown on a culture medium. A **culture medium** is a mixture of nutrients on which microorganisms are grown in the laboratory. The culture medium and the environment in which it is placed must meet the requirements to support and encourage the growth of the suspected pathogen. These growth requirements include the presence or the absence of oxygen (depending on the microorganism), proper nutrition, temperature, pH, and moisture.

The culture medium may be solid or liquid. Blood agar is one of the most frequently used solid culture media. It is prepared by adding sheep's blood to a substance known as *agar*, which is transparent and colorless. Blood added to the agar provides nutrients that support the growth of a variety of bacteria. When heated, it melts and becomes a liquid. On cooling, agar solidifies, forming a firm surface on which microorganisms can be grown. A liquid culture medium is often referred to as a *broth* and is usually contained in a tube; an example is nutrient broth. Culture media must be stored in the refrigerator and warmed to room temperature before use. A cold culture medium must not be used because the cold temperature results in the death of microorganisms placed on it.

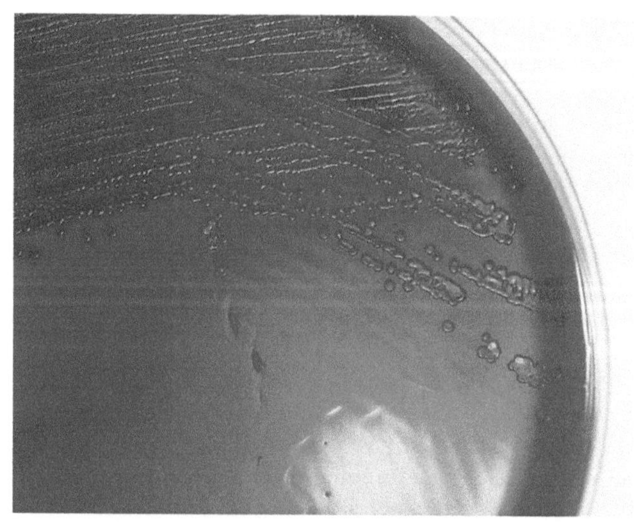

Fig. 20.8 Streptococcal colonies growing on a blood agar culture medium contained in a Petri plate. (From Mahon CR, Lehman DC, Manuselis G Jr.: *Textbook of diagnostic microbiology,* ed 4, Philadelphia: Elsevier; 2010.)

A *Petri plate* is frequently used to hold a solid culture medium. The plate consists of a shallow circular dish made of glass or clear plastic with a cover, the diameter of which is greater than that of the base. Microorganisms can be cultured on the surface of the medium in the plate (Fig. 20.8). Petri plates allow examination of a culture while preventing microorganisms from entering or escaping. A **culture** is a mass of microorganisms growing in a laboratory culture medium.

The solid culture medium in a Petri plate is inoculated by lightly rolling the swab containing the specimen over the surface of the medium. **Inoculate** is defined as the introduction of microorganisms into a culture medium for growth and multiplication. The cover of the Petri plate should be removed only when the specimen is being spread on the culture medium. Unnecessary removal of the cover results in contamination of the medium with extraneous microorganisms. The culture is **incubated** for 24 to 48 hours in conditions that encourage the growth of the suspected pathogen.

Most specimens taken for analysis contain a mixture of organisms because of the presence of normal flora in most parts of the body. When this is the case, the resulting culture is known as a *mixed culture,* or one that contains two or more types of microorganisms. To analyze most microbiologic specimens, the suspected pathogen must be separated from the mixed culture and permitted to grow alone. This establishes a *pure culture,* or a culture that contains only one type of microorganism. After the culture has grown sufficiently, the appropriate tests are performed to identify the pathogen. It is impossible to grow viruses by this method; rather, they must be cultured on living tissue or identified using serologic tests.

SENSITIVITY TESTING

The provider may request not only that the laboratory identify the infecting pathogen, but also that a sensitivity test be performed on it to determine the best antibiotic to treat the condition. The test is always performed on a pure rather than a mixed culture. A sensitivity test determines the susceptibility of pathogenic bacteria to various antibiotics; only the growth of the infectious pathogen is desired on the culture.

A common method for sensitivity testing is the *disc-diffusion method* (Fig. 20.9). Commercially prepared disks impregnated with known concentrations of various antibiotics are dropped on the surface of a solid culture medium in a Petri plate inoculated with the pathogen. The culture is incubated, allowing the antibiotics to diffuse into the culture medium. If the pathogen is susceptible or sensitive to an antibiotic, a clear zone without bacterial growth surrounds the disk. This indicates that the antibiotic was effective in destroying the pathogen. If the pathogen is unaffected by or resistant to the antibiotic, no clear zone is seen around the disk, indicating that the antibiotic was unable to kill the pathogen. Sensitivity testing enables the provider to decide which antibiotics would most likely be effective against the infectious disease in question.

PREVENTION AND CONTROL OF INFECTIOUS DISEASES

Individuals in the community can help prevent and control infectious diseases by practicing good techniques of medical asepsis, obtaining proper nutrition and rest, and using good hygienic measures. In addition, infected individuals should contact their providers in an effort to ensure early diagnosis and treatment of the infectious disease. Immunizations are available to prevent a wide range of infectious diseases. The medical assistant has a responsibility to help educate community members about practices that reduce the transmission of pathogens and help control and prevent infectious diseases.

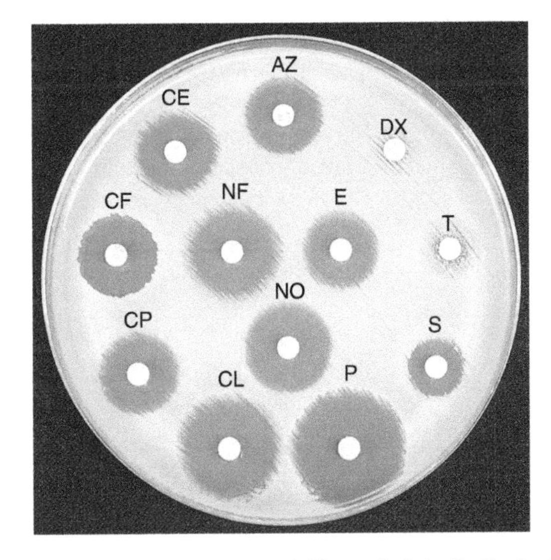

AZ:	Azithromycin
CE:	Cephalothin
CF:	Ciprofloxacin
CL:	Clarithromycin
CP:	Ciprozil
DX:	Doxycycline
E:	Erythromycin
NF:	Nitrofurantoin
NO:	Norfloxacin
P:	Penicillin
S:	Sulfisoxazole
T:	Tetracycline

Fig. 20.9 Sensitivity testing. (From Mahon CR, Lehman DC, Manuselis G Jr.: *Textbook of diagnostic microbiology,* ed 4, Philadelphia: Elsevier; 2010.)

What Would You Do? What Would You *Not* Do? RESPONSES

Case Study 1
Page 691

What Did Alexandra Do?

- ❑ Empathized with John and told him that a lot of people do not like coming to see the doctor. Told him that the doctor could not legally or ethically prescribe medication for him without seeing him.
- ❑ Told John that the office could not bill him for an appointment that he did not have.
- ❑ Asked John whether he wanted to make an appointment to see the doctor.

What Did Alexandra Not Do?

- ❑ Did not tell John he should not be diagnosing himself with information he found on the internet.

Case Study 2
Page 699

What Did Alexandra Do?

- ❑ Told Paula that it is important that the physician find out whether Caitlin has strep throat because strep can sometimes develop into a more serious infection. Explained that if Caitlin

Continued

What Would You Do? What Would You *Not* Do? RESPONSES—cont'd

does have strep throat, the doctor would want to prescribe the best antibiotic to treat the infection.

- ❑ Talked with Caitlin about the reason for the test. Explained that it will help the doctor find the best way to treat her so that she starts feeling better as soon as possible.
- ❑ Reassured Caitlin that the procedure would be quick and it would be over before she knew it. Told Caitlin that after the specimen was obtained, she could choose a prize from the treasure box.
- ❑ Explained to Paula that the physician must first determine if Caitlin has strep throat before antibiotics can be prescribed.

What Did A Not Do?

- ❑ Did not force the collection swab into Caitlin's mouth.

Case Study 3

Page 702

What Did A Do?

- ❑ Explained to Hollie that it takes approximately 2 weeks following vaccination for the flu vaccine to be effective.
- ❑ Explained to Hollie that influenza is caused by a virus and that antibiotics do not work against viruses.
- ❑ Empathized with Hollie and made sure she understood the home measures she could take to treat the symptoms of influenza.

What Did Alexandra Not Do?

- ❑ Did not ignore or minimize Hollie's concerns ■

TERMINOLOGY REVIEW

Medical Term	Word Parts	Definition
Bacilli (*sing.* bacillus)		Bacteria that have a rod shape.
Cocci (*sing.* coccus)	*-cocci:* berry-shaped	Bacteria that have a round shape.
Contagious		Capable of being transmitted directly or indirectly from one person to another.
Culture		The propagation of a mass of microorganisms in a laboratory culture medium.
Culture medium		A mixture of nutrients on which microorganisms are grown in the laboratory.
False-negative result		A test result denoting that a condition is absent when it is actually present.
Incubate		In microbiology, the act of placing a culture in a chamber (incubator) that provides optimal growth requirements for the multiplication of the organisms, such as the proper temperature, humidity, and darkness.
Incubation period		The interval of time between the invasion by a pathogenic microorganism and the appearance of the first symptoms of the disease.
Infection		The condition in which the body, or part of it, is invaded by a pathogen.
Infectious disease		A disease caused by a pathogen that produces harmful effects on its host (also known as a communicable disease).
Inoculate		To introduce microorganisms into a culture medium for growth and multiplication.
Microbiology	*micro-:* small *bi/o:* life *-ology:* study of	The scientific study of microorganisms and their activities.
Mucous membrane		A membrane lining body passages or cavities that open to the outside.
Normal flora		Harmless, nonpathogenic microorganisms that normally reside in many parts of the body but do not cause disease.
Specimen		A small sample or part taken from the body to represent the whole.
Spirilla (*sing.* spirillum)		Bacteria that have a spiral or curved shape.

PROCEDURE 20.1 Operate a Microscope

Outcome Operate a compound microscope.

Equipment/Supplies

- Compound microscope with mechanical stage
- Lens paper
- Specimen slide
- Tissue or gauze
- Immersion oil
- Xylene
- Soft cloth

1. **Procedural Step.** Clean the ocular and objective lenses with lens paper using a circular motion.

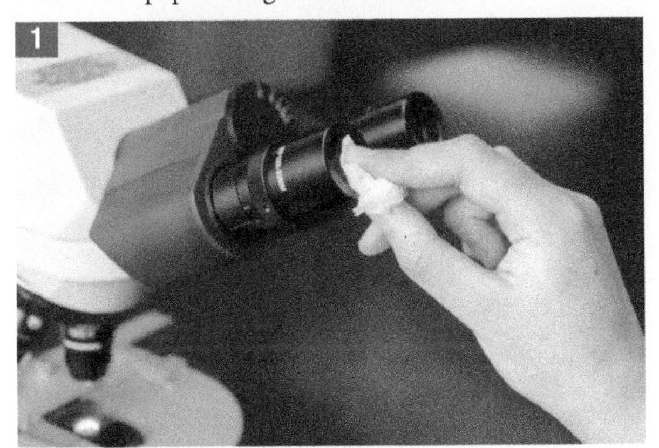

Clean the lens.

2. **Procedural Step.** Turn on the light source.
3. **Procedural Step.** Rotate the nosepiece to the low-power objective (10×), and click it into place. Lower the stage all the way down using the coarse adjustment knob. Lowering the stage all the way down provides sufficient working space for placing the slide on the stage and also avoids damaging the objective lens.
4. **Procedural Step.** Place the slide on the mechanical stage specimen side up, and use the slide holder to secure it.

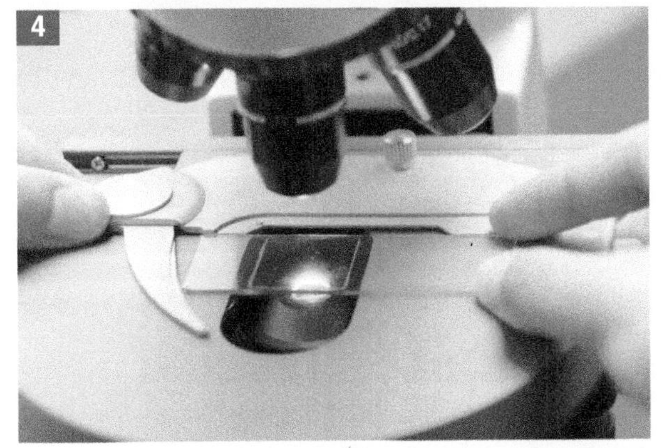

Place the slide on the stage.

5. **Procedural Step.** Using the coarse adjustment knob, raise the stage as far as it will go without touching the low-power objective. Be sure to observe this step to prevent the objective from striking the slide.
6. **Procedural Step.** Look through the eyepiece(s). If a monocular microscope is being used, keep both eyes open to prevent eyestrain. With a binocular microscope, adjust the two eyepieces to the width between your eyes until a single circular field of vision is obtained.
7. **Procedural Step.** Slowly lower the stage using the coarse adjustment knob. Observe the specimen through the eyepieces until it comes into focus.

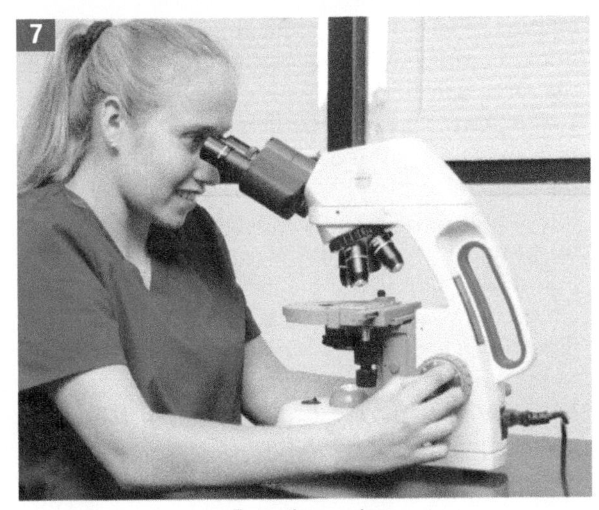

Focus the specimen.

8. **Procedural Step.** Use the fine adjustment knob to bring the specimen into a sharp, clear focus. Use the mechanical stage adjustment knobs to center the specimen as needed for optimal viewing.
9. **Procedural Step.** Adjust the light as needed, using the intensity dial of the illuminator and the diaphragm lever to provide maximal focus and contrast.

PROCEDURE 20.1

Continued

PROCEDURE 20.1 Using the Microscope—cont'd

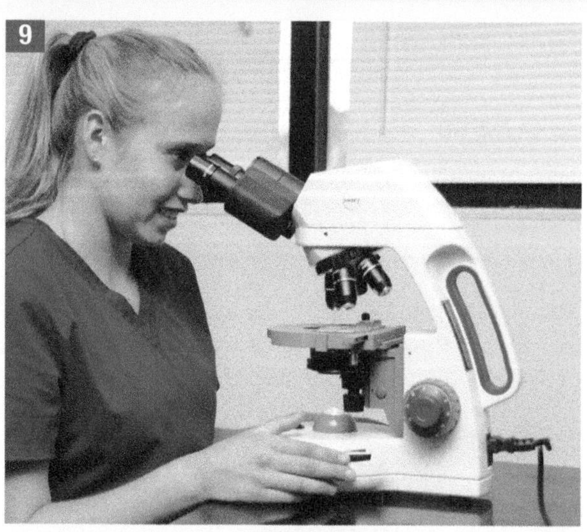

Adjust the light.

10. **Procedural Step.** Rotate the nosepiece to the high-power objective, making sure it clicks into place. Proper focusing with the low-power objective ensures that the objective does not hit the slide during this operation. Use only the fine adjustment knob to bring the specimen into a precise focus. Do not use the coarse adjustment to focus the high-power objective to prevent the objective from moving too far and striking the slide. This can break the slide and damage the objective lens.
11. **Procedural Step.** Examine the specimen as required by the test or procedure being performed.
12. **Procedural Step.** Turn off the light after use, and remove the slide from the stage.
13. **Procedural Step.** Clean the stage with a tissue or gauze.
14. **Procedural Step.** Properly care for and store the microscope.

Using the Oil-Immersion Objective

1. **Procedural Step.** Perform the steps listed above to bring the specimen into focus with first the low-power objective and then with the high-power objective. Rotate the nosepiece to the oil-immersion objective. Do not click it into place, but move it to one side.
2. **Procedural Step.** Place a drop of immersion oil on the slide directly over the center opening on the stage.

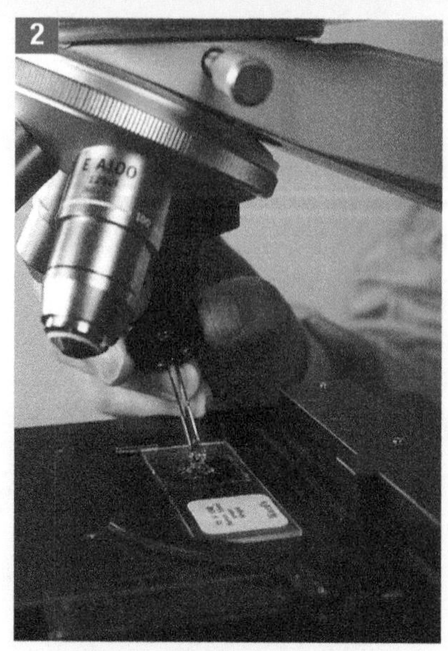

Place a drop of oil on the slide.

3. **Procedural Step.** Move the oil-immersion objective into place until a click is heard.
4. **Procedural Step.** Using the fine adjustment knob, slowly position the oil-immersion objective until the tip of the lens touches the oil but does not come in contact with the slide. A "pop" of light is observed. Be sure to observe carefully this step of the procedure.

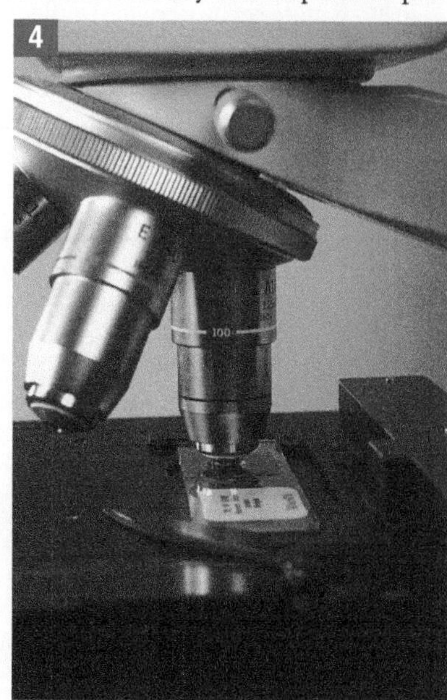

Move the lens until it just touches the oil.

5. **Procedural Step.** Look through the eyepieces, and focus slowly using the fine adjustment. Bring the specimen into a sharp clear focus to view fine details.

PROCEDURE 20.1 Using the Microscope—cont'd

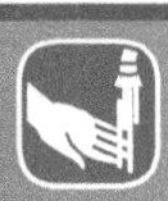

6. **Procedural Step.** Adjust the light as needed, using the diaphragm lever to provide maximal focus and contrast. Increased light intensity is required for good visualization of the specimen with the oil-immersion objective.
7. **Procedural Step.** Examine the specimen as required by the test or procedure being performed.
8. **Procedural Step.** Turn off the light after use. Remove the slide from the stage, being careful not to get oil on the high-power objective. Immersion oil can damage the lens of the high-power objective.
9. **Procedural Step.** Using a piece of clean, dry lens paper, gently clean the oil-immersion objective. The lens must be cleaned immediately after use to prevent oil from drying on the lens surface. In addition, the oil may seep into the lens and perhaps loosen it.

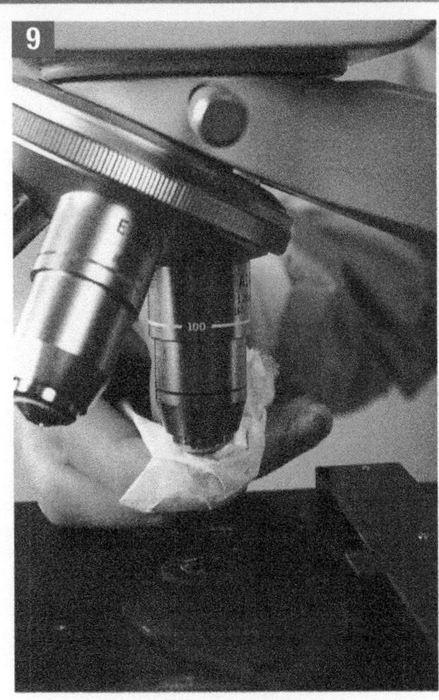

Clean the oil from the lens.

10. **Procedural Step.** Clean the oil from the slide by immersing it in xylene and wiping it off with a soft cloth.

PROCEDURE 20.2

PROCEDURE 20.2 Collecting a Throat Specimen

Outcome

Collect a throat specimen for transport to an outside laboratory.

A throat specimen is obtained by using a sterile swab. It is commonly collected to aid in the diagnosis of infections such as streptococcal sore throat, pharyngitis, and tonsillitis. Less frequently, it is used to diagnose whooping cough and diphtheria. These latter diseases are not prevalent today because of the availability of immunizations against them. This procedure outlines the steps necessary to obtain a throat specimen for transport to an outside laboratory.

Equipment/Supplies

- Disposable gloves
- Tongue depressor
- Sterile swab
- Sterile transport container
- Laboratory request form
- Biohazard specimen bag
- Waste container

1. **Procedural Step.** Sanitize your hands and assemble the equipment. Check the expiration date of the peel-apart swab envelope. Label the transport container with the patient's name and date of birth, the date, the source of the specimen, your initials, and any other required information. Complete a laboratory requisition.
2. **Procedural Step.** Greet the patient and introduce yourself. Identify the patient by full name and date of birth and explain the procedure.
3. **Procedural Step.** Position the patient and adjust the light to provide clear visualization of the throat.
   Principle. The throat must be clearly visible so that the medical assistant is able to determine the proper area for obtaining the specimen.

Continued

PROCEDURE 20.2 Collecting a Throat Specimen—cont'd

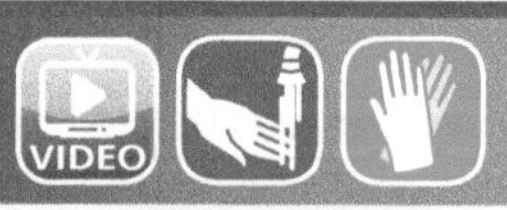

4. Procedural Step. Apply gloves. Remove the sterile swab from its peel-apart package, being careful not to contaminate it.

Principle. Contamination of the swab may lead to inaccurate test results.

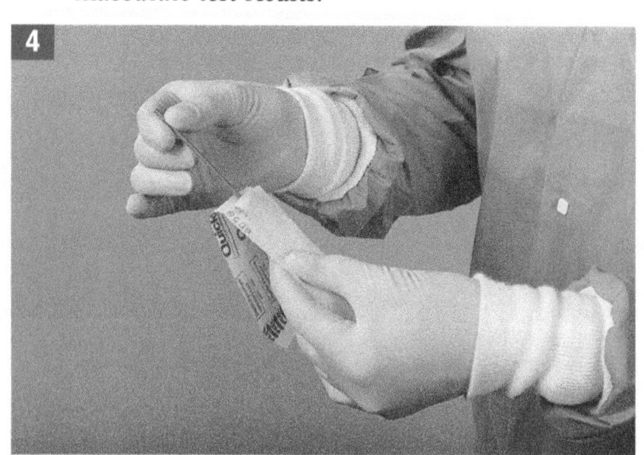

Remove the swab.

5. Procedural Step. Depress the tongue with the tongue depressor.

Principle. The tongue depressor holds the tongue down and facilitates access to the throat.

6. Procedural Step. Place the swab at the back of the throat (posterior pharynx), and firmly rub it over any lesions or white or inflamed areas of the mucous membrane of the tonsillar area and posterior pharyngeal wall. Rotate the swab constantly as you collect the specimen, making sure there is good contact with the tonsillar area. Do not allow the swab to touch any areas other than the throat, such as the inside of the mouth.

Principle. The swab should be rubbed over suspicious-looking areas where pathogens are likely to be found. A rotating motion is used to deposit the maximal amount of material possible on the swab. Touching it to any areas other than the throat contaminates the specimen with extraneous microorganisms.

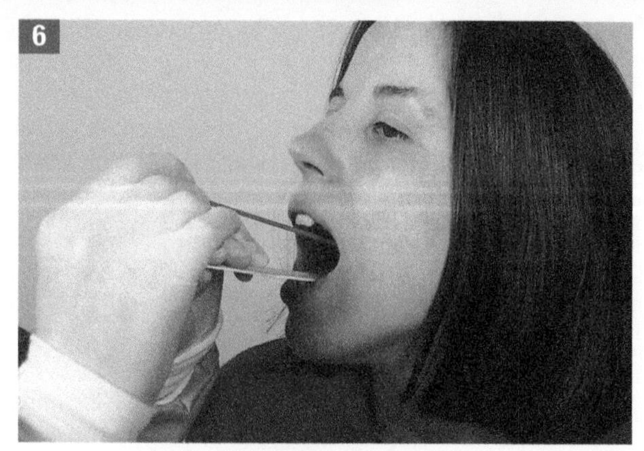

Collect the specimen.

7. Procedural Step. Keeping the patient's tongue depressed, withdraw the swab, and remove the tongue depressor from the patient's mouth.

8. Procedural Step. Properly dispose of the tongue depressor in a regular waste container to prevent transmission of microorganisms.

9. Procedural Step. Properly handle and prepare the specimen for transport to an outside laboratory.

10. Procedural Step. Remove gloves and sanitize your hands.

11. Procedural Step. Document the information.

a. *Electronic health record (EHR):* Document the type and source of the specimen, the laboratory test(s) ordered by the provider, and information indicating its transport to the outside laboratory using the appropriate radio buttons, drop-down menus, and free-text entry.

b. *Paper-based patient record:* Document the date and time of collection, the type and source of the specimen, the laboratory test(s) ordered by the provider, and information indicating its transport to the outside laboratory, including the date the specimen was sent (refer to the PPR charting example).

PPR Documentation Example

Date	
7/12/XX	10:30 a.m. Throat specimen collected for
	culture and sensitivity. Picked up by Medical
	Center Laboratory on 7/12/XX. ____________
	____________ A. Schostek, CMA (AAMA)

PROCEDURE 20.3 Perform a CLIA-Waived Rapid Strep Test

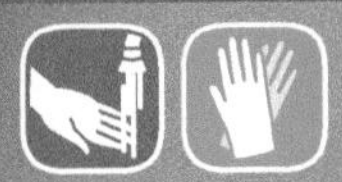

Outcome Collect a throat specimen and perform a CLIA-waived rapid strep test.

Equipment/Supplies

- CLIA-waived QuickVue rapid strep test kit
- Sterile throat swab
- Disposable gloves
- Tongue depressor
- External controls
- Manufacturer's instructions
- Quality control log
- Biohazard waste container

1. **Procedural Step.** Sanitize your hands, and assemble the equipment. Check the expiration date on the testing kit. It should not be used if the expiration date has passed.
   Principle. An expired strep test may produce inaccurate test results.
2. **Procedural Step.** If necessary, apply gloves, and perform an external positive and negative control procedure. When a new testing kit is opened (and thereafter on a monthly basis), external positive and negative controls should be performed according to the instructions in the product insert accompanying the controls. If the controls do not perform as expected, patient testing should not be conducted until the problem is identified and resolved.
   Principle. Running positive and negative external controls ensures that the test results are valid and reliable. Factors that can cause abnormal external control results include outdated controls or testing reagents, improper storage of testing components, and an error in the technique used to perform the procedure.
3. **Procedural Step.** Dispose of the test cassettes and control swabs in a biohazard waste container. Remove gloves and sanitize hands.
4. **Procedural Step.** Document the control results in a quality control log.
5. **Procedural Step.** Greet the patient and introduce yourself. Identify the patient by full name and date of birth and explain the procedure.
6. **Procedural Step.** Position the patient in a sitting position and adjust the light to provide clear visualization of the throat.
   Principle. The throat must be clearly visible so that the medical assistant is able to determine the proper area for obtaining the specimen.
7. **Procedural Step.** Sanitize the hands and apply gloves. Remove the test cassette from its foil pouch and place it on a clean, dry, level surface.
   Principle. The foil pouch should not be opened until it is time to perform the test.

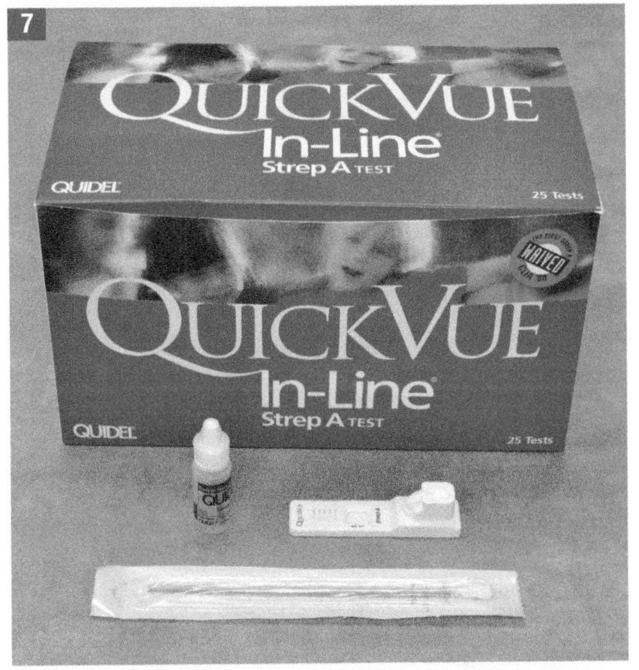

Remove the test cassette from its foil pouch. (From Niedzwiecki B, Pepper J, Weaver PA: *Kinn's the medical assistant: an applied learning approach,* ed 14, St Louis: Elsevier; 2020.)

8. **Procedural Step.** Check the expiration date of the sterile swab and remove it from its peel-apart package being careful not to contaminate it.
   Principle. Contamination of the swab may lead to inaccurate test results.
9. **Procedural Step.** Depress the tongue with the tongue depressor and collect a throat specimen (following the steps outlined in Procedure 20.2: Collecting a Throat Specimen).
10. **Procedural Step.** Using the notch at the back of the chamber as a guide, insert the swab completely into the swab chamber.

PROCEDURE 20.3

Continued

PROCEDURE 20.3 Perform a CLIA-Waived Rapid Strep Test—cont'd

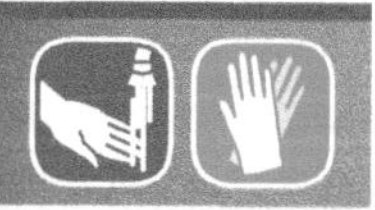

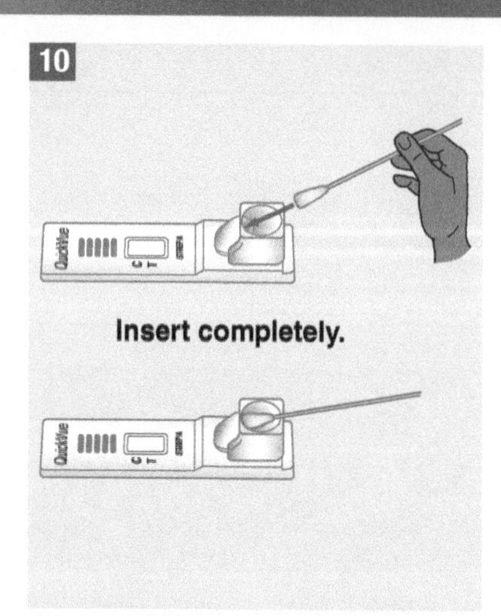

Insert the swab completely into the swab chamber. (Courtesy Quidel Corporation, San Diego, CA.)

11. **Procedural Step.** Squeeze the extraction bottle once to break the glass ampule inside the bottle. Vigorously shake the bottle five times to mix the solutions in the bottle. The solution should turn green after the ampule is broken. (*Note:* Do not use the extraction solution if it is green prior to breaking the ampule.)

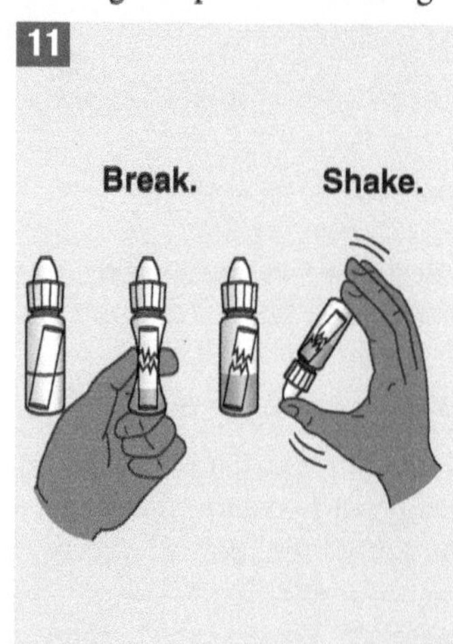

(A) Break the glass ampule inside the bottle. (B) Vigorously shake the bottle five times. (Courtesy Quidel Corporation, San Diego, CA.)

12. **Procedural Step.** Remove the cap of the extraction bottle. Hold the bottle in a vertical position and quickly fill the swab chamber to the rim with the extraction solution (approximately 8 drops).
Principle. The purpose of the extraction solution is to extract the specimen from the swab. Invalid results may occur if too little sample is added to the chamber.

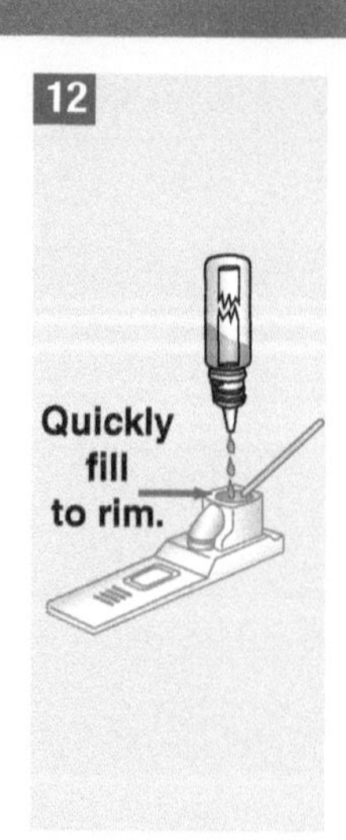

Quickly fill the swab chamber to the rim. (Courtesy Quidel Corporation, San Diego, CA.)

13. **Procedural Step.** Start the timer for 5 min. Do not move the test cassette until the procedure is completed. If the liquid has not moved across the result window in 1 min, completely remove the swab and reinsert it into the chamber. If the liquid still does not move across, repeat the test with a new specimen, test cassette, and bottle of extraction solution.
14. **Procedural Step.** Wait 5 min, and read the results by observing the test result window.
Principle. Reading the results before or after 5 min has elapsed may result in inaccurate test results.
15. **Procedural Step.** Interpret the test results as follows:

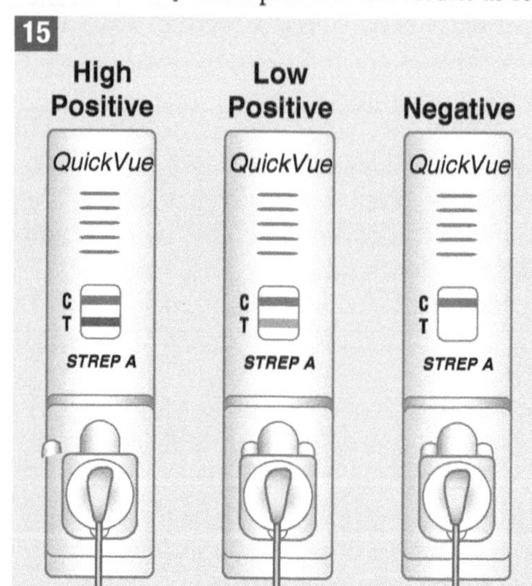

Interpret the test results. (Courtesy Quidel Corporation, San Diego, CA.)

Negative: The test result window exhibits a blue procedural control line next to the letter "C." It is presumed that the test is negative for strep but the provider may order further testing to verify this. In addition, there should be a clearing of the background color in the test result window.

PROCEDURE 20.3 Perform a CLIA-Waived Rapid Strep Test—cont'd

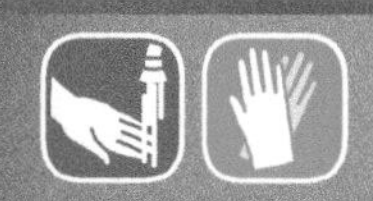

This area should be white to light pink within 5 min and not interfere with the ability to read test results.

Positive: The test result window exhibits any shade of a pink to red test line next to the letter "T" along with a blue procedural control line next to the letter "C." This means the test is positive for group A streptococcus. In addition, there should be a clearing of the background color in the test result window. This area should be white to light pink within 5 min and not interfere with the ability to read test results.

Invalid results: The blue procedural control line does not appear next to the letter "C" at 5 min or the background of the test result window interferes with reading the results. This means the test result is invalid. The test should be repeated with a new specimen and test cassette. ***Principle.*** The blue control line is a positive internal quality control indicator designating that a sufficient sample was added to the test device and that the test is working properly. A background in the test result window that is clear and does not interfere with reading the test results is a negative internal quality control indicator and signifies that the test has been performed properly.

16. **Procedural Step.** Dispose of the test cassette in a biohazard waste container. Remove gloves and sanitize your hands.
17. **Procedural Step.** Document the results in the patient's medical record.
    a. *Electronic health record (EHR):* Document the name of the test and the test results using the appropriate radio buttons, drop-down menus, and free text fields.
    b. *Paper-based patient record:* Document the date and time, the name of the test, and the test results as positive or negative.

PPR Documentation Example

Date	
7/12/XX	10:30 a.m. QuickVue Strep Test: Positive. ___
	___________ A. Schostek, CMA (AAMA)

PROCEDURE 20.4 Perform a CLIA-Waived Rapid Influenza Test

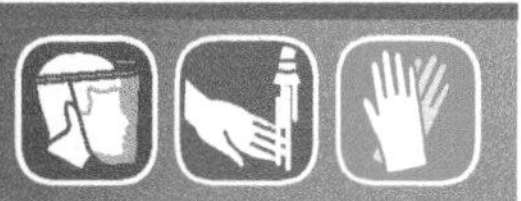

Outcome Collect a nasopharyngeal specimen and perform a CLIA-waived rapid influenza test.

Equipment/Supplies

- CLIA-waived BinaxNOW Influenza A and B test kit
- Sterile nasopharyngeal flocked swab
- Disposable gloves
- Face mask
- Protective eyewear
- External controls
- Manufacturer's instructions
- Quality control log
- Tissues
- Biohazard waste container

Perform the Control Procedure

1. **Procedural Step.** Sanitize your hands, and assemble the equipment. Check the expiration date on the testing kit. It should not be used if the expiration date has passed.
   Principle. An expired influenza test may produce inaccurate test results.
2. **Procedural Step.** If necessary, apply gloves, and perform an external positive and negative control procedure. When a new testing kit is opened (and thereafter on a monthly basis), external positive and negative controls should be performed according to the instructions in the product insert accompanying the controls. If the controls do not perform as expected, patient testing should not be conducted until the problem is identified and resolved.
   Principle. Running positive and negative external controls ensures that the test results are valid and reliable. Factors that can cause abnormal external control results include outdated controls or testing reagents, improper storage of testing components, and an error in the technique used to perform the procedure.

Continued

PROCEDURE 20.4

PROCEDURE 20.4 Perform a CLIA-Waived Rapid Influenza Test—cont'd

3. **Procedural Step.** Dispose of test devices and swabs used to perform the control procedure in a biohazard waste container. Remove gloves and sanitize hands.
4. **Procedural Step.** Document the control results in a quality control log.

Collect the Nasopharyngeal Swab Specimen

5. **Procedural Step.** Greet the patient and introduce yourself. Identify the patient by full name and date of birth and explain the collection procedure. Explain to the patient that the collection procedure may cause coughing, sneezing, or tearing of the eyes.
6. **Procedural Step.** Position the patient in a sitting position. Ask the patient to blow his or her nose to remove excess mucus secretions from the nasal passages.
   Principle. The nasal passages should be clear of mucus, prior to the insertion of the swab.
7. **Procedural Step.** Sanitize the hands and apply personal protective equipment including a face mask, protective eyewear, and clean disposable gloves.
   Principle. Personal protective equipment shields the medical assistant from pathogens that may be released into the environment if the patient coughs or sneezes during the collection procedure.
8. **Procedural Step.** Tilt the patient' s head back slightly (about 70 degrees).
   Principle. Tilting the head back makes the nasal passages more accessible and straightens the passage from the front of the nose to the nasopharynx, making insertion of the swab easier.
9. **Procedural Step.** Remove the cap from the extraction vial using a twisting motion and place it in its cardboard holder. Check the expiration date of the nasopharyngeal swab. Remove the sterile swab from its peel-apart package, being careful not to contaminate it.
   Principle. A swab past its expiration date should not be used. Contamination of the swab may lead to inaccurate test results.
10. **Procedural Step.** Estimate the distance for insertion of the swab by visually determining the distance from the corner of the nose to the earlobe. The swab should be inserted approximately one-half this distance.
    Principle. Estimating the distance helps to ensure that the swab is inserted to the proper depth for adequate specimen collection.
11. **Procedural Step.** Gently insert the swab into one nostril along the floor of the nasal passage. The swab should be inserted straight back and not in an upward direction. Slowly push the swab forward into the nasal passage until resistance is encountered, indicating the swab has reached the nasopharyngeal mucosa. The depth of insertion should be equal to approximately one-half the distance from the corner of the nose to the ear lobe (as previously estimated). Do not force the swab. If an obstruction or resistance is encountered before reaching the nasopharynx, remove the swab. Obtain a new sterile swab and try the other nostril.
    Principle. The swab must reach the nasopharyngeal mucosa in order to obtain an adequate specimen.

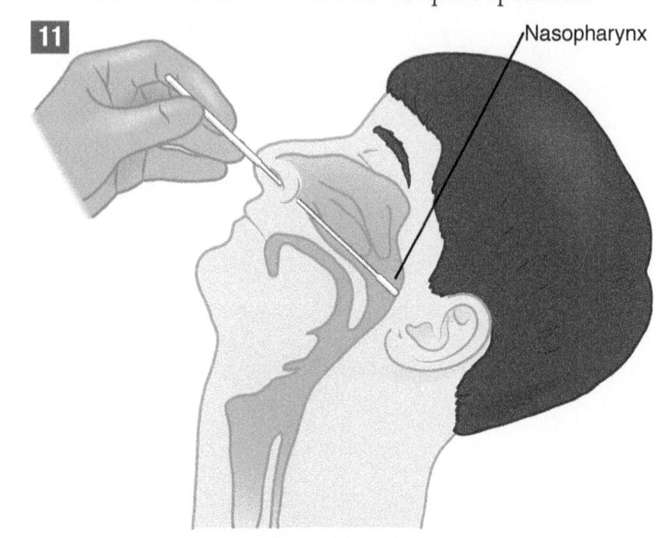

Insert the swab.

12. **Procedural Step.** Rotate the swab against the mucosa of the nasopharynx 3 –5 times to dislodge and collect epithelial cells on the swab. Leave the swab in place for a few seconds to ensure maximum absorption of cells on the swab.
    Principle. A rotating motion is used to deposit the maximal amount of material possible on the swab. Failure to collect a sufficient amount of cells may cause a false-negative test result
13. **Procedural Step.** Gently remove the swab from the patient's nose with a rotating motion. Provide the patient with tissues, as required.

Perform the BinaxNOW Influenza A and B Test

14. **Procedural Step.** Insert the swab into the solution in the extraction vial. Rinse the swab in the extraction solution by vigorously rotating it three times without creating a lot of bubbles.
    Principle. The purpose of the extraction solution is to extract or remove the specimen from the swab. Vigorous rotation of the swab facilitates the removal of the specimen from the swab.

PROCEDURE 20.4 Perform a CLIA-Waived Rapid Influenza Test—cont'd

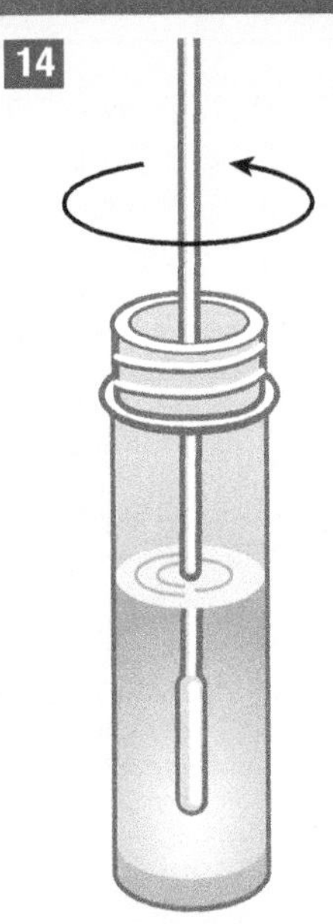

Rinse the swab in the extraction solution.

15. **Procedural Step.** Remove the swab from the vial by rolling it with pressure against the inside of the vial to further extract as much of the specimen as possible from the swab to ensure adequate specimen collection. Properly dispose of the swab in a biohazard waste container.
    Principle. Inadequate specimen collection may lead to a false-negative test result.
16. **Procedural Step.** Remove the cardboard test device from its foil pouch and lay it on a clean, dry, level surface.
    Principle. The foil pouch should not be opened until it is time to perform the test.
17. **Procedural Step.** Fill the pipette by firmly squeezing the top bulb and then placing the pipette tip into the extraction solution. Fill the pipette by slowly releasing pressure from the bulb while the tip is still in the solution.

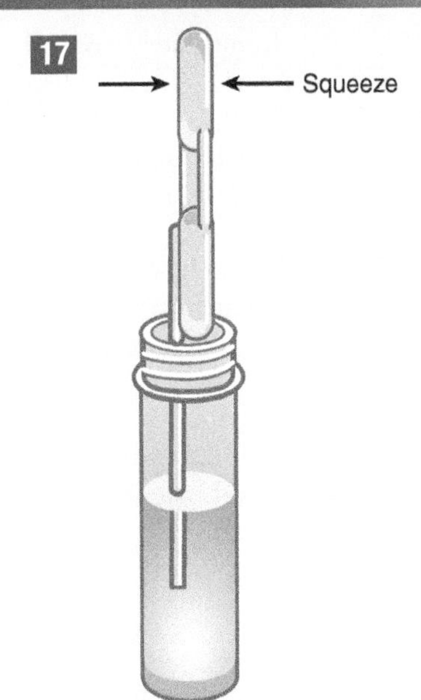

Fill the pipette.

18. **Procedural Step.** Check to make sure the pipette is full and that there are no air spaces in the lower part of the pipette. If air spaces occur, squeeze the sample back into the specimen container and redraw the sample from the vial. Air spaces take up space that the sample should occupy.
    Principle. Invalid results may occur if too little sample is added to the test.
19. **Procedural Step.** Locate the arrow on the test device to find the white pad at the top of the test strip. Slowly (drop by drop) add the contents of the pipette to the middle of this pad by squeezing the bulb until the entire sample is absorbed into the pad. Do not allow the pipette to touch the pad.

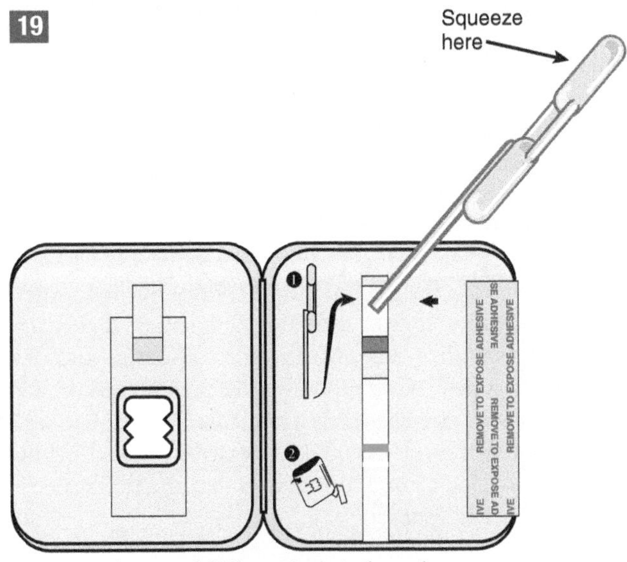

Add the contents to the pad.

Continued

PROCEDURE 20.4 Perform a CLIA-Waived Rapid Influenza Test—cont'd

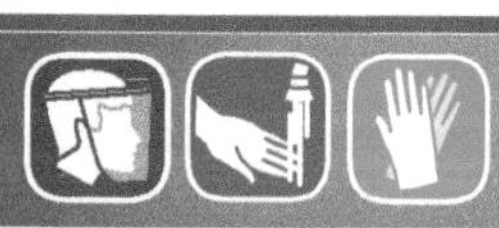

20. **Procedural Step.** Immediately peel off the adhesive liner from the test device. Close and securely seal the test device.
21. **Procedural Step.** Wait 15 min, and read the results by observing the test result window.
    Principle. Reading the results before or after 15 min has elapsed may result in inaccurate test results.
22. **Procedural Step.** Interpret the test results as follows:
    Negative: The test result window exhibits a pink to purple procedural control line next to the word "CONTROL" with no other lines appearing in the test window. (*Note:* An untested test device has a blue line at the "CONTROL" position.) In addition, the background color in the test result window should change from light pink to white within 15 min.

    Positive:
    a. ***Influenza type A:*** The test result window exhibits any shade of a pink to purple test line next to the word "FLU A" along with a pink to purple procedural control line next to the word "CONTROL." In addition, the background of the test result window should be clear and should not interfere with the ability to read test results.
    b. ***Influenza type B:*** The test result window exhibits any shade of a pink to purple test line next to the word "FLU B" along with a pink to purple procedural control line next to the word "CONTROL." In addition, the background of the test result window should be clear and should not interfere with the ability to read test results.
    c. ***Influenza types A and B:*** The test result window exhibits any shade of a pink to purple test line next to the words "FLU A" and "FLU B" along with a pink to purple procedural control line next to the word "CONTROL." In addition, the background of the test result window should be clear and should not interfere with the ability to read test results.

    Invalid results: If the procedural control line remains blue or is not present at all, or if the background of the test result window interferes with reading the results, the test result is invalid. The test should be repeated with a new specimen and test device.
    Principle. The pink to purple control line is an internal quality control indicator designating that a sufficient sample was added to the test device and that the test is working properly. A background in the test result window that is clear and does not interfere with reading the test results is a negative internal quality control indicator and indicates that the test has been performed properly.

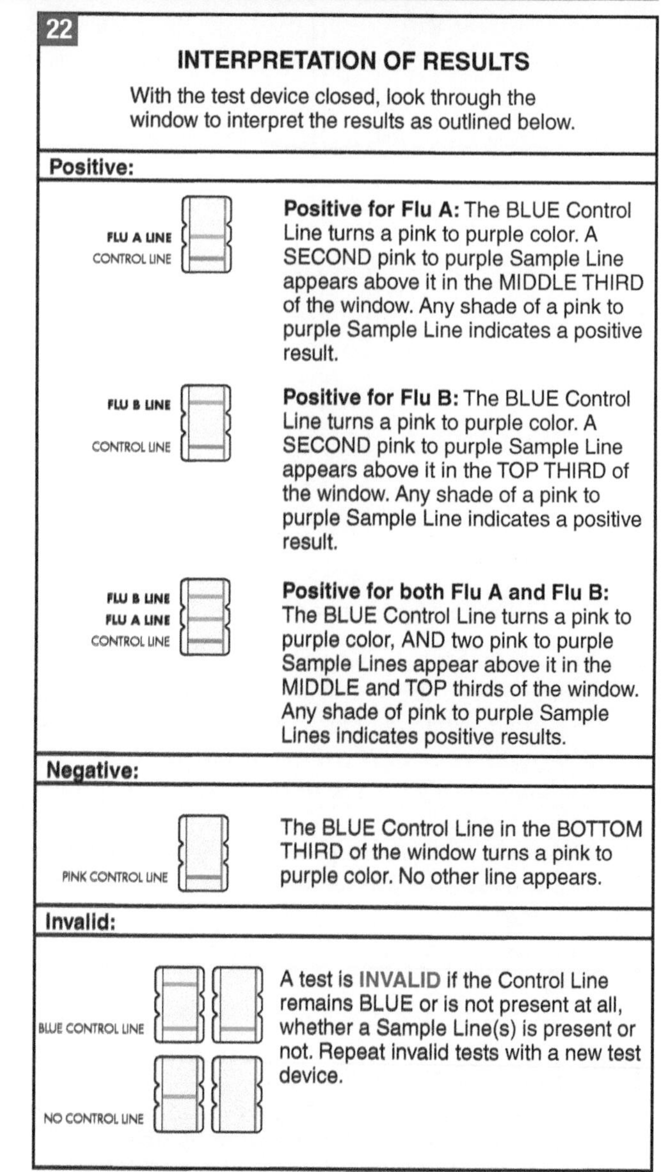

23. **Procedural Step.** Dispose of the test device in a biohazard waste container. Remove personal protective equipment and sanitize your hands.
24. **Procedural Step.** Document the results in the patient's medical record.
    a. *Electronic health record (EHR):* Document the name of the test and the test results using the appropriate radio buttons, drop-down menus, and free-text fields.
    b. *Paper-based patient record:* Document the date and time, the name of the test, and the results as follows:

    For negative results: Influenza A and B virus not detected.

PROCEDURE 20.4 Perform a CLIA-Waived Rapid Influenza Test—cont'd

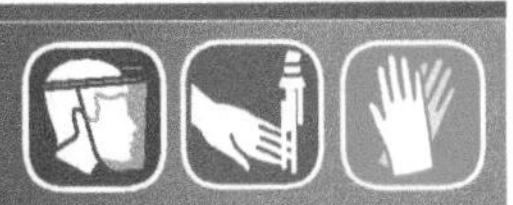

For positive results:

Depending on the results, document one of the following:

- Positive for influenza A.
- Positive for influenza B.
- Positive for influenza A and B.

PPR Documentation Example

Date	
3/25/XX	11:30 a.m. BinaxNOW influenza A and B
	test: Positive for influenza A ____________
	____________ A, CMA (AAMA)

Nutrition

 Check out the Evolve site at http://evolve.elsevier.com/Bonewit/today/ to access additional interactive activities and exercises to help you study and prepare for success.

LEARNING OUTCOMES

Nutrients

1. List the six classes of nutrients.
2. Explain the difference between a macronutrient and a micronutrient.
3. State the number of kilocalories provided by 1 g of each of the following: carbohydrate, fat, and protein.
4. Explain the difference between simple carbohydrates and complex carbohydrates. List food sources of each.
5. State the function of fat in the body.
6. Describe the different types of fat found in food.
7. State the function of protein in the body.
8. Explain the difference between essential amino acids and nonessential amino acids.
9. Describe the difference between complete protein and incomplete protein. List food sources of each.
10. Identify the water-soluble vitamins and state the function, food sources, and deficiency diseases of each.
11. Identify the fat-soluble vitamins and state the function, food sources, and deficiency diseases of each.
12. Identify the major minerals and state the function, food sources, and deficiency diseases of each.
13. Identify the trace minerals and state the function, food sources, and deficiency diseases of each.
14. State the function of water in the body.
15. Identify methods by which water is lost from the body.

Tools for Healthy Nutrition

16. Identify the MyPlate food groups and their recommended proportions on the plate.
17. State the purpose of the Dietary Guidelines for Americans.
18. List the key recommendations included in the Dietary Guidelines for Americans.
19. State the purpose of food labeling.
20. List and describe the seven basic sections of the Nutrition Facts panel.

Nutrition Therapy

21. Explain the purpose of weight management.
22. List and describe the three components included in a treatment plan for obesity.
23. Identify the elements of the TLC eating plan for a heart-healthy diet.
24. Identify the elements of the DASH eating plan to lower hypertension.
25. List examples of foods that are high and low in sodium.
26. Explain the difference between type 1 and type 2 diabetes.
27. Explain the recommended nutrition therapy for type 1 and type 2 diabetes.
28. List the symptoms of lactose intolerance and identify the recommended nutrition therapy.
29. Explain the difference between celiac disease and non-celiac gluten sensitivity.
30. Identify the symptoms and describe the recommended treatment for gluten intolerance.
31. List the common food allergens.
32. Describe the common methods of treatment for food allergies.

PROCEDURES

Instruct a patient according to the patient's special dietary needs.

CHAPTER OUTLINE

Introduction to Nutrition
- Definition of Terms

Nutrients
- Classification of Nutrients
- Carbohydrates
- Fats
- Proteins
- Vitamins
- Minerals
- Water

Dietary Supplements

Tools for Healthy Nutrition
- Nutrition Guides
- Food Labels

Nutrition Therapy
- Weight Management
- Cardiovascular Disease
- Hypertension
- Diabetes
- Lactose Intolerance
- Gluten Intolerance
- Food Allergies

KEY TERMS

added sugars
antioxidant (an-tee-OCKS-i-dent)
atherosclerosis (ath-er-oh-skleh-ROH-sis)
bariatrics
cholesterol (ko-LES-ter-ol)
complete protein
disaccharide (die-SAK-a-ride)
eating pattern
empty-calorie food
essential amino acid
gluten (GLOO-ten)
glycogen (GLIE-koe-jen)
incomplete protein
kilocalorie (KIL-o-cal-or-ee)
lactose (LAK-tos)
macronutrient (MAK-ro-noo-tree-ent)
micronutrient (MY-crow-noo-tree-ent)
mineral
monosaccharide (mah-no-SAK-a-ride)
natural sugars
nonessential amino acid
nutrient (NOO-tree-ent)
nutrition (noo-TRI-shun)
nutrition therapy
obesity (oh-BEE-si-tee)
percent daily value
polysaccharide
saturated fat
triglycerides (tri-GLIS-eh-rides)
unsaturated fat
vitamin

INTRODUCTION TO NUTRITION

Nutrition is the study of nutrients in food including how the body uses them and their relationship to health. A **nutrient** is a chemical substance found in food that is needed by the body for survival and well-being. Good nutrition is an important component of the health and well-being of an individual. Inadequate nutrition can result in poor health and even disease. Some of the specific benefits derived from good nutrition include the following:

- Supports good physical and mental well-being
- Helps to maintain a healthy weight
- Boosts the functioning of the immune system
- Delays the effects of aging
- Lowers the risk of certain conditions and diseases (e.g., obesity, heart disease, cancer, diabetes)

The medical assistant should have a knowledge of basic nutrition principles and the recommended nutrition therapy for common conditions and diseases. The medical assistant uses this information when scheduling a patient for an appointment with a dietitian, relaying information to patients on dietary restrictions required for tests and procedures, providing patients with nutrition education handouts, and answering basic questions a patient may have regarding nutrition.

Medical assistants are not qualified to conduct nutritional assessments or recommend nutrition therapy. This is the responsibility of a registered dietitian. Medical assistants should make sure to adhere to these guidelines to stay within the scope of practice for a medical assistant.

DEFINITION OF TERMS

Terms that aid in understanding this chapter are listed and defined here.

Diet: A diet consists of the food and drinks an individual consumes each day. To promote sound nutrition, an individual's diet should include the proper balance of nutrients.

Dietitian: A dietitian is a professional specially trained to assess the nutritional status of an individual and recommend appropriate nutrition therapy.

Digestion: The process by which food is broken down in the gastrointestinal tract into smaller components that can be absorbed by the bloodstream for use by the body.

Empty-calorie food: A food that provides calories but few or no nutrients.

Enriched food: A food to which vitamins and minerals have been added to replace those lost during the processing of that food.

Fortified food: A food to which vitamins and minerals that were not there originally have been added to increase the nutritional quality of the food.

Malnutrition (or poor nutrition): A condition caused by a deficiency of one or more nutrients (undernutrition) or an

TABLE 21.1 Energy Value of the Macronutrients

Macronutrient	Energy Value
Carbohydrate	4 kcal/g
Fat	9 kcal/g
Protein	4 kcal/g

overconsumption of nutrients (overnutrition) resulting in an overweight or obese individual.

Nutrient density: Refers to the amount of nutrients in a food compared with the number of calories. A food with a high nutrient density is low in calories and high in nutrients. A food with a low nutrient density (known as an *empty-calorie food*) is high in calories and low in nutrients.

NUTRIENTS

Nutrients can be categorized into six classes according to their chemical structure and the role they play in nourishing the body. The six classes of nutrients include carbohydrates, fat, protein, vitamins, minerals, and water and are described in more detail in this section.

Each of the six classes of nutrients plays an important role in supporting good nutritional health. Nutrients provide three primary functions in the body as follows:

- Provide energy for the body
- Build, repair, and maintain body tissue
- Assist in the regulation of body processes

The National Academy of Medicine developed Dietary Reference Intake (DRI) tables to assist individuals in determining their recommended daily intake of essential nutrients. Nutrient recommendations in the DRI tables are based on gender, age, and life stage and also allow for individual variation. The DRI tables can be accessed on the National Academies website (www.nationalacademies.org).

CLASSIFICATION OF NUTRIENTS

Nutrients can be further classified as macronutrients or micronutrients.

Macronutrients

Macronutrients are nutrients needed in relatively large amounts by the body and include carbohydrates, fats, and proteins. Macronutrients provide kilocalories to the body to yield energy in addition to performing other important body functions, which are discussed in this chapter. A **kilocalorie** (kcal), often referred to simply as a *calorie,* is a measurement unit of energy. A kilocalorie is defined as the amount of heat needed to raise the temperature of 1 kg of water 1° Celsius. The energy value provided by each of the macronutrients is outlined in Table 21.1.

The body uses carbohydrates as short-term energy fuel and uses fat as long-term fuel. Although protein provides 4 kcal of energy per gram and can be used as an energy source, the body would rather *not* use protein as an energy source. Instead, the body prefers to use carbohydrates as an energy source to "spare" protein for its more important functions of building, maintaining, and repairing body tissues. Refer to the chart below which outlines the function and food sources of the macronutrients.

Macronutrient	Function	Food Sources
Carbohydrate	Chief source of energy for the body Primary source of energy for the central nervous system	Pasta, rice, bread, cereal, fruits, vegetables
Fat	Provides energy for the body Transports fat-soluble vitamins in the body Provides essential fatty acids for the body	Fatty meats, butter, cheese, cream, whole milk, egg yolk, vegetable oils, nuts, avocados
Protein	Builds, maintains, and repairs body tissue Makes up enzymes, antibodies, and most hormones	Meat, fish, poultry, potatoes, eggs, milk, cheese, legumes, nuts

Micronutrients

Micronutrients are nutrients required in very small amounts by the body and include vitamins and minerals. Vitamins and minerals are not broken down by the body and are used in the form in which they are absorbed. Micronutrients do not provide calories to yield energy for the body; however, they do perform a variety of other very important functions, which are discussed in this chapter.

CARBOHYDRATES

Carbohydrates are organic compounds that consist of carbon, hydrogen, and oxygen. According to the Acceptable Macronutrient Distribution Ranges (AMDR), approximately 45% to 65% of the total daily caloric intake of an individual should come from carbohydrates.

Through the process of digestion, carbohydrates are broken down into sugar units and converted into glucose by the body. Glucose is the chief source of energy for the body and the preferred source of energy for the central nervous system. Energy is needed to perform all body functions such as breathing, contraction of the heart, blood circulation, digestion, maintenance of body temperature, and voluntary muscle movement such as walking, running, and lifting.

The body must maintain a constant blood glucose level to ensure a continuous source of energy for the body. Ingested glucose that is not needed for energy is stored for later use in the form of **glycogen** in muscle and liver tissue. Insulin is a hormone secreted by the beta cells of the pancreas that is required for the normal use of glucose in the body. Insulin enables glucose to enter the body cells and be converted to energy. Insulin also is needed for the proper storage of glycogen in muscle and liver tissue.

Classification of Carbohydrates

Carbohydrates are classified into simple and complex carbohydrates.

Simple Carbohydrates

Simple carbohydrates are made of just one or two sugar units. Simple carbohydrates consisting of one sugar unit are termed **monosaccharides**; they include glucose, fructose (fruit sugar), and galactose. Simple carbohydrates consisting of two sugar units are known as **disaccharides**; they include sucrose (table sugar), lactose (milk sugar), and maltose. Simple carbohydrates provide an immediate source of energy for the body because they can be quickly converted to glucose for use as energy. Simple carbohydrates are found in processed foods and refined sugars such as candy, cake, cookies, pastries, sweetened beverages, table sugar, syrup, and honey (Fig. 21.1A). Such simple carbohydrates are known as **empty-calorie foods** (or *low-nutrient density foods*) because they provide calories but very few or no nutrients. Simple carbohydrates are also found naturally in foods such as milk, fruits, and vegetables. These simple carbohydrates are considered a healthier food choice because they are also rich in vitamins, minerals, and fiber.

Complex Carbohydrates

Complex carbohydrates, also known as **polysaccharides**, are made up of many sugar units strung together into a long chain. Because complex carbohydrates consist of many sugar units, they take more time for the body to break down. This leads to a less dramatic rise in the blood sugar level and provides a more steady supply of energy for the body. Complex carbohydrates come from plant-based foods; examples include pasta, rice, bread, cereal, potatoes, and legumes (see Fig. 21.1B). It is recommended that complex carbohydrates be eaten in their whole-grain form (e.g., whole-grain breads and cereals) about half of the time.

Dietary Fiber

Dietary fiber is also a complex carbohydrate consisting of many sugar units; however, fiber does not provide calories for the body. This is because the human body lacks the enzymes necessary to break fiber down so that it can be used as an energy source. Fiber serves some very important functions in the body, which are discussed in this section. The daily recommended amount of fiber and the fiber content of common foods are presented in Table 21.2.

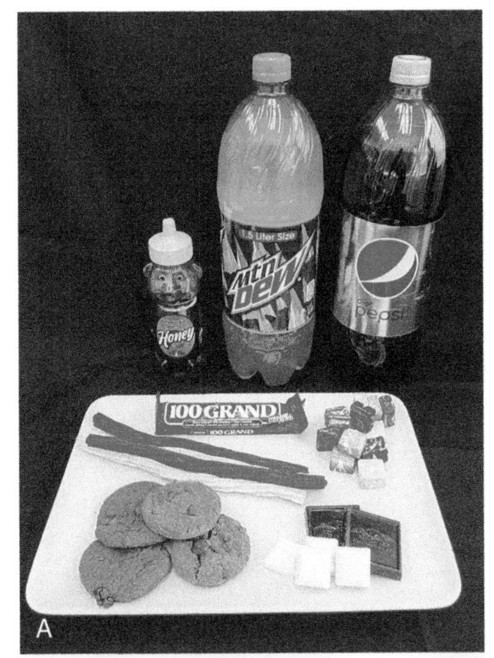

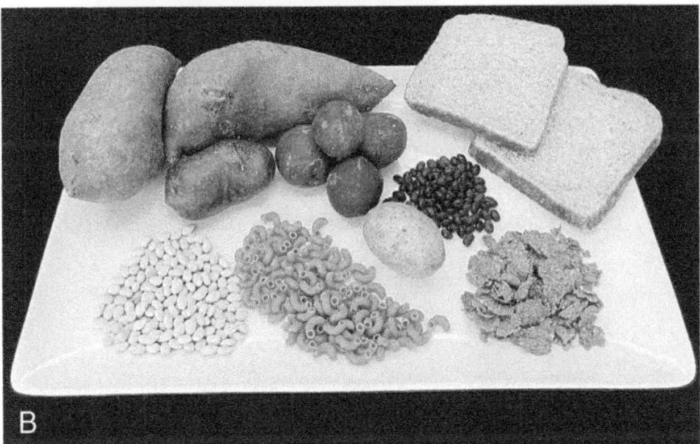

Fig. 21.1 (A) Simple carbohydrate food sources. (B) Complex carbohydrate food sources.

Based on chemical, physical, and functional properties, fiber can be classified as soluble or insoluble.

Soluble Fiber

Soluble fiber dissolves in water after it has been consumed, forming a gel-like material that slows down digestion. This delays the emptying of the stomach and makes an individual feel full longer, which assists in weight control. Soluble fiber also functions to lower blood cholesterol, which helps to protect against heart disease. Good sources of soluble fiber include oatmeal, oat bran, barley, some fruits (e.g., apples, pears, oranges), broccoli, and legumes (Fig. 21.2A).

Insoluble Fiber

Insoluble fiber is found in the rough, fibrous structures of plants such as the outer coverings, seeds, and strings of plants. It does not dissolve in water and passes through the gastrointestinal (GI) tract relatively intact. Because of this, insoluble fiber provides roughage or bulk to the diet, which helps promote normal elimination and prevents constipation. It may

TABLE 21.2 Fiber Recommendations and Food Sources

Age	Women	Men
Under age 50	25 g/day	38 g/day
Over age 50	21 g/day	30 g/day

Fiber Content of Common Foods

Food	Serving Size	Grams of Fiber
Navy beans (cooked)	1 cup	19.2
Split peas (cooked)	1 cup	16.3
Black beans (cooked)	1 cup	15
Bran flakes	¾ cup	5.3
Broccoli (boiled)	1 cup	5.1
Apple with skin	1 medium	4.4
Oatmeal (instant, cooked)	1 cup	4.0
Popcorn (air-popped)	3 cups	3.5
Brown rice (cooked)	1 cup	3.5
Almonds	1 ounce	3.5
Banana	1 medium	3.1
Potato (with skin, baked)	1 medium	2.9
Carrot (raw)	1 medium	1.7

also reduce the risk of diverticular disease and some forms of cancer. Good food sources of insoluble fiber include whole grains, wheat and corn bran, legumes, most fruits and vegetables, and nuts and seeds (see Fig. 21.2B).

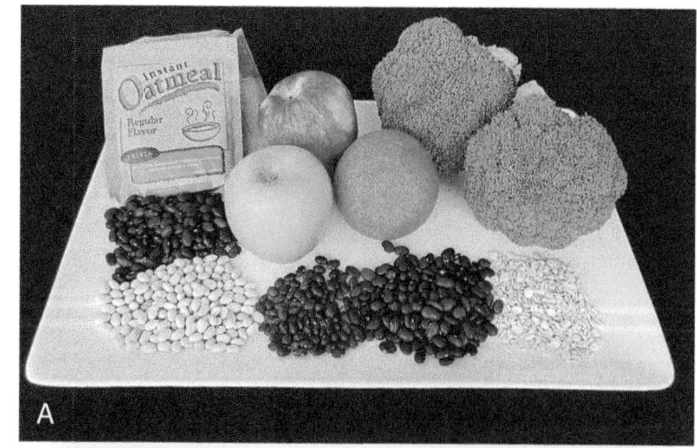

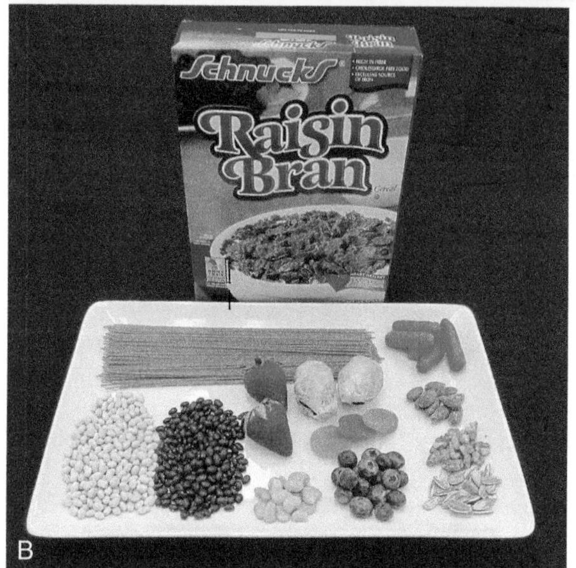

Fig. 21.2 (A) Soluble fiber food sources. (B) Insoluble fiber food sources.

FATS

Fats, also known as lipids, are organic compounds that do not dissolve in water. Fats are composed of carbon, hydrogen, and oxygen. These are the same elements that make up carbohydrates; however, fats are lower in oxygen content than carbohydrates. The body uses fat as long-term energy fuel and can store it in unlimited quantities in the body.

Despite the misconception that fat is bad for the body and only leads to weight gain, fat serves a number of very important functions. In addition to providing energy for the body, fat functions in transporting fat-soluble vitamins, providing essential fatty acids for the body, assisting in the transmission of nerve impulses, and insulating and cushioning the body. Because fat contains the most calories per gram (9 kcal/g) among the macronutrients, moderation should be practiced to maintain a healthy weight and a healthy heart. According to the AMDR, no more than 20% to 35% of the total daily caloric intake of an individual should come from fat.

Types of Dietary Fat

Different types of fat are found in foods (dietary fat) and can be classified as follows.

Saturated Fat

Saturated fat is a type of fat that is solid at room temperature and comes primarily from animal sources. It can be found in high amounts in fatty animal products such as bacon, sausage, heavily marbled beef and pork, and the skin of poultry. Whole-fat milk products such as cheese, butter, heavy cream, cream cheese, and ice cream are also high in saturated fat (Fig. 21.3A). Plant sources that are high in saturated fat include palm oil and coconut oil. Saturated fat raises the total blood cholesterol level, which can increase the risk of heart disease. Because of this, the American Heart Association (AHA) recommends limiting saturated fat to no more than 7% of the total calories consumed each day.

Unsaturated Fat

Unsaturated fat is a type of fat that is liquid at room temperature and comes primarily from plant sources. Unsaturated fat tends to have a protective effect against heart disease and should make up approximately two-thirds or more of the total fat percentage consumed each day. Unsaturated fat includes monounsaturated fat and polyunsaturated fat. *Monounsaturated* fat is considered to be the most protective against heart disease. Good food sources of monounsaturated fat include olives and olive oil, canola oil, peanut oil, nuts, and avocados. *Polyunsaturated* fat is found primarily in plant-based foods and oils. Good food sources include

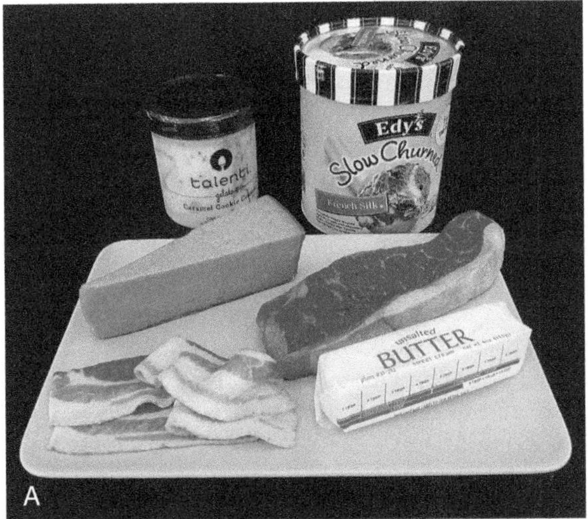

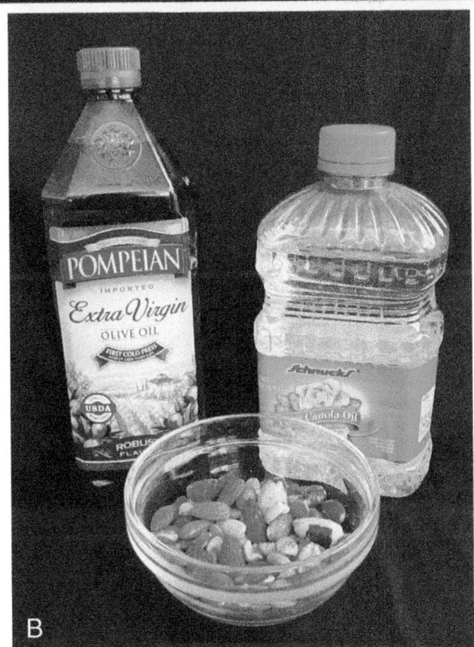

Fig. 21.3 (A) Saturated fat food sources. (B) Unsaturated fat food sources.

walnuts, flax seeds, corn oil, soybean oil, sunflower oil, and vegetable oil (see Fig. 21.3B). Vegetable oil typically consists of a blend of corn oil and soybean oil. Fatty fish and fish oils are polyunsaturated fats that are high in omega-3 fatty acids.

Trans Fat

Trans fat is a form of unsaturated fat. There are two types of trans fat, including natural trans fat and artificial trans fat. *Natural trans fat* is found in small amounts in certain foods such as beef, lamb, and butter. *Artificial trans fat* is formed as a result of a food-processing method known as hydrogenation. Hydrogenation works by adding hydrogen ions to unsaturated fat to form a semi-solid product known as *partially hydrogenated oil.* Artificial trans fat is more stable and less likely to turn rancid and was developed to preserve food items and increase their shelf-life. It also gives food a more desirable taste and texture. However, studies showed that artificial trans fat increases the level of low-density lipoprotein (LDL) (bad) cholesterol and decreases the level of high-density lipoprotein (HDL) (good) cholesterol in the body which, in turn, increases the risk of cardiovascular disease (CVD). Based on these findings, the Food and Drug Administration (FDA) ruled that artificial trans fat was not generally recognized as safe and banned the use of it in all foods sold in grocery stores and restaurants after June 18, 2018.

TABLE 21.3 Interpretation of Total Blood Cholesterol Levels

Total Blood Cholesterol Level	Interpretation
Less than 200 mg/dL	Desirable
200–239 mg/dL	Borderline high
240 mg/dL or above	High

Cholesterol

Cholesterol is not a true fat, but rather a white, waxy, fat-like substance that is essential for the normal functioning of the body. It is an important component of cell membranes and is used in the production of hormones and bile. Most of the cholesterol circulating in the blood is manufactured by the liver; however, a portion of it comes from an individual's diet and is known as *dietary cholesterol.* Dietary cholesterol is found only in animal products, such as organ meats, egg yolks, and dairy products. Although cholesterol serves some very important functions in the body, a high blood cholesterol level may cause fatty deposits, or plaque, to build up on the walls of the arteries, a condition known as **atherosclerosis.** As atherosclerosis progresses, the arteries become more occluded, which eventually could lead to a heart attack or stroke. Because of this, high blood cholesterol is considered a risk factor for CVD. Total blood cholesterol levels are interpreted as outlined in Table 21.3.

Triglycerides

Triglycerides are the *chemical form* in which most fat exists in food, as well as in the body. Triglycerides are derived from two sources. The first is synthesis by the body. As previously discussed, ingested glucose that is not needed for energy can be stored in the form of glycogen in muscle and liver tissue for later use. When no more tissue storage is possible, excess glucose is synthesized by the body into triglycerides and stored as adipose tissue. Excess protein not needed by the body is also converted to triglycerides and stored as adipose tissue. The second source of triglycerides is food. Excess triglycerides consumed by eating foods containing fat are also stored as adipose tissue.

Some of the triglycerides in the body are not stored as adipose tissue but remain in the bloodstream, specifically in the plasma. Most triglycerides in the bloodstream are carried by a lipoprotein known as *very-low-density lipoprotein* (VLDL). In normal amounts, triglycerides are essential to good health. Triglycerides carried by the blood serve as an important source of energy for the body. An excess of blood triglycerides, however, places an individual at increased risk for CVD, particularly when the "bad" LDL cholesterol is

TABLE 21.4 Interpretation of Blood Triglycerides Levels

Blood Triglycerides Level	Interpretation
Less than 150 mg/dL	Normal
150–199 mg/dL	Borderline high
200–499 mg/dL	High
500 mg/dL or above	Very high

high and the "good" HDL cholesterol is low. Triglycerides levels in the blood are interpreted as outlined in Table 21.4. Conditions that result in elevated blood triglycerides levels include obesity, type 2 diabetes, a physically inactive lifestyle, excessive alcohol consumption, smoking, hypothyroidism, kidney disease, and liver disease.

PROTEINS

Protein is often considered the "special force" macronutrient. Protein contains not only carbon, hydrogen, and oxygen (like carbohydrates and fats), but also nitrogen. The nitrogen provides protein with a special force that enables it to build, maintain, and repair body tissue.

Protein has many important functions in the body. Protein is the primary structural material making up all body tissues such as muscle, bone, skin, and hair. In addition, protein is a major component of enzymes, antibodies, and many hormones that are essential to the proper functioning of the body. Protein also plays a role in fluid balance and muscle contractions. According to the AMDR, 10% to 35% of the total daily caloric intake of an individual should come from protein. Rich food sources of protein include meat, fish, poultry, milk, cheese, eggs, legumes, soybeans, and nuts. Grains and soy products also contain moderate amounts of protein and are very useful in a vegetarian diet.

Protein plays an important role in physical activity because exercise breaks down muscle protein, which then requires repair and restoration. The amount of activity performed in a day assists in determining how much protein is needed by an individual. The average adult requires approximately 0.8 g of protein per kilogram of body weight per day. For a 160-pound man, this translates to about 58 g of protein. That amount of protein could be easily obtained by consuming 2 cups of milk; 5 ounces of meat, fish, or poultry; and three servings of grain. Protein needs for athletes increase to about 1.2 to 1.8 g/kg of body weight per day. The additional protein needed by an athlete can easily be obtained by an adequate, balanced diet, and the addition of protein supplements is not necessary. In fact, the American diet typically contains too much dietary protein, leading to adverse effects. The consequences of excessive protein intake include calcium loss in the urine, increased risk of kidney stones, and dehydration.

HIGHLIGHT on Vegetarianism

Answer questions that patients have about vegetarianism.

What is a vegetarian?

A vegetarian is an individual who adopts a style of eating in which one or more types of animal protein are omitted from the diet. An individual may choose to become vegetarian for a variety of reasons, including religious beliefs, concerns about animal cruelty, or a desire to conserve the earth's resources. Additional factors that influence an individual's decision to become a vegetarian include the healthfulness of a vegetarian diet or simply a dislike of animal protein. The foundation of a vegetarian diet includes plant-based foods such as grains, legumes, nuts, seeds, and fruits and vegetables. Research shows that there are many health benefits to be derived from a vegetarian diet. Vegetarians have a lower risk of developing chronic diseases such as CVD, diabetes, and certain types of cancer. Vegetarians also tend to maintain a healthy weight range throughout their lives. Health professionals recognize that a vegetarian diet may not be suitable for everyone but will encourage the general population to lean in that direction when possible because of the proven health benefits.

What are the different types of vegetarians?

There are different types of vegetarianism, as follows:

- *Vegan*: A vegetarian who does not consume any type of animal products including meat, eggs, and dairy. Many vegans also avoid using anything made from animal products, such as leather, fur, and wool.
- *Lacto vegetarian*: A vegetarian who consumes dairy products.
- *Ovo vegetarian:* A vegetarian who consumes eggs.
- *Lacto-ovo vegetarian:* A vegetarian who consumes dairy products and eggs.
- *Pescetarian*: A vegetarian who consumes fish and shellfish.
- *Pollo vegetarian:* A vegetarian who consumes poultry.
- *Fruitarian:* An individual who consumes only fruits, nuts, and seeds.
- *Flexitarian:* An individual who primarily follows a vegetarian diet but occasionally makes exceptions.

For what nutrient deficiencies is a vegetarian at risk?

Vegetarians (particularly vegans) should have a knowledge of menu planning principles so that their nutritional status remains optimal. Careful menu planning is of particular importance for the following nutrients:

- *Calcium*: Individuals who omit dairy products from their diet may consume marginal levels of calcium. Good alternatives

HIGHLIGHT on Vegetarianism—cont'd

to include in the diet include some green vegetables such as broccoli and kale, legumes, and calcium-fortified products such as orange juice.

- *Vitamin D:* Vegetarians who omit cow's milk from their diet may have a low intake of vitamin D. This can be avoided by supplementing the diet with soy milk that is fortified with vitamin D. The body also manufactures vitamin D when it is exposed to the ultraviolet rays of the sun.
- *Vitamin B_{12}:* Vitamin B_{12} is found only in animal-based foods. The old saying "If it doesn't oink, it doesn't cluck, or it doesn't moo, it doesn't have any B_{12}" holds true. A vitamin B_{12} deficiency can be avoided by supplementing the diet with vitamin B_{12}–fortified soy milk, almond milk, and rice milk. Fortified breakfast cereals are also an excellent source of vitamin B_{12}.
- *Iron:* Iron is found in a variety of foods including red meat, poultry, fish, legumes, dark greens, and dried fruit. Even though a plant-based diet does provide some iron to the diet, the body is unable to absorb it as well as the iron found in animal products. Vitamin C helps to increase the absorption of iron. It is recommended that a vegetarian consumes foods rich in vitamin C (e.g., citrus fruits) along with plant-based foods containing iron (e.g., dark green leafy vegetables). ■

Amino Acids

Protein is made up of smaller units known as *amino acids.* The dietary protein consumed by an individual is broken down into amino acids through the process of digestion. These amino acids are then arranged into different combinations to create the various proteins needed by the body (e.g., by cells, tissues, hormones, and enzymes). This can be compared to forming different words using the letters of the alphabet; because of this, amino acids are known as the "building blocks" of life. There are 20 different amino acids that join together to make all types of protein in the body.

Classification of Amino Acids

Amino acids can be classified into two categories: essential and nonessential amino acids.

Essential Amino Acids

Essential amino acids are required by the body; however, they cannot be manufactured by the body and must be obtained from food. Of the 20 amino acids that make up the proteins in the body, nine of these are essential amino acids.

Nonessential Amino Acids

Nonessential amino acids are required by the body; however, they can be synthesized by the body in sufficient quantities to meet its needs. Although nonessential amino acids are required for good health, it is not necessary that they be obtained from food because the body can manufacture them.

Classification of Protein

Proteins can be classified as complete or incomplete.

Complete Protein

A **complete protein** is a protein that contains all the essential amino acids needed by the body. Food sources that contain complete protein include animal-based foods such as meat, poultry, fish, milk, eggs, and cheese (Fig. 21.4A).

Incomplete Protein

An **incomplete protein** is a protein that lacks one or more of the essential amino acids needed by the body. Food sources that contain incomplete protein include plant-based foods such as fruits, vegetables, grains, legumes, and nuts (see Fig. 21.4B). *Complementary proteins* are two or more incomplete protein sources that together provide adequate amounts of all the essential amino acids. Examples of complementary proteins include beans and rice, tofu and rice, and humus and pita bread. Vegetarians can obtain all of their essential amino acids through careful planning and the use of complementary proteins.

VITAMINS

A **vitamin** is an organic compound that is required in small amounts by the body for normal growth and development. Vitamins occur naturally in foods and may be added to processed foods to increase their nutritional value. Most vitamins cannot be produced by the body and therefore must be obtained from food.

Classification of Vitamins

Vitamins can be classified into two groups: water-soluble vitamins and fat-soluble vitamins.

Water-Soluble Vitamins

Water-soluble vitamins derive their name because they dissolve in water. They cannot be stored by the body; water-soluble vitamins consumed in excess of the body's needs are removed through the urine. To maintain good nutritional health, these vitamins should be consumed daily. Water-soluble vitamins include vitamins B_1, B_2, B_3, B_5, B_6, B_7, B_9, B_{12}, and C.

The overall function of the B vitamins is to regulate metabolism, facilitate nervous system functions, and

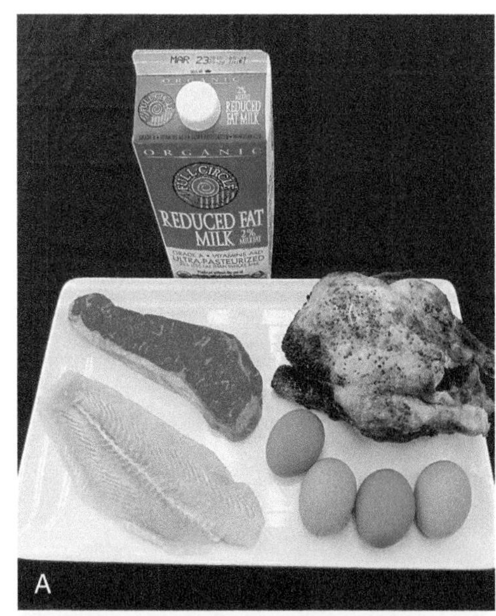

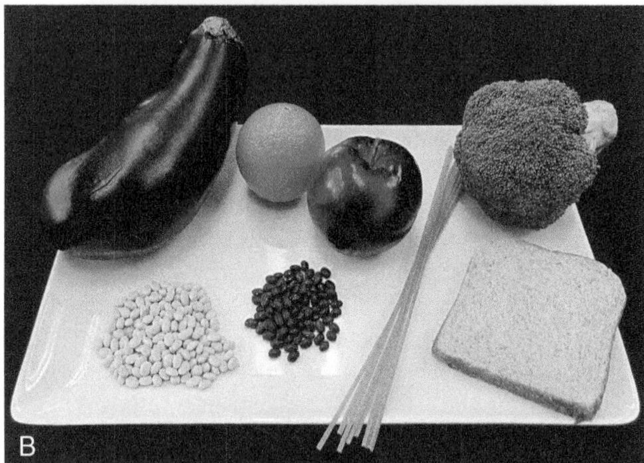

Fig. 21.4 (A) Complete protein food sources. (B) Incomplete protein food sources.

maintain healthy skin. Many of the B vitamins function as coenzymes in energy metabolism. This means that they assist important enzymes in converting food into fuel or energy for the body. Rich food sources of many of the B vitamins include whole grains, legumes, dark green leafy vegetables, pork, beef, and liver (Fig. 21.5). Refer to Table 21.5 for the specific function, food sources, and deficiency diseases of the water-soluble vitamins.

Fat-Soluble Vitamins

Fat-soluble vitamins dissolve in fat. They can be stored by the body; because of this, they do not need to be consumed as often as water-soluble vitamins. In fact, consuming an excessive amount of fat-soluble vitamins can result in toxicity symptoms leading to health problems. The fat-soluble vitamins include A, D, E, and K. Refer to Table 21.6 for the specific function, food sources, deficiency diseases, and toxicity symptoms (caused by an excessive intake) of the fat-soluble vitamins.

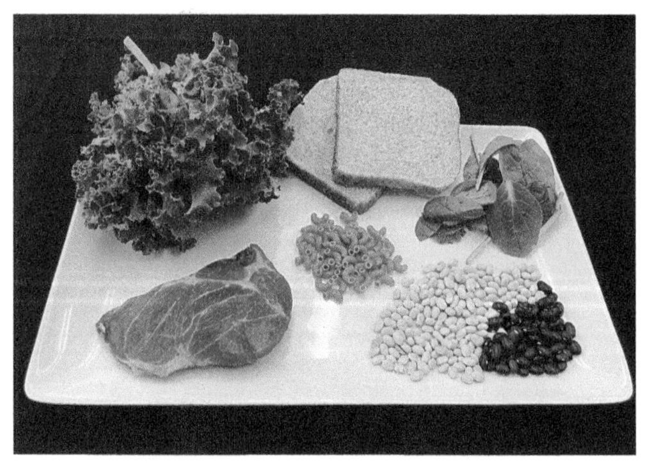

Fig. 21.5 Food sources of the B vitamins.

Antioxidant Vitamins

Vitamins A, C, and E are known as antioxidant vitamins. An **antioxidant** is a molecule that inhibits the oxidation of other molecules. Oxidation reactions can produce free radicals that can damage body cells. These damaged cells are thought to contribute to aging and certain diseases such as cancer and heart disease. Rich food sources of vitamins A and C include brightly colored fruits and vegetables such as sweet potatoes, citrus fruits, tomatoes, and spinach (Fig. 21.6), while margarine, nuts, and vegetable oils are rich in vitamin E.

MINERALS

A **mineral** is a naturally occurring inorganic substance that is essential to the proper functioning of the body. Minerals tend to be highly concentrated in foods of animal origin and are absorbed better by the body in this form. Vegetarians can obtain an adequate intake of minerals and avoid a mineral deficiency by emphasizing the following foods in their diet: grains, nuts, and dark green leafy vegetables. A mineral deficiency can lead to poor health and serious illness that affects numerous body systems.

Classification of Minerals

Minerals are divided into two classifications based on the amount required by the body; these classifications include major minerals and trace minerals. Major minerals are required in the body in larger quantities, whereas trace minerals are required in very small amounts. Each of these mineral classifications is described in more detail in the following sections.

Major Minerals

Major minerals are required in the adult diet in amounts greater than 100 mg/day and are found in the body in levels of 5 g or higher. They play important roles in bone and tooth health, blood pressure regulation, and water and acid-base balance. The major minerals include calcium (Fig. 21.7), magnesium phosphorus, potassium, chloride, and sodium.

TABLE 21.5 Water-Soluble Vitamins

Vitamin	Function	Food Sources	Deficiency Diseases and Conditions
Vitamin B_1 (thiamine)	Coenzyme in energy metabolism Normal functioning of the nervous system	Pork, beef, liver, eggs, fish, whole-grain and enriched breads, legumes	Beriberi Problems with the GI tract, nervous system, and cardiovascular system
Vitamin B_2 (riboflavin)	Coenzyme in energy metabolism Normal vision and skin health	Milk, meats, green leafy green vegetables, whole-grain and enriched bread and cereals	Cheilosis Eye sensitivity Dermatitis Glossitis
Vitamin B_3 (niacin)	Coenzyme in energy metabolism Healthy skin Healthy nervous and digestive systems Skin health	Milk, eggs, meat, fish, poultry, whole-grain and enriched breads and cereals	Pellagra (dermatitis, neuritis, diarrhea)
Vitamin B_5 (pantothenic acid)	Coenzyme in energy metabolism Synthesis of fatty acids, cholesterol, steroid hormones	Eggs, liver, salmon, poultry, mushrooms, cauliflower, peanuts	Burning feet and other neurologic symptoms
Vitamin B_6 (pyridoxine)	Coenzyme in protein metabolism Assists in making red blood cells	Meat, fish, poultry, liver, milk, eggs, whole grains, legumes, soy products	Cheilosis Glossitis Dermatitis Confusion Depression Irritability
Vitamin B_7 (biotin)	Coenzyme in carbohydrate and protein metabolism	Milk, liver, egg yolk, legumes, yeast, soy flour, cereals, fruit	Dermatitis Nausea Anorexia Depression Hair loss
Vitamin B_9 (folic acid)	Synthesis of red blood cells Synthesis of DNA Development of the fetal nervous system	Liver, leafy green vegetables, legumes, seeds, fruit, cereal and bread fortified with folate	Megaloblastic anemia Neural tube birth defects (anencephaly and spina bifida)
Vitamin B_{12} (cobalamin)	Synthesis of red blood cells Maintenance of myelin sheaths	Meat, poultry, fish seafood, liver, eggs, milk, cheese	Pernicious anemia Degeneration of myelin sheaths Sore mouth and tongue Neurologic disorders
Vitamin C (ascorbic acid)	Building and maintenance of strong tissues through collagen synthesis Wound healing Assists in the absorption of iron Resistance to infection Antioxidant	Citrus fruits, broccoli, melons, strawberries, tomatoes, Brussels sprouts, potatoes, cabbage, green peppers	Scurvy Muscle cramps Bleeding and loose gums Tendency to bruise easily Poor wound healing Weakened bones

GI, Gastrointestinal.

TABLE 21.6 Fat-Soluble Vitamins

Vitamin	Function	Food Sources	Deficiency Diseases and Conditions, and Toxicity Symptoms
Vitamin A (retinol)	Maintenance of vision in dim light Maintenance of mucous membranes and healthy skin Antioxidant	Liver, whole milk, butter, cream, fish liver oils, dark green leafy vegetables, deep orange fruits and vegetables	*Deficiency:* Night blindness Xerosis Xerophthalmia *Toxicity Symptoms:* Bone pain Dry skin Loss of hair Fatigue Anorexia

Continued

TABLE 21.6 Fat-Soluble Vitamins—cont'd

Vitamin	Function	Food Sources	Deficiency Diseases and Conditions, and Toxicity Symptoms
Vitamin D (calciferol)	Regulation of the absorption of calcium and phosphorus Calcification of bones and teeth	Fortified milk and margarine, liver, oily fish, fish liver oils Synthesized by the body using the ultraviolet rays of the sun	*Deficiency:* Rickets (in children) Osteomalacia Poorly developed bones and teeth Muscle spasms *Toxicity Symptoms:* Kidney stones Fragile bones Calcification of soft tissue
Vitamin E (tocopherol)	Protection of red blood cells Antioxidant	Vegetable oils, margarine, salad dressing, wheat germ, nuts, avocados	*Deficiency:* Hemolysis of red blood cells
Vitamin K (phylloquinone)	Formation of prothrombin for normal blood clotting Bone development	Green leafy vegetables, milk, meats, cabbage, broccoli, Brussels sprouts Synthesized by intestinal bacterial	*Deficiency:* Bleeding tendencies Poor bone growth *Toxicity Symptoms:* Prolonged blood clotting

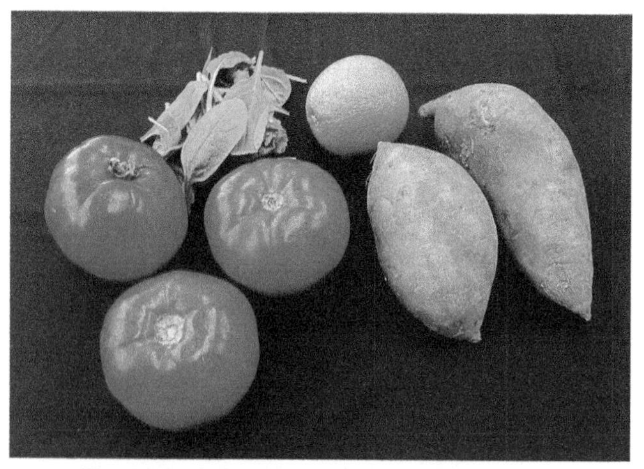

Fig. 21.6 Antioxidant vitamins A and C food sources.

Refer to Table 21.7 for the specific function, food sources, and deficiency diseases of major minerals.

Trace Minerals

Trace minerals are required in the adult diet in amounts less than 50 mg/day and are found in the body in levels of less than 5 g. They are a diverse group of minerals that assist in proper metabolism and structure as well as immune and blood system functions. Trace minerals include iron, copper, zinc, manganese, fluoride, selenium, iodine, chromium, and molybdenum. Refer to Table 21.8 for the specific function, food sources, and deficiency diseases of trace minerals.

WATER

Water is essential to the survival of an individual. This old adage still holds true: man can survive in the desert without

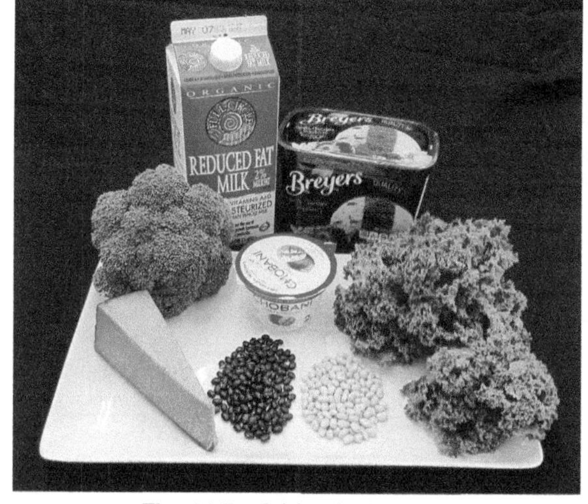

Fig. 21.7 Calcium food sources.

food for more than 30 days but can live only about 3 days without water. Water makes up approximately 60% to 65% of an adult's total body weight, and that percentage is even higher in young children.

Water serves many important functions in the body. Water is the universal solvent of the body; it allows nutrients such as glucose, vitamins, and minerals to dissolve in water and be transported by the circulatory system to the cells of the body. Water allows for the transport of substances in and out of cells and is the basis of many chemical reactions in the body. In addition, water provides a solvent for ridding the body of waste products in the form of urine. Water also cushions the shock to bones and joints and functions to cool the body's internal temperature through perspiration.

Balancing the amount of water coming into and going out of the body is extremely important to life. Water is obtained primarily from the consumption of fluids and foods. It is also

TABLE 21.7 Major Minerals

Mineral	Function	Food Sources	Deficiency Diseases and Conditions
Calcium	Healthy bones and teeth Muscle and nerve functioning Proper blood clotting Blood pressure regulation	Milk and milk products, canned fish containing bones (salmon, sardines), some green vegetables such as broccoli and kale, legumes	Osteomalacia Osteoporosis Muscle cramps
Magnesium	Healthy bones and teeth Building protein Muscle and nerve functioning Blood pressure regulation Healthy immune system	Nuts and seeds, whole grains, legumes, dark green vegetables, seafood, chocolate	Muscle weakness and twitching Irritability Fatigue
Phosphorus	Healthy bones and teeth Normal cell membranes Energy production	Meats, milk, nuts, seeds, and legumes	Bone weakness Loss of appetite
Potassium	Normal fluid and electrolyte balance Muscle and nerve functioning Normal cardiac rhythms	Fruits (especially bananas, dried fruit, fruit juices, orange juice), vegetables, grains, legumes	Muscle weakness, twitching, or spasms Cardiac arrhythmias Respiratory failure
Chloride	Normal fluid and electrolyte balance Component of gastric juice (hydrochloric acid in the stomach)	Salt, soy sauce, processed foods	Loss of appetite Muscle weakness and cramps
Sodium	Normal fluid and electrolyte balance Muscle and nerve functioning	Salt, soy sauce, processed foods	Muscle weakness and cramps Nausea and vomiting Dizziness Apathy

TABLE 21.8 Trace Minerals

Mineral	Function	Food Sources	Deficiency Diseases and Conditions
Iron	Makes up hemoglobin (carries oxygen to the body) Makes up myoglobin (carries oxygen to muscles) Assists in energy metabolism	Red meat, liver, dark green leafy vegetables, egg yolk, whole grains, dried fruits	Anemia Irritability Inability to concentrate Pallor Cold sensitivity Lethargy
Copper	Helps form hemoglobin Part of many enzymes	Organ meats, seafood, whole grains, legumes, nuts, seeds, drinking water	Anemia Bone abnormalities
Zinc	Part of many enzymes Functions in taste perception, wound healing, sperm production, normal fetal development, healthy immune system	Meat, fish, poultry, seafood, egg yolk, whole-grain and enriched breads and cereals	Decreased wound healing Decreased taste perception Impaired immune function Growth failure in children
Manganese	Part of many enzymes involved in protein and energy metabolism Bone growth Healthy immune system	Whole-grain breads and cereals, legumes, fruits, vegetables, tea	Impaired bone growth Skeletal abnormalities Depressed growth of hair and nails
Fluoride	Helps to make bones and teeth stronger Increased resistance to cavities	Seafood Fluoridated drinking water, tea	Badly formed or weak teeth Increase in dental cavities
Selenium	Antioxidant Proper functioning of the thyroid gland	Brazil nuts, seafood, organ meats, whole grains	Impaired thyroid function Muscle weakness and tenderness Poor heart function Weakened immune system
Iodine	Proper functioning of the thyroid gland Synthesis of thyroid hormones Energy metabolism	Seafood Iodized salt	Goiter Hypothyroidism Cretinism
Chromium	Normal glucose metabolism	Insulin resistance Glucose intolerance Meat, poultry, fish, whole grains, egg yolks, mushrooms, onions	Insulin resistance Glucose intolerance

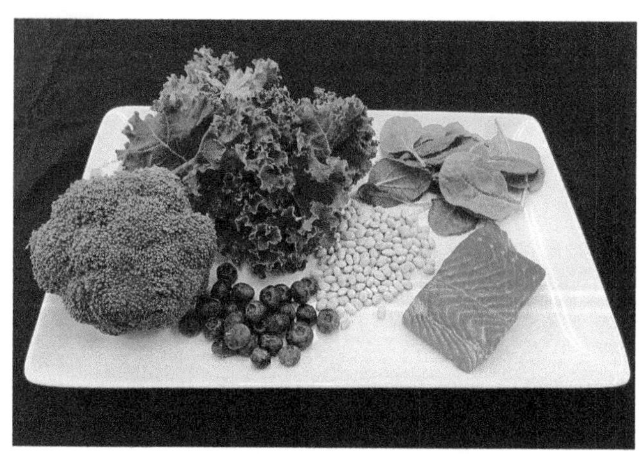

Fig. 21.8 High-nutrient density foods.

obtained from chemical reactions that take place in the body that produce water as a by-product. Daily fluid needs can be met by drinking water or beverages such as tea, coffee, juices, and milk. A portion of the body's fluid needs can be met by consuming foods that have a high water content such as fresh fruits and vegetables and dairy products.

The hypothalamus is the hunger and thirst regulator of the body and is now recognized as a reliable indicator of fluid balance. One way in which health professionals calculate an individual's fluid needs is as follows: An individual should consume 1 mL of water for every kilocalorie consumed. For example, an individual who requires about 2000 kcal/day should consume 2000 mL of water (approximately 2 1/2 quarts) each day.

Water is lost from the body primarily through urine but can also be lost through other means including perspiration, breathing, and defecation. Illness can cause an individual to lose an excessive amount of water through perspiration (associated with a fever), diarrhea, and vomiting. Signs and symptoms of dehydration may begin to occur when the amount of fluid lost reaches 2% of the body weight. Dehydration can be fatal when 9% to 12% of the body weight is lost through water. Symptoms of dehydration in the adult include increased thirst, dry mouth, decreased urine output, dry skin, headache, weakness, and dizziness.

DIETARY SUPPLEMENTS

The best way to obtain all the nutrients needed by the body is to consume a balanced, healthy diet consisting of foods with a high nutrient density and adequate calories. A food with a high nutrient density is a food that is low in calories and high in nutrients; examples include fruits, vegetables, whole grains, low-fat or fat-free dairy products, lean cuts of meat, beans, nuts, and seeds (Fig. 21.8).

Approximately half of the American population takes a dietary supplement, the most common one being a multivitamin and mineral (MVM) supplement. Although MVM supplements can help to fill minor nutritional gaps in the American diet, they do not serve as a substitute for an unhealthy diet. This is because MVM supplements do not compare with the wide variety of vitamins, minerals, phytochemicals, and fiber found in foods. On the other hand, there are certain conditions or diseases that may warrant the use of a vitamin and mineral supplement, as follows:

- *Individuals consuming less than 1200 kcal/day.* A calorie intake of 1200 kcal/day is the lowest calorie level that an individual can consume and still obtain all their necessary nutrients. Individuals who consume less than this amount may need an MVM supplement to ensure adequate nutrition.
- *Individuals with conditions or diseases that interfere with the absorption of vitamins and minerals.* Certain diseases, such as Crohn's disease, celiac disease, chronic liver disease, cystic fibrosis, and chronic pancreatitis, may interfere with the proper absorption of vitamins and minerals from food. A vitamin and mineral supplement may be prescribed by the provider for patients with these diseases. Smoking can interfere with the absorption of some vitamins such as vitamin C and D.
- *Individuals who are pregnant or lactating.* Pregnant and lactating women benefit from taking an MVM supplement because of their increased need for vitamins and minerals. It is important for a pregnant woman to obtain an adequate amount of folic acid to help prevent neural tube defects in the infant. The MVM supplement is prescribed by a provider and is specially formulated to meet the requirements of the pregnant or lactating woman.
- *Individuals who practice a vegetarian lifestyle.* Vegetarians may be at risk for an inadequate intake of certain nutrients and therefore may benefit from an MVM supplement.
- *Elderly individuals.* Elderly individuals often experience a decrease in the absorption of nutrients because of an aging GI tract and therefore may require an MVM supplement. The elderly may also be at risk for an inadequate intake of nutrients because of illness or socioeconomic factors.

There are certain disadvantages to taking an excessive amount of a vitamin supplement. As previously discussed, water-soluble vitamins consumed in excess of the body's needs are removed from the body through the urine. On the other hand, fat-soluble vitamins (A, D, E, and K) can be stored by the body. Consuming an excessive amount of fat-soluble vitamins can cause a buildup of these vitamins in the body, resulting in toxicity symptoms. These symptoms may be relatively mild such as itching, headache, flushed skin, and nausea. They may also be more severe and include symptoms such as loss of hair, bone pain, kidney stones, hemolysis of blood cells, and prolonged blood clotting. (Refer to Table 21.6 for a list of the fat-soluble vitamins and the toxicity symptoms that can occur from an excessive intake of these vitamins.)

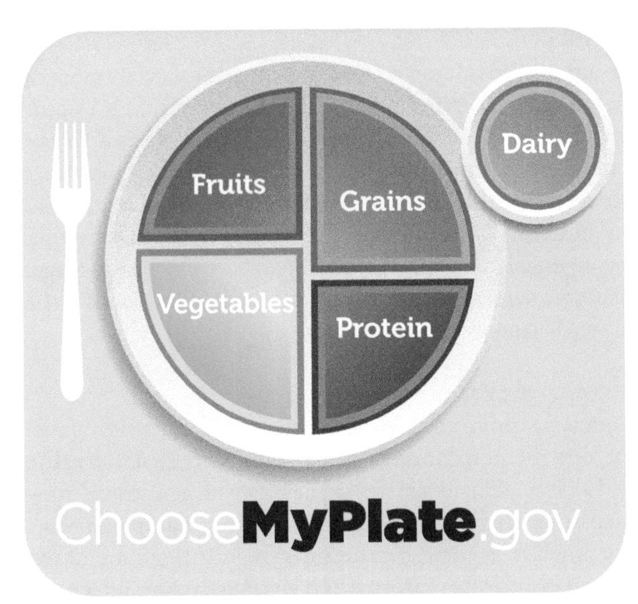

Fig. 21.9 MyPlate nutrition guide. (From US Department of Agriculture: MyPlate, 2011, www.myplate.gov.)

TOOLS FOR HEALTHY NUTRITION

NUTRITION GUIDES

MyPlate and the *Dietary Guidelines for Americans* (DGA) are nutrition guides developed by the US Department of Agriculture (USDA) and the US Department of Health and Human Services (HHS). The major objective of these guides is to achieve and maintain a healthy weight through a balanced nutritious diet that assists in preventing and reducing chronic diseases and conditions such as diabetes, heart disease, and obesity. Studies show that approximately half of all American adults have one or more preventable chronic diseases relating to poor-quality eating and physical inactivity. The MyPlate and the DGA nutrition guides are described in more detail in this section.

MyPlate

MyPlate is an easy-to-follow nutrition guide (published by the USDA) that is available online at www.myplate.gov. MyPlate consists of a food circle or pie chart that illustrates a place setting with a plate and glass divided into five food groups (Fig. 21.9). The MyPlate nutrition guide encourages Americans to practice portion control by including specific proportions of the following food groups on their plate:

- ***Fruits and vegetables:*** Half the plate should include fruits and vegetables, with the vegetable portion being a bit bigger. Fruits and vegetables contribute carbohydrates, vitamins A and C, potassium, folate, and fiber to the diet.
- ***Protein:*** One-quarter of the plate should be made up of the protein group. Dried beans, peas, nuts, and seafood should be incorporated into this group, which reduces a heavy reliance on animal-based proteins. This food group provides protein, iron, vitamins B_6 and B_{12}, zinc, and magnesium to the diet.
- ***Grains:*** One-quarter of the plate should consist of grains. Whole-grain breads and cereals should make up at least half of the total grain intake. This food group provides rich sources of carbohydrates, fiber, B vitamins, and iron to the diet.
- ***Dairy:*** One serving of low-fat dairy foods such as skim milk or yogurt should accompany the meal. This food group contributes protein, calcium, vitamin D, riboflavin, and vitamin B_{12} to the diet.

Numerous resources are available on the MyPlate website. It provides the user with individualized nutritional guidance that allows tracking of daily food intake and physical activity (SuperTracker), access to calorie and food group information for specific foods (Food-A-Pedia), and a personalized nutrition plan based on gender, age, and physical activity (My Plan). One of the most important messages promoted by the MyPlate guide is to avoid oversized portions. It can often be difficult to understand what standard serving sizes for specific foods are. The MyPlate website features a section that contains an extensive reference about the specific food groups and related serving sizes.

Dietary Guidelines for Americans

The Dietary Guidelines for Americans (www.dietaryguidelines.gov) works hand-in-hand with MyPlate to provide important recommendations that support sound nutrition. The information in the DGA is also used in developing and implementing food and nutrition programs and policies in the United States. These guidelines are intended for Americans ages 2 years and older, including those at increased risk of chronic disease. They are issued and updated every five years by the USDA and HHS to reflect the most recent scientific research about nutrition and health.

The DGA focuses on achieving and maintaining a healthy eating pattern along with paying attention to caloric limits and obtaining regular physical activity. An **eating pattern** is defined as the combination of food and beverages that constitute an individual's complete dietary intake over time. It has been determined that an eating pattern is more predictive of overall health status than a focus on individual nutrients. Specific examples of eating patterns include the MyPlate eating plan, the Therapeutic Lifestyle Changes (TLC) eating plan, and the Dietary Approaches to Stop Hypertension (DASH) eating plan.

For most individuals, achieving a healthy eating pattern may require adjustments in food and beverage choices. A healthy eating pattern is not intended to be a rigid prescription but rather an adaptable framework within which individuals can enjoy foods that meet their personal, cultural, and traditional preferences and fit within their budget.

The DGA for 2015–2020 consists of five primary dietary guidelines and a number of key recommendations for healthier living. A recommendation on the amount of cholesterol to consume each day is not included in the 2015–2020 DGA; however, this does not mean that dietary cholesterol is no longer important to consider in developing a healthy eating pattern. Individuals should consume as little dietary cholesterol as possible while consuming a healthy eating pattern. The DGAf and Summary of Key Recommendations for Healthier Living are presented in Box 21.1.

FOOD LABELS

Food labels are required by the FDA for most packaged foods such as breads, cereals, canned and frozen foods, snacks, desserts, and beverages. Food labels for raw produce such as fruits and vegetables are not required but rather are voluntary.

The purpose of food labeling is to provide consumers with accurate and valid information about the nutrients and ingredients in packaged food. Each packaged food is required to state the following information:

- The common or usual name of the product
- The name and address of the manufacturer, packer, or distributor
- The net quantity of contents in terms of weight, measure, or numeric count
- The nutrient contents of the food item (Nutrition Facts panel)
- The ingredients in descending order of predominance by weight

Two important components of the food label are the Nutrition Facts panel and the ingredients list. These components provide guidance to the consumer for making healthy food choices and are discussed in more detail in the following sections.

Nutrition Facts Panel

The Nutrition Facts panel (Fig. 21.10) provides detailed information about the nutrient content of a food, which serves as a nutrition guide to consumers when purchasing packaged foods. The Nutrition Facts panel is especially beneficial to individuals with health conditions that require them to follow a specialized diet such as hypertension and diabetes.

The Nutrition Facts panel can be divided into sections, which are listed and described here.

Serving per Package and Serving Size

The serving section indicates the total number of servings included in the package and the size of a single serving. The serving size reflects the amount that people typically eat or drink. It is not a recommendation of how much a person should eat or drink. A packaged food frequently contains more than one serving. The serving size is presented in common household measures, such as cup, tablespoon, piece, or slice, followed by the metric amount in grams. The amount of calories and nutrients listed on the panel are based on one serving. This section assists consumers in comparing similar foods with the same serving size to determine which is a healthier choice.

Amount of Calories

The amount of calories section indicates the total number of calories in one serving in large, bold numbers. It is important to note that an individual must pay attention to the number of servings consumed. If an individual consumes two servings, this in turn doubles the amount of calories and nutrients consumed. For example, if the calories per serving equals 250 but there are two servings per package, the consumer would actually be taking in 500 calories if the entire package was consumed.

Percent Daily Value

There is a column on the right side of the nutrition panel that lists the percent daily value. The **percent daily value** (% DV) is defined as the percentage of a nutrient provided by a single serving of a food item compared with how much is required for the entire day. This section of the food label provides information on whether a nutrient in one serving of food contributes "a little" or "a lot" of that nutrient to the total daily diet.

The % DV is based on a 2000-kcal/day diet, and each nutrient is based on 100% of the recommended daily amount for that nutrient. For example, a food item with a 20% DV of iron provides 20% of the daily iron needed by an individual on a 2000-kcal diet. For the individual to meet the recommended daily goal of 100%, the remaining 80% DV of iron would need to come from other foods containing iron. These percentages should be modified appropriately if an individual consumes more or less than 2000 kcal/day.

The % DV also allows consumers to make informed food choices to meet their specific dietary requirements by following these interpretation guidelines:

- Low nutrient level: 5% DV or less
- Good nutrient level: 10% to 19% DV
- High or rich nutrient level: 20% DV or more

For example, if individuals want to include foods in their diet to assist them in decreasing their risk of osteoporosis, they should look for labels that indicate a 20% DV or more for calcium. Other individuals might be trying to lower their risk of heart disease and should look for labels that indicate a 5% DV or less in total fat and saturated fat.

Nutrients that Should Be Limited

There are certain nutrients presented on the nutrition label that should be limited in the diet because they contribute to health problems such as heart disease, some cancers, obesity, and hypertension. These nutrients include saturated fat, trans fat, cholesterol, sodium, and added sugars. Added sugars includes sugars that are either added during the processing of foods, or are packaged as sweetners (e.g., table sugar), and also includes sugars from syrups and honey, and sugars from concentrated fruit or vegetable juices. To consume less of these nutrients, individuals should select foods with a low % DV of these nutrients; 5% DV or less is considered low. There is no recommended % DV for *trans* fat on a food label since artificial trans fat is now banned in all foods sold

BOX 21.1 2015–2020 Dietary Guidelines and Summary of Key Recommendations for Healthier Living

2015–2020 Dietary Guidelines

Guidelines that encourage healthy eating patterns include the following:

1. **Follow a healthy eating pattern across the lifespan.** All food and beverage voices matter. Choose a healthy eating pattern at an appropriate calorie level to help achieve and maintain a healthy body weight, support nutrient adequacy, and reduce the risk of chronic disease.
2. **Focus on variety, nutrient density, and amount.** To meet nutrient needs within calorie limits, choose a variety of nutrient-dense foods across and within all food groups in recommended amounts.
3. **Limit calories from added sugars and saturated fats and reduce sodium intake.** Consume an eating pattern low in added sugars, saturated fats, and sodium. Cut back on foods and beverages higher in these components to amounts that fit within healthy eating patterns.
4. **Shift to healthier food and beverage choices.** Choose nutrient-dense foods and beverages across and within all food groups in place of less healthy choices. Consider cultural and personal preferences to make these shifts easier to accomplish and maintain.
5. **Support healthy eating patterns for all.** Everyone has a role in helping to create and support healthy eating patterns in multiple settings nationwide, from home to school to work to communities.

Summary of Key Recommendations for Healthier Living

The Dietary Guidelines' Key Recommendations for healthy eating patterns should be applied in their entirety, given the interconnected relationship that each dietary component can have with others. Consume a healthy eating pattern that accounts for all foods and beverages within an appropriate calorie level.

A healthy eating pattern includes:

- A variety of vegetables from all of the subgroups—dark green, red and orange, legumes (beans and peas), starchy, and other.
- Fruits, especially whole fruits.
- Grains, at least half of which are whole grains.
- Fat-free or low-fat dairy, including milk, yogurt, cheese, and/or fortified soy beverages.
- A variety of protein foods, including seafood, lean meats and poultry, eggs, legumes (beans and peas), and nuts, seeds, and soy products.
- Oils.

A healthy eating pattern limits:

- Saturated fats and *trans* fats, added sugars, and sodium.

Quantitative Recommendations: Key Recommendations that are quantitative are provided for several components of the diet that should be limited. These components are of particular public health concern in the United States, and the specified limits can help individuals achieve healthy eating patterns within calorie limits:

- Consume less than 10% of calories per day from added sugars.
- Consume less than 10% of calories per day from saturated fats.
- Consume less than 2300 mg per day of sodium.
- If alcohol is consumed, it should be consumed in moderation—up to one drink per day for women and up to two drinks per day for men—and only by adults of legal drinking age.

Additional Key Recommendations are as Follows:

- Meet the Physical Activity Guidelines for Americans: The Physical Activity Guidelines for healthy American adults between the ages of 18–65 state that a minimum of 150 min each week be spent in moderate-intensity aerobic activity, and that resistance exercise should be performed at least 2 days per week. Children between the ages of 6–17 should be physically active for at least 60 min each day including aerobic, muscle-strengthening, and bone-strengthening activities.
- Individuals should aim to achieve and maintain a healthy body weight.
- Individuals should strive to consume more foods and beverages with a high nutrient density.

in grocery stores and restaurants. Because natural trans fat is found in small amounts in certain foods, the grams of *trans* fat in a food item must be listed on the label.

Nutrients That Should Be Obtained in Adequate Amounts

There are certain nutrients that that are especially important to health and should be obtained in adequate amounts. These nutrients include dietary fiber, vitamin D, calcium, iron, and potassium. The actual amount (in mg or mcg) and the % DV must be listed for each of these nutrients. An individual should strive to achieve a 100% DV of these nutrients. Consuming adequate amounts of these nutrients improves health and helps reduce the risk of certain diseases and conditions. To consume adequate amounts of these nutrients, individuals should select foods with a high % DV of these nutrients; 20% DV or more is considered high.

Footnote With Daily Values

The footnote explains the meaning of % Daily Value and identifies the number of calories used (2000) for general nutrition advice.

Nutrition Facts	
2 servings per container	
Serving size 1 1/2 cup (208g)	
Amount per serving	
Calories	**240**
	% Daily Value*
Total Fat 4g	**5%**
Saturated Fat 1.5g	**8%**
Trans Fat 0g	
Cholesterol 5mg	**2%**
Sodium 430mg	**19%**
Total Carbohydrate 46g	**17%**
Dietary Fiber 7g	**25%**
Total Sugars 4g	
Includes 2g Added Sugars	**4%**
Protein 11g	
Vitamin D 2mcg	10%
Calcium 260mg	20%
Iron 6mg	35%
Potassium 240mg	6%

* The % Daily Value (DV) tells you how much a nutrient in a serving of food contributes to a daily diet. 2,000 calories a day is used for general nutrition advice.

Fig. 21.10 Nutrition Facts panel. (From Niedzwiecki B, Pepper J, Weaver PA: *Kinn's The medical assistant*, ed 14, St. Louis: Elsevier; 2020.)

Additional Nutrients

Additional nutrients presented on the label include carbohydrates and proteins.

Carbohydrates

The total carbohydrate value featured on the food label consists of both simple and complex types. "Sugars" include simple carbohydrates, whereas dietary fiber is classified as a complex carbohydrate. The remaining carbohydrates come from starches.

Proteins

Most Americans consume more protein than they need; therefore a % DV for protein is not required on the Nutrition Facts panel. Individuals are encouraged to consume moderate portions of foods containing protein such as meat, poultry, milk, eggs, cheese, legumes, and nuts.

Ingredients List

The ingredients list is an important component of food labeling. Ingredients are listed in descending order of weight from highest to lowest (Fig. 21.11). This means that the first ingredient makes up the largest proportion of the food by weight compared with any other ingredients.

Consumers can use the information in the ingredients list to make healthy food choices. For example, the AHA recommends limiting the amount of added sugars in the diet to reduce the incidence of obesity and heart disease. A good guideline to follow is to avoid food items that list added sugar as the first or second ingredient. Added sugar appears in the ingredients list under a number of different terms. Refer to Fig. 21.12 for a list of names used to describe sugar and to the Highlight on Added Sugars box for more detailed information on added sugars.

A
Ingredients: Whole grain wheat, wheat bran, raisins, oat fiber, sugar, sea salt.

B
Ingredients: Corn flour, high-fructose corn syrup, oat flour, brown sugar, partially hydrogenated vegetable oil, salt, sodium citrate, natural and artificial flavor, trisodium phosphate, fruit juice concentrate, malic acid, red 40, niacinamide, yellow 5, blue 1, thiamin mononitrate, pyridoxine hydrochloride, BHT.

Fig. 21.11 Ingredients list. (A) Short ingredients list. (B) Lengthy ingredients list.

The ingredients list also allows consumers to quickly scan for ingredients that may cause food allergies (e.g., peanuts) or food intolerances (e.g., lactose) or that should be avoided for religious or cultural reasons.

Another benefit of the ingredients list is to assist individuals in selecting fresh or unprocessed foods that promote good health and prevent disease. These foods typically have an ingredients list that is short and simple (see Fig. 21.11A), and "fresh" terms are found in the list of ingredients such as *whole oats, whole-grain flour, diced tomatoes, chicken broth,* and *vegetable oil.* On the other hand, processed foods typically have a lengthy list of ingredients (see Fig. 21.11B) and include chemical terms such as *sodium citrate, trisodium phosphate, benzoic acid, sodium nitrate,* and *monosodium glutamate.*

HIGHLIGHT on Added Sugars

Answer questions patients have on added sugars.

What is the difference between natural sugars and added sugars?

Natural sugars are sugars that occur naturally in foods and beverages; examples include fructose in fruit and lactose in milk and dairy products. **Added sugars** include sugars and syrups that are added to foods and beverages at home or during the commercial preparation of food known as *processing.* Examples include the sugar individuals add to their coffee or cereal at home and the sugar added to ketchup during commercial food processing.

What role does sugar play in the diet?

All sugar—whether natural or added–is classified as a simple carbohydrate. Simple carbohydrate is used as a source of energy by the body. Natural sugars are considered a healthier food choice because they typically occur in foods that are also rich in vitamins, minerals, and fiber such as fruits and vegetables. Added sugars contribute "empty calories" to foods because they provide additional calories to a food without adding any nutritional value. Added sugars are often found in processed foods such as baked goods, sauces, and salad dressing.

Why is sugar added to foods and beverages?

Sugar is added to foods for a variety of reasons which include the following:

- **Taste:** Sugar provides sweetness to improve the taste of foods such as breakfast cereal.
- **Color and Flavor:** Sugar improves the color and flavor of many foods such as baked goods and chocolate.
- **Bulk and Texture:** Sugar contributes bulk to certain foods, improving the texture of the food such as baked goods and ice cream.
- **Fermentation**: Sugar assists in the fermentation of many common foods such as yogurt, vinegar, sour cream, cheese, soy sauce, sauerkraut, wine, and beer. Sugar is also involved in a chemical reaction (along with yeast) that allows bread to rise.
- **Preservation**: Sugar assists in preserving and extending the shelf-life of certain foods such as jams, jellies, and baked goods.

What are the primary sources of added sugars consumed by Americans?

According to the American Cancer Society, the sources of sugar in the typical American diet are broken down as follows:

1. Approximately 50% of sugar consumed in the typical American diet comes from sweetened beverages such as:
   - Regular (non-diet) soft drinks
   - Sweetened fruit drinks
   - Sugary specialty coffees and teas
   - Sports and energy drinks
2. Another 25% of sugar in the American diet comes from sweet treats such as:
   - Candy
   - Pies and cakes
   - Cookies
   - Doughnuts, pastries, and sweet rolls
   - Ice cream and sweetened yogurt
   - Sugary breakfast cereal
3. The remaining 25% of sugar in the American diet comes from:
   - Sugar used in cooking
   - Sugar added at the table
   - Sugar present in processed foods such as crackers, salad dressing, and spaghetti sauce

Why should added sugars be limited?

Consuming added sugar can make it difficult for individuals to meet their nutrient requirements while staying within their caloric limits. The new 2015–2020 Dietary Guidelines for Americans recommend that individuals should limit total daily consumption of added sugars to less than 10% of calories per day from added sugars. This equates to no more than 200 calories of added sugars each day for an individual following a 2000 calories per day eating pattern. Studies suggest that consuming too much added sugar can lead to the following health problems:

- Obesity
- Increased risk of heart disease
- Suppression of the immune system
- Increased risk of hypertension
- Difficulty in controlling type 2 diabetes
- Tooth decay

How can I reduce added sugar in my diet?

Tips for reducing added sugar in the diet include the following:

- Drink water instead of sugary beverages such as regular (non-diet) soft drinks, sports drinks, and specialty coffees and teas.
- Limit foods that are high in added sugar such as sugary breakfast cereals, candy, baked goods, and sweet desserts.
- Cut back on the amount of sugar added to foods and beverages such as cereal, pancakes, coffee, and tea.
- Buy fresh fruit or fruit packed in water or natural juice. Avoid those packed in syrup.
- Limit condiments that are high in added sugar such as ketchup, barbecue sauce, relish, and salad dressing. Instead, use herbs and spices to provide flavor.
- Choose heart-healthy snacks such as fruits, vegetables, and low-fat cheese instead of candy, pastries, and cookies.
- Reduce the amount of sugar used in recipes for foods prepared at home such as cookies, cakes, and brownies.
- Choose fruit for dessert instead of cakes, cookies, pies, ice cream, and other sweets.

Continued

TERMS FOR ADDED SUGAR	
• Anhydrous dextrose • Brown sugar • Cane crystals • Confectioner's powdered sugar • Corn sweetener • Corn syrup • Dextrose • Evaporated cane juice • Fructose • Fruit juice concentrate	• Granulated sugar • High-fructose corn syrup • Honey • Lactose • Malt syrup • Maple syrup • Molasses • Raw sugar • Sucrose • Sugar

Fig. 21.12 Names that describe sugar.

NUTRITION THERAPY

Nutrition therapy is the application of the science of nutrition to promote optimal health and treat illness. Nutrition therapy is an important component of the medical treatment plan for managing certain diseases and conditions. As previously discussed, the medical assistant should have a basic knowledge of the type of nutrition therapy prescribed for common conditions and diseases; however, the medical assistant is not qualified to recommend or provide nutrition therapy to patients. This is the responsibility of a registered dietitian, who is specially trained to assess the nutritional status of a patient and recommend appropriate nutrition therapy.

Common conditions and diseases that require nutrition therapy are discussed in this section.

WEIGHT MANAGEMENT

Weight management involves following a set of practices and behaviors that keep an individual's weight at a healthy level. The basis of weight management depends on the number of calories consumed ("calories in") compared with the number of calories used ("calories out") over a period of time. Individuals who consume roughly the same number of calories that they use will remain at the same weight. On the other hand, individuals who consume more calories than they use over a period of time will gain weight, and individuals who consume fewer calories than they use over a period of time will lose weight. Weight management is particularly important in the prevention and treatment of obesity.

HIGHLIGHT on Eating Disorders

Answer questions that patients have on eating disorders.

What is an eating disorder?

Eating disorders are characterized by severe disturbances in eating behaviors, thoughts, and emotions. They can cause serious health problems and may even become life-threatening. Eating disorders affect approximately 24 million people in the United States. Eating disorders include anorexia nervosa (AN), bulimia nervosa (BN), orthorexia, and compulsive overeating. Despite having significant nutritional implications, all of these conditions have been classified as psychological disorders. Some of the underlying problems that may be associated with an eating disorder include low self-esteem, depression, feelings of worthlessness and loss of control, troubled family and personal relationships, and a history of physical and sexual abuse.

Anorexia Nervosa

What is anorexia nervosa?

AN is characterized by a distorted body image, self-starvation, and extreme weight loss that usually stem from underlying emotional problems. Girls and young women aged 15–19 years are most commonly affected by AN.

Individuals diagnosed with AN often become preoccupied with weight and an intense fear of becoming fat. Rituals surrounding food are common with AN—for example, where food is positioned on the plate and how the napkin is folded. Affected individuals often spend a lot of time cutting and rearranging the food on the plate. They typically are very knowledgeable about the caloric and nutritional content of food and may exclude themselves from social gatherings or activities where food is served. Individuals with AN are often high achievers who experience anxiety and depression. They are also typically raised in families where the pressure to succeed exists and where criticism (particularly of physical appearance) is commonplace.

What are the signs and symptoms of anorexia nervosa?

The physical signs and symptoms of AN include very thin arms and legs, dry skin, loss of muscle, brittle pluckable hair, frequently being cold, sunken dark eyes, and amenorrhea. The presence of lanugo or fine "peach fuzz" hair may develop as the body attempts to trap heat and maintain an adequate body temperature. Other symptoms may include irregular heart rhythms, low blood pressure, a decreased heart and respiratory rate, abdominal pain, and an impaired immune response.

What is the treatment for anorexia nervosa?

Treatment for AN is best provided by a team of professionals (provider, nurse, dietitian, counselor, and social worker) in a specialized

Continued

HIGHLIGHT on Eating Disorders—cont'd

treatment facility. Cognitive behavior therapy (CBT) is considered the counseling method of choice for AN. This counseling technique encourages the individual to carefully explore her or his beliefs surrounding body image, food, and self-esteem. Once these irrational beliefs are identified, healthful eating behaviors may then be pursued and reinforced. Counseling related to the patient's family dynamics is also considered a vital part of the recovery process. Nutrition therapy focuses on a gradual increase in the caloric intake that includes mandatory nutrition supplements. Meals and snacks are frequent and small to minimize feelings of fullness.

Bulimia Nervosa

What is bulimia nervosa?

BN is an eating disorder characterized by the consumption of a large amount of food at one time (binging) and then immediately ridding the body (purging) of that food through self-induced vomiting, laxative abuse, or over-exercising. The binge-purge cycle may occur anywhere from several times per week to many times each day.

Individuals with BN often come from families where emotional connections are minimal and criticism is common. As a result, bulimics frequently exhibit a negative self-image, which triggers the binge-purge cycle. In addition, individuals diagnosed with BN may have a history of physical or sexual abuse. Bulimia is similar to AN in that individuals may be overachievers and may have obsessive-compulsive tendencies. Bulimics often have feelings of shame and guilt after a binge episode, which stimulates the desire to purge. The body weight of an individual with BN is usually within the normal range; however, intense dissatisfaction about body weight and shape is usually present.

What are the dangers of purging?

Continued purging results in damage and irritation to the lining of the esophagus as well as erosion of the tooth enamel. Self-induced vomiting also causes broken capillaries of the face and eyes and swollen salivary glands or "chipmunk cheeks." Individuals with BN may also develop sores, scars, or calluses on their knuckles from self-induced vomiting. Excessive loss of fluid from vomiting and diarrhea (from laxative abuse) can lead to an electrolyte imbalance and dehydration.

What is the treatment for bulimia nervosa?

Treatment of BN consists of a multidisciplinary team approach of medical, nutritional, individual, and family counseling. The goal of recovery is to explore the underlying causes of the binge-purge cycle and to identify any irrational beliefs that may be present. Nutrition therapy focuses on returning the individual to normal eating behaviors. Patients are taught to focus on their "hunger and fullness signals" and to pay attention to proper portion control. Meals and snacks should be consumed by the patient at a relaxed pace.

Other Eating Disorders

Are there other types of disorders involved with eating?

There are several other types of disordered eating, including orthorexia and compulsive overeating.

Orthorexia

Orthorexia is defined as an extreme preoccupation with the healthfulness of food. It is a "proposed" eating disorder, meaning it has not yet been classified as a true eating disorder. Individuals with orthorexia often impose strict eating rules on themselves such as consuming only organic, raw, or plant-based foods. Ironically, such restrictive behavior often leads to an unbalanced and inadequate intake of nutrients. Patients with this disorder typically exhibit low self-esteem and a negative body image and often become increasingly socially isolated.

Compulsive Overeating

Compulsive overeating, also known as "food addiction," occurs when an individual engages in binging behaviors without purging. Compulsive overeaters report feeling "out of control" during eating binges. They spend large amounts of time thinking about food, planning their binge, and shopping for it. Uncontrolled eating behaviors typically occur in a frenzied manner and in private. Compulsive overeaters may continue to eat even after they become uncomfortably full. Like the bulimic, an overeater feels shame, embarrassment, and guilt after a binge episode. If left untreated, food addiction can lead to obesity and increase the risk of chronic diseases such as diabetes, high blood pressure, and heart disease. Depression and sleep apnea are also seen in these individuals.

Recovery and Prevention

What is the prognosis for eating disorders?

Recovery from an eating disorder is a gradual process with relapses often occurring. Approximately 50% of individuals with an eating disorder recover completely, and another 30% attain partial recovery. The remaining 20% continue to struggle with disordered eating throughout their lives. Suicide rates are more common in individuals with eating disorders than in the general population. If the medical assistant observes that a patient is exhibiting any of the physical or psychological symptoms of an eating disorder, he or she should inform the provider.

Are there methods for preventing eating disorders?

There are many strategies that help to decrease the risk of developing an eating disorder. These include the following:

- Strive for body acceptance. Focus on what your body can do, not how it looks.
- Avoid physical comparisons with others.
- Be mindful of your genetic influences on body type and embrace them.
- Avoid caloric restrictions that are below 1200 kcal daily.
- Be realistic with weight loss goals. The rate of healthy weight loss is 1–2 pounds weekly.
- Adopt a grazing type of eating style. Avoid going more than 4 hours without a meal or snack.
- Listen to your body. Eat when you are hungry and stop when you are full.■

TABLE 21.9 Interpretation of Body Mass Index

Body Mass Index	Weight Status Category
Less than 15	Very severely underweight
15–15.9	Severely underweight
16–8.49	Underweight
18.5–24.9	Healthy weight
25–29.9	Overweight
30–34.9	Obese Class I (Moderately obese)
35.0–39.9	Obese Class II (Severely obese)
40 or more	Obese Class III (Very severely obese)

Obesity

Obesity is a medical condition in which there is an excessive accumulation of body fat to the extent where it may have an adverse effect on the health and well-being of an individual.

The incidence of obesity in the United States has increased markedly, and obesity is now one of the most common chronic health problems encountered by primary care providers. Almost 69% of adults in the United States are either overweight or obese. That means that nearly two of every three Americans are overweight or obese. Obesity is not just an appearance or body image concern. It is associated with premature death and, after smoking, is the second leading cause of preventable death in the United States today. The primary causes of obesity include an excessive food intake and a lack of physical exercise.

The body mass index (BMI) strongly correlates with total body fat and therefore is used as a screening tool to identify patients who may be at risk for diseases that occur with overweight and obesity. As previously discussed in Chapter 5, an adult patient's weight and height are used to determine his or her BMI. Refer to *Highlight on Body Mass Index* in Chapter 5 to review the methods for determining the BMI. The BMI of an adult is then interpreted using the weight status categories outlined in Table 21.9. It has been determined that as the BMI increases to greater than 25, there is an increased risk of developing certain diseases associated with overweight and obesity such as hypertension, heart disease, stroke, type 2 diabetes, sleep apnea and respiratory problems, and osteoarthritis.

Treatment of Obesity

Obesity is considered a chronic condition that requires a multiple treatment approach consisting of the following three components: nutrition therapy, a physical exercise program, and a behavior modification plan. These three components are also key elements for the long-term maintenance of weight loss. Additional methods of the treatment for obesity include prescription weight loss medications and bariatric surgery. Studies show that even a modest loss of weight results in improved health and the prevention of problems associated with obesity.

It should be emphasized that it is important for an individual to consult with his or her provider before beginning treatment for obesity. Primary care providers often manage individuals with Class I obesity and Class II obesity, but patients with Class III obesity are usually referred to a bariatric specialist. **Bariatrics** is the branch of medicine that deals with the treatment and control of obesity and diseases associated with obesity.

Nutrition Therapy

Nutrition therapy for obesity involves the selection of an appropriate eating plan for weight loss. It is essential that the eating plan selected ensure an adequate intake of nutrients. The MyPlate nutrition guide and the Dietary Guidelines for Americans (previously discussed in this chapter) provide valuable recommendations for a healthy and balanced eating plan.

Before beginning a weight reduction program, it is important to first set reasonable and safe weight loss goals. Most weight loss authorities recommend a slow steady weight loss of no more than 1 to 2 pounds per week. This is accomplished by a moderate reduction in the total number of calories consumed to create what is known as a *caloric deficit.* A caloric deficit occurs when more calories are used for energy by the body (calories out) than are consumed (calories in), resulting in the burning of body fat, which leads to a loss of weight.

To completely understand the concept of a caloric deficit, it is important to have knowledge of the relationship between calories and body fat. One pound of body fat is equal to 3500 kilocalories. Therefore, a decrease of 500 kilocalories each day typically results in a loss of 1 pound each week (500 × 7 = 3500 kilocalories, or 1 pound). A decrease of 1000 kilocalories each day is needed to lose about 2 pounds each week (1000 × 7 = 7000 kilocalories, or 2 pounds). The total number of kilocalories consumed each day, however, should not fall below 12,000 kilocalories to ensure an individual is obtaining all the required nutrients. Most women lose weight safely on an eating plan consisting of 1200 to 1500 kcal/day, and most men lose weight safely by consuming 1500 to 1800 kcal/day.

Numerous weight loss programs are available to assist individuals in achieving their weight loss goals; examples include the DASH eating plan, Weight Watchers, the Mediterranean Diet, and the Mayo Clinic diet. When choosing a weight loss program, it is important for individuals to choose a program that is medically proven and is best suited to their particular needs and lifestyle. Fad diets should be avoided because they can be harmful to health and do not typically result in good long-term results; examples include the grapefruit diet, the cabbage soup diet, and the Scarsdale diet. Characteristics of fad diets typically include no exercise, a promise of quick and easy weight loss, a guarantee of a large amount of weight loss, and the elimination of one or more food groups.

Physical Exercise Program

Physical exercise plays a key role in the treatment of obesity. Exercise increases the number of calories the body burns for energy (calories out), contributing to a caloric deficit and loss of weight. Physical exercise offers additional benefits such as increased lean body mass, improved cardiorespiratory functioning, and an improved quality of life and general well-being. Studies show that individuals who exercise are also less likely to regain their weight after having lost it.

The AHA recommends that healthy adults spend at least 150 minutes per week in moderate-intensity physical exercise. The AHA further recommends that adults perform muscle-strengthening activities at least 2 days per week. Refer to the Patient Coaching box *Aerobic Exercise* in Chapter 4 for a more thorough discussion of physical exercise recommendations for adults.

Behavior Modification Plan

A behavior modification plan is an important component in the treatment of obesity. The purpose of such a plan is to assist individuals in changing behaviors that have contributed to their weight gain. An individual must first identify the behaviors that have contributed to his or her weight gain; examples include eating too fast, eating when not hungry, using food as a reward, eating while standing or watching television, and eating to relieve stress or boredom. Once an individual identifies these behaviors, he or she can then take steps to replace these unhealthy behaviors with behaviors that encourage weight loss such as chewing food more slowly, keeping tempting foods out of the house, using nonfood incentives as a reward, eating only while sitting at a table, and using techniques other than food to relieve stress and boredom.

CARDIOVASCULAR DISEASE

The leading cause of death in the United States is CVD. The most common cause of CVD is atherosclerosis of the coronary arteries. As previously described, atherosclerosis of the coronary arteries is a condition in which fibrous plaques of fatty deposits and cholesterol builds up on the inner walls of the coronary arteries. This causes narrowing and partial blockage of the lumen of these arteries, along with hardening of the arterial wall, leading to coronary artery disease (CAD). As the atherosclerosis progresses, the coronary arteries become more occluded, which eventually could lead to a heart attack.

Research has shown, beyond doubt, that high total blood cholesterol is a major risk factor for CAD, and the higher the cholesterol, the greater the risk. The National Cholesterol Educational Program (NCEP) was established by the federal government to reduce the prevalence of elevated blood cholesterol levels in the United States by educating the public about the health risks associated with high blood cholesterol and to make recommendations for helping individuals reduce their cholesterol levels. It has been shown that for every 1% that an individual lowers his or her total blood cholesterol, the risk of CAD is reduced by 2%. The NCEP recommendations are published as a set of guidelines known as the TLC eating plan. The TLC plan provides numeric recommendations for a heart-healthy diet, which is presented in Table 21.10 and is described in more detail in the following section.

TABLE 21.10 TLC Eating Plan

Nutrient	Daily Recommended Intake
Total fat	25%–35% of total calories
Saturated Fat	Less than 7% of total calories
Polyunsaturated fat	Up to 10% of total calories
Monounsaturated fat	Up to 20% of total calories
Carbohydrate	50%–60% of total calories
Dietary fiber	20–30 g/day (10–25 g/day should consist of soluble fiber)
Protein	15%–25% of total calories
Cholesterol	Less than 200 mg/day
Sodium	Less than 2300 mg/day

Nutrition Therapy

TLC Eating Plan

Nutrition therapy is the first line of treatment for high blood cholesterol. The TLC eating plan recommends that all individuals older than 2 years reduce dietary cholesterol and saturated fats and increase their dietary fiber (refer to Table 21.10). Many foods high in fat tend to be high in cholesterol. Nutrition labels on packaged products provide information on the cholesterol, fat, and fiber content of a food. Following the nutrition therapy measures discussed later can help individuals reduce their level of "bad" LDL cholesterol and increase their level of "good" HDL cholesterol.

Dietary Cholesterol

The body manufactures all the cholesterol it needs for normal functioning, and dietary intake of cholesterol (in foods) serves only to increase the blood cholesterol. According to the TLC plan, dietary cholesterol should be limited to less than 200 mg each day. Cholesterol is found only in animal foods and shellfish. Egg yolks, dairy products, and organ meats such as liver and kidneys are especially high in cholesterol.

Saturated Fat

The intake of saturated fat is the most important dietary factor leading to high blood cholesterol, even more so than consuming dietary cholesterol. This is because a diet that is high in saturated fat raises the LDL cholesterol and lowers the HDL cholesterol. In general, the more saturated a fat is, the harder and more solid it is at room temperature. The main source of saturated fat is animal products, including meat fat, poultry skin, and the fat in dairy products (butter, cream, ice cream, cheese, whole milk). Plant sources that are high in saturated fat include palm oil and coconut oil.

The TLC eating plan recommends that no more than 25% to 35% of the calories consumed each day come from total fat, with less than 7% of calories coming from saturated fat and with the remaining fat coming from unsaturated (monounsaturated and polyunsaturated) fat. Refer to Table 21.10 for a summary of the TLC recommendations for daily fat consumption.

Soluble Fiber

Soluble fiber, in particular, has been shown to lower the cholesterol level by keeping the cholesterol consumed in food from being absorbed through the intestinal wall and into the body. Examples of foods high in soluble fiber include oatmeal, oat bran, barley, some fruits (e.g., apples and oranges), broccoli, and legumes. The TLC eating plan recommends that an individual consume 20 to 30 g of dietary fiber each day, with 10 to 25 g of that amount consisting of soluble fiber.

In general, the cholesterol level begins to decrease 2 to 3 weeks after a cholesterol-lowering diet and other cholesterol-lowering measures (such as exercise and weight loss) are begun. Over time, it is possible to reduce the total cholesterol level by 30 to 55 mg/dL or even more through these lifestyle changes. If the blood cholesterol level cannot be lowered to an acceptable level, the provider may prescribe cholesterol-lowering medications along with continuation of the aforementioned measures.

HYPERTENSION

Hypertension is the most common life-threatening disease among Americans. It is estimated that 78 million Americans age 18 and older (one in three adults) have high blood pressure. Another 70 million Americans have blood pressure in the prehypertension range. Without lifestyle modifications, individuals with prehypertension have an increased risk of developing hypertension. The incidence of hypertension in the United States has increased dramatically as a result of an aging population and an increased incidence of obesity.

If high blood pressure is not brought under control, it can cause severe damage to vital organs, such as the heart, brain, kidneys, and eyes. This damage can result in a heart attack or heart failure, stroke, kidney damage, or damaged vision. Early detection and treatment of hypertension can prevent these complications.

Nutrition Therapy

DASH Eating Plan

Hypertension can be prevented and controlled by following the DASH eating plan (Table 21.11). Studies performed by the National Heart, Lung, and Blood Institute (NHLBI) show that individuals with normal blood pressure who follow the DASH eating plan can lower their systolic pressure by 6 mm and their diastolic pressure by 3 mm. Furthermore, prehypertensive and hypertensive patients following the DASH plan can actually lower their systolic pressure by 11 mm and their diastolic pressure by 6 mm.

TABLE 21.11 DASH Eating Plan

Food Group	Frequency
Whole grains	6–8 servings per day
Vegetables	4–5 servings per day
Fruits	4–5 servings per day
Low-fat or fat-free milk and milk products	2–3 servings per day
Lean meats, poultry, and fish	6 or fewer servings per day
Nuts, seeds, and beans	4–5 servings per week
Fats and oils	2–3 servings per day
Sweets (preferably low-fat or fat-free)	5 or fewer per week
Sodium	Limit sodium intake to 1500–2300 mg daily

DASH Recommendations

The DASH eating plan is a lifelong approach to healthy eating that is recommended not only for individuals who have hypertension or prehypertension but for all individuals. The DASH plan consists of a balanced diet that is low in saturated fat, total fat, cholesterol, and sodium. The DASH plan focuses on fruits, vegetables, whole grains, legumes, and low-fat dairy products. In addition to lowering blood pressure, the DASH eating plan can help prevent the development of certain conditions such as obesity, osteoporosis, diabetes, cancer, heart disease, and stroke. The comprehensive DASH diet plan is available on the National Heart, Lung, and Blood Institute website and is summarized in Table 21.11.

Sodium Intake

A small amount of sodium is needed in the diet; however, most Americans consume too much sodium. It is particularly important for individuals with hypertension to limit the amount of sodium in their diet, which assists in lowering blood pressure.

The relationship between sodium and water can be summarized as follows: "Where sodium goes, water follows." Because the plasma of the blood consists primarily of water, a decrease in sodium in the diet causes a decrease in the blood volume. When the blood volume is reduced, there is less resistance or force of the blood against artery walls. Less resistance translates into a lowered blood pressure. Refer to Box 21.2 for a list of foods that are high and low in sodium content.

DIABETES

Diabetes is a lifelong condition that occurs when the body is not able to use glucose for energy because of a problem with

BOX 21.2 Sodium Content of Food

High-Sodium Foods

- Many restaurant and fast food meals
- Cured meats such as ham, bologna, and hot dogs
- Canned foods such as soups, vegetables, vegetable juices, and meats
- Frozen meals
- Snack foods including pretzels, potato chips, salted crackers, and nuts
- Many condiments such as soy sauce, steak sauce, onion salt, garlic salt, salad dressings, marinades, and catsup
- Pickled foods such as pickles, relish, and sauerkraut

Low-Sodium Foods

- Fresh or frozen fruits and vegetables
- Dried beans, peas, and legumes
- Whole-grain products
- Fresh meat, fish, and poultry
- Dairy products including milk, yogurt, hard cheeses, and ice cream and frozen yogurt
- Most beverages including fruit juices and carbonated beverages
- Unsalted nuts and seeds

Condiments such as herbs, spices, citrus, Tabasco, salsa, mustard, and chili sauce

insulin. Diabetes develops when the body produces little or no insulin, or when the body cannot use the insulin it does produce effectively (known as *insulin resistance*). According to the American Diabetes Association, more than 34 million Americans have diabetes; of these, nearly 7 million are not yet diagnosed and are unaware that they have diabetes. An additional 88 million people have prediabetes. Prediabetes is a condition in which the glucose levels of an individual are higher than normal but not high enough to be classified as diabetes. An individual with prediabetes has an increased risk of developing type 2 diabetes.

Type 1 Diabetes

Type 1 diabetes is caused by an autoimmune defect that destroys the insulin-producing cells or beta cells of the pancreas. As a result, the body can no longer produce insulin and therefore it must be administered by injection. Refer to Chapter 19 for a more in-depth discussion of type 1 diabetes.

Nutrition Therapy

The nutrition therapy for type 1 diabetes focuses on maintaining good control of the blood glucose level. This is accomplished by keeping track of the amount and type of carbohydrate consumed and when (time of day) the carbohydrate is consumed. Nutrition therapy for controlling a patient's blood glucose level includes the following methods: exchange lists, carbohydrate counting, and MyPlate. These methods are described here.

Exchange List System

The exchange list system categorizes foods into six groups according to their carbohydrate, protein, and fat content. The six food groups include starch, fruits, vegetables, meat, milk, and fat. Each food group lists examples of specifically portioned foods belonging to that group. An example of an exchange list for fruits is illustrated in Fig. 21.13.

The term *exchange* is actually the same as a food serving. Each exchange or serving has a known or predictable blood glucose response. Any food within a given food group can be exchanged for another one in that group. For example, in the fruit group, a small orange is equivalent to or can be exchanged with one small banana (refer to Fig. 21.13). Because of this, patients following the exchange system must become familiar with food serving sizes. The patient is provided with an individualized plan that specifies the number and type of exchanges that should be included for both meals and snacks. The exchange method provides a balanced and portion-controlled nutrition plan that assists in nourishing the individual while controlling his or her blood glucose level.

Carbohydrate Counting Method

The carbohydrate counting method offers more flexibility in meal planning than the exchange method. With this method, the carbohydrate content of a food measured in grams is balanced against the amount of insulin administered. Typically, 1 unit of insulin helps to process or metabolize 15 g of carbohydrate. To balance the amount of insulin administered, women usually need to consume 45 to 60 g of carbohydrate at each meal and men need 60 to 75 g at each meal.

Individuals following the carbohydrate counting method must determine the carbohydrate content (in grams) of all of the foods they consume. This information can be obtained by referring to the data provided in the diabetic exchange lists or by referring to food labels and noting the total carbohydrate content of each food item consumed.

MyPlate Method

The MyPlate method (discussed earlier in this chapter) is the most basic dietary approach for controlling blood glucose (refer to Fig. 21.9). It is ideal for the patient who has low literacy skills or may be mentally challenged. Patients are taught to visually divide their dinner plate in half. Fruits and vegetables should occupy 50% of the plate. The remaining 50% of the plate is then divided into two parts, one for the protein group, and the other for the starchy foods (grains). Starchy foods produce the highest blood glucose response and include grain-based foods such as pasta, rice, and bread. Starchy vegetables such as corn, peas, potatoes, winter squash, and lima beans are also included under this classification. By limiting the intake of starchy foods to one-quarter of the plate, the individual can control the blood glucose level.

Fruit Each fruit exchange (one serving) contains about 15 grams of carbohydrate.	Serving Size
Apple with skin (fresh)	1 small
Applesauce (unsweetened)	½ cup
Apricots (fresh)	4 apricots
Banana (fresh)	1 small
Blackberries (fresh)	¾ cup
Blueberries (fresh)	¾ cup
Cantaloupe (fresh)	1 cup
Cherries (fresh)	12 cherries
Grapefruit (fresh)	½ medium
Grapes	17 grapes
Orange (fresh)	1 small
Peaches (fresh)	1 medium
Peaches (canned)	½ cup
Pear (fresh)	½ large
Pears (canned)	½ cup
Pineapple (fresh)	¾ cup
Plums (fresh)	2 small
Raspberries (fresh)	1 cup
Strawberries (fresh)	1¼ cups
Tangerine	2 small
Watermelon (cubes)	1¼ cups

Fig. 21.13 Diabetic exchange list for fruit.

Type 2 Diabetes

Type 2 diabetes can affect people at any age, but the chance of developing it increases with age, and it is more likely to occur in individuals who are 40 years of age or older. The biggest risk factor for developing type 2 diabetes is excess body weight. As a result of the recent increase in childhood obesity combined with a sedentary lifestyle, type 2 diabetes is starting to appear in younger age groups. Individuals with type 2 diabetes may not produce enough insulin or they may have a condition known as *insulin resistance.*

Insulin resistance is a condition in which the body produces insulin but does not use it effectively. Normally, when the blood glucose level rises in the body, insulin is released by the pancreas. Insulin binds to the surface of the cells at a special receptor site, similar to a lock-and-key system. The cell recognizes the insulin and opens up so that the glucose in the blood can flow into the cell and be converted to energy. Obesity can interfere with this lock-and-key system, causing the cell to become insensitive or resistant to the presence of insulin. When this occurs, the pancreas produces more insulin in an attempt to lower the blood glucose level. Over time, the pancreas is unable to keep up with the increased demand for insulin. Without enough insulin, the blood glucose level rises above normal, resulting in hyperglycemia.

Nutrition Therapy

Weight management and carbohydrate control are the keys for the dietary management of type 2 diabetes. Individuals with type 2 diabetes should consume well-balanced meals and snacks that provide an even distribution of carbohydrates throughout the day. These individuals can also maintain good blood glucose levels by controlling portion size, limiting concentrated sweets, emphasizing low glycemic index foods, and increasing the amount of soluble fiber in the diet. Soluble fiber slows down the absorption of glucose, which helps in controlling blood glucose levels.

Another very important aspect of blood glucose management in individuals with type 2 diabetes is attaining a healthy body weight through caloric restriction and daily exercise. Lowering the calorie intake by 500 kcal each day usually results in a weight loss of about 1 pound each week. Caloric restriction should not fall lower than 1200 kcal/day, however, to ensure an adequate intake of nutrients.

LACTOSE INTOLERANCE

Lactose intolerance is not a food allergy but rather a condition in which the body is unable to fully digest lactose. **Lactose** (milk sugar) is a disaccharide that consists of two sugar units and is found in milk and milk products.

Lactose intolerance is caused by a deficiency of lactase, which is an enzyme produced by the lining of the small intestine. Lactase is needed to break down lactose into glucose and galactose, which are then absorbed into the bloodstream for use by the body. When the small intestine does not produce enough of the lactase enzyme, lactose is unable to be broken down and moves through the intestines in an undigested form. When this undigested lactose reaches the large intestine, it is broken down and used as a food source by bacteria normally found in the large intestine. The by-products that result from this breakdown include copious amounts of gas that cause the symptoms of lactose intolerance.

Lactose intolerance usually begins during late adolescence or adulthood. This is because the amount of lactase produced by the body gradually declines after childhood. Lactose intolerance can also be caused by intestinal disease or injury. Lactose intolerance is most common in individuals of Asian, African American, and Hispanic descent and much less common in individuals of European descent.

The symptoms of lactose intolerance vary based on the amount of lactose an individual can tolerate. Some individuals may be able to tolerate only very small amounts of lactose before they begin experiencing symptoms, whereas others may be able to consume larger amounts of lactose before experiencing symptoms. The symptoms of lactose intolerance can range from mild to severe and usually begin 30 minutes to 2 hours after consumption of foods containing lactose.

Common signs and symptoms of lactose intolerance include the following:

- Abdominal bloating and cramping
- Flatulence
- Diarrhea
- Borborygmi (gurgling or rumbling sounds in the abdomen)
- Nausea

Nutrition Therapy

Lactose intolerance is treated by limiting or avoiding foods containing lactose such as milk and milk products (Fig. 21.14). Consuming a food containing lactose with a meal instead of by itself may help prevent or reduce symptoms.

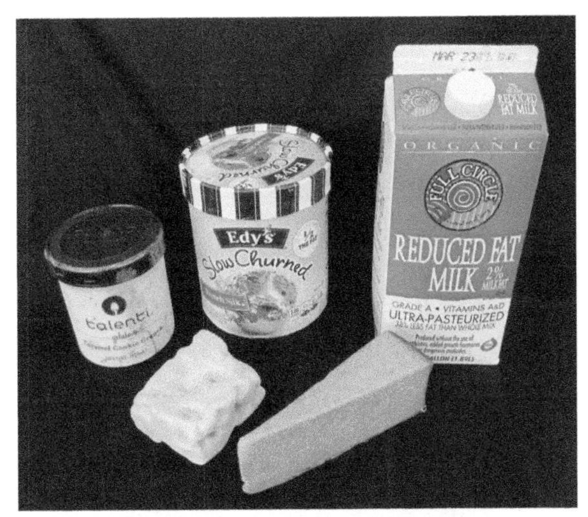

Fig. 21.14 Foods containing lactose.

Other forms of treatment include consuming lactose-free dairy products (Fig. 21.15) and substituting rice milk, soy milk, and soy cheese for milk and milk products. Cultured milk products such as yogurt contain bacteria that produce the enzyme for breaking down lactose. These products can usually be consumed by a lactose-intolerant individual without triggering symptoms. There are also over-the-counter lactase enzyme supplements available (e.g., Dairy Ease capsules, Lactaid Chewables) that assist in digesting lactose. These supplements must be taken before consuming foods that contain lactose. Although there is no cure for lactose intolerance, it is not a serious condition and can be treated effectively through careful dietary planning.

Consuming milk and milk products provides a convenient way to obtain enough calcium and vitamin D in the diet. Individuals who are lactose intolerant may need to ensure they are obtaining enough of these nutrients through careful menu planning. Nondairy foods that contain calcium include canned fish containing bones (e.g., salmon, sardines), broccoli, spinach, legumes, and calcium-fortified breads and cereals. Nondairy foods that contain vitamin D include fish liver oil, liver, and fortified cereals. The body also manufactures vitamin D when it is exposed to the ultraviolet rays of the sun.

GLUTEN INTOLERANCE

Gluten intolerance is a condition in which an individual cannot tolerate the ingestion of a substance known as gluten. **Gluten** consists of a protein found in certain grains such as wheat, rye, barley, and triticale (a cross between wheat and rye). Gluten intolerance most commonly occurs with celiac disease and non-celiac gluten sensitivity (NCGS), which are discussed in more detail in the following sections.

Celiac Disease

Celiac disease is an autoimmune disorder of the digestive tract in which the immune system launches an attack against gluten. The ingestion of gluten irritates the small

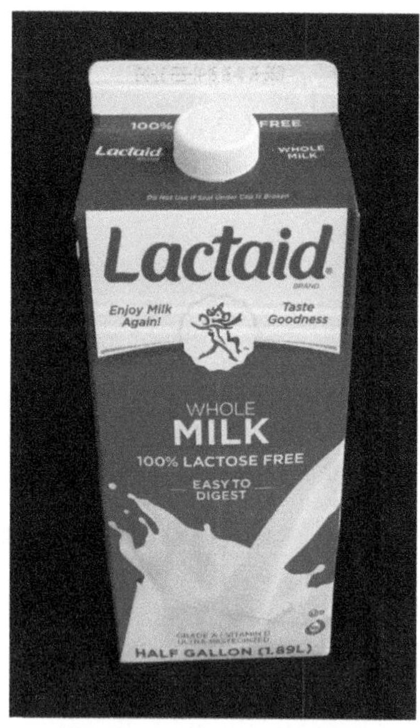

Fig. 21.15 Lactose-free milk.

intestine, which causes damage to the villi. Villi are finger-like extensions that line the small intestine and increase its surface area, providing for increased absorption of nutrients into the bloodstream. Damage to the villi results in a decreased surface area for absorption, leading to malabsorption of nutrients.

Non-Celiac Gluten Sensitivity

NCGS is also a disorder in which the body cannot tolerate gluten. Unlike celiac disease, however, NCGS does not cause damage to the villi of the small intestine. Before a diagnosis of NCGS is made, the patient is first tested for celiac disease to rule out that condition. Research estimates that approximately 18 million individuals in the United States have NCGS, which is six times the number of individuals with celiac disease.

Symptoms of Gluten Intolerance

Celiac disease and NCGS share many of the same symptoms; however, the symptoms of NCGS are usually less severe. Symptoms of gluten intolerance tend to vary widely among patients and can include the following:

- Abdominal bloating
- Abdominal pain
- Weight loss
- Flatulence
- Diarrhea
- Constipation
- Foul-smelling stools
- Headache
- Fatigue
- Joint pain
- Brain fog
- Depression

Nutrition Therapy

The treatment for gluten intolerance is to follow a gluten-free diet, which excludes the consumption of all foods containing wheat, barley, rye, and triticale. Foods that frequently contain gluten include bread, cereal, crackers, pasta, salad dressing, baked goods, soups, sauces, and beer (Fig. 21.16A). Foods that are gluten free include beans, seeds, nuts, eggs, meat, poultry, fish, seafood, fruits, vegetables, and dairy products (see Fig. 21.16B). Grains that are gluten free include buckwheat, cornmeal, flax, quinoa, rice, soy, and gluten-free oats. There are also many gluten-free food products available that can be used as alternatives to foods that contain gluten.

FOOD ALLERGIES

In the United States, food allergies affect approximately 6% to 8% of young children and about 4% of adults. Common food allergens include milk, eggs, wheat, fish and shellfish, peanuts, soybeans, and tree nuts (Fig. 21.17). Examples of tree nuts include cashews, pecans, walnuts, Brazil nuts, hazelnuts, almonds, and coconut. Food allergies may also be triggered by certain fruits and vegetables such as strawberries, tomatoes, and peppers.

It is important to recognize the signs and symptoms of food allergies so that proper treatment can be obtained. The symptoms of a food allergy commonly occur within 2 hours after ingestion of the food. The skin and the respiratory and GI systems are often affected. Common symptoms include skin rash, hives, and swelling. In addition, swelling and itching of the face, tongue, ears, eyelids, and lips may occur. Respiratory symptoms include wheezing, shortness of breath, or difficulty breathing. GI symptoms may occur, such as abdominal cramping and pain, nausea, vomiting, or diarrhea.

Nutrition Therapy

Food allergies are most commonly treated with special diets. The response of the body to a food allergen can range from mild to moderate to severe. The specific treatment recommended depends, in large part, on the severity of the allergy.

Common methods of treatment for food allergies are as follows.

Elimination Diet

An elimination diet involves removing the offending food from the diet and is typically recommended when an individual is allergic to only one or two foods. Removing the offending food(s) from the diet is an easy way to prevent an allergic reaction. An elimination diet is also necessary when an individual has a very severe allergy to a food (e.g., peanuts) that might result in an anaphylactic reaction if the food were consumed. Food allergies are typically more severe earlier in life and tend to diminish in intensity as aging occurs. Reintroduction of that food allergen should be conducted only under a provider's guidance.

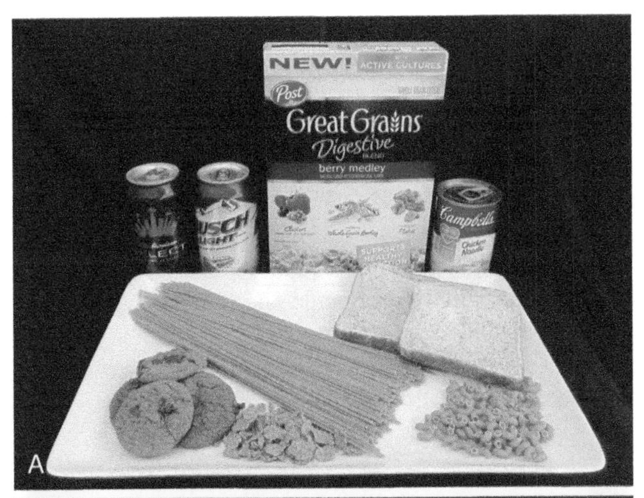

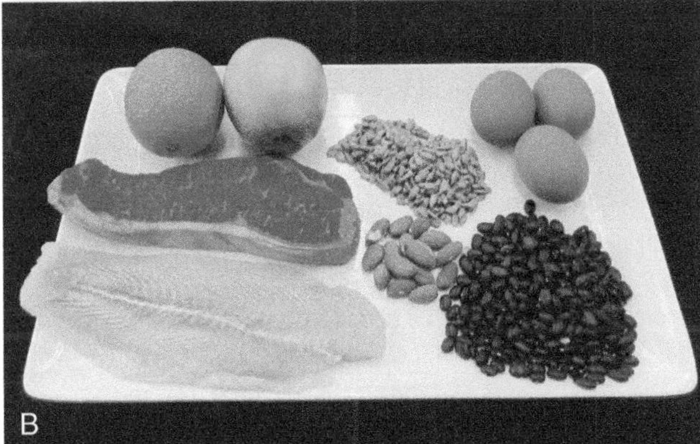

Fig. 21.16 (A) Foods containing gluten. (B) Gluten-free foods.

Rotation Diet

The allergic response to a food is often increased when a food is repeatedly consumed. A rotation diet (use of a rotation schedule) limits the number of times a food is ingested. This typically leads to a gradual desensitization to the food allergen, which lowers the allergic response to that food. A rotation diet is usually recommended for mild or moderate food allergies.

The most commonly used food rotation interval is 4 to 5 days. This means that the problem food (as well as foods belonging to the same food family) is consumed only every 4 to 5 days. A rotational schedule not only allows for the consumption of a known food allergen on a rotational basis but may also minimize the development of a new food allergy.

Denaturation

Exposing a food to heat will denature or alter the chemical structure of the food allergen protein so that the body no longer recognizes it as an invader. A child who is allergic to milk may be able to tolerate milk if it is heated in hot chocolate because of this denaturing process. An individual's tolerance to cooked or canned fruits and vegetables is typically much better than to fresh fruits and vegetables. Exposing the food allergen to acid has the same result. For example, adding tomato or lemon juice to food allergens may significantly reduce the allergic response.

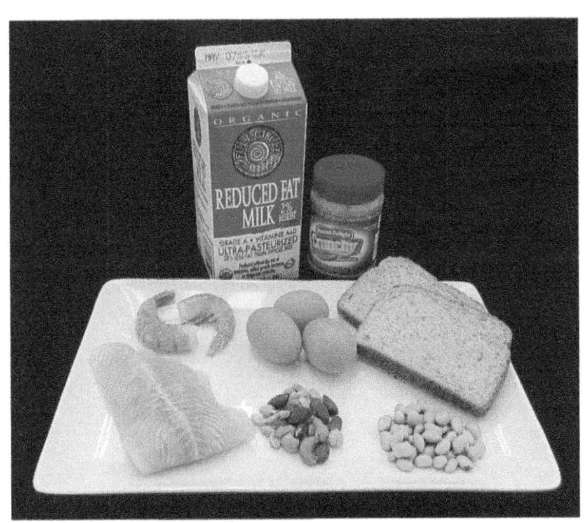

Fig. 21.17 Common food allergens.

Medication and Supplements

Medications that suppress the allergic response may be prescribed to treat the food allergy. Because such medications treat only the symptoms and not the cause of the allergy, the food allergy may actually become worse over time.

The oral intake of supplemental digestive enzymes can assist in treating food allergies. Digestive enzymes help break down the food into smaller, less allergenic molecules. This, in turn, decreases the allergenic response of the body. With continued intake, however, the individual may actually become allergic to the enzymes themselves.

Antacids that contain bicarbonate are used to treat food reactions. The pH of the blood becomes more acidic during an allergic reaction. Bicarbonate antacids cause the blood to become more alkaline, which works to neutralize the acid pH and helps to relieve the allergic symptoms.

There are several vitamins that assist in controlling food allergies; they include vitamin C and vitamin B_5 (pantothenic acid). Vitamin C exerts a stabilizing effect on mast cells, resulting in a reduction in the amount of histamine released by the body. Vitamin B_5 (pantothenic acid) functions in steroidal hormone production, which can lower the allergic response. Both of these vitamins are water soluble and therefore can be administered as a supplement without the danger of toxicity or overdose.

TERMINOLOGY REVIEW

Key Term	Word Parts	Definition
Added sugars		Sugar and syrups that are added to food and beverages at home or during commercial preparation of food.
Antioxidant	*anti-:* against *ox/i:* oxygen	A molecule that inhibits the oxidation of other molecules.
Atherosclerosis	*ather/o:* yellowish, fatty plaque *-sclerosis:* hardening	Buildup of fibrous plaques of fatty deposits and cholesterol on the inner walls of an artery that causes narrowing, obstruction, and hardening of the artery.
Bariatrics	*bar/o:* weight *-iatrics:* a branch of medicine	The branch of medicine that deals with the treatment and control of obesity and diseases associated with obesity.
Cholesterol		A white, waxy, fatlike substance that is essential for the normal functioning of the body.
Complete protein		A protein that contains all the essential amino acids needed by the body.
Disaccharide	*di-:* two *-saccharide:* containing sugar	A simple carbohydrate consisting of two sugar units.
Eating pattern		The combination of food and beverages that constitute an individual's complete dietary intake over time.
Empty-calorie food		A food that provides calories but few or no nutrients. Also known as a low-nutrient density food.
Essential amino acid		An amino acid that is required by the body but cannot be manufactured by the body and must be obtained from food.
Gluten		A type of protein found in certain grains such as wheat, rye, and barley.
Glycogen	*glyc/o-:* sugar *-gen:* substance or agent that produces or causes	The form in which carbohydrate is stored in the body.
Incomplete protein		A protein that lacks one or more of the essential amino acids needed by the body.
Kilocalorie	*kilo-:* thousand	The amount of heat needed to raise the temperature of 1 kg of water 1 degree Celsius. (Often referred to as a *calorie.*)
Lactose	*lact/o:* milk *-ose:* full of (sugar)	A disaccharide that consists of two sugar units and is found in milk and milk products.
Macronutrient	*macro-:* large *nutriti/o:* nourishing	A nutrient required in relatively large amounts by the body. Includes carbohydrates, fat, and protein.
Micronutrient	*micro-:* small *nutriti/o:* nourishing	A nutrient required in very small amounts by the body. Includes vitamins and minerals.
Mineral		A naturally occurring inorganic substance that is essential to the proper functioning of the body.
Monosaccharide	*mono-:* one	A simple carbohydrate consisting of one sugar unit.
Natural sugars		Sugars that occur naturally in foods and beverages.
Nonessential amino acid	*non-:* not	An amino acid required by the body that can be synthesized by the body in sufficient quantities to meet its needs.
Nutrient	*nutriti/o:* nourishing	A chemical substance found in food that is needed by the body for survival and well-being.
Nutrition	*nutriti/o:* nourishing *-ion:* condition of	Nutrition is the study of nutrients in food including how the body uses them and their relationship to health.
Nutrition therapy	*nutriti/o:* nourishing *-ion:* condition of	The application of the science of nutrition to promote optimal health and treat illness.

TERMINOLOGY REVIEW—cont'd

Key Term	Word Parts	Definition
Obesity		A medical condition in which there is an excessive accumulation of body fat to the extent to which it may have an adverse effect on the health and well-being of an individual.
Percent daily value		The percentage of a nutrient provided by a single serving of a food item compared with how much is required for the entire day.
Polysaccharide	*poly-*: many	A complex carbohydrate made up of many sugar units strung together in a long chain.
Saturated fat	*satur-:* full, well-fed	A type of fat that is solid at room temperature and comes primarily from animal sources.
Triglycerides	*tri-:* three	The chemical form in which most fat exists in food, as well as in the body.
Unsaturated fat	*un-:* not *satur-:* full, well-fed	A type of fat that is liquid at room temperature and comes primarily from plant sources.
Vitamin	*vit/a:* life	An organic compound that is required in small amounts by the body for normal growth and development.

22 Emergency Preparedness and Protective Practices

Check out the Evolve site at http://evolve.elsevier.com/Bonewit/today/ to access additional interactive activities and exercises to help you study and prepare for success.

LEARNING OUTCOMES

Disasters

1. State the effects a disaster or serious emergency can have on a health care facility.
2. Explain the difference between a natural disaster and a man-made disaster and list examples of each.

Psychological Effects of Emergencies

3. List the characteristics of a disaster that tend to cause the most serious psychological effects.
4. List and describe the three phases of the generalized adaptation syndrome.
5. List and describe the stages of anxiety and the intervention that should be employed for each.

Emergency Preparedness

6. State the purpose of an emergency action plan.
7. List and describe the six elements that must be included in an emergency action plan.
8. List and describe the three components of an emergency evacuation plan.
9. Identify the information that should be included on an evacuation floor plan.
10. State the duties that may be performed by evacuation wardens in the medical office.

Fire Safety and Prevention

11. List and describe the elements of a fire.
12. State the five elements that must be included in a fire prevention plan.
13. Identify methods of fire prevention for the medical office.
14. List and describe safety measures used for fire protection in the medical office.
15. List and describe the five classes of fire.
16. Identify the steps included in the RACE response.

Employee Training

17. Identify the education and training that must be provided to medical assistants related to medical office emergency situations.
18. State the purpose of emergency practice drills.
19. Describe the role of the medical assistant in disasters and serious emergencies.

PROCEDURES

Develop an emergency action plan for a natural or man-made disaster.

Demonstrate methods of fire prevention in the health care setting.

Demonstrate proper use of a fire extinguisher.

Participate in a mock exposure event, and document the steps taken.

CHAPTER OUTLINE

Introduction to Disaster and Emergency Planning
Categories of Disasters
- Natural Disasters
- Man-Made Disasters

Psychological Effects of Emergencies
- The Stress Response
- Managing Anxiety

Emergency Preparedness in the Medical Office
- Emergency Action Plan

Fire Safety in the Medical Office
- Elements of a Fire
- Fire Prevention Plan
- Emergency Response to a Fire

Employee Education and Training
Emergency Practice Drills
- Fire Drills
- Disaster Drills

Medical Assistant's Role

KEY TERMS

anxiety
disaster
emergency action plan
emergency preparedness
evacuation
evacuation procedures
exit route
fire extinguisher
fire prevention plan
fire protection
HAZMAT
man-made disaster
natural disaster
stress

INTRODUCTION TO DISASTER AND EMERGENCY PLANNING

Every health care facility faces the possibility that a disaster or serious emergency may occur, resulting in injuries, loss of life, property damage, and the inability to provide usual services. Medical offices must plan ahead to minimize the damage from any disaster or serious emergency and facilitate recovery so that services can be restored as efficiently as possible.

This chapter presents an overview of the various types of disasters and serious emergencies that may affect the medical office along with the psychological effects that emergency situations can have on an individual. Also presented in this chapter is a discussion of emergency preparedness and protective practice guidelines, including the OSHA requirements for developing an emergency action plan (EAP) and a fire prevention plan.

CATEGORIES OF DISASTERS

A **disaster** is defined as a sudden adverse event that can cause damage or loss of life. Disasters can be categorized as natural or man-made.

NATURAL DISASTERS

A **natural disaster** is a catastrophic event that is caused by nature or the natural processes of the earth (Fig. 22.1). Examples of natural disasters include floods, tornados, hurricanes, earthquakes, tsunamis, blizzards, volcanic eruptions, and epidemics. Natural disasters may cause injuries and loss of life as well as significant damage to the environment. Natural disasters may occur with or with or without warning. For example, a hurricane develops over a period of days, which allows for some preparation. On the other hand, an earthquake usually occurs without warning. The

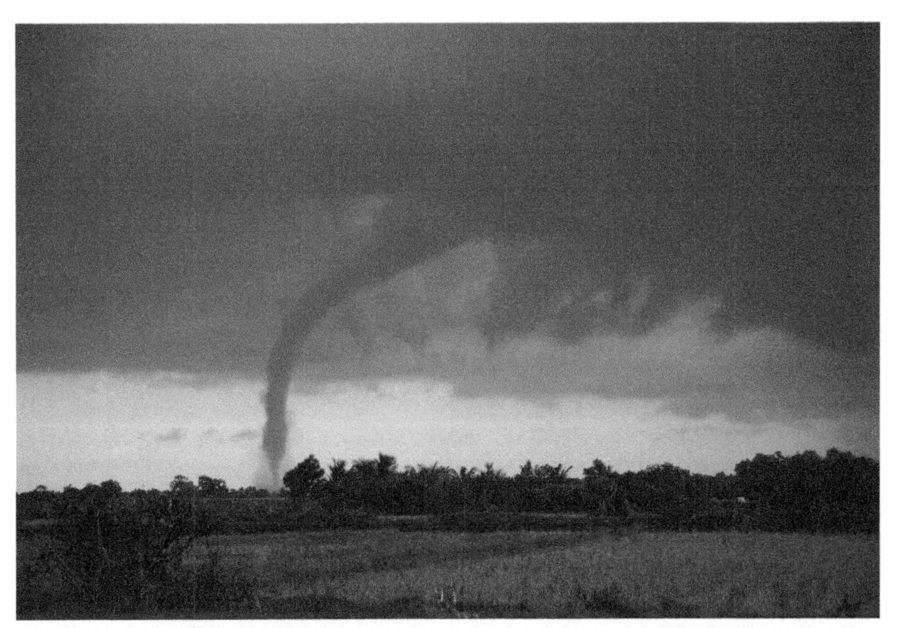

Fig. 22.1 A tornado is an example of a natural disaster. (Copyright © 2015 PhanXuanHuong, iStock, Thinkstock.com. All rights reserved.)

impact of a natural disaster may be random. For example, the exact strength and path of a hurricane are difficult to predict. This often requires numerous communities to prepare for this type of disaster in the event the hurricane hits their community.

MAN-MADE DISASTERS

A **man-made disaster** is an event that causes serious damage through intentional or negligent human actions or the failure of a man-made system (Fig. 22.2). Examples of man-made disasters include fire, power outages, bomb explosions, terrorism, structural collapse, radiation accidents, chemical spills, and bioterrorism.

The amount of threat or damage from man-made disasters can vary considerably. For example, a fire in a wastebasket is usually quickly contained. On the other hand, a hazardous chemical spill may involve an entire city or area. The type of emergency personnel who respond to a man-made disaster depends on the nature of the disaster. Municipal fire departments and police departments provide rapid assistance for fires, injury, structural collapse, and criminal activity. The National Response Center of the Environmental Protection Agency (EPA) responds to the release, or potential release, of oil, radioactive materials, or hazardous chemicals into the air, land, or water (Fig. 22.3).

PSYCHOLOGICAL EFFECTS OF EMERGENCIES

Whenever an emergency situation occurs that causes serious damage or interruption of the normal daily routine, individuals react positively and negatively to the loss of property or disruption of service. Positive reactions involve the triggering of resources, both internal and external, to meet the challenges. For example, when a serious flood threatens an area, individuals usually mobilize quickly to fill and place sandbags to minimize the anticipated damage. When physical and emotional resources are depleted, however, individuals react negatively. Disasters that tend to cause the most serious psychological effects include those with the following characteristics:

- Occur without warning
- Pose a serious threat to personal safety or have unknown health effects
- Have an uncertain duration (such as serious floods of major rivers)
- Result from malicious intent or human error
- Have symbolic significance (such as the 9/11 attacks)

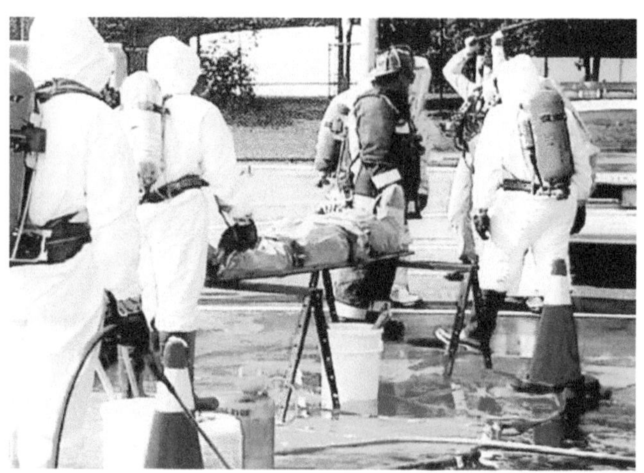

Fig. 22.3 Teams responding to disasters involving a hazardous material (HAZMAT) must wear protective clothing and initiate decontamination of casualties.

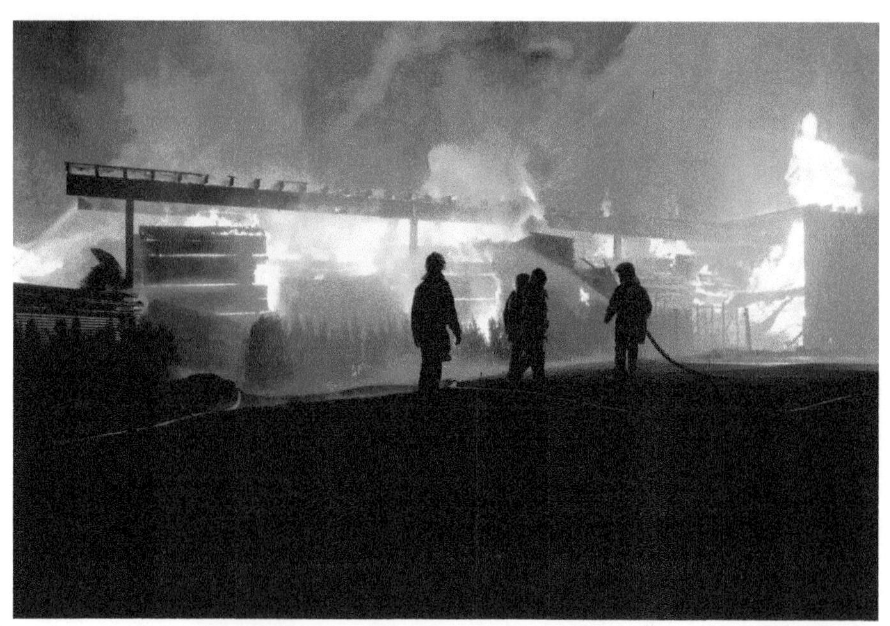

Fig. 22.2 A fire is an example of a man-made disaster. (Copyright © 2015 Steinbergpix, iStock, Thinkstock.com. All rights reserved.)

THE STRESS RESPONSE

Stress is the body's response to threat or change. When a disaster or serious emergency occurs, individuals who are affected by it frequently experience stress. Hans Selye, an Austrian physician who practiced medicine in the middle of the twentieth century, described the body's reaction to stress as a three-part general adaptation syndrome (GAS), which is illustrated in Fig. 22.4. The three stages of GAS include the alarm phase, the resistance phase, and the recovery or exhaustion phase.

Alarm Phase

This phase is often called the *fight-or-flight response*. In this phase, the body senses a stressor and begins to react to combat it. Epinephrine is released from the adrenal medulla, which stimulates the sympathetic nervous system, triggering the following changes in the body: dilation of the pupils and increase in heart rate, respirations, perspiration, and increase in the blood pressure. These changes prepare the body to fight or to run away. In addition, the muscles tense in preparation for action, and the attention becomes narrowly focused on the perceived threat or significant task. This phase does not last very long; in some instances, it may only last a matter of seconds. Some people experience the alarm phase as energizing, whereas others quickly become extremely anxious.

Example: If a serious fire erupts in a medical office, employees typically experience the alarm phase. The fight-or-flight response helps employees remain focused and allows them to quickly and effectively evacuate themselves and others from the burning building and perform other types of rescue duties.

Resistance Phase

The resistance phase begins almost immediately after the alarm phase. In this phase, the stress remains but the body adapts in an effort to cope with the stressor. The resistance phase may last hours, days, or even months depending on the circumstances. During this phase, the adrenal cortex secretes cortisol. Cortisol increases the blood glucose level to sustain energy because more energy is required to maintain the stage of resistance than the normal state. The body constantly remains "on guard" and is not in a state of balance (homeostasis) but is able to carry on its normal functions. Individuals may experience a number of stress-related symptoms during this phase such as fatigue, irritability, lethargy, and lapses in concentration.

Example: If a medical office employee temporarily becomes trapped by the fire (described in the earlier example), he or she may be unable to cope with the stress of that experience. In this case, the employee enters the resistance phase and constantly feels on guard but is still able to function normally. If the resistance phase lasts for a period of time, the employee may begin experiencing stress-related symptoms.

Recovery or Exhaustion Phase

If the stress is removed, the body enters the recovery phase. However, if the stress continues, the body's ability to resist stress is lost and the individual enters the exhaustion phase.

a. *Recovery phase*: In the recovery phase, the stress has been removed and the parasympathetic nervous system begins to regain control. Eventually the body returns to its normal level of function (homeostasis).
b. *Exhaustion phase*: If stress is chronic and excessive, the body's resources to combat it become depleted. Eventually the immune system is compromised, and the individual becomes more susceptible to a variety of illnesses ranging all the way from colds and flu to cancer.

Example: If the employee learns to cope with the stress of being trapped in the fire, the body enters the recovery phase and returns to a normal level of functioning. If the employee is unable to cope, the stress becomes chronic, and he or she will enter the exhaustion phase and begin to experience stress-related illnesses (Fig. 22.5).

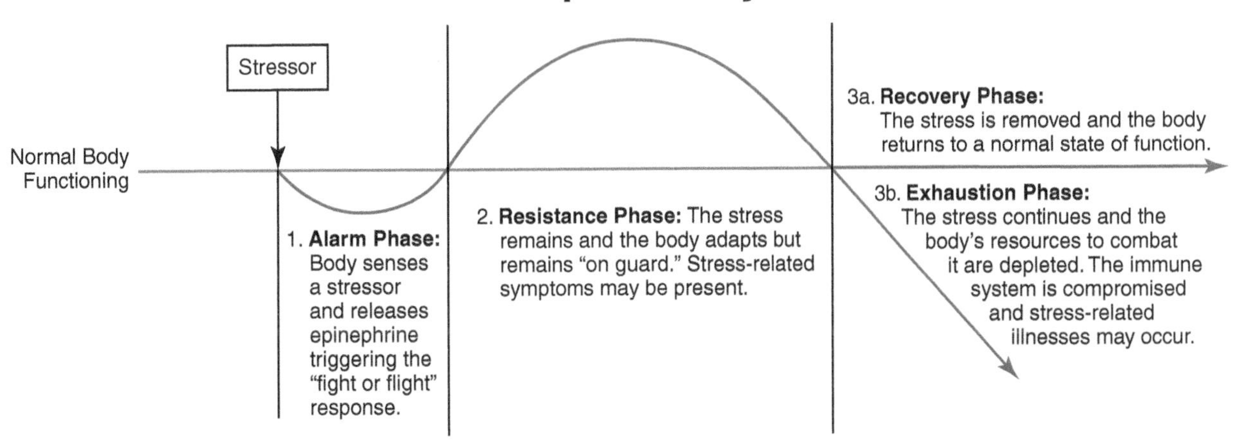

Fig. 22.4 The general adaptation syndrome (GAS) developed by Hans Selye.

MANAGING ANXIETY

Anxiety is defined as a feeling of worry or uneasiness, often triggered by an event that is perceived as having an uncertain outcome. There are four levels of anxiety that range in degree from fleeting worried thoughts to a full-blown panic attack. The four levels of anxiety are outlined in Fig. 22.6.

An individual's level of anxiety has a direct influence on his or her ability to function effectively in an emergency situation. For example, a medical assistant with moderate anxiety is not able to notice details and think as clearly in an emergency situation. However, emergency procedures that have been thoroughly learned through practice drills help the medical assistant decide what to do without having to think through all the possibilities. In addition, practice drills tend to keep the anxiety level from rising because he or she feels more confident when there is a structured plan to respond to in an emergency situation.

Severe anxiety can be problematic in an emergency situation because it tends to immobilize an individual and stimulate anxiety in others. Symptoms of severe anxiety include the following: hyperventilation, rapid pulse rate, excessive perspiration, and confused speech. In an emergency situation, a patient with severe anxiety may lose control of his or her emotions and cry or scream. This behavior can be minimized by the medical assistant giving the patient directions in a calm and reassuring voice. It may first be necessary to touch the patient to gain his or her attention, and then directions should be given in short sentences, speaking a little more slowly than usual. Helping the patient to breathe deeply helps to reduce anxiety, but it is also important to direct the person exactly where to go if a dangerous area must be evacuated.

If an emergency occurs in the workplace, the medical assistant should immediately focus on responding to the immediate situation, implementing established procedures, and helping others. Deep breaths will help to control anxiety, which should be seen as a normal response. Even in disasters that have caused enormous amounts of damage, lives have been saved and injury has been minimized when people have been able to stay reasonably calm and follow established emergency procedures.

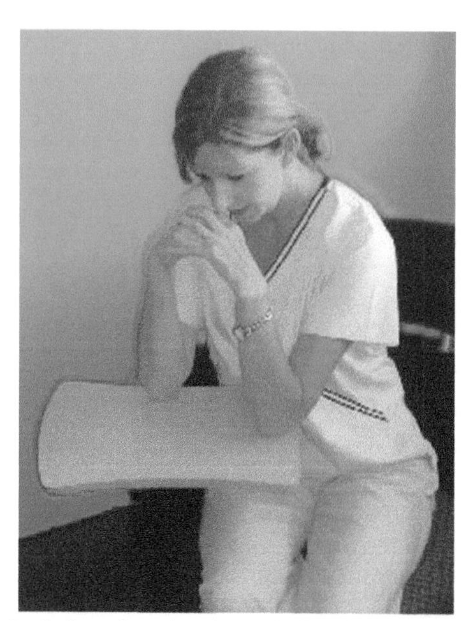

Fig. 22.5 In the exhaustion phase, the body's resources to combat stress become depleted.

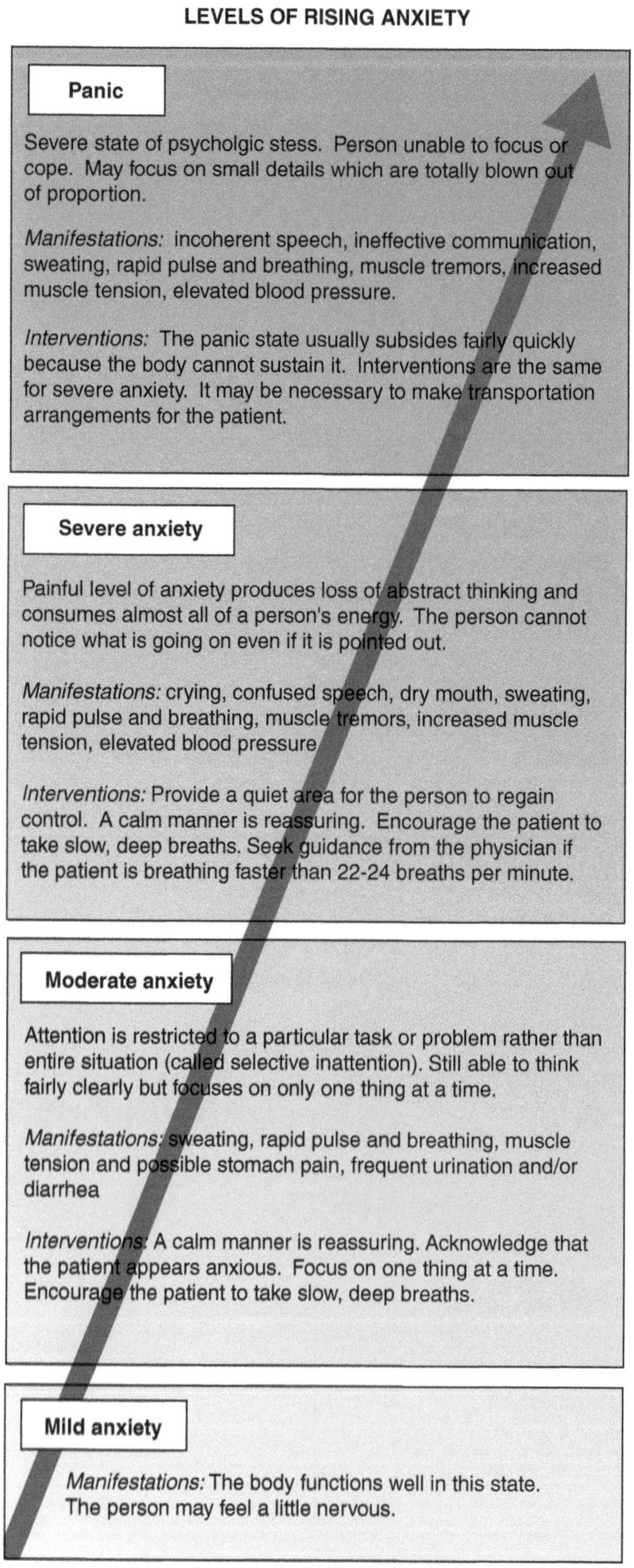

LEVELS OF RISING ANXIETY

Panic

Severe state of psycholgic stess. Person unable to focus or cope. May focus on small details which are totally blown out of proportion.

Manifestations: incoherent speech, ineffective communication, sweating, rapid pulse and breathing, muscle tremors, increased muscle tension, elevated blood pressure.

Interventions: The panic state usually subsides fairly quickly because the body cannot sustain it. Interventions are the same for severe anxiety. It may be necessary to make transportation arrangements for the patient.

Severe anxiety

Painful level of anxiety produces loss of abstract thinking and consumes almost all of a person's energy. The person cannot notice what is going on even if it is pointed out.

Manifestations: crying, confused speech, dry mouth, sweating, rapid pulse and breathing, muscle tremors, increased muscle tension, elevated blood pressure.

Interventions: Provide a quiet area for the person to regain control. A calm manner is reassuring. Encourage the patient to take slow, deep breaths. Seek guidance from the physician if the patient is breathing faster than 22-24 breaths per minute.

Moderate anxiety

Attention is restricted to a particular task or problem rather than entire situation (called selective inattention). Still able to think fairly clearly but focuses on only one thing at a time.

Manifestations: sweating, rapid pulse and breathing, muscle tension and possible stomach pain, frequent urination and/or diarrhea

Interventions: A calm manner is reassuring. Acknowledge that the patient appears anxious. Focus on one thing at a time. Encourage the patient to take slow, deep breaths.

Mild anxiety

Manifestations: The body functions well in this state. The person may feel a little nervous.

Fig. 22.6 Levels of anxiety.

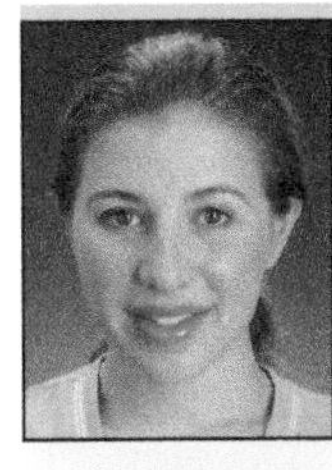

Putting It All Into Practice

My name is Beth Ann Wilson, and I am a Certified Medical Assistant. I have been assisting the office manager in updating the equipment in our office that might be used in case of fire or natural disaster. We recently purchased an additional fire extinguisher for the staff break room, where we have a microwave and coffee maker. In addition, we have purchased an office disaster kit which has emergency supplies for 10 people for a few days including food, water, a flashlight, a radio, batteries, a first aid kit, and other supplies that might be useful in a building collapse. Of course, we hope that we will never have to use these things. I was also one of the staff members from our office who participated recently as a "victim" in a mock disaster drill that was held for emergency personnel in our town. I pretended to be a victim with fractures of my arm and leg. I had never been in a situation where there were many people injured or transported in an ambulance. The experience increased my understanding of the problems that emergency personnel face, and now I have a more personal understanding of how important it is to be prepared with training and equipment. ■

What Would You Do? What Would You *Not* Do?

Case Study 1

Julie Manning, who is sitting in the waiting room, receives a telephone call, speaks on the telephone for a few minutes, and rushes to the front desk window. She tells Beth Ann that she has to leave immediately because she has just learned that there is a fire at her son's school. Mrs. Manning speaks very quickly, but her story seems disconnected. It is also clear that she is breathing very rapidly and is perspiring excessively. ■

EMERGENCY PREPAREDNESS IN THE MEDICAL OFFICE

Large clinics and small medical offices alike may experience emergencies such as fires, floods, earthquakes, power outages, workplace violence, and a variety of other emergency situations. **Emergency preparedness** is the process of making plans to prevent, respond, and recover from an emergency situation. To protect employees from fire and other emergencies and to prevent property loss, medical offices should develop emergency preparedness plans. Emergency preparedness plans, as stipulated by OSHA, must include an EAP and a fire prevention plan. These plans are discussed in more detail on the following pages.

EMERGENCY ACTION PLAN

An **emergency action plan** is a written document that describes the actions that employees should take to ensure their safety if a fire or other emergency situation occurs. The purpose of an EAP is to prevent fatalities, injuries, and property damage during an emergency situation. Almost all medical offices are required by OSHA to develop an EAP, which must be in writing, kept in in the workplace, and available for employee review.

Before development of the EAP, an assessment must be performed by the medical office to determine the potential emergencies that could affect the office. Some emergencies may occur within the medical office; examples include a fire, workplace violence, or a medical emergency (e.g., patient having a heart attack). Other emergencies may arise from situations occurring outside of the facility; examples include a flood, tornado, and earthquake. The EAP should outline the actions that should be taken for each of the potential emergency situations identified by the office.

Components of an Emergency Action Plan

There are six elements (as required by OSHA) that must be included in an EAP; these are listed and described in the following paragraphs. Other EAP elements that are recommended by OSHA (but not required) include a description of the alarm system to notify employees to evacuate, the site of an alternative communication center to be used in the event of a fire or explosion, and a secure location to store originals or duplicate copies of essential records.

The six elements required in an EAP are as follows:

1. *The preferred means of reporting fires and other emergencies:* In the event of an emergency situation, it is important to report the situation and alert employees immediately. Emergency situations, such as fires, can reach dangerous levels very quickly, and a delay in summoning emergency responders and alerting employees may result in the loss of life and property. One or more of the following methods are typically used to report the emergency and/or alert employees to the presence of an emergency situation:
   a. *Dialing 911:* This is a common and preferred method for reporting emergencies.
   b. *Dialing an internal emergency phone number:* If internal ("in-house") numbers are used for reporting emergencies, they should be posted on or near each phone. Internal emergency numbers are sometimes connected to an intercom system so that coded announcements may be made throughout the facility. For example, a facility may indicate a patient is having a heart attack by an announcement of "Code Blue" or that there is a fire in the facility by an announcement of "Code Red."
   c. *Activation of a manual alarm system:* OSHA requires that employers provide an early warning system so that employees can safely escape the workplace. The most common means to alert employees (and other building occupants) are audible and visual alarms. In offices with 10 or fewer employees, it is acceptable to use direct voice communication for alerting employees, provided that all employees can hear the voice alarm. OSHA requires that the alarm be distinctive

and recognized by all employees as a signal to evacuate the workplace or to begin implementing emergency actions.

2. *Emergency evacuation plan:* An **evacuation** is a planned systematic retreat of people to safety in an emergency situation. According to OSHA, the emergency evacuation plan for the medical office must include the following three components:
   a. *Emergency evacuation procedures:* **Evacuation procedures** consist of clear step-by-step procedures for the rapid, efficient, and safe removal of individuals from a building during an emergency. It is recommended that an *emergency evacuation coordinator* be assigned to take charge of and manage the evacuation procedures during an emergency. In high-rise buildings, the office evacuation procedures should coordinate with the building evacuation procedures. Evacuation procedures should include the following:
      - The conditions that would require evacuation of the area
      - The chain of command showing who can authorize an evacuation
      - The actions employees should take during the evacuation (e.g., shutting windows, turning off equipment, closing doors)
      - Procedures for evacuating individuals with disabilities or who do not speak English
   b. *Type of evacuation:* The type of evacuation ordered during an emergency depends on the type of emergency situation. For example, the immediate and complete evacuation of a building to a safe area is typically required in the event of a large fire. On the other hand, a small fire in a wastebasket may require only a partial evacuation of employees from the immediate area. In some instances, the evacuation of occupants from the building may not be the best response. In the event of a tornado, for example, employees are typically required to evacuate to a safe part of the building such as a designated shelter area (known as a *shelter-in-place* evacuation). The EAP should specify the type of evacuation recommended for each type of emergency identified in the plan.
   c. *Exit routes:* An **exit route** is a continuous and unobstructed path of travel from any point within a workplace to a place of safety. OSHA requires that specific guidelines be followed with respect to exit routes. Some of these guidelines (that most affect the medical office) are as follows:
      - Exits should be clearly marked and well lit.
      - Exit routes must be at least 28 inches wide at all points.
      - Exit routes should be unobstructed and free of clutter at all times.
      - Exit signs should be posted indicating the nearest emergency exit.
      - Exit doors must be free of decorations or signs that obscure visibility of the exit route door.
      - Doors that cannot be used to leave the facility should be clearly labeled "Not an Exit" or identified by a sign indicating the door's actual use (e.g., "Storeroom").
      - An exit door must be unlocked from the inside.
      - An exit door must open outward.
   d. *Evacuation floor plan:* Exit routes should be clearly identified and marked on an evacuation floor plan (Fig. 22.7). It is recommended (if possible) that both a primary and a secondary exit route be identified on the floor plan. A *primary exit route* is the quickest and easiest way to exit a building during an evacuation and is usually represented on the floor plan by a continuous solid red line with a directional arrow. A *secondary exit route* provides a secondary means of escape in the event the primary route becomes blocked by smoke or fire. It is often represented by a continuous dashed blue line with a directional arrow on the evacuation floor plan.

      The floor plan of a multiple-story building should show the locations of stairways and elevators and must indicate that the stairs (not the elevators) should be used as a means of exit in an emergency. Evacuation floor plans should be posted in multiple locations throughout the medical office, including each examination room, waiting room, rest rooms, break room, and offices.

      An evacuation floor plan should include the location of the following:
      - Employee's current location
      - Primary and secondary exit routes
      - Manual fire alarm boxes
      - Portable fire extinguishers
      - Emergency exit doors
      - Wheelchair accessible exits
      - Shelter-in-place areas
      - Assembly areas
3. *Procedures for employees who remain behind to perform critical operations before evacuation:* If necessary, some employees may be designated to stay behind briefly to operate fire extinguishers or shut down electrical equipment or special equipment that could be damaged if left operating or create additional hazards to emergency responders. The EAP should identify each of these employees and describe in detail the procedure that he or she is to perform. Any employee remaining behind must be capable of recognizing when to abandon the operation or task and evacuate to a safe area.
4. *Procedures to account for all employees after an evacuation*: The EAP should identify an assembly area for employees to meet after an evacuation. The assembly area should be a safe distance from the building and have enough space to accommodate all of the employees. Assembly areas typically include parking lots and other open areas away from busy streets. The EAP should include a mechanism for accounting for all

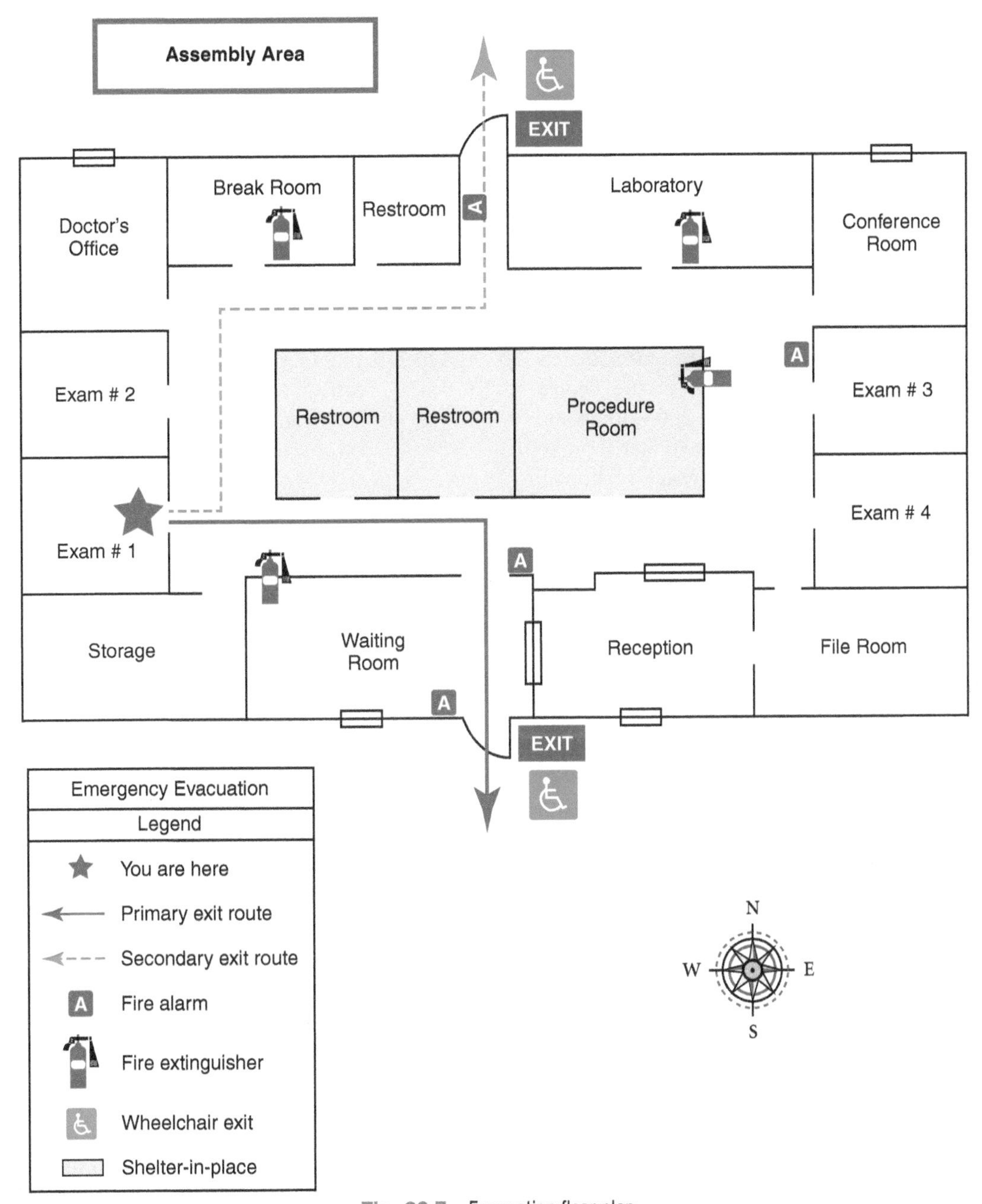

Fig. 22.7 Evacuation floor plan.

employees after an evacuation. The purpose of accounting for building occupants following an evacuation is to help determine if someone is still in the building in need of rescue. This can be accomplished by taking a head count or through the use of an employee roster checklist. A mechanism also needs to be established for accounting for non-employees such as patients and visitors (e.g., pharmaceutical company representatives). Most offices designate the patient log-in sheet as a means of accounting for patients in the event of an evacuation. The name and last known location of any individual not accounted for need to be relayed to an emergency official. It is important that the building occupants be instructed not to leave the assembly area until everyone has been accounted for and dismissed.

5. *Procedures for employees performing rescue or medical duties:* During an emergency situation, various rescue or medical duties may need to be performed by employees. These employees are often referred to as *evacuation wardens.* The type of duties varies depending on the emergency situation. The EAP should specify these duties, including the type of duty to be performed and the name of the employee who is to perform it. Each employee evacuation warden must be thoroughly trained in the duty he or she is to perform. Duties that need to be performed by evacuation wardens during a fire are discussed later in this chapter.
6. The names or job titles of individuals who can be contacted for further information or explanation of duties

under the plan. At times, an employee may need additional information or further clarification of the duties to perform under the plan. The EAP should list the names or job titles of the individuals, both within and outside of the facility, who can be contacted to provide this information.

FIRE SAFETY IN THE MEDICAL OFFICE

Fire is the most common type of emergency situation that occurs in the workplace. Each year there are approximately 70,000 to 80,000 serious workplace fires in the United States that result in the deaths of more than 200 workers and injures 5000 more workers. It has been shown that approximately 85% of workplace fires are the result of human behavior, whereas only 15% are caused by catastrophic failure of equipment. Overall, fire is the third leading cause of accidental death in the United States. In addition to the human cost, a fire can also cause structural damage to the medical facility as well as the loss of valuable documents and information.

There are numerous ways for fires to start in the medical office. Examples include overloaded electrical outlets; heat-producing equipment that is too close to combustible materials; improper use of appliances (e.g., coffee makers, microwave ovens, stoves); improper handling and storage of chemicals, cleaning supplies, and other combustible materials; and arson. If the medical office processes its own laundry, poorly maintained washers and dryers can also cause fires, especially if the dryer is vented improperly or if the lint trap is not kept clean.

ELEMENTS OF A FIRE

A fire is a chemical reaction that involves the rapid burning of a fuel. A fire needs three elements to occur: a fuel source, an ignition source (heat), and oxygen. Once a fire has started, it will grow hotter, and it will not stop until at least one of these three elements has been removed.

Fuel Source

A fuel source consists of any flammable or combustible material. A *flammable* material catches on fire easily (e.g., propane, gasoline), whereas a *combustible* material is any material that will burn (e.g., paper, wood). All flammable materials are combustible, but not all combustible materials are flammable. A tiny spark may cause a flammable material to ignite but would not cause a combustible material to ignite. Many items can provide fuel for a fire, such as paper, cardboard, wood, plastic, fabric, and flammable liquids. Common examples of fuel sources found in the medical office include the following:

- Patient medical records
- Furniture
- Drapes and rugs
- Office equipment
- Chemicals used for sterilization and disinfection
- Laboratory testing chemicals
- Trash

Ignition Source (Heat)

An ignition source provides the energy necessary to increase the temperature of the fuel source to a point at which it ignites. Once the fuel source has ignited, it produces heat. As long as enough fuel and oxygen are present, the heat generated by the fuel source will continue the combustion process. Examples of common ignition sources include the following:

- Open flames (e.g., burning candle)
- Faulty electrical equipment
- Hot surfaces (e.g., examination light)
- Sparks (e.g., burning cigarette)

Oxygen

The air around us has about a 21% oxygen content, and most fires only require an atmosphere of 16% to burn. Many medical offices store oxygen in their facilities to administer to patients if necessary. This stored oxygen is a safe gas as long as it is stored and used properly. Oxygen stored in the medical office is not flammable, nor will it explode; however, it greatly increases the combustion rate of a fire. If something catches fire, oxygen will make the flame hotter and cause it to burn faster and more vigorously. The result is that a fire involving stored oxygen can appear explosive-like.

FIRE PREVENTION PLAN

A **fire prevention plan** is a written document that identifies flammable and combustible materials stored in the workplace and ways to control workplace fire hazards. A fire prevention plan reduces the probability that a workplace fire will ignite or spread, which helps prevent injury or death, keeps the workplace safe, and helps to prevent financial losses to the medical office. Almost all medical offices are required by OSHA to develop a fire prevention plan. The fire prevention plan must be in writing, kept in the workplace, and available for employee review.

Components of a Fire Prevention Plan

Five elements (as required by OSHA) must be included in a fire prevention plan; these are as follows:

1. A list of all major fire hazards including:
   a. Proper handling and storage of fire hazards
   b. Potential ignition sources and controls
   c. Type of fire protection equipment necessary to control each fire hazard
2. Procedures to control accumulation of flammable and combustible waste materials
3. Procedures for regular maintenance of safeguards installed on heat-producing equipment to prevent accidental ignition of combustible materials
4. Name or job title of employees responsible for maintaining equipment to prevent or control ignition sources or fires

BOX 22.1 Methods of Fire Prevention in the Medical Office

Flammable and Combustible Materials

1. Keep the medical office free of clutter.
2. Keep flammable and combustible materials away from ignition sources.
3. Read the label and safety data sheet (SDS) accompanying medical office supplies (e.g., laboratory testing kits, hazardous chemicals, printer toner cartridges) to determine how to properly handle, store, and use these items.
4. Do not allow trash to accumulate.
5. Store trash awaiting removal in a safe location away from heat-producing equipment.
6. Safely dispose of flammable and combustible waste.
7. Clean up any spill of flammable liquids immediately.
8. Do not allow the use of open flames (e.g., burning candles) in the medical office.
9. Ensure that smoking bans are enforced in the workplace.
10. Designate an area outside the building for smoking with fire-resistant containers.

Electrical Equipment and Appliances

1. Make sure equipment and appliances are properly plugged into wall outlets.
2. Use only grounded appliances plugged into grounded outlets (three-prong plug).
3. Do not overload electrical outlets.
4. Promptly disconnect and replace cracked, frayed, or broken electrical cords.
5. Keep heat-producing equipment (e.g., coffee makers, copy machines) away from flammable or combustible materials.
6. Turn off all heat-producing equipment (e.g., examination lights, autoclave) and appliances (e.g., coffee makers) at the end of each workday.
7. Shut down electrical equipment that malfunctions or gives off a strange odor.
8. Avoid the use of extension cords.
9. Avoid the use of space heaters.

Inspection and Maintenance

1. Store oxygen in a clean, dry, well-ventilated room.
2. Keep compressed oxygen cylinders and liquid oxygen tanks upright at all times.
3. Ensure that fire alarms and fire extinguishers are clearly visible and not blocked by equipment, decorations, coats, or other objects.
4. Ensure that fire extinguishers are properly stored in their designated locations.
5. Ensure that authorized personnel perform yearly inspections and maintenance of medical equipment (e.g., autoclave, electrocardiograph).
6. Test smoke detectors every month and replace batteries every 6 months.
7. Have authorized personnel perform regular inspections, maintenance, and testing of fire alarms, sprinkler systems, and fire extinguishers.
8. Report fire hazards you cannot correct yourself.

5. Name or job title of employees responsible for the control of fuel source hazards

Methods of fire prevention for the medical office (which incorporate many of the elements listed above) are presented in Box 22.1.

Fire Protection in the Medical Office

Fire protection involves the implementation of safety measures to reduce the unwanted effects of fire. The purpose of fire protection is to prevent the spread of fire from one area of a building to another, allow for the safe exit of building occupants, and prevent or reduce the amount of property damage. Fire protection for an office building is specified by fire code requirements and is the responsibility of the owner of the building; however, fire protection for the contents of the office is the responsibility of office staff. Some of the important safety measures employed in fire protection are listed and described in the following paragraphs.

Sprinkler Systems

Sprinkler systems are one of the best measures available to extinguish a fire in its early stages. Sprinkler systems are usually located at ceiling level and use water to put out or slow the progress of a fire. Sprinklers are activated by the build-up of heat in the fire area, which causes a glass component in the sprinkler head to melt or break, releasing water from the sprinkler. Only those sprinklers closest to the fire area are activated, which reduces water damage to the contents of the building. For example, just one or two activated sprinklers may be able to quickly extinguish a fire that has just started in an office laboratory. Most sprinkler systems include an alarm system that alerts both building occupants and emergency responders when sprinkler activation occurs.

Many states require sprinkler systems in commercial and office buildings. Some states that require sprinklers for larger office buildings do not require them for smaller offices (e.g., provider's office that has been converted from a house).

Fire Doors

A fire door is a fire-resistant door that is designed to prevent the spread of fire from one area of a building to another (Fig. 22.8). Fire doors assist in the safe escape of occupants from a building during a fire and help to reduce property damage. In a large office or freestanding clinic, fire doors are typically located at certain points in the corridors. Fire doors should never be propped open; instead, they should be allowed to shut to their naturally closed position.

KEEP CLOSED
FIRE DOOR
DO NOT BLOCK

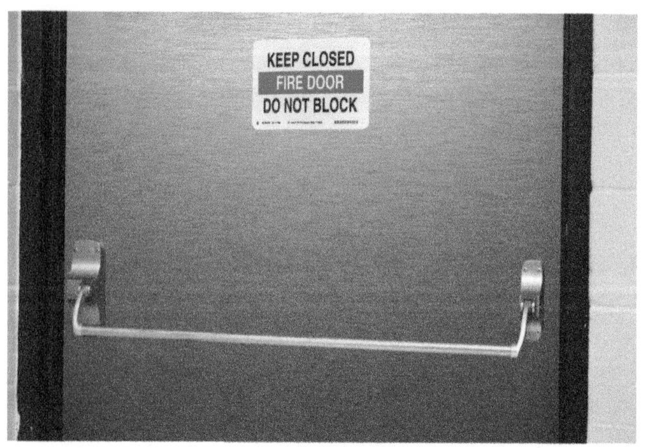

Fig. 22.8 A fire door prevents the spread of fire from one area of a building to another.

Fire-Resistant Cabinets

Whenever possible, records should be stored in fire-resistant file cabinets. If the office uses a physical system to back up computer files (instead of a network or an Internet system), the backup drives should be stored in a fire-resistant file cabinet or fire-resistant box-type safe. It is always preferable to store a backup copy on the Internet or at another location.

Fire Alarms

A fire alarm is a device that warns building occupants of the presence of a fire (Fig. 22.9). Once a fire alarm has been activated, a loud noise and flashing lights are broadcasted to alert building occupants of the fire and to provide them with enough time to safely evacuate the building. The alarm also notifies the fire department so that firefighters can quickly respond to the fire. Fire alarm pull stations are frequently located in the corridors of buildings. It is important for employees to be trained in the proper activation of a fire alarm and what conditions necessitate activating the alarm.

Smoke Detectors

A smoke detector is a device that detects and automatically provides a warning of the presence of smoke. Smoke detector laws vary by state in terms of how many must be in an office and where they must be located. In many buildings, smoke detectors are wired into the building's security and fire alarm system. If the office has battery-operated smoke detectors, these should be tested monthly by pressing the test button. Batteries should be changed every 6 months, and the date should be noted on the detector.

Fire Extinguisher

A **fire extinguisher** is a portable device that discharges an agent designed to extinguish a fire (Fig. 22.10A). Common examples of extinguishing agents include dry chemicals, foam, carbon dioxide, and water. Portable fire extinguishers are considered a first line of defense in the early stages of a fire and have two primary functions: to control or extinguish a small fire that has just started and to protect an evacuation route that a fire may block with smoke or burning

LIFT THEN
PULL HANDLE
PULL FOR
FIRE
EDWARDS

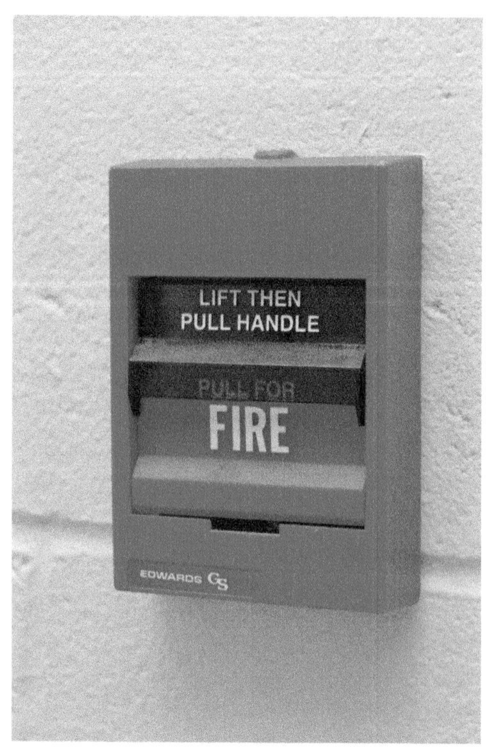

Fig. 22.9 Fire alarm pull stations are commonly found in the corridors of an office building.

materials. A fire extinguisher should never be used to fight a large fire that is out of control; instead, the building occupants should evacuate the premises immediately and call the fire department.

Fires are classified into five categories according to the type of fuel that is burning. For example, a class A fire involves the burning of ordinary combustible materials. Fire extinguishers are marked with a label indicating the type of fire classification they are designed to handle. Newer types of fire extinguishers are labeled with a pictogram illustrating the type of fuel that can be extinguished by that particular extinguisher. Older types of extinguishers are labeled with colored geometric shapes with letter designations. Table 22.1 lists and describes the five fire classifications along with the type of extinguisher (by label) that can be used to extinguish each class of fire. Most fire extinguishers are designed to handle more than one fire classification. For example, a multipurpose fire extinguisher is labeled with three pictograms (see Fig. 22.10B) and is designed to extinguish class A, B, and C fires. Most medical offices have multipurpose fire extinguishers in their facilities because this type of extinguisher can put out most types of fire.

Fire extinguishers must be properly identified (Fig. 22.11) and readily accessible in an emergency situation. Fire code requirements specify the size, number, location, and type of fire extinguishers within a facility. These requirements are based on the protection level that is appropriate for the hazard class of the building and the types (classes) of fire most likely to occur in that facility. Fire extinguishers are mounted on brackets or installed in wall cabinets (see Fig. 22.11) and are usually located along normal paths of travel and near

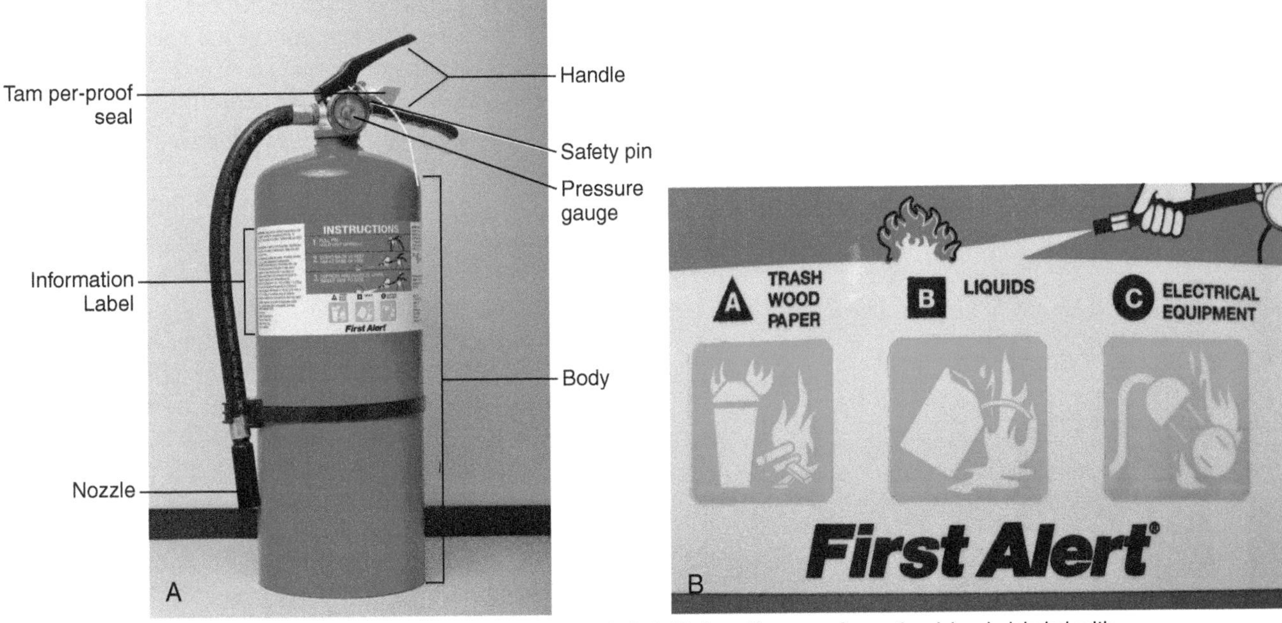

Fig. 22.10 (A) Fire extinguisher with parts labeled. (B) A multipurpose fire extinguisher is labeled with three pictograms indicating the A, B, and C fire classifications it is designed to extinguish.

Table 22.1 Extinguishers Used to Extinguish Various Classifications of Fire

Extinguisher Label: Pictogram	Extinguisher Label: Geometric Symbol	Works on: Fire Classification
	A	**Class A: Ordinary Combustibles** Paper, wood, cloth, rubber, many plastics
	B	**Class B: Flammable Liquids** Gasoline, oil, grease, tar, oil-based paints, solvents, lacquers, alcohols, flammable gases
	C	**Class C: Electrical Equipment** Equipment and appliances that are plugged into an outlet, wiring, circuit breakers, electrical outlets
	D	**Class D: Combustible Metals** Magnesium, titanium, zirconium, sodium, lithium, potassium
	K	**Class K: Cooking Media** Vegetable oil, animal oil, fats in cooking appliances involving these substances

building exits. If a fire extinguisher is mounted in a room, it is placed near the door so that the fire does not get between an individual and an exit. There should always be a fire extinguisher within a 50-foot travel distance of flammable liquids that are stored in containers. Fire extinguishers must be stored in their designated place at all times except during operation.

Fire extinguishers must be properly maintained to ensure that they are safe to use and will operate properly when needed. Most medical offices use maintenance personnel and a certified fire extinguisher agency to inspect, maintain, and test their fire extinguishers on a regular basis (monthly and yearly). A durable tag is attached to each fire

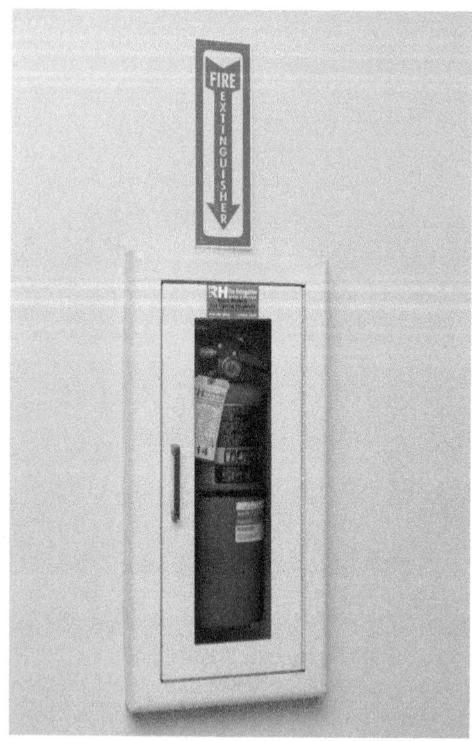

Fig. 22.11 A fire extinguisher installed in a wall cabinet.

extinguisher to document each service check, including the date of the service and the signature of the individual performing the service.

Small fires can often be put out quickly by an employee using a portable fire extinguisher, ending the threat of a major fire. To do this safely, however, the employee must know how to properly operate a fire extinguisher. OSHA requires that any employee responsible for operating a portable fire extinguisher be thoroughly trained in the use of the fire extinguisher as well as the hazards associated with fighting a fire. The acronym *PASS* is used to help remember the steps involved in operating a fire extinguisher:

P: Pull out the pin.
A: Aim the nozzle at the base of the fire.
S: Squeeze the handle.
S: Sweep the nozzle from side to side at the base of the fire.

Procedure 22.1 outlines in more detail the procedure for operating a fire extinguisher.

EMERGENCY RESPONSE TO A FIRE

It is important to respond immediately to a fire. Most fires start out small but can quickly increase in size and intensity and become life-threatening in just a matter of minutes. The heat, smoke, and toxic gases from a fire that is spreading are often more dangerous than the flames.

The acronym *RACE* can be used to identify the basic steps to follow in responding to a fire (RACE against fire). These steps are as follows:

R: Rescue anyone in immediate danger of the fire.
A: Activate the alarm.
C: Confine the fire by closing doors and windows.
E: Extinguish the fire or evacuate the area. If the fire is small, use a fire extinguisher to put the fire out. If the fire cannot be extinguished, evacuate the area.

Procedure 22.2 presents a more detailed emergency plan for responding to a fire, incorporating the RACE response outlined previously.

What Would You Do? What Would You *Not* Do?

Case Study 2

Brie Matthews is at the medical office for an evaluation of her diabetes. Mary Beth enters the examining room to measure Brie's vital signs. As Mary Beth enters the room, she notices that Brie is studying the fire extinguisher mounted on brackets near the door and turning the service tag over to read the information on it. Brie indicates that she needs to get a fire extinguisher for her home and wants to know the meaning of the three pictures on the extinguisher and why the extinguisher has a tag attached to it. Brie wants to know who is allowed to operate the fire extinguisher and how long the extinguisher lasts before it gets "used up." Brie also wants to know why there are fire extinguishers in the office, because she noticed that the office has sprinklers in the ceiling. ■

EMPLOYEE EDUCATION AND TRAINING

Medical assisting employees must know what types of emergencies may occur in their medical office and what course of action they should take. OSHA requires that employees be provided with education and training on the EAP. The training should include the following:

- Individual roles and responsibilities
- Threats, hazards, and protective actions
- Location and operation of manually activated pull stations and communication equipment
- Emergency response procedures
- Evacuation, shelter, and accountability procedures
- Location and use of common emergency equipment
- Emergency shutdown procedures

The EAP must be reviewed with each employee at the following times:

- When the initial plan is developed
- When new employees are hired
- When the employee's responsibilities or designated actions under the plan change
- Whenever the plan is changed

EMERGENCY PRACTICE DRILLS

Once employees have reviewed and been trained in the EAP, it is important to hold emergency practice drills. The purpose of a practice drill is to provide employees with the opportunity to practice their assigned duties in a simulated emergency situation. This increases the probability that employees

TABLE 22.2 Duties Performed by Evacuation Wardens During a Fire

Duties	Guidelines and Key Points
Activate the nearest fire alarm pull station	The employee who first discovers the fire should activate the nearest fire alarm pull station.
Operate a fire extinguisher	A fire extinguisher can be used to extinguish a small fire in the beginning stages. *Do not* attempt to extinguish a fire if it is too large or if there is excessive smoke or heat.
Alert patients to the presence of a fire	Alert patients using a calm and firm manner so as not to cause panic. Use a clear and distinct voice to instruct patients during the evacuation.
Evacuate patients and visitors from each room and close windows and doors in each room	Closing windows and doors reduces the amount of oxygen that is able to get to the fire and helps to limit the spread of smoke and fire throughout the building.
Escort patients and visitors to the nearest exit and assembly area according to the evacuation floor plan	Use the primary exit route if available. If the primary exit route is blocked, use the secondary exit route. If smoke is present, stay low and close to the floor while evacuating because the air is fresher nearer to the ground. Proceed (walk, do not run) through the escape route in a quiet, orderly manner.
Assist patients with disabilities	If it is not possible to evacuate a disabled patient, take the patient to a shelter-in-place area and notify emergency personnel of the patient's location.
Direct patients to stairways that are free of smoke	Instruct individuals to not push, rush, or jostle other individuals when exiting by way of a stairway.
Keep people out of elevators	Elevators should not be used during a fire because: a. Elevator may fail during a fire, trapping the occupants. b. Elevator shafts may fill with smoke. c. Elevators need to be available to emergency responders.
Perform a final check of each room (examining rooms, rest rooms, offices, break room, storage rooms) to make sure everyone has been evacuated	A final check ensures that all occupants have been evacuated from the building.
Make sure fire doors are closed when exiting	Fire doors prevent spread of fire from one area to another.
Instruct building occupants not to leave the assembly area or to go back into the building	Building occupants need to remain in the assembly area so that they can be accounted for by the emergency evacuation coordinator. Occupants should not go back into the building until given permission to do so by emergency officials.
Direct emergency responders to the location of the fire	Use a clear and distinct voice to direct emergency responders to the location of the fire.
Notify emergency responders of hazardous materials (e.g., oxygen tanks, hazardous chemicals) in the building	Providing information on hazardous materials is essential to the safety of emergency responders.

will perform their duties safely and effectively in the event of an actual disaster or serious emergency. Emergency practice drills also provide the opportunity to evaluate the effectiveness of the EAP and determine any necessary changes or adjustments needed for improving performance. There are two types of emergency practice drills—fire drills and disaster drills—which are discussed in more detail in the following sections.

FIRE DRILLS

Fire drills may be required at specific intervals depending on the municipal or state laws for the type of building and insurance requirements. Fire drills may be announced or unannounced. They assist employees of a medical facility to review emergency escape routes and procedures to respond to a fire. Fire drills provide employees with the opportunity to become familiar with exit routes under nonthreatening conditions. This increases the probability of an organized and smooth evacuation during an actual emergency. The type of duties that need to be performed by evacuation wardens during a fire are outlined in Table 22.2.

DISASTER DRILLS

Disaster drills are usually more comprehensive than fire drills. Disaster drills often involve several community agencies depending on the severity of the disaster scenario that will be simulated. Disaster drills are time-consuming, but they allow all participants to practice skills that would be needed in the event of a disaster. In addition, they allow organizations and communities to evaluate the effectiveness of their systems and identify potential weaknesses in the ability to respond to an actual disaster.

MEDICAL ASSISTANT'S ROLE

The medical assistant is an important team member in developing and implementing the EAP for a health care setting and can also contribute to emergency preparedness in the community. He or she may make recommendations to supplement emergency equipment or facilities in the office, serve on a committee to review or revise the emergency plan, participate actively in all fire drills and disaster drills, and participate in the review of the effectiveness of any drill. In addition, the medical assistant must be prepared to provide emergency first aid or cardiopulmonary resuscitation (CPR), both in the workplace and in the community (see Chapter 23). In an actual disaster, medical assistants might assist by providing emergency first aid, conducting patient interviews, helping to calm victims, documenting services provided, and performing phlebotomy or other procedures as directed.

The medical assistant should be aware of community resources for emergency preparedness. The medical office may keep a list of local organizations with telephone numbers or other contact information in the following areas:

- Emergency Medical Services (911)
- Poison Control Center
- Telephone numbers of local hospitals
- Telephone numbers of local and state health departments
- Telephone number for the state HAZMAT response team (**HAZMAT** is an acronym constructed from "*haz*ardous *mat*erials." It refers to materials that pose a danger to health or the environment and for which protective clothing is required for cleanup.)

The medical assistant should also be aware of community disaster plans and community organizations that might assist in a disaster. The website of the state emergency medical agency often includes helpful articles related to the disasters that occur most frequently in that state. It is helpful to develop a list of useful resources for the medical office and update it regularly.

What Would You Do? What Would You *Not* Do?

Case Study 3

Jordan Mendels, 32 years of age, is at the medical office complaining of headaches, fatigue, and insomnia. Jordan tearfully relays that her brother's house burned down 2 weeks ago. Jordan is now concerned about a fire in her own home. She wants to know the best way to prevent that from happening and also wants to know if her family should hold fire drills. Jordan says that she knows she should get a fire extinguisher, but she doesn't know how to use one. ■

Memories *from* Practicum

Beth Ann Wilson: The office where I did my practicum was a clinic in a large city hospital. While I was there, I was allowed to attend a hands-on fire training session for hospital employees. We met at a training facility at the fire department where we saw two training videos. One of them showed how to test a door for warmth and emphasized that a warm door or a door with smoke leaking around the edge should never be opened. In the film, a fireman did open the door, and we saw how the flames and smoke gushed out when the fire received the new supply of oxygen. Someone asked what you should do if you knew there was a patient in the room behind a warm door. The fireman answered that, if possible, you should wait for a firefighter, who would be prepared to handle the flame and smoke. After the videos, we were dressed in protective equipment and allowed to discharge fire extinguishers to put out small fires. Even though the fires were small, it was still a scary experience. I hope I never have to deal with a fire, even a small one, but I know that this experience helped to prepare me if it ever happens. ■

What Would You Do? What Would You *Not* Do? RESPONSES

Case Study 1

Page 751

What Did Beth Ann Do?

- ❑ Told Mrs. Manning to stop and breathe, encouraging her to take several deep breaths.
- ❑ Recognized that Mrs. Manning was showing signs of severe anxiety, which would make it difficult for her to focus on driving safely.
- ❑ Told Mrs. Manning that she seemed very upset by the news, reassured her that the fire department would respond promptly, and encouraged her to sit down and relax for a minute until she collects herself.
- ❑ Asked Mrs. Manning if there was a family member or friend she could call to pick her up and drive her to her son's school.
- ❑ Listened attentively to Mrs. Manning's concerns.

What Did Beth Ann Not Do?

- ❑ Did not allow Mrs. Manning to leave and drive an automobile while in a state of severe anxiety.
- ❑ Did not tell Mrs. Manning to calm down because she was overreacting.
- ❑ Did not give Mrs. Manning a detailed explanation of the effects of anxiety.

Case Study 2

Page 758

What Would You Do? What Would You *Not* Do? RESPONSES—cont'd

What Did Beth Ann Do?

- ❑ Told Brie that the pictures indicate the type of fires the extinguisher can handle, and that this extinguisher is a multipurpose extinguisher and can put out fires caused by ordinary combustibles, such as paper or wood, flammable liquids, and electrical equipment.
- ❑ Explained to Brie that each fire extinguisher must be inspected and maintained on a regular basis and the tag documents the date of each service check.
- ❑ Informed Brie that only employees with the proper training and knowledge are permitted to operate the fire extinguishers in the office in the event of a fire.
- ❑ Told Brie that fire extinguishers use up their extinguishing agent within 10 to 30 seconds depending on the size of the extinguisher.
- ❑ Relayed to Brie that fire code requirements, which often include a variety of safety measures, specify the type of fire protection safety measures that must be present in a building.

What Did Beth Ann Not Do?

- ❑ Did not let Brie remove the fire extinguisher from its mounting brackets.
- ❑ Did not scold Brie for not already having a fire extinguisher in her home.

Case Study 3
Page 760

What Did Beth Ann Do?

- ❑ Listened empathetically to Jordan and allow her to express her fears and concerns.
- ❑ Reassured Jordan that practicing fire prevention methods in the home is the best way to reduce the possibility of a fire.
- ❑ Provided Jordan with the names of websites (FEMA, American Red Cross, National Fire Protection Association, ready.gov) that she could use to access information on fire prevention and protective measures in the home.
- ❑ Told Jordan that it is a very good idea to hold fire drills in the home to make sure everyone knows what to do in the event of a fire and how to evacuate quickly and safely.
- ❑ Explained to Jordan that fire extinguishers are not difficult to operate and that each fire extinguisher comes with step-by-step instructions.
- ❑ Informed the physician of the situation so that he could provide the best treatment for Jordan.
- ❑ Reminded Jordan that fires in the home do happen, but they are not regular occurrences.

What Did Beth Ann Not Do?

- ❑ Did not say or imply that Jordan was overreacting or worrying for no reason.
- ❑ Did not push Jordan to accept her suggestions, but rather just offered information.
- ❑ Did not alarm Jordan about the possibility of a home fire.

TERMINOLOGY REVIEW

Key Term	Definition
Anxiety	A feeling of worry or uneasiness, often triggered by an event that is perceived as having an uncertain outcome.
Disaster	A sudden event that causes damage or loss of life.
Emergency action plan	A written document that describes the actions that employees should take to ensure their safety if a fire or other emergency situation occurs.
Emergency preparedness	The process of making plans to prevent, respond to, and recover from an emergency situation.
Evacuation	A planned systematic retreat of people to safety in an emergency situation.
Evacuation procedures	Clear step-by-step procedures for the rapid, efficient, and safe removal of individuals from a building during an emergency.
Exit route	A continuous and unobstructed path of travel from any point within a workplace to a place of safety.
Fire extinguisher	A portable device that discharges an agent designed to extinguish a fire.
Fire prevention plan	A written document that identifies flammable and combustible materials stored in the workplace and ways to control workplace fire hazards.
Fire protection	The implementation of safety measures to reduce the unwanted effects of fire.
HAZMAT	An acronym constructed from the beginnings of the two words "*haz*ardous *mat*erials." It refers to materials that pose a danger to health or the environment and must be handled with protective equipment.
Man-made disaster	An event that causes serious damage through intentional or negligent human actions or the failure of a man-made system.
Natural disaster	A catastrophic event that is caused by nature or the natural process of the earth.
Stress	The body's response to threat or change.

PROCEDURE 22.1 Demonstrating Proper Use of a Fire Extinguisher

Outcome Demonstrate proper use of a fire extinguisher in a role-playing situation

Equipment/Supplies

- Portable office-size multipurpose (ABC) fire extinguisher that has been discharged

1. **Procedural Step.** Identify a safe evacuation route before approaching the fire.
   Principle. A clear evacuation route allows for immediate escape if the fire gets worse.
2. **Procedural Step.** Remove the multipurpose fire extinguisher from its mounting device and hold it upright with the nozzle pointing away from you. Stand 6–8 feet from the fire, keeping your back to the exit at all times.
   Principle. Standing at 6–8 feet prevents being burned or being hit by splattering material or sparks. Keeping the back to the exit allows for constant monitoring of the situation and immediate awareness if the fire begins to flare up or spread.
3. **Procedural Step.** Perform a quick assessment of the fire to determine if it is small enough to extinguish with a fire extinguisher (while continuing to stand at a distance of 6–8 feet). *Do not* attempt to extinguish the fire if it is too large or if there is excessive smoke or heat. In these instances, close the door to contain the fire then evacuate immediately.
   Principle. A fire extinguisher is designed to handle only small fires in the beginning stages.
4. **Procedural Step.** Operate the fire extinguisher using the PASS technique:
   a. *Pull* the safety pin straight out from the handle located at the top of the extinguisher. This will also break the tamper-proof seal. Make sure the fire extinguisher is held in an upright position at all times.
   Principle. The tamper-proof seal holds the safety pin in place. The safety pin provides a locking mechanism that prevents the fire extinguisher from accidentally discharging.

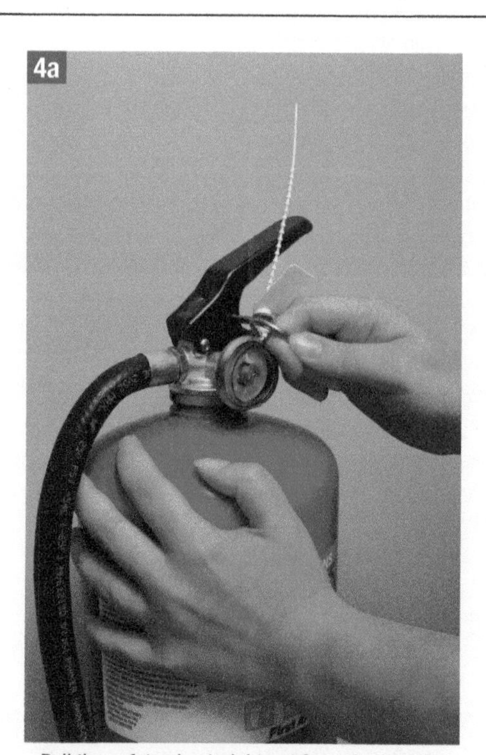

Pull the safety pin straight out from the handle.

   b. *Aim* the nozzle at the base of the fire (not the flames) with your dominant hand.
   Principle. Aiming the nozzle at the base of the fire allows the extinguishing agent to deprive the fire of fuel. Aiming the nozzle at the flames causes the extinguishing agent to pass through the flames without stopping the fire.
   c. *Squeeze* the handle slowly and continuously to release the extinguishing agent. Letting go of the pressure on the handle causes the discharge of the extinguishing to cease.
   Principle. Squeezing the handle opens a valve that releases the pressurized extinguishing agent from the fire extinguisher.

PROCEDURE 22.1 Demonstrating Proper Use of a Fire Extinguisher—cont'd

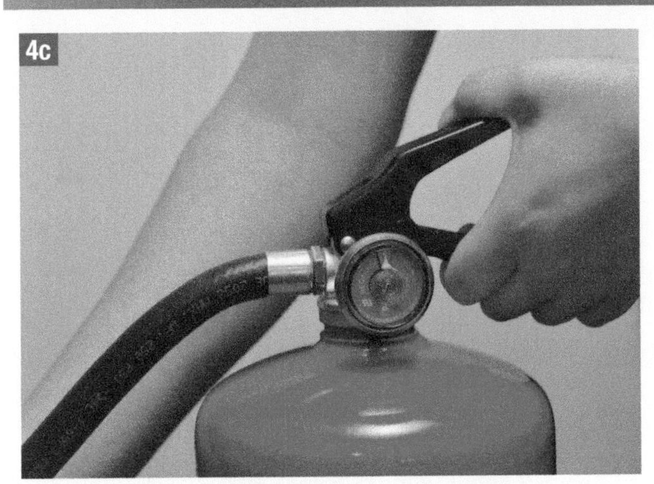

Squeeze the handle slowly and continuously.

d. *Sweep* the nozzle of the extinguisher evenly from side to side at the base of the fire. Gradually move closer to the fire as it begins to smolder. Continue to discharge the extinguishing agent until the fire is completely out. Evacuate immediately if the fire grows larger or if the extinguisher is empty and the fire is not out. Fire extinguishers use up their extinguishing agent within 10–30 s, depending on the size of the extinguisher.

Principle. A sweeping motion helps to extinguish the fire. Even distribution of the agent helps to put out the fire at a faster rate.

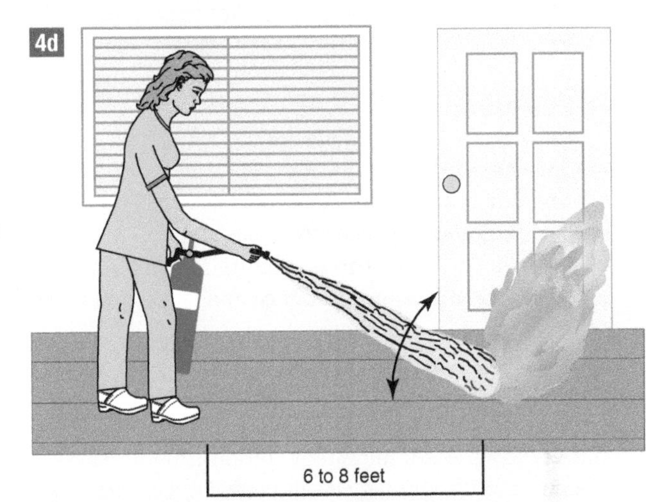

Sweep the nozzle of the extinguisher at the base of the fire.

5. **Procedural Step.** Back away from the extinguished fire in case it flares up again. Continue to watch the area to be sure that flames do not recur after having been extinguished.
   Principle. Material that has been burning can remain hot enough that flames will reignite.

PROCEDURE 22.2

PROCEDURE 22.2 Participating in a Mock Exposure Event

Outcome Participate in a mock environmental exposure event and document the steps taken

Scenario

A fire has erupted in an examining room at your medical office. The fire, caused by faulty electrical wiring, has ignited several boxes of disposable drapes. (Place a poster, flashing light, or other indicator at the location of the "fire.") A disabled patient in a wheelchair is located in the room where the fire erupts. The emergency evacuation coordinator determines that an evacuation of the facility is necessary.

Equipment/Supplies

- Scenario
- Emergency evacuation floor plan
- Employee roster
- Patient log-in sheet
- Pen and paper

Predrill Activities

1. **Procedural Step.** Make a list of the names and phone numbers of the following resources that may be needed in the event of a fire:
   a. Emergency responders (911)
   b. Fire department
   c. Police department
   d. Local hospital
   e. Insurance carrier

Continued

PROCEDURE 22.2 Participating in a Mock Exposure Event—cont'd

2. Procedural Step. Review the location and purpose of fire protection safety measures.

a. Locate and review the purpose of the following in your facility using the evacuation floor plan as a reference:
- The path of the primary exit route
- The path of the secondary exit route
- Manual fire alarm pull stations
- Portable fire extinguishers
- Emergency exit doors
- Wheelchair accessible exits
- Assembly area
- Shelter-in-place areas

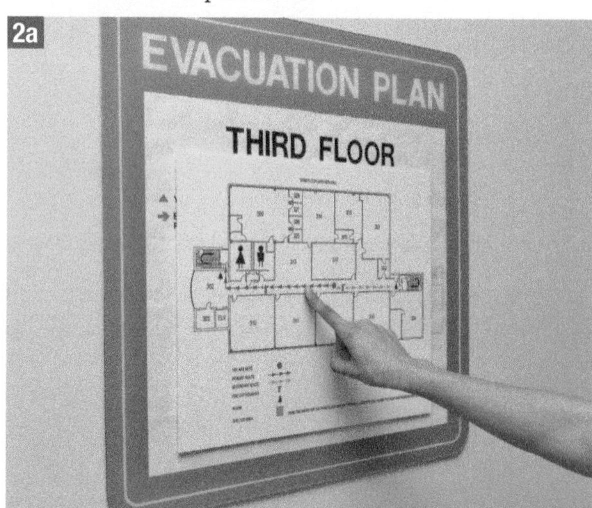

Locate the path of the primary and secondary exit routes.

b. Locate and review the purpose of the following through visual inspection of the facility:
- Sprinklers
- Smoke detectors
- Fire doors
- Exit signs

Principle. The medical assistant should know the location and purpose of the fire protection safety measures in his or her facility.

3. Procedural Step. Evaluate primary and secondary exit routes for the following:
a. Exits are clearly marked and well lit.
b. Exit routes are unobstructed and free of clutter.
c. Exit doors are free of decorations or signs that obscure the visibility of the exit.
d. Exit doors are unlocked from the inside.
e. Exit doors open outward.
f. Fire extinguishers are in place and clearly identified.
g. Evacuation floor plans are posted in multiple locations throughout the facility.

4. Procedural Step. Assign an emergency evacuation coordinator to assume overall charge and responsibility for the evacuation process including the following:
a. Calling emergency responders (911)
b. Identifying safe evacuation routes
c. Ensuring that evacuation wardens are performing their duties
d. Coordinating with the emergency responders

Principle. The emergency evacuation coordinator is responsible for taking charge of the evacuation process.

5. Procedural Step. Compile an employee roster and assign evacuation wardens to perform one or more of the duties outlined in Table 22.2. Make sure each evacuation warden understands his or her roles and responsibilities and is well trained in his or her assigned duties.

Principle. Evacuation wardens are responsible for performing rescue duties during an evacuation.

6. Procedural Step. Assign individuals to play the role of patients and compile a patient log-in sheet. Patients with special needs should be included, such as:
a. Mother with a young child with an illness
b. Patient with emphysema on oxygen
c. Pregnant patient in the last trimester of pregnancy
d. Patient with crutches wearing a leg cast
e. Elderly patient with a heart condition
f. Patient with dementia
g. Disabled patient in a wheelchair
h. Patient with severe anxiety
i. Hearing-impaired patient
j. Patient with a visual impairment

Conduct the Fire Drill

(The emergency evacuation coordinator and evacuation wardens should perform their assigned duties during the fire drill.)

1. Procedural Step. Rescue anyone in immediate danger of the fire. If an individual's clothes catch on fire, the following can be performed to extinguish the flames:
a. Instruct the person to stop, drop, and roll.
b. Cover the person with a blanket or clothing to help extinguish the flames.

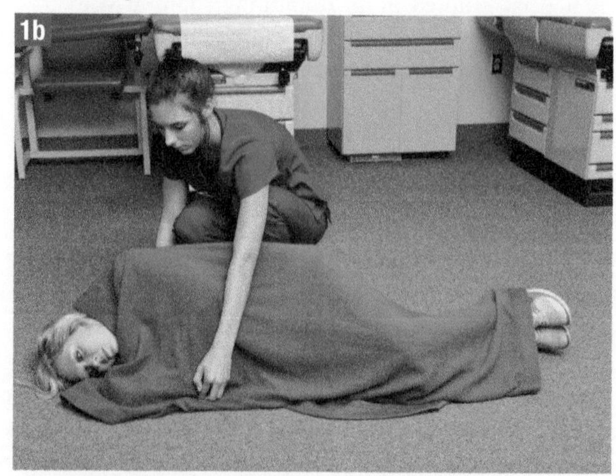

Cover the person with a blanket or clothing to extinguish flames.

PROCEDURE 22.2

PROCEDURE 22.2 Participating in a Mock Exposure Event—cont'd

2. Procedural Step. Activate the alarm. The employee who first discovers the fire should activate the nearest fire alarm pull station by pulling down on the lever.
Principle. Activating the alarm warns building occupants of the presence of a fire to provide them with enough time to safely evacuate the building.

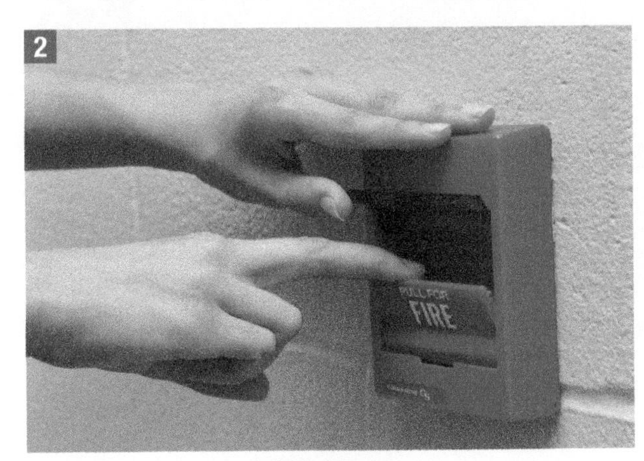

Activate the alarm.

3. Procedural Step. Immediately notify emergency responders by dialing 911. Speak clearly and calmly to the emergency medical dispatcher. Identify the problem as accurately and concisely as possible so that proper equipment and personnel can be sent. Do not hang up until the dispatcher gives you permission to do so. Information that should be relayed (if known) to the emergency dispatcher includes the following:
a. Type of fire (e.g., electrical, combustibles, flammable liquids)
b. Exact location of the fire
c. Extent of the fire
d. Whether an evacuation is in process
e. Other information requested by the dispatcher
Principle. Calling 911 allows the fire department to be on its way while other activities are being performed. Any delay may allow the fire to grow and further endanger the building occupants and property.

4. Procedural Step. Confine the fire by closing doors and windows in the immediate area of the fire.
Principle. Closing doors and windows helps prevent the spread of smoke and fire throughout the building.

5. Procedural Step. Extinguish the fire with a portable fire extinguisher if it is small and confined, following the steps outlined in Procedure 22.1. *Do not* attempt to extinguish the fire if it is too large or if there is excessive smoke or heat. In these instances, close the door to contain the fire then evacuate immediately.

6. Procedural Step. Evacuate the area immediately. The evacuation wardens should perform their evacuation duties as assigned in Table 22.2. Important evacuation guidelines include the following:
a. Shut down all electrical equipment and appliances in the immediate area
b. Before exiting a room, feel the door with the back of your hand. If the door is warm:
- Do not open the door.
- Call 911 to report your location or place a signal in the window.
- Place clothing or towels along the bottom of the door to keep out smoke.
- Stay calm and wait to be rescued.
- Do not break the window. Smoke entering from the outside may hamper rescue.

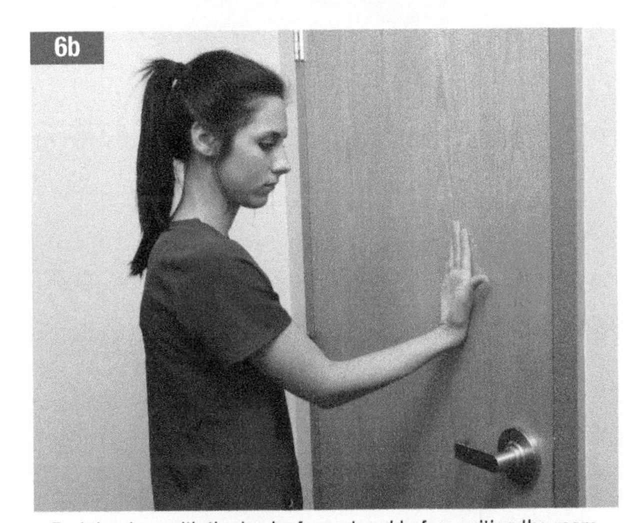

Feel the door with the back of your hand before exiting the room.

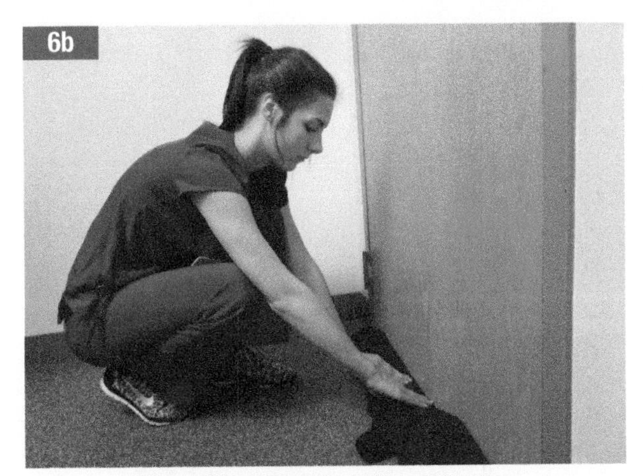

Place clothing along the bottom of the door.

c. Use the primary exit route if possible. If the primary exit route is blocked by fire or smoke, use the secondary exit route.

Continued

PROCEDURE 22.2 Participating in a Mock Exposure Event—cont'd

d. Exit by stairways only. Do not use elevators.

6d
3
In case of fire
do not use elevators
Use stairways

Do not use elevators.

e. Close doors after a room is evacuated and place an X on the door with chalk or a marker to indicate the room has been evacuated

Principle: The size of a fire can double every 30 s; therefore, it is important to evacuate immediately. The primary exit route is the quickest and easiest way to exit a building during an evacuation. Elevators may fail during a fire, trapping occupants.

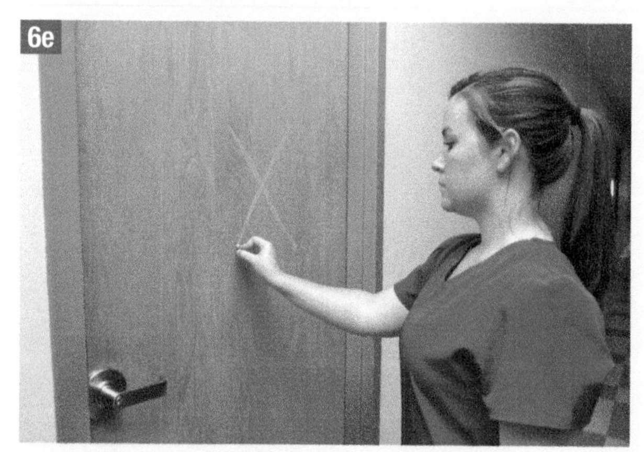

Place an X on the door.

7. **Procedural Step.** Escort patients to the designated assembly area. Check to make sure everyone is accounted for by completing the following:

a. Account for all employees using the employee roster checklist.

b. Account for all patients using the patient log-in sheet.

Principle. Accounting for building occupants helps to determine if someone is still in the building and in need of rescue.

7a

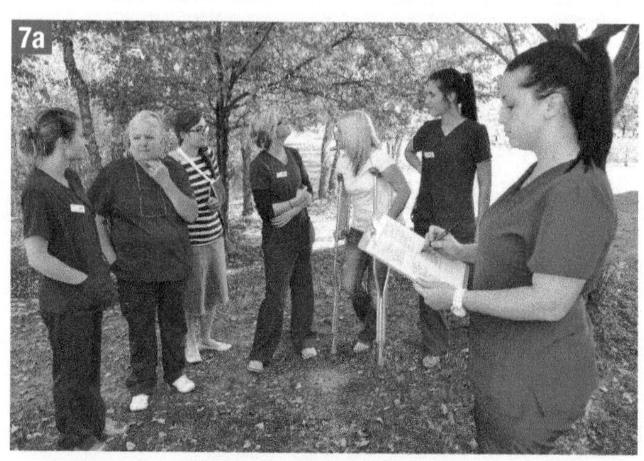

Account for all employees.

7b

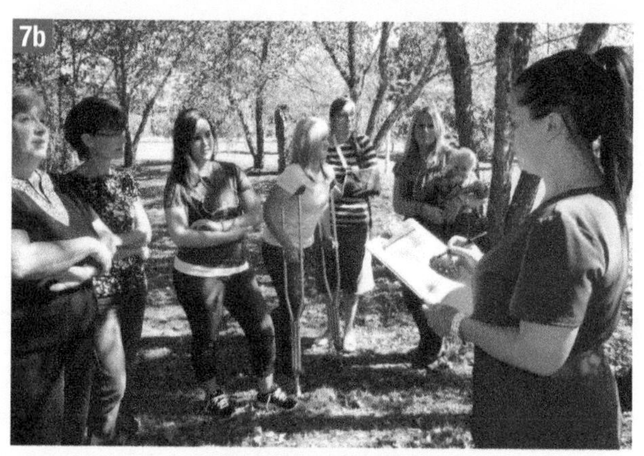

Account for all patients.

8. **Procedural Step.** Keep the building occupants together in the assembly area at a safe distance from the building. Make sure that occupants do not block access to the building by emergency responders. Do not allow anyone to re-enter the building unless directed to do so by emergency officials. Instruct occupants not to leave until everyone has been accounted for and dismissed.

9. **Procedural Step. Provide emergency responders with the following information:**
   a. The name and last known location of any individual not accounted for during the head count
   b. Special hazards in the building that may endanger emergency responders such as oxygen tanks and hazardous chemicals

PROCEDURE 22.2 Participating in a Mock Exposure Event—cont'd

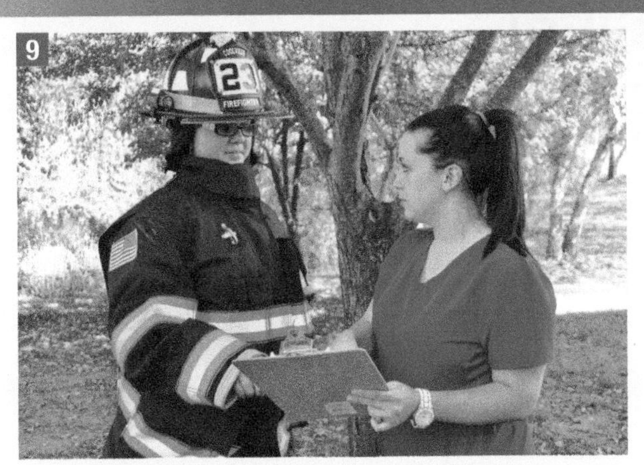

Provide emergency responders with information.

Post-drill Activities

1. **Procedural Step. Critique the effectiveness of the fire drill (in terms of strengths, concerns, and means of improvement) by evaluating the following:**
   a. The evacuation was completed in an orderly, efficient, and timely manner.
   b. Building occupants and emergency responders were immediately alerted of the situation.
   c. Evacuation wardens effectively completed their duties.
   d. Patients and visitors were escorted to the nearest exit and assembly area.
   e. Each building occupant was accounted for after the evacuation.
   f. Emergency responders were provided with appropriate information.
2. **Procedural Step.** Document the results of the fire drill including your role and the effectiveness of the group as a whole in carrying out the evacuation.
   Principle. Evaluation of the fire drill identifies strengths, concerns, and means of improvement.

Emergency Medical Procedures and First Aid

 Check out the Evolve site at http://evolve.elsevier.com/Bonewit/today/ to access additional interactive activities and exercises to help you study and prepare for success.

LEARNING OUTCOMES

First Aid

1. State the purpose of first aid.
2. Explain the purpose of the emergency medical services (EMS) system.
3. List the OSHA standards for administering first aid.
4. List the guidelines that should be followed when providing emergency care.

Common Emergency Situations

5. List and describe conditions that cause respiratory distress.
6. List the symptoms of a heart attack and a stroke.
7. Explain the causes of each of the following types of shock: cardiogenic, neurogenic, anaphylactic, and psychogenic.
8. Identify and describe the three classifications of external bleeding.
9. Explain the difference between an open wound and a closed wound.
10. Describe the characteristics of each of the following fractures: impacted, greenstick, transverse, oblique, comminuted, and spiral.
11. Identify the characteristics of each of the following burns: superficial, partial thickness, and full thickness.
12. Explain the difference between a partial seizure and a generalized seizure.
13. List examples of each of the following types of poisoning: ingested, inhaled, absorbed, and injected.
14. Identify factors that place an individual at higher risk for developing heat-related and cold-related injuries.
15. Describe the differences between type 1 and type 2 diabetes mellitus.
16. Explain the causes of insulin shock and diabetic coma.
17. Identify the symptoms and describe emergency care for each of the following conditions: respiratory distress, heart attack, stroke, shock, bleeding, wounds, musculoskeletal injuries, burns, seizures, poisoning, heat and cold exposure, and diabetic emergencies.

PROCEDURES

Respond to common emergency situations.

CHAPTER OUTLINE

KEY TERMS

burn
crash cart
crepitus (KREP-it-us)
dislocation
emergency medical services (EMS) system
first aid
fracture (FRAK-shur)
hypothermia (hie-poe-THER-mee-ah)
poison
pressure point
seizure (SEE-zhur)
shock
splint
sprain
strain
wound

INTRODUCTION TO EMERGENCY MEDICAL PROCEDURES

Medical emergencies often arise inside and outside of the workplace that can result in sudden loss of life or permanent disability. If an emergency situation occurs in the medical office, the provider provides immediate medical care for the patient. Some medical offices maintain a crash cart for this purpose. In these situations, the medical assistant may be required to assist the provider in providing emergency medical care.

The medical assistant may need to administer first aid for medical emergencies that occur outside of the medical office environment. **First aid** is defined as the immediate care administered before complete medical care can be obtained to an individual who is injured or suddenly becomes ill. The medical assistant is most likely to administer first aid to a family member or friend. The purposes of first aid are to save a life, reduce pain and suffering, prevent further injury, reduce the incidence of permanent disability, and increase the opportunity for an early recovery.

This chapter focuses on common emergency situations that the medical assistant may encounter and the first aid required for each. It is not intended, however, as a substitute for thorough first aid instruction through the American Red Cross, National Safety Council, or American Heart Association.

OFFICE CRASH CART

A **crash cart** is a specially equipped cart for holding and transporting medications, equipment, and supplies needed to perform lifesaving procedures in an emergency. A growing number of providers are incorporating crash carts into their medical offices. Patients who are injured or suddenly become ill might be brought to the medical office for emergency medical care. In addition, a patient might develop a sudden illness at the medical office that requires emergency medical care. Examples of these situations include life-threatening cardiac dysrhythmias, shock, cardiac arrest, poisoning, and traumatic injury.

The items on an office crash cart vary widely among medical offices depending on the extent of the emergency medical care that is likely to be administered. This is directly related to the time it takes for emergency medical personnel to arrive and the location of the nearest hospital. The medical assistant may be responsible for regularly checking the crash cart to replenish supplies and to check the expiration dates on medications.

EMERGENCY MEDICAL SERVICES SYSTEM

The **emergency medical services (EMS) system** is a network of community resources, equipment, and emergency medical technicians (EMTs) that provides emergency care to victims of injury or sudden illness. An *EMT* is a professional provider of prehospital emergency care, which includes care at the scene and during transportation to the hospital. An EMT-Basic (EMT-B) has received formal training and is certified to provide basic life support measures. An *EMT-Paramedic* (EMT-P) is qualified to provide advanced life support care, including advanced airway maintenance, initiation of intravenous drips, administration of medication, cardiac monitoring and interpretation, and cardiac defibrillation.

Activating the EMS system is often the most important step in an emergency. Rapid arrival of EMTs increases the patient's chances of surviving a life-threatening emergency. In most urban and in some rural areas in the United States, the medical assistant can activate the local EMS system by dialing 911 on the telephone. Other areas have a local seven-digit number, in which case it is important to keep the number at hand.

When calling local EMS, the medical assistant speaks with an *emergency medical dispatcher* (EMD). An EMD has had formal training in handling emergency situations over the phone. The responsibility of the EMD is to answer the emergency call, listen to the caller, obtain critical information, determine what help is needed, and send the appropriate personnel and equipment. The EMD also is responsible for relaying instructions to the caller about providing emergency care until the EMTs arrive.

These guidelines should be followed when calling EMS:

- Speak clearly and calmly to the EMD. Identify the problem as accurately and concisely as possible so that proper equipment and personnel can be sent. The EMD needs to know the number of victims, the condition of the victim or victims, and the emergency care that has already been administered.

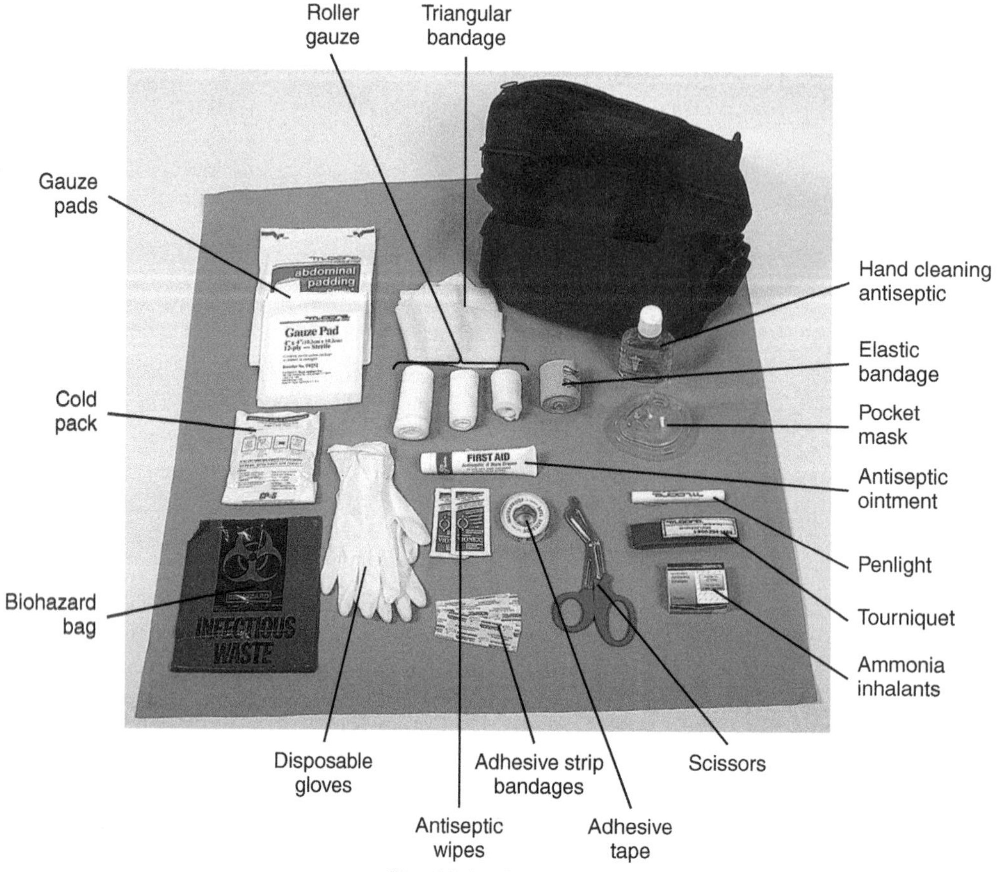

Fig. 23.1 First aid kit.

- The EMD will ask you for your phone number and address. In responding, relay to the dispatcher the exact location of the victim, including the correct street name and house number and (if applicable) the building name, floor, and room number. With the 911 enhanced emergency system, the address automatically appears on a monitor; however, there is a chance that the address will not show up on the monitor. In addition, the emergency may not be happening in the same location as the caller. If possible, have someone meet the ambulance personnel and direct them to the scene.
- Do not hang up until the EMD gives you permission to do so. The dispatcher may need additional information or may give you instructions on treating the patient until EMTs arrive.

FIRST AID KIT

The medical office should acquire and maintain a first aid kit. A first aid kit contains basic supplies to provide emergency care to individuals who have been injured or become suddenly ill (Fig. 23.1). It is recommended that a first aid kit be kept at home and in the car.

First aid kits are available at most drug stores. It also is possible to make your own. Along with the items shown in Fig. 23.1, the first aid kit should include the phone numbers of the local EMS, the Poison Help center, and the police and fire departments. It is important to check the first aid kit regularly and replace supplies as needed.

OSHA SAFETY PRECAUTIONS

To prevent exposure to bloodborne pathogens and other potentially infectious materials, the OSHA Bloodborne Pathogens Standard presented in Chapter 2 should be followed when performing first aid. The following guidelines help reduce or eliminate the risk of infection:

1. Make sure that your first aid kit contains personal protective equipment, such as gloves, a face shield and mask, and a pocket mask.
2. Wear gloves when it is reasonably anticipated that your hands will come into contact with the following: blood and other potentially infectious materials, mucous membranes, nonintact skin, and contaminated articles or surfaces.
3. Perform all first aid procedures involving blood or other potentially infectious materials in a manner that minimizes splashing, spraying, spattering, and generation of droplets of these substances.
4. Wear protective clothing and gloves to cover cuts or other lesions of the skin.

5. Sanitize your hands as soon as possible after removing gloves.
6. Avoid touching objects that may be contaminated with blood or other potentially infectious materials.
7. If your hands or other skin surfaces come in contact with blood or other potentially infectious materials, wash the area as soon as possible with soap and water.
8. If your mucous membranes (in eyes, nose, and mouth) come in contact with blood or other potentially infectious materials, flush them with water as soon as possible.
9. Avoid eating, drinking, and touching your mouth, eyes, and nose while providing emergency care or before you sanitize your hands.
10. If you are exposed to blood or other potentially infectious materials, report the incident as soon as possible to your provider so that post-exposure procedures can be instituted.

GUIDELINES FOR PROVIDING EMERGENCY CARE

The remainder of this chapter presents specific emergency situations that may be encountered by the medical assistant and the emergency care required for each. These guidelines should be followed when providing emergency care:

1. Remain calm and speak in a normal tone of voice. These measures help calm and reassure the patient.
2. Make sure that the scene is safe before approaching the patient. It is important that you protect yourself from harm in an emergency situation.
3. Before administering emergency care to a conscious patient, you must first have permission or consent. To obtain consent, you must inform the patient who you are, your level of training, and what you are going to do to help. *Never* administer care to a conscious patient who refuses it. When a life-threatening condition exists and the patient is unconscious or otherwise unable to give consent, consent is assumed or implied. Under law, it is implied that if the patient could give consent to care, he or she would.
4. Follow the OSHA standards when providing emergency care to reduce or eliminate exposure to bloodborne pathogens or other potentially infectious materials.
5. Know how to activate your local EMS system. Activating the EMS is often the most important step you can take to help a patient who has experienced an injury or sudden illness.
6. Do not move the patient unnecessarily. Unnecessary movement can result in further injury or can be life-threatening to a patient with a serious condition.
7. Obtain information as to what happened from the patient, family members, co-workers, or bystanders.
8. Look for a medical alert tag on the patient's wrist, neck, or ankle. A medical alert tag provides information on a medical condition the patient may have.
9. Continue caring for the patient until more highly trained personnel arrive. On the arrival of emergency medical personnel or a provider, relay the condition in which you found the patient and the emergency care that has been administered.

HIGHLIGHT on Good Samaritan Laws

In most states, Good Samaritan laws have been enacted to provide immunity to individuals, such as the medical assistant who administers first aid at the scene of an emergency. These laws were enacted to encourage individuals to help others in an emergency. They assume that an individual would do her or his best to save a life or prevent further injury.

The legal immunity provided by Good Samaritan laws protects an individual from being sued and found financially responsible for a patient's injury. The individual is immune from liability (except for "gross negligence") if he or she acts in good faith and uses a reasonable level of skill that does not exceed the scope of the individual's training.

Good Samaritan laws do not mean that an individual cannot be sued for administering first aid. An individual is not protected from liability if he or she is grossly careless or reckless in handling the situation. Because the components of Good Samaritan laws vary from state to state, the medical assistant must become familiar with the laws that govern his or her state. ■

RESPIRATORY DISTRESS

Respiratory distress indicates that the patient is breathing but is having great difficulty doing so. Respiratory distress sometimes may lead to respiratory arrest. It is important that the medical assistant be alert for the signs and symptoms of respiratory distress, which may include noisy breathing, such as gasping for air or rasping, gurgling, or whistling sounds; breathing that is unusually fast or slow; and breathing that is painful. The general care for respiratory distress is to place the patient in a comfortable position that facilitates breathing. Most patients prefer a sitting or semireclining position. Remain calm and reassure the patient to help reduce anxiety. Calming the patient may help the patient breathe easier. If the patient's condition worsens or does not resolve within a few minutes, activate the local EMS system. Examples of conditions that frequently cause respiratory distress are described next.

Asthma

Asthma is a condition characterized by wheezing, coughing, and dyspnea. During an asthmatic attack, the bronchioles constrict and become clogged with mucus, which accounts for many of the symptoms of asthma.

Asthma may occur at any age, but it is more common in children and young adults. If the condition is not treated, it can lead to serious complications, such as permanent lung damage. It is frequently, but not always, associated with a family history of allergies. Any of the common allergens, such as house dust, pollens, molds, or animal danders, may trigger an asthmatic attack. Asthmatic attacks also may be caused by nonspecific factors, such as air pollutants, tobacco smoke, chemical fumes, vigorous exercise, respiratory infections, exposure to cold, and emotional stress. In normal circumstances an individual with asthma easily controls attacks with medications. These medications stop the muscle spasms and open the airway, making breathing easier.

Some patients may develop a severe prolonged asthmatic attack that is life-threatening, which is known as *status asthmaticus.* These patients can move only a small amount of air. Because so little air is being moved, the typical breathing sounds associated with asthma may not be audible. The patient may have a bluish discoloration of the skin and extremely labored breathing. Status asthmaticus is a true emergency and requires immediate transportation of the patient to an emergency care facility by the fastest way possible.

Emphysema

Emphysema is a progressive lung disorder in which the terminal bronchioles that lead into the alveoli become plugged with mucus. Because of this problem, the alveoli become damaged, resulting in less surface area to diffuse oxygen into the blood. Eventually this condition results in loss of elasticity of the alveoli, causing inhaled air to become trapped in the lungs. This makes breathing difficult, particularly during exhalation.

Emphysema usually develops over many years and is found most frequently in heavy smokers. It also occurs in patients with chronic bronchitis and in elderly patients whose lungs have lost their natural elasticity. Chronic emphysema is one of the major causes of death in the United States. As the lungs progressively become less efficient, breathing becomes more and more difficult. Patients with advanced cases may go into respiratory or cardiac arrest.

Hyperventilation

Hyperventilation literally means "overbreathing." Hyperventilation is a manner of breathing in which the respirations become rapid and deep, causing an individual to exhale too much carbon dioxide. Low carbon dioxide levels in the body account for many of the symptoms of hyperventilation. Hyperventilation is often the result of fear or anxiety and is more likely to occur in individuals who are tense and nervous. It also is caused by serious organic conditions, such as diabetic coma, pneumonia, pulmonary edema, pulmonary embolism, head injury, high fever, and aspirin poisoning.

In addition to rapid and deep respirations, the signs and symptoms of hyperventilation include dizziness, faintness, and light-headedness; visual disturbances; chest pain; tachycardia; palpitations; fullness in the throat; and numbness and tingling of the fingers, toes, and the area around the mouth. Despite their rapid breathing efforts, patients complain that they cannot get enough air. They often think they are having a heart attack.

Treatment for hyperventilation caused by emotional factors is as follows: Calm and reassure the patient, and encourage him or her to slow the respirations, allowing the carbon dioxide level to return to normal. In the past, breathing into a paper bag was advocated as a remedy for hyperventilation. More recent studies no longer recommend this practice because it could be harmful if an underlying medical condition exists or if the patient is not actually hyperventilating. If the medical assistant suspects that hyperventilation has been caused by an organic problem, EMS should be activated immediately.

HEART ATTACK

A heart attack, also known as a *myocardial infarction* (MI), is caused by partial or complete obstruction of one or both of the coronary arteries or their branches. In most cases, the severity of the attack depends on the size of the obstructed artery and the amount of myocardial tissue nourished by that artery. If a small branch of a coronary artery is obstructed, myocardial damage and symptoms may be mild, whereas the damage is usually extensive and the symptoms intense if a coronary artery is completely blocked.

The principal symptom of a heart attack is chest pain or discomfort. Patients describe the chest pain as squeezing or crushing pressure, severe indigestion or burning, heaviness, or aching. Chest discomfort can range in severity from only mildly uncomfortable to intense and accompanied by a feeling of suffocation and doom. The pain is usually felt behind the sternum and may radiate to the neck, throat, or jaw or to both shoulders and both arms. The pain associated with a heart attack is prolonged and usually is not relieved by resting or taking nitroglycerin. Other signs and symptoms of a heart attack include shortness of breath, profuse perspiration, nausea, and fainting.

If the medical assistant suspects that the patient is having a heart attack, EMS should be activated immediately. Meanwhile, loosen tight clothing and have the patient rest in a comfortable position that facilitates breathing. If cardiac arrest occurs, the medical assistant should begin cardiopulmonary resuscitation (CPR) immediately.

STROKE

A stroke, also called a *cerebrovascular accident* (CVA), results when an artery to the brain is blocked or ruptures, causing an interruption of blood flow to the brain. The signs and symptoms of a stroke include sudden weakness or numbness of the face, arm, or leg on one side of the body; difficulty in speaking; dimmed vision or loss of vision in one eye; double vision; dizziness; confusion; severe headache; and loss of consciousness.

If the medical assistant suspects that the patient is having a stroke, EMS should be activated immediately. Meanwhile, loosen tight clothing and have the patient rest in a comfortable position. If respiratory arrest, cardiac arrest, or both occur, begin rescue breathing and CPR as required.

SHOCK

For the body to function properly, adequate blood flow must be maintained to all of the vital organs. This is accomplished by the three important cardiovascular functions, as follows:

- Adequate pumping action of the heart
- Sufficient blood circulating in the blood vessels
- Blood vessels being able to respond to blood flow

When an individual experiences a severe injury or illness, one or more of these cardiovascular functions may be affected, which can lead to shock.

Shock is defined as the failure of the cardiovascular system to deliver enough blood to all of the body's vital organs. Shock accompanies different types of emergency situations, such as hemorrhaging, MI, and severe allergic reaction. The five major types of shock are categorized according to cause: hypovolemic, cardiogenic, neurogenic, anaphylactic, and psychogenic. Each type of shock is described in this section. If not treated, most types of shock become life-threatening. This is because shock is progressive—when it reaches a certain point, it becomes irreversible, and the patient's life cannot be saved.

The signs and symptoms of shock are caused by the failure of the vital organs to receive enough oxygen and nutrients. The organs most affected are the heart, brain, and lungs, which can be irreparably damaged in 4 to 6 minutes. The general signs and symptoms of shock are weakness, restlessness, anxiety, disorientation, pallor, cold and clammy skin, rapid breathing, and rapid pulse.

If not treated, these symptoms can progress rapidly to a significant drop in blood pressure, cyanosis, loss of consciousness, and death. The signs and symptoms of shock may be subtle or pronounced. In addition, no single sign or symptom determines accurately the presence or severity of the shock. Because of this, it is crucial to consider the nature of the illness or injury in determining whether the patient is a possible victim of shock. If a patient has a traumatic injury to the abdomen, shock should be considered a possibility, even if the patient's signs and symptoms do not suggest shock.

Shock (with the exception of psychogenic shock) requires immediate medical care. The medical assistant should activate EMS without delay so that proper medical care can be obtained as soon as possible.

Hypovolemic Shock

Hypovolemic shock is caused by loss of blood or other body fluids. Conditions that result in this type of shock include external and internal hemorrhaging; plasma loss from severe burns; and severe dehydration from vomiting, diarrhea, or profuse perspiration. The first priority in hypovolemic shock is to control bleeding. A patient in hypovolemic shock must have the volume of fluid that was lost replaced and must be transported to an emergency care facility immediately.

Cardiogenic Shock

Cardiogenic shock is caused by the failure of the heart to pump blood adequately to all of the body's vital organs. This type of shock occurs when the heart has been injured or damaged. Cardiogenic shock is most frequently seen with MI. Other causes include dysrhythmias, severe congestive heart failure, acute valvular damage, and pulmonary embolism. When a patient develops cardiogenic shock, it is difficult to reverse and has a high fatality rate (80% to 90%).

Neurogenic Shock

Neurogenic shock occurs when the nervous system is unable to control the diameter of the blood vessels. In normal situations, the nervous system instructs the blood vessels to constrict or dilate, which controls blood pressure. In neurogenic shock, that control is lost, and the blood vessels dilate, causing the blood to pool in peripheral areas of the body away from vital organs.

This type of shock is most often seen with brain and spinal injuries. The blood vessels become dilated, and not enough blood is present in the circulatory system to fill the dilated vessels, which causes the blood pressure to drop significantly.

Anaphylactic Shock

Anaphylactic shock is a life-threatening reaction of the body to a substance to which an individual is highly allergic. Allergens that are most apt to result in anaphylaxis are drugs (e.g., penicillin), insect venoms, foods, and allergen extracts used in hyposensitization injections.

An anaphylactic reaction causes the release of large amounts of histamine, resulting in dilation of the blood vessels throughout the entire body and a decrease in blood pressure. The symptoms of anaphylactic shock begin with sneezing, hives, itching, angioedema, erythema, and disorientation and progress to difficulty in breathing, dizziness, fainting, and loss of consciousness. Medical care should be obtained immediately because most fatalities occur within the first 2 hours.

The emergency care for anaphylactic shock is the administration of epinephrine. Because time is a factor, individuals known to have a severe allergy carry an anaphylactic emergency treatment kit that contains injectable epinephrine (Fig. 23.2) and oral antihistamines. With the kit, treatment for a severe allergic reaction can be started immediately.

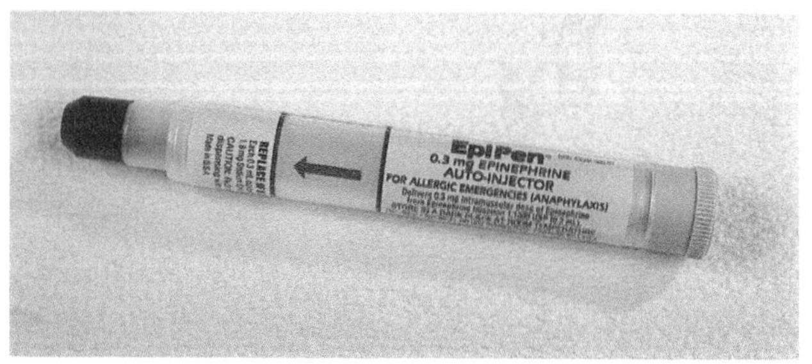

Fig. 23.2 Anaphylactic emergency epinephrine injector.

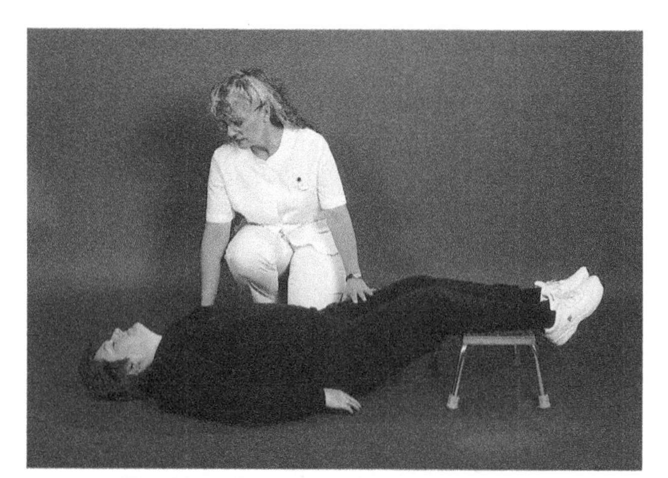

Fig. 23.3 Prevention and treatment of fainting.

Psychogenic Shock

Psychogenic shock is the least serious type of shock. It is caused by unpleasant physical or emotional stimuli, such as pain, fright, and the sight of blood. With psychogenic shock, sudden dilation of the blood vessels causes blood to pool in the abdomen and extremities. This temporarily deprives the brain of blood, causing a temporary loss of consciousness (fainting), usually lasting 1 to 2 minutes. In general, fainting occurs when an individual is in an upright position. Before fainting, the patient usually experiences some warning signals such as sudden lightheadedness, pallor, nausea, weakness, yawning, blurred vision, a feeling of warmth, and sweating.

An individual who is about to faint should be placed in a position that facilitates blood flow to the brain and told to breathe deeply. The preferred position is to move the patient into a supine position with the legs elevated approximately 12 inches and the collar and clothing loosened (Fig. 23.3). This position is not always possible, such as when a patient is seated; in this case, the patient's head should be lowered between the legs (Fig. 23.4). A patient who has fainted should be placed in the supine position with the legs elevated. It is recommended that a patient who has fainted should contact her or his provider for further evaluation.

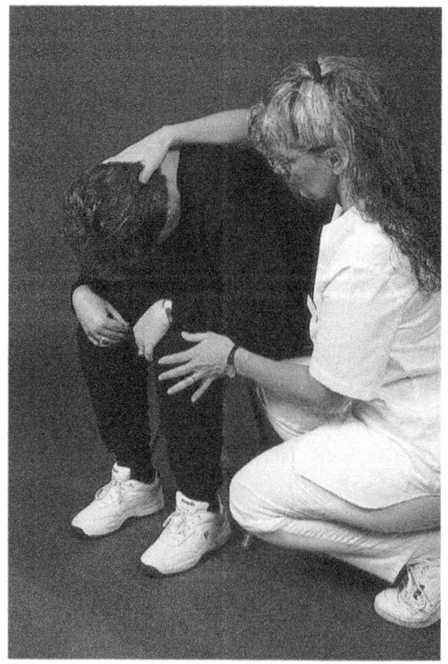

Fig. 23.4 Prevention of fainting.

BLEEDING

Bleeding, or hemorrhaging, is the escape of blood from a severed blood vessel. Bleeding can range from very minor to very serious, leading to shock and death. The amount of blood that can be lost before bleeding becomes life-threatening varies according to each individual. In general, loss of 25% to 40% of an individual's total blood volume can be fatal. This equates to approximately 2 to 4 pints of blood for the average adult.

External Bleeding

External bleeding is bleeding that can be seen coming from a wound. Common examples of external bleeding include bleeding from open fractures, lacerations, and the nose. Individuals with serious external bleeding exhibit the following symptoms: obvious bleeding, restlessness, cold and clammy skin, thirst, increased and thready pulse, rapid and shallow respirations, a drop in blood pressure (a late symptom), and decreasing levels of consciousness. Three types of external bleeding can be classified according to the type of blood vessel that has been injured: capillary, venous, and arterial.

Capillary Bleeding

Capillary bleeding, the most common type of external bleeding, consists of a slow oozing of bright red blood. This type of bleeding occurs with minor cuts, scratches, and abrasions.

Venous Bleeding

Venous bleeding occurs when a vein has been punctured or severed. This type of bleeding is characterized by a slow and steady flow of dark red blood.

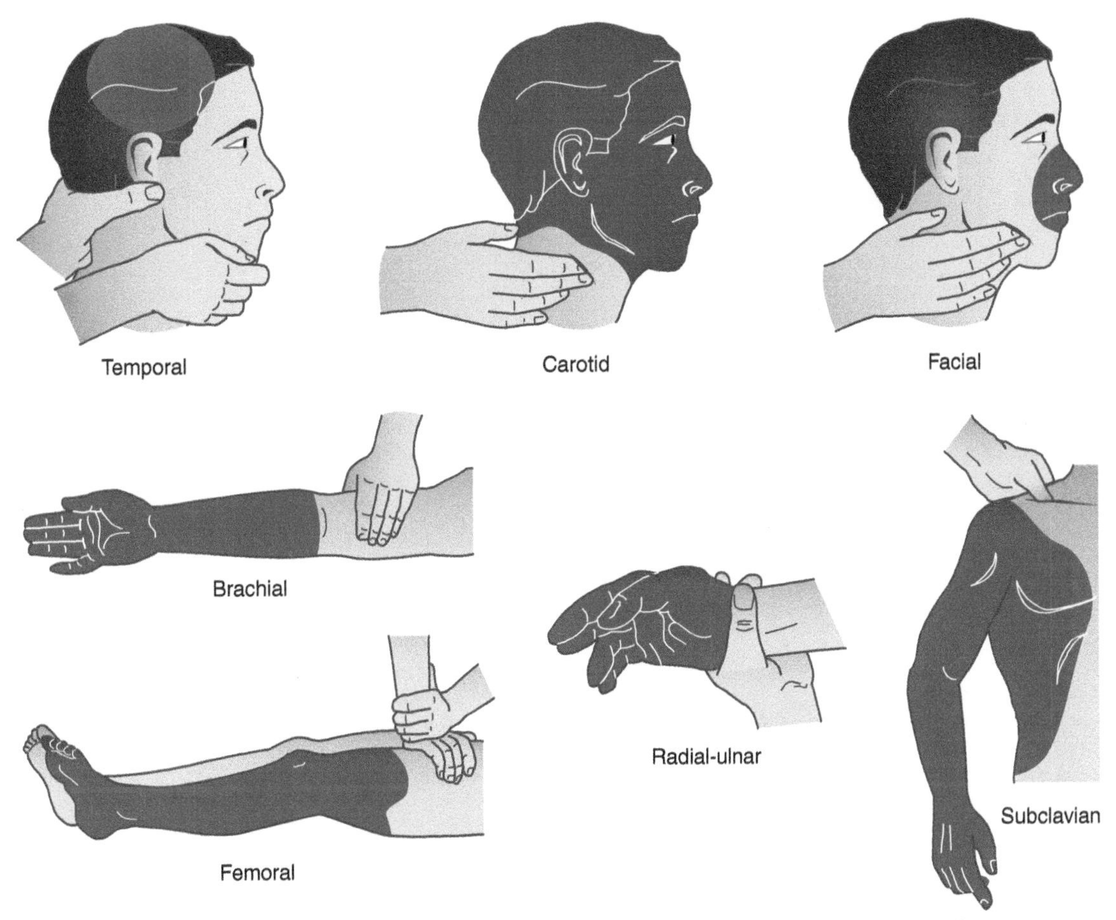

Fig. 23.5 Locations of pressure points. Shaded areas show the regions in which bleeding may be controlled by pressure at the points indicated. (From Miller BF, Keane CB: *Encyclopedia and dictionary of medicine, nursing, and allied health*, ed 7, Philadelphia: Elsevier; 2003.)

Arterial Bleeding

Arterial bleeding, the most serious type of external bleeding, occurs when an artery is punctured or severed. It is the least common type of bleeding because arteries are situated deeper in the body and are protected by bone. Arterial bleeding is characterized by bright red blood that spurts. The arteries most frequently involved in accidents are the carotid, brachial, radial, and femoral arteries.

Emergency Care for External Bleeding

The most effective way to control bleeding is to apply direct pressure to the bleeding site. The pressure functions by slowing down or stopping the flow of blood. The amount of pressure required depends on the type of bleeding. A small amount of pressure is usually sufficient to control capillary bleeding, whereas significant pressure is often required to control arterial bleeding.

If bleeding cannot be controlled with direct pressure, a pressure point can be used. A **pressure point** is a site on the body where an artery lies close to the surface of the skin and can be compressed against an underlying bone. Fig. 23.5 illustrates pressure points. Using a pressure point helps slow or stop the flow of blood from the wound. The pressure points used most often are found on the brachial and femoral arteries. The brachial artery is located on the inside of the upper arm midway between the elbow and the shoulder. Squeezing the brachial artery helps control severe bleeding in the arm. The femoral artery is located in the groin, and squeezing helps control severe bleeding in the leg.

The specific steps for controlling bleeding are as follows:

1. Apply direct pressure to the wound with a clean covering such as a large, thick gauze dressing (Fig. 23.6A). If gauze is unavailable, a clean material such as a sanitary napkin, washcloth, handkerchief, or sock can be used. If the wound is located on an extremity, elevate the limb while continuing to apply direct pressure.
2. Apply additional dressings if needed. If the dressing soaks through, apply another dressing over the first one, and continue to apply pressure (see Fig. 23.6B). (Never remove a dressing after it has been applied because this could result in more bleeding.) If bleeding cannot be controlled with direct pressure, apply pressure to the appropriate pressure point while continuing to apply direct local pressure.
3. Apply a pressure bandage. When bleeding has been controlled, apply a bandage snugly over the dressing to maintain pressure on the wound (see Fig. 23.6C).
4. Transport the patient to an emergency care facility, or, if the case is serious enough, activate the local EMS system.

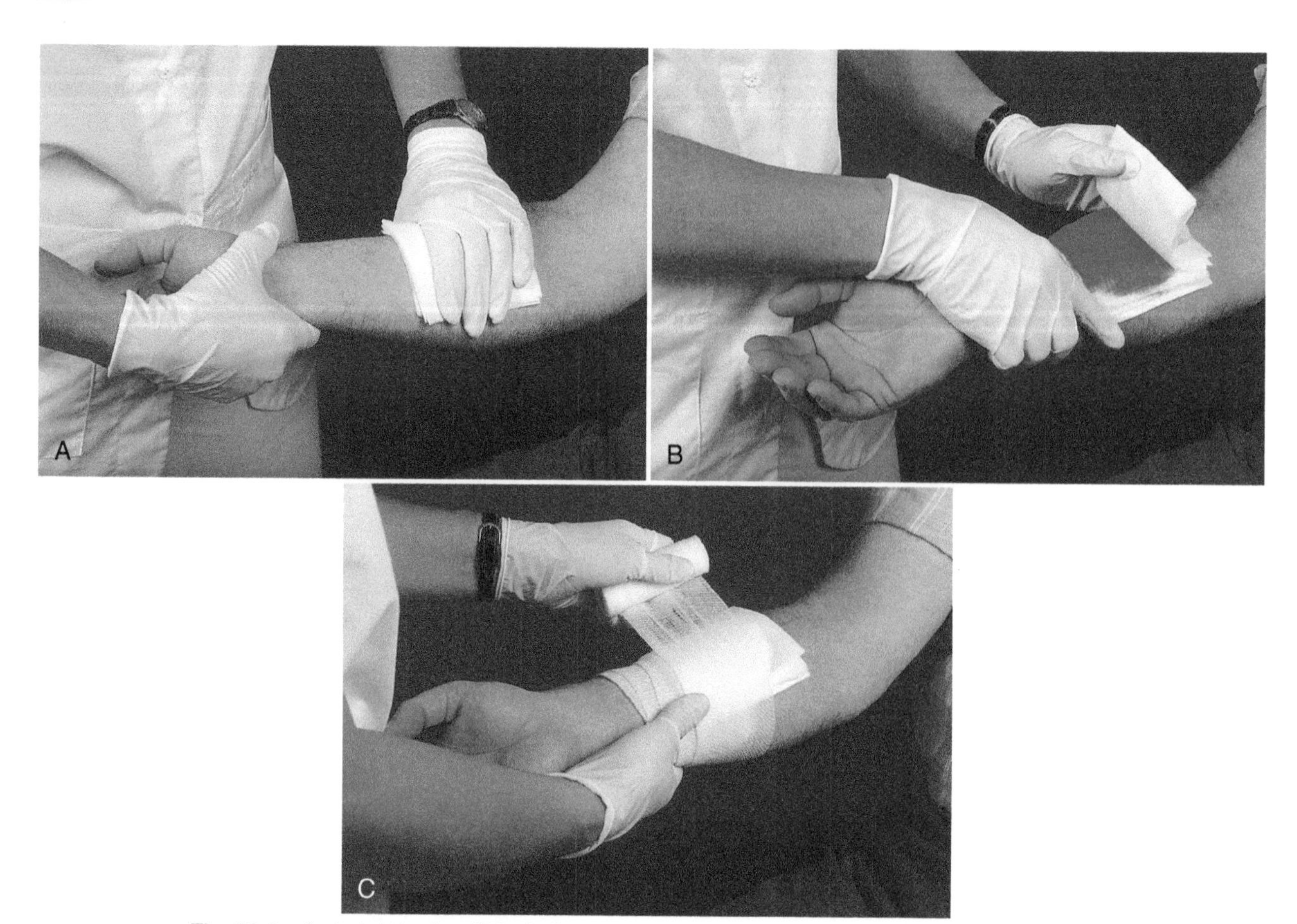

Fig. 23.6 Control of bleeding. (A) Apply direct pressure to the wound with a large, thick gauze dressing. (B) If blood soaks through the dressing, apply another dressing over the first one, and continue to apply pressure. (C) When bleeding has been controlled, apply a pressure bandage.

Nosebleeds

A nosebleed, or epistaxis, is a common form of external bleeding that usually is not serious but is more of a nuisance. Nosebleeds are usually caused by an upper respiratory infection but can result from a direct blow from a blunt object, hypertension, strenuous activity, and exposure to high altitudes.

Emergency Care for a Nosebleed

1. Position the patient in a sitting position with the head tilted forward. This prevents the blood from running down the back of the throat, which may result in nausea.
2. Apply direct pressure by pinching the nostrils together (Fig. 23.7A). Do not release the pressure too soon because the bleeding may resume. Adequate clot formation usually takes about 15 minutes. An ice pack can be applied to the bridge of the nose to help control the bleeding (see Fig. 23.7B). After the bleeding has stopped, tell the patient not to blow the nose for several hours because this could loosen the clot, causing the bleeding to start again.
3. If bleeding cannot be controlled, transport the patient to an emergency care facility for further treatment.

Internal Bleeding

Internal bleeding is bleeding that flows into a body cavity or an organ, or between tissues. It may be minor, as in the

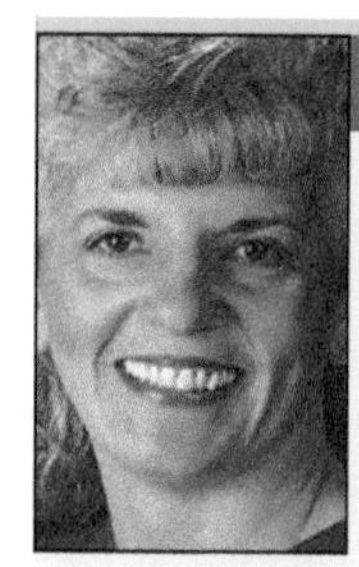

Putting It All Into Practice

My name is Judy Markins, and I work at a large clinic in the family medicine department with 12 physicians. We also have 6–10 physicians who do their internships and residency programs with us.

One day as I was performing my usual morning duties of getting the office ready for that day's patients, the office door opened. There stood a mother with her very ill child. I immediately took them back to a room. When I took the boy's temperature, it was 104 °F. I asked the mother if she had been giving him any type of fever reducer. She said she had, but that it was not helping. Under the direction of our physician, I immediately started trying to reduce the fever. The fever started to come down, and the look of relief on the mother's face was beyond words. That was one of the many days that reinforced how satisfied I am with my career choice. ■

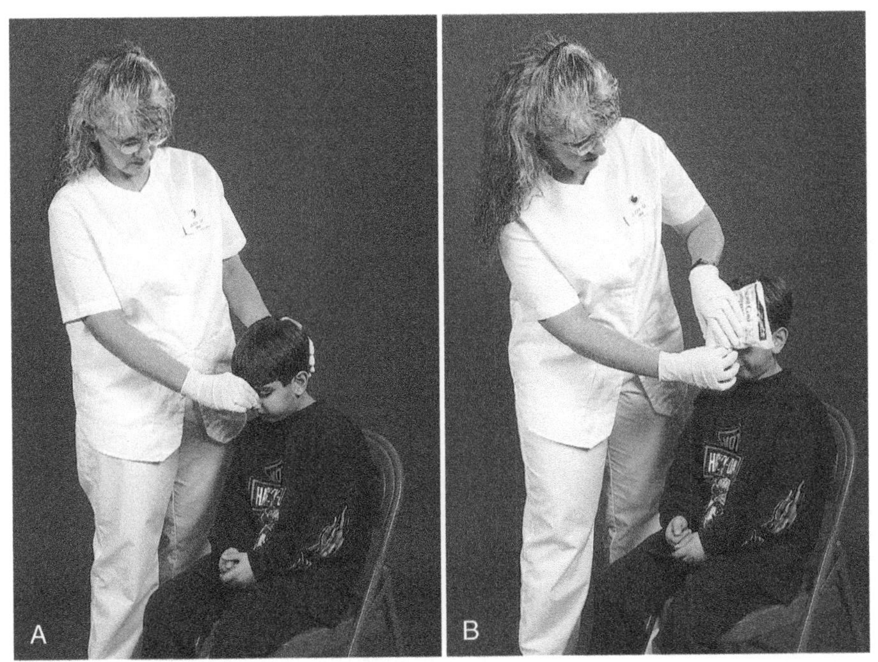

Fig. 23.7 Care of a nosebleed. (A) Apply direct pressure by pinching the nostrils together. (B) An ice pack can be applied to the bridge of the nose to help control the bleeding.

case of a contusion, or it may be very serious, such as with a severe, blunt blow to the abdomen.

Severe internal bleeding is a life-threatening emergency. Because no obvious blood flow occurs, the nature of the injury and the signs and symptoms of bleeding must be used to recognize internal bleeding. Signs and symptoms include bruises, pain, tenderness, or swelling at the site of the injury; rapid weak pulse; cold, clammy skin; nausea and vomiting; excessive thirst; a drop in blood pressure; and a decreased level of consciousness.

If a patient is suspected to have internal bleeding, the local EMS system should be activated immediately. Until emergency medical personnel arrive, the patient should be kept quiet and treated for shock.

WOUNDS

A **wound** is a break in the continuity of an external or internal surface, caused by physical means. Wounds may be open or closed.

Open Wounds

An open wound is a break in the skin surface or mucous membrane that exposes the underlying tissues. Because the skin is broken, hemorrhaging and wound contamination are primary concerns with open wounds. Open wounds include incisions, lacerations, punctures, and abrasions (Fig. 23.8). An individual with an open wound should receive prompt medical attention from a provider if any of the following occur: spurting blood; bleeding that cannot be controlled; a break in the skin that is deeper than just the outer skin layers; embedded debris or an embedded object in the wound; involvement of nerves, muscles, or tendons; and occurrence on the mouth, tongue, face, genitals, or other area where scarring would be apparent.

Incisions and Lacerations

An incision is a clean, smooth cut caused by a sharp cutting instrument, such as a knife, a razor, or a piece of glass. Deep incisions are accompanied by profuse bleeding; in addition, damage to muscles, tendons, and nerves may occur. Because the edges of the wound are smooth and straight, incisions usually heal better than lacerations.

A laceration is a wound in which the tissues are torn apart, rather than cut, leaving ragged and irregular edges. Lacerations are caused by dull knives, large objects that have been driven into the skin, and heavy machinery. Deep lacerations result in profuse bleeding, and a scar often results from jagged tearing of the tissues.

Emergency Care for Incisions and Lacerations

Minor Incisions and Lacerations

1. Assess the length, depth, and location of the wound.
2. Control bleeding by covering the wound with a dressing and applying firm pressure.
3. Clean the wound with soap and water to remove dirt and other debris (Fig. 23.9).
4. Cover the wound with a dry, sterile dressing. Instruct the patient to check the wound for redness, swelling, discharge, or an increase in pain and to contact a provider if any of these problems occur.

Serious Incisions and Lacerations

1. Control bleeding by covering the wound with a large, thick gauze dressing and applying firm pressure. Do not

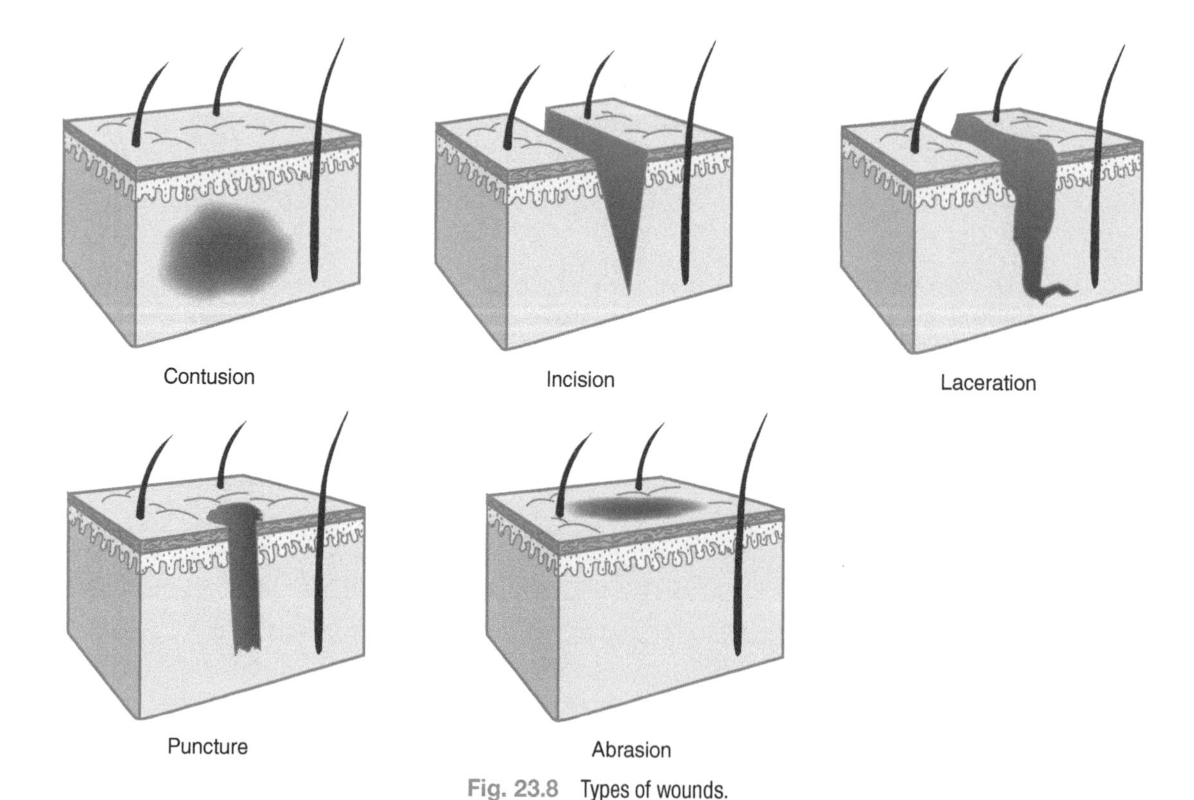

Fig. 23.8 Types of wounds.

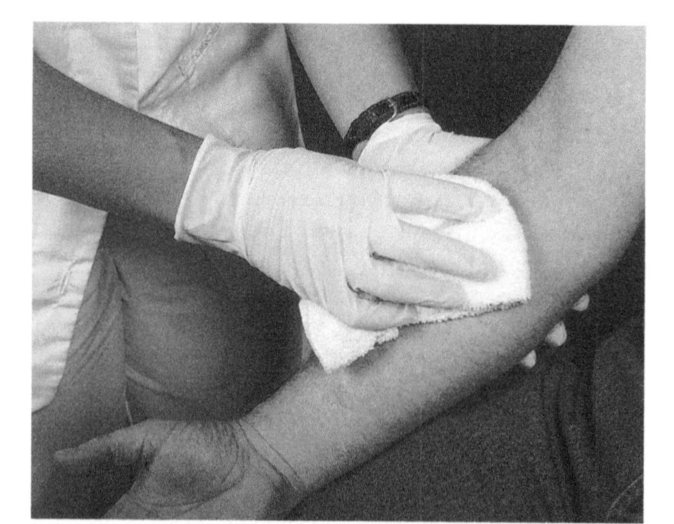
Fig. 23.9 Minor incisions and lacerations should be cleaned with soap and water to remove dirt and other debris.

clean or probe the wound because this may result in more bleeding.
2. Transport the individual to a provider, or, if the wound is serious enough, activate the local EMS system.

Punctures

A puncture is a wound made by a sharp, pointed object piercing the skin layers and sometimes the underlying structures. Objects that cause a puncture wound include a nail, splinter, needle, wire, knife, bullet, and animal bite. A puncture wound has a very small external skin opening, and for this reason bleeding is usually minor. A tetanus booster may be administered because the tetanus bacteria grow best in a warm, anaerobic environment, as would be found in a puncture wound.

Emergency Care for Puncture Wounds

1. Allow the wound to bleed freely for a few minutes to help wash out bacteria.
2. Clean the wound with soap and water.
3. Apply a dry, sterile dressing to prevent contamination.
4. Transport the individual to a provider so that medical care can be provided to prevent infection and to ensure that the patient's tetanus toxoid immunization is up to date.

Abrasions

An abrasion, or scrape, is a wound in which the outer layers of the skin are scraped or rubbed off. Blood may ooze from ruptured capillaries; however, the bleeding usually is not severe. Abrasions are caused by falls, resulting in floor burns and skinned knees and elbows. Dirt and other debris are frequently rubbed into the wound; it is important to clean scrapes thoroughly to prevent infection.

Emergency Care for Abrasions

1. Rinse the wound with cold running water.
2. Wash the wound gently with soap and water to remove dirt and other debris. A provider should remove embedded debris.
3. Cover large abrasions with a dry, sterile dressing. Small minor abrasions do not require a dressing.
4. Instruct the patient to check the wound for signs of inflammation, including redness, swelling, discharge, or increased pain, and to contact a provider if they occur.

Closed Wounds

A closed wound involves an injury to the underlying tissues of the body without a break in the skin surface or mucous membrane; an example is a contusion or a bruise. A contusion results when the tissues under the skin are injured (see Fig. 23.8); it is often caused by a sudden blow or force from a blunt object. Blood vessels rupture, allowing blood to seep into the tissues, which results in a bluish discoloration of the skin and swelling. Most contusions heal without special treatment, but cold compresses may reduce bleeding, reduce swelling and discoloration, and relieve pain. After several days, the color of the contusion turns greenish or yellow owing to oxidation of blood pigments. Contusions commonly occur with injuries such as fractures, sprains, strains, and black eyes. These injuries, along with the corresponding emergency care, are discussed next.

MUSCULOSKELETAL INJURIES

The musculoskeletal system consists of all the bones, muscles, tendons, and ligaments of the body. Injuries that affect the musculoskeletal system include fractures, dislocations, sprains, and strains.

Fracture

A **fracture** is any break in a bone. The break may range in severity from a simple chip or a crack to a complete break or shattering of the bone. Fractures can occur anywhere on the surface of the bone, including across the surface of a joint such as the wrist or ankle. Fractures result from a direct blow, a fall, bone disease, or a twisting force as may occur in a sports injury. Although fractures often cause severe pain, they are seldom life-threatening.

The two basic types of fracture are closed fractures and open fractures (Fig. 23.10). A *closed fracture,* the most common type, occurs when there is a break in a bone but no break in the skin over the fracture site. An *open fracture* involves a break in the bone along with penetration of the overlying skin surface. Open fractures are more serious owing to the risk of blood loss and contamination leading to infection.

The signs and symptoms of a fracture include pain and tenderness, deformity, swelling and discoloration, loss of function of the body part, and numbness or tingling. The patient usually guards the injured part and may relay to you that he or she heard the bone break or snap or felt a grating sensation. This grating sensation, known as **crepitus**, is caused by the bone fragments rubbing against each other.

Fractures also can be classified according to the nature of the break: impacted, greenstick, transverse, oblique, comminuted, and spiral. Fig. 23.11 illustrates and describes these types of fracture.

Dislocation

A **dislocation** is an injury in which one end of a bone making up a joint is separated or displaced from its normal position.

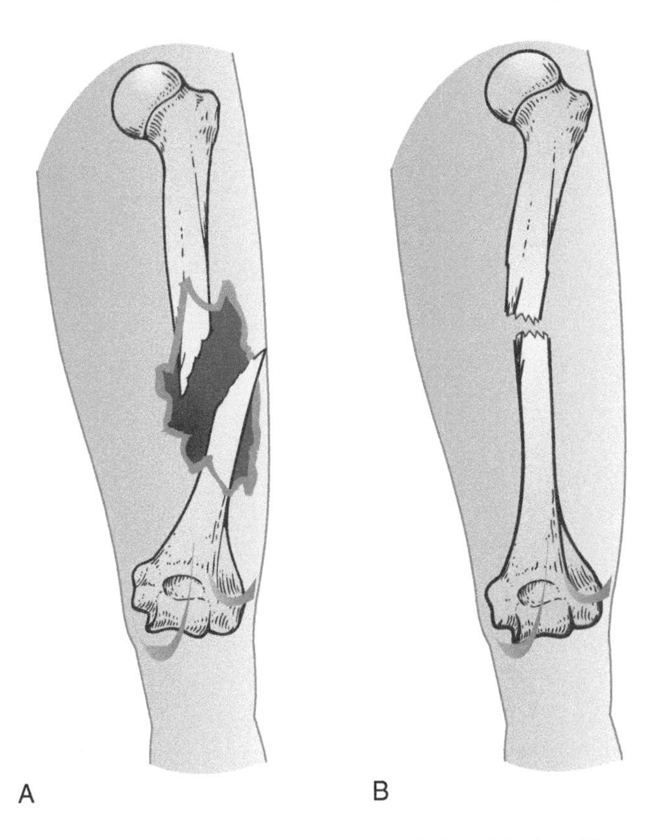

Fig. 23.10 Fractures. (A) Open fracture. (B) Closed fracture. (From Connolly JF: *DePalma's The management of fractures and dislocations: an atlas*, Philadelphia: WB Saunders; 1981.)

A dislocation is caused by a violent pulling or pushing force that tears the ligaments. Dislocations usually result from falls, sports injuries, and motor vehicle accidents. Signs and symptoms of a dislocation include significant deformity of the joint, pain and swelling, and loss of function.

Sprain

A **sprain** is the tearing of ligaments at a joint. Sprains may result from a fall, a sports injury, or a motor vehicle accident. The joints most often sprained are the ankle, knee, wrist, and fingers. Signs and symptoms of a sprain include pain, swelling, and discoloration. Sprains can vary in seriousness from mild to severe, depending on the amount of damage to the ligaments.

Strain

A **strain** is the stretching and tearing of muscles or tendons. Strains are most likely to occur when an individual lifts a heavy object or overworks a muscle, as during exercise. The muscles most commonly strained are those of the neck, back, thigh, and calf. Signs and symptoms of a strain are pain and swelling. Strains do not usually cause the intense symptoms associated with fractures, dislocations, and sprains.

Emergency Care for a Fracture

It is often difficult to determine whether a patient has a fracture, a dislocation, or a sprain because the symptoms of these injuries are similar. Because of this, any serious

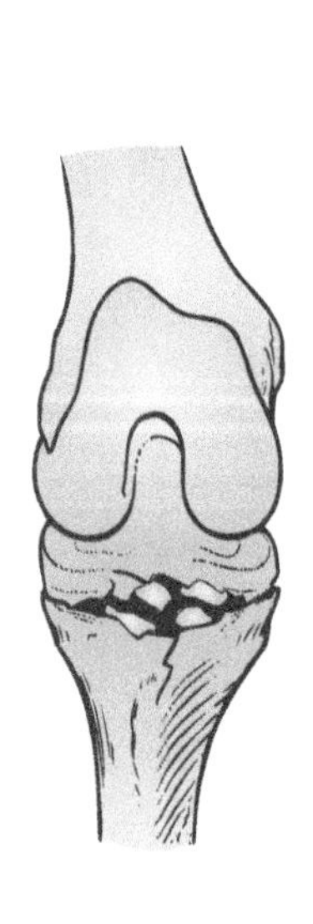

Impacted Fracture
The broken ends of the bones are forcefully jammed together.

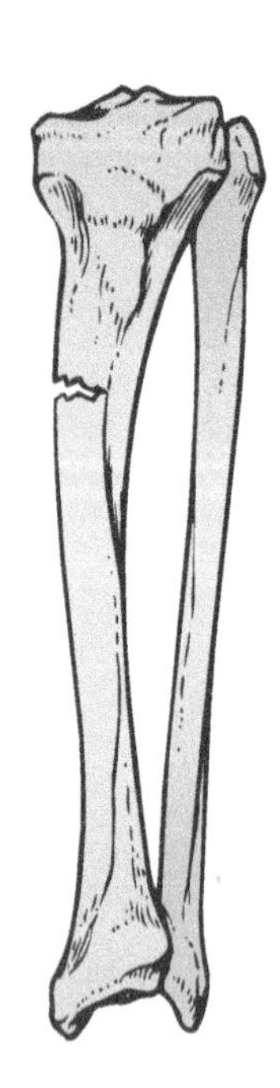

Greenstick Fracture
The bone remains intact on one side, but broken on the other, in much the same way that a "green stick" bends; common in children, whose bones are more flexible than those of adults.

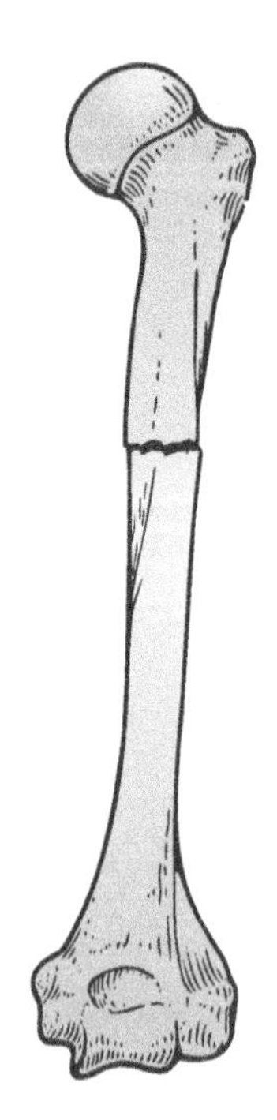

Transverse Fracture
The break occurs perpendicular to the long axis of the bone.

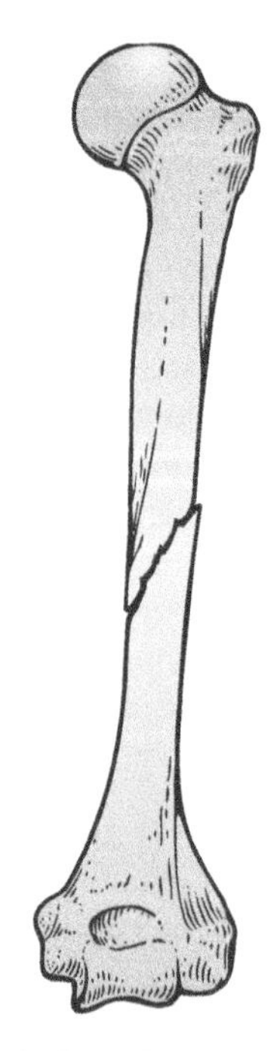

Oblique Fracture
The break occurs diagonally across the bone; generally the result of a twisting force.

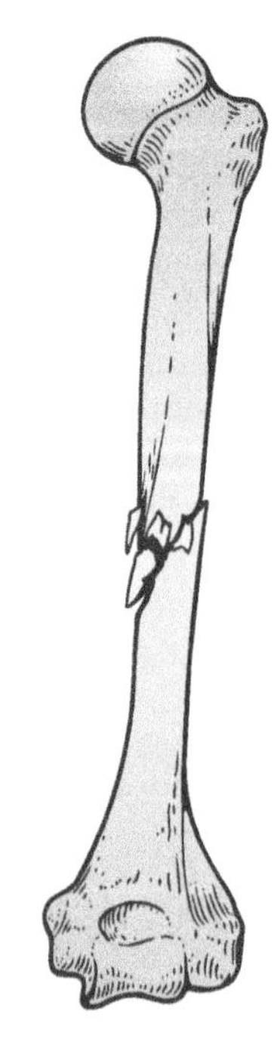

Comminuted Fracture
The bone is splintered or shattered into three or more fragments; usually caused by an extremely traumatic direct force.

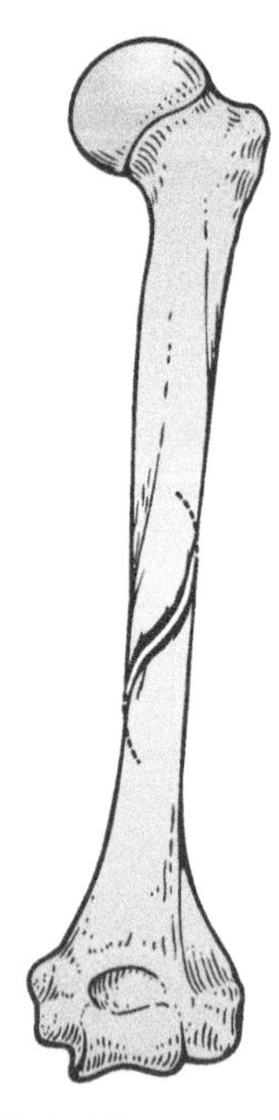

Spiral Fracture
The bone is broken into a spiral or S-shape; caused by a twisting force.

Fig. 23.11 Types of fractures.

musculoskeletal injury to an extremity should be treated as though it were a fracture.

The primary goal of emergency care for a fracture is to immobilize the body part. Immobilization reduces pain and prevents further damage. A **splint** is any item that immobilizes a body part. In an emergency situation, items such as a length of wood, cardboard, or rolled newspapers or magazines can be used for splinting. The splint should be padded with a soft material such as a rolled-up towel.

The body part should be splinted in the position in which you found it. Severely angulated fractures may have to be straightened before splinting, however. If you attempt to straighten an angulated fracture, be careful not to force the affected part. A dislocated bone end can become "locked" and would have to be realigned at the hospital. If you straighten an angulated bone and encounter pain, stop and splint it in the position in which you found it. The splint also should immobilize the area above and below the injury. In splinting an injured wrist, the hand and forearm also should be immobilized (Fig. 23.12A). In splinting an injury to the shaft of the bone, the joints above and below the injury should be immobilized. In splinting the forearm, the elbow joint and the wrist joint should be immobilized.

The splint should be held in place with a roller gauze bandage or other suitable material, such as neckties, scarves, or strips of cloth (see Fig. 23.12B). The splint should be applied snugly, but not so tightly that it interferes with proper circulation. After applying the splint, check the pulse below the splint to ensure the splint has not been applied too tightly. If you cannot detect a pulse, immediately loosen the splint until you can feel the pulse (see Fig. 23.12C).

Whenever possible, elevate an injured extremity after it has been immobilized to reduce swelling (see Fig. 23.12D). An ice pack also can be applied to the injured part. Cold limits the accumulation of fluid in the body tissues by constricting blood vessels and reducing leakage of fluid into the tissues. In addition, cold temporarily relieves pain through its anesthetic or numbing effect, which reduces stimulation of nerve receptors.

After you have properly immobilized the injury, transport the patient to an emergency care facility, or if the injury is serious enough, activate the local EMS system. In any situation in which an injury to the spine is suspected, activate EMS.

BURNS

A **burn** is an injury to the tissues caused by exposure to thermal, chemical, electrical, or radioactive agents. The severity of a burn depends on the depth of the burn, the percentage of the body involved, the type of agent causing the burn, the duration and intensity of the agent, and the part of the body

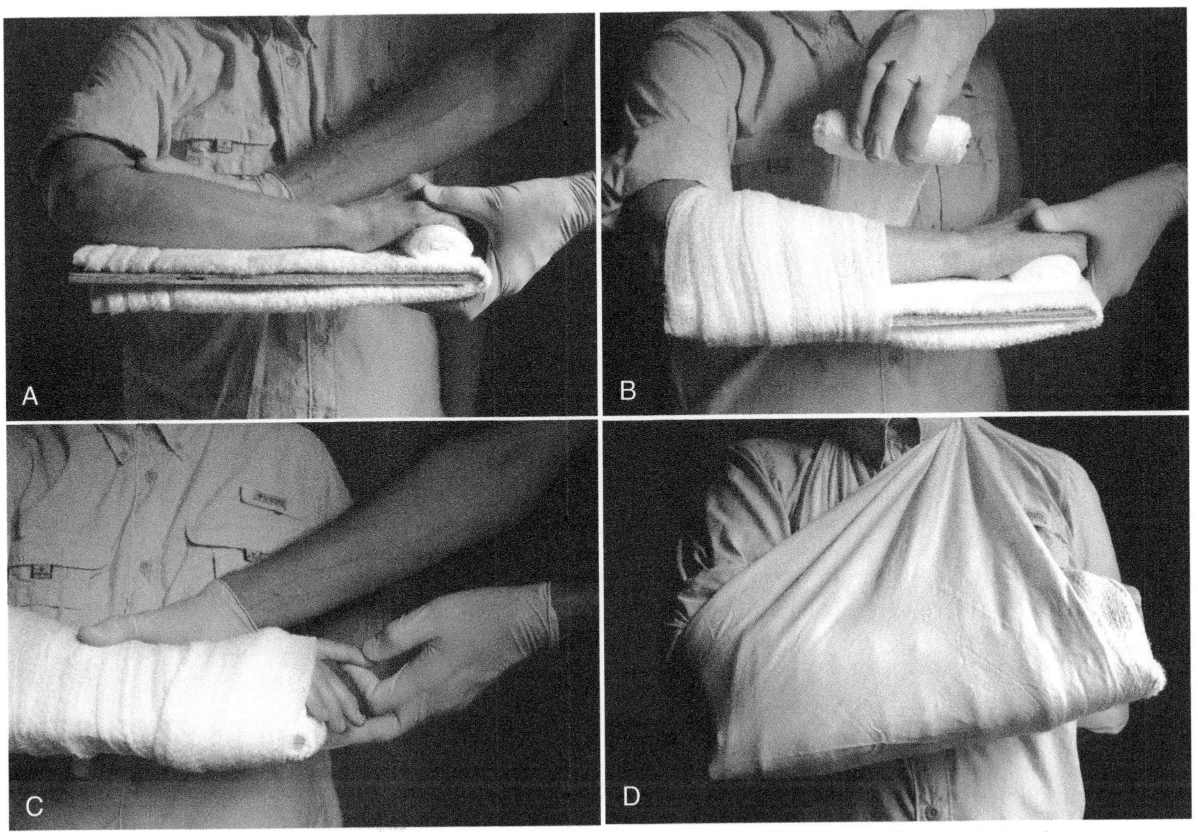

Fig. 23.12 Emergency care of a fracture. (A) The splint should immobilize the area above and below the injury. (B) The splint is held in place with a roller gauze bandage. (C) After the splint is applied, the pulse below the splint should be checked to ensure that the splint has not been applied too tightly. (D) A sling can be used to elevate the extremity to reduce swelling.

affected. Burns are classified according to the depth of tissue injury, as illustrated in Fig. 23.13.

Superficial (First-Degree) Burn

A superficial burn is the most common type of burn. It involves only the top layer of skin, the epidermis. With this type of burn, the skin appears red, is warm and dry to the touch, and is usually painful. Sunburn is a common example of a superficial burn. A superficial burn heals in 2 to 5 days of its own accord and does not cause scarring.

Partial-Thickness (Second-Degree) Burn

A partial-thickness burn involves the epidermis and extends into the dermis but does not pass through the dermis to the underlying tissues. The burned area usually appears red, mottled, and blistered. In most cases, the blisters should not be broken because they provide a protective barrier against infection. Partial-thickness burns are usually very painful, and the area often swells. This type of burn usually heals within 3 to 4 weeks and may result in some scarring.

Full-Thickness (Third-Degree) Burn

A full-thickness burn completely destroys the epidermis and the dermis and extends into the underlying tissues, such as fat, muscle, bone, and nerves. The affected area appears charred black, brown, and cherry red, with the damaged tissues underneath often pearly white. The patient may experience intense pain; however, if damage to the nerve endings is substantial, the patient may feel no pain at all. During the healing process, dense scars typically result. Infection is a major concern, and the patient must be carefully monitored.

Thermal Burns

Thermal burns usually occur in the home, often as a result of fire, scalding water, or coming into contact with a hot object such as a stove or curling iron.

Emergency Care for Major Thermal Burns

1. Stop the burning process to prevent further injury. If the individual is on fire, wrap him or her in a blanket, rug, or heavy coat and push him or her to the ground to help smother the flames. If a covering is unavailable, shout at the individual to drop to the ground and roll around to smother the flames.
2. Cool the burn, using large amounts of cool water from a faucet or garden hose. Do not use ice or ice water because this may result in further tissue damage; it also causes heat loss from the body. If the burn covers a large surface area (greater than 20%), do not use water. The loss of a large amount of skin surface places the patient at risk for hypothermia (generalized body cooling). With large

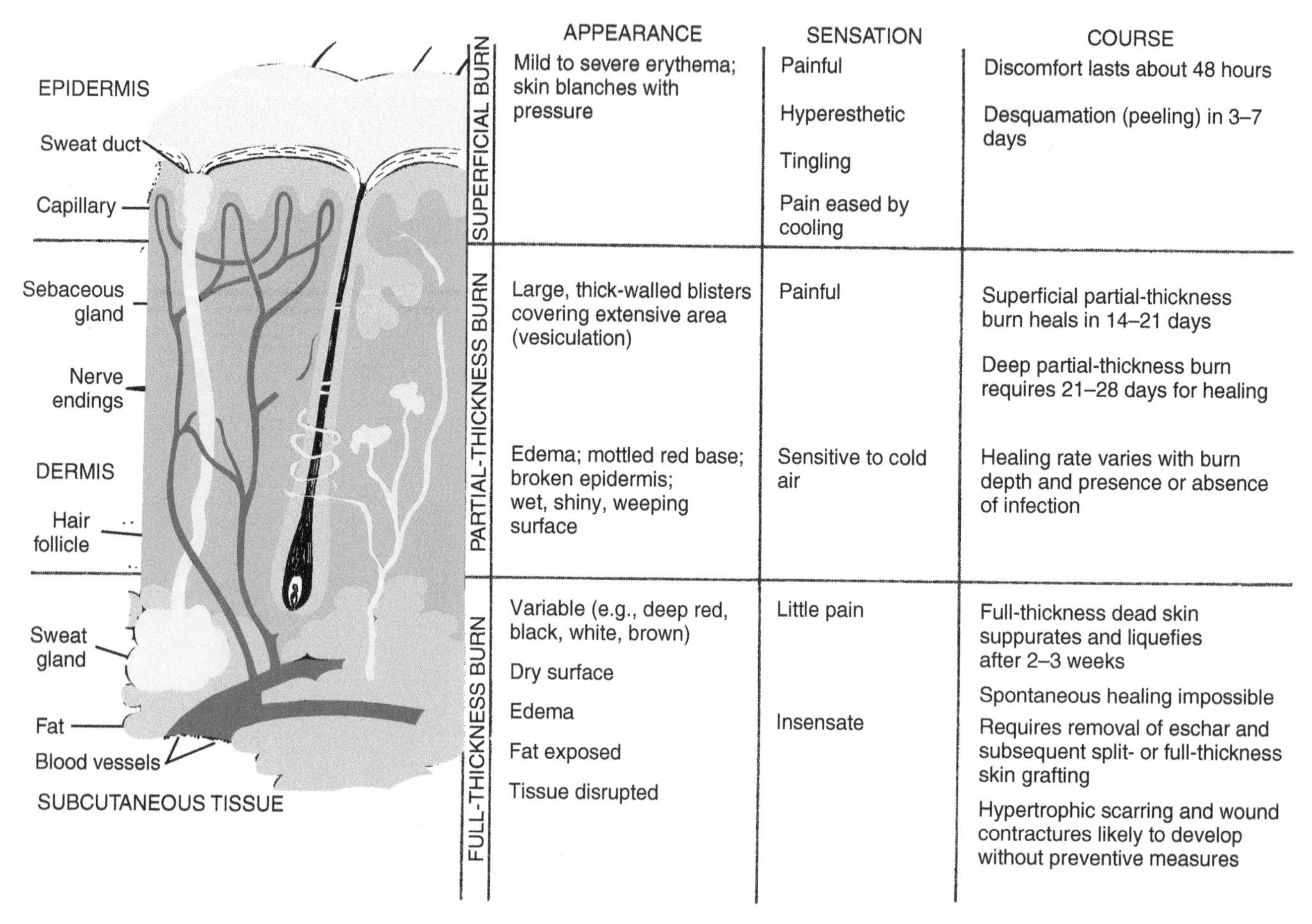

Fig. 23.13 Types of burns. (From Polaski AL, Tatro SE: *Luckmann's Core principles and practice of medical-surgical nursing*, Philadelphia: WB Saunders; 1996.)

surface area burns, you may cool the most painful areas, but not an area greater than 20% of the body (e.g., two arms, one leg).
3. Activate the local EMS system.
4. Cover the patient with a clean, nonfuzzy material such as a tablecloth or sheet. The cover maintains warmth, reduces pain, and reduces the risk of contamination. Do not apply any type of ointment, antiseptic, or other substance to the burned area.

Emergency Care for Minor Thermal Burns

1. Immerse the affected area in cool water for 2 to 5 minutes. Be careful not to break any blisters because they provide a protective barrier against infection.
2. Cover the burn with a dry sterile dressing.

Chemical Burns

Chemical burns occur in the workplace and at home. The severity of the burn depends on the type and strength of the chemical and the duration of exposure to the chemical. The main difference between a chemical burn and a thermal burn is that the chemical continues to burn the patient's tissues as long as it is on the skin. Because of this factor, it is important to remove the chemical from the skin as quickly as possible and then to activate the local EMS system.

Liquid chemical burns should be treated by flooding the area with large amounts of cool running water until emergency personnel arrive. If a solid substance such as lime has been spilled on the patient, it should be brushed off before flooding the area with water. This is because a dry chemical may be activated by contact with water.

SEIZURES

A **seizure** is a sudden episode of involuntary muscular contractions and relaxation, often accompanied by changes in sensation, behavior, and level of consciousness. A seizure results when the normal electrical activity of the brain is disturbed, causing the brain cells to become irritated and overactive. Specific conditions that trigger a seizure include epilepsy, encephalitis, a recent or old head injury, high fever in infants and young children, drug and alcohol abuse or withdrawal, eclampsia associated with toxemia of pregnancy, diabetic conditions, and heatstroke.

Seizures are classified as partial or generalized according to the location of the abnormal electrical activity in the brain. *Partial seizures* are the most common type, occurring in approximately 80% of individuals who have seizures. With a partial seizure the abnormal electrical activity is localized into specific areas of the brain; only the brain functions in those areas are affected.

Partial seizures are further classified as simple or complex, depending on whether the patient's level of consciousness is affected. The symptoms of a *simple partial seizure* include twitching or jerking in just one part of the body. This type of seizure lasts less than 1 minute, and the patient remains awake and alert during the seizure. With a *complex partial seizure,* the patient's level of consciousness is affected, and the patient has little or no memory of the seizure afterward. Symptoms of this type of seizure include abnormal behavior such as confusion, a glassy stare, aimless wandering, lip smacking or chewing, and fidgeting with clothing, which lasts from a few seconds to a minute or two. A simple and a complex partial seizure can progress to a generalized seizure.

With a *generalized seizure,* the abnormal electrical activity spreads through the entire brain. The best-known type of generalized seizure is a *tonic-clonic seizure* (formerly known as a *grand mal seizure*). With this type of seizure, the patient exhibits tonic-clonic activity followed by a postictal state. During the tonic phase, the patient suddenly loses consciousness and exhibits rigid muscular contractions, which result in odd posturing of the body. Respirations are inhibited, which may cause cyanosis around the mouth and lips. The patient may lose control of the bladder or bowels, resulting in involuntary urination and defecation. The tonic phase lasts 30 seconds, followed by the clonic phase. During the clonic phase, the patient's body jerks about violently. The patient's jaw muscles contract, which may cause the patient to bite the tongue or lips. The final phase of the seizure is the postictal state, lasting 10 to 30 minutes, in which the patient exhibits a depressed level of consciousness, is disoriented, and often has a headache. The patient typically has little or no memory of the seizure and feels confused and exhausted for several hours after the seizure.

In some instances of seizures, particularly in patients with epilepsy, an aura precedes the seizure. An *aura* is a sensation perceived by the patient that something is about to happen; examples include a strange taste, smell, or sound; a twitch; or a feeling of dizziness or anxiety. An aura provides the patient with a warning signal that a seizure is about to begin.

Although seizures are frightening to observe, they usually are not as bad as they look. Most patients fully recover within a few minutes after the seizure begins. An exception to this is *status epilepticus,* in which seizures are prolonged or come in rapid succession without full recovery of consciousness between them. Status epilepticus is a potentially life-threatening situation that requires immediate medical care.

Emergency Care for Seizures

The most important criterion in caring for a patient in a seizure is to protect the patient from harm. Remove hazards from the immediate area to protect the patient from injury sustained by striking a surrounding object. Do not restrain the patient. Loosen restrictive clothing that may interfere with breathing, such as collars, neckties, scarves, and jewelry. The seizure will occur no matter what you do; restraining the patient could seriously injure the patient's muscles, bones, or joints. Do not insert anything into the patient's mouth during the seizure because this could damage the teeth or mouth or interfere with breathing. In addition, it could trigger the gag reflex, causing the patient to vomit and possibly aspirate the vomitus into the lungs. If the patient vomits, roll him or her onto one side so that the vomitus can drain from the mouth.

If you are uncertain as to the cause of the seizure, or if you suspect that the patient is having status epilepticus, activate your local EMS system immediately. Otherwise, transport the patient to an emergency medical care facility for further evaluation and treatment after the seizure is over.

POISONING

A **poison** is any substance that causes illness, injury, or death if it enters the body. Most poisoning episodes occur in the home, are accidental, and occur in children younger than 5 years. Poisoning usually involves common substances, such as cleaning agents, medications, and pesticides. For most poisonous substances, the reaction is more serious in children and the elderly than in adults. A poison can enter the body in four ways: ingestion, inhalation, absorption, or injection.

Poison control centers are valuable resources that are easily accessible to medical personnel and the community. More than 500 regional poison control centers have been established across the United States; most are located in the emergency departments of large hospitals. These centers are staffed by personnel who have access to information about almost all poisonous substances. Most centers are staffed 24 hours a day, and calls are toll-free. In addition, a national Poison Help number (1-800-222-1222) can be called 24 hours a day.

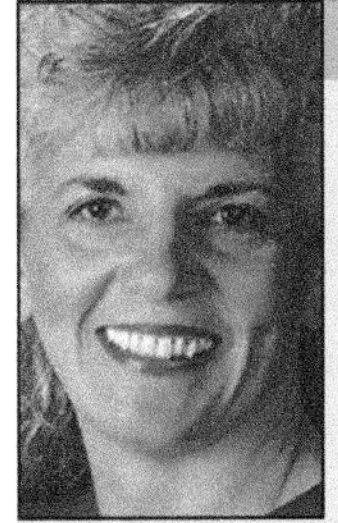

Memories *from* Practicum

Judy Markins: As it turned out, one of my most terrible moments during my practicum was a great learning experience. I was drawing blood (which was not my favorite procedure) and missed the vein—not once, but twice. You could see the sweat under my gloves. My stomach was in my throat, and I did not want to try again. Thank goodness my patient was understanding, and I had an excellent practicum supervisor. She insisted that I try again, encouraging me that I could do it and suggesting some techniques that she had learned from her many years of experience. I got the blood specimen, along with some new-found confidence.

In most situations, someone can help you if you have questions. Use your resources when you need to. Be honest, know your procedure, and have confidence in yourself. ■

What Would You Do? What Would You *Not* Do?

Case Study 1

Beth Eaton calls the office. She says that she thinks her 3-year-old daughter, Olivia, has eaten some chewable vitamins. Beth was taking a shower, and when she came out, Olivia was holding an empty vitamin bottle and saying "Good candy." Beth says she does not know how Olivia got the childproof top off. She thinks the bottle was about a third of the way full. Beth says that Olivia is complaining that her tummy hurts. Beth says she has syrup of ipecac and wants to know whether she should give some to Olivia. ■

Ingested Poisons

Poisons that are ingested enter the body by being swallowed. Ingestion is the most common route of entry for poisons. Examples of poisons that are often ingested include cleaning products, pesticides, contaminated food, petroleum products (e.g., gasoline, kerosene), and poisonous plants. Abuse of drugs, alcohol, or both also can result in poisoning from an accidental or intentional overdose. Signs and symptoms of poisoning by ingestion are based on the specific substance that has been consumed but often include strange odors, burns or stains around the mouth, nausea, vomiting, abdominal pain, diarrhea, difficulty in breathing, profuse perspiration, excessive salivation, dilated or constricted pupils, unconsciousness, and convulsions.

Emergency Care for Poisoning by Ingestion

1. Acquire as much information as possible about the type of poison, the amount ingested, and when it was ingested.
2. Call your poison control center or local EMS. *Never* induce vomiting unless directed to do so by a medical authority. Vomiting is often contraindicated—for instance, when an individual is unconscious, has swallowed a petroleum product, or has swallowed a corrosive poison such as a strong acid or base. Corrosive poisons may cause more injury to the esophagus, throat, and mouth if they are vomited back up. If it is available, you may be directed by the poison control center to administer activated charcoal. Activated charcoal is used to absorb the poison that remains in the stomach and prevents absorption by the intestine.
3. If the individual vomits, collect some of the vomitus for transport with the patient to the hospital for analysis by a toxicologist, if necessary. In addition, bring along containers of any substances ingested, such as empty medication bottles and household cleaner containers, because the label of the container often lists the ingredients in the product.

Inhaled Poisons

A poison that is inhaled is breathed into the body in the form of gas, vapor, or spray. The most commonly inhaled poison is carbon monoxide, such as from car exhausts, malfunctioning furnaces, and fires. Other inhaled poisons include carbon dioxide from wells and sewers and fumes from household products such as glues, paints, insect sprays, and cleaners (e.g., ammonia, chlorine). Signs and symptoms of inhaled poisoning often include severe headache; nausea and vomiting; coughing or wheezing; shortness of breath; chest pain or tightness; facial burns; burning of the mouth, nose, eyes, throat, or chest; cyanosis; confusion; dizziness; and unconsciousness.

Emergency Care for Inhaled Poisons

1. Determine whether it is safe to approach the patient. Toxic gases and fumes also can be dangerous to individuals helping the patient.
2. Remove the individual from the source of the poison and into fresh air as quickly as possible.
3. Call your poison control center or local EMS.
4. If oxygen is available, you may be directed to administer it under the supervision of a provider. Oxygen is the primary antidote for carbon monoxide poisoning.

Absorbed Poisons

A poison that is absorbed enters the body through the skin. Examples of absorbed poisons include fertilizers and pesticides used for lawn and garden care. Signs and symptoms of absorbed poisoning include irritation, burning and itching, burning of the skin or eyes, headache, and abnormal pulse or respiration or both.

Emergency Care for Absorbed Poisons

1. Remove the patient from the source of the poison. Avoid contact with the toxic substance.
2. Call your poison control center or local EMS. In most cases, you will be instructed to flood the area that has been exposed to the poison with water. Dry chemicals should be brushed from the skin before flooding with water.

What Would You Do? What Would You *Not* Do?

Case Study 2

Anita Alland calls the office and says that her son, Garon, was stung by a yellow jacket about an hour ago while mowing the grass. She says that his entire arm and back are red and swollen, and that he has a lot of redness and swelling around his eyes. Garon is itching all over and seems fuzzy headed. Anita says she has never seen anyone do this after being stung. She says she had Garon take a cold shower to see if it would help. After the shower, he started feeling faint and dizzy, and now he is having trouble breathing. Anita wants to know whether she can bring him to the office so that he can be seen by the physician. ■

Injected Poisons

An injected poison enters the body through bites, through stings, or from a needle. Examples of injected poisons include the venom of insects, spiders, snakes, and marine creatures such as jellyfish and substances from the bite of a rabid animal. The poison also may be a drug that is self-administered with a hypodermic needle, such as heroin. General signs and symptoms of injected poisoning include an altered state of awareness; evidence of stings, bites, or puncture marks on the skin; mottled skin; localized pain or itching; burning, swelling, or blistering at the site; difficulty in breathing; abnormal pulse rate; nausea and vomiting; and anaphylactic shock.

Insect Stings

It is estimated that 1 of every 125 Americans is allergic to insect stings. Approximately 40 people in the United States die every year from a severe allergic reaction to insect stings. The incidence of deaths is low because most people know they need to obtain medical attention immediately if an allergic reaction begins.

Almost all of the insects whose venom can cause allergic reactions belong to a group called *Hymenoptera,* which includes honeybees and bumblebees, wasps, yellow jackets, and hornets. When a honeybee stings, its stinger remains embedded in the victim's skin, causing the bee to die as it tries to tear itself away. Wasps, yellow jackets, and hornets are more aggressive than bees and can sting repeatedly. Hornets are the most aggressive of the group and may sting even when not provoked. Yellow jackets are close behind in aggressiveness, and wasps usually sting only if someone interferes with them near their nest.

If an insect sting does not cause an allergic reaction within 30 minutes, chances are excellent that no problem will occur. A normal reaction to an insect sting includes localized pain, redness, swelling, and itching lasting 1 to 2 days. Any generalized reaction not arising directly from the area of the sting is almost certain to be an allergic reaction, which begins with symptoms such as sneezing, hives, itching, angioedema, erythema, and disorientation and progresses to difficulty in breathing, dizziness, faintness, and loss of consciousness.

Medical care should be sought immediately because these are the symptoms of an anaphylactic reaction, and most fatalities occur within 2 hours of the sting. Because time is a factor, individuals known to have a severe allergy to insect stings carry an anaphylactic emergency treatment kit containing injectable epinephrine and oral antihistamines (see Fig. 23.2). With this kit, treatment for a severe allergic reaction can be started immediately.

Emergency Care for Insect Stings

1. Remove the stinger and attached venom sac. Scrape the stinger off the patient's skin with your fingernail or a plastic card such as a credit card (Fig. 23.14). Do not use tweezers or forceps because squeezing the venom sac may cause more venom to be injected into the patient's tissues.
2. Wash the site with soap and water.

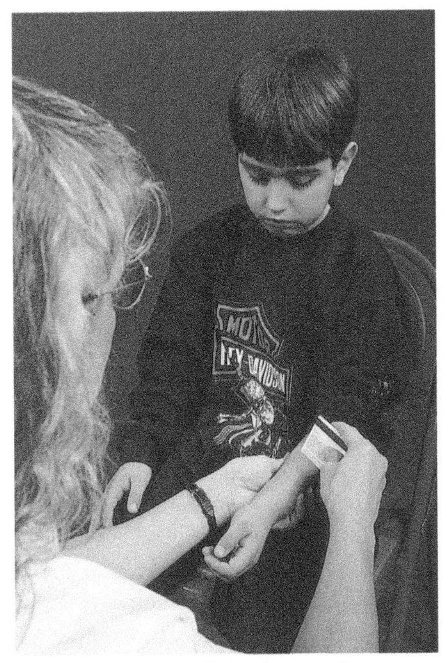

Fig. 23.14 Removing a honeybee stinger and venom sac using the edge of a credit card.

3. Apply a cold pack to the affected area to reduce pain and swelling.
4. Observe the patient for signs of an anaphylactic reaction.

Spider Bites

Although spiders are numerous throughout the United States, most do not cause injuries or serious complications. Only two spiders have bites that cause serious or life-threatening reactions: the black widow spider and the brown recluse spider. Both of these spiders prefer dark, out-of-the-way places such as in woodpiles, in brush piles, under rocks, and in dark garages and attics. Because of this, bites usually occur on the hands and arms of individuals reaching into places where the spiders are hiding. Often the individual does not know that he or she has been bitten until he or she begins to feel ill or notices swelling and a bite mark on the skin.

The black widow spider is approximately 1 inch long and is black with a distinctive bright-red hourglass shape on its abdomen. The venom injected when this spider bites an individual is toxic to the central nervous system. Signs and symptoms of a black widow bite include swelling and a dull pain at the injection site; nausea and vomiting; a rigid, boardlike abdomen; fever; rash; and difficulty in breathing or swallowing. Although the symptoms are severe, they are not usually fatal. An antivenin is available; however, because of its undesirable and frequent side effects, it usually is administered only to individuals with severe bites and to those who may have a heightened reaction, such as elderly individuals and children younger than 5 years.

The brown recluse spider is light brown with a dark-brown violin-shaped mark on its back. The bite of a brown recluse causes severe local effects, including tenderness, redness, and swelling at the injection site. Systemic effects, such as difficulty in breathing or swallowing, seldom occur.

Emergency Care for Spider Bites

1. Wash the wound.
2. Apply a cold pack to the affected area to reduce pain and swelling.
3. Obtain medical help immediately if you suspect the individual has been bitten by a black widow spider or a brown recluse spider, or if a severe reaction begins to occur.

Snakebites

Snakebites kill very few people in the United States. Every year, approximately 45,000 persons are bitten by a snake; however, only 7000 of these bites involve a poisonous snake, and fewer than 15 of the individuals die. Species of poisonous snakes in the United States include rattlesnakes, copperheads, cottonmouths (water moccasins), and coral snakes. Individuals, zoos, or laboratories may own other poisonous species, however. Rattlesnakes account for most snakebites and nearly all fatalities from snakebites. Most snakebites occur near the home, as opposed to in the wild. Because it is often difficult to identify a snake, any unidentified snake should be considered poisonous. General signs and symptoms of a bite from a poisonous snake include puncture marks on the skin, pain and swelling at the puncture site, rapid pulse, nausea, vomiting, unconsciousness, and convulsions.

Emergency Care for Snakebites

1. Wash the bite area gently with soap and water.
2. Immobilize the injured part, and position it below the level of the heart.
3. Call emergency personnel. Do not apply ice to a snakebite. Do not apply a tourniquet, and do not cut or suction the wound.
4. If the snake is dead, inform emergency personnel of its location so that it can be transported to the hospital for identification.

Animal Bites

Bites and other injuries from animals range in severity from minor to serious and fatal. Most people who are bitten by animals do not report the bite to a provider. Because of this factor, the incidence of animal bites in the United States each year is unknown but has been estimated at approximately 1 to 2 million for dog bites and 400,000 for cat bites.

The most serious type of bite is one from an animal with rabies. Rabies is a viral infection transmitted through the saliva of an infected animal. If the condition is not treated, rabies is usually fatal. Certain animals tend to have a higher incidence of rabies than others. These include skunks, bats, raccoons, cats, dogs, cattle, and foxes. Hamsters, gerbils, guinea pigs, chipmunks, rats, mice, gophers, and rabbits are rarely infected with the rabies virus.

An individual who has been bitten by an animal that has rabies or is suspected of having rabies must obtain medical care. To prevent rabies, a rabies vaccine, which produces antibodies to fight the rabies virus, is administered to the individual.

Emergency Care for Animal Bites

Minor Animal Bites

Wash the wound with soap and water. Apply an antibiotic ointment and a dry sterile dressing. Transport the individual to a provider so that medical care can be provided to prevent infection and to ensure that the patient's tetanus toxoid immunization is up-to-date.

Serious Bites

If the wound is bleeding heavily, first control the bleeding with direct pressure. Do not clean the wound because this may result in more bleeding. Transport the patient to a provider, or if the bite is serious enough, call the local EMS system.

All Animal Bites

If you suspect that the animal has rabies, relay this information to the appropriate authorities, such as medical personnel, the police, or animal control personnel. If possible, try to remember what the animal looked like and the area in which you last saw it.

HEAT AND COLD EXPOSURE

Exposure to excessive environmental heat or cold can result in injury to the body ranging in severity from minor to life-threatening. Heat-related injuries are most apt to occur on very hot days that are accompanied by high humidity with little or no air movement. The three conditions caused by overexposure to heat are heat cramps, heat exhaustion, and heatstroke.

The two major types of cold-related injury are frostbite and hypothermia. Although cold-related injuries are most apt to occur in the winter months, they can occur at other times of the year, such as when an individual is exposed to cold water in a near-drowning incident.

Certain individuals are at higher risk for developing heat-related and cold-related injuries, as follows:

- Elderly individuals
- Young children, particularly infants
- Individuals who work or exercise outdoors
- Individuals with medical conditions that cause poor blood circulation, such as diabetes mellitus and cardiovascular disease
- Individuals who have had heat-related or cold-related injuries in the past
- Individuals under the influence of drugs or alcohol

Heat Cramps

Heat cramps are the least serious of the three types of heat-related injury. Heat cramps are most apt to occur when an individual is exercising or working in a hot environment and fails to replace lost fluids and electrolytes. Lost

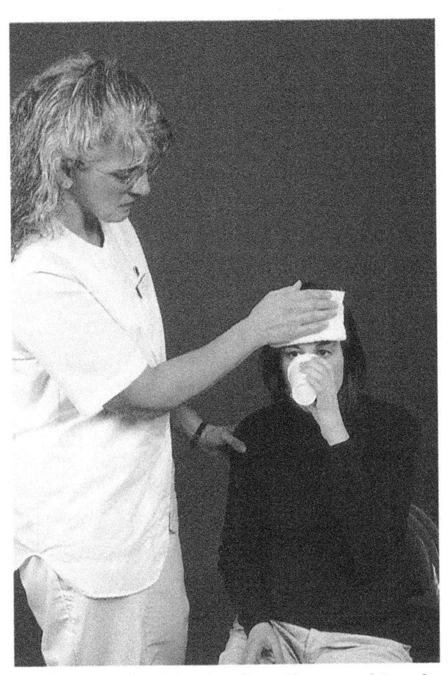

Fig. 23.15 Treatment of heat exhaustion consists of moving the patient to a cool environment, replacing fluids and electrolytes, and applying a cold compress to the forehead; the patient should then rest.

electrolytes can be replaced with a commercial sports drink (e.g., Gatorade).

Signs and symptoms of heat cramps include painful muscle spasms, particularly of the legs, calves, and abdomen; hot, sweaty skin; weakness; and a rapid pulse. These symptoms are a warning that an individual is having a problem with the heat. If the problem is ignored, heat cramps may progress to a more serious condition, such as heat exhaustion or heatstroke.

Treatment of heat cramps consists of removal of the patient to a cool environment, rest, and replacement of fluids and electrolytes. If the patient's condition does not improve, he or she should be transported to an emergency care facility for further treatment.

Heat Exhaustion

Heat exhaustion is the most common heat-related injury. It occurs most often in individuals involved in vigorous physical activity on a hot and humid day, such as athletes and construction workers. It also can occur in people who are wearing too much clothing on a hot and humid day. Signs and symptoms of heat exhaustion are similar to those of influenza: cold and clammy skin that is pale or gray, profuse sweating, headache, nausea, dizziness, weakness, and diarrhea.

Treatment of heat exhaustion consists of removal of the patient to a cool environment, replacement of fluids and electrolytes, application of a cold compress to the forehead, and rest (Fig. 23.15). Tight clothing should be loosened, and excessive layers of clothing should be removed. In most cases, these measures improve the patient's condition in approximately 30 minutes. If the patient's condition does not improve, however, he or she should be transported to an emergency care facility.

Heatstroke

Heatstroke is the least common, but most serious, of the three heat-related injuries. Heatstroke is most apt to occur in elderly people during a heat wave and in athletes who overexert in a hot and humid environment. Heatstroke can occur in a very short time, as when a child has been left to wait in a closed car on a hot day.

During heatstroke, the body becomes so overheated that the heat-regulating mechanism breaks down and is unable to cool the body. The body temperature increases to a dangerous level, causing destruction of tissues. Signs and symptoms of heatstroke include a body temperature of 105 °F (40 °C) or greater; red, hot, dry skin; a rapid, weak pulse; dizziness and weakness; rapid, shallow breathing; decreased levels of consciousness; and seizures.

Heatstroke is a life-threatening emergency that requires immediate transport of the patient to an emergency care facility by the fastest way possible. If not treated, heatstroke is always fatal. During transport, every attempt should be made to lower the body temperature, such as setting the air conditioner to its maximal capacity; covering the victim with cool, wet sheets; and fanning the victim.

What Would You Do? What Would You *Not* Do?

Case Study 3

David Brently has come to the medical office. He is a member of Kiwanis, and this year it was his turn to deliver Easter candy and flowers to patients at the local hospital and nursing home while wearing a bunny costume. It is a very warm day, and David says that he got really hot and sweaty in his costume and then started feeling dizzy and nauseous. He got a little worried and decided to drive himself to the medical office. David says he cannot get his costume off because the zipper is stuck. He does not want to cut it off because that would ruin it and Kiwanis would not be able to use it next year. He is hoping the physician can fix him up well enough so that he can drive home. David says he is sure his wife can get the costume off without damaging it. ■

Frostbite

Frostbite is the localized freezing of body tissue as a result of exposure to cold. The severity of frostbite depends on the environmental temperature, the duration of exposure, and the wind-chill factor. Frostbite most commonly affects the hands, fingers, feet, toes, ears, nose, and cheeks. Although frostbite is not life-threatening, it can cause severe tissue damage that may require amputation of the affected body part. Signs and symptoms of frostbite include loss of feeling in the affected area; cold and waxy skin; and white, yellow, or blue discoloration of the skin.

Treatment of frostbite requires rewarming of the affected body part to prevent permanent damage. This is best accomplished in an emergency care facility because improper rewarming can result in further tissue damage. To transport the patient, loosely wrap warm clothing or blankets around the affected body part. The frozen area also can be placed in contact with another body part that is warm. It is important to handle the affected area gently. Do not rub or massage the affected area because this can damage frozen tissue further.

Hypothermia

Hypothermia is a life-threatening emergency in which the temperature of the entire body falls to a dangerously low level. Hypothermia can occur rapidly, such as when an individual falls through the ice on a frozen lake. It also can occur slowly when an individual is exposed to a cold environment for a long time, such as when a hiker is lost in the woods.

When the core body temperature decreases too much, the body loses its ability to regulate its temperature and to generate body heat. Signs and symptoms of hypothermia include shivering, numbness, drowsiness, apathy, a glassy stare, and decreased levels of consciousness.

Treatment of hypothermia should focus on preventing further heat loss. Remove the patient from the cold, or, if this is impossible, wrap him or her in blankets. Do not attempt to rewarm the patient such as through immersion in warm water. Rapid rewarming can result in serious respiratory and cardiac problems. The patient should be transported immediately to an emergency care facility.

DIABETIC EMERGENCIES

Glucose is the end product of carbohydrate metabolism. It serves as the chief source of energy to perform normal body functions and to assist in maintaining body temperature. The body maintains a constant blood glucose level to ensure a continuous source of energy for the body. Glucose that is not needed for energy can be stored in the form of glycogen in muscle and liver tissue for later use. When no more tissue storage is possible, excess glucose is converted to fat and stored as adipose tissue.

Insulin, a hormone secreted by the beta cells of the pancreas, is required for normal use of glucose in the body. Insulin enables glucose to enter the body's cells and be converted to energy. Insulin also is needed for proper storage of glycogen in liver and muscle cells.

Diabetes mellitus is a disease in which the body is unable to use glucose for energy because of a lack of insulin in the body. There are two types of diabetes—a severe form, usually appearing in childhood, known as *type 1 diabetes,* and a mild form, usually appearing in adulthood, known as *type 2 diabetes.* Most individuals with diabetes (90%) have type 2 diabetes. No cure for diabetes mellitus is known, but significant advances have been made in controlling the disease through a combination of drug therapy, diet therapy, and activity. The goal for the diabetic patient is to balance food intake and level of activity with the body's insulin.

A diabetic patient can experience two types of emergency: *hypoglycemia,* commonly referred to as "insulin shock," and *diabetic ketoacidosis,* commonly known as "diabetic coma." Insulin shock (hypoglycemia) occurs when there is too much insulin in the body and not enough glucose. Insulin shock can be caused by administration of too much insulin, skipping meals, and unexpected or unusual exercise. Symptoms of insulin shock include normal or rapid respirations; pale, cold, and clammy skin; sweating; dizziness and headache; full, rapid pulse; normal or high blood pressure; extreme hunger; aggressive or unusual behavior; fainting; and seizure or coma. The onset of insulin shock occurs rapidly, usually over 5 to 20 minutes, after the blood glucose level begins to decrease. Because the brain requires a constant supply of glucose for proper functioning, permanent brain damage or death can result from severe hypoglycemia.

Diabetic coma (diabetic ketoacidosis) occurs when there is not enough insulin in the body. This causes the blood glucose level to increase, resulting in hyperglycemia. When glucose cannot be used for energy, fat is broken down. This results in a buildup of acid waste products in the blood, known as *ketoacidosis.* The combined effect of the hyperglycemia and the ketoacidosis causes the following symptoms: polyuria; excessive thirst and hunger; vomiting; abdominal pain; dry, warm skin; rapid, deep sighing respirations; a sweet or fruity (acetone) odor to the breath; and a rapid, weak pulse.

If the condition is not treated, diabetic coma can progress to dehydration, hypotension, coma, and death. In contrast to insulin shock, however, the onset of diabetic coma is gradual, usually developing over 12 to 48 hours. Diabetic coma can be caused by illness and infection, overeating, forgetting to administer an insulin injection, or administering an insufficient amount of insulin.

Most individuals with diabetes have a thorough knowledge of their disease and manage it effectively. Because of this, diabetic emergencies are most apt to occur when there is an unusual upset in the insulin-glucose balance in the body, such as might be caused by illness or infection. An emergency situation also may arise in an individual who has diabetes but in whom the condition has not yet been diagnosed.

It may be difficult to tell the difference between insulin shock and diabetic coma because the symptoms are similar. Often a patient with either of these conditions seems to be intoxicated. If he or she is conscious, the diabetic patient usually knows what the trouble is; you should listen carefully to the patient to determine what may have caused the problem (e.g., not eating, forgetting to administer an insulin injection). If the patient is unconscious and unable to communicate, you should observe the patient's respirations. A patient in insulin shock has normal or rapid respirations,

DIABETIC
A
ALERT
I HAVE TYPE I DIABETES
If I appear to be intoxicated or am unconscious, I may be having a reaction to diabetes or its treatment.
EMERGENCY TREATMENT
If I am able to swallow, please give me a beverage that contains sugar, such as orange juice, cola or even sugar in water. Then please send me to the nearest hospital IMMEDIATELY.
B

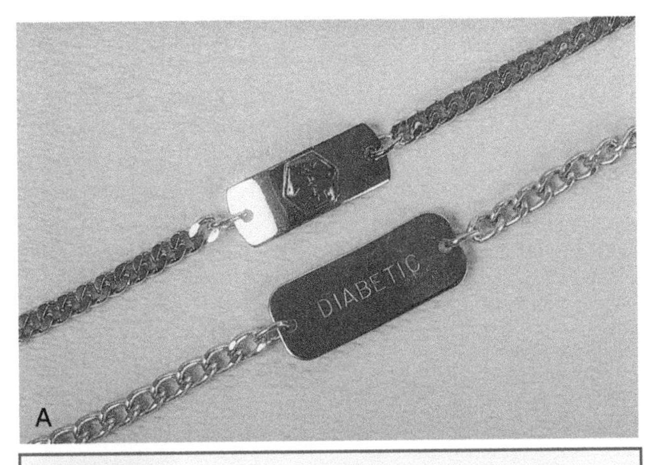

Fig. 23.16 Diabetic medical identification. (A) Diabetic medical alert bracelet. (B) Diabetic wallet card.

whereas a patient in diabetic coma has deep, labored respirations. Most diabetic patients carry an emergency medical identification, such as a medical alert bracelet or necklace and a wallet card (Fig. 23.16), to alert others to their condition when they cannot.

Emergency Care in Diabetes

Insulin Shock (Hypoglycemia)

A patient in insulin shock needs sugar immediately. For a conscious patient, glucose should be administered by mouth in the form of fruit juice (e.g., orange juice), non-diet soft drinks, candy, honey, or table sugar dissolved in water (Fig. 23.17). Improvement is usually rapid after the glucose has been consumed. If the patient is unconscious, do not give anything by mouth because it may be aspirated into the lungs. Instead, provide the fastest possible transportation of the patient to an emergency care facility.

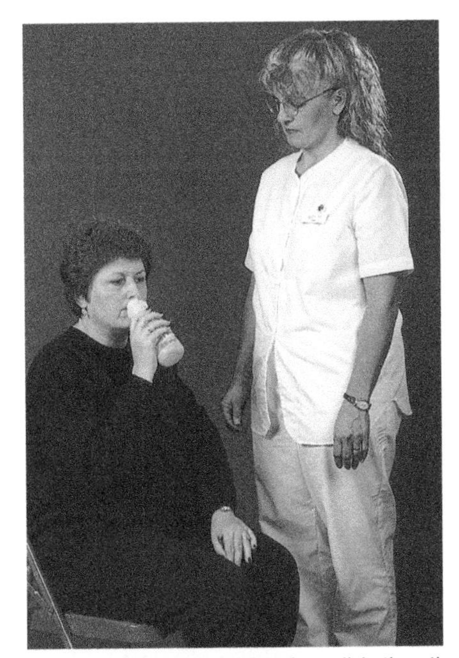

Fig. 23.17 Orange juice is administered to a diabetic patient showing signs and symptoms of insulin shock.

Diabetic Coma (Diabetic Ketoacidosis)

A patient in diabetic coma needs insulin and must be transported as soon as possible to an emergency care facility.

Doubtful Situations

If you are ever in doubt as to whether a patient is developing insulin shock or diabetic coma, give sugar, even though the final diagnosis may be diabetic coma. This is because insulin shock develops much more rapidly than diabetic coma and can quickly cause permanent brain damage or death. If you give sugar to a patient in diabetic coma, there is little risk of making the condition worse because a patient can withstand a high blood glucose level longer than he or she can tolerate a low blood glucose level.

What Would You Do? What Would You *Not* Do? RESPONSES

Case Study 1
Page 784

What Did Judy Do?

- ❑ Gave Beth the national Poison Help number (1-800-222-1222) and told her to call it immediately. Explained that was the fastest way to obtain information on what to do.
- ❑ Told Beth not to give the syrup of ipecac to Olivia unless she was told to do so by the Poison Help operator.
- ❑ Told Beth to have the vitamin bottle in her hand when she calls. Told her that the Poison Help operator would want to know information from the label and would especially want to know whether the vitamins contained iron.
- ❑ Told Beth to call the office back if she needs any more help after talking with Poison Help.

What Did Judy Not Do?

- ❑ Did not tell Beth she should give Olivia syrup of ipecac, because some poisons can cause additional problems if they are brought back up.

Case Study 2
Page 784

What Did Judy Do?

- ❑ Told Anita that Garon needs to get to the hospital as soon as possible. Explained that he is having a very serious allergic reaction that could be life-threatening.
- ❑ Told her to stay calm and call 911 immediately.
- ❑ Notified the physician of the situation.

What Did Judy Not Do?

- ❑ Told her to bring Garon to the office because he may need special life-support equipment available at the hospital.

Case Study 3
Page 787

What Did Judy Do?

- ❑ Took David to an examining room that was cool and gave him a glass of water.
- ❑ Told David she needed to get his costume off as soon as possible. Explained that if his condition gets worse, it could become life-threatening.
- ❑ Helped David out of the costume and gave him another glass of water.

What Did Judy Not Do?

- ❑ Did not tell David keep the costume on.

TERMINOLOGY REVIEW

Key Term	Word Parts	Definition
Burn		An injury to the tissues caused by exposure to thermal, chemical, electrical, or radioactive agents.
Crash cart		A specially equipped cart for holding and transporting medications, equipment, and supplies needed for lifesaving procedures in an emergency.
Crepitus		A grating sensation caused by fractured bone fragments rubbing against each other.
Dislocation	*dis-:* to undo, free from	An injury in which one end of a bone making up a joint is separated or displaced from its normal anatomic position.
Emergency medical services (EMS) system		A network of community resources, equipment, and personnel that provides care to victims of injury or sudden illness.
First aid		The immediate care administered before complete medical care can be provided to an individual who is injured or suddenly becomes ill.
Fracture		Any break in a bone.
Hypothermia	*hypo-:* below, deficient *therm/o:* heat *-ia:* condition of diseased or abnormal state	A life-threatening condition in which the temperature of the entire body falls to a dangerously low level.
Poison		Any substance that causes illness, injury, or death if it enters the body.
Pressure point		A site on the body where an artery lies close to the surface of the skin and can be compressed against an underlying bone to control bleeding.

TERMINOLOGY REVIEW—cont'd

Key Term	Word Parts	Definition
Seizure		A sudden episode of involuntary muscular contractions and relaxation, often accompanied by changes in sensation, behavior, and level of consciousness.
Shock		The failure of the cardiovascular system to deliver enough blood to all of the vital organs of the body.
Splint		Any device that immobilizes a body part.
Sprain		Trauma to a joint that causes tearing of ligaments.
Strain		A stretching or tearing of muscles or tendons caused by trauma.
Wound		A break in the continuity of an external or internal surface, caused by physical means.

On the Web

For information on emergency medicine:

American Red Cross: www.redcross.org

Federal Emergency Management Agency: www.fema.gov

Glossary

A

Abortion The termination of the pregnancy before the fetus has reached the stage of viability (20 weeks).

Abrasion A wound in which the outer layers of the skin are damaged; a scrape.

Abscess A collection of pus in a cavity surrounded by inflamed tissue.

Absorbable suture Suture material that is gradually digested by tissue enzymes and absorbed by the body.

Acute infection An infection that develops suddenly and lasts for a short period of time.

Added sugars Sugar and syrups that are added to food and beverages at home or during the commercial preparation of food.

Adolescent An individual from 12 to 18 years old.

Adventitious sounds Abnormal breath sounds.

Adverse reaction An unintended and undesirable effect produced by a drug.

Aerobe A microorganism that needs oxygen to live and grow.

Afebrile Without fever; the body temperature is normal.

Agglutination (As it pertains to blood)Clumping of blood cells.

Allergen A substance that is capable of causing an allergic reaction.

Allergy An abnormal hypersensitivity of the body to substances that are ordinarily harmless.

Alveolus (*pl.* alveoli) A thin-walled air sac of the lungs in which the exchange of oxygen and carbon dioxide takes place.

Ambulation Walking or moving from one place to another.

Ambulatory Able to walk, as opposed to being confined to bed or a wheelchair.

Ameboid movement Movement used by leukocytes that permits them to propel themselves from the capillaries into the tissues.

Amenorrhea The absence or cessation of the menstrual period. Amenorrhea occurs normally before puberty, during pregnancy, and after menopause.

Amplitude Refers to amount, extent, size, abundance, or fullness.

Ampule A small sealed glass container that holds a single dose of medication.

Anaerobe A microorganism that grows best in the absence of oxygen.

Analyte A body substance that is being identified or measured by a laboratory test.

Anaphylactic reaction A serious allergic reaction that requires immediate treatment.

Anemia A condition in which there is a decrease in the number of erythrocytes or in the amount of hemoglobin in the blood.

Anisocytosis A variation in the size of red blood cells.

Antecubital space The surface of the arm in front of the elbow.

Antibody A substance capable of combining with an antigen, resulting in an antigen-antibody reaction.

Anticoagulant A substance that inhibits blood clotting.

Antigen A substance capable of stimulating the formation of antibodies.

Antioxidant A molecule that inhibits the oxidation of other molecules.

Antipyretic An agent that reduces fever.

Antiseptic An agent that kills inhibits the growth of or kills microorganisms. An antiseptic is usually applied to living tissue.

Antiserum (*pl.* antisera) A serum that contains antibodies.

Anuria Failure of the kidneys to produce urine.

Anxiety A feeling of worry or uneasiness, often triggered by an event that is perceived as having an uncertain outcome.

Aorta The major trunk of the arterial system of the body. The aorta arises from the upper surface of the left ventricle.

Apnea The temporary cessation of breathing.

Approximation The process of bringing two parts, such as tissue, together, through the use of sutures or other means.

Artifact Additional electrical activity picked up by the electrocardiograph that interferes with the normal appearance of the electrocardiogram (ECG) cycles.

Astigmatism A refractive error that causes distorted and blurred vision for both near and far objects due to a cornea that is oval shaped.

Atherosclerosis Buildup of fibrous plaques of fatty deposits and cholesterol on the inner walls of an artery that causes narrowing, obstruction, and hardening of the artery.

Audiometer An instrument used to measure hearing acuity quantitatively for the various frequencies of sound waves.

Auscultation The process of listening to the sounds produced within the body to detect signs of disease.

Autoclave An apparatus for the sterilization of materials, using steam under pressure.

Axilla The area under the shoulder or armpit.

B

Bacilli (*sing.* bacillus) Bacteria that have a rod shape.

Bandage A strip of woven material used to wrap or cover a part of the body.

Bariatrics The branch of medicine that deals with the treatment and control of obesity and diseases associated with obesity.

Baseline The flat horizontal line that separates the various waves of the ECG cycle.

Bilirubin An orange-colored bile pigment that is a by-product of heme destruction from the hemoglobin molecule.

Bilirubinuria The presence of bilirubin in the urine.

Biopsy The surgical removal and examination of tissue from the living body. Biopsies are generally performed to determine whether a tumor is benign or malignant.

Bladder catheterization The passing of a sterile catheter through the urethra and into the bladder to remove urine.

Blood antibody A protein in blood plasma that is capable of combining with its corresponding blood antigen to produce an antigen-antibody reaction.

Blood antigen A protein present on the surface of red blood cells that determines a person's blood type.

Blood pressure The pressure or force exerted by the circulating blood on the walls of the arteries.

Body mechanics Use of the correct muscles to maintain proper balance, posture, and body alignment to accomplish a task safely and efficiently without undue strain on any muscle or joint.

Bounding pulse A pulse with an increased volume that feels very strong and full.

Brace An orthopedic device used to support and hold a part of the body in the correct position to allow functioning of the body part while healing takes place.

Bradycardia An abnormally slow heart rate (fewer than 60 beats per minute).

Bradypnea An abnormal decrease in the respiratory rate of fewer than 10 respirations per minute.

Braxton Hicks contractions Intermittent and irregular painless uterine contractions that occur throughout pregnancy. They occur more frequently toward the end of pregnancy and are sometimes mistaken for true labor pains.

Buffy coat A thin, light-colored layer of white blood cells and platelets that lays between a top layer of plasma and a bottom layer of red blood cells when an anticoagulant has been added to a blood specimen.

Burn An injury to the tissues caused by exposure to thermal, chemical, electrical, or radioactive agents.

C

Calibration A mechanism to check the precision and accuracy of an automated analyzer, to determine if the system is providing accurate results. Calibration is typically performed using a calibration device, often called a *standard.*

Canthus The junction of the eyelids at either corner of the eye.

Capillary action The action that causes liquid to rise along a wick, a tube, or a gauze dressing.

Cardiac arrest A condition in which the heart has stopped beating or beats too irregularly to circulate blood effectively through the body.

Cardiac cycle One complete heartbeat.

Cast A stiff cylindrical casing that is used to immobilize a body part until healing occurs.

Celsius scale A temperature scale on which the freezing point of water is 0 ° and the boiling point of water is 100 °; also called the centigrade scale.

Cerumen A yellowish waxy substance secreted by glands in the ear canal that functions to lubricate and protect the ear canal. Ear wax.

Cervix The lower narrow end of the uterus that opens into the vagina.

Chemotherapy The use of chemicals to treat disease. *The term chemotherapy* is most often used to refer to the treatment of cancer using antineoplastic medications.

Cholesterol A white, waxy, fatlike substance (lipid) that is essential for normal functioning of the body.

Chronic infection An infection that develops slowly and may worsen over an extended period of time.

Cilia Slender, hairlike projections that constantly beat toward the outside to remove microorganisms from the body.

CLIA-nonwaived test A complex laboratory test that does not meet the criteria for waiver and is subject to the CLIA regulations.

CLIA-waived test A laboratory test that meets the CLIA criteria for being a simple procedure that is easy to perform and has a low risk of erroneous test results. Waived tests include tests that have been US Food and Drug Administration (FDA) approved for use by patients at home.

Clinical diagnosis A tentative diagnosis of a patient's condition obtained through evaluation of the health history and the physical examination, without the benefit of laboratory or diagnostic tests.

Clinical laboratory A facility in which tests are performed on biologic specimens to obtain information regarding the health of a patient.

Cocci (*sing.* coccus) Bacteria that have a round shape.

Colonoscope An endoscope that is specially designed for passage through the anus to permit visualization of the rectum and the entire length of the colon.

Colonoscopy The visualization of the rectum and the entire colon using a colonoscope.

Colposcope A lighted instrument with a binocular magnifying lens used to examine the vagina and cervix.

Colposcopy The visual examination of the vagina and cervix using a colposcope (a lighted instrument with a magnifying lens).

Complete protein A protein that contains all the essential amino acids needed by the body.

Compress A soft, moist, absorbent cloth that is folded in several layers and applied to a part of the body in the local application of heat or cold.

Conduction The transfer of energy, such as heat, from one object to another by direct contact.

Contagious Capable of being transmitted directly or indirectly from one person to another.

Contaminate As it relates to sterile technique, to cause a sterile object or surface to become unsterile.

Contrast medium A substance that is used to make a particular structure visible on a radiograph.
Control A solution that is used to monitor a test system to ensure reliable and accurate test results.
Controlled drug A drug that has restrictions placed on it by the federal government because of its potential for abuse.
Contusion An injury to the tissues under the skin causing blood vessels to rupture, allowing blood to seep into the tissues; a bruise.
Convection The transfer of energy, such as heat, through air currents.
Conversion Changing from one system of measurement to another.
Crash cart A specially equipped cart for holding and transporting medications, equipment, and supplies needed for performing lifesaving procedures in an emergency.
Crepitus A grating sensation caused by fractured bone fragments rubbing against each other.
Crisis (pertaining to fever) A sudden falling of an elevated body temperature to normal.
Critical item An item that comes in contact with sterile tissue or the vascular system.
Cross-contamination The process by which microorganisms are unintentionally transferred from one person, object, or place to another.
Critical value A patient test results that is dangerously abnormal and is life-threatening requiring immediate attention.
Cryosurgery The therapeutic use of freezing temperatures to destroy abnormal tissue.
Cubic centimeter The amount of space occupied by 1 milliliter (1 mL = The amount of space occupied by 1 milliliter (1 mL = 1 cc).
Culture The propagation of a mass of microorganisms in a laboratory culture medium.
Culture medium A mixture of nutrients in which microorganisms are grown in the laboratory.
Cyanosis A bluish discoloration of the skin and mucous membranes.
Cytology The science that deals with the study of cells, including their origin, structure, function, and pathology.

D

DEA number A registration number assigned to providers by the US Drug Enforcement Administration (DEA) for prescribing or dispensing controlled drugs.
Decontamination The use of physical or chemical means to remove pathogens from an item so that it is no longer capable of transmitting disease.
Detergent An agent that cleanses by emulsifying dirt and oil.
Diagnosis The scientific method of determining and identifying a patient's condition.
Diagnostic procedure A procedure performed to assist in the diagnosis, management, or treatment of a patient's condition.
Diapedesis The ameboid movement of blood cells (especially leukocytes) through the wall of a capillary and out into the tissues.
Diastole The phase in the cardiac cycle in which the heart relaxes between contractions.
Diastolic pressure The point of less pressure on the arterial wall, which is recorded during diastole.
Differential diagnosis A determination of which of two or more diseases with similar symptoms is producing a patient's symptoms.
Dilation (of the cervix) The stretching of the external os from an opening a few millimeters wide to an opening large enough to allow the passage of an infant (approximately 10 cm).
Disaccharide A simple carbohydrate consisting of two sugar units.
Disaster A sudden event that causes damage or loss of life.
Disinfectant An agent used to destroy pathogenic microorganisms but not necessarily their spores. Disinfectants are usually applied to inanimate objects.
Dislocation An injury in which one end of a bone making up a joint is separated or displaced from its normal anatomic position.
Diuresis Secretion and passage of large amounts of urine.
Documenting The process of recording information about a patient in the medical record.
Donor One who furnishes something such as blood, tissue, or organs to be used in another individual.
Dose The quantity of a drug to be administered at one time.
Drug A chemical used for the treatment, prevention, or diagnosis of disease.
Dysmenorrhea Pain associated with the menstrual period.
Dyspareunia Pain in the vagina or pelvis experienced by a woman during sexual intercourse.
Dysplasia The growth of abnormal cells. Dysplasia is a precancerous condition that may or may not develop into cancer.
Dyspnea Shortness of breath or difficulty in breathing.
Dysrhythmia An irregular heart rhythm; also termed arrhythmia.
Dysuria Difficult or painful urination.

E

Eating pattern The combination of food and beverages that constitute an individual's complete dietary intake over time.
ECG cycle The graphic representation of the electrical activity of a heartbeat.
Echocardiogram An ultrasound examination of the heart.
Ectocervix The part of the cervix that projects into the vagina consisting of stratified squamous epithelium.
Edema The retention of fluid in the tissues, resulting in swelling.
Effacement The thinning and shortening of the cervical canal from its normal length of 1 to 2 cm to a structure with paper-thin edges in which there is no canal at all. Effacement occurs late in pregnancy or during labor, or both. The purpose of effacement along with dilation is to permit passage of the infant into the birth canal.
Electrocardiogram (ECG) The graphic representation of the electrical activity of the heart.

Electrocardiograph The instrument used to record the electrical activity of the heart.
Electrode A conductor of electricity which is used to promote contact between the body and the electrocardiograph.
Electrolyte A chemical substance that promotes conduction of an electrical current.
Electronic health record (EHR) A medical record that is stored on a computer.
Embryo The child in utero from the time of conception through the first 8 weeks of development.
Emergency action plan A written document that describes the actions that employees should take to ensure their safety if a fire or other emergency situation occurs.
Emergency medical services (EMS) system A network of community resources, equipment, and personnel that provides care to victims of injury or sudden illness.
Emergency preparedness The process of making plans to prevent, respond to, and recover from an emergency situation.
Empty calorie food A food that provides calories but few or no nutrients. Also known as a low–nutrient density food.
Endocervix The inner part of the cervix that forms a narrow canal that connects the vagina to the uterus.
Endoscope An instrument that consists of a tube and an optical system that is used for direct visual inspection of organs or cavities.
Enema An injection of fluid into the rectum to aid in the elimination of feces from the colon.
Engagement The entrance of the fetal head or the presenting part into the pelvic inlet.
Enteral nutrition The delivery of nutrients through a tube inserted into the gastrointestinal tract.
Erythema Reddening of the skin caused by dilation of superficial blood vessels in the skin.
Erythrocyte Red blood cell (RBC). RBCs are responsible for transporting oxygen and carbon dioxide in the body.
Essential amino acid An amino acid that is required by the body but cannot be manufactured by the body and must be obtained from food.
Eupnea Normal respiration. The rate is 16 to 20 respirations per minute, the rhythm is even and regular, and the depth is normal.
Evacuated collection tube A sterile glass or plastic blood collection tube with a color-coded closure that contains a vacuum.
Evacuation A planned systematic retreat of people to safety in an emergency situation.
Evacuation procedures Clear step-by-step procedures for the rapid, efficient, and safe removal of individuals from a building during an emergency.
Exhalation The act of breathing out.
Exit route A continuous and unobstructed path of travel from any point within a workplace to a place of safety.
Expected date of delivery (EDD) Projected birth date of the infant.
External os The opening of the cervical canal of the uterus into the vagina.
Exudate A discharge produced by the body's tissues.

F

Fahrenheit scale A temperature scale on which the freezing point of water is 32 ° and the boiling point of water is 212 °.
False-negative result A test result denoting that a condition is absent when it is actually present.
False-positive result A test result indicating that a condition is present when, in actuality, it is absent.
Familial disease A condition that occurs in or affects blood relatives more frequently than would be expected by chance.
Fasting Abstaining from food or fluids (except water) for a specified amount of time before the collection of a specimen.
Febrile Pertaining to fever.
Fetal heart rate The number of times per minute the fetal heart beats.
Fetal heart tones The sounds of the heartbeat of the fetus heard through the mother's abdominal wall.
Fetus The child in utero, from the third month after conception to birth; during the first 2 months of development, it is called an embryo.
Fever A body temperature that is above normal. Synonym for pyrexia.
Fibroblast An immature cell from which connective tissue can develop.
Fire extinguisher A portable device that discharges an agent designed to extinguish a fire.
Fire prevention plan A written document that identifies flammable and combustible materials stored in the workplace and ways to control workplace fire hazards.
Fire protection The implementation of safety measures to reduce the unwanted effects of fire.
First aid The immediate care administered before complete medical care can be provided to an individual who is injured or suddenly becomes ill.
Flow rate The number of liters of oxygen per minute that comes out of an oxygen delivery system.
Fluoroscope An instrument used to view internal organs and structures directly.
Fluoroscopy An x-ray procedure for viewing internal organs and structures directly in real time.
Forceps A two-pronged instrument for grasping and squeezing.
Fracture Any break in a bone.
Frenulum linguae The midline fold that connects the undersurface of the tongue with the floor of the mouth.
Frequency The condition of having to urinate often.
Fundus The dome-shaped upper portion of the uterus between the fallopian tubes.
Furuncle A localized staphylococcal infection that originates deep within a hair follicle; also known as a boil.

G

Gauge The diameter of the lumen of a needle used to administer medication.
Gene A unit of heredity.

Gestation The period of intrauterine development from conception to birth; the period of pregnancy. The average pregnancy lasts approximately 280 days, or 40 weeks, from the date of conception to childbirth.
Gestational age The age of the fetus between conception and birth.
Glucose The end product of carbohydrate metabolism which serves as the chief source of energy for the body.
Gluten A type of protein found in certain grains such as wheat, rye, and barley.
Glycogen A polysaccharide deposited in muscle and liver tissue which is the principal form in which glucose is stored for later use.
Glycosuria The presence of sugar in the urine.
Glycosylation The process of glucose attaching to hemoglobin.
Gravidity The total number of pregnancies a woman has had regardless of duration, including a current pregnancy.
Gynecology The branch of medicine that deals with health maintenance and diseases of the female reproductive system.

H

Hand hygiene The process of cleansing or sanitizing the hands.
Hazardous chemical Any chemical that is classified as a health or physical hazard.
HAZMAT An acronym constructed from the beginnings of the two words "*haz*ardous *mat*erials." It refers to materials that pose a danger to health or the environment and must be handled with protective equipment.
HDL cholesterol A lipoprotein consisting of protein and cholesterol that removes excess cholesterol from the cells and carries it to the liver to be excreted.
Health hazard The potential of a chemical to cause acute toxicity, skin corrosion or irritation, serious eye damage or irritation, respiratory or skin sensitization, germ cell mutagenicity, cancer, or reproductive toxicity or is an aspiration hazard.
Health history report A collection of subjective data about a patient.
Hematology The study of blood and blood-forming tissues.
Hematoma A swelling or mass of coagulated blood caused by a break in a blood vessel.
Hematopoiesis The process of blood cell formation.
Hematuria Blood present in the urine.
Hemoconcentration An increase in the concentration of nonfilterable blood components in the blood vessels, such as red blood cells, enzymes, iron, and calcium as a result of a decrease in the fluid content of the blood.
Hemoglobin The protein and iron-containing pigment of erythrocytes that carries oxygen to the tissues of the body.
Hemoglobin A_{1c} The compound formed when glucose attaches or glycosylates to the protein in hemoglobin.
Hemolysis The breakdown of erythrocytes with the release of hemoglobin into the plasma.
Hemophilia An inherited bleeding disorder caused by a deficiency of a clotting factor needed for proper coagulation of the blood.
Hemostasis The arrest of bleeding by natural or artificial means.
Homeostasis The state in which body systems are functioning normally and the internal environment of the body is in equilibrium; the body is in a healthy state.
Hyperglycemia An abnormally high level of glucose in the blood.
Hyperopia A refractive error in which the light rays are brought to a focus behind the retina resulting in difficulty viewing objects at a reading or working distance. Farsightedness.
Hyperpnea An abnormal increase in the rate and depth of respiration.
Hyperpyrexia An extremely high fever.
Hypertension The force of the circulating blood against the walls of the blood vessels is consistently above normal.
Hyperventilation An abnormally fast and deep type of breathing usually associated with acute anxiety conditions.
Hypochromic A red blood cell with a decreased concentration of hemoglobin.
Hypoglycemia An abnormally low level of glucose in the blood.
Hypopnea An abnormal decrease in the rate and depth of respiration.
Hypotension The pressure of the circulating blood against the walls of the blood vessels is less than normal.
Hypothermia A body temperature that is less than normal.
Hypoxemia A decrease in the oxygen saturation of the blood. Hypoxemia may lead to hypoxia.
Hypoxia A reduction in the oxygen supply to the tissues of the body.

I

Immune globulin A blood product consisting of pooled human plasma containing antibodies.
Immunity The resistance of the body to the effects of a harmful agent such as a pathogenic microorganism and its toxins.
Immunization (active, artificial) The process of becoming immune or of rendering an individual immune through the use of a vaccine or toxoid.
Immunology The scientific study of antigen and antibody reactions.
Impacted cerumen Cerumen that is wedged firmly together in the ear canal so as to be immovable.
Incision A clean cut caused by a cutting instrument.
Incomplete protein A protein that lacks one or more of the essential amino acids needed by the body.
Incubate In microbiology, the act of placing a culture in a chamber (incubator) that meets optimal growth requirements for multiplication of the organisms, such as the proper temperature, humidity, and darkness.

Incubation period The interval of time between invasion by a pathogenic microorganism and the appearance of first symptoms of the disease.
Induration An abnormally raised hardened area of the skin with clearly defined margins.
Infant A child from birth to 12 months of age.
Infection The condition in which the body, or part of it, is invaded by a pathogen.
Infectious disease A disease caused by a pathogen that produces harmful effects on its host.
Infiltration The process by which a substance passes into and is deposited within the substance of a cell, tissue, or organ.
Inflammation A protective response of the body to trauma and the entrance of foreign matter. The purpose of inflammation is to destroy invading microorganisms and to remove damaged tissue debris from the area so that proper healing can occur. Symptoms at the site of inflammation include pain, swelling, redness, and warmth.
Infusion The administration of fluids, medications, or nutrients into a vein.
Inhalation The act of breathing in.
Inhalation administration The administration of medication by way of air or other vapor being drawn into the lungs.
Inoculate To introduce microorganisms into a culture medium for growth and multiplication.
Inscription The part of a prescription that indicates the name of the drug and the drug dosage.
Inspection The process of observing a patient to detect signs of disease.
Instillation The dropping of a liquid into a body cavity.
Insufflate To blow a powder, vapor, or gas (e.g., air) into a body cavity.
Intercostal Between the ribs.
Internal os The internal opening of the cervical canal into the uterus.
Interval The length of one or more waves and a segment.
Intradermal injection The introduction of medication into the dermal layer of the skin.
Intramuscular injection The introduction of medication into the muscular layer of the body.
Intravenous (IV) therapy The administration of a liquid agent directly into a patient's vein, where it is distributed throughout the body by way of the circulatory system.
In vitro Occurring in glass. Refers to tests performed under artificial conditions, as in the laboratory.
In vivo Occurring in the living body or organism.
Irrigation The washing of a body canal with a flowing solution.
Ischemia Deficiency of blood in a body part.

K

Ketonuria The presence of ketone bodies in the urine.
Ketosis An accumulation of large amounts of ketone bodies in the tissues and body fluids.
Kilocalorie The amount of heat needed to raise the temperature of 1 kilogram of water 1 degree Celsius. (Often referred to as a *calorie.*)
Korotkoff sounds Sounds heard during the measurement of blood pressure that are used to determine the systolic and diastolic blood pressure readings.

L

Laboratory test The clinical analysis and study of a body substance to obtain objective data for the diagnosis, treatment, and management of a patient's condition.
Laceration A wound in which the tissues are torn apart, leaving ragged and irregular edges.
Lactose A disaccharide that consists of two sugar units and is found in milk and milk products.
LDL cholesterol A lipoprotein, consisting of protein and cholesterol that picks up cholesterol and delivers it to blood vessels and muscles.
Length (recumbent) The measurement from the vertex of the head to the heel of the foot of a patient in a supine position.
Leukocyte White blood cell (WBC). WBCs function in defending the body against infection and foreign materials.
Leukocytosis An abnormal increase in the number of leukocytes (greater than 11,000 per cubic millimeter of blood).
Leukopenia An abnormal decrease in the number of leukocytes (less than 4500 per cubic millimeter of blood).
Ligate To tie off and close a structure such as a severed blood vessel.
Lipoprotein A complex molecule consisting of protein and a lipid fraction such as cholesterol. Lipoproteins function in transporting lipids in the blood.
Load The articles that are being sterilized.
Local anesthetic A drug that produces a loss of feeling and an inability to perceive pain in only a specific part of the body.
Lochia A discharge from the uterus after delivery, that consists of blood, tissue, white blood cells, and some bacteria.
Long arm cast A cast that extends from the axilla to the fingers, usually with a bend in the elbow.
Long leg cast A cast that extends from the midthigh to the toes.

M

Maceration The softening and breaking down of the skin as a result of prolonged exposure to moisture.
Macrocytic An abnormally large red blood cell.
Macronutrient A nutrient required in relatively large amounts by the body. Includes carbohydrates, fats, and proteins.
Malaise A vague sense of body discomfort, weakness, and fatigue that often marks the onset of a disease and continues through the course of the illness.
Man-made disaster An event that causes serious damage through intentional or negligent human actions or the failure of a human-made system.
Manometer An instrument for measuring pressure.
Mayo tray A broad, flat metal tray placed on a stand and used to hold sterile instruments and supplies when it has been covered with a sterile towel.

Medical asepsis Practices that are employed to inhibit the growth and hinder the transmission of pathogenic microorganisms to prevent the spread of infection.

Medical record A written record of important information regarding a patient, including the care of that individual and the progress of the patient's condition.

Menopause The permanent cessation of menstruation, which usually occurs between the ages of 45 and 55 years.

Menorrhagia Excessive bleeding during a menstrual period, in the number of days or the amount of blood or both; also called dysfunctional uterine bleeding (DUB).

Mensuration The process of measuring a patient.

Metrorrhagia Bleeding between menstrual periods.

Microbiology The scientific study of microorganisms and their activities.

Microcytic An abnormally small red blood cell.

Micronutrient A nutrient required in very small amounts by the body. Includes vitamins and minerals.

Microorganism A microscopic plant or animal.

Micturition The act of voiding urine.

Mineral A naturally occurring inorganic substance that is essential to the proper functioning of the body.

Monosaccharide A simple carbohydrate consisting of one sugar unit.

Morphology (of blood cells) The study of the size, shape, and structure of a blood cell.

Mucous membrane A membrane lining body passages or cavities that open to the outside.

Multigravida A woman who has been pregnant more than once.

Multipara A woman who has completed two or more pregnancies to the age of fetal viability regardless of whether they ended in live infants or stillbirths.

Myopia A refractive error in which the light rays are brought to a focus in front of the retina resulting in difficulty viewing objects at a distance. Nearsightedness.

N

Natural disaster A catastrophic event that is caused by nature or the natural process of the earth.

Natural sugars Sugars that occur naturally in foods and beverages.

Needle biopsy A type of biopsy in which tissue from deep within the body is obtained by the insertion of a biopsy needle through the skin.

Nephron The functional unit of the kidney that filters waste substances from the blood and dilutes them with water to produce urine.

Nocturia Excessive (voluntary) urination during the night.

Nocturnal enuresis Inability of an individual to control urination at night during sleep (bedwetting).

Nonabsorbable suture Suture material that is not absorbed by the body and either remains permanently in the body tissue and becomes encapsulated by fibrous tissue or is removed.

Noncritical item An item that comes into contact with intact skin but not with mucous membranes.

Nonessential amino acid An amino acid required by the body that can be synthesized by the body in sufficient quantities to meet its needs.

Nonintact skin Skin that has a break in the surface. It includes, but is not limited to, abrasions, cuts, hangnails, paper cuts, and burns.

Nonpathogen A microorganism that does not normally produce disease.

Normal flora Harmless, nonpathogenic microorganisms that normally reside in many parts of the body but do not cause disease.

Normal sinus rhythm Refers to an ECG that is within normal limits.

Normochromic A red blood cell with a normal concentration of hemoglobin.

Normocytic A normal-sized red blood cell.

Nullipara A woman who has not carried a pregnancy to the point of fetal viability (20 weeks of gestation).

Nutrient A chemical substance found in food that is needed by the body for survival and well-being.

Nutrition The study of nutrients in food including how the body uses them and their relationship to health.

Nutrition therapy The application of the science of nutrition to promote optimal heath and treat illness.

O

Obesity A medical condition in which there is an excessive accumulation of body fat to the extent to which it may have an adverse effect on the health and well-being of an individual.

Objective symptom A symptom that can be observed by an examiner.

Obstetrics The branch of medicine concerned with the care of the woman during pregnancy, childbirth, and the postpartal period.

Occult blood Blood in such a small amount that it is not detectable by the unaided eye.

Oliguria Decreased or scanty output of urine.

Ophthalmoscope An instrument for examining the interior of the eye.

Opportunistic infection An infection that takes advantage of an opportunity not normally available such as the weakened immune system of an HIV-infected individual.

Optimum growth temperature The temperature at which an organism grows best.

Oral administration Administration of medication by mouth.

Orthopedist A physician who specializes in the diagnosis and treatment of disorders of the musculoskeletal system, which includes the bones, joints, ligaments, tendons, muscles, and nerves.

Orthopnea The condition in which breathing is easier when an individual is in a sitting or standing position.

Osteochondritis Inflammation of bone and cartilage.

Osteomyelitis Inflammation of the bone or bone marrow as a result of a bacterial infection.

Otoscope An instrument used to examine the external ear canal and tympanic membrane.

Oxygen therapy The administration of supplemental oxygen at concentrations greater than room air to treat or prevent hypoxemia.

Oxyhemoglobin Hemoglobin that has combined with oxygen.

P

Package insert A printed document developed by the manufacturer of a laboratory test that provides detailed information on the use of the test and how to perform the test.

Palpation The process of feeling with the hands to detect signs of disease.

Panel A combination of laboratory tests that have been determined to be the most sensitive and specific means of identifying a disease state or evaluating a particular organ or organ system.

Paper-based patient record (PPR) A medical record in paper form.

Parenteral Taken into the body through piercing of the skin barrier or mucous membranes, such as through needlesticks, human bites, cuts, and abrasions. Administration of medication by injection.

Parity The condition of having borne offspring regardless of the outcome.

Pathogen A disease-producing microorganism.

Peak flow rate The maximum volume of air that can be exhaled when the patient blows into a peak flow meter as forcefully and as rapidly as possible.

Pediatrician A physician who specializes in the care and development of children and the diagnosis and treatment of children's diseases.

Pediatrics The branch of medicine that deals with the care and development of children and the diagnosis and treatment of children's diseases.

Percent daily value The percentage of a nutrient provided by a single serving of a food item compared with how much is required for the entire day.

Percussion The process of tapping the body to detect signs of disease.

Percussion hammer An instrument with a rubber head, used for testing reflexes.

Perimenopause Before the onset of menopause, the phase during which the woman with regular periods changes to irregular cycles and increased periods of amenorrhea.

Perineum The external region between the vaginal orifice and the anus in a female and between the scrotum and the anus in a male.

Peroxidase (As it pertains to the guaiac-based fecal occult blood test [gFOBT]) A substance that is able to transfer oxygen from hydrogen peroxide to oxidize guaiac, causing the guaiac to turn blue.

pH The unit that describes the acidity or alkalinity of a solution.

Phagocytosis The engulfing and destruction of foreign particles, such as pathogens and damaged cells.

Pharmacology The study of drugs.

Phlebotomist A health professional trained in the collection of blood specimens.

Phlebotomy Incision of a vein for the removal of blood; the collection of blood.

Physical hazard The potential of a chemical to catch fire, explode, or react with other chemicals.

Plasma The liquid part of the blood, consisting of a clear, straw-colored fluid that makes up approximately 55% of the total blood volume.

Poison Any substance that causes illness, injury, or death if it enters the body.

Polycythemia A disorder in which there is an increase in the number of red blood cells or the amount of hemoglobin.

Polyp (colorectal) An abnormal noncancerous growth that protrudes from the mucous membrane of the large intestine.

Polysaccharide A complex carbohydrate made up of many sugar units strung together in a long chain.

Polyuria Increased output of urine.

Position The relation of the presenting part of the fetus to the maternal pelvis.

Postexposure prophylaxis (PEP) Treatment administered to an individual after exposure to an infectious disease to prevent the disease.

Postoperative After a surgical operation.

Postpartum Occurring after childbirth.

Prediabetes A condition in which glucose levels are higher than normal, but not high enough to be classified as diabetes.

Preeclampsia A major complication of pregnancy, the cause of which is unknown, characterized by increasing hypertension, albuminuria, and edema. If this condition is neglected or is not treated properly, it may develop into eclampsia, which could cause maternal convulsions and coma. Preeclampsia generally occurs between the 20th week of pregnancy and the end of the first week postpartum.

Prenatal Before birth.

Preoperative Preceding a surgical operation.

Presbyopia A decrease in the elasticity of the lens that occurs with aging, resulting in a decreased ability to focus on close objects.

Preschool child A child from 3 to 6 years old.

Prescription An order from a licensed provider authorizing the dispensing of a drug by a pharmacist.

Presentation Indication of the part of the fetus that is closest to the cervix and will be delivered first. A cephalic presentation is a delivery in which the fetal head is presenting against the cervix. A breech presentation is a delivery in which the buttocks or feet are presented instead of the head.

Pressure point A site on the body where an artery lies close to the surface of the skin and can be compressed against an underlying bone to control bleeding.

Preterm birth Delivery occurring between 20 and 37 weeks gestation regardless of whether the child was born alive or stillborn.
Primigravida A woman who is pregnant for the first time.
Primipara A woman who has carried a pregnancy to viability (20 weeks of gestation) for the first time, regardless of whether the infant was stillborn or alive at birth.
Prognosis The probable course and outcome of a patient's condition and the patient's prospects for recovery.
Proteinuria The presence of protein in the urine.
Puerperium The period of time, usually 4 to 6 weeks after delivery, in which the uterus and the body systems are returning to normal.
Pulse oximeter A device used to measure the oxygen saturation of arterial blood.
Pulse oximetry The use of a pulse oximeter to measure the oxygen saturation of arterial blood.
Pulse pressure The difference between the systolic and diastolic pressures.
Pulse rhythm The time interval between heartbeats.
Pulse volume The strength of the heartbeat.
Puncture A wound made by a sharp pointed object piercing the skin.
Pyuria The presence of pus in the urine.

Q

Qualitative test A test that indicates whether or not a particular analyte is present in a specimen and may also provide an approximate indication of the amount of the analyte present.
Quality control The application of methods to ensure that test results are reliable and valid and that errors are detected and eliminated.
Quantitative test A test that indicates the exact amount of an analyte that is present in the body with the results being reported in measurable units.
Quickening The first movements of the fetus in utero as felt by the mother, which usually occurs between 16 and 20 weeks of gestation, and are felt consistently thereafter.

R

Radiation The transfer of energy, such as heat, in the form of waves.
Radiograph The permanent image produced by x-rays acting on a radiosensitive receptor device such as a digital detector or radiographic film.
Radiography The taking of permanent records (radiographs) of internal body organs and structures by passing x-rays through the body to act on a radiosensitive receptor device.
Radiologist A provider who specializes in the diagnosis and treatment of disease using radiation and other imaging techniques.
Radiology The branch of medicine that uses radiation and other imaging techniques to diagnose and treat disease.
Radiolucent Describing a structure that permits the passage of x-rays.
Radiopaque Describing a structure that obstructs the passage of x-rays.
Reagent A chemical that reacts with a specimen to allow the detection or measurement of an analyte.
Recipient One who receives something, such as a blood transfusion, from a donor.
Reference range A certain established and acceptable range within which the laboratory test results of a healthy individual are expected to fall.
Refraction The deflection or bending of light rays by a lens.
Regulated medical waste Medical waste that may contain infectious materials posing a threat to health and safety.
Renal threshold The concentration at which a substance in the blood that is not normally excreted by the kidneys begins to appear in the urine.
Resident flora Harmless, nonpathogenic microorganisms that normally reside on the skin and usually do not cause disease; also known as *normal flora*.
Retention The inability to empty the bladder. The urine is being produced normally but is not being voided.
Risk factor Anything that increases an individual's chance of developing a disease. Some risk factors (e.g., smoking) can be avoided, but others (e.g., age, family history) cannot (e.g., age, family history).

S

Safety Data Sheet A document that provides information on a chemical, its hazards, and measures to take to prevent injury and illness when handling the chemical.
Sanitization A series of steps designed to remove debris from an item and reduce the number of microorganisms to a safe level.
SaO_2 (saturation of arterial oxygen) Abbreviation for the percentage of hemoglobin that is saturated with oxygen in arterial blood.
Saturated fat A type of fat that is solid at room temperature and comes primarily from animal sources.
Scalpel A surgical knife used to divide tissues.
School-age child A child from 6 to 12 years of age.
Scissors A cutting instrument.
Screening That process of testing to detect disease in an individual who is not yet experiencing symptoms.
Screening test (laboratory) A laboratory test performed routinely on apparently healthy individuals to assist in the early detection of disease.
Sebaceous cyst A thin, closed sac or capsule that contains fatty secretions from a sebaceous gland.
Segment The portion of the ECG between two waves.
Seizure A sudden episode of involuntary muscular contractions and relaxation, often accompanied by a change in sensation, behavior, and level of consciousness.
Semicritical item An item that comes into contact with nonintact skin or intact mucous membranes.
Serum The clear, straw-colored part of the blood that remains after the solid elements and the clotting factor fibrinogen have been separated out of it.
Shock The failure of the cardiovascular system to deliver enough blood to all the vital organs of the body.

Short arm cast A cast that extends from below the elbow to the fingers.

Short leg cast A cast that begins just below the knee and extends to the toes.

Sigmoidoscope An endoscope that is specially designed for passage through the anus to permit visualization of the rectum and sigmoid colon.

Sigmoidoscopy The visual examination of the rectum and sigmoid colon using a sigmoidoscope.

Signatura The part of a prescription that indicates the information to print on the medication label.

Soak The direct immersion of a body part in water or a medicated solution.

Sonogram The record obtained with ultrasonography.

Specific gravity The weight of a substance compared with the weight of an equal volume of distilled water. In urinalysis, the specific gravity refers to the measurement of the amount of dissolved substances present in the urine compared with the same amount of distilled water.

Specimen A small sample taken from the body to represent the nature of the whole.

Speculum An instrument for opening a body orifice or cavity for viewing.

Sphygmomanometer A device that measures the pressure of blood within an artery.

Spirilla (*sing.* spirillum) Bacteria that have a spiral or curved shape.

Spirometer An instrument for measuring air taken into and expelled from the lungs.

Spirometry Measurement of an individual's breathing capacity by means of a spirometer.

Splint An orthopedic device used to support and immobilize a part of the body.

SpO_2 (saturation of peripheral oxygen) Abbreviation for the percentage of hemoglobin that is saturated with oxygen in arterial blood as measured by a pulse oximeter.

Spore A hard, thick-walled capsule formed by some bacteria that contains only the essential parts of the protoplasm of the bacterial cell.

Sprain Trauma to a joint that causes injury to the ligaments.

Sterile Free of all living microorganisms and bacterial spores.

Sterilization The process of destroying all forms of microbial life, including bacterial spores.

Stethoscope An instrument for amplifying and hearing sounds produced by the body.

Strain A stretching or tearing of muscles or tendons caused by trauma.

Stress The body's response to threat or change.

Subcutaneous injection Introduction of medication beneath the skin, into the subcutaneous or fatty layer of the body.

Subjective symptom A symptom that is felt by the patient but is not observable by an examiner.

Sublingual administration Administration of medication by placing it under the tongue, where it dissolves and is absorbed through the mucous membrane.

Subscription The part of the prescription that gives directions to the pharmacist and usually designates the number of doses to be dispensed.

Supernatant The clear liquid that remains at the top after a precipitate settles.

Superscription The part of a prescription consisting of the abbreviation Rx (from the Latin word *recipe,* meaning "take").

Suppuration The process of pus formation.

Suprapubic aspiration The passing of a sterile needle through the abdominal wall into the bladder to remove urine.

Surgery The branch of medicine that deals with operative and manual procedures for correction of deformities and defects, repair of injuries, and diagnosis and treatment of certain diseases.

Surgical asepsis Practices that keep objects and areas sterile or free from microorganisms.

Susceptible Easily affected; lacking resistance.

Sutures Material used to approximate tissues with surgical stitches.

Swaged needle A needle with suturing material permanently attached to its end.

Symptom Any change in the body or its functioning that indicates the presence of disease.

Systole The phase in the cardiac cycle in which the ventricles contract, sending blood out of the heart and into the aorta and pulmonary trunk.

Systolic pressure The point of maximum pressure on the arterial walls, which is recorded during systole.

T

Tachycardia An abnormally fast heart rate (more than 100 beats/min).

Tachypnea An abnormal increase in the respiratory rate of more than 20 respirations per minute.

Term birth Delivery occurring after 37 weeks, regardless of whether the child was born alive or stillborn.

Test system A setup that includes all of the test components required to perform a laboratory test such as testing devices, controls, and test reagents.

Thready pulse A pulse with a decreased volume that feels weak and thin.

Thrombocyte Platelets. Thrombocytes function by participating in the blood clotting mechanism of the body.

Thrombocytopenia An abnormal decrease in the number of thrombocytes (less than 150,000 per cubic millimeter of blood).

Thrombocytosis An abnormal increase in the number of thrombocytes (greater than 150,000 per cubic millimeter of blood).

Toddler A child from 1 to 3 years old.

Topical administration Application of a drug to a particular spot, usually for a local action.

Toxemia A condition that can occur in pregnant women that includes preeclampsia and eclampsia. If preeclampsia goes undiagnosed or is not satisfactorily controlled, it could develop into eclampsia, characterized by convulsions and coma.

Toxoid A toxin (poisonous substance produced by a bacterium) that has been treated by heat or chemicals to destroy its harmful properties. It is administered to an individual to prevent an infectious disease by stimulating the production of antibodies in that individual.

Transfusion The administration of whole blood or blood products by the intravenous route.

Transient flora Microorganisms that reside on the superficial skin layers and are picked up in the course of daily activities. They are often pathogenic but can be removed easily from the skin by sanitizing the hands.

Triglycerides The chemical form in which most fat exists in food, as well as in the body.

Trimester Three months, or one third, of the gestational period of pregnancy.

Tympanic membrane A thin, semitransparent membrane located between the external ear canal and the middle ear that receives and transmits sound waves; also known as the eardrum.

U

Ultrasonography The use of high-frequency sound waves to produce an image of an organ or tissue.

Unique identifier Information directly associated with an individual that reliably identifies the individual as the person for whom the service or treatment is intended.

Unsaturated fat A type of fat that is liquid at room temperature and comes primarily from plant sources.

Urgency The immediate need to urinate.

Urinalysis The physical, chemical, and microscopic analyses of urine.

Urinary incontinence The inability to retain urine.

V

Vaccine A suspension of attenuated (weakened) or killed microorganisms administered to an individual to prevent an infectious disease by stimulating the production of antibodies in that individual.

Venipuncture Puncturing of a vein.

Venous reflux The backflow of blood (from a collection tube) into the patient's vein.

Venous stasis The temporary cessation or slowing of the venous blood flow.

Vertex The top of the head.

Vial A closed glass container with a rubber stopper that holds medication.

Visual acuity Acuteness or sharpness of vision. A person with normal visual acuity can see clearly and is able to distinguish fine details close up and at some distance.

Vitamin An organic compound that is required in small amounts by the body for normal growth and development.

Void To empty the bladder.

Vulva The region of the external female genital organs.

W

Wheal A tense, pale, raised area of the skin.

Wheezing A continuous high-pitched whistling musical sound heard particularly during exhalation and sometimes during inhalation.

Wound A break in the continuity of an external or internal surface caused by physical means.

Index

Page numbers followed by "*f*" refer to illustrations; page numbers followed by "*t*" refer to tables; page numbers followed by "*b*" refer to boxes.

D

Q

R